OXFORD MEDICAL PUBLICATIONS

Oxford Desk Reference
Critical Care

▶ Except where otherwise stated, drug doses and recommendations are for the non-pregnant adult who is not breast-feeding.

Oxford Desk Reference
Critical Care

Carl Waldmann

Consultant in Anaesthesia and Intensive Care
Royal Berkshire Hospital
Reading

Neil Soni

Honorary Clinical Senior Lecturer
Division of Surgery, Oncology,
Reproductive Biology and Anaesthetics
Imperial College
London

and

Andrew Rhodes

Consultant in Intensive Care
St George's Hospital
London

OXFORD
UNIVERSITY PRESS

OXFORD
UNIVERSITY PRESS

Great Clarendon Street, Oxford OX2 6DP

Oxford University Press is a department of the University of Oxford.
It furthers the University's objective of excellence in research, scholarship,
and education by publishing worldwide in

Oxford New York

Auckland Cape Town Dar es Salaam Hong Kong Karachi
Kuala Lumpur Madrid Melbourne Mexico City Nairobi
New Delhi Shanghai Taipei Toronto

With offices in

Argentina Austria Brazil Chile Czech Republic France Greece
Guatemala Hungary Italy Japan Poland Portugal Singapore
South Korea Switzerland Thailand Turkey Ukraine Vietnam

Oxford is a registered trade mark of Oxford University Press
in the UK and in certain other countries

Published in the United States
by Oxford University Press Inc., New York

First published 2008

British Library Cataloguing in Publication Data
Data available

Library of Congress Cataloguing in Publication Data
Data available

Typeset by Cepha Imaging Private Ltd., Bangalore, India
Printed in Great Britain
on acid-free paper by
CPI Antony Rowe,
Chippenham, Wiltshire

ISBN 978–0–19–922958–1

10 9 8 7 6 5 4 3 2 1

Preface

Intensive care medicine is an evolving speciality in which the amount of available information is growing daily and increasingly, textbooks reflect this in terms of their size. Size and immediate clinical utility are often inversely related and 'bottom line' practicality is drowned in comprehensive discussion. The natural habitat of this new textbook of critical care and emergency medicine is on the desktops of Intensive Care units, High Dependency units, acute medical or surgical wards, Accident & Emergency departments and maybe even operating theatres where it is easily accessible with useful and relevant information.

While aimed primarily at a specialist readership including clinicians, nurses, and other allied health professionals in Critical Care, Anaesthesia and the acute specialities, we hope it will find a niche with anyone involved in care of the critically ill, whether in specialist areas or in the wards.

It is intended that the key feature of this book is ease of access to up-to-date relevant evidenced-based information regarding the management of commonly encountered conditions, techniques, and problems in those who are critically ill. Most importantly that it is practical and useful. The content of the book is based, wherever possible and useful, upon the latest sets of guidelines from national or international bodies (e.g. Society of Critical Care Medicine, European Society of Intensive Care Medicine). We hope the book will be useful not only in the United Kingdom, but to anyone using international guidelines. Indeed, the range of invited authors incorporates a large number of countries but for all, the common theme is management of the critically ill.

To facilitate the key aim of rapid and easy access to information, the book is designed such that each subject will form a self-contained topic in its own right, laid out across two (or, for larger subjects, up to four) pages. This format facilitates the use of the book as a desk reference and we envisage that it will be consulted in the clinic or ward setting for information on the optimum management of a particular condition.

It is the fervent wish of the editors that this book, one in a series of desk top books from Oxford University Press, becomes a valuable tool in the management of critically ill patients.

CW, NS, and AR

Brief contents

Detailed contents

Abbreviations

±	plus or minus
≤	less than or equal to
≥	more than or equal to
~	approximatley
°	degrees
↑	increase
↓	decrease
–ve	negative
+ve	positive
AAC	acute acalculous cholecystitis
AAFB	acid- and alcohol-fast bacilli
ABG	arterial blood gas
ABPA	allergic bronchopulmonary aspergillosis
AC	activated charcoal
ACS	acute coronary syndrome
ACTH	adrenocorticotrophic hormone
ACE	angiotension-converting enzyme
AChR	acetylcholine receptor
ACTH	adrenocorticotrophic hormone
ADH	antidiuretic hormone
AECOPD	acute exacerbations of chronic obstructive airways disease
AED	automated external defibrillator/ antiepileptic drug
AF	atrial fibrillation
AFE	amniotic fluid embolism
AG	anion gap
AHF	acute heart failure
AI	acoustic impedance
AIDP	acute inflammatory demyelinating polyneuropathy
AIDS	autoimmune deficiency syndrome
AKI	acute kidney injury
ALI	acute lung injury
ALS	advanced life support
AMAN	acute motor axonal neuropathy
AMI	acute myocardial infarction
AMSAN	acute motor sensory axonal neuropathy
ANC	absolute neutrophil count
ANCA	antineutrophil cytoplasmic antibody
ANP	atrial natriuretic peptide
APACHE	Acute Physiology and Chronic Health Evaluation
APC	activated protein C
APH	antepartum haemorrhage
APP	abdominal perfusion pressure
aPPT	activated partial prothrombin time
AR	aortic regurgitation
ARB	angiotensin II receptor blocker
ARDS	acute respiratory distress syndrome
ARF	acute respiratory failure
ARV	antiretroviral
AS	aortic stenosis
ASA	acetylsalicylic acid (aspirin)
aSAH	aneurysmal subarachnoid haemorrhage
AST	aspartate aminotransferase
ATLS	Advanced Trauma Life Support
ATP	adenosine triphosphate
AV	atrioventricular
AVP	arginine vasopressin
AXR	abdominal X-ray
BAE	bronchial artery embolization
BAL	bronchoalveolar lavage
BAEP	brainstem auditory evoked potential
BBB	blood–brain barrier
bd	twice a day
BiPAP	bilevel positive airway pressure
BLS	basic life support
BMI	body mass index
BMP	bone morphogenetic protein
BMPR2	bone morphogenetic protein receptor II
BMS	bone marrow suppression
BP	blood pressure
BPF	bronchopleural fistula
bpm	beats per minute
BNP	brain natriuretic peptide
BTF	Brain Trauma Foundation
CABG	coronary artery bypass graft
CAD	coronary artery disease
cAMB	conventional amphotericin B
CAP	community-acquired pneumonia
CAPD	continuous ambulatory peritoneal dialysis
CBF	cerebral blood flow
CCB	calcium channel blocker
CCC	Comprehensive Critical Care
CCCP	Critical Care Contingency Planning
CCN	critical care nurse
CDAD	*Clostridium difficile*-associated disease
CDT	*Clostridium difficile* toxin
CEA	cost-effective analysis
CEMCH	Confidential Enquiry into Maternal and Child Health
CFAM	cerebral function analysing monitor
CFM	colour flow mapping
CHF	chronic heart failure
CI	confidence interval
CIM	critical illness myopathy
CIN	contrast-induced nephropathy

CINM	critical illness neuromyopathy
CIP	critical illness polyneuropathy
CK	creatine kinase
CMAP	compound muscle action potential
CMR	cerebral metabolic rate
CMV	conventional mechanical ventilation/ cytomegalovirus
cNOS	constitutive nitric oxide synthase
CNS	central nervous system
COMT	catechol-o-methyltransferase
COPD	chronic obstructive pulmonary disease
COX	cyclo-oxygenase
CPAP	continuous positive airway pressure
CPIS	Clinical Pulmonary Infection Score
CPP	cerebral perfusion pressure
CPR	cardiopulmonary resuscitation
CPT	chest physiotherapy
CrAg	cryptococcal antigen
CR-BSI	catheter-related bloodstream infection
CRP	C-reactive protein
Crs	respiratory compliance
CSF	cerebrospinal fluid
CSS	Churg–Strauss syndrome
CT	computed tomography
CTA	CT angiogram
CTV	CT venogram
CTZ	chemoreceptor trigger zone
CVA	cerebrovascular accident
CVC	central venous catheter
CVP	central venous pressure
CV ratio	compression:ventilation ratio
CVVH	continuous venovenous haemofiltration
CVVHD	continuous venovenous haemodialysis
CVVHDF	continuous venovenous haemodiafiltration
CXR	chest X-ray
DBP	diastolic blood pressure
DCCV	direct current cardioversion
DAH	diffuse alveolar haemorrhage
DAI	diffuse axonal injury
DD	deep dermal
DDAVP	1-deamino-D-arginine vasopressin
DGLA	di-homo-γ-linolenic acid
DHA	docosohexanoic acid
DIC	disseminated intravascular coagulation
DIND	delayed ischaemic neurological deficit
DKA	diabetic ketoacidosis
DMS	direct muscle stimulation
DNAR	do not attempt resuscitation
2,3-DPG	2,3-diphosphoglycerate
DPPC	dipalmitoylphosphatidylcholine
DrotAA	drotrecogin alfa (activated)
DSA	digital subtraction angiogram
DVT	deep vein thrombosis
EACA	ε-aminocaproic acid
EBV	Epstein–Barr virus
ECG	electrocardiograph
ECMO	extracorporeal membrane oxygenation
EDA	end-diastolic area
EDV	end-diastolic volume
EEG	electroencephalograph
EF	ejection fraction
ELISA	enzyme-linked immunosorbent assay
EMG	electromyograph
EN	enteral nutrition
ENT	ear, nose and throat
EPA	eicosopentanoic acid
EPCR	endothelial protein C receptor
EPO	erythropoietin
EPUAP	European Pressure Ulcer Advisory Panel
ERCP	endoscopic retrograde cholangiopancreatography
ESBL	extended-spectrum β-lactamase
ESD	end-systolic volume
ESRD	end-stage renal disease
ESR	erythrocyte sedimentation rate
$ETCO_2$	end-tidal CO_2
ETT	endotracheal tube
EVLW	extravascular lung water
FBC	full blood count
FDA	Food and Drug Administration
FDP	fibrinogen degradation product
FEV	forced expiratory volume
FFP	fresh frozen plasma
FiO_2	fractional inspired oxygen concentration
FNA	fine needle aspiration
FRC	functional residual capacity
FT	full thickness
FTc	corrected flow time
FVC	forced vital capacity
GABA	γ-aminobutyric acid
GAVE	gastric antral vascular ectasia
GBS	Guillain–Barre syndrome
GCS	Glasgow Coma Score (Scale)
G-CSF	granulocyte colony-stimulating factor
GDP	Gross Domestic Product
GEDVI	global end-diastolic volume index
GFR	glomerular filtration rate
GI	gastrointestinal
GIST	gastrointrestinal stromal tumour
GLA	γ-linolenic acid
GNC	General Medical Council
GM-CSF	granulocyte–macrophage colony-stimulating factor
GOJ	gastro-oesophageal junction
G-6-PD	glucose-6-phospate dehydrogenase
γGT	γ-glutamyltransferase

GTN	glyceryl trinitrate
GvHD	graft vs host disease
HAART	highly active antiretroviral therapy
HAP	hospital-acquired pneumonia
HAS	human albumin solution
HAV	hepatitis A virus
Hb	haemoglobin
H2B	histamine receptor 2 blocker
HBO	hyperbaric oxygen
HBV	hepatitis B virus
HCA	healthcare assistant
HCT	haematopoetic cell transplantation
HCV	hepatitis C virus
HDU	High Dependency Unit
HELLP	haemolysis, elevated liver enzymes, low platelets
HEPA	high efficiency particulate air
HF	haemofiltration/heart failure
HFJV	high-frequency jet ventilation
HFOV	high-frequency oscillatory ventilation
HFV	high-frequency ventilation
HIT	heparin-induced thrombocytopenia
HIV	human immunodeficiency virus
HLA	human leucocyte antigen
HME	heated membrane exchange
HNS	hyperosmolar non-ketotic state
HO	heterotopic ossification
HOCM	hypertrophic obstructive cardiomyopathy
HPA	hypothalamo-pituitary–adrenal
HRCT	high resolution CT
HRS	hepatorenal syndrome
HSCT	haematopoietic stem cell transplantation
HSV	herpes simplex virus
5-HT	5-hydroxytryptamine
HT	health technology assessment
HTS	hypertonic saline
HU	hydroxyurea
HUS	haemolytic–uraemic syndrome
HVAC	heating, ventilation and air conditioning
HVHF	high volume haemofiltration
IABP	intra-aortic balloon pump
IAH	intra-abdominal hypertension
IAP	intra-abdominal pressure
IBD	irritable bowel disease
IBTICM	Intercollegiate Board for Training in Intensive Care Medicine
IBW	ideal body weight
ICG	indocyanine green
ICH	intracranial (intracerebral) haemorrhage
ICNSS	Intensive Care Nursing Scoring System
ICP	intracranial pressure
ICS	inhaled corticosteroid/Intensive Care Society
ICU	Intensive Care Unit
IE	infective endocarditis
IEN	immune-enhancing nutrition
I:E ratio	inspiratory:expiratory ratio
IGF-1	insulin-like growth factor-1
IL	interleukin
ILMA	intubating laryngeal mask airway
IM	intramuscular
iNO	inhaled nitric oxide
iNOS	inducible nitric oxide synthase
INR	international normalized ratio
IPPV	intermittent positive pressure ventilation
IPV	intrapulmonary percussive ventilator
IRDS	infant respiratory distress syndrome
IRIS	immune reconstitution inflammatory syndrome
IS	incentive spyrometry
ITBVI	intrathoracic blood volume index
ITP	intrathoracic pressure
ITT	intention-to-treat
ITU	Intensive Therapy Unit
IV	intravenous
IVC	inferior vena cava
IVIG	intravenous immunoglobulin
JVP	jugular venous pressure
LA	left atrium
LABA	long-acting β_2 agonist
LBBB	left bundle branch block
LDH	lactate dehydrogenase
LEMS	Lambert–Eaton myasthenia syndrome
LFT	liver function test
LIP	lower inflection point
LMA	laryngeal mask airway
LMWH	low molecular weight heparin
LOLA	L-ornithine l-aspartate
LOS	length of stay
LP	lumbar puncture
LPA	Lasting Power of Attorney
LPS	lipopolysaccharide
LTB	leukotriene B
LTOT	long-term oxygen therapy
LV	left ventricle
LVAD	left ventricular assist device
LVH	left ventricular hypertrophy
LVOT	left ventricular outflow tract
MAO	monoamine oxidase
MAOI	monoamine oxidase inhibitor
MAP	mean arterial pressure
MCA	middle cerebral artery
MDI	metered-dose inhalation
MDR	multiple drug-resistant
MEG-X	monoethylglycinxylidide
MET	medical emergency team

MetHb	methaemoglobin
MG	myasthenia gravis
MH	malignant hyperthermia
MHI	manual hyperinflation
MI	myocardial infarction
MOD	multi-organ dysfunction
MODS	multi-organ dysfunction syndrome
MOF	multi-organ failure
MPA	microscopic polyangitis
MPM	Mortality Probability Model
MPO	myeloperoxidase
MR	mitral regurgitation
MRCP	magnetic resonance cholangiopancreatography
MRI	magnetic resonance imaging
MRSA	methicillin-resistant *Staphylococcus aureus*
MS	mitral stenosis
MuSK	muscle-specific receptor kinase
NAC	*N*-acetylcysteine
nAChR	nicotinic acetylcholine receptor
NAECC	North American–European Consensus Conference
NAG	*N*-acetylglucosaminidase
NAPQI	*N*-acetyl-*p*-benzoquinone imine
NCEPOD	National Confidential Enquiry into Patient Outcome and Death
NCSE	non-convulsive status epilepticus
NF-κB	nuclear factor-κB
NG	nasogastric
NHBD	non-heart-beating donor
NICE	National Institute for Health and Clinical Excellence
NIPPV	non-invasive positive pressure ventilation
NIRS	near-infrared spectroscopy
NIV	non-invasive ventilation
NJ	nasojejunal
NK	neurokinin
NMDA	*N*-methyl-D-aspartate
NO	nitric oxide
NOS	nitric oxide synthase
NRT	nicotine replacement therapy
NSAID	non-steroidal anti-inflammatory drug
NSTEMI	non-ST-segment elevation myocardial infarction
nv-CJD	new variant Creutzfeld–Jacob disease
NYHA	New York Heart Association
od	once daily
OHCA	out-of-hospital cardiac arrest
OJEU	*Official Journal of the European Union*
OP	opening pressure
OR	odds ratio
OSAHS	obstructive sleep apnoea hypopnoea syndrome
$PaCO_2$	arterial partial pressure of carbon dioxide
PAH	pulmonary arterial hypertension
PAMP	pathogen-associated molecular pattern
PAN	polyarteritis nodosa
Pao	pressure at airway opening
PaO_2	arterial partial pressure of oxygen
PAoP	pulmonary artery occlusion pressure
PAR1	protease-activated receptor 1
PAWP	pulmonary artery wedge pressure
PBV	pulmonary blood volume
PBW	predicted body weight
PCA	patient-controlled anaesthesia
PCC	prothrombin complex concentrate
PCI	percutaneous coronary intervention
PCP	*Pneumocystis carinii* pneumonia
PCR	polymerase chain reaction
PCT	procalcitonin
PD	peritoneal dialysis
PDE	phosphodiesterase
PDH	pyruvate dehydrogenase
PE	pulmonary embolism
PEA	pulseless electrical activity
$PECO_2$	partial pressure of expired CO_2
PEEP	positive end-expiratory pressure
PEFR	peak expiratory flow rate
PEG	percutaneous endoscopic gastrostomy
PEJ	percutaneous endoscopic jejunostomy
PEP	positive expiratory pressure
PET	positron emission tomography
$PetCO_2$	end-tidal CO_2 partial pressure
PG	prostaglandin
PIE	pulmonary interstitial emphysema
PIP	positive inspiratory pressure
PLR	passive leg raising
PN	parenteral nutrition
PO	per os
PONV	post-operative nausea and vomiting
PP	partial pressure
PPA	plexogenic pulmonary arteriopathy
PPH	postpartum haemorrhage
PPHN	persistent pulmonary hypertension of the newborn
PPI	proton pump inhibitor
PPM	potentially pathogenic microorganism
PPV	pulse pressure variation
PR3	proteinase 3
PRA	plasma renin activity
PRF	pulse repetition frequency
PSV	pressure support ventilation
PT	prothrombin time
PTC	percutaneous transhepatic cholecystotomy
PTCA	percutaneous transluminal coronary angioplasty

PTSD	post-traumatic stress disorder
PUFA	polyunsaturated fatty acid
P/V	pressure–volume
PVR	pulmonary vascular resistance
QALY	quality-adjusted life year
qds	four times a day
RA	right atrium
RAAS	renin–angiotensin–aldosterone system
Raw	airway resistance
RBBB	right bundle branch block
RCT	randomized controlled trial
RDS	respiratory distress syndrome
REM	rapid eye movement
RH	relative humidity
ROSC	return (restoration) of spontaneous circulation
RPGN	rapidly progressive glomerulonephritis
RR	relative risk
Rrs	respiratory resistance
RRT	renal replacement therapy
RV	right ventricle
RVAD	right ventricular assist device
RV EDVI	right ventricular end-diastolic volume index
RWMA	regional wall motion abnormality
SA	sinoatrial
SABA	short-acting β agonist
SAH	subarachnoid haemorrhage
SAP	severe acute pancreatitis
SAPS	Simplified Acute Physiology Score
SB	spontaneous breathing
SBE	standard base excess
SBP	systolic blood pressure
SBT	spontaneous breathing trial
SBT-CO_2	single breath test for CO_2
SC	subcutaneous/seiving coefficient
SCD	sickle cell disease
SCI	spinal cord injury
SCUF	slow continuous ultrafiltration
SD	superficial dermal
SDB	sleep-disoderded breathing
SDD	selective decontamination of the digestive tract
SE	status elipticus
SEP	sensory evoked potential
SIADH	syndrome of inappropriate ADH secretion
SID	strong ion difference
SIG	strong ion gap
SIMV	synchronized intermittent mandatory ventilation
SIRS	systemic inflammatory response syndrome
SLE	systemic lupus erythematosus
SLED	sustained low efficiency dialysis
SNP	sodium nitroprusside
SOFA	Sequential Organ Failure Assessment
SP	surfactant protein
SRH	stigmata of recent haemorrhage
SSEP	somatosensory evoked potential
STEMI	ST-segment elevation myocardial infarction
SV	stroke volume
SVC	superior vena cava
SVR	systemic vascular resistance
SVT	supraventricular tachycardia
SVV	stroke volume variation
T_3	triiodothyronine
T_4	thyroxine
TB	tuberculosis
TBI	traumatic brain injury
TBSA	total body surface area
TCA	tricyclic antidepressant
TCD	transcranial Doppler
Tds	three times a day
TED	thromboembolism deterrent
TEG	thromboelastogram
TENS	transcutaneous electrical nerve stimulation
TGF	transforming growth factor
TIA	transient ischaemic attack
TIPS	transjugular intrahepatic portosystemic shunt
TK	thymidine kinase
TLC	total lung capacity
TLR	Toll-like receptor
TLS	tumour lysis syndrome
TMP	transmembrane pressure
TNF	tumour necrosis factor
TOD	target organ damage
TOE	transoesophageal echocardiography
tPA	tissue plasminogen activator
TPN	total parenteral nutrition
TR	tricuspid regurgitation
TSH	thyroid-stimulating hormone
TT	thrombin time
TTE	transthoracic echocardiography
TTP	thrombotic thrombocytopenic purpura
TURP	transurethral resection of prostate
UA	unstable angina
UAO	upper airway obstruction
UC	ulcerative colitis
U&E	urea and electrolyte
UF	ultrafiltration
UFH	unfractionated heparin
UIP	upper inflection point
UKOSS	UK Obstetric Surveillance System
URR	urea reduction ratio

UTI	urinary tract infection
VA ECMO	venoarterial extracorporeal membrane oxygenation
VV ECMO	venovenous extracorporeal membrane oxygenation
VAD	ventricular assist device
VAP	ventilator-associated pneumonia
VATS	video-assisted thoracoscopy
VC	vital capacity
VEP	visual evoked potential
VF	ventricular fibrillation
VHI	ventilator hyperinflation
VIE	vacuum-insulated evaporator
VILI	ventilator-induced lung injury
V/Q	ventilation/perfusion
VRE	vancomycin-resistant enterococci
VSD	ventricular septal defect
VT	ventricular tachycardia
VTEC	verocytotoxin-producing *Escherichia coli*
vWF	von Willebrand factor
VZV	varicella-zoster virus
WA	Welfare Attorney
WBC	white blood cell
WCC	white cell count
WG	Wagner's granulomatosis
WOB	work of breathing
WPW	Wolff–Parkinson-White

Contributors

Dr. Jane Adcock
Consultant Neurologist
John Radcliffe Hospital, Oxford
Royal Berkshire Hospital, Reading

Dr Imran Ahmad
Specialist Registrar in Anaesthesia
John Radcliffe Hospital
Oxford

Dr Peter Anderson
Specialist Registrar in Critical Care
St. Georges Hospital
London

Professor Peter JD Andrews
Anaesthetics, Intensive Care & Pain Medicine
University of Edinburgh & Lothian University Hospitals Division

Professor Djillali Annane
General Intensive Care Unit,
Department of Acute Medicine
Raymond Poincaré hospital (AP-HP)
University of Versailles SQY (UniverSud Paris)
104 boulevard Raymond Poincaré,
92380 Garches, France

Dr Tarek F Antonios
Senior Lecturer & Consultant Physician
Blood Pressure Unit,
St. George's, University of London
London

Dr Elizabeth Ashley
The Intensive Care Unit
The Heart hospital,
Westmoreland Street,
London

Dr Jonathan Ball
Consultant in Intensive Care
General Intensive Care Unit
St George's Hospital
London

Dr Nicholas Barrett
Consultant in Intensive Care Medicine
Guy's and St Thomas' Hospital
Westminster Bridge Road
London

Dr Anthony Bastin
Specialist Registrar in Intensive Care Medicine
Royal Brompton Hospital
London

Dr Anna Batchelor
Consultant in Anaesthesia and Intensive Care Medicine
Royal Victoria Infirmary Newcastle
Newcastle

Dr Rafik Bedair
Department of Critical Care
Manchester Royal Infirmary
Manchester

Dr Geoff Bellingan
Director of Intensive Care
University College Hospital
London

Dr Dennis CJJ Bergmans
Intensive Care Center Maastricht
Maastricht University Medical Center+
The Netherlands

Professor Julian Bion
Professor of Intensive Care Medicine
University Department of Anaesthesia & Intensive Care Medicine,
N5 Queen Elizabeth Hospital,
Edgbaston,
Birmingham

Dr Andrew Bodenham
Anaesthetic Department
Leeds General Infirmary
Leeds

Dr Jonathan Booth
Consultant Gastroenterologist
Royal Berkshire Hospital
Reading

Mr Michael Booth FRCS
Consultant Upper GI Surgeon,
Royal Berkshire Hospital
Reading

Mr Mark Borthwick,
Consultant Pharmacist, Critical Care
John Radcliffe Hospital
Oxford

Mr Richard Bourne,
Lead Critical Care Pharmacist
Sheffield Teaching Hospital
Sheffield

Ms Gillian Bradbury
Matron, Intensive Care Unit
The Royal London Hospital
Whitechapel Road
London

Dr Aimee Brame
Specialist Registrar in Intensive Care Medicine
Adult Intensive Care Unit,
Royal Brompton Hospital
London

Dr Stephen Brett
Consultant in Intensive Care Medicine
Imperial College London
Hammersmith Hospital
Du Cane Road, London

Dr Kate Brignall,
Specialist Registrar in critical care
Guy's and St Thomas' Hospital Trust
London

Dr Matthew A Butkus
The CRISMA (Clinical Research, Investigation, and Systems Modeling of Acute Illness) Laboratory,
Department of Critical Care Medicine,
University of Pittsburgh,
Pittsburgh, PA, USA

Dr Luigi Camporota
Specialist Registrar in Intensive Care Medicine
Department of Adult Intensive Care
Guy's and St Thomas' NHS Foundation Trust
London, UK

Dr Jean Carlet
Directeur médical,
Direction de l'Amélioration et de la Qualité et de la Sécurité des Soins (DAQSS)
HAS, 2 avenue du Stade de France
93218 Saint-Denis La Plaine Cedex
France

Dr Susana Afonso de Carvalho
Unidade de Cuidados Intensivos Polivalente
Hospital de St. António dos Capuchos
Centro Hospitalar de Lisboa Central, E.P.E.
Lisboa Portugal

Dr Maurizio Cecconi
Consultant in Anaesthesia and Intensive Care Medicine
Dept. of Anaesthesia and Intensive Care,
University of Udine Italy

Dr. Felix Chua
Consultant in Respiratory Medicine
St. George's Healthcare NHS Trust
Blackshaw Road
London

Dr Jerome Cockings
Consultant in Intensive Care Medicine and Anaesthesia
Royal Berkshire Hospital
Reading

Dr Andrew Cohen
Consultant, Anaesthesia and Intensive Care Medicine
St James's University Hospital
Leeds

Professor Christine Collin
Neurorehabilitation
Royal Berkshire Hospital
Reading

Ms Catherine Collins
Dept of Nutrition and Dietetics
St Georges Hospital
London

Mr P Conaghan
Specialist Registrar
John Radcliffe Hospital
Oxford

Dr Daniel Conway
Dept of Anaesthesia
Manchester Royal Infirmary
Manchester

Dr Jeremy Cordingley
Consultant in Intensive Care Medicine
Royal Brompton Hospital
London

Dr Matthew Cowan,
Specialist Registrar & NIH Research Fellow
St. George's,
University of London,
London

Dr Agnieszka Crerar-Gilbert
Consultant in Cardiothoracic Intensive Care & Anaesthesia
St George's Cardiothoracic Intensive Care Unit
London

Dr Chris Danbury
Consultant Intensivist
Royal Berkshire Hospital
Reading

Dr Craig Davidson
Director Lane Fox Respiratory Unit
Guys & St Thomas' Foundation Trust
London

Dr Rebecca Davis
Microbiology department
Chelsea and Westminster Hospital
Fulham Road
London

Dr Jamil Darrouj
Pulmonary/Critical Care Division
Cooper University Hospital
Robert Wood Johnson Medical School
393 Dorrance
Camden
USA

Dr Daniel De Backer
Dpt of Intensive Care
Erasme University Hospital
Université Libre de Bruxelles
808 Route de Lennik
B-1070 Brussels (Belgium)

Dr Kayann Dell
John Radcliffe Hospitals
Oxford

Prof. Giorgio Della Rocca
Professor of Anesthesia and Intensive Care
Chair of the Dept of Anesthesia and Intensive Care
University of Udine.
Udine, Italy

Dr Phil Dellinger
Critical Care Division
Cooper University Hospital
Robert Wood Johnson Medical School
393 Dorrance
Camden USA

Dr James Down
Consultant in Intensive care and Anaesthesia
University College Hospital
London

Dr Martin Dresner
Consultant Obstetrics
Leeds Royal Infirmary
Leeds

Dr Robert T Duncan
Senior Trainee in Burns
Wythenshawe Hospital
Manchester

Miss N Dunne
Specialist Registrar
John Radcliffe Hospital,
Oxford

Dr Andy Eynon
Director of Neurosciences Intensive Care
Wessex Neurological Centre
Southampton General Hospital
Southampton

Dr Paul Ferris
Advanced Trainee in Intensive Care
Wythenshawe Hospital
Manchester

Dr Simon Finney
Consultant in Intensive Care Medicine
The Royal Brompton Hospital
London

Dr Robert Galland
Royal Berkshire Hospital
Reading

Dr Magnus Garrioch
Dept of Anaesthesia and Critical Care,
Manchester Royal Infirmary,
Manchester

Anis el Ghorch
Département d'Anesthésie et Réanimation
Hôpital Lariboisière
Paris France

Dr Phil Gillen
Specialist Registrar in Anaesthesia and Intensive Care
Royal Berkshire Hospital
Reading

Dr David Goldhill
Consultant, Department of Anaesthesia and Critical Care
The Royal National Orthopaedic Hospital
Stanmore
Middlesex

Dr Andrew Gratrix
Consultant in Intensive Care and Anaesthesia
Hull Royal Infirmary
Hull

Dr Mark Griffiths
Consultant in Intensive Care Medicine
The Royal Brompton Hospital
London

Prof Richard D Griffiths
Professor of Medicine (Intensive Care),
Unit of Pathophysiology
School of Clinical Science
University of Liverpool
Liverpool

Dr Mark Hamilton
Consultant in Anaesthesia &
Intensive Care Medicine
St. George's Hospital,
London,

Dr Olfa Hamzaoui
Réanimation médicale
CHU Bicêtre
Université Paris-Sud, 11
France

Dr Jonathan M Handy
Consultant in Intensive Care Medicine
Chelsea & Westminster Hospital
Honorary Senior Lecturer
Imperial College
London

Dr Derek Hausenloy
Clinical Lecturer,
The Hatter Cardiovascular Institute,
University College London Hospital,
London

Professor Ken Hillman
Professor of Intensive Care,
University of New South Wales
Sydney
Australia

Dr Steven Hollenberg
Professor of Medicine
Robert Wood Johnson Medical School/UMDNJ
Director, Coronary Care Unit
Cooper University Hospital
Camden, NJ

Dr Simon Hughes
RAF Consultant in Intensive Care Medicine and Anaesthesia
John Radcliffe Hospital,
Oxford

Professor Beverley J Hunt
Consultant, Depts of Haematology,
Pathology & Rheumatology Lead in Blood Sciences,
Guy's & St Thomas' Trust
London

Dr Shabnam Iyer
Dept Microbiology
Royal Berkshire Hospital

Dr Ana Luisa Jardim
Unidade de Cuidados Intensivos Polivalente
Hospital de St. António dos Capuchos
Centro Hospitalar de Lisboa Central, E.P.E.
Lisboa
Portugal

Dr. Michael Joannidis,
Professor
Director, Medical Intensive Care Unit
Department of Internal Medicine
Medical University of Innsbruck
Innsbruck,
Austria

Dr Max Jonas
Consultant in Intensive Care
Intensive Care Unit
Southampton General Hospital
Southampton

Dr Andrew Jones
Consultant Critical Care and Respiratory Medicine
Guy's and St Thomas's NHS Foundation Trust
Department of Intensive Care
St Thomas's Hospital
London

Dr Christina Jones
Nurse Consultant Critical Care Follow-up
Whiston Hospital
Warrington Road
Prescot
Liverpool

Dr Rachael Jones
Department of HIV/GU Medicine,
St Stephens Centre,
Chelsea & Westminster Healthcare NHS Trust,
London

Dr Atul Kapila
Consultant Anaesthetist
Royal Berkshire Hospital
Reading

Dr Juliane Kause
Department of Critical Care
Queen Alexandra Hospital
Portsmouth

Dr Richard Keays
Consultant in Intensive Care Medicine
Chelsea & Westminster Hospital
London

Dr John A Kellum
The CRISMA (Clinical Research, Investigation, and Systems Modeling of Acute Illness) Laboratory,
Department of Critical Care Medicine,
University of Pittsburgh,
Pittsburgh, PA, USA

Dr Chris Kirwan
Clinical Research Fellow,
Intensive Care Medicine
St George's NHS Trust

Dr Roop Kishen,
Consultant in Intensive Care Medicine & Anaesthesia,
Hon Lecturer,
Salford Royal NHS Foundation Trust,
Salford, Manchester

Dr John Knighton
Consultant in Critical Care & Anaesthesia
Portsmouth Hospitals NHS Trust
Portsmouth

Dr Martin Kuper
Consultant in Anaesthesia and Intensive Care.
The Whittington Hospital NHS Trust,
London

Professor Richard Langford
Professor of Inflammation Science
William Harvey Research Institute
Barts and The London,
Queen Mary's School of Medicine and Dentistry
London

Dr Smaoui Lassäad
Département d'Anesthésie et Réanimation
Hôpital Lariboisière
Paris France

Dawn Lau
Specialist Registrar in Respiratory Medicine
Osler Chest Unit
Churchill Hospital
Oxford

Dr Jonathan Lightfoot
Anaesthetic Trainee Bristol Rotation
Department of Anaesthetics
Weston-Super-Mare General Hospital

Dr Thiago Lisboa,
CIBER Respiratory Diseases.
Tarragona,
Spain

Professor Richard Langford
Director, Anaesthetic Laboratory
Barts and the London NHS Trust
London

Dr. Lies Langouche
Department of Intensive Care Medicine
University Hospital
Katholieke Universiteit Leuven
Belgium

Dr Andrew Lawson
Consultant in Pain Medicine & Anaesthesia
Royal Berkshire Hospital
Reading

Dr Peter MacNaughten
Clinical Director Critical Care
Intensive Care Unit
Derriford Hospital
Plymouth

Professor Brendan Madden
Professor of Cardiothoracic Medicine
St George's Hospital, Cardiothoracic Unit
Blackshaw Road
London

Dr Hilary Madder
Clinical Director, Neurosciences Intensive Care Unit
John Radcliffe Hospital
Oxford

Dr Nicholas Madden
The CRISMA (Clinical Research, Investigation, and
Systems Modeling of Acute Illness) Laboratory,
Department of Critical Care Medicine,
University of Pittsburgh,
Pittsburgh, PA,
USA

Dr. Michael MacMahon
Anaesthetic Trainee South East Scotland Rotation
Intensive Care Unit
Western General Hospital
Edinburgh

Alexander R. Manara
Consultant in Anaesthesia and Intensive Care.
The Intensive Care Unit,
Frenchay Hospital,
Frenchay Park Road,
Bristol

Dr Luciana Mascia
Department of Anesthesia and Intensive Care Medicine
University of Turin,
Italy

Alexandre Mebazaa
Université Paris 7 Denis Diderot
Département d'Anesthésie et Réanimation
Hôpital Lariboisière
Paris
France

Mr S Middleton
Royal Berkshire Hospital
Reading

Dr Rui Moreno
Unidade de Cuidados Intensivos Polivalente
Hospital de St. António dos Capuchos
Centro Hospitalar de Lisboa Central, E.P.E.
Lisboa Portugal

Dr Giles Morgan
Queen Alexandra Hospital
Portsmouth

Mr Satvinder Mudan
Consultant Surgeon
Royal Marsden Hospital
Fulham Road London

Raghavan Murugan,
The CRISMA (Clinical Research, Investigation,
and Systems Modelling of Acute Illness)
Laboratory Department of Critical Care Medicine
University of Pittsburgh
Pittsburgh PA, USA

Dr Mark Nelson
Director of HIV Services
Chelsea and Westminster Hospital
London

Dr Peter Nightingale
Consultant in Anaesthesia
Wythenshawe Hospital
Manchester

Dr Jerry Nolan
Consultant in Anaesthesia and
Intensive Care Medicine
Royal United Hospital
Bath

Mrs Michelle Norrenberg
Head of ICU physiotherapist
Dept of Intensive Care
Erasme University Hospital
Brussels

Dr Pauline O'Neil
Aberdeen Royal Infirmary
Foresterhill
Aberdeen

Dr Mark Palazzo
Consultant Critical Care Medicine
Imperial College Healthcare NHS Trust
Charing Cross Hospital
London

Dr Tim Palfreman
Specialist Registrar in Intensive Care Medicine
Adult Intensive Care Unit,
Royal Brompton Hospital
London

Dr John Park
Specialist Registrar in Intensive Care Medicine
The Royal Brompton Hospital
London

Dr Tim Parke
Consultant in Intensive Care Medicine and Anaesthesia
Royal Berkshire Hospital
Reading

Dr Hina Pattani
Specialist Registrar in Critical Care
Queens Medical Centre
Nottingham

Dr Rupert Pearse
Senior Lecturer and Honorary Consultant in Intensive Care Medicine
Barts and The London School of Medicine and Dentistry
Queen Mary's, University of London

Dr Barbara Philips
Senior Lecturer, Intensive Care Medicine
Department of Cardiac and Vascular Sciences
St Georges Hospital Medical School
London

Mr Giles Peek
Consultant in Cardiothoracic Surgery & ECMO
Glenfield Hospital
Groby Road
Leicester

Dr Amanda Pinder
Consultant Obstetric Anaesthetist,
Leeds Teaching Hospitals

Dr Alison Pittard
Consultant in Anaesthesia and Intensive Care
Leeds General Infirmary
Leeds

Professor Michael R Pinsky
Professor of Critical Care Medicine,
Bioengineering and Anesthesiology
University of Pittburgh
Pittsburgh USA

Dr Kees Polderman
Associate Professor in Intensive Care Medicine,
Department of Intensive Care
University medical center Utrecht
Heidelberglaan 100
Utrecht 3584 CX
The Netherlands

Dr Susanna Price
Consultant Cardiologist and Intensivist,
Royal Brompton Hospital,
London

Dr Caroline Pritchard
Clinical Research Fellow
Department of Neuroanesthesia and Neurocritical Care
The National Hospital for Neurology and Neurosurgery
Queen Square London

Dr Paul Quinton
Consultant in Cardiothoracic Intensive Care & Anaesthesia
St George's Cardiothoracic Intensive Care Unit
London

Dr Tony Rahman
Consultant Gastroenterologist & ICU Physician
Honorary Senior Lecturer,
St. George's,
University of London,
London

Professor Marco Ranieri
President of ESICM
Professor of Anesthesia and Intensive Care
University of Turin, Italy

Dr Ravishankar Rao Baikady
Consultant in Anaesthesia
The Royal Marsden NHS Foundation Trust
London

Dr Charlotte FJ Rayner
Consultant Physician
Parkside Hospital, London

Dr Ian Rechner
Consultant in Intensive Care Medicine and Anaesthesia
Royal Berkshire Hospital
Reading

Dr Jennie Rechner
Specialist Registrar is Anaesthesia
John Radcliffe Hospital
Oxford

Dr A Reece-Smith
Clinical Fellow in Surgery
Addenbrookes Hospital
Cambridge

Mr Howard Reece-Smith
Consultant Surgeon
Royal Berkshire Hospital
Reading

Prof. Dr. Konrad Reinhart
Director of Clinic for Anaesthesiology and Intensive Care
University of Jena
Erlanger Allee 101
07747 Jena
Germany

Jordi Rello,
Critical Care Department.
Joan XXIII University Hospital
University Rovira & Virgili.
Tarragona, Spain

Dr Andrew Retter
Specialist Registrar in Intensive Care and Haematology
Department of Haematology
Guy's & St Thomas' Trust
London

Dr Andrew Rhodes
Consultant in Intensive Care
St George's Hospital
London

Dr Zaccaria Ricci,
Dept of Pediatric Cardiac Surgery,
Bambino Gesù Hospital,
Rome, Italy

Dr Angela Riga
Specialist Registrar Upper GI/HPB
Academic Surgery Department
Royal Marsden Hospital
London

Dr Claudio Ronco,
Dept of Nephrology,
Dialysis and Transplantation,
S.Bortolo Hospital,
Vicenza Italy

Dr Hendrick KF van Saene,
Department of Clinical Microbiology and
Infection Control
Royal Liverpool Children's NHS Trust of Alder Hey
Liverpool

Dr Som Sarkar
Specialist Registrar in Anaesthesia
Leicester

Dr Karnan Satkunam
Specialist Registrar in Respiratory Medicine
Royal London Hospital
London

Pallav Shah
Consultant Physician
Royal Brompton Hospital
Chelsea & Westminster Hospital
London

Dr Manu Shankar Hari
Specialist Registrar Anaesthesia and
Intensive Care Medicine.
Guy's and St Thomas Hospital
NHS foundation trust,
London

Dr Alasdair Short
Director, Critical Care
Broomfield Hospital
Chelmsford
Essex

Dr Jeroen Schouten,
Internist/Intensivist
Intensive Care Unit
Canisius Wilhelmina Hospital
Nijmegen,
The Netherlands

Dr Kevin Sim
Aberdeen Royal Infirmary
Foresterhill
Aberdeen

Dr Suveer Singh
Consultant Intensive Care and Respiratory Medicine
Chelsea and Westminster Hospital
London

Dr Andrew Smith
Consultant in Anaesthesia & Intensive Care
The Heart Hospital
Westmoreland Street
London

Dr Martin Smith
Consultant in Neuroanaesthesia and Neurocritical Care
Department of Neuroanaesthesia and Neurocritical Care
The National Hospital for Neurology
and Neurosurgery
University College London Hospitals
Queen Square
London

Dr Neil Soni
Honorary Clin Senior Lecturer
Division of Surgery, Oncology, Reproductive Biology and
Anaesthetics
Imperial College
London

Professor Charles L. Sprung
General Intensive Care Unit,
Department of Anesthesiology and
Critical Care Medicine,
Hadassah Hebrew University
Medical Center, P.O. Box 12000, Jerusalem,
Israel 91120

Dr Paul Stevens
Department of Renal Medicine
Kent and Canterbury Hospital
Ethelbert Road
Canterbury

Dr Sarah Stirling
Specialist Registrar Intensive Care Medicine and
Anaesthesia
Barts and The London NHS Trust
London

Dr Stephanie Strachan
Specialist Registrar in Anaesthesia
Chelsea and Westminster,
London

Dr Gustav Strandvik
Specialist Registrar in Intensive Care Medicine
Adult Intensive Care Unit,
Royal Brompton Hospital
London

Dr Daniel Tarditi,
Cardiovascular Associates of the Delaware Valley
Camden, NJ

Dr Bruce Taylor
Dept of Critical Care
Portsmouth Hospitals NHS Trust
Queen Alexandra Hospital
Cosham Hants

Miguel Tavares
Departmento de Anestesia e Cuidados Intensivos
Hospital Geral de Santo António
Porto Portugal

Prof. Jean-Louis Teboul
Réanimation médicale
CHU Bicêtre
Université Paris-Sud, 11 France

Chris Theaker
Royal Brompton Hospital
Sydney Street London

Dafydd Thomas
Consultant in Intensive Care
Morriston Hospital
Abertawe Bro Morganwwg
University NHS Trust Swansea

Dr Ian Thomas
Advanced Trainee in Intensive Care Medicine
The Intensive Care Unit,
Frenchay Hospital,
Frenchay Park Road,
Bristol

Dr Sam Thomson,
Specialist Registrar & Clinical Research Fellow
St. George's,
University of London,
London

Dr Louise Thwaites
Specialist in Musculoskeletal Medicine
Oxford University Clinical Research Unit
Oxford

Dr David Treacher
Department of Intensive Care
St Thomas' Hospital
Guy's & St Thomas' NHS Foundation Trust
London

Dr W James N Uprichard
Clinical Lecturer in Haematology
Imperial College London
Hammersmith Hospital
Du Cane Road
London

Prof. Dr. Greet Van den Berghe
Department of Intensive Care Medicine
University Hospital
Katholieke Universiteit Leuven
Belgium

Dr. Ilse Vanhorebeek
Department of Intensive Care Medicine
University Hospital
Katholieke Universiteit Leuven
Belgium

Dr Nilangi Virgincar
Royal Berkshire Hospital
Reading

Dr Gorazd Voga
Department of Intensive Internal Medicine,
General Hospital,
Celje, Slovenia

Dr Sam Waddy
Consultant in Intensive Care and Acute Medicine
Derriford Hospital
Plymouth

Dr Adrian Wagstaff
Magill Department of Anaesthesia
Chelsea and Westminster
London

Dr Andrew Walden
Specialist Registrar in intensive care
John Radcliffe hospital
Oxford

Dr Carl Waldmann
Consultant in Anaesthesia and Intensive Care
Royal Berkshire Hospital
Reading

Dr Colin Webb
Intensive care Registrar
Royal Berkshire Hospital
Reading

Professor Nigel R Webster
Anaesthesia and Intensive Care
Institute of Medical Sciences
Foresterhill
Aberdeen

Dr Jan Wernerman
Dept of Anaesthesia
University Hospital
Stockholm
S-141 86 HUDDINGE

Dr Bob Winter
Adult Intensive Care
Queens Medical Centre
Nottingham

Dr Duncan Wyncoll
Dept of Intensive Care
St Thomas' Hospital
Lambeth Palace Road
London

Dr Gary Yap
Intensive care Registrar
Royal Berkshire Hospital
Reading

Professor Dr DF Zandstra
Professor of Intensive Care
Faculty of Medicine
Universiteit van Amsterdam
Amsterdam Netherlands

Dr Andrew Zurek
Consultant Respiratory Physician
Royal Berkshire Hospital
Reading

Chapter 1

Respiratory therapy techniques

Chapter contents

Oxygen therapy

Aerobic respiration is the most efficient method of energy production in the mammalian cell. It utilizes oxygen to produce adenosine triphosphate (ATP). The absence of oxygen or low oxygen levels result in more inefficient anaerobic respiration. Cellular energy levels become inadequate, and this can lead to loss of cellular homeostasis, which in turn can lead to cellular death and very possibly organism death. A substantial part of critical care is targeted at treating and/or preventing hypoxia.

Pathophysiology of oxygen delivery

In critical illness the delivery (DO_2) and uptake (VO_2) of oxygen are often abnormal. Currently there are few therapeutic strategies for improvement of VO_2. Most methods of oxygen therapy target improvement in DO_2.

Delivery of oxygen from the environment is necessary to provide for cellular metabolism. In single-celled organisms (e.g. amoeba), simple diffusion suffices. However, in the multi-cellular, multi-organ human, more sophisticated mechanisms have evolved, each with their problems in illness.

Transport of oxygen to the cells follows six stages reliant only on the laws of physics.

1 Convection from the environment (ventilation).
2 Diffusion into the blood.
3 Reversible chemical bonding with haemoglobin.
4 Convective transport to the tissues (cardiac output).
5 Diffusion into the cells and organelles.
6 The redox state of the cell.

This chain of events is DO_2. Failure of DO_2 to match VO_2 leads to shock. This occurs when DO_2 declines to below approximately 300ml/min. Shock is defined loosely as failure of delivery of oxygen to match tissue demand. Commonly this refers to circulatory failure, but low DO_2 can result from several pathological mechanisms which can occur as a single problem or in combination (Table 1.1.1).

The impact of low DO_2 can be made worse by an increase in VO_2. Metabolic rate increases with exercise, inflammation, sepsis, pyrexia, thryotoxicosis, shivering, seizures, agitation, anxiety and pain. This mismatch leads to the need for early detection of shock and prompt treatment. This has been shown to be beneficial in surviving sepsis.

Clinical signs such as heart rate, blood pressure and urine output can be misleading, especially in the young. This therefore requires the concept of an effective cardiac output (ECO). This couples the clinical signs with evidence of normal DO_2 and VO_2 balance. The assessment includes peripheral temperature, oxygen haemoglobin saturation and arterial partial pressure, the presence of acidosis with a base excess greater than −2, lactataemia and abnormal SvO_2 or $ScvO_2$. These more technical measures of adequacy of oxygen delivery and uptake must always be taken in the clinical context. For example, in cyanide poisoning, both circulatory and ventilatory indices appear normal, yet the severe acidosis and lactataemia seen in this condition demonstrates tissue hypoxia. Manipulating DO_2 by increasing the environmental oxygen fraction (FiO_2) or cardiac output in this setting is unlikely to be helpful, and, even in sepsis and other more common types of shock, achieving supranormal values for DO_2 is not thought to be beneficial.

Strategies for increasing DO_2

By assessing the type of hypoxia and its likely cause, the correct choice of DO_2-improving strategy can be chosen. In the critically ill, the commonly seen combination of mechanisms leading to hypoxia may require several techniques to be instigated in parallel. The methods for improving oxygen delivery to the tissues are based on reversing problems seen at each of the six stages of oxygen delivery. Improving the transport of oxygen once in the body will be covered later in this book. This chapter is concerned with improving oxygen delivery from the environment to the bloodstream. Oxygen delivery at this stage should be considered a support mechanism, and treatment of the underlying cause is most important to reverse hypoxia.

Oxygen therapy apparatus

Principles

In the hypoxic self-ventilating patient, delivery of oxygen to the alveoli is usually achieved by increasing the FiO_2. Commonly this involves the application of one of the many varieties of oxygen masks to the face, such that it covers the mouth and/or nose. Each type of delivery system consists of broadly the same six components:

1 **Oxygen supply**. Delivery of oxygen can be from pressurized cylinders, hospital supply from cylinder banks or

Table 1.1.1 Types of hypoxia

Type of hypoxia	Pathophysiology	Examples
Hypoxic hypoxia	Reduced supply of oxygen to the body leading to a low arterial oxygen tension	**1.** Low environmental oxygen (e.g altitude) **2.** Ventilatory failure (respiratory arrest, drug overdose, neuromuscular disease) **3.** Pulmonary shunt **a.** Anatomical—ventricular septal defect with right to left flow **b.** Physiological—pneumonia, pneumothorax, pulmonary oedema, asthma
Anaemic hypoxia	Normal arterial oxygen tension, but circulating haemoglobin is reduced or functionally impaired	Massive haemorrhage, severe anaemia, carbon monoxide poisoning, methaemoglobinaemia
Stagnant hypoxia	Failure of oxygen transport due to inadequate circulation.	Left ventricular failure, pulmonary embolism, hypovolaemia, hypothermia
Histotoxic hypoxia	Impaired cellular metabolism of oxygen despite adequate delivery.	Cyanide poisoning, arsenic poisoning, alcohol intoxication

a vacuum-insulated evaporator (VIE), or an oxygen concentrator.

2 **Oxygen flow control.** For example an OHE ball valve flow meter.

3 **Connecting tubing.** Both from supply to control, and from control to patient. The bore of the tubing is important as it has effects on the oxygen flow rate. In some systems it can also act as a reservoir.

4 **Reservoir.** All have reservoirs. In the simple oxygen mask it is the mask itself. Nasal cannulae use the nasopharynx as the reservoir. An oxygen tent is a large-volume reservoir. The reservoir serves to store oxygen, but must not allow significant storage of exhaled gases leading to rebreathing of carbon dioxide.

5 **Patient attachment.** This permits delivery of oxygen to the airway. This is achieved either by directly covering the upper airway, e.g. plastic mask/head box, or by increasing the oxygen concentration in the wider environment, e.g. oxygen tent.

6 **Expired gas facility.** Expired gas needs to dissipate to the environment. This can be achieved by having a small reservoir with holes, one-way valves as in the non-rebreather masks, or high oxygen flows as seen in some of the continuous positive airway pressure (CPAP) systems.

Additional features of oxygen breathing systems are the presence of humidification such as a water bath, to prevent drying of the mucosal membranes. Some devices have an oxygen monitor incorporated into the apparatus to permit more accurate defining of the FiO_2.

Factors that affect the performance of oxygen delivery systems

Most of the simpler oxygen delivery devices, e.g. plastic masks, nasal cannulae, etc., deliver oxygen at relatively low oxygen flow rates. The patient inspiratory flow rate varies throughout inspiration (25–100+L.min^{-1}) and exceeds the oxygen flow rate. This drains the small reservoir and causes entrainment of environmental air. The effect is to dilute the oxygen concentration to the final FiO_2. The actual FiO_2 that reaches the alveolus is therefore unpredictable and is dependent on the interaction of patent factors and device factors (Table 1.1.2). In the hypoxic patient it is common to find significant increases in inspiratory flow rates as well as the loss of the respiratory pause. This causes significant entrainment of air, lowering the alveolar FiO_2. This is particularly true of the variable performance masks, but is also seen in Venturi-type masks, particularly when higher FiO_2 inserts are used. The presence of a valve-controlled reservoir bag on a non-rebreather mask should compensate for high inspiratory flows, hence the belief that such devices can deliver an FiO_2 of 1.0 which does not actually happen. This is not seen in models of human ventilation (Fig. 1.1.1)

Table 1.1.2 Factors that influence the FiO_2 delivered to a patient by oxygen delivery devices[5]

Patient factors	Device factors
Inspiratory flow rate	Oxygen flow rate
Presence of a respiratory pause	Volume of mask
Tidal volume	Air vent size
	Tightness of fit

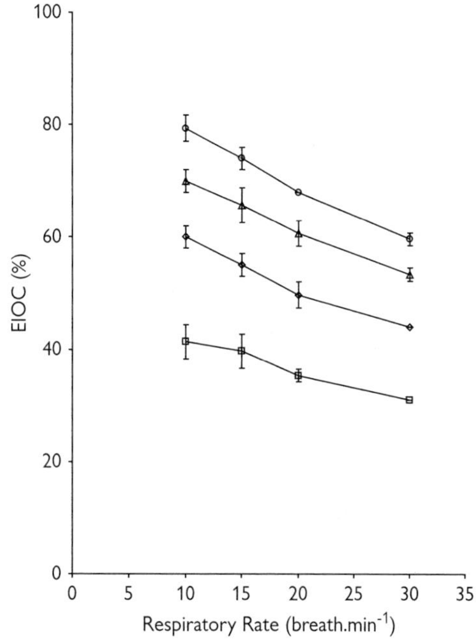

Fig. 1.1.1 The performance of a Hudson non-rebreather mask on a model of human ventilation. Tidal volume of 500ml and four oxygen flow rates (2l/min (□), 6l/min (◇), 10l/min (△) and 15l/min (○)). As the respiratory rate increases, so the effective inspired oxygen concentration (EIOC) deteriorates.

Classification of oxygen delivery devices

Methods of delivering oxygen to the conscious patient with no airway instrumentation can be broadly divided into the following categories.

- Variable performance systems
- Fixed performance systems
- High flow systems
- Others

Variable performance systems are so called because their FiO_2 can vary as described above. Fixed performance systems cannot. High flow systems use high oxygen flows to maintain a fixed performance. The common types and their properties are summarized in Table 1.1.3.

Hazards of oxygen therapy

Oxygen is a drug and, like most drugs, its use is not without risk. It is also a gas and commonly delivered from compressed sources.

Supply

Medical oxygen is supplied at 137bar from a cylinder, and 4bar from hospital pipelines. Direct administration at delivery pressures is highly dangerous and requires properly functioning pressure-limiting valves. Oxygen supports combustion. Patients must not smoke cigarettes when receiving oxygen therapy, and oxygen should be removed from the environment when sparking may occur, e.g. during defibrillation.

Table 1.1.3 Classification of oxygen delivery systems

Oxygen delivery system	Types used	Properties
Variable performance	Nasal cannulae, semi-rigid masks (Hudson, MC), non-rebreathing masks, tracheostomy mask, T-piece systems	Non-sealed masks or nasal cannulae. Oxygen at low flow (2–15l.min^{-1}). Small reservoir. Significant entrainment of environmental air. Accurate FiO_2 not possible. Comfortable and simple to use.
Fixed performance	Venturi-type masks, anaesthetic breathing circuits (waters circuit, Ambu-bag)	Venturi-type masks rely on the Venturi principle to dilute oxygen predictably to FiO_2. Need to change valve to alter FiO_2. Higher FiO_2 valves have larger orifices, so behave more like a variable performance system. Comfortable. Simple to use, but needs attention to detail
		Anaesthetic breathing systems require sealing mask to prevent entrainment. Valves prevent rebreathing. Large reservoir. Accurate FiO_2. Sealed mask can be uncomfortable. Knowledge of breathing systems required.
High flow systems	T-piece systems, Vapotherm® (humidified high flow nasal cannulae)	Rely on high oxygen flows to match patient's inspiratory flow rate. Small reservoirs and sealed mask or naso-pharynx. Requires humidification. Accurate FiO_2. Sealed mask uncomfortable with risk of mucosal dryness. More complicated to set up.
Others	Intravascular oxygenation (cardiopulmonary bypass, interventional lung assist devices (Novolung®), ECMO)	Unusual in the self-ventilating patient. Oxygenation achieved across synthetic membrane. CO_2 removal can be an issue. FiO_2 can be difficult to measure. Complicated and limited to specialist centres.

Oxygen toxicity

CNS toxicity (Paul Bert effect)

Seen in diving, oxygen delivered at high pressures (>3atm) can lead to acute central nervous system (CNS) signs and seizures.

Lung toxicity (Lorraine Smith effect)

Prolonged exposure to a high FiO_2 results in pulmonary injury. Possibly mediated by free oxygen radicals, there is a progressive reduction in lung compliance, associated with interstitial oedema and fibrosis. Avoidance of long periods of high oxygen concentrations reduces this effect. Clinically it can be difficult to prevent long exposure times; however, in general, patients should remain below an FiO_2 of 0.5 where possible and not remain above this value for much longer than 30h.

Broncho-pulmonary dysplasia (BPD)

A condition concerning neonates, it is a chronic fibrotic lung disease associated with ventilation at high FiO_2. Pathologically it is similar to the adult condition above, but with the additional effect of immaturity. Surfactant and maternal steroid therapies have lowered the incidence and severity.

Retinopathy of prematurity

This is a vasoproliferative disorder of the eye affecting premature neonates. Initially thought to be solely due to the use of high FiO_2, its continued incidence despite tighter oxygen control suggests that other factors associated with prematurity are involved.

Hyperbaric oxygen therapy

Oxygen can be delivered to patients at higher than atmospheric pressures (2–3atm). This serves to increase the amount of oxygen dissolved in the plasma, rather than that bound to haemoglobin. At rest, the metabolic demands of an average person can be met by dissolved oxygen alone when breathing an FiO_2 of 1.0 at 3atm.

Hyperbaric oxygen is delivered in a sealed chamber. The gas is warmed and humidified. The common indications for hyperbaric oxygen therapy are listed in Table 1.1.4. High pressure therapy also has important side effects. Whilst clearly of value in these situations, the availability of a hyperbaric chamber often reduces its use, particularly in carbon monoxide poisoning.

Table 1.1.4 Suggested indications for hyperbaric oxygen therapy

Primary therapy	Adjunctive therapy
Carbon monoxide poisoning	Radiation tissue damage
Air or gas embolism	Crush injuries
Decompression sickness (the 'bends')	Acute blood loss
Osteoreadionecrosis	Compromised skin flaps or grafts
Clostridial myositis and myonecrosis	Refractory osteomyelitis Intracranial abscess Enhancement of healing of problem wounds

Further reading

Dellinger RP, Carlet JM, Masur H, *et al.* Surviving Sepsis Campaign guidelines for management of severe sepsis and septic shock. *Crit Care Med* 2004; 32: 858–73.

Gattinoni L, Brazzi L, Pelosi P, *et al.* A trial of goal-oriented hemodynamic therapy in critically ill patients. SvO_2 Collaborative Group. *N Engl J Med* 1995; 333: 1025–32.

Grocott M, Montgomery H, Vercueil A. High-altitude physiology and pathophysiology: implications and relevance for intensive care medicine. *Crit Care* 2007; 11: 203.

Hayes MA, Timmins AC, Yau EH, *et al.* Elevation of systemic oxygen delivery in the treatment of critically ill patients. *N Engl J Med* 1994; 330: 1717–22.

Leigh J. Variation in performance of oxygen therapy devices. *Anaesthesia* 1970; 25: 210–22.

Stoller KP. Hyperbaric oxygen and carbon monoxide poisoning: a critical review. *Neurol Res* 2007; 29: 146–55.

Tibbles PM, Edelsberg JS. Hyperbaric-oxygen therapy. *N Engl J Med* 1996; 334: 1642–8.

Wagstaff TAJ, Soni N. Performance of six types of oxygen delivery devices at varying respiratory rates. *Anaesthesia* 2007; 62, 492–503.

Ventilatory support: indications

The requirement for ventilatory support is the most common reason that patients are admitted to an Intensive Care Unit (ICU).

The aims of ventilatory support are to:

- Improve gas exchange by correcting hypoxaemia and reversing acute respiratory acidosis.
- Relieve respiratory distress by reducing the work of breathing and reducing the oxygen cost of breathing.
- Change the pressure–volume relationships of lungs including improving compliance and reversing or preventing atelectasis.
- Ensure patient comfort.
- Avoid complications and permit lung healing.

Use of ventilatory support

In addition to the treatment of acute respiratory failure, ventilatory support is also used in circulatory shock (e.g. cardiogenic shock, septic shock) and in the management of cerebral injury. In a study of 1638 patients from eight countries, the indications for ventilatory support were as follows:

- Acute respiratory failure (66%) (including acute respiratory distress syndrome) ARDS, sepsis, cardiac failure, pneumonia, post-operative respiratory failure, trauma)
- Coma (15%)
- Acute exacerbation of chronic obstructive pulmonary disease (COPD) (13%)
- Neuromuscular disease (5%)

Physiology

Respiratory failure: is defined as the failure to maintain normal arterial blood gases breathing room air:

- Hypoxaemic (type 1)—arbitrarily defined as a PaO_2 of <6.7kPa (50mm Hg) breathing room air
- Hypercapnic (type 2)—defined as a $PaCO_2$ of >6.7kPa (50mm Hg).

Respiratory failure may be acute, chronic or acute on chronic. Patients with chronic type 2 respiratory failure develop a compensatory metabolic alkalosis and maintain a normal pH despite an elevated $PaCO_2$. An acidaemia (pH <7.30) rather than the $PaCO_2$ value indicates the need for ventilatory support.

The most important mechanisms of hypoxaemia are ventilation–perfusion mismatch and shunt (cardiac and intrapulmonary). Diffusion impairment and reduced inspired oxygen tension (e.g. high altitude) are less relevant.

Ventilation–perfusion mismatch: describes areas of the lung which have excessive perfusion compared with ventilation (shunt-like effect) and areas which have excessive ventilation compared with perfusion (dead space effect). Hypoxaemia due to ventilation–perfusion mismatch is usually easily corrected by increasing the inspired oxygen tension. As long as the patient is able to increase minute ventilation by increasing tidal volume and respiratory rate, an increase in carbon dioxide tension is prevented.

Pulmonary shunt: describes the most severe form of ventilation–perfusion mismatch where venous blood passes through the lungs without any involvement in gas exchange. It occurs if there are areas of the lung which are not ventilated (e.g. atelectasis, air spaces full of fluid, blood or inflammatory exudate). The hypoxaemia associated with shunt is not reversed by increasing the inspired oxygen tension, and treatment needs to be directed towards opening up the non-ventilated parts of the lung by the application of positive pressure ventilatory support.

Intracardiac shunt: results in profound hypoxaemia that is not reversed by 100% oxygen or positive pressure ventilation. Although usually associated with congenital heart disease, intracardiac shunt may develop through a patent foramen ovale (present in 25% of the population). The foramen ovale remains closed as long as left atrial pressure is higher than right atrial pressure. In right ventricular failure (e.g. pulmonary hypertension secondary to pulmonary embolus, ARDS, etc.), right atrial pressure is elevated above left atrial pressure which may open the foramen ovale causing a right to left shunt and severe hypoxaemia. Echocardiography can be invaluable in confirming right to left intracardiac shunts as a cause for profound hypoxaemia that is not corrected by conventional ventilatory management.

Ventilatory support and cardiac failure

Positive pressure ventilation may have adverse and beneficial effects on cardiac function.

- Hypotension is common after commencing intermittent positive pressure ventilation (IPPV) due to the reduction in venous return. This may precipitate myocardial ischaemia in a patient with critical coronary artery disease.
- Left ventricular function may be improved. An increase in intrathoracic pressure results in a reduction in left ventricular transmural pressure and left ventricular afterload. This improves function of the failing ventricle as it moves to a more favourable position on the left ventricular function (Starling) curve.
- Right ventricular function may be impaired. In addition to reduced preload, right ventricular function may be impaired from an increase in pulmonary vascular resistance from alveolar vessel compression associated with alveolar overdistension.
- Correction of hypoxaemia and respiratory acidosis is associated with improved cardiac function. Mechanisms include a direct effect on cellular function and from reversal of pulmonary vasoconstriction caused by hypoxaemia and respiratory acidosis.

The application of raised intrathoracic pressure with continuous positive airways pressure typically results in a rapid clinical improvement in patients with acute left ventricular failure. In right ventricular failure (e.g. massive pulmonary embolus), positive pressure ventilation with high intrathoracic pressures should be avoided in order that right ventricular function is not compromised further.

Ventilatory support and septic shock

Severe sepsis may result in hypoxaemic respiratory failure and is a common indication for ventilatory support. Severe sepsis is also associated with a severe metabolic acidosis and a markedly increased work of breathing. The high work of breathing increases demand for oxygen consumption in a shocked patient with inadequate utilization of oxygen. In patients with septic shock, ventilatory support may be commenced due to a deteriorating metabolic acidosis without respiratory failure in order to reduce the work of breathing and the oxygen cost of breathing.

Assessment of a patient with respiratory failure

Severe hypoxaemia (PaO_2 <8kPa) despite high flow oxygen or a deteriorating respiratory acidosis (pH <7.30) are common indications for commencing ventilatory support. Blood gas values reflect on both the severity of the acute episode and the degree of chronic impairment of respiratory function. Clinical assessment is more important than arbitrary arterial blood gas values when considering ventilatory support. Clinical signs of severe respiratory failure indicating the need for ventilatory support may include:

- Altered conscious level (from agitation to coma)
- Increased work of breathing including tachypnoea (respiratory rate >30), use of accessory muscles and nasal flaring
- Paradoxical breathing pattern reflecting diaphragmatic fatigue when the flaccid diaphragm paradoxically moves cephalad during inspiration causing inward movement of the abdominal wall
- Central cyanosis
- Signs of excessive catecholamine release including diaphoresis, tachycardia, cardiac arrhythmias and hypertension.

Lung function tests may be of value in indicating the need for ventilatory support in selected patients at risk of respiratory failure due to neuromuscular disease. A vital capacity of <10ml/kg is associated with a markedly impaired ability to cough and, if untreated, a progressive decline in respiratory capacity occurs due to atelectasis, ending with respiratory arrest. Serial measurements of vital capacity are helpful in predicting the need for ventilatory support in the Guillian–Barre syndrome. Ventilatory support should be instituted when vital capacity falls to between 10 and 15ml/kg and before there is deterioration in arterial blood gases. Measurements of vital capacity appear to be less predictive of the need for ventilatory support in myasthenia gravis, probably due to the unpredictable and variable course of muscle function in this condition.

Complications of ventilatory support

These relate either to the requirement for tracheal intubation or to the effects of positive pressure ventilation.

Upper airway trauma is not infrequent and increases with the duration of intubation. Complications of endotracheal intubation include laryngeal swelling, prolonged larygneal dysfunction (dysphonia and impaired swallowing) and, rarely, tracheal stenosis.

Pulmonary oxygen toxicity describes airway and lung parenchyma damage secondary to prolonged exposure to high inspired oxygen tensions. Prolonged (>24h) exposure of the normal lung to a partial pressure of oxygen of >0.5bar has been associated with damage in previously normal lungs (atelectasis, reduced CO transfer factor). The priority is to correct hypoxaemia in the patient with acute respiratory failure, but unnecessary exposure to high inspired oxygen concentrations should be avoided. A PaO_2 of >8kPa is an acceptable target in the majority of patients.

Nosocomial pneumonia (ventilator-associated pneumonia or VAP) is the most common complication of mechanical ventilation and is thought to arise due to micro-aspiration of colonized upper airway secretions. Mechanical ventilation should be discontinued and the patient extubated at the earliest opportunity in order to reduce the risk of developing VAP (see 'Hospital-acquired pneumonia' in Chapter 125).

Hypotension is common after commencing positive pressure ventilation due to the reduction in venous return. It may be severe if the patient is hypovolaemic.

Barotrauma describes pressure-related damage to the lungs resulting in extrapulmonary air which may cause pneumothorax, subcutaneous emphysema, mediastinal emphysema and systemic air embolism. Incidence is ~10% of patients with acute lung injury receiving mechanical ventilation. Although recent studies have suggested that barotrauma is more related to the degree of damage to the underlying lung than the use of high airway pressures, it is prudent to avoid high airway pressures (e.g. peak pressure <45cm H_2O and plateau pressure <35cm H_2O).

Ventilator-associated lung injury

Laboratory studies and recent clinical trials have demonstrated that exposing already injured lungs to high tidal volumes and pressures results in an insidious and progressive worsening of the underlying lung injury. Overdistension ('volutrauma') and tidal lung recruitment–derecruitment ('atelectrauma') appear to be the important mechanisms. Selecting an inappropriately high tidal volume increases mortality in patients with acute lung injury

Outcome from mechanical ventilation

The outcome of mechanical ventilation was reported in an international study of 361 ICUs. Over 5000 patients received ventilation for a mean of duration if 5.9 days. The mortality of patients receiving ventilation for acute respiratory distress syndrome was 52%, and 22% in patients being treated for an acute exacerbation of COPD. The survival of unselected patients receiving ventilation for >12h was 69%.

Further reading

Esteban A, Anzueto A, Alia I, *et al.* How is mechanical ventilation employed in the intensive care unit. *Am J Resp Crit Care Med* 2000; 161: 1450–8.

Marples IL, Heap MJ, Suvarna SK, Mills GH. Acute right to left interatrial shunt: an important cause of profound hypoxaemia. *Br J Anaesthes* 2000: 85: 921–5.

Esteban A, Anzueto A, Frutos F, *et al.* Characteristics and outcomes in adult patients receiving mechanical ventilation. A 28-day international study. *JAMA* 2002; 287: 345–55.

IPPV—description of ventilators

Ventilators generate a pressure gradient between the upper airway and the alveoli that results in a controlled flow of gas (air and or oxygen) into the lungs. This can be achieved either by creating a negative pressure around the chest wall whilst the upper airway remains at atmospheric pressure (e.g. tank ventilator or a curaiss) or more commonly by creating a positive pressure in the airway. Negative pressure ventilators are rarely used in modern intensive care practice. Positive pressure ventilation may be applied via an artificial airway (invasive ventilation) or by a mask (non=invasive ventilation)

ICU ventilators

Positive pressure ventilators used in the ICU are complex microprocessor-controlled pieces of equipment. They require a high pressure (4bar) source of oxygen and air, and a power source from mains electricity. There may be a battery as a short-term (e.g. 10–30min) back-up power source in case of failure of the mains supply.

Inspiration is the active phase of mechanical ventilation that is controlled by the ventilator. Expiration is passive and occurs when the expiratory valve is opened, with gas flow depending on the elastic recoil forces of the lungs and chest wall combined with the expiratory airway resistance.

Ventilator circuit

The ventilator circuit (Fig. 1.3.1) comprises inspiratory and expiratory limbs which connect to the relevant ventilator port. The two limbs are joined close to the patient by the 'Y' piece. The Y piece may be attached directly to the airway (endotracheal tube (ETT) or tracheostomy) or with the aid of a catheter mount. A humidifier must be included in the circuit. An active humidifier (heated water bath) or a passive heat and moisture exchanger (HME) may be used. Any additional tubing (e.g. catheter mount, heat and moisture exchanger/bacterial filter) between the airway and the Y piece is termed equipment dead space as it results in rebreathing of exhaled CO_2, reducing the effective tidal volume.

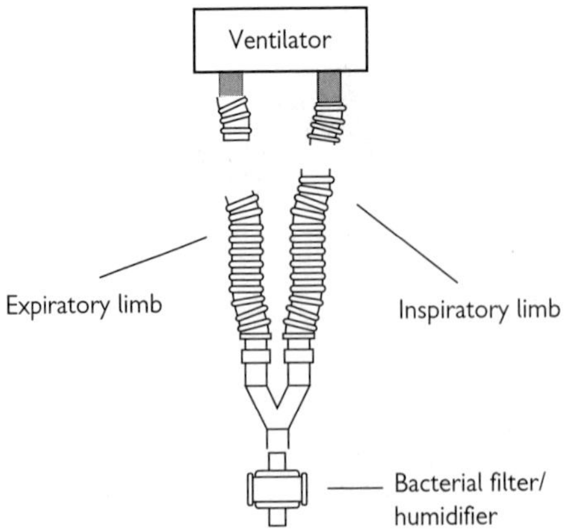

Fig. 1.3.1 Diagram of a ventilator circuit.

Classification of positive pressure ventilation

The wide and often confusing modes of ventilation offered by an ICU ventilator can be simplified by considering the following:

- Are the breaths volume or pressure targeted (or both)?
- Are the breaths initiated by the ventilator or by the patient's efforts (or both)?
- How is the duration of inspiration controlled?

Volume- or pressure-targeted breaths

In volume-controlled ventilation the tidal volume is set, and the airway pressure generated depends upon the compliance and resistance of the respiratory system (lungs and respiratory circuit). The inspiratory flow waveform is constant during volume ventilation whilst the airway pressure gradually increases to a peak (see below).

In pressure-controlled ventilation the ventilator delivers a set inspiratory airway pressure and the tidal volume that is delivered will depend upon the compliance and resistance of the respiratory system. The inspiratory flow waveform has a decelerating envelope whilst airway pressure remains constant throughout inspiration (see below).

Many modern ICU ventilators now offer dual control of the inspiratory phase where the breath is both volume targeted and pressure limited. This results in a breath with the characteristics of a pressure breath (constant pressure, decelerating flow) together with a predictable tidal volume.

Triggering: time, pressure or flow triggered

Breaths may be delivered according to a set frequency (ventilator or mandatory breaths) or in response to the patient making an attempt to inhale (spontaneous or supported breaths). Some modes allow a mixture of mandatory and spontaneous breaths.

Triggering describes what parameter the ventilator uses to initiate a breath and cycle to inspiration.

In ***time triggering,*** breaths are delivered according to a pre-set frequency. This is also termed controlled ventilation (e.g. controlled mechanical ventilation) as there is no interaction between ventilator and spontaneous respiratory efforts.

Pressure or flow triggering are used to detect spontaneous respiratory efforts to allow supported breaths. In ***pressure triggering,*** the ventilator detects the drop in airway pressure that occurs when the patient makes a spontaneous inspiratory effort with the inspiratory valve closed. As soon as the pressure drop exceeds the trigger limit, the ventilator will cycle to inspiration. The sensitivity of the trigger may be adjustable by setting the pressure drop that will initiate inspiration (e.g. 0.5–2cm H_2O).

In ***flow triggering,*** the patient's inspiratory effort is detected from a change in flow in the ventilator circuit. This is usually achieved by maintaining a flow rate in the ventilator circuit during the expiratory phase and monitoring the flow returning to the expiratory valve. If the patient makes an inspiratory effort, the flow returning to the expiratory valve falls below the background flow rate and the ventilator cycles to inspiration.

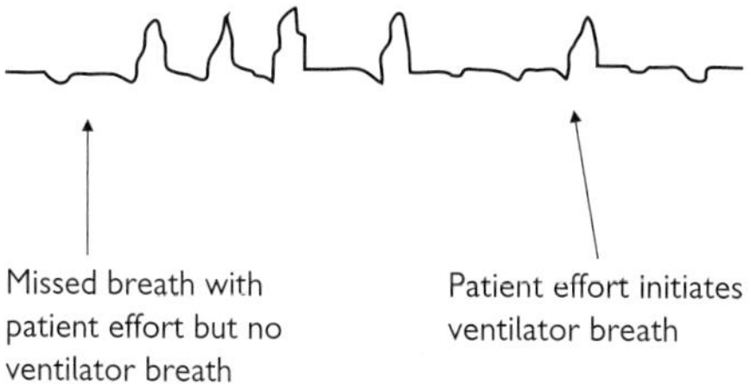

Fig. 1.3.2 An airway pressure trace from a ventilator showing poor triggering with 'missed breaths'.

Flow triggering is considered the most sensitive method of triggering that improves synchrony between patient and ventilator. Optimal setting of the trigger ensures that all patient efforts are detected by the ventilator and that auto-triggering does not occur.

Autotriggering describes the ventilator incorrectly cycling to inspiration when the patient has not made an inspiratory effort. It occurs due to the trigger being set at a too sensitive level with the result that small changes in pressure or flow within the ventilator circuit that are not due to patient effort (e.g. movement) erroneously initiate inspiration.

Cycling: time, flow or time

The ventilator can use volume, time or flow to dictate when the inspiratory phase is complete and when cycling to expiration should occur.

Volume cycling: expiration occurs as soon as the set tidal volume is delivered. There is no end-inspiratory pause. If a pause is added, the tidal volume is held within the lungs for a short period at the end of inspiration before expiration, then cycling can be considered to be by both volume and time.

Time cycling is most common and describes the inspiratory method used in most ICU ventilators. The inspiratory time is either set directly or derived from the set frequency and inspiratory to expiratory time ratio. Pressure-controlled breaths are always time cycled.

Flow cycling is used in pressure support ventilation to terminate the inspiratory phase. The inspiratory flow has a decelerating flow profile and when inspiratory flow falls to a predetermined percentage of the peak flow rate the ventilator cycles to expiration. In most ventilators this flow rate is set at 25% of the peak flow rate although some ventilators now have the facility for the user to choose the flow rate at which cycling occurs (e.g. between 10 and 90% of peak flow rate).

Graphic waveforms

Most ICU ventilators display continuous graphical displays of airway pressure, gas flow and volume plotted against time.

Observation of these displays can provide useful information regarding the mode of ventilation and ventilator settings, adequacy of patient ventilator synchrony, evidence of gas trapping and an indication of the mechanical properties of the respiratory system.

In volume-controlled ventilation with a constant inspiratory flow rate, the airway pressure gradually increases to a

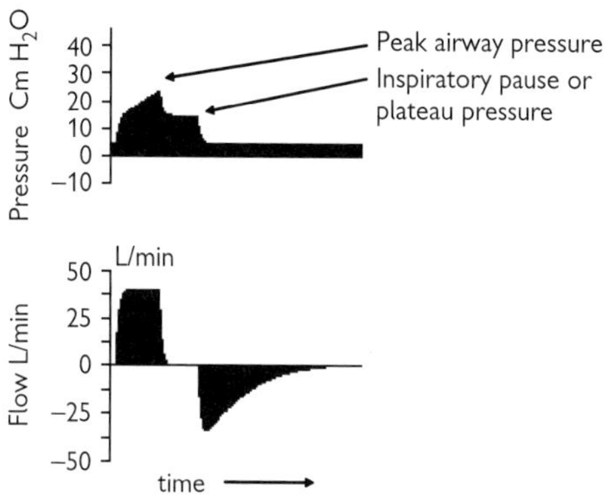

Fig. 1.3.3 Diagram of volume-controlled ventilation.

peak during inspiration. If an end-inspiratory pause has been set, the plateau pressure can be observed.

The difference in the peak and plateau pressure reflects the pressure required to overcome resistive forces and increases as inspiratory flow rate or airway resistance increase. If inspiratory flow rate remains constant, the peak to plateau gradient changes proportionately with changes in airway resistance. The plateau pressure reflects the pressure required to overcome elastic forces during inspiration and depends upon tidal volume and respiratory system compliance (lung and chest wall). Inspection of the airway pressure trace during volume-controlled ventilation can therefore provide useful information about the elastic and resistive properties of the respiratory system.

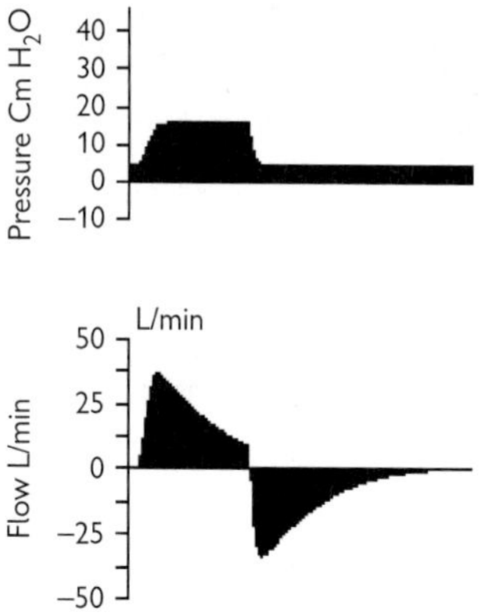

Fig. 1.3.4 Diagram of pressure-controlled ventilation.

In pressure-controlled ventilation (and in dual modes) the inspiratory pressure is constant throughout the inspiratory phase and it is not possible to differentiate the elastic and resistive properties of the lung from observation of the airway pressure trace. However, many modern ICU ventilators will calculate and display continuously values of respiratory system resistance and compliance.

IPPV—modes of ventilation

The modern ICU ventilator offers a complex and wide range of ventilation modes. Unfortunately, there is little standardization of terminology between the different ventilator manufacturers, and modes that are essentially the same may have different names depending upon the particular ventilator. To understand how a particular mode functions and interacts with the patient the following should be considered:

- Are the breaths volume or pressure targeted (or a combination)?
- Is inspiration initiated by ventilator (controlled mode) or following patient effort (spontaneous or assist mode) or are there a combination of ventilator and spontaneous breaths (synchronized intermittent mandatory ventilation)?
- How is the duration of inspiration controlled (cycling)?

Although there are a large number of modes available, there is little evidence that one mode improves clinical outcomes compared with another mode. The majority of patients can be managed with two modes: one controlled mode and one spontaneous mode.

Controlled modes

Controlled mandatory ventilation (other terms CMV, IPPV, volume control)

This describes a fully controlled mode where the respiratory rate is set by the ventilator and the breaths are usually volume targeted. Cycling from the inspiratory to expiratory phase is usually by time or by volume. There is no interaction or synchronization with the patient's efforts, and additional breaths cannot be triggered. CMV is typically used when patients are anaesthetized and paralysed (e.g. in the operating theatre). CMV may also be applied with a pressure-targeted breath (pressure control).

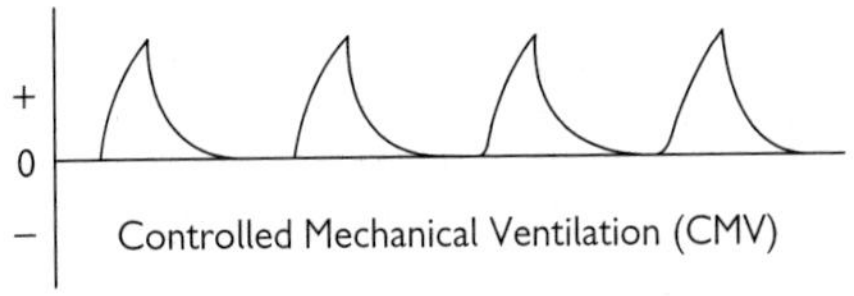

Fig. 1.4.1 Pressure–time plot of controlled mechanical ventilation (CMV).

Assist volume control (other terms CMV assist, IPPV assist)

This is similar to CMV but the patient is able to trigger ventilator breaths. All breaths are volume targeted. If the patient does not make any respiratory efforts the respiratory rate remains at the set frequency and the mode is effectively identical to CMV. Any spontaneous effort will trigger a ventilator breath of the pre-set tidal volume. If the patient's respiratory rate is above the pre-set frequency, the mandatory breaths are inhibited and the mode functions as a spontaneous mode with all breaths being patient triggered. Cycling may be by volume or time.

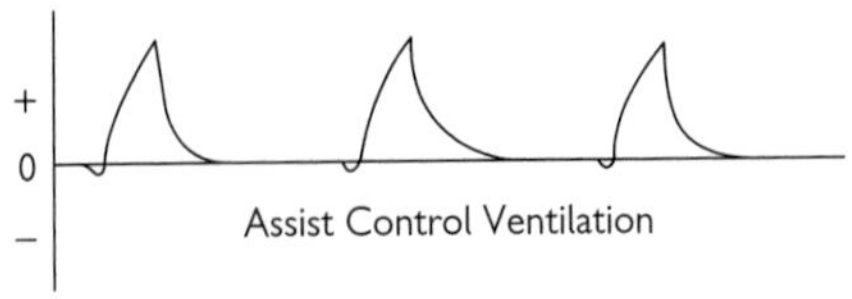

Fig. 1.4.2 Pressure–time plot of assist volume control.

Assist pressure control is analogous to assist volume control but with a pressure-targeted breath. An inspiratory pressure is set and the delivered tidal volume will depend upon the respiratory system compliance and resistance. Cycling is always by time, which differentiates this mode from pressure support (see below) where cycling is by flow.

Synchronized intermittent mandatory ventilation (SIMV)

In this mode a mandatory frequency of breaths is delivered which will be synchronized to any spontaneous patient effort occurring within a time window that follows the preceding breath (trigger window). If the patient breaths at a rate greater than the set rate, the additional breaths will be allowed but unsupported unless pressure support is also set. Thus a mixture of two breaths is delivered, mandatory ventilator breaths and pressure-supported breaths for any efforts above the mandatory frequency. Cycling of the mandatory breaths is by time, while the pressure-supported breaths are flow cycled. When first developed, the mandatory breaths in SIMV were volume targeted. This mode is now available with pressure-targeted breaths (SIMV pressure control).

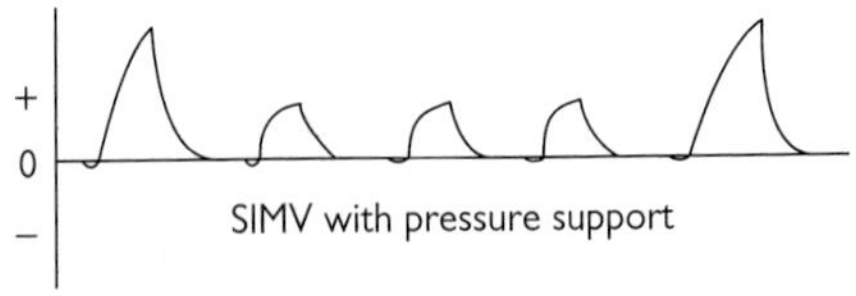

Fig. 1.4.3 Pressure–time plot of SIMV with pressure support.

Dual control modes

This term is used to describe modes that deliver breaths that are both volume and pressure targeted. A range of names are used by the manufacturers, including Autoflow®, Pressure Regulated Volume Control®, volume assured pressure control and volume control plus®.

The ventilator delivers a breath with the characteristics of a pressure-targeted breath (constant inspiratory pressure and decelerating flow profile) combined with a guaranteed tidal volume (within certain pressure limits). On commencing a dual mode, a volume-targeted test breath is delivered first to assess the compliance and resistance. Subsequent breaths are pressure controlled using an inspiratory pressure that ensures delivery of the set tidal volume. The ventilator monitors the tidal volume on a breath-by-breath basis and can automatically change the inspiratory pressure (usually in 2–3cm H_2O increments) to ensure that the desired tidal volume is delivered. In dual modes, the maximum inspiratory pressure that may be delivered is a function of the high airway pressure alarm setting. This varies between manufacturers but is usually 5 or 10cm H_2O less than the high pressure alarm limit setting. Dual control can be applied to a wide range of modes including volume control, assist volume control, SIMV and pressure support.

Spontaneous modes

Continuous positive airways pressure (CPAP)

This is the simplest mode of respiratory support for spontaneously breathing patients where a constant pressure above atmospheric is maintained throughout inspiration and expiration.

Pressure support (other terms assisted spontaneous breathing)

This is a spontaneous mode where the ventilator provides an inspiratory assist by increasing airway pressure to a set level following each patient effort. The pressure support equals the difference in pressure during inspiration and expiration (PEEP). In this mode there is no set rate and the ventilator will only deliver inspiratory assistance in response to patient efforts. It may be combined with a back-up mandatory mode (apnoea ventilation) that will take over if the patient has a prolonged period without any inspiratory effort (e.g. >15s).

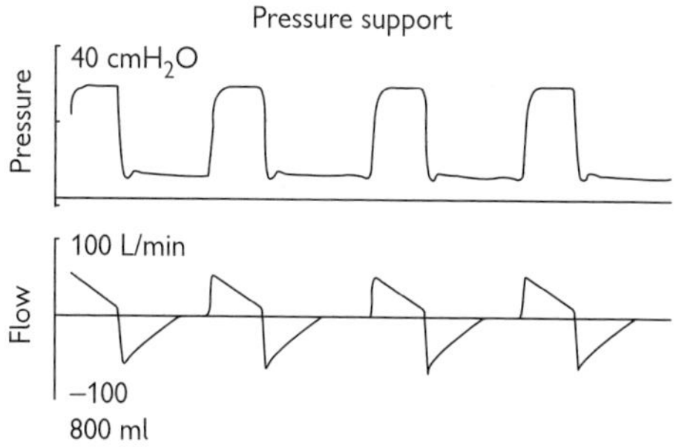

Fig. 1.4.4 Pressure and flow waveforms with pressure support.

In pressure support, cycling is by flow. The inspiratory flow follows a decelerating profile that is monitored by the ventilator. In most ventilators, cycling to expiration occurs when inspiratory flow has fallen to 25% of the peak inspiratory flow. Some ventilators offer the facility to adjust the flow at which cycling occurs (e.g. 10–90% of peak flow). This may be useful for improving patient ventilator synchrony when the duration of the inspiratory phase is either longer or shorter than desired by the patient.

Bilevel ventilation (BIPAP, DuoPAP)

This can be considered as a mode of ventilatory support where there is cycling between two different levels of CPAP at the set ventilator frequency. There is no synchronization with spontaneous respiratory efforts although the patient is able to breath without support at any time. An adaptation of this mode may offer pressure support for spontaneous breaths during the lower pressure phase. If the patient makes no spontaneous efforts, bilevel ventilation functions in an identical manner to pressure control. Proposed advantages of bilevel ventilation are improved patient comfort, as spontaneous breathing is allowed at any point of the respiratory cycle, and better gas exchange, as maintaining spontaneous breathing enhances ventilation–perfusion matching.

Airway pressure release ventilation is a variant of bilevel ventilation where the higher airway pressure is maintained for a relatively prolonged period (e.g. 10s) with brief episodes when the pressure falls to the lower value (0.5s). Spontaneous breathing is maintained throughout. It may be used in acute lung injury and ARDS where the high mean airway pressure improves oxygenation, the transient fall in airway pressure assists CO_2 clearance and the small tidal volumes ensure a lung protective mode of support.

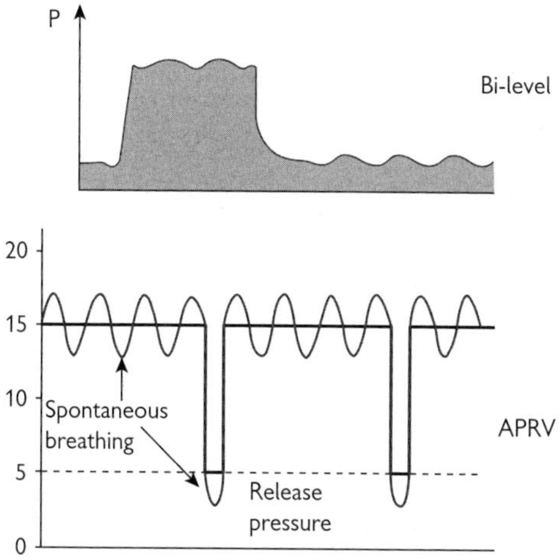

Fig. 1.4.5 Bilevel and assisted pressure release ventilation (APRV).

Automatic tube compensation (ATC)

The resistance of the endotracheal or tracheostomy tube increases the work of breathing that is reflected by a pressure gradient across the tracheal tube. This pressure drop, which changes during the respiratory cycle in proportion to the gas flow, can be estimated continuously by the ventilator. With automatic tube compensation, the ventilator increases airway pressure during inspiration and reduces airway pressure during expiration to offset the estimated pressure gradient across the breathing tube. ATC effectively removes the imposed work of breathing from the ETT and can be used during spontaneous breathing trials to assess readiness for extubation.

Automated modes

Some manufacturers offer modes that may automatically adjust certain ventilator parameters that would normally be set by the operator. Modes that switch between controlled and spontaneous modes according to patient effort are available (e.g. adaptive support ventilation, automode). A mode that automatically adjusts the level of pressure support (Smart care®) has been developed with the aim of weaning the patient as long as the patient does not have signs of respiratory distress.

IPPV—adjusting the ventilator

Initial settings

Chose a mode of ventilation that is familiar and appropriate for the clinical situation. This will usually be a controlled mode (e.g. volume or pressure control) as the patient will often have received sedative agents and muscle relaxants to assist intubation.

The following parameters are set:

Tidal volume

Regardless of mode used, the desirable tidal volume should be based on the patient's ideal body weight (IBW). This can be calculated from the patient's height using the following formulae:

Males IBW = 50 + 0.91 (height in cm – 152.4)

Females IBW = 45.5 + 0.81 (height in cm – 152.4)

In normal lungs, a tidal volume of 8–10ml/kg is acceptable, while in patients with acute lung injury a lung protective strategy with a reduced tidal volume of 6–8ml/kg is appropriate.

When using pressure control modes, the inspiratory pressure is adjusted once ventilation is commenced to achieve the desired tidal volume.

Respiratory rate

An initial rate between 10 and 20 breaths/min is set to achieve the required minute ventilation in order to maintain pH within normal limits (7.35–7.45). A patient with underlying metabolic acidosis (e.g. septic shock or cardiogenic shock) will require a high respiratory rate to ensure respiratory compensation with a low $PaCO_2$. The patient with a metabolic alkalosis secondary to chronic CO_2 retention will maintain a normal pH with a low rate and high $PaCO_2$. As the underlying metabolic abnormality improves, the respiratory rate will need to be adjusted to ensure that pH remains within the normal range.

Inspiratory phase

In controlled modes of ventilation the duration of the inspiratory phase is pre-set. How this is achieved varies according to the individual ventilator and may be by setting total inspiratory time, by selecting the inspiratory:expiratory time ratio (I:E) or from the inspiratory flow rate (volume control modes). Appropriate initial settings are:

- Inspiratory time 1.0–1.5s
- I:E ratio 1:2–1:3
- Inspiratory flow rate 30–60l/min

If using a ventilator where the I:E ratio is directly set, this may need to be adjusted following changes to the respiratory rate in order to ensure an inspiratory time >1s. Inspiratory times if <1s may not allow adequate time for ventilation of lung units with long time constants, resulting in impaired gas exchange.

In volume modes, inspiration is divided into an active inspiratory phase and the end-inspiratory pause. Setting an inspiratory pause during volume-controlled modes allows the plateau (end-inspiratory pause) pressure to be measured. An inspiratory pause may improve gas exchange.

Inspiratory waveform

Some ventilators allow the profile of the inspiratory flow waveform to be changed in volume-controlled modes. Options may include constant, decelerating and sinusoidal flow patterns. Constant flow ventilation is the most commonly used, although decelerating flows are increasingly available and have the advantage of reduced peak airway pressure and improved patient ventilator synchrony. Sinusoidal flow mimics the normal flow pattern during spontaneous breathing although it is unknown if it is associated with any clinical benefits

Inspired oxygen tension

In an unstable patient, ventilatory support should be commenced with an FiO_2 of 1.0. This can then be adjusted according to arterial saturations recorded by pulse oximetry and from blood gas analysis. A saturation >92% and a PaO_2 >8kPa are appropriate targets in the majority of patients. To avoid oxygen toxicity, inspired oxygen tension should be adjusted to the lowest level that maintains these values.

Positive end-expiratory pressure

The initial PEEP setting is 5cm H_2O in the majority of patients. This maintains the 'physiological PEEP' that occurs in spontaneous breathing due to exhalation through a partially closed glottis.

Trigger

There is no advantage to preventing the patient initiating spontaneous breaths, and the trigger should always be switched on unless the patient is sedated and receiving muscle relaxants. The mode of triggering (pressure or flow) and sensitivity may be adjustable according to the ventilator used. The trigger sensitivity should be set to ensure that all spontaneous patient efforts are detected by the ventilator. Auto-triggering occurs if the trigger is too sensitive when the ventilator delivers a breath in response to minor fluctuations in airway pressure caused by patient movement, airway manipulation, etc., and not from patient inspiratory effort. Careful patient observation allows appropriate trigger setting.

Alarms

The alarm parameters vary according to the individual ventilator. Usually there will be alarms to monitor the following:

- Exhaled tidal volume
- Minute ventilation (high and low)
- Airway pressure (high and low)
- Respiratory rate (high and low)

An appropriate alarm setting for each parameter is when the measured value deviates by 25% from the desired setting. Patient disconnection will activate a number of alarms including low pressure, low tidal volume, low minute ventilation or low rate (or apnoea). The high pressure alarm limit is usually set to activate at between 30 and 40cm H_2O. If set too close to the peak airway pressure, it will activate frequently, which could result in an inadequate minute ventilation as the ventilator will cycle to expiration as soon as the alarm is triggered.

Commencing ventilation

The ventilator should be checked before connecting to the patient. Many ventilators include an automatic pre-use test that occurs whenever first switched on. Typically this includes a circuit check (leak and compliance) and sensor (pressure, flow and oxygen) calibration. Once the initial settings have been set, the ventilator can be connected to the patient. Clinical assessment after commencing ventilatory support should include:

- Adequacy and symmetry of chest wall movement,
- Synchronization of the ventilator with the patient's efforts
- Vital signs including heart rate and blood pressure
- Gas exchange (pulse oximetry, capnography and arterial blood gases)

The expired tidal volume displayed by the ventilator should be checked and should be similar to the set tidal volume. Airway pressures should be monitored with the aim of keeping inspiratory plateau pressure as low as possible and certainly <30cm H_2O in the majority of patients.

Hypoxaemia

Only two parameters directly influence arterial oxygen tension, the inspired oxygen concentration and the mean airway pressure.

Mean airway pressure can be adjusted by prolonging the inspiratory time (adding an inspiratory pause) or by applying PEEP. Increasing mean airway pressure may increase haemodynamic instability as it may reduce venous return. Increasing PEEP will increase peak airway pressures and increase the risk of barotrauma. Increasing inspiratory time may result in gas trapping due to the reduction in expiratory time. Prolonged exposure of normal lungs to high inspired oxygen concentrations is damaging and, although it is unknown whether oxygen has the same effect on abnormal lungs, it would seem prudent to minimize the inspired oxygen concentration. A PaO_2 of >8 kPa (SaO_2 >92%) is a satisfactory target in the majority of patients and is achieved by a combination of selecting an appropriate FiO_2 and level of PEEP.

When assessing a patient with hypoxaemia during mechanical ventilation, reversible causes should always be considered such as endobronchial intubation, atelectasis secondary to sputum plugs, and pulmonary oedema.

Hypercapnia

The CO_2 tension is influenced by minute ventilation, dead space and CO_2 production. Minute ventilation is adjusted by changing the tidal volume and/or respiratory rate in order to maintain pH within the normal range (7.35–7.45). If this cannot be achieved without exposing the patient to excessive tidal volumes (>6–10ml/kg depending on underlying lung diagnosis) or high airway pressures (plateau pressure >30cm H_2O), it is invariably safer to limit tidal volumes and accept the associated respiratory acidosis. This permissive hypercapnia is well tolerated unless the patient has raised intracranial pressure (e.g. head injury) and is associated with an improved outcome in acute lung injury and acute severe asthma.

An increase in dead space will raise $PaCO_2$. Reversible causes of increased pulmonary dead space include low cardiac output, hypovolaemia and high intrathoracic pressures (secondary to externally applied PEEP or intrinsic PEEP from gas trapping). Equipment dead space may be minimized by removing the catheter mount and using a water bath humidifier rather than an HME. Reducing CO_2 production with therapeutic hypothermia combined with deep sedation and muscle relaxation may be of value in managing severe respiratory acidosis in the difficult to ventilate patient (e.g. severe asthma).

High airway pressures

When the high airway pressure alarm is activated, the ventilator immediately cycles to expiration that will reduce the inspired tidal volume and rapidly results in the patient receiving inadequate ventilation.

Causes of high airway pressures include:

- Low lung compliance (e.g. ARDS)
- Hyperinflation
  - gas trapping
  - excessive tidal volumes
- Low chest wall compliance
  - morbid obesity
  - intra-abdominal distension
  - chest wall rigidity (e.g. secondary to high dose opiates)
- Increased airway resistance
  - bronchospasm
  - airway obstruction (secretions)
  - airway occlusion due to compression/kinking
- Patient 'fighting the ventilator'
  - agitation, coughing, straining

Reversible causes of high airway pressures should be treated if possible (e.g. removal of secretions, administration of bronchodilator).

Patient ventilator asynchrony

This describes poor synchronization between the patient's inspiratory efforts and inspiration applied by the ventilator. It is common and has a number of adverse effects including increased work of breathing, impaired gas exchange, increased requirement for sedation and prolonged weaning from mechanical ventilation.

When severe, it presents as the patient 'fighting the ventilator' with failure to settle, frequent coughing, straining and agitation. It is more common when first commencing a patient on ventilatory support and results in poor gas exchange as minute ventilation is not maintained due to frequent activation of the high pressure alarm.

A number of factors may contribute to asynchrony:

Ventilator factors

- Inadequate trigger sensitivty (missed breaths)
- Autotriggering
- Inspiratory flow waveform (e.g. constant flow)
- Inspiratory flow rate does not match patient effort
- Rise time setting (time to reach maximum inspiratory pressure)

Patient factors

- Lung pathology (e.g. high resistance and compliance
- AutoPEEP (impairs ability to trigger)
- High inspiratory effort/drive (e.g. metabolic acidosis)
- Sedation level, inadequate pain control

Asynchrony may occur at different times in the respiratory cycle:

- Triggering of inspiration
- During active inspiratory flow
- Termination of inspiratory flow

Treatment of patient–ventilator asynchrony requires recognition and correction of the underlying cause(s) with optimal setting of the ventilator. However, increasing the levels of sedation and the administration of a non-depolarizing muscle relaxant is often required.

IPPV—barotrauma

Introduction

Mechanical ventilation, particularly in the setting of acute lung injury, although life-saving, has been shown also to cause significant lung injury. Only in recent times has the significance of ventilator-induced lung injury (VILI) been more widely acknowledged. The incidence of barotrauma complicating the management of ARDS; recent figures include 6.5% by Anzueto *et al.*, 11% in the ARDS network, and 13% by Brochard *et al.* These contrast with figures of between 40 and 60% 10–15yrs ago.

Gross barotrauma manifesting as pneumothorax is the most frequently and easily recognized complication of mechanical ventilation. Barotrauma is, however, only one manifestation of VILI. Other types of injury are described:

Volutrauma—direct injury to the alveoli from overdistension of the lung.

Atelectrauma—shearing injury to the alveoli resulting from repetitive collapse and opening of distal airways or alveoli.

Biotrauma—injury to the lung (and distant organs) resulting from the release of inflammatory mediators into the airspaces and systemic circulation.

Pathophysiology

A mechanism for the development of extra-alveolar air has been described whereby an initial site of disruption occurs in the base of the perivascular alveoli. The risk of such a disruption is consequent to the pressure gradient between the alveolus and the vascular sheath. Air in the vascular sheath, which was termed pulmonary interstitial emphysema (PIE), is the first manifestation of barotrauma. In the mediastinum, air can track along the tissue planes creating a pneumomediastinum, or the increased pressure can rupture through the mediastinal pleura to produce a pneumothorax.

Clinical

History

Often mechanically ventilated patients are unable to communicate, but the history can often be gleaned from their medical records or from other staff. Those at highest risk of barotraumas from mechanical ventilation are those with acute lung injury (ALI) or ARDS.

Co-existing lung pathology such as interstitial lung disease, COPD, *Pneumocystis carinii* pneumonia (PCP) or blunt thoracic injuries increases the risk.

Thoracic

The manifestations of barotrauma span from the asymptomatic to cardiac arrest from an unrecognized tension pneumothorax. The severity depends on the degree of extra-alveolar air present. Signs of respiratory distress, e.g. ventilator–patient dys-synchrony, use of accessory muscles, etc., may be the earliest clinical manifestation in the patient unable to communicate. The earliest clinical signs of a pneumothorax may be decreased breath sounds and hyper-resonance on percussion. These signs are often less apparent in the mechanically ventilated compared with the conscious self-ventilating patient.

Extrathoracic

A systemic gas embolus is the most dramatic extrathoracic manifestation of barotrauma. These may cause cerebral air emboli, myocardial infarction and livido reticularis.

The increased intrathoracic pressures from mechanical ventilation affect venous drainage from other sites, with reduction in venous return and increased venous pressures from the brain and abdomen.

Biotrauma in the lung increases leukocytes, tumour necrosis factor, interleukin-6 (IL-6) and IL-8. These are the same cytokines implicated in the systemic inflammatory response syndrome and in sepsis.

Imaging studies

A high clinical index of suspicion with radiological confirmation is often required for diagnosis in an asymptomatic patient.

Chest radiographs

Radiological findings in PIE include:

- Parenchymal cysts
- Lucent lines directed towards the hilum
- Subpleural air cysts
- Presence of gas around large vessels
- Pneumatoceoles
- Pneumomediastinum outling the great vessels
- Pneumopericardium outlining the pericardium and contiguous diaphragm

Pneumothoraces especially small ones may be difficult to diagnose on portable chest radiographs.

CT scanning

Computed tomography (CT) scanning is rarely indicated to establish the diagnosis of barotraumas but it may be helpful in determining the size of a pneumothorax and is often an incidental finding when imaging for other indications. It is also easier to appreciate pneumothoraces that are primarily anterior or basilar than on a two-dimensional chest radiograph. CT scans may be useful in guiding the placement of thoracostomy tube(s) in loculated pneumothoraces or where draining more than one tube is required.

Protective mechanical ventilation

Protective mechanical ventilation is the practice of adjusting ventilator parameters to minimize lung injury. There is no agreed single approach to protective ventilation, yet most authorities now share the basic principles of low tidal volumes and permissive hypercapnea as long as arterial pH remains in an acceptable range.

PEEP

The pressure–volume curve of the lung has both upper and lower inflection points. The upper inflection point is the pressure at which the lung volume ceases to increase sharply with rising airway pressure. The lower inflection point is the pressure at which the lung volume begins to decline sharply with falling airway pressure. Lung injury might be avoided by ventilating the lung at a PEEP above the lower inflection point to prevent atelectrauma while restricting tidal volumes so that the end-inspiratory pressure does not exceed the upper inflection point.

Eisner *et al.* in the ARDSNetwork trial showed that by decreasing tidal volume from 12 to 6ml/kg the mortality rate fell from 40 to 30% in ARDS patients. An important component of this trial was the selection of PEEP and FiO_2 parameters.

Plateau pressure

This provides the best approximation of transalveolar pressure. Amato *et al.* have shown that failure to limit plateau pressures is associated with a high incidence of barotraumas and an increased mortality. It is widely agreed that plateau pressures >35mm H_2O leads to increase incidence of barotraumas.

Surgical treatment

Only rarely is surgical repair of the lung required for the treatment of barotrauma. However, the effective management of pneumothorax requires evacuation of pleural air and placement of a pleural drain to permit the gas to escape. The urgency and type of tube placement depends on the patient's clinical status. In most instances, leaks associated with ventilator-induced barotrauma are small, and tension pnuemothoraces develop slowly.

Tube thoracostomy

Many commercial kits are available using a Seldinger technique as an alternative to the traditional intercostal drain insertion using blunt dissection.

Emergency needle thoracostomy

This is indicated for patients with a tension pneumothorax and cardiovascular compromise requiring immediate decompression. In mechanically ventilated patients, the ventilator should be removed and replaced with a bag valve device connected to oxygen. In this way the clinician can assess the lung compliance and eliminate the deleterious effect of PEEP on the cardiovascular system. Following emergency needle decompression, a thoracostomy tube placement is required.

Further reading

Amato MBP, Barbas CS, Medeiros DM, *et al.* Beneficial effects of the open lung approach with low distending pressure in acute respiratory distress syndrome; a prospective randomised study on mechanical ventilation. *Am J Respir Crit Care Med* 1995; 23: 1–15.

Amato MBP, Barbas CSV, Medeiros D, *et al.* Improved survival in ARDS: beneficial effects of a lung protective strategy. *Am J Respir Crit Care Med* 1996; 153 suppl: A531.

Anzueto A, Frutos-Vivar F, Esteban A. *et al.* Incidence, risk factors and outcome of barotraumas in mechanically ventilated patients. *Intensive Care Med* 2004; 30: 612–9.

Brochard L, Roudot-Thoraval F, Roupie E, *et al.* Tidal volume reduction for the prevention of ventilator-induced lung injury in acute respiratory distress syndrome. *Am J Respir Crit Care Med* 1998; 158: 1831–8.

Eisner MD, Thompson BT, Schoenfeld D, *et al.*; Acute Respiratory Distress Syndrome Network. Airway pressures and early barotrauma in patients with acute lung injury and acute respiratory distress syndrome. *Am J Respir Crit Care Med* 2002; 165: 978–82.

Fuhrman BP. Avoidance of ventilator induced lung injury. *Acta Pharmacol Sin* 2002; Suppl 23: 44–7.

Gammon RB, Shin MS, Buchalter SE. Pulmonary barotraumas in mechanical ventilation. Patterns and risk factors. *Chest* 1992; 102: 568–72.

Gropper MA. New approaches to mechanical ventilatory support. 56th Annual Refresher Course Lectures and Basic Science Reviews. Presented in October 2005 during the Meeting of the American Society of Anaesthesiologist.

Hoo GWS. Emedicine.com/topic209.htm

Ricard J-D. Editorial. *Intensive Care Med* 2004; 30: 533–5.

IPPV—weaning techniques

The weaning process

The progressive reduction in the degree of ventilatory support that leads to the re-establishment of spontaneous breathing (SB) is conventionally termed weaning. Liberation might be a better descriptive as we now better appreciate the potential risks of invasive mechanical ventilation (IPPV) such as ventilator-induced lung injury (VILI) and ventilator-associated pneumonia (VAP). The start of weaning coincides with clinical stability and the beginnings of recovery from the critical illness that precipitated ICU admission. When weaning is prolonged, it extends into the period of general rehabilitation, e.g. sitting out of bed or even ambulatory mechanical ventilation. Weaning is unnecessary when mechanical ventilation is employed, for instance, to manage major elective surgery. In such circumstances, controlled ventilation may be employed to allow for the initial recovery from surgery and is followed by cessation of sedation, establishment on low level pressure support and rapid extubation.

Weaning occupies >40% of ICU stay and therefore is of major economic importance. Weaning delay is associated with a high mortality, 51% in one large US report, and is not uncommon. Patient case mix determines how common but, in one large UK report, weaning delay (>3 days but <2 weeks) occurred in 8% of all ICU patients, and in a further 7% weaning failed as defined by the requirement of >6h per day ventilatory assistance >3 weeks after treatment of the initiating illness.

Skeletal myopathy is almost universal in critical illness, and involvement of the respiratory muscles is a major factor in weaning delay. The role of disuse atrophy vs diaphragmatic dysfunction is uncertain. The link between paralytic agents, steroids and critical illness neuropathy/myopathy (CINM) may be more an indicator of severity of illness rather than purely a causative factor. The balance between reduced respiratory pump function and an increased ventilatory load, arising as a result of airflow obstruction and reduced lung, chest and abdominal wall compliance, will determine whether weaning can successfully proceed or whether improvement is required before progress can be made.

Causes of weaning delay/failure

- Unresolved primary illness
- Pre-morbid (neuromuscular disease or severe COPD)
- Sepsis
- Weak muscles ± ineffective cough (bulbar disease or depressed respiratory drive, CINM, malnutrition)
- CNS (brain injury, sedation, anxiety depression)
- Physician related (failure to recognize imbalance between pump and load, ventilator–patient dys-synchrony).

Weaning techniques

Two contrasting philosophies lie behind the strategies that can be adopted. When the load/capacity ratio is unfavourable, a slowly progressive reduction in pressure support is appropriate. If disuse atrophy and diaphragm retraining is required, intermittent T-tube SB or CPAP trials might be a better strategy. Direct measurements of diaphragm strength and ventilatory load are, however, technically demanding and have not yet been shown to influence outcome. What evidence is there for choosing the right strategy?

Trails of SIMV with pressure support of SB (and a gradual reduction in the number of mandatory breaths and in degree of pressure support) vs either progressive reduction in pressure support or intermittent CPAP/T-tube SB trials (SBTs) have demonstrated that SIMV is a poor weaning strategy. The relative merits between progressive pressure support reduction and intermittent SBTs have not yet been established. The value of periods of unsupported ventilation is to detect when patients can wean faster than their carers believe possible!

Non-ventilatory aspects of weaning

Optimal fluid balance, treatment of heart failure, ensuring adequate nutrition and avoiding, or treating, nosocomial infection are all important. Psychological and rehabilitation aspects are equally so. For instance, improving communication, with a speaking valve in the ventilator tubing, managing anxiety and delirium, and re-establishing the sleep/wake cycle are crucial steps in rehabilitation. Feelings of dependency and fear may need to be addressed.

Weaning centres

Economic pressure has led to the development of specialist weaning centres in the USA. The benefits may be more than simply economic.

IPPV/assessment of weaning

Weaning stages

The initial step in weaning is the decision to allow/encourage supported SB. This coincides with evidence of a response to treatment such as a reduction in inotrope requirement or FiO_2.

Suggested pre-requisites for stage 1

- Respiratory variables:
  - FiO_2 <0.5
  - PEEP ≤10cm H_2O
  - pH >7.3 or $PaCO_2$ <6.5kPa
- Cardiovascular variables:
  - Heart rate ≤120bpm
  - Mean arterial blood pressure stable (with or without inotropes)
- Neurological variables:
  - Adequate analgesia
  - Awake and cooperative
- Nutrition:
  - Potassium and phosphate levels normalized
  - No severe abdominal distension

VILI remains a consideration. Pressure support should be titrated to limit the tidal volume to between 6 and 8ml/kg whilst monitoring for signs of fatigue as indicated by a rising respiratory rate, blood pressure or heart rate, or the development of agitation or a change in conscious level.

Stage 2 is characterized by a period during which pressure support and PEEP are reduced. This may be a continual and progressive process or be associated with setbacks when more support will be required, e.g. a septic episode. Initially controlled ventilatory modes may be better at night to ensure that the gains by day are not compromised by inadequate support during sleep.

Stage 3 involves assessment for extubation or self-ventilation in the case of a patient with a tracheostomy. It usually employs a trial of SB. Clinical stability over 30–60min in the absence of signs of fatigue or distress is required before proceeding to extubation. Whilst the SBT is valuable, ~10% of patients will fail post-extubation usually due to an inability to clear secretions, CNS factors or unexpected upper airways obstruction due to glottic oedema. The SBT is a conservative indicator. Many COPD patients will wean despite a respiratory rate during the SBT of >35 breaths/min.

Inclusion criteria for spontaneous breathing trial:

- Cooperative patient requiring no sedation (score ≥ –2), adequate analgesia
- Pressure support ≤5cm H_2O
- PEEP ≤5, FiO_2 ≤40%,
- Minute volume <15l/min
- No or low dose inotropes
- Adequate cough; secretions not excessive

Weaning protocols

Some patients are capable of proceeding quickly and are held back inappropriately. Weaning protocols are effective by the earlier detection of such patients. 'Smart' ventilators capable of adjusting the degree of pressure support to the arterial carbon dioxide tension and tidal volume targets may be more effective than simple protocols.

Non-invasive ventilation (NIV)

NIV speeds weaning by acting as a bridge to spontaneous breathing in COPD and is probably effective in neuromuscular causes of respiratory failure. As NIV may lead to delayed re-intubation, its value in post-extubation respiratory failure in the general ICU population is uncertain.

Further reading

Baudouin SV, Davidson AC *et al.* National Patients Access Team Critical Care Programme: weaning and long term ventilation, London: Department of Health. 2002. `www.modern.nhs.uk/critical care`

Ely EW, Meade M, Haponik EF, *et al.* Mechanical ventilation weaning protocols driven by non-physician health care professionals: evidence based clinical practice guidelines. *Chest* 2001; 120: 454–635.

Esterban A, Frutos-Vivar F, Ferguson ND, *et al.* Non invasive positive pressure ventilation for respiratory failure after extubation. *N Eng J Med* 2004; 350: 2452–60.

Ferrer M, Esquinhas A, Arancibia F, *et al.* Non invasive ventilation during persistent weaning failure: a randomised controlled trial. *Am J Resp Crit Care Med* 2003; 168: 5–6.

Laghi F, Tobin MJ. Disorders of the respiratory muscles. *Am J Resp Crit Care Med* 2003; 168 : 10–48.

Lellouche F, Mancebo J, Jolliet P, *et al.* A multicentre randomised trial of computer driven protocolised weaning from mechanical ventilation. *Am J Resp Crit Care Med* 2006; 174: 894–900.

Pilcher DV, Bailey MJ, Treacher DF, *et al.* Outcomes, cost and long-term survival of patients referred to a regional weaning centre. *Thorax* 2005; 60: 187–92.

High-frequency ventilation

Definition

High-frequency ventilation (HFV) encompasses a family of modes of mechanical ventilation that deliver small tidal volumes (near to or less than the anatomical dead space) at respiratory rates in excess of normal physiological rates (60–3000 breaths/min).

Background

In 1915, Henderson and colleagues described their observation that sufficient ventilation occurred in panting dogs with tidal volumes less than the anatomical dead space.

In the 1980s, the first commercial high-frequency oscillatory ventilator was produced for use in neonates.

Types of high-frequency ventilation

High-frequency jet ventilation (HFJV) and high-frequency oscillatory ventilation (HFOV) are the modes most commonly used in clinical practice.

High-frequency jet ventilators are time-cycled flow generators, delivering a high-pressure jet (10–50psi) into the airway via a small bore cannula. Air is entrained and exhalation occurs passively

High-frequency oscillators use a piston or reciprocating diaphragm to push gas actively into and subsequently draw gas out of the airway.

High-frequency ventilation can be classified according to its expiratory phase as passive or active.

Passive	Active
High-frequency jet ventilation (HFJV)	High-frequency oscillatory ventilation (HFOV)
High-frequency positive pressure ventilation (HFPPV)	High-frequency chest wall oscillation (HFCWO)
High-frequency percussive ventilation (HFPV)	
High-frequency flow interruption (HFFI)	

Theory of high-frequency ventilation

HFV, especially HFOV, is theoretically suited to lung protective mechanical ventilation:

- Small tidal volumes limit cyclic overdistension (volutrauma)
- Intrinsic/extrinsic PEEP prevents shear stress from repetitive opening and closing of atelectatic lung units (atelectrauma) and increases functional residual capacity. Mean airway pressure is maintained, correlating well with oxygenation for a given FiO_2.
- Peak airway pressures are reduced, minimizing potential for barotrauma.
- The lung is maintained on its deflation limb on the static pressure–volume curve, thereby improving lung compliance and increasing the number of aerated alveoli.
- HFOV has the added advantage that oxygenation and carbon dioxide elimination are decoupled.

Physiology of high-frequency ventilation

Gas transport

Conventional mechanical ventilation aims to duplicate the normal bulk flow gas exchange pattern. For effective alveolar ventilation (VA), tidal volume must exceed dead space (VD). VA = f x (VT – VD).

As the tidal volumes (VT) are near to or less than the anatomical dead space (VD) during HFV, alternative mechanisms of gas transport are required:

- Convection—a small amount of bulk flow occurs in the proximal airways/alveoli.
- Molecular diffusion—this is the principle mechanism of gas transport in the terminal airways.
- Streaming (asymmetric velocity profiles)—during laminar flow, a central current delivers gas distally whereas a peripheral current returns gas proximally.
- Taylor dispersion—the interplay between convective forces and molecular diffusion causes laminar and radial gas dispersion.
- Pendelluft—this is the exchange of gas between adjacent lung units due to their differing time constants. Gas flows from fast to slow filling units at end inspiration. The reverse occurs at end expiration.
- Cardiogenic mixing—agitation of lung units near to the heart increases molecular diffusion along concentration gradients by up to 5-fold.

Gas exchange

Oxygenation

Oxygenation is directly proportional to lung volume.

The sigmoid shape of the oxygen dissociation curve means that no amount of hyperventilation can compensate directly for shunt.

The important focus is to limit ventilation–perfusion mismatch by recruitment of the maximum number of gas exchange units and then to keep them open and available for gas exchange.

Carbon dioxide elimination

$PaCO_2$ is inversely proportional to fa x VTb, where a is ~1 and b is ~2.

Although tidal volumes are much smaller in HFV than in conventional mechanical ventilation (CMV), the product of tidal volume (VT) and frequency (f) is much higher.

The linear shape of the carbon dioxide dissociation curve throughout the physiological range makes it possible to achieve normocapnia through regional hyperventilation, even with a substantial proportion of the alveoli remaining under- or non-ventilated.

Practical aspects of high-frequency ventilation

Fessler *et al.* describe guidelines for the use of HFV in adults with ARDS, including initial settings and weaning strategies. As yet there is no grade A evidence available to determine optimal parameters.

	CMV	HFJV	HFOV
f	2–60	<600	300–3000
VT	>VD	<VD or >VD	<VD
PEEP manipulated by	Extrinsic PEEP valve	Extrinsic PEEP valve	Bias flow
mPaw manipulated by	Pinsp	P	Bias flow
	PEEP	PEEP	
CO_2 elimination manipulated	f x (VT – VD)	P	ΔP
Oxygenation manipulated by	f x (VT – VD)	P	mPaw
	PEEP	PEEP	FiO_2
	FiO_2	FiO_2	

CMV, conventional mechanical ventilation; HFJV, high-frequency jet ventilation; HFOV, high-frequency oscillatory ventilation; f, frequency/tidal volume; VT, tidal volume; VD, anatomical dead space; VA, alveolar ventilation; PEEP, positive end-expiratory pressure; FiO_2, fractional inspired oxygen; ΔP, amplitude of oscillations (determines VT); Pinsp, peak airway pressure; mPaw, mean airway pressure; P, driving pressure (determines VT).

Indications for high-frequency ventilation

- Acute respiratory distress syndrome (ARDS)[1]
- Low resistance large volume airway leak, e.g. bronchopulmonary fistula
- Upper airway surgery

[1]There are significant data to support the use of HFOV in infants and children, albeit few, if any, studies comparing it with CMV using a low tidal volume strategy. There is currently no evidence supporting the use of HFV in adults with ARDS over low tidal volume conventional ventilation. Animal studies demonstrate advantages of HFOV compared with CMV provided an open-lung technique is used.

Advantages and disadvantages of high-frequency ventilation

Advantages

Respiratory

- Minimal vocal cord/surgical field movement
- Improved visibility and surgical access

Cardiovascular

- Cardiac output may be augmented using ECG synchronization

Renal

- Reduced antidiuretic hormone production and fluid retention

Disadvantages

Respiratory

- Suctioning causes loss of mean airway pressure
- Cannot meaure end-tidal carbon dioxide[2]
- Inaccurate measurement of FiO2[2]
- Inaccurate measurement of tidal volume
- Cooling and drying of inspiratory gases[2]
- Inhalational anaesthesia impractical
- Contamination of operating room air if anaesthetic gases are used*
- Pressure measurements may be unrepresentative
- High gas flow required
- Potential for lower airway soiling in ENT surgery[2]
- Contamination of expired gas flow by surgical debris[2]

[2]Associated with HFJV, not HFOV.

CNS

- Increased sedation requirement

Miscellaneous

- Training
- Familiarity
- Cost
- Ventilators not portable so cannot transfer patients on HFV

Complications of high-frequency ventilation

All complications associated with HFV can occur in any mode of positive pressure mechanical ventilation that uses high airway pressures or a low I:E ratio that does not allow sufficient time for expiration.

Cardiovascular

- Increased vagal activity
- Decreased venous return
- Decreased cardiac output
- Increased pulmonary vascular resistance
- Dysrrhythmias

Optimizing blood volume and myocardial function before the HFV treatment may limit these problems.

Respiratory

- Pulmonary overinflation (gas-trapping)
- Barotrauma (pneumothorax, pneumomediastinum, pneumoperitoneum, pneumopericardium)
- Shearing at the interface of different lung regions with differing impedances
- Necrotizing tracheobronchitis[3]
- Increased secretions[3]
- Air embolism

[3]More likely in HFJV where humidification of the fresh gas flow is difficult.

Miscellaneous

- Intracranial haemorrhages in neonates
- Necrotizng enterocolitis in neonates
- Malposition of catheters (gastric distension, gastric rupture)

Adjunctive strategies

The following strategies are advocated in conjunction with HFV:

- Permissive hypercapnoea
- Prone ventilation to recruit lung and improve distribution of ventilation (may also improve removal of secretions)
- Nitric oxide to improve oxygenation and reduce vascular stress
- Positioning—lateral rotation therapy
- Extracorporeal carbon dioxide removal

Future developments

- A multi-centre randomized controlled trial (RCT) (i.e. the OSCAR trial) comparing the use of HFOV with CMV using a low tidal volume strategy commenced in 2007.
- The Canadian Critical Care Trials Group (CCCTG) is funding a national pilot study of HFOV.
- The National Heart, Lung and Blood Institute (USA) has funded a phase II study of HFOV as a prelude to a full clinical trial.

Further reading

High-frequency ventilation. *Resp Care Clin North Am* 2001; 7: 523–695 (compilation of 10 review articles).

Fessler HE, Derdak S, Ferguson ND, *et al.* A protocol for high-frequency oscillatory ventilation in adults: Results from a roundtable discussion *Crit Care Med* 2007; 35: 1649–54.

Stachow R. High frequency ventilation basics and practical application. *Draeger*, 1995

Positive end-respiratory pressure

Positive end-expiratory pressure (PEEP) is the positive pressure applied at the end of expiration during mechanical ventilation. When PEEP is applied to a spontaneous breathing cycle it is named 'continuous positive airway pressure' (CPAP). Physiological consequences of the application of PEEP depend on its effects on gas exchange, pulmonary compliance and systemic haemodynamics.

Effects of PEEP on gas exchange

Hypoxaemic acute respiratory failure (ARF) is characterized by an acute reduction of lung volume due to pulmonary oedema, atelectasis and pneumonia; alveolar units tend to collapse at the end of expiration particularly in gravitationally dependent regions. The use of PEEP improves gas exchange by recruiting functionally closed alveoli, redistributing lung water and therefore reducing ventilation–perfusion (V/Q) mismatch.

Alveolar recruitment, defined as the amount of non-inflated tissue that is re-expanded by a given level of PEEP, results in a more homogeneous distribution of tidal volume and in an increased functional residual capacity (FRC). Moreover, application of PEEP leads to the redistribution of lung water from the alveolar space to the perivascular interstitial space and improves V/Q mismatch by diverting blood flow from shunt regions to normal V/Q regions.

All these effects are strongly conditioned by whether or not PEEP recruits previously collapsed alveoli. If PEEP induces alveolar recruitment, a reduction in shunt with improvement in oxygenation and reduction in dead space is expected. If hyperinflation of normal alveoli is the predominant effect, a rise in $PaCO_2$ due to the increase in dead space is expected, while PaO_2 will slightly change according to the variations in cardiac output.

Effects of PEEP on respiratory mechanics

The analysis of volume–pressure curves (V/P) of the respiratory system is a key point to understand the physiological effects of PEEP on respiratory mechanics. In patients with ARF, reduced compliance of the respiratory system corresponds to small variations in volume occurring for unit of change in pressure.

The inflation limb of the V/P curve shows: (1) a 'lower inflection point' (LIP) where compliance suddenly improves and (2) an 'upper inflection point' (UIP) corresponding to the pressure where compliance starts to deteriorate. In normal subjects, the LIP occurs below the volume at FRC and the UIP occurs at a volume close to total lung capacity. In patients with ARDS, both occur within tidal ventilation and indicate the pressure at which recruitment of collapsed alveoli and at which hyperinflation start to occur, respectively. Ventilation using levels of PEEP lower than the LIP may exacerbate lung injury by shear forces applied during repeated opening and closing alveoli; therefore, tidal excursion during mechanical ventilation should occur between LIP and UIP.

Compliance of the respiratory system (i.e. tidal volume divided by plateau pressure minus PEEP) represents a good estimate of the elastic properties of the respiratory system.

Effects of PEEP on compliance

- Increase in compliance suggests recruitment
- No change in compliance indicates that ventilation is occurring on the linear portion of the V/P curve
- Decrease in compliance indicates lung over distension and risk of barotrauma

The interpretation of the effects of PEEP requires assessment of both lung and chest wall mechanics. In patients with a stiff chest wall due to increased intra-abdominal pressure, underestimation of LIP is expected and consequently relatively higher levels of PEEP should be applied. Conversely, in the presence of a stiff chest wall, the pressure required to expand the lung may exceed the limit of 30cm H_2O without risk of alveolar overdistension.

Effects of PEEP on systemic haemodynamics

Application of PEEP increases intrathoracic pressure diminishing venous return to the right heart and increasing the right ventricular afterload. These haemodynamic consequences depend on previous ventricular loading conditions and function, and respiratory system compliance. An adequate circulating blood volume is required before application of PEEP to prevent this depression of right ventricular output.

Application of PEEP decreases left ventricular stroke volume, while heart rate does not change significantly. The reduction in stroke volume is mainly due to a decrease in left ventricular preload. This effect may be explained by different mechanisms: decreased venous return to the right heart; increased right ventricular afterload; decreased ventricular compliance; and decreased ventricular contractility.

In patients with normal cardiac function, the main consequence of increased intrathoracic pressure is the reduction of venous return; in patients with poor left ventricular function or congestive heart failure, the increase in intrathoracic pressure reduces the left ventricular transmural pressure leading to a reduction in left ventricular afterload and improving left ventricular function. In these patients, cardiac output is relatively insensitive to reduction in venous return because diastolic volume is elevated.

PEEP in the clinical setting

ALI/ARDS

The application of PEEP in ALI/ARDS is aimed at preventing the end-expiratory collapse of the lung in order to reverse severe hypoxaemia resulting from pulmonary shunting. Moreover, since mechanical ventilation with a high tidal volume and a low level of PEEP is associated with pulmonary injury (VILI) indistinguishable from ARDS, the use of PEEP may reduce VILI by preventing the cyclical opening and closing of the alveoli. The potential benefit of the 'open lung approach' lies in the avoidance of recruitment–derecruitment of partially consolidated areas, avoiding their exposure to shear stress and miminizing the local inflammatory reaction.

A protective ventilatory strategy, limiting the Vt to 6ml/kg and the plateau pressure to <30cm H_2O, is the gold standard of ventilatory strategy in patient with ALI/ARDS. Titration of the optimal level of PEEP has been a compromise between the minimal PEEP providing maximum oxygen delivery at the lowest airway pressure, and high PEEP keeping the lung fully recruited at end expiration.

Chronic obstructive pulmonary disease (COPD)

In patients with an exacerbation of COPD, the rate of lung emptying is impaired because of increased respiratory resistance and expiratory flow limitation. End-expiratory lung volume is expected to be higher than resting volume: a condition named dynamic hyperinflation. As a consequence a positive pressure named intrinsic PEEP (PEEPi) is present at the end of expiration. PEEPi represents an inspiratory threshold load to be counterbalanced by the patient's inspiratory muscles in order to initiate inspiration or to trigger the ventilator. In the presence of PEEPi due to expiratory flow limitation, externally applied PEEP below measured PEEPi (85% of total PEEP) does not cause hyperinflation or an increase in intrathoracic pressure and does not affect respiratory mechanics and haemodynamics. During the assisted mode of ventilation, application of PEEP reduces inspiratory muscle effort and improves patient–ventilator interaction.

Acute severe asthma

The main cause of dynamic hyperinflation and PEEPi during acute exacerbation of asthma is the increased expiratory resistance in the absence of flow limitation. Consequently flow continues to the very end of expiration, driven by the difference in pressure between the alveoli and the airway opening. In this situation, use of external PEEP provides a back pressure to respiratory airflow, causing parallel increases in lung volume and airway, alveolar and thoracic pressure. In these patients undergoing mechanical ventilation, the use of external PEEP is often detrimental and should be eventually used only if expiratory flow limitation is proved.

Adverse effects of PEEP

Hepatic and renal perfusion

PEEP decreases splanchnic blood flow and may compromise hepatic perfusion and portal venous drainage. This effect may be explained by a reduction in cardiac output, coupled with elevation of central venous pressure (CVP) and an increased outflow resistance due to a direct compressive effect of the diaphragm on the liver. The resulting passive hepatic congestion can cause moderate elevation of bilirubin and hepatic enzymes. PEEP may also interfere with renal function, even when cardiac output is preserved, by reducing renal blood flow depending on the volaemic state and the amount of applied pressure.

Cerebral perfusion

The application of PEEP may affect the cerebral circulation by haemodynamic and CO_2-mediated mechanisms. The haemodynamic mechanism may alter cerebral circulation both on the arterial side, reducing arterial pressure, and on the venous side, reducing cerebral venous drainage. According to the concept of the vasodilatory cascade, the decrease in arterial pressure caused by PEEP may diminish cerebral blood flow in patients whose cerebral autoregulation is impaired, while may cause a compensatory vaso-dilation if auto-regulation is preserved. In the latter case, vasodilation will lead to an increase in cerebral blood volume and intracranial pressure (ICP), given a reduced intracranial compliance. However, application of PEEP does not induce a significant reduction in arterial and cerebral perfusion pressure if euvolaemia is ensured.

Reduced oxygen delivery (DO_2)

Application of PEEP may worsen global oxygen delivery through three mechanisms: decreased cardiac output, increase venous admixture and increased intracranial shunt.

Further reading

Brower RG, Lanken PN, MacIntyre N, *et al.* Higher versus lower positive end-expiratory pressures in patients with acute respiratiry distress syndrome. *N Engl J Med* 2004; 351: 327–36.

Pinsky MR. The hemodynamic consequences of mechanical ventilation: an evolving story. *Intensive Care Med* 1997; 23: 493–503.

Ranieri VM, Giuliani R, Fiore T, *et al.* Volume–pressure curve of the respiratory system predicts effects of PEEP in ARDS: 'occlusion' versus 'constant flow' tecnhique. *Am J Respir Crit Care* 1994; 149: 19–27.

Suter PM, Fairlay B, Isemberg MD. Optimum end-expiratory pressure in patients with acute pulmonary failure. *N Engl J Med* 1975; 292: 284–9.

The Acute Respiratory Distress Syndrome Network. Ventilation with lower tidal volumes as compared with traditional tidal volumes for acute lung injury and the acute respiratory distress syndrome. *N Engl J Med* 2000; 342: 1301–8.

Continuous positive airway pressure ventilation (CPAP)

Introduction

Continuous positive airway pressure ventilation (CPAP) is the application of a positive pressure throughout the respiratory cycle, non-invasively, in spontaneously breathing patients. It is applied by generating a constant flow of an oxygen/air mixture, with a resistance applied in the circuit to create PEEP. It is primarily used to improve oxygenation in patients with distal airways collapse for a variety of reasons, thereby improving oxygen exchange in selected patients whose hypoxaemia does not respond to merely increasing fractional inspired oxygen concentration (FiO_2). There may also be a beneficial reduction in the work of breathing, and an increase in minute ventilation through lung expansion and a small inspiratory positive pressure support effect. Thus, it may even correct acute respiratory hypercapnia associated with cardiorespiratory insufficiency in selected patients with cardiogenic pulmonary oedema.

Alternatively, CPAP is also effective for maintaining patency of the collapsible upper airway in obstructive sleep apnoea hypopnoea syndrome (OSAHS), and related sleep disordered breathing (SDB).

CPAP increases intrathoracic pressure, which may reduce venous return and preload to the heart. However, this may also be beneficial in offloading the left atrium/ventricle in cardiogenic pulmonary oedema associated with acute left ventricular failure. Conversely, in patients with relative intravascular depletion, the application of CPAP may cause a further reduction in ventricular preload, stroke volume, cardiac output and blood pressure.

Indications

1 *Acute respiratory failure (ARF)* (usually normocapnic but even in acute hypercapnic ARF if due to reversible basal atelectasis/collapse).
   - a *Post-operative*—for assisted ventilation as an adjunct to lung expansion manoeuvres and analgesia (i.e. physiotherapy, incentive spirometry, intermittent positive pressure breathing)
   - b *Acute respiratory insufficiency* (e.g. pneumonia, inflammatory lung diseases, acute lobar collapse)—when simply increasing FiO_2 is insufficient to maintain adequate oxygenation.
   - c *Inadequate oxygenation* but adequate ventilatory drive.
   - d *Chest wall trauma with persistent hypoxaemia*, despite high FiO_2 and analgesia (care with potential pneumothorax).

2 *Cardiogenic pulmonary oedema*—unresponsive to initial medical management (i.e. increased FiO_2, nitrate containing venodilators, diuretics).

3 Obstructive sleep apnoea/hypopnoea syndrome (OSAHS) and related conditions of SDB.

4 Weaning from mechanical ventilation—prior to extubation /tracheostomy decannulation or prior to step down to oxygenation only.

Contraindications

1 Coma/impaired consciousness
2 Inability to maintain/protect own airway
3 Fixed upper airway obstruction
4 Haemodynamic instability/severe co-morbidity (relative)
5 Head/facial trauma.
6 High risk of aspiration—including patients with gastrointestinal bleeding. A nasogastric tube reduces the risk.
7 Mechanical bowel obstruction
8 Recent upper gastrointestinal surgery
9 Copious secretions—risk of inability to clear with tight-fitting mask.

Equipment

CPAP machine, circuit, PEEP valves, heated membrane exchange (HME) filter, heated humidifier, full facial mask, straps, Oxygen analyser and alarm, power supply and oxygen source (Fig. 1.10.1).

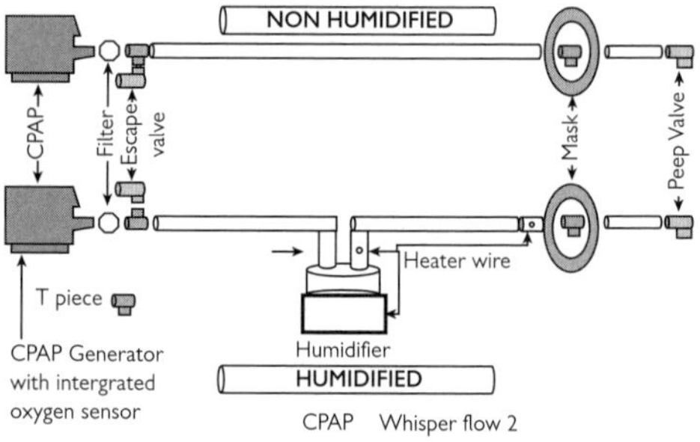

Fig. 1.10.1 CPAP set-up.

Venturi devices (i.e. WhisperFlow 2™ or Vital Signs™ CPAP systems, Figs 1.10.2 and 1.10.3) use an oxygen supply in conjunction with entrained air to generate an output. It can generate flows >140l/min with a minimal FiO_2 of 28%. These systems have internal pressure relief safety valves for pressures >28cm H_2O. The use of pressure and oxygen monitors ensures measured pressures approximate to the specified PEEP and FiO2.

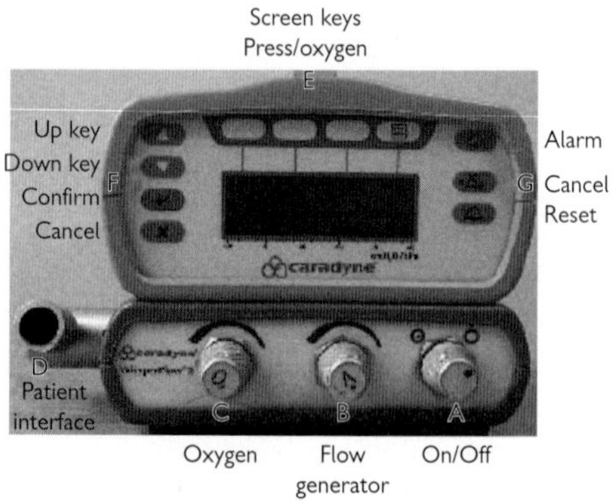

Fig. 1.10.2 WhisperFlow 2™ CPAP with Cardyne's Criterion Monior™—front view. A, on–off; B, flowmeter; C, oxygen flowmeter; D, patient interface-tubing-PEEP valve; E, monitor; F, settings; G, alarm.

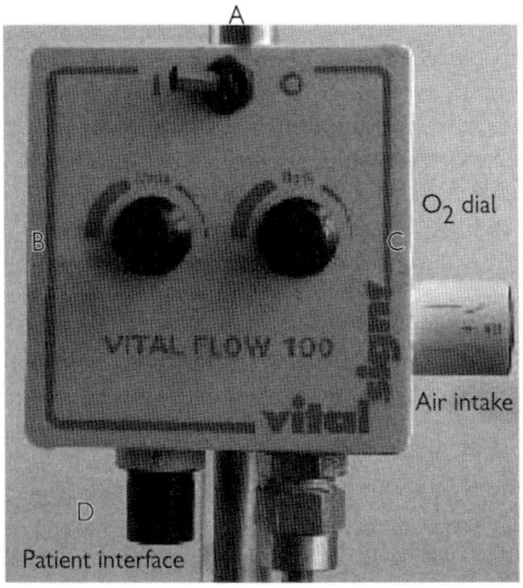

Fig. 1.10.3 Vital Signs™ CPAPA. A, on–off; B, flowmeter; C, oxygen flowmeter; D, patient interface-tubing-PEEP valve.

Portable CPAP flow generators used in the treatment of OSAHS produce lower flow rates (i.e. 30l/min).

Masks and headgear

In the acute hospital/ICU setting, full face masks are preferred to maintain a closed system. In contrast, the outpatient population with OSAHS generally prefer nasal interfaces with mouth closure. Careful daily inspection is required to prevent skin sores. Use of a sponge or grani-flex is advised. Dentures are maintained *in situ* if possible. Special attention should be paid to leaks into the eyes, and around the mouth. Pressure monitoring is advisable to check the delivered PEEP.

Checklist prior to commencement

- Refractory hypoxaemia? No hypercapnia?
- Contraindications?
- Optimization of standard management
- Reversible component?/Need for further step-up care
- Correct setting for CPAP delivery, i.e. High Dependecny Unit (HDU)/ICU
- Check and set up equipment
- Initial settings, e.g. PEEP 5 cmH_2O, FiO_2 maximum
- Nasogastric tube necessary?
- Explanation to patient
- Monitoring clinical/physiological parameters.

Application of CPAP in clinical settings

Acute respiratory insufficiency—as a bridge to recovery.

Early clinico-physiological improvement, based upon subjective parameters, respiratory rate and oxygenation improve, as compared with face mask oxygen alone. However, CPAP may not reduce intubation rates in acute lung injury. There remains some debate as to the minimum effective PEEP level to produce a CPAP effect on oxygenation that is not merely a high flow phenomenon. This is particularly so with the availability of high=flow humidified oxygen systems through nasal cannulae.

Weaning from mechanical ventilation

The time spent on weaning as a percentage of total ventilator time remains the same, and can vary from one to several days. CPAP has been used as part of spontaneous breathing trials (SBTs) prior to extubation. Flow-based CPAP is deemed superior to ventilator-delivered CPAP, although both provide a degree of inspiratory support to compensate for tube-related airway resistance during SBT (however, it may be argued that this reduces the sensitivity of the SBT). There is no published robust evidence demonstrating an outcome benefit of CPAP used pre-emptively in post-operative patients. Nevertheless, intuitively and anecdotally, successes and reassurance are apparent, so the adage 'absence of evidence does not mean evidence of absence' is applicable in this setting.

CPAP as an adjunct to physiotherapy

There are a number of techniques used to support the active cycle of breathing by physiotherapists; to promote lung expansion manoeuvres. These include IPPV, CPAP, positive expiratory pressure (PEP) devices (e.g. flutter valve) and cough in-exsufflators. The literature would suggest there is little to choose between them, and personal preference/patient comfort are their determinants.

CPAP in OSAHS

OSAHS is the periodic reduction (hypopnea) or cessation (apnoea) of airflow through repetitive closure of the upper airway during sleep. CPAP, delivered by a portable flow generator and mask, overcomes this periodic obstruction, thereby reducing episodic hypoxia and fragmented sleep. Since its first use in this setting in 1981, it has become the standard of care for domiciliary management of laboratory-diagnosed OSAHS. There is compelling evidence emerging of its short- and mid-term benefits, in those with moderate to severe OSAHS, in improving daily function and cardiovascular/cerebrovascular/metabolic risk profiles. The evidence in mild OSAHS is less apparent, although a trial of treatment is suggested if clinical symptoms persist in spite of a low apneoa/hypopnoea index. Patients' tolerability of mask interfaces is sometimes problematic. This has driven the technical development of newer machines and masks for ease of increased nocturnal use.

Further reading

Delclaux C, L'Her E, Alberti C, *et al.* Treatment of acute hypoxemic nonhypercapnic respiratory insufficiency with continuous positive airway pressure delivered by a face mask: a randomized controlled trial. *JAMA* 2000; 284: 2352–60.

Giles TL, Lasserson TJ, Smith BJ, *et al* Continuous positive airways pressure for obstructive sleep apnoea in adults. *Cochrane Database Syst Rev* 2006; (1): CD001106.

Placidi G, Cornacchia M, Polese G, *et al.* Chest physiotherapy with positive airway pressure: a pilot study of short-term effects on sputum clearance in patients with cystic fibrosis and severe airway obstruction. *Respir Care* 2006; 51: 1145–53.

Richardson A, Killen A. How long do patients spend weaning from CPAP in critical care? *Intens Crit Care Nurs* 2006; 22: 206–13.

Sullivan CE, Issa FG, Berthon-Jones M, *et al.* Reversal of obstructive sleep apnoea by continuous positive airway pressure applied through the nares. *Lancet* 1981;1: 862–5.

Recruitment manoeuvres

The mechanism underlying hypoxaemia in acute lung injury is intrapulmonary shunt due to non-ventilated but perfused alveoli. Any manoeuvre that recruits lung volume and increases the amount of aerated lung can be expected to improve gas exchange. However, the challenge is to recruit atelectatic alveoli without overdistending normal lung units. Although PEEP is the most commonly used method to achieve or maintain recruitment, others techniques have been evaluated: volume recruitment manoeuvres, prone position and HFOV. Volume recruitment manoeuvres, periodic inflations to airways pressures of 35–45cm H_2O sustained for 5–30s, are used to reverse alveolar derecruitment and to improve gas exchange while allowing acceptable ventilator pressure.

In ALI/ARDS, inadequate levels of PEEP may cause tidal recruitment/derecruitment of part of the consolidated lung and may expose these regions to shear stress. The combined use of low tidal volume and PEEP may minimize VILI. Recruitment manoeuvres are procedures specifically designed to reach an opening pressure sufficient to open the collapsed lung regions that, in association with an increased level of PEEP post- recruitment manoeuvre, may improve gas exchange, reducing intrapulmonary shunt. However, the effectiveness of recruiting manoeuvres to improve oxygenation is also influenced by elastic properties of the chest wall since part of the pressure applied to the respiratory system during the recruiting manoeuvres can be dissipated against a stiff chest wall. Moreover, the response to recruitment manoeuvres is a function of the potential for recruitment (unstable units), the phase and extent of lung injury, the level of PEEP and the characteristics of the recruiting technique.

In clinical practice, RM may play a role in the lung-protective ventilatory strategies based on the so-called 'open lung approach'; however, their utility has not been confirmed by large clinical trials. Lung recruitment manoeuvres have also been successfully used in patients during general anaesthesia, to restore the decreased respiratory system compliance and oxygenation.

Techniques

Several approaches have been used to perform the recruitment manoeuvres:

- Sustained inflation by application of CPAP at 30–40cm H_2O for 40s.
- Incremental PEEP on maximum pressure: PEEP is increased in increments of 5cm H_2O from a baseline PEEP to 35cm H_2O, reducing tidal volume to limit peak inspiratory pressure to 35cm H_2O. CPAP of 35cm H_2O is maintained for 30s.
- Intermittent higher tidal volume in pressure-controlled ventilation applied with escalating PEEP and constant driving pressure: peak pressure of 45cm H_2O, I:E ratio of 1:2 and PEEP level of 16cm H_2O for 2min.

If gas exchange and lung mechanics improve substantially with recruitment manoeuvres, the patients should be considered to have 'high potential for recruitment'. However, in gauging response to PEEP, it is important to consider the oxygenation response as well as CO_2 exchange: when PEEP is applied, PaO_2 tends to increase and CO_2 exchange may improve, reflecting increased alveolar ventilation.

If gas exchange and lung mechanics do not improve substantially with recruitment manoeuvres, the patients are considered to have a 'low potential for recruitment', and the use of higher level of PEEP may provide little benefit and actually be harmful since application of PEEP may cause overdistention.

Data suggest that patients with 'high potential for recruitment' are those ventilated for not more than 48–72h, while patients with 'low potential for recruitment' are those ventilated for >3 days; the underlying disease responsible for ARDS (primary vs secondary ARDS) seems not to have a role in identifying responders or non-responders to recruitment manoeuvres.

Monitoring

Clinical evaluation of the response to recruitment manoeuvres and of its potential use can be evaluated at the bedside. More accurate evaluation of the percentage of potentially recruitable lung may be obtained by analysis of CT images or of respiratory mechanics.

Clinical evaluation

After performing a recruitment manoeuvre, its efficacy can be evaluated at the bedside by looking at the values of plateau pressure (or tidal volume if the patient is ventilated in a pressure-controlled mode), PaO_2 and $PaCO_2$. If the recruitment manoeuvre: (1) decreases plateau pressure (or increases tidal volume if the patient is ventilated in a pressure-controlled mode); (2) increases PaO_2; and (3) decreases $PaCO_2$ (even if only few mm Hg), the patients may be considered as a responder.

CT scanning

Analysis of CT findings can identify the distribution of normally aerated lung regions in the non-dependent regions, and poorly aerated lung regions distributed in the dependent lung region. The CT analysis can assess the effects of the recruitment manoeuvres as well as its safety, and most importantly the adequate PEEP levels to keep the lungs opened after the recruitment manoeuvres. With an inspiratory and expiratory pause image acquisition of the lung, the regional tidal volume distribution can be assessed.

Respiratory mechanics

Pressure–volume (P/V) curve

Analysis of P/V curves can confirm that the lower inflection point and upper inflection point correspond to CT scan evidence of atelectasis and overdistension. Alveolar recruitment is confirmed to occur continuously and along the inspiratory limb of the P/V curve, while the critical point for lung derecruitment is identified below the point of maximum curvature of the deflation limb.

Stress index

The analysis of the dynamic pressure/time (P/T) curve during constant flow ventilation (stress index) is a new parameter to identify clinically the best compromise between alveolar recruitment and overdistention. The stress index is the exponent of the equation correlating the airway pressure profile and time during each tidal volume. A stress index <1 is associated with recruitment, assessed by CT scan, whereas a stress index >1 is associated with hyperinflation. Modern ventilators are able to deliver square-wave inspiratory flow profiles and are equipped with monitoring that provides on-line dynamic P/T curves.

Risks

The potential risks of the recruitment manoeuvres are barotrauma (high transpulmonary pressure) and haemodynamic derangement (high pleural pressure). In patients with 'low potential for recruitment' (non-responders), application of recruiting manoeuvres may result in a substantial haemodynamic impairment. These effects are due a reduced preload secondary to transmission of pleural pressure to intrathoracic structures and an increased afterload due to increased lung volume. The degree of pleural pressure transmitted is higher in patients with a stiff chest wall than in patients with a normal chest wall. Therefore, the use of recruitment manoeuvres may be indicated only in patients with high potential for recruitment, keeping in mind that after the manoeuvre, the level of PEEP has to be increased otherwise its beneficial effects on gas exchange and respiratory mechanics will be lost in a few minutes.

Further reading

Gattinoni L, Caironi P, Cressoni M, *et al.* Lung recruitment in patients with the acute respiratory distress syndrome. *N Engl J Med* 2006; 354: 1775–86.

Grasso S, Mascia L, Del Turco M, *et al.* Effects of recruiting maneuvers in patients with acute respiratory distress syndrome ventilated with protective ventilatory strategy. *Anesthesiology* 2002; 96: 795–802.

Grasso S, Terragni P, Mascia L, *et al.* Airway pressure–time curve profile (stress index) detects tidal recruitment/hyperinflation in experimental acute lung injury. *Crit Care Med* 2004; 32: 1018–27.

Lachmann B. Open up the lung and keep the lung open. *Intensive Care Med* 1992; 18: 319–21.

Lim S-C, Adams AB, Simson DA, *et al.* Intercoparison of recruitment maneuvers efficacy in three models of acute injury. *Crit Care Med* 2004: 32: 2371–7.

Prone position ventilation

Acute lung injury (ALI) occurs in 7.1% of ICU admissions, with 55% of these patients progressing to ARDS within 72h. The population-based incidence of ALI is estimated to be 78.9 per 100 000 person-years. Interestingly, respiratory failure is thought to be the primary cause of death in only 16% of patients with ARDS. However, it is now recognized that mechanical ventilation may itself be directly harmful to the injured lung, so-called ventilator induced lung injury (VILI), and contribute to the development of multi-organ dysfunction. As such, the present literature supports a lung-protective approach to ventilation in patients with ARDS, via limitations on plateau pressure and tidal volume.

Prone position ventilation is one of several adjuncts employed by clinicians when adequate gas exchange cannot be achieved with conventional ventilatory strategies, and has been used effectively to improve oxygenation in patients with both ALI and ARDS from a wide range of aetiologies.

Oxygenation response to prone position

In numerous observational and randomized studies in ALI/ARDS, prone positioning results in improved oxygenation (increased PaO_2/FiO_2 of 10–30%) in ~70–80% of patients. Three oxygenation response patterns have been described.

- Non-responders (20%)—no improvement in oxygenation
- Responders (80%)
  - Persistent: improve oxygenation and maintain improved oxygenation on turning supine (50%)
  - Non-persistent: improvement in oxygenation is not sustained on returning to supine position (30%)

Attempts have been to define factors that predict a favourable response to oxygenation. Although in an individual subject response to prone positioning may vary from one episode to another, the following have generally been associated with a more favourable oxygenation response.

- Higher baseline $PaCO_2$
- Improved $PaCO_2$ clearance during prone positioning
- More severe lung injury
- Early vs late lung injury
- Extrapulmonary vs pulmonary lung injury
- Lobar radiological pattern of lung injury.

Physiological effects of prone position

The improvement in oxygenation and respiratory mechanics observed during prone positioning result from a synergistic interaction of the effects of the prone position on the lung parenchyma, chest and abdominal wall, and the pulmonary circulation.

The physiological effects of prone position

Ventilation-related effects

- More homogenous distribution of ventilation due to favourable changes in thoraco-abdominal compliance
- Improved alveolar recruitment
- Sustained effect of recruitment manoeuvres
- Better drainage of secretions

Perfusion-related effects

- More homogenous distribution of perfusion

Other effects

- Reduction in VILI
- Reduction in extravascular lung water (EVLW)

Effect on alveolar ventilation

Prone positioning results in a more homogenous distribution of alveolar pressure and ventilation, due a reduction in thoraco-abdominal compliance secondary to restriction of the anterior thoracic and abdominal walls. The more uniform distribution of alveolar pressure also prevents collapse of vulnerable lung units on expiration, maintaining alveolar recruitment. In addition, in the prone position, the heart is dependent and the diaphragm is caudally displaced, reducing posterior compression of the lung parenchyma and improving regional ventilation in these areas. The net result of these effects is a reduction in intrapulmonary shunt and an improvement in hypoxaemia. There is emerging evidence that relative to the semi-recumbent position, indices of lung stress are reduced in the prone position, offering the potential for prone positioning to attenuate VILI.

Effects on pulmonary perfusion

Traditionally, the effect of gravity has been used to explain the heterogeneity in regional pulmonary perfusion. As such, in ALI, perfusion and atelectasis are both greater in the dependent lung, resulting in shunt and hypoxaemia. It was suggested that prone positioning would allow redistribution of perfusion to aerated lung regions and thus improve shunt and oxygenation. Experimental studies have had conflicting results, and the effect of the prone position on perfusion distribution, independent of changes in ventilation, are thought to be minimal. Prolonged prone position (18h) may also reduce EVLW .

Technique of prone position

Prone positioning requires a concerted effort from all members of the multi-disciplinary team. Although there is no standard approach to the prone manoeuvre, detailed descriptions of appropriate algorithms have been published. Specialist beds do exist, but are not commonplace, with most units using a modified two-step 'logroll', with specific individuals assigned to manage the ETT, vascular access devices and surgical drains. At least one of those present must be competent to undertake re-intubation if required. Prone positioning requires no additional monitoring, although ECG leads must be placed on the back. The need for endotracheal suctioning may increase in frequency and there needs to be strict attention to potential pressure areas, including regular repositioning of the patient, padding to vulnerable areas and specific attention to ETT and catheter entry sites. As with the standard supine position, elevation of the head of the bed (reverse Trendelenberg) may reduce the risk of pharyngeal aspiration as well as help minimize ocular and facial oedema whilst prone. Despite this, however, enteral feeding may be more problematic in the prone position, and a reduction in the target rate may need to be considered to minimize potential complications. In the presence of adequate levels of sedation, paralysis is not usually required, and may have detrimental effects on diaphragm-related benefits. The optimal duration of prone positioning is unknown. Whilst most earlier studies used repeated periods of up to 6–8h/day, more recent studies have preferred more prolonged periods (up to 20h day), in an attempt to make use of the persisting oxygenation benefit via application of a lung-protective ventilatory approach. Although manually onerous, with appropriate equipment, guidelines and training in place, prone positioning is a relatively simple and safe procedure with a low economic burden.

Contraindications

Contraindications to prone positioning detailed in previous studies include;

- severe haemodynamic instability/arrythmias
- spinal instability
- pelvic fractures/multiple trauma
- pregnancy
- raised ICP
- recent tracheal surgery or sternotomy
- abdominal surgey/raised intra-abdominal pressure

Spinal instability is the main absolute contraindication, although haemodynamic instability and arrythmias are strong relative contraindications due to the inherent difficulties in immediate access for CPR (cardiopulmonary resuscitation) in the prone position. Prone positioning in patients with wounds/surgical intervention to the face or ventral body surface, or in obese individuals, may cause special problems, but can be possible on an individual patient basis.

Complications

Prone positioning is associated with complications which have both immediate and long term effects for the patient. Marked facial oedema is almost ubiquitous, and pressure sores to the face, anterior chest wall, and iliac crests are common unless specifically targeted. Displacement or malfunction of the ETT, chest drains and vascular access are potentially serious complications during the proning manoeuvre.

Complications observed with prone positioning

During turning

- Loss of airway and vascular access
- Injury to cervical spine, shoulder
- Increased sedation requirements
- Transient hypoxaemia
- Cardiac arrhythmia
- Haemodynamic instability

During prone position ventilation

- Oedema and pressure sores of the face, thorax and iliac crests
- Conjuctival oedema and haemorrhage
- Retinal damage
- Airway obstruction
- Malfunction of vascular access, bladder catheter, enteral feeding tubes, chest drains
- Intolerance to enteral feeding
- Nerve compression
- Persistent hypoxaemia
- Haemodynamic instability

Outcome with prone position ventilation

There have been four randomized controlled trials on prone positioning, and none has shown a survival advantage. However, one small study was confined to patients with polytrauma, and a second larger study considered patients with acute hypoxaemic respiratory failure of all causes, of whom only 45% had ALI/ARDS. In the largest study in unselected patients with ALI/ARDS, 304 patients were randomized to receive supine vs prone ventilation (>6h) for 10 days. Although oxygenation improved during prone positioning, there was no difference in 10-day, ICU and 6-month mortality, non-pulmonary organ failure or iatrogenic complications, between the two groups. A *post hoc* analysis implied improved 10-day survival with prone ventilation in the sickest patients (PaO_2/FiO_2 <88; Simplified Acute Physiology Score II (SAPS II) >49), but this did not persist to ICU discharge. However, this study employed relatively short periods of prone ventilation and a ventilatory strategy (Vt >10ml/kg and relatively low levels of PEEP) that preceded present lung-protective approaches. In a more recent study, 136 patients with early severe ARDS were randomized to supine or prolonged prone ventilation (20h/day), with an established protective ventilatory approach. Although there no difference in overall mortality, the 12–15% and 20–25% reduction in ICU and hospital mortality in the prone group is clinically intriguing, especially as they were deemed to be sicker at study entry.

Conclusions

Prone positioning improves oxygenation but not outcome in unselected patients with ARDS. With appropriate education and training, it can be safely performed in most patients. At present it should be considered an adjunct for those patients with severe ARDS failing to progress or deteriorating with conventional ventilatory approaches. We advocate more prolonged periods of prone position, incorporating existing lung-protective approaches to mechanical ventilation.

Further reading

Gattinoni L, Tognoni G, Pesenti A, *et al.* Effect of prone positioning on the survival of patients with acute respiratory failure. *N Eng J Med* 2001; 345: 568–73.

Guerin C, Gaillard S, Lemasson S et al Effects of systematic prone positioning in hypoxemic acute respiratory failure: a randomized controlled trial. *JAMA* 2004; 292: 2379–87.

Mancebo J, Fernandez R, Blanch L *et al.* A Multicenter Trial Of Prolonged Prone Ventilation In Severe Acute Respiratory Distress Syndrome. *Am J Resp Crit Care Med* 2006; 173: 1233–9.

Voggenreiter G, Aufmkolk M, Stiletto R *et al.* Prone positioning improves oxygenation in post-traumatic lung injury—a prospective randomized trial. *J Trauma* 2005; 59: 333–41.

Non-invasive positive pressure ventilation (NIPPV)

Introduction

Non-invasive positive pressure ventilation (NIPPV) is the delivery of mechanically assisted or generated breaths through a facial interface, without the placement of an artificial airway, such as an ETT or a tracheostomy. It is an established alternative to invasive mechanical ventilation, for selected patients with ARF, and as a weaning mode following extubation or tracheostomy decannulation. However, it does not replace invasive mechanical ventilation in patients requiring emergent endotracheal intubation.

Benefits

NIPPV is a safe, effective technique that can avoid the side effects associated with endotracheal intubation. It is primarily used to avert invasive mechanical ventilation in patients with early acute respiratory failure, and prevent re-intubation in patients with recurrent weaning failure. NIPPV preserves upper airway defence mechanisms, speech and swallowing.

NIPPV improves alveolar ventilation, decreases work of breathing and reduces intubation rates, length of hospital stay morbidity (i.e. pneumonia) and mortality. These are greatest for patients with acute exacerbations of COPD associated with hypercapnic respiratory failure. There is also benefit in cardiogenic pulmonary oedema complicated by hypercapnia. Conversely, failure of NIPPV to prevent intubation has been associated with a higher mortality in patients with respiratory failure due to other causes, emphasizing the need for careful patient selection and monitoring for markers of early of treatment failure.

Contraindications

Other than the need for emergent intubation, contraindications for NIPPV include cardiorespiratory arrest, non-respiratory system organ failure (e.g. severe encephalopathy, haemodynamic instability, severe gastrointestinal bleeding), facial or upper airway trauma, post-neurosurgery to the head, loss of airway patency, excessive airway secretions or lack of cooperation with a high aspiration risk.

Severe respiratory acidosis is not a contraindication to NIPPV, so long as intubation is available in an ICU setting if the NIPPV trial fails. In a case–control study of 64 patients with COPD and severe hypercapnic respiratory failure (mean pH 7.18) who received NIPPV, 38% never required an ETT. Those who failed NIPPV and required intubation were not harmed by the delayed intubation and prolonged acidaemia.

Technical considerations

Pressure-cycled modes (pressure support or bilevel, BiPAP) are preferred for patient comfort, although volume-cycled modes may further reduce the work of breathing. Delivery through standard ventilators can offer time-cycled options to improve synchrony, precise O_2 concentrations and enhanced CO_2 clearance. Full face masks, nasal masks or alternatives such as helmets are available. Initiation requires dedicated staff, awareness of mask-related complications and troubleshooting skills. Early clinico-physiological assessment of success/failure by blood gases and respiratory rate at 1h is vital.

Complications

Complications associated with invasive ventilation (e.g. nosocomial pneumonia, barotrauma, haemodynamic instability) are less common in NIPPV. Local skin damage is related to pressure effects of the mask and straps. Cushioning the forehead and the bridge of the nose helps. Mask leaks are common and do not preclude NIPPV. Consider using different masks or ventilator settings. Eye irritation and sinus congestion may occur and may necessitate lower inspiratory pressures or the use of a facial mask rather than a nasal mask. Gastric distension occurs with some frequency but is rarely significant. Routine use of a nasogastric tube is not warranted. Barotrauma is uncommon in NIPPV when administered in the pressure support or bilevel modes. Adverse haemodynamic effects due to NIPPV are unusual.

Indications

The success of NIPPV depends on several factors, such as type of ARF, the underlying disease, location of treatment, experience of the team. The timing of initiation and duration of use are also important for outcomes. Guidelines for the use of NIPPV improve the utilization and process of care, without changing clinical outcomes

Acute hypercapnic respiratory failure

Patients with acute hypercapnic respiratory acidosis secondary to an exacerbation of COPD benefit the most from NIPPV, and are the best studied group in the context of randomized controlled trials, and systematic reviews of NIPPV for ARF. Medical treatment failure rates vary between 27 and 74% from studies. The successful use of NIPPV can reduce mortality (relative risk (RR) 0.41), intubation rates (RR 0.42) and treatment failure rates (RR 0.51). It can also reduce length of hospital stay, and may be cost-effective through reduced ICU admissions/tracheostomy rates. These benefits are for patients with mild to moderate ARF (i.e. pH <7.3 and >7.25), who can be managed on a dedicated general ward/intermediate care setting with trained staff. The benefits are less and potentially harmful (i.e. through delayed intubation) in the more severely ill patients, who should be managed in a higher dependency setting, with greater staffing and monitoring, thus allowing intubation without delay if deemed necessary. There is no evidence to suggest that NIPPV can prevent acute respiratory distress/failure in mild exacerbations (i.e. pH >7.35, respiratory rate RR <20).

There are no robust, easily reproducible clinical predictors of success/failure in acute exacerbations of COPD. Poor signs include an increase in respiratory rate and/or worse pH at 1–2h post-initiation. A Glasgow Coma Score below 11, and/or an APACHE II index of >29 can predict increasing need for intubation.

Hypoxaemic respiratory failure

The efficacy of NIPPV in patients with hypoxaemic respiratory failure has been demonstrated in pneumonia, immunosuppression, and following single lung resection. However, the studies have generally enrolled patients with moderate ARF, in whom emergent endotracheal intubation was not necessary. In a heterogeneous population of 105 ICU patients, bilevel NIPPV decreased the need for intubation (25 vs 52%) and the incidence of septic shock (12 vs 31%), improved ICU mortality (18 vs 39%) and increased 90-day survival vs high concentration oxygen. The benefits of NIPPV in ARF (PaO_2/FiO_2 <33kPa) due to pneumonia may be limited, to those with underlying COPD, although a trial in all comers is justified.

Alternative to invasive ventilation

Weaning off invasive ventilation

Patients with COPD receiving invasive mechanical ventilation for >48h and failing SBTs can be safely extubated to NIPPV, shortening ICU stay and reducing mortality.

Extubation failure

NIPPV reduces re-intubation rates when used early in patients at risk of post-extubation failure (i.e. previous extubation failure, high APACHE score >12, hypercapnia, chronic heart failure, poor cough, stridor, co-morbidities). However, it is ineffective, and potentially harmful in post-extubation respiratory failure 48h on, due to delayed re-intubation. Thus the early use of NIPPV is once again emphasized for best efficacy. It has been used successfully to pre-oxygenate patients prior to endotracheal intubation, compared with bag-valve-mask ventilation.

Other specific indications

Cardiogenic pulmonary oedema.

NIPPV reduces the incidence of intubation compared with standard medical therapy and oxygen alone. It is equivalent to CPAP, but may be more advantageous in patients with associated hypercapnia. There appears to be no additional risk of acute myocardial infarction associated with the use of NIPPV in this setting.

Patients with 'do not intubate' orders.

In patients unsuitable for, or declining intubation for ARF, NIPPV can act as a bridge to recovery in >40%. It may also be used as palliation for breathlessness if tolerated.

Asthma

Only one prospective trial has adequately assessed the value of NIPPV in acute asthma (not requiring emergent intubation). Using sham (subtherapeutic BiPAP) as the control arm, NIPPV improved lung function and reduced admission rates from the emergency room.

ARDS

There is insufficient information to recommend the use of NIPPV in this setting. If used, then an ICU setting with early recognition of failure and intubation is advisable.

Neuromuscular disease

NIPPV has been used successfully to support decompensated neuromuscular diseases such Guillan–Barre syndrome and muscular dystrophies to recovery, while it is also a bridge to transplantation in cystic fibrosis, avoiding intubation.

Further reading

Demoule A, Girou E, Richard JC, *et al.* Benefits and risks of success or failure of noninvasive ventilation. *Intensive Care Med* 2006; 32: 1756.

Evans TW. International Consensus Conferences in Intensive Care Medicine: non-invasive positive pressure ventilation in acute respiratory failure. *Intensive Care Med* 2000; 27: 166–78.

Liesching T, Kwok H, Hill NS. Acute applications of noninvasive positive pressure ventilation. *Chest* 2003; 124: 699.

Lightowler J, Wedzicha J, Elliott M, *et al.* Non-invasive positive pressure ventilation to treat respiratory failure resulting from exacerbations of chronic obstructive pulmonary disease. *BMJ* 2003; 326: 185.

Sinuff, T, Cook, DJ, Randall, J, *et al.* Evaluation of a practice guideline for noninvasive positive-pressure ventilation for acute respiratory failure. *Chest* 2003; 123: 2062.

Extracorporeal membrane oxygenation (ECMO) for adults in respiratory failure

Introduction

Extracorporeal membrane oxygenation (ECMO) uses modified cardiopulmonary bypass technology to provide prolonged respiratory or cardiorespiratory support to patients of all ages who have failed conventional intensive care. Venous blood is drained into the ECMO circuit where it is oxygenated, carbon dioxide is removed and it is rewarmed before being returned to the body. ECMO can be used to support any patient with severe but potentially reversible respiratory, cardiac or multi-organ failure who does not have a contraindication to limited heparinization.

Types of ECMO

There are two types: venoarterial ECMO (VA ECMO) and venovenous ECMO (VV ECMO).

VA ECMO drains deoxygenated blood from a central vein or right atrium and returns it to a central artery. This flow is in addition to the native cardiac output, hence there is partial cardiac support.

VV ECMO drains blood from a central vein or right atrium and returns the oxygenated blood back to a large vein. The volumes of blood drained from and re-infused into the venous system are equal, therefore there is no change in CVP or ventricular filling; the pulmonary artery pressure usually falls due to the increased venous oxygen tension. Native cardiac output provides the full systemic blood flow, which usually improves with the reduction in airway pressure.

VV ECMO is preferred to VA ECMO in the treatment of respiratory failure as normal pulmonary blood flow is maintained.

The ECMO circuit

The ECMO circuit consists of cannulae, pump, membrane lung, servo-regulator, heat exchanger, pressure transducers and a bridge. It is designed to eliminate areas of stasis so that only small amounts of anticoagulation are required.

Oxygenator

The key component of the circuit is the oxygenator or membrane lung. Modern circuits use non-porous hollow fibre oxygenators (polymethylpentene). They have much better gas exchange, lower priming volume and resistance, and are more biocompatible than previous silicone devices.

Cannulae

The amount of oxygen delivered by the ECMO circuit is related to the oxygen content of the blood and the ECMO circuit flow. This is limited by the size and number of venous drainage cannulae. The shortest widest cannula possible should be used.

Pump

The pump pulls bloods either from a small compliance chamber (bladder) or directly from the patient, pumps it through the oxygenator and then back to the patient. It is vital to have a mechanism preventing negative pressure developing proximally when the venous flow is inadequate as this pressure, if unchecked, can cause damage to the atrium and vessel wall as it is 'sucked in'. It can also cause haemolysis and cavitation as gas is pulled out of solution.

Heat exchanger

There is considerable heat loss from the circuit. Normothermia is maintained with a heat exchanger which is usually integral to the oxygenator.

Pressure transducers

Pressure transducers constantly measure pre- and post-oxygenator pressures. A high post-oxygenator pressure signifies a cannula obstruction, and an increasing pressure drop across the oxygenator implies membrane lung failure.

Cannulation

Cannulation for VV is percutaneous. The patient must be anaesthetized and paralysed to reduce the risk of air embolism.

ECMO patient management

Maintain haemostasis

The principle is to balance the anticoagulation so as to prevent significant circuit thrombus formation without causing major haemorrhage. The main agent used is heparin. Anticoagulation is initiated with a bolus of 75 units/kg of heparin IV followed by an infusion to achieve an activated clotting time of 180–200s. The international normalized ratio (INR), fibrinogen levels and platelet count should also be monitored and corrected. Progressive elevation of D-dimers can indicate thrombolytic activity related to the circuit or patient.

Allow lung recovery by use of gentle ventilation.

Once on ECMO, the high pre-ECMO ventilator settings are gradually decreased to 'rest settings' which is positive inspiratory presure (PIP) 20–25, PEEP 10–15cm H_2O, FiO_2 0.3, and rate 10/min. The aim is to reduce ventilator-induced barotrauma and oxygen toxicity.

Provide adequate systemic oxygen delivery

Oxygen delivery is dependent on :

- Capacity (rated flow) of membrane oxygenator
- Oxygen binding capacity of blood
- Flow through circuit
- Oxygen uptake through native lung
- Cardiac output

> Oxygen content of blood = (1.39 x Hb x % saturations) + dissolved Hb (minimal and usually ignored)

On ECMO, to maximize oxygen delivery, the oxygen content of blood needs to be optimized by maintaining a normal Hb concentration of 12–14g/dl. Within the range of the rated flow (design maximum for the oxygenator), increasing the flow can increase oxygenation. Oxygenation is assessed during VV ECMO using the arterial PaO_2 and SpO_2.

Carbon dioxide removal

Carbon dioxide clearance is more efficient than oxygen uptake because unlike oxygen it is diffusion dependent. As the sweep gas contains no carbon dioxide, the diffusion gradient is highest at the inlet end of the oxygenator. Increasing the sweep gas flow will clear more carbon dioxide.

Though carbon dioxide removal is relatively independent of blood flow rate it is dependent on the surface area of the gas-exchanging membrane. When the effective gas exchange area decreases, CO_2 clearance is affected before oxygenation is.

Intensive care

Normal intensive care principles apply to ECMO patients. Full nutrition and appropriate use of antibiotics, steroids and other drugs are essential. In addition to an Intensive Care Nurse, there is an ECMO specialist with the patient and circuit at all times. The ECMO specialist is trained in the management of ECMO circuit and any potential complications.

Weaning, 'trial off' and decannulation

The ECMO flow rate is reduced as the patient gets better. This is shown by improved gas exchange, lung compliance and radiological appearance. Once the flow has come down to 1l/min the patient is usually ready to come off ECMO. To trial off VV ECMO, the patient is ventilated using optimum settings and the oxygen supply to the membrane oxygenator is disconnected. If the patient is stable for 2h, the cannulae can be removed.

Complications

The main complication of ECMO is bleeding. The main potential areas for bleeding are gastrointestinal, intracranial and pulmonary, as well as cannulation sites. Bleeding should be anticipated and actively prevented. Experienced medical staff should be involved in all procedures.

Other complications are associated with cannulation, which includes pneumothorax, haemothorax, pericardial tamponade, vascular tears, embolization and complications associated with the circuit, including cannula obstruction, clots or air in the circuit, oxygenator failure and tubing rupture.

Indications of ECMO

1 Severe respiratory failure.
2 Potentially reversible underlying condition.
3 Failed or failing conventional treatment.

The reversibility of respiratory failure is difficult to determine in adults. Patients ventilated with high pressure, PIP >30cm H_2O and high FiO_2 >0.8 for more than 7 days, patients with advanced chronic lung disease and irreversible conditions such as pulmonary fibrosis are excluded as they are unlikely to recover with ECMO support.

Evidence

The CESAR (Conventional Ventilation or ECMO for Severe Adult Respiratory failure) trial is a multi-centre RCT conducted in the UK

It evaluates survival without severe disability at 6 months and the cost–benefits of ECMO vs conventional ventilation. A total of 180 patients were recruited and the result is currently awaited. The only other trial dates back to the 1970s. This was a multi-centre trial sponsored by the National Institutes of Health and it compared VA ECMO with conventional ventilation in adults. This trial did not show any difference in outcome, but case selection, ECMO techniques and technology, and ventilation strategies in this trial have been superseded by modern protocols. ECMO is an evidence-based therapy for neonates with severe respiratory failure.

The ELSO registry (1990–2006) shows a 59% survival for adult ECMO patients with respiratory failure, and our experience in Glenfield (Leicester UK) is similar, with a survival of 66%.

Conclusion

ECMO is a rational treatment for adult respiratory failure in patients who have failed conventional treatment. The CESAR trial will further define the role of ECMO in these patients.

Further reading

ELSO. Extracorporeal cardiopulmonary support in critical care, 3rd edn. Extracorporeal Life Support Organization, *Ann Arbor, MI*, 2005.

Kolla S, Awad SS, Rich PB, *et al*. Extracorporeal life support for 100 adult patients with severe respiratory failure. *Ann Surg* 1997; 226: 544–66.

Peek GJ, Moore HM, Moore N, *et al*. Extracorporeal membrane oxygenation for adult respiratory failure. *Chest* 1997; 112: 759–64.

UK Collaborative Trial Group. UK Collaborative randomized trail of neonatal extra corporeal membrane oxygenation. *Lancet* 1996; 348: 75–82.

Zapol WM, Snider MT, Hill JD *et al/* Extracorporeal membrane oxygenation in severe respiratory failure. A randomized prospective study. *JAMA* 1979; B: 2193–6.

Tracheostomy

Minitracheostomy/cricothyroidotomy

Introduction

Mini-tracheostomy is a term used to describe the insertion of a small-bore non-cuffed tube through the cricothyroid membrane (usually 4mm internal diameter), principally to aid the clearance of secretions. The passage of suction catheters stimulates coughing and allows secretions to be aspirated. As a short-term measure these devices may help to prevent the need for naso/orotracheal intubation and assisted ventilation. The small size of the tube limits its value, and the use of mini-tracheostomy has declined in many centres in recent years.

Cricothyroidotomy is a life-saving procedure used to provide emergency access to the airway (e.g. following obstruction of the upper airway) when measures such as bag and mask ventilation and translaryngeal intubation have failed. It involves the insertion of a small tube through the cricothyroid membrane, through which oxygen/ventilation can be provided until a definitive airway is obtained. A cuffed device is desirable, and a 6mm rather than 4mm internal diameter greatly improves suctioning and ventilation capacity.

Both cricothyroidotomy and mini-tracheostomy kits are commercially available. The technique for the insertion of each is essentially the same.

Relative contraindications

- Coagulopathy
- Abnormal neck anatomy
- Uncooperative patient

Technique

Explain to the patient what you are going to do. Get written or verbal consent if appropriate. Check the patient's coagulation status. Position the patient comfortably with the head and neck extended over a pillow.

- Palpate anatomy to identify the cricothyroid membrane.
- Clean the neck with antiseptic solution.
- Infiltrate over the cricothyroid membrane with 2–3ml of local anaesthetic.
- Warn the patient that you are going to make him or her cough and perform cricothyroid puncture with a green 21-gauge needle. Aspirate air to confirm the tracheal position of the needle and rapidly inject 2ml of lidocaine (lignocaine). Wait for coughing to subside.
- Perform a superficial skin incision.
- Pass the introducing needle into the trachea and aspirate air.
- Pass the guide wire through the needle and then remove the needle.
- Pass the introducing dilator(s) over the guide wire and then slide the cricothyroidotomy/mini-tracheostomy tube off the introducer. Remove the introducer and guide wire together, leaving the cricothyroidotomy/mini-tracheostomy in place. Suction to remove any blood.
- Obtain a chest X-ray (CXR) to verify the position, appreciating the limitations of such imaging.

Complications

The complications of mini-tracheostomy are the same as for formal tracheostomy. Misplacement and bleeding are particular problems.

Early complications

- Bleeding (may lead to total airway obstruction)
- Pneumothorax
- Tube misplacement or dislodgement
- Emphysema
- Mucus plugging/obstruction
- Stomal inefection

Late complications

- Tracheal stenosis
- Tracheo-oesophageal fistula
- Skin tethering/scarring
- Haemorrhage from innominate vessels

Tracheostomy

Introduction

Tracheostomy is a common procedure in intensive care. The most common problems, in both general wards and critical care, are related to obstruction or displacement. The indications for temporary tracheostomy in intensive care include treatment for upper airway obstruction, the avoidance of the laryngeal complications of prolonged endotracheal intubation and the continued need to protect and maintain the airway in patients with severe neurological injury. The development of percutaneous techniques that enable a tracheostomy tube to be inserted by the critical care physician as a bedside procedure has resulted in temporary tracheostomy becoming more commonplace.

Insertion

A tracheostomy may be performed surgically or percutaneously, and as an emergency or elective procedure.

Indications for a tracheostomy

- Aid to weaning from assisted ventilation
- Tracheal access to remove thick pulmonary secretions (easier suction than translaryngeal intubation)
- Long-term airway management
- Bypass of upper airway obstruction (e.g. patients with trauma, infection, malignancy, laryngeal or subglottic stenosis, bilateral recurrent laryngeal nerve palsy, severe sleep apnoea)
- Prevention of pulmonary aspiration (e.g. patients with laryngeal incompetence, bulbar dysfunction (e.g. cerebrovascular accidents, Parkinson disease))
- Neuromuscular disorders (e.g. Guillain–Barre syndrome, critical illness neuromyopathy)
- Severe brain injury, reversible or irreversible
- Trauma or surgery in the face/neck region

Relative contraindications for percutaneous dilatational tracheostomy (PDT)

- Children <12yrs old
- Uncorrectable coagulopathy
- Active infection over the anterior neck
- Local malignancy in trachea
- Unstable cervical spine fracture
- Morbid obesity (BMI >35)
- Gross anatomical distortion of the neck
- Previous neck surgery or tracheostomy

- Previous radiotherapy to the neck
- Extensive burns to the neck
- Requirement for high PEEP >15cm H_2O or FiO_2 >0.6.
- Haemodynamic instability
- Raised ICP
- Patient unlikely to survive >48h

Provision of information and consent/assent

Few patients within intensive care have the capacity to give informed consent, but attempts should be made to seek their understanding and approval where this is possible. The role of the next of kin in healthcare decision making is being formalized under the new Mental Capacity Act (England and Wales) and the Adults with Incapacity Act (Scotland). Current directives from the GMC and Department of Health specify their involvement using Consent Form 4; *'Form for Adults who are Unable to Consent to Investigation or Treatment'*. This process requires provision of information on the nature of the procedure, proposed benefits, potential hazards and alternatives.

Monitoring

Routine monitoring of ECG and oxygen saturation, and invasive blood pressure monitoring should be in place given the potential for abrupt changes in blood pressure with either administration of anaesthetic agents or the stimulation of the procedure. An arterial line is also indicated for arterila blood gas analysis, since capnography may be unreliable in the presence of inadequate ventilation due to obstruction of the ETT by the bronchoscope or loss of tidal volume by the inevitable leak as the stoma is created.

Capnography should be considered mandatory given the potential for accidental extubation, and subsequent need for re-intubation, assessment of the adequacy of ventilation with obstruction of the airway by a bronchoscope or as a leak develops, as well as for confirmation of correct needle and subsequent tracheostomy placement.

Ultrasound

Ultrasound scanning of the neck prior to percutaneous tracheostomy allows visualization of anterior neck structures, particularly the assessment of blood vessels, of and depth, level of rings and angulation of the trachea. Useful information about adjacent structures helps with the risk-benefit analysis of an open vs percutaneous tracheostomy. Imaging can guide needles and dilators away from at-risk structures.

Endoscopy

A flexible fibreoptic scope passed through the tracheal tube may be used to guide correct placement of the introducer needle, guide wire and tracheostomy tube. Direct visualization should reduce tracheal wall damage and tube misplacement. The presence of a scope may hinder ventilation, increasing the risk of hypoxia and hypercarbia with associated increase in ICP in susceptible patients. It should be appreciated that bleeding, distortion of structures and obstruction of the visual field with larger dilators may prevent endoscopic visualization of damage until after it has occurred. Also the section of trachea adjacent to the tracheostomy tube cannot be easily visualized after tube insertion. Alternative approaches include the use of a semi-rigid, small-diameter scope, such as a Bonfil's laryngoscope or optical stylets, which interferes less with ventilation and avoids potential expensive damage to a flexible bronchoscope by needle puncture.

Post-procedure CXR?

The usefulness of a CXR is debatable. It should be appreciated that tracheal placement cannot be inferred from a plain X-ray. A tube that is partially kinked or too short may be identified from plain film.

Aftercare of the patient with a tracheostomy

Aftercare

Meticulous skin care at the stoma site has been suggested to decrease bacterial contamination and the inflammatory response leading to granulation tissue. Adequate humidification, tracheal suctioning and physiotherapy are essential to avoid obstruction of tracheostomy tubes. The obstruction of tracheostomy tubes can be static, due to thick tenacious secretion, or dynamic, due to partial obstruction by the membranous posterior wall encroaching on the tracheostomy tube lumen. The degree of dynamic obstruction appears to increase when the intrathoracic pressure increases. Dynamic obstruction can be prevented by a properly designed tube with optimum length and angle to ensure correct tracheostomy tube positioning within the trachea.

Tracheostomy tubes with an inner cannula require them to be regularly removed for cleaning, to maintain tube patency. Tubes without inner cannulae should be exchanged every 7–14 days, or more frequently if secretions build up. A tracheostomy tube blocked with tenacious secretions renders the patient at risk of progressive hypoxia and possibly cardiorespiratory arrest. Resuscitation attempts will be unsuccessful unless the airway obstruction is recognized and treated promptly. Removal of the tracheostomy tube may be required if suctioning fails to clear the obstruction. In the short term, spontaneously breathing patients will usually manage to breathe through their own upper airway or the stoma. If the tracheostomy is >1 week old, the stoma is generally well established to allow early tube replacement if required.

For patients dependent on assisted ventilation, re-intubation by the oral route may be needed in the interim if difficulties occur in replacing the tracheostomy tube.

When caring for a tracheostomy patient, the following equipment should always remain with the patient:

- Tracheostomy tubes (same size as *in situ* and one size smaller)
- Tracheal dilators
- Suction unit, catheters and gloves
- Self-inflating bag-valve mask device and tubing
- A 10ml syringe for cuff inflation and deflation
- Translaryngeal intubation equipment
- Portable oxygen

Choice of tracheostomy tube

There is a wide range of tubes commercially available:

- Rigid and flexible
- Plain and cuffed (profile vs non-profile cuff)
- Fixed length vs longer length adjustable flange
- Inner liner for ease of cleaning
- Fenestrations for communication
- PVC/silver/silastic materials
- Flexible, metallic reinforced tubes for distorted airway anatomy
- Contoured tip for ease of percutaneous insertion
- Thin walled to reduce external diameter

Soft and flexible tubes provide maximum patient comfort, minimizing any trauma to the trachea and associated structures. Rigid tubes are used more commonly in the longer term as they are thought to keep the stoma open and are easier to change.

Cuffed tubes provide airway protection and facilitate IPPV. Disadvantages are risk of excessive cuff pressure, and difficulty in swallowing and communication. High-volume low-pressure cuffs reduce the incidence of cuff-related mucosal damage by providing a wider surface area of the trachea for the pressure to be dissipated. The cuff pressure should not exceed 25cm H_2O (18mm Hg) to reduce the risk of impaired mucosal perfusion, tissue necrosis and tracheal stenosis.

Adjustable longer length flange tubes are designed for patients whose trachea is deeper than usual below the skin and soft tissues in the neck, e.g. obese patients. The depth of the stoma should be considered at the outset, during the insertion procedure and by visualizing the tube position within the trachea at endoscopy via the glottis and through the tube.

Tracheostomy tubes with an inner tube may remain in place up to 30 days or more as the inner cannula can be cleaned and changed regularly.

A fenestrated tube allows airflow through the vocal cords when the tube is occluded or a speaking valve is attached. A disadvantage is that the diameter of the inner lumen will be reduced by 1–2mm, increasing work of breathing and potential for aspiration of gastric contents. It is unsuitable for patients dependent on positive pressure ventilation unless a non-fenestrated inner cannula is used. There have been problems with surgical emphysema when the fenestrations lie within the stoma and air under positive pressure tracks up between the inner liner and the tube itself.

Changing tracheostomy tubes

Basic principles for changing a tracheostomy tube

- Tracheostomy tubes without an inner cannula should be changed every 7–14 days, the frequency then decreasing once the patient is free of pulmonary secretions and has a well-formed clean stoma.
- A European Economic Community Directive (1993) states that tracheostomy tubes with an inner cannula can remain in place for a maximum of 30 days.
- The first routine tracheostomy tube change:
  - Should not be performed within 72h following a surgical tracheostomy and not before 3–5 (and ideally 7–10) days after a percutaneous tracheostomy to allow the stoma to become established.
  - The decision to change the tube must be made by a medical practitioner competent in the care of tracheostomies.
  - Must be carried out by a medical practitioner with appropriate, advanced airway skills.
- Subsequent changes can be made by experienced personnel trained in tracheostomy tube changes (e.g. specialist tracheostomy nurse).

In practice, the frequency with which the tube needs to be changed will be affected by the individual patient's condition and the type of tube used. Elective changes are inherently safer than those done in a crisis.

Initiation of oral intake

- Confirm that patient can tolerate cuff deflation
- Sit patient up with head slightly flexed and deflate cuff
- Start with sips of water, moving on to thickened fluids and then a soft diet providing patient shows no signs of respiratory distress (coughing, de-saturation, increased tracheal secretions, etc.)

In problematic cases, consider referral to speech and language therapy.

Risk factors for swallowing problems in patients with a tracheostomy

- Neurological injury, e.g. bulbar palsy
- Head and neck surgery
- Evidence of aspiration of enteral feed or oral secretions on tracheal suctioning
- Increased secretion load, or persistent wet/weak voice, when cuff is deflated
- Coughing and/or desaturation following oral intake
- Patient anxiety or distress during oral intake

De-cannulation

De-cannulation should be considered when patients demonstrate a satisfactory respiratory drive, a good cough and the ability to protect their own airway. Patients who show no signs of tiring on cCPAP or a T-piece with low flow oxygen therapy are potential candidates for de-cannulation. Coughing secretions up into the tracheostomy tube is a good sign, whereas generalized weakness and inability to hold the head up are negative predictors of successful de-cannulation. An impaired conscious level also reduces the chance of success. There is a common tendency to leave tubes in too long whilst clinicians await the perfect time to de-cannulate, and time-consuming referrals to speech or physiotherapy are made. If left too long, it can stimulate mucus production and affects the mucociliary system. It should be appreciated that an effective cough relies on build up of positive pressure within the trachea against a closed glottis and then sudden release to generate a cough. This cannot be achieved with a large bore cannula open within the trachea. So you may be doing your patient a disservice by leaving the tube *in situ* for too long.

Following de-cannulation, most tracheostomy stomas are allowed to granulate without suturing. They achieve a functional seal within 2–3 days. These partially healed wounds can be quickly re-opened with artery forceps in the first few weeks after closure if necessary. Occasional patients will require ENT referral for tethered scars or a sinus. At longer term follow-up, clinicians should be aware of the rare significant tracheal or laryngeal stenosis giving rise to respiratory symptoms of stridor, persistent cough and voice changes. Such cases require specialist ENT or thoracic referral.

Further reading

Paw H, Bodenham A. Percutaneous tracheostomy. *Greenwich Medical*, 2004.

Standards for care of adult patients with temporary tracheostomies. *Intensive Care Society* 2007. www.ics.ac.uk.

Chest drain insertion

Indications

- Treatment of a pneumothorax in a patient requiring positive pressure ventilation
- Treatment of a large pneumo/hydro/haemo thorax
- Following needle decompression of a tension pneumothorax
- Management of broncho-pleural fistula
- Management of empyema
- Management of localized pneumothorax causing ventilatory compromise (this usually requires CT guidance)

Equipment preparation

Depending upon the size, site and anticipated nature of the pleural collection, select an appropriate drain. Smaller drains are preferable for most indications. The exceptions requiring larger drains with multiple (>3) holes are:

- Bronchopleural fistulas with a large gas leak
- Haemothoraces with ongoing bleeding
- Viscous/highly purulent empyemas

This procedure should always be performed with strict adherence to aseptic precautions.

Suggested items:

- 2% chlorhexidine-based skin cleaning fluid and reservoir.
- Sterile gauze
- Local anaesthetic, syringe and needle. Consider adjunctive systemic analgesia and sedation.
- For Seldinger technique:
  - Bedside ultrasound
  - Needle and syringe
  - J-wire
  - Scalpel
  - Dilator
  - Drain with stiffener
  - 3-way tap
- For blunt dissection/thoracostomy technique
  - Scalpel
  - Blunt dissection forceps (e.g. curved Robert's)
  - Drain
- Collection bag/underwater seal drainage bottle/Heimlich valve
- Suture
- Appropriate dressing

Patient preparation

Whenever practical, inform the patient regarding the proposed procedure and gain their consent.

Position the patient such that they are comfortable and the area in which the procedure is to be performed is easily accessible and, for fluid collections, is gravitationally dependent. This may be difficult in sedated and intubated patients on positive pressure ventilation. Sitting the patient in as near an upright posture as possible with unhindered access to the posterior and/or lateral chest walls is ideal. Ensure that whatever the position, the operator is in an ergonomic position with access to the equipment.

Procedure

Seldinger technique

Though not obligatory, it is undoubtedly best practice to perform a thoracic ultrasound immediately prior to aspiration to define the anatomy and avoid visceral injury. When aspirating small or complex collections, continuous ultrasound guidance is essential.

Clean the area and apply sterile towels.

Infiltrate a small volume of local anaesthetic into the subcutaneous and intradermal spaces, avoiding the neurovascular bundle which runs along the inferior border of the rib.

Insert the needle, whilst aspirating using a syringe, until air/fluid is freely withdrawn. Having entered the pleural space, disconnect the syringe and gently insert the J-wire through the needle. Be aware, that the J-wire, despite its soft tip, can puncture and damage visceral organs, in particular consolidated lung. Withdraw the needle, leaving the wire **in situ**. Make a small stabbing incision through the skin at the exit site of the wire. This is most easily performed by placing the flat surface of a no. 11 blade on the wire and sliding it into the skin. Insert the dilator into the pleural cavity over the wire; be cautious not to insert this too far and angle the tract formed towards the desired location (apical for simple pneumothorax; posterior-basal for fluid). Leave the dilator in place for a few moments, then remove, again leaving the wire *in situ*. Depending upon the drain design (straight, curved or pigtail), ensure it is mounted on its stiffener (if required) and gently insert, over the wire, directing the tip as required. Withdraw the wire and stiffener then connect to a closed 3-way tap. Aspirate via the tap to ensure adequate placement and anchor with a holding suture. Connect to the appropriate drainage device, having first obtained any desired specimens (see Chapter 1.18). Pad and stick to the skin using a small dressing, ensuring that the drain will not kink and that the 3-way tap is accessible and will not cause a pressure injury. One possible technique is to stick the drain in line with the ribs directed anteriorly.

Blunt dissection/thoracostomy technique

Clean the area and apply sterile towels.

The site of drain insertion should usually be in the so-called 'safe triangle'. This is made up of the anterior border of latissimus dorsi, the lateral border of pectoralis major, a line superior to the horizontal level of the nipple, and an apex below the axilla.

Infiltrate a small volume of local anaesthetic into the subcutaneous and intradermal spaces, avoiding the neurovascular bundle which runs along the inferior border of the rib. As an alternative, consider performing an intercostal nerve block in the relevant space and the spaces above and below. Perform a diagnostic aspiration to ensure air/fluid can be drained from the intended insertion site.

Make a 2–3cm incision along the upper edge of the rib that makes the inferior border of the relevant rib space. Using forceps, bluntly dissect into the pleural cavity. Insert a finger into the pleural cavity and perform a sweep. This acts as a diagnostic examination, enhances the blunt dissection and can potentially break down loculations, if present. Take hold of the drain tip with the forceps by placing them in through the distal side hole and out through the end hole. Prior to drain insertion consider disconnecting the patient from any positive pressure ventilation to reduce the chance of intrapulmonary lung placement. Gently insert the drain with the forceps and release. Try to position the drain apically for a pneumothorax and posterior-basally for fluid. Be cautious of intrapulmonary and mediastinal drain placement. To ensure adequate position and to obtain any desired specimens, aspirate using a bladder-tipped syringe and/or connect to an underwater sealed drainage bottle. Suture one end of the incision and place an anchoring suture around the drain. Avoid purse string sutures and use monofilament suture material. Pad and stick to the skin using a small dressing, ensuring that the drain will not kink. One possible technique is to stick the drain in line with the ribs directed anteriorly.

Management

Following insertion, obtain a CXR to assess the position. If functionally inadequate, regardless of radiological position, manipulate the drain accordingly or remove and, if necessary, re-insert. In difficult circumstances, seek radiological advice and consider CT guidance or thoracic surgical assistance.

Draining fluid off at too high a rate can result in re-expansion pulmonary oedema. This is rare, especially in patients receiving positive pressure ventilation. The risk can be minimized by limiting drainage to a maximum of 1500ml/h by clamping the drain. In all other instances, clamping of the drain, except transiently, should be avoided. Clamping has no place in the management of pneumothoraces.

For small drains, consider flushing 6–12 hourly with 5–10ml of 0.9% saline to assess and maintain patency.

If connected to an underwater seal drainage bottle, the meniscus in the tube should transduce intrapleural pressure and swing with respiratory phase. If it does not, the drain is blocked, kinked or has become mislocated. Examine, flush and re-image as necessary.

Removal

Remove the drain as soon as it is no longer required or has failed. Close the drain site with a suture if required. If there continues to be a leak through the drain site, place a stoma bag over it. If this fails to contain the situation, then either insert a new drain or seek surgical advice.

Complications

- Bleeding from an intercostal vessel or a damaged viscous/organ. This is rare, but can be fatal.
- Trauma to lung (including formation of bronchopleural fistula), heart, liver, spleen or kidney. Again serious trauma is rare, but can be fatal.
- Infection: from superficial drain site infection to empyema and lung abcess.

Further reading

Bouhemad B, Zhang M, Lu Q, *et al.* Clinical review: bedside lung ultrasound in critical care practice. *Crit Care* 2007; 11: 205.

Laws D, Neville E, Duffy J, *et al.* BTS guidelines for the insertion of a chest drain. *Thorax* 2003; B Suppl 2: ii53–9.

Pleural aspiration

Pleural aspiration or thoracocentesis is the removal of air or fluid from the pleural space (see also Chapter 1.17).

Indications

- Diagnosis of the nature of a pleural effusion
- Treatment of a simple pneumothorax
- Treatment of pleural effusion of sufficient size to impair or compromise respiratory mechanics
- Treatment of an empyema

Equipment preparation

Depending upon the size, site and anticipated nature of the pleural collection, select an appropriately sized needle or cannula.

This procedure should always be performed with strict adherence to aseptic precautions.

Suggested items:

- Bedside ultrasound
- 2% chlorhexidine-based skin cleaning fluid and reservoir.
- Sterile gauze
- Local anaesthetic, syringe and needle.
- Chosen needle/cannula, t3-way tap on a short extension, an appropriately sized syringe for sampling/aspiration (20–60ml).
- Sterile sample pots, blood gas syringe, glucose testing strip or blood glucose (fluoride) sample bottle, blood culture bottles (aerobic and anaerobic), blood chemistry/enzyme assay sample bottle
- Small dressing

Patient preparation

Whenever practical, inform the patient regarding the proposed procedure and gain their consent.

Position the patient such that they are comfortable and the area in which the procedure is to be performed is easily accessible and, for fluid collections, is gravitationally dependent. This may be difficult in sedated and intubated patients on positive pressure ventilation. Sitting the patient in as near an upright posture as possible with unhindered access to the posterior and/or lateral chest walls is ideal. Ensure that whatever the position, the operator is in an ergonomic position with access to the equipment.

Procedure

Though not obligatory, it is undoubtedly best practice to perform a thoracic ultrasound immediately prior to aspiration to define the anatomy and avoid visceral injury. When aspirating small or complex collections, continuous ultrasound guidance is essential. For further information on thoracic ultrasound, see Bouhemad *et al.* (2007). A classic image of a significant pleural effusion is shown in Fig. 1.18.1.

Clean the area and apply sterile towels.

Infiltrate a small volume of local anaesthetic into the subcutaneous and intradermal spaces, avoiding the neurovascular bundle which runs along the inferior border of the rib.

Insert the needle/cannula, whilst aspirating using a syringe, until air/fluid is freely withdrawn. Having entered the pleural space, if there is a significant volume of air/fluid to be aspirated, attach a 3-way tap on a short extension to facilitate syringe change over.

If no fluid/air is aspirated, remove the needle/cannula and re-image with ultrasound. If necessary, reposition the patient.

For a simple pneumothorax, aspirate as much air as possible, making note of the volume. If, having drained 1000ml, air is still freely aspiratable, consider inserting a pleural drain. If in doubt, re-image with X-ray or ultrasound.

For a pleural effusion, aspirate sufficient fluid for all diagnostic tests. Continue to aspirate further fluid if there is a significant residual volume. Measure the total volume removed and be conscious of the possibility of re-expansion pulmonary oedema.

Once completed, remove the needle/cannula and cover the puncture site with a simple dressing if required. If fluid starts to leak through the puncture site, cover with a small stoma bag or consider inserting a drain.

Specimens

For microbiology, send raw fluid for microscopy, culture and sensitivities. If suspicious, also request staining and culture for mycobacteria. To increase the sensitivity of bacterial culture, inoculate a set of blood culture bottles with 10ml of fluid per bottle.

Unless the fluid is frankly purulent, take a specimen in a blood gas syringe and put it through a blood gas analyser to measure the pH. A pH <7.20 is consistent with an empyema and probably the most sensitive test. The two other assays consistent with this diagnosis is a fluid glucose of <3.35mmol/l and/or a lactate dehydrogenase level >3 times the upper limit of normal for serum.

Determination of the fluid total protein to establish whether the effusion is a transudate or exudate is not of any great value and is unreliable in diagnosing empyema.

Complications and their management

The most common complication of pleural aspiration is a small pneumothorax. This requires no action other than vigilance for increasing size, which is rare unless the lung has been punctured. If this has occurred, it is usually obvious, as air is unexpectedly aspirated during the procedure. The risk of an enlarging.significant pneumothorax is increased if the patient is on positive pressure ventilation. Under these circumstances, watch for an evolving tension pneumothorax and be prepared for immediate decompression and chest drain insertion.

The second most common complication is damage to the intercostal neurovascul;ar bundle. To avoid this, use the superior border of the rib as the landmark for the puncture site and maintain an insertion angle that minimizes the risk of damage to the bundle associated with the rib above. Be aware that damage to the intercostal artery can result in a significant haemothorax and require surgical ligation.

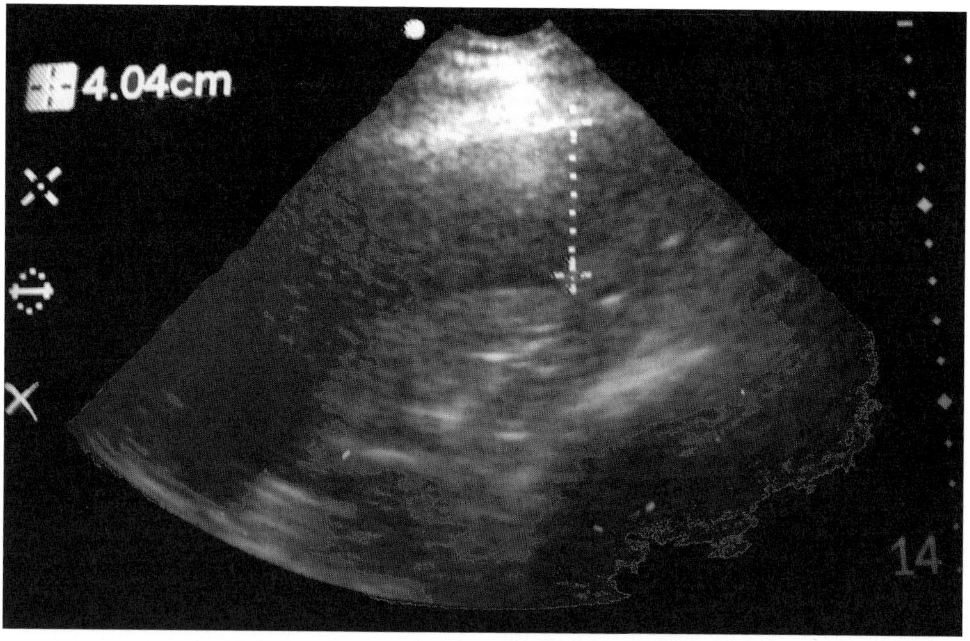

Fig 1.18.1 Ultrasound still image demonstrating a 4.04cm rim of pleural fluid between the chest wall (apex of image) and underlying consolidated lung. The value of ultrasound assessment and, where necessary, ultrasound guidance in pleural aspiration cannot be overstated.

Puncture of and/or damage to adjacent structures is easily avoided by ultrasound guidance. There are case reports of serious complications from pleural aspiration procedures in which the liver, spleen, kidneys, diaphragm and myocardium have been injured. Such iatrogenic injuries are rare with this procedure but have a significantly higher incidence associated with pleural drain insertion.

Further reading

Bouhemad B, Zhang M, Lu Q, *et al.* Clinical review: bedside lung ultrasound in critical care practice. *Crit Care* 2007; 11: 205.

Light RW. Parapneumonic effusions and empyema. *Proc Am Thorac Soc* 2006; 3: 75–80.

Flexible bronchoscopy

Flexible bronchoscopy is an essential diagnostic and therapeutic procedure in the ICU. The majority of procedures are performed in intubated patients receiving mechanical ventilation.

ICU indications

- Direct visualization of the upper airway in difficult endotracheal intubation.
- Direct endotracheal visualization and guidance during percutaneous tracheostomy.
- Inspection of the distal portion of an endotracheal or tracheostomy tube to assess patency and position.
- Inspection of the distal trachea and proximal bronchial tree for mucosal pathology/extrinsic compression.
- Removal of material obstructing one or more major bronchi.
- Performing sampling of distal airways for microbiological and/or cytological specimens.
- Guiding the placement of an endobronchial blocking/isolation catheter.

Equipment preparation and aftercare

Prior to use, the bronchoscope should be thoroughly cleaned and disinfected. Cross-infection between patients is a serious hazard. If stored, this should be in a dedicated clean environment. The scope should be handled aseptically and transported in an appropriate enclosed container. All the remaining equipment should be clean or sterile single use. Essential equipment:

- Light source
- Camera/videoscope stack (optional)
- Cleaning brush for working channel
- A packet of sterile gauze
- A sterile 1 litre jug.
- A 500ml bag of 0.9% sodium chloride
- A 20ml syringe
- Sputum traps
- Dedicated suction
- A bronchoscopy catheter mount

The scope should be checked for clear vision and a functioning suction system immediately prior to use. The outside of the scope should be wiped with saline-soaked gauze. Avoid water-based gel lubricants as these can dry out and become sticky rather that lubricate. In situations where there is problematic sticking of the scope to the inside of an endotracheal or tracheostomy tube, use sterile liquid paraffin.

The bronchoscopist and any assistants should wear full protective clothing including gowns, gloves and face/eye cover. Appropriate and sensible precautions should be made regarding the potential aerosolization of infected material.

At the end of the procedure, the suction channel of the scope should be immediately brushed through and then rinsed. The outside of the scope should be cleaned. The scope should then be sent for full decontamination. Any other reusable equipment should be cleaned and stored appropriately.

Patient preparation

Whenever practical, inform the patient regarding the proposed procedure and gain their consent. Depending upon the indication, likely duration and clinical condition of the patient, an appropriate plan regarding topical anaesthesia, sedation and neuromuscular blockade should be made. At a minimum, continuous ECG and SpO_2 monitoring together with intermittent, automated non-invasive blood pressure should be used. The FiO_2 should be increased to 100% (or as high as possible). If ventilated, a pressure control mode is preferable although a strictly pressure-limited volume control mode can be used. Hypoventilation is an inevitable occurrence during the procedure. In patients in whom even transient hypercapnia needs to be avoided, a series of timed, short bronchoscopies can usually be safely performed. In such circumstances, continuous end-tidal capnography is essential. Alternatively, consider using HFV.

Procedure

Before starting, ensure all necessary equipment is available and working, the patient is comfortable and the bronchoscopist is ergonomically positioned. Consider slowly injecting 3–5ml of sterile saline into the endotracheal/tracheostomy tube to lubricate the passage of the scope. At least one assistant must be present to watch the patient, the ventilator and the monitoring, in addition to being able to assist the bronchoscopist.

First navigate the endotracheal/tracheostomy tube and ascertain whether the tube is encrusted with secretions. If so, this may both inhibit the procedure and present the patient with unwanted additional resistance. It may be possible to clean the tube effectively using the scope; however, electively changing the tube is usually preferable.

Next, consider whether the tube opens centrally within the trachea and is a sufficient distance from the main carina. If this is not so, reposition the tube under bronchoscopic guidance and make note of the optimal position using the visible reference markers on the tube. Always consider whether moving the patient will adversely affect the position of the distal end of the tube, and leave a detailed description in the patient's notes.

Then go on to examine the distal trachea, in particular, looking for mucosal trauma caused by the distal tip of the tube and blind suction catheter insertion. Continue by inspecting the remainder of the accessible bronchial tree in a logical order. It should be possible to visualize the first 2–5 divisions of each lobar bronchus.

For visible secretions, try to sample/remove without causing trauma to the mucosa and without using saline lavage. If required, collect a specimen for microbiological examination. Difficult to clear secretions can often be removed piecemeal. Large pieces can often be held against the tip of the scope by application of continuous suction. The scope, together with the offending mass, can then be removed *en masse*, by slowly withdrawing the scope whilst maintaining suction. Obstructing aggregations of inspissated secretions, blood clots or mucosal sloughing may require prolonged or multiple procedures. The use of biopsy forceps and cytology brushes may be useful but require skill and patience. Should flexible bronchoscopy fail, consider using a rigid scope. Nebulized 0.9% saline, 3% saline, *N*-acetyl cysteine (10–20%), unfractionated heparin (10 000–25 000IU 4–12 hourly), 4.2% sodium bicarbonate and dornase alfa have all been described as useful adjuncts, but none has been proven to have superior efficacy over the others in ventilated patients. There is also no evidence to suggest a superior efficacy for direct instillation vs nebulization.

For visible mucosal bleeding, haemostasis will usually occur spontaneously. Haemostasis can be augmented by topical vasoconstriction using adrenaline (epinephrine). Gently instil/irrigate with a 1 in 10 000 (0.1mg/ml) solution. Topical antifibrinolytics, such as neat tranexamic acid (100mg/ml) can also be useful.

If the bleeding is distal to the main carina and unstoppable and/or distal to the limit of visualization, temporary isolation and tamponade can be achieved by wedging the tip of the bronchoscope into the origin of the identified bronchus. The efficacy of instilling vasoconstrictors and/or antifibrinolytics is uncertain. The value of prolonged continuous suction is also debatable. If this fails to achieve haemostasis, then a balloon-tipped bronchial isolation catheter can be inserted parallel to the bronchoscope, which can then be used to guide catheter placement. This can be a difficult procedure due to the aerosolization of blood within the airway masking any vision. Be careful not to dislodge the blocking catheter when withdrawing the scope. Consider paralysing the patient and applying a high level of PEEP. If practical, turn the patient bleeding side down. As a further adjunct, connect and instil oxygen through the bronchoscope suction channel at a high flow rate. Definitive treatment for persistent haemorrhage is either selective bronchial angiography and embolisation or surgery.

Specimens

Whenever possible, send undiluted secretions for microbiological investigation. To obtain a specimen from a region of interest beyond visualization, first locate the nearest lobar, segmental or subsegmental division, then gently wedge the tip of the bronchoscope into it. Before any sampling, ensure that the suction channel is clear of any proximal secretions, which might contaminate the specimen. This may require the scope to be fully withdrawn, the channel cleaned with a brush and rinsed with clean saline, and the scope reinserted and positioned. Next, apply the specimen trap as close to the bronchoscope as possible. Slowly instil 20–60ml of 0.9% sterile saline, wait for a few seconds, then apply continuous suction. If the airway completely collapses, ask an assistant gently to turn the strength of the suction down until some fluid is drawn into the specimen trap. When no further fluid flows, slowly withdraw the scope whilst maintaining continuous suction. Make a note of the volume instilled and the volume of the specimen. Examine the specimen for adequacy, looking for the presence of mucoid or infected airway secretions. It is worth discussing the optimal handling of specimens with the labs receiving them, in particular if qualitative or semi-quantative microscopy are required or specific pathogens are suspected. If a good quality, large volume specimen is obtained, this can often be divided in the laboratory for both microbiological and cytological examination if required. This prevents repeated saline lavage and scope trauma, both of which are injurious

Blind brush specimens may be useful in both cytological and microbiological testing. Brush and biopsy specimens of visible lesions can also be taken. In patients receiving positive pressure ventilation, transbronchial biopsy and transbronchial needle aspiration specimens carry a significant risk of pneumothorax and pneumomediastinum and are best avoided.

Protected lavage and brush catheters are available, but are of questionable value. There is conflicting evidence regarding the value of bronchoscopic specimens over and above those obtained by blind endotracheal suctioning, most especially in the diagnosis of ventilator-associated pneumonia.

Complications

The following complications can occur and should be prepared for:

- Displacement of the endotracheal/tracheostomy tube out of the trachea.
- Obstruction of the endotracheal/tracheostomy tube.
- Obstruction of the trachea or major bronchus
- Hypoxia/derecruitment/increasing ventilatory requirements post-procedure
- Hypercapnia/underventilation
- Coughing
- Bronchospasm
- Haemorrhage
- Pneumothorax
- Pneumomediastinum
- Sepsis secondary to translocation (bacteraemia) (see Yigla *et al.*, 1999)
- Hypo- or hypertension/cardiac arrhythmias

Further reading

BTS. British Thoracic Society guidelines on diagnostic flexible bronchoscopy. *Thorax* 2001; 56 Suppl 1: i1–21.

Ernst A, Silvestri GA, Johnstone D, *et al.* Interventional pulmonary procedures: guidelines from the American College of Chest Physicians. *Chest* 2003; 123: 1693–717.

Mehta AC, Prakash UB, Garland R, *et al.* American College of Chest Physicians and American Association for Bronchology [corrected] consensus statement: prevention of flexible bronchoscopy-associated infection. *Chest* 2005; 128: 1742–55.

Yigla M, Oren I, Bentur L, *et al.* Incidence of bacteraemia following fibreoptic bronchoscopy. *Eur Respir J* 1999; 14: 789–91.

Chest physiotherapy

Critical illness is associated with high morbidity and mortality rates, and the associated care is a major determinant of healthcare costs. Critically ill patients cared for on the ICU can have prolonged periods of immobility, with critical illness lasting from hours to months, depending on the underlying pathophysiology and the patient's response to treatment.

Respiratory dysfunction is one of the most common causes of critical illness necessitating ICU admission. The aims of chest physiotherapy (CPT) are to clear secretions, to prevent pulmonary complications, to improve ventilation and/or regional ventilation and lung compliance, and to reduce airway resistance and the work of breathing.

CPT in mechanically ventilated patients

Such patients are especially at risk of complications. They are generally sedated, with an artificial airway and sometimes inadequate humidification. These three components alter mucociliary clearance.

Increase of expiratory flow

CPT manoeuvres involve inspiratory and expiratory techniques, with and without the aid of positive pressure devices. The physiotherapist applies external forces during expiration, inducing an increase in expiratory flow and therefore an increase in mucus transport. These techniques of increased expiratory flow can be used passively in ventilated, sedated patients or actively in more alert, cooperative patients. Patients are often placed in the lateral decubitus position for these manoeuvres. To evacuate the sputum, physiotherapists perform tracheal suctioning. Some may also add manual hyperinflations, manual vibrations, etc.

Manual hyperinflation (MHI) or ventilator hyperinflation (VHI)

The aims of hyperinflation are to prevent pulmonary atelectasis, re-expand collapsed alveoli, improve oxygenation, improve lung compliance and facilitate movement of pulmonary secretions towards the central airways. MHI is performed by delivering a large tidal volume combined with an expiratory plateau and a fast release of the resuscitator bag. The quick release of the bag enhances expiratory flow and mimics a forced expiration. MHI can result in marked haemodynamic changes associated with a decreased cardiac output, which result from large fluctuations in intrathoracic pressure. A pressure of 40cm H_2O has been recommended as an upper limit. MHI can also ICP and mean arterial pressure (MAP) which has implications for patients with brain injury. These increases are usually limited, however, so that the cerebral perfusion pressure commonly remains stable.

Prevention of pulmonary complications in mechanically ventilated patients

In mechanically ventilated patients there is a decrease in VAP in patients treated with physiotherapy and standard nursing care in comparison with those managed with standard nursing care alone.

CPT in patients without endotracheal intubation

Breathing exercises

Inspiratory breathing exercises coupled with mobilization and body positioning are used to increase lung volumes and improve ventilation for patients with reduced inspiratory volumes, e.g. following surgery. Expiratory breathing techniques (forced expirations, huffing and coughing) are used to increase expiratory flow rates and, thereby, enhance airway clearance and mobilize secretions from the peripheral to upper airways. Thus, expiratory breathing exercises may need to be accompanied by interventions that increase inspiratory volume, if reduced inspiratory volumes are contributing to an ineffective cough. To evacuate the sputum, physiotherapists help the patient with cough techniques or perform tracheal suctioning. Forced expiratory manoeuvres should be used with caution in patients with bronchospasm, to avoid exacerbation of spasm, or cardiac dysfunction.

Instrumental techniques

Manually assisted cough, using thoracic or abdominal compression, may be indicated for patients with expiratory muscle weakness or fatigue (e.g. neuromuscular conditions)

An inspiratory/expiratory insufflator is a device that delivers inspiratory pressure followed by a high negative expiratory force, via a mouthpiece or face mask. It is indicated when a patient is unable to clear secretions using other interventions. It has been applied with success in the management of patients with retained secretions secondary to respiratory muscle weakness (e.g. muscular dystrophy).

Incentive spirometry (IS) can be used to encourage improved lung volumes and flow rates. IS is believed to improve the distribution of ventilation by increasing lung volumes and encouraging prolonged slow inspiration. IS may be prescribed for patients after major surgery to either prevent or treat post-operative pulmonary complications; however, it has not been shown to be of added benefit (beyond body position and early mobilization) in the management of routine post-operative patients.

An intrapulmonary percussive ventilator (IPV) is a mode of ventilation that can be used in the management of intubated or non-intubated patients using a mouthpiece. IPV is believed to increase mucociliary clearance. A recent review has shown that this technique has no effect on sputum weight, mucociliary transport or pulmonary function. Adverse effects include bronchospasm, haemoptysis, hypoxaemia and bradycardia, thus appropriate monitoring is indicated.

Positive expiratory pressure (PEP) refers to a device to augment oxygenation and airway clearance in non-intubated patients and can be applied with a face mask or mouthpiece. PEP is used mostly for medical patients with excessive airway secretions (e.g. cystic fibrosis). PEP in critical care could assist in secretion removal in COPD patients requiring NIPPV.

Flutter® valve device. The Flutter® valve is contained within a pipe-shaped device with an opening at the mouthpiece and small outlets at the top of the bowl. As the patient exhales, a steel ball is displaced, generating PEP and oscillating waves of pressure within the airways (high-frequency oscillations). The Flutter® device is indicated in spontaneously breathing patients who have excessive airway secretions (e.g. cystic fibrosis). The role of the Flutter® device in critically ill patients has not been studied, but may be limited by the patient's capacity to cooperate.

Respiratory muscle training

Comparably with other skeletal muscles, respiratory muscles can be trained to enhance contraction performance (force, endurance, velocity of shortening and metabolic efficiency). Because ventilatory failure can be related to respiratory muscle dysfunction, improving the function of the respiratory muscles is a rational treatment goal. Recent uncontrolled trials of inspiratory muscle training in critically ill patients suggest that it improves inspiratory muscle function and, hence, may contribute to successful weaning.

Positioning

Patient positioning can be used to increase gravitational stress and associated fluid shifts, through head tilt and other positions that approximate the upright position. The upright position increases lung volumes and gas exchange, stimulates autonomic activity and can reduce cardiac stress from compression.

The semi-recumbent, prone and lateral position are used, respectively, to decrease the risk of nosocomial pneumonia, and to improve gas exchange in ARDS and in unilateral lung disease. It has been suggested that good positioning combined with CPT in the treatment of acute lobar atelectasis is as effective as fibreoptic bronchoscopy.

Mobilization

Although part of physiotherapy, mobilization cannot be included as part of CPT, but it can influence ventilation and can play a role in pulmonary complications. Mobilization has been part of the physiotherapy management of acutely ill patients for several decades and refers to physical activity sufficient to elicit acute physiological effects that enhance ventilation, central and peripheral perfusion, circulation, muscle metabolism and alertness.

Conclusions

CPT clears secretions, prevents pulmonary complications, and improves ventilation and lung compliance. Physiotherapists must choose their therapeutic interventions as a function of a preliminary clinical examination to be sure that their treatment will be therapeutic and safe. Unstable patients should be monitored continuously during physiotherapy. Finally, physiotherapists can contribute to the patient's overall well-being by providing emotional support and enhancing communication.

Further reading

Denehy L. The use of manual hyperinflation in airway clearance. *Eur Respir J* 1999; 14: 958–65.

Devroey M. Percussion intrapulmonaire: une aide pour le kinésithérapeute? In: Actualités en kinésithérapie de réanimation. Elsevier,2000; 74–7.

Gosselink R.K, Schrever P, Cops H, *et al.* Incentive spirometry does not enhance recovery after thoracic surgery. *Crit Care Med* 2000; 28: 679–83.

Martin AD, Davenport PD, Franceschi AC, *et al.* Use of inspiratory muscle strength training to facilitate ventilator weaning: a series of 10 consecutive patients. *Chest* 2002; 122: 192–6.

Stiller K. Physiotherapy in Intensive Care. Towards an evidence based practice. *Chest* 2000; 118: 1801–13.

Van der Schans CP, Postma DS, Koeter BK. Physiotherapy and bronchial mucustransport. *Eur Respir J* 1999; 13: 1477–86.

Humidification

Introduction

Water vapour is contained in the air and its amount is influenced by atmospheric conditions. While the normal temperature of the atmosphere never reaches the boiling point of water (100°C), variation in air temperature is certainly the most important parameter influencing water vapour content. Water vapour capacity is the maximum amount of water that a gas can hold at a particular temperature. Two other concepts are important concerning water vapour content: one is the absolute humidity (AH) defined as the weight of water vapour contained in a given volume of gas. The second is the relative humidity (RH), defined as the relationship between the content of water in air at a specific temperature and the capacity of water that air can hold at the same temperature

RH = (content/capacity) × 100

Humidification during spontaneous breathing and mechanical ventilation

With natural airways

The upper airways ensure that inspired gases are heated or cooled to body temperature (37°C) and humidified to an RH of ~100% at body temperature.

More specifically, when inspired gases arrive at the conchae, turbulent flow is created. The architecture of the conchae consists of three turbinates covered by a folded mucous membrane, representing a volume of only 20ml but a surface area of 160cm^2. Therefore, each gas molecule is likely to come into contact with the surface area of the vascular nasal mucous membrane. The moist mucous membrane heats inspired gases to body temperature and, producing up 650–1000ml of H_2O per day, brings inspired gases to an RH of 80% on leaving the nose to enter the nasopharynx. Mucus produced in the nasal cavity is also responsible for the humidification of inspired gases

With artificial airways

The gas arriving from the ventilator is cold (15°C) and dry (2% RH), and the ETT bypasses the physiological humidification and heating of inspired gases. Absence of humidification induces alterations in mucus transport, decreased mucus clearance, lesions of the epithelium and mucosa, and changes in ventilatory parameters (decreased compliance and functional residual capacity, increased resistance). Therefore, artificial devices must be installed during mechanical ventilation. There is a relationship between airway mucosal dysfunction and the combination of inspired gas humidity and temperature with exposure time to a given humidity

An artificial humidifier replaces the humidifying function of the upper airways by increasing the water vapour content of a dry gas.

Humidifiers

There are two types of humidifier: active and passive.

Active humidifiers add water vapour to inspired gases, whereas passive humidifiers exchange heat and moisture by preserving the moisture and heat in the gas exhaled by the patient.

Active humidifiers

Active humidifiers consist of a humidity generator (or water reservoir) and humidity delivery system (or breathing circuit). An ideal system generates the required amount of humidity, in the form of water vapour, at the correct temperature, and transports it to the patient without the loss of either heat or moisture.

The most effective way to achieve this is to use a large heated water surface for the generator, and heating elements within the delivery system to prevent condensation.

There are three types of active humidifiers:

Bubble: unheated humidifiers most generally dedicated to simple oxygen therapy. At body temperature, the RH of the inspired gas never exceeds 40%. Humidification with this device is a function of the temperature in the room, the volume of water in the humidifier and the gas flow (most efficient with flows <5l/min).

Passover and wick: these two heated humidifiers are used for patients being treated by mechanical ventilation. They are designed to bring the gas in the airways to a temperature between 34 and 37°C with an RH of 100%. Nevertheless, ventilatory settings may influence the humidity of the inspired gas.

Condensation in ventilator circuits is limited by using heated circuits.

Heat and moisture exchangers (HMEs)

This system, which is placed close to the patient at the end of the dead space, preserves the water vapour contained in the gas exhaled by the patient. During the subsequent inspiration, the water maintained in the HME is used to humidify the inspired gas.

There are two types of HME: hygroscopic and hydrophobic. The efficiency of these two types of HME is quite similar, close to 70%. Hydrophobic HMEs can filter bacteria.

Contraindications of HME

- Thick, copious or bloody secretions
- Leaks in the circuit creating an expired tidal volume <70% of the inspired tidal volume.
- Patients with a body temperature <32°C
- High minute volumes (>10l/min)

Comparison between active and passive humidifiers

Le Bourdellès *et al.* observed a significant decrease in alveolar ventilation with HMEs (as indicated by an increase in minute ventilation and respiratory rate, but an increase in $PaCO_2$) in comparison with heated humidifiers during weaning from mechanical ventilation in a pressure support mode. These observations should be taken into account during difficult weaning .

Other authors reached the same conclusions. HME sincrease work of breathing (WOB), respiratory rate and minute ventilation in pressure support in comparison with heated humidifiers. On the basis of these observations, one may recommend increasing the level of pressure support (by 5–10cm H_2O) to maintain the WOB constant. For all these reasons, HME is not recommended for patients with COPD.

In non-COPD patients receiving prolonged mechanical ventilation, Ricard *et al.* compared a group of patients where the HME was changed every 48h with a group with a change after 7 days. There was no difference in resistance in the ETT or in infection, indicating that the HME can be changed only once a week, which represents a substantial cost saving.

Nevertheless, few studies have studied the problem of the reduction in diameter of the ETT. Two different methods have been used (measurement of internal pressure and flow along the tube, and an acoustic reflection method), and both concluded that there was a progressive reduction in ETT patency with active and passive humidification, but this occurred to a greater extent with HMEs than with active humidifiers.

The effect of these systems on the incidence of VAP is controversial. Three recent reviews or meta-analyses reached different conclusions: Ricard *et al.* and Niël-Weise *et al.* concluded that the type of humidification device does not influence the incidence of VAP. If an active humidifier is used, Niël-Weise *et al.* recommended using a heated wire circuit because less condensate reduces colonization. On the other hand, Kola *et al.* reported a significant reduction in the occurrence of VAP with HMEs, particularly for patients ventilated for >7 days, but they excluded patients at high risk of airway occlusion (COPD).

Finally, in NIV, if humidification is mandatory (i.e. with an ICU ventilator using cold and dry gases), a heated humidifier is recommended over HMEs because HMEs decrease the beneficial effects of NIV on WOB.

Conclusions

Regardless of their type, humidifiers are essential for mechanically ventilated patients. For at risk patients (e.g. COPD, copious secretions, etc.), one may prefer active humidifiers with heated wire circuits.

During weaning from mechanical ventilation in pressure support mode and in NIV, HMEs are not recommended because of increases in dead space, $PaCO_2$ and WOB, unless one significantly increases the pressure support level. Passive and active devices seem to be equivalent in terms of efficacy and prevention of infection.

Further reading

Jaber S, Pigeot J, Fodil R, *et al.* Long-term effects of different humidification systems on endotracheal tube patency: evaluation by the acoustic reflection method. *Anesthesiology* 2004; 100: 782–8.

Kola A, Echmanns T, Gastmeier P. Efficacy of heat and moisture exchangers in preventing ventilator-associated pneumonia: meta-analysis of randomized controlled trials. *Intensive Care Med* 2005; 31: 5–11.

Le Bourdellès G, MierL, Fiquet B, et al. Comparison of the effects of heat and moisture exchangers and heated humidifiers on ventilation and gas exchange during weaning trials from mechanical ventilation. *Chest* 1996; 110: 1294–8.

Niël-Weise BS, Wille JC, van den Broeck PJ. Humidification policies for mechanically ventilated intensive care patients and prevention of ventilator-associated pneumonia: a systematic review of randomized controlled trials. *J Hosp Infect* 2007; 65: 285–91.

Ricard JD, Boyer A, Dreyfuss D. The effect of humidification on the incidence of ventilator-associated pneumonia. *Respir Care Clin N Am* 2006; 12: 263–73.

Ricard JD, Le Mière E, Markowicz P, *et al.* Efficiency and safety of mechanical ventilation with a heat and moisture exchanger changed only once a week. *Am J Respir Crit Care Med* 2000; 161: 104–9.

Villafane MC, Cinnella G, Lofaso F, et al. Gradual reduction of endotracheal tube diameter during mechanical ventilation via different humidification devices. *Anesthesiology* 1996; 85: 1341–9.

Heart–lung interactions

Introduction

The respiratory system and the cardiovascular systems are not separate, but tightly integrated. ARF can directly alter cardiovascular function, and vice versa. Many of these effects are predictable from knowledge of cardiovascular function. Both lung underinflation and hyperinflation increase pulmonary vascular resistance, heart–lung interactions and the work of breathing. Both spontaneous inspiratory efforts during acute bronchospasm and acute lung injury induce markedly negative swings in intrathoracic pressure (ITP). Artificial ventilatory support increases ITP during inspiration, in contradistinction to spontaneous ventilation which will decrease ITP for the same tidal breath. Heart–lung interactions involve four basic concepts: inspiration increases lung volume, spontaneous inspiration decreases ITP, positive pressure ventilation increases ITP, and ventilation is exercise, i.e. it consumes O_2 and produces CO_2.

Haemodynamic effects of changes in lung volume

Lung inflation alters autonomic tone and pulmonary vascular resistance, and, at high lung volumes, compresses the heart, limiting filling, similar to cardiac tamponade. The associated diaphragmatic dissent increases abdominal pressure, compressing the liver and altering venous return. Each of these processes may predominate in determining the final cardiovascular state. Small tidal volume (<10ml/kg) inspiration increase heart rate by vagal withdrawal, called respiratory sinus arrhythmia. Larger tidal volumes (>15ml/kg) decrease heart rate, arterial tone and cardiac contractility by sympathetic withdrawal.

The major determinants of the haemodynamic response to increases in lung volume are mechanical in nature. Lung inflation, independently of changes in ITP, primarily alters right ventricular (RV) preload and afterload and left ventricular (LV) preload. First, inspiration induces diaphragmatic dissent which increases abdominal pressure. Venous return is a function of the ratio of the pressure difference between the right atrium and the systemic venous reservoirs and the resistance to venous return. Since a large proportion of the venous blood volume is in the abdomen, abdominal pressure increases should augment venous blood flow. Diaphragmatic descent also compresses the liver, increasing hepatic outflow resistance thus decreasing venous blood flow. Thus, inspiration shifts venous flow from high resistance splanchnic circuits draining through the liver, to low resistance systemic venous circuits, making venous return greater for the same blood volume. Thus, increasing lung volume may increase or decrease venous return depending on which factors predominate. Usually, inspiration increases venous return in volume-overloaded states and decreases venous return in hypovolaemic and hepatic cirrhotic states.

End-expiratory lung volume also determines alveolar stability. Alveolar collapse increases pulmonary vasomotor tone by hypoxic pulmonary vasoconstriction. Alveolar recruitment reverses this process, although during the recruitment manoeuvres, the associated hyperinflation may impair RV function. Increasing lung volume above the FRC also increases RV outflow resistance by increasing transpulmonary pressure more than pulmonary artery pressure. Reversing hyperinflation by any means decreases pulmonary arterial pressure, improving RV ejection. The use of smaller tidal volumes and less positive end-expiratory pressure has reduced the incidence of acute cor pulmonale seen in critically ill patients. LV end-diastolic volume (preload) can be altered by ventilation by decreasing venous return, RV dilation-induced decreased LV diastolic compliance (ventricular interdependence) and by cardiac compression by the expanding lungs.

Haemodynamic effects of changes in intrathoracic pressure

The heart within the chest is a pressure chamber within a pressure chamber. Changes in ITP affect the pressure gradients for systemic venous return to the RV and systemic outflow from the LV independent of the heart itself. Increases in ITP reduce these pressure gradients decreasing intrathoracic blood volume. Decreases in ITP augment venous return and impede LV ejection, increasing intrathoracic blood volume. Variations in right atrial pressure represent the major factor determining the fluctuation in pressure gradient for systemic venous return during ventilation. Increases in ITP with positive-pressure ventilation or hyperinflation during spontaneous ventilation decrease venous return, whereas decreases in ITP during spontaneous inspiration increase venous return.

LV afterload or systolic wall tension is proportional to the product of transmural systolic LV pressure and LV volume. Thus, increasing ITP will decrease transmural LV pressure if arterial pressure is constant; increases in ITP unload the LV, whereas decreases in ITP have the opposite effect. Increases in ITP actually may increase cardiac output in congestive heart failure states. Spontaneous ventilatory efforts against a resistive (bronchospasm) or elastic (acute lung injury) load decrease LV stroke volume manifest as pulsus paradoxus by ventricular interdependence and increased LV afterload. Increases in ITP have the opposite effect, decreasing LV afterload. Although increases in ITP should augment LV ejection by decreasing LV afterload, this effect is limited because of the obligatory decrease in venous return.

There is no difference from a mechanical perspective between increasing ITP from a basal end-expiratory level

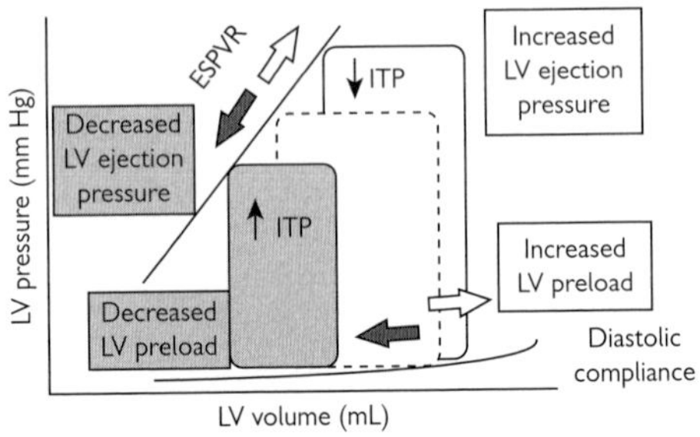

Fig 1.22.1 Normal cardiac function.

and eliminating negative end-inspiratory ITP swings seen in spontaneous ventilation. Removing negative swings in ITP may be more clinically relevant than increasing ITP for many reasons. First, many pulmonary diseases are associated with exaggerated decreases in ITP during inspiration. In restrictive lung disease states, such as interstitial fibrosis or acute hypoxaemic respiratory failure, ITP must decrease greatly to generate a large enough transpulmonary pressure to ventilate the alveoli. Similarly, in obstructive diseases, such as upper airway obstruction or asthma, large decreases in ITP occur owing to increased resistance to inspiratory airflow. Secondly, exaggerated decreases in ITP require increased respiratory efforts that increase the work of breathing, taxing a potentially stressed circulation. Finally, the exaggerated decreases in ITP can only increase venous blood flow so much before venous collapse limits blood flow. The level to which ITP must decrease to induce venous flow limitation is different in different circulatory conditions but occurs in most patients below an ITP of –10cm H_2O. Thus, further decreases in ITP will further increase only LV afterload without increasing venous return. Abolishing these markedly negative swings in ITP reduces LV afterload more than venous return (LV preload). These concepts of a differential effect of increasing and decreasing ITP on cardiac function are illustrated for both normal and failing hearts in Figs 1.22.1 and 1.22.2 using the LV pressure–volume relationship during one cardiac cycle

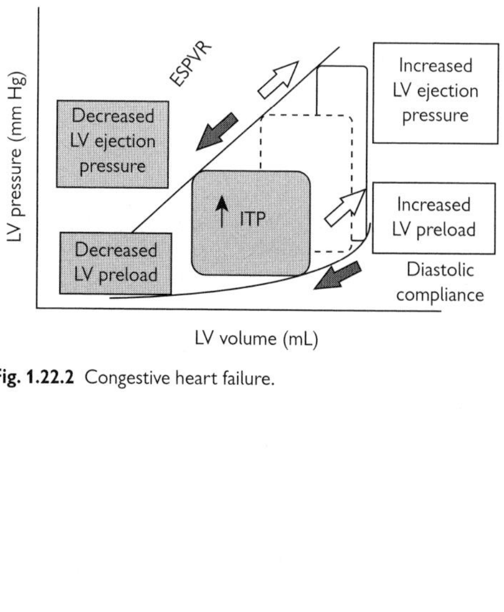

Fig. 1.22.2 Congestive heart failure.

to interpose venous return (end-diastolic volume) and afterload (end-systolic volume). Thus, performing an endotracheal intubation in patients with obstructive breathing abolishes the markedly negative swings in ITP without reducing venous return.

Ventilation as exercise

Spontaneous ventilatory efforts are exercise, requiring increased blood flow and O_2, and produce CO_2. In lung disease states where the work of breathing is increased, the work cost of breathing may increase to 25% or more of total O_2 delivery, limiting exercise capacity, inducing coronary ischaemia and leading to weaning failure. Starting artificial ventilation will decrease O_2 extraction, increasing SvO_2 for a constant cardiac output and CaO_2. Under conditions in which fixed right-to-left shunts exist, the obligatory increase in SvO_2 will result in an increase in the PaO_2, despite no change in the ratio of shunt blood flow to cardiac output.

Further reading

Buda AJ, Pinsky MR, Ingels NB, *et al.* Effect of intrathoracic pressure on left ventricular performance. *N Engl J Med* 1979; 301: 453–9.

Butler J. The heart is in good hands. *Circulation* 1983; 67: 1163–8.

Kaneko Y, Floras JS, Usui K, *et al.* Cardiovascular effects of continuous positive airway pressure in patients with heart failure and obstructive sleep apnea. *N Engl J Med* 2003; 348: 1233–41.

Nielson J, Ostergaard M, Kjaegaad J, *et al.* Lung recruitment maneuver decreases central haemodynamics in patients after cardiac surgery. *Intensive Care Med* 2005; 31: 1189–94.

Pinsky MR, Matuschak GM, Klain M. Determinants of cardiac augmentation by increases in intrathoracic pressure. *J Appl Physiol* 1985; 58: 1189–98.

Taylor RR, Covell JW, Sonnenblick EH, *et al.* Dependence of ventricular distensibility on filling the opposite ventricle. *Am J Physiol* 1967; 213: 711–8.

Van den Berg P, Jansen JRC, Pinsky MR. The effect of positive-pressure inspiration on venous return in volume loaded post-operative cardiac surgical patients. *J Appl Physiol* 2002; 92: 1223–31.

Viellard-Baron A, Schmitt JM, Augarde R, *et al.* Acute cor pulmonale in acute respiratory distress syndrome submitted to protective ventilation: incidence, clinical implications, and prognosis. *Intensive Care Med* 2001; 29: 1551–8.

Chapter 2

Cardiovascular therapy techniques

Chapter contents

Defibrillation

Defibrillation is the delivery of sufficient electrical current to depolarize a critical mass of myocardium and enable restoration of coordinated electrical activity. All defibrillators have three features in common:

- a power source capable of providing direct current
- a capacitor that can be charged to a pre-determined energy level
- two electrodes which are placed on the patient's chest through which the capacitor is discharged.

Defibrillation is defined as the termination of fibrillation or, more precisely, the absence of ventricular fibrillation/ventricular tachycardia (VF/VT) at 5s after shock delivery; however, the goal of attempted defibrillation is to restore spontaneous circulation.

Defibrillation is a key link in the chain of survival and is one of the few interventions that have been shown to improve outcome from VF/VT cardiac arrest. The likelihood of successful defibrillation diminishes rapidly with any delay in shock delivery. Automated external defibrillators (AEDs) have microprocessors that analyse several features of the ECG, including frequency and amplitude—the user does not need to be able to interpret the ECG. Manual defibrillators rely on the user interpreting the rhythm and determining if a shock is appropriate.

Quality of CPR

By incorporating a force transducer in a sternal compression pad and measuring transthoracic impedance, some defibrillators can provide real-time feedback on compression depth and rate, and ventilation volume and rate. This improves the quality of CPR and may improve outcome.

Strategies before defibrillation

Safe use of oxygen during defibrillation

In an oxygen-enriched atmosphere, sparking from poorly applied defibrillator paddles can cause a fire. This can be minimized by taking the following precautions.

- Take off any oxygen mask or nasal cannulae and place them at least 1m away from the patient's chest.
- Leave the ventilation bag connected to the tracheal tube or disconnect and remove it at least 1m from the patient's chest during defibrillation.
- If the patient is connected to a ventilator, leave the ventilator tubing connected to the tracheal tube unless chest compressions prevent the ventilator from delivering adequate tidal volumes.
- Minimize the risk of sparks during defibrillation. Theoretically, self-adhesive defibrillation pads are less likely to cause sparks than manual paddles.

The technique for electrode contact with the chest

An optimal defibrillation technique aims to deliver current across the fibrillating myocardium in the presence of minimal transthoracic impedance. Transthoracic impedance varies considerably with body mass, but is ~70–80Ω in adults.

- A very hairy chest may cause poor electrode–skin electrical contact and high impedance—with minimal delay, rapidly shave off excess hair.
- If using manual paddles, apply firm force (8kg) to reduce impedance.
- For ventricular arrhythmias, place electrodes (either pads or paddles) in the conventional sternal–apical (AP) position. Anteroposterior electrode placement may be more effective than the AP position in elective cardioversion of atrial fibrillation (AF).
- Self-adhesive defibrillation pads are preferable to standard defibrillation paddles.

CPR vs defibrillation as the initial treatment

After out-of-hospital cardiac arrest, if response times exceed 4–5min, a period of 2min of CPR before shock delivery may improve survival compared with immediate defibrillation. After in-hospital cardiac arrest, response times should be much less than 5min—if a shockable rhythm is identified, give a shock immediately.

One-shock vs three-shock sequence

There are no published human studies comparing a single-shock protocol with a three-stacked-shock protocol for treatment of VF cardiac arrest. The 2005 CPR guidelines included a single-shock protocol followed by immediate resumption of CPR for the following reasons:

- The time taken to deliver three shocks (up to 1min) results in prolonged interruptions to chest compressions, which affects outcome adversely.
- Modern, biphasic defibrillators have a first shock efficacy of >90%—failure to defibrillate implies that the quality of VF is poor. Two minutes of high-quality CPR may make the VF 'more shockable'.
- Immediately after a successful shock, despite ROSC (return of spontaneous circulation), the pulse may not be palpable—at this stage, 2min of CPR will maintain some coronary and cerebral blood flow while the myocardial contractility picks up. If the shock has not been successful, any time spent feeling for a pulse represents a period of zero blood flow.

Waveforms and energy levels

- All modern defibrillators deliver a biphasic shock: the current direction is reversed midway through shock delivery. First-shock efficacy for long duration VF/VT is greater with biphasic (86–98%) than monophasic waveforms (54–91%); however, a long-term survival advantage with biphasic defibrillators has yet to be demonstrated.
- Biphasic devices have smaller capacitors and need less battery power. They are smaller, lighter and easily portable.
- Many biphasic defibrillators are impedance-compensating. i.e. the output is adjusted depending on the transthoracic impedance.
- Although energy levels are selected for defibrillation, it is the transmyocardial current flow that achieves defibrillation. Current correlates well with the successful defibrillation and cardioversion. The optimal current for defibrillation using a monophasic waveform is in the range of 30–40amps. Indirect evidence from measurements during cardioversion for AF suggests that the current during defibrillation using biphasic waveforms is in the range of 15–20amps.
- Optimal energy levels for both monophasic and biphasic waveforms are unknown. The recommended energy levels vary between manufacturers, partly because the

precise waveform varies between different defibrillators. Although higher energy levels might cause more myocardial injury, the earlier conversion to a perfusing rhythm may outweigh this risk.

- In general, the energy level for the first shock with a biphasic defibrillator should be 150–200J. If using a monophasic defibrillator, deliver the first and subsequent shocks at 360J.
- Subsequent shocks can be given at the same energy level (fixed) or at a higher (escalating) energy level. The strategy used will depend on the manufacturer's recommendations and the setting available on the defibrillator. Both strategies are acceptable; however, if the first shock is not successful and the defibrillator is capable of delivering shocks of higher energy, it is rational to increase the energy for subsequent shocks.

Manual defibrillation

The sequence for using a defibrillator in manual mode is described. Because of the interruption in chest compressions caused by automatic rhythm analysis, shock advisory or AED mode should be used only by those unfamiliar with rhythm interpretation.

1. Confirm cardiac arrest clinically and confirm VF from the monitor or from adhesive pads or the defibrillator paddles.
2. Place self-adhesive pads or defibrillator gel pads on patient's chest—one below the right clavicle and one in the V6 position in the midaxillary line. If using defibrillator paddles, place them firmly on gel pads.
3. Select correct energy level: 150–200J biphasic (360J monophasic) for first shock and 150–360J biphasic (360J monophasic) for subsequent shocks.
4. Ensure that high flow oxygen is not passing across the zone of defibrillation
5. Charge self-adhesive pads or defibrillator paddles.
6. Warn everyone to 'stand clear' and deliver shock.
7. Without reassessing the rhythm or feeling for a pulse, start CPR using a ratio of 30:2, starting with chest compressions.
8. Continue CPR for 2min, then pause briefly to check the monitor.
9. If VF/VT, deliver a second shock.
10. Continue CPR for 2min, then pause briefly to check the monitor.
11. If VF/VT persists, give adrenaline 1mg IV followed by a third shock and 2min CPR. If the adrenaline is not ready, do not delay the shock—the adrenaline can be given after the shock.
12. Repeat this sequence if VF/VT persists.
13. Give further adrenaline 1mg IV after alternate shocks (i.e. approximately every 3–5min).
14. After three shocks, consider amiodarone 300mg IV.
15. If organized electrical activity is seen during the pause to check the monitor, feel for a pulse.
    a. If pulse is present, start post-resuscitation care.
    b. If no pulse is present, continue CPR and switch to the non-shockable algorithm.
16. If asystole is seen, continue CPR and switch to the non-shockable algorithm.

Cardioversion

If electrical cardioversion is used to convert atrial or ventricular tachyarrhythmias, the shock must be synchronized to occur with the R wave of the electrocardiogram rather than with the T wave: VF can be induced if a shock is delivered during the relative refractory portion of the cardiac cycle. Synchronization can be difficult in VT because of the wide-complex and variable forms of ventricular arrhythmia. If synchronization fails, give unsynchronized shocks to the unstable patient in VT to avoid prolonged delay in restoring sinus rhythm.

Atrial fibrillation

Biphasic waveforms are more effective than monophasic waveforms for cardioversion of AF.

- When using a monophasic defibrillator for cardioversion of AF, start with 200J, and increase stepwise as necessary.
- With a biphasic defibrillator, use an initial shock of 120–150J, escalating if necessary.

Atrial flutter and paroxysmal supraventricular tachycardia

Atrial flutter and paroxysmal supraventricular tachycardia generally require less energy than AF for cardioversion. Give an initial shock of 100J monophasic or 70–120J biphasic waveform. Give subsequent shocks using stepwise increases in energy.

Ventricular tachycardia

The energy required for cardioversion of VT depends on the morphological characteristics and rate of the arrhythmia.

- Ventricular tachycardia with a pulse responds well to cardioversion using initial monophasic energies of 200J.
- Use biphasic energy levels of 120–150J for the initial shock. Increase stepwise if the first shock fails to achieve sinus rhythm.

Further reading

Anonymous. 2005 International Consensus on Cardiopulmonary Resuscitation and Emergency Cardiovascular Care Science with Treatment Recommendations. Part 3: defibrillation. *Resuscitation* 2005; 67, 203–11.

Deakin CD, Nolan JP. European Resuscitation Council guidelines for resuscitation 2005. Section 3. Electrical therapies: automated external defibrillators, defibrillation, cardioversion and pacing. *Resuscitation* 2005; 67 Suppl 1: S25–37.

Nolan J, Soar J, Lockey A, *et al.*. Advanced life support, 5th edn. Resuscitation Council (UK), London, 2006.

Wik L, Hansen TB, Fylling F, *et al.* Delaying defibrillation to give basic cardiopulmonary resuscitation to patients with out-of-hospital ventricular fibrillation: a randomized trial. *JAMA* 2003; 289: 1389–95.

Temporary cardiac pacing

Temporary cardiac pacing provides a potentially life-saving measure for supporting the heart in patients with haemodynamic compromise due to a disturbed conducting system. Depending on the particular indication for temporary cardiac pacing and the availability of suitable equipment and skilled personnel, there exist several types of temporary cardiac pacing.

Indications for temporary cardiac pacing

The setting of an acute myocardial infarction (AMI)

- Asystole,
- 2nd or 3rd degree atrioventricular (AV) block with symptoms ,
- New trifascicular block,.
- 2nd or 3rd degree AV block without symptoms but following an anterior AMI.

Not related to an AMI

- Asystole.
- 2nd or 3rd degree AV block with symptoms.
- Sinus or junctional bradycardia with symptoms.
- Tachyarrhythmias secondary to bradycardia.

Overdrive suppression of tachyarrhythmias

- To prevent or treat Torsade de Pointes.

Prophylactic temporary cardiac pacing

Pre-operative patient with symptoms and:

- Sinus node disease or 2nd degree AV block (type I).
- Bifascicular/trifascicular block.

Pre-operative patient without symptoms and:

- 2nd degree (type II) or 3rd degree AV block.

The setting of cardiac surgery

- Valvular surgery (especially tricuspid and aortic).
- Ventricular septal defect (VSD) closure or ostium primum repair.
- Biatrial pacing to reduce post-operative AF.

During the replacement of a permanent pacemaker and rarely for right coronary artery angioplasty.

Types of temporary cardiac pacing

Temporary transcutaneous cardiac pacing

This non-invasive approach is used if temporary transvenous cardiac pacing is not immediately available. Self-adhesive electrode pads are placed on the left anterior chest between the xiphoid process and the left nipple, and posteriorly below the left scapula and spine. These are attached to the external pulse generator. Conscious patients should be given sedation to minimize discomfort.

Temporary transvenous cardiac pacing

This procedure requires suitable equipment and skilled personnel as stipulated by American Heart Association guidelines. Cannulation of a central vein allows a pacing wire to be placed in the right ventricle and/or the right atrium under fluoroscopic guidance. Where fluoroscopy is unavailable, pacing wires can be placed using balloon-tipped catheters.

The procedure

- Check that the fluoroscopy equipment, pacemaker box and defibrillator are functioning properly.
- Put on a lead apron, and a sterile gown and gloves.
- Obtain central venous access (see Chapter 7.3). The right internal jugular vein offers easiest access to the right ventricle and is the recommended approach. The right subclavian vein is the most comfortable for the patient. The right femoral vein should be considered if the above fail.
- Insert a venous sheath that is one size larger than the pacing wire, which is usually 5F or 6F in size.
- Right ventricular lead placement: from the right atrium, advance the pacing wire across the tricuspid valve and into the right ventricle. If it does not cross the tricuspid valve, rotate it so that it faces the lateral wall of the right atrium and forms a loop, and then prolapse the loop into the right ventricle. Entering the right ventricular outflow tract and then withdrawing the pacing wire will allow the tip to position in the apex. Maintain some slack in the pacing wire.
- Right atrial lead placement: on entering the right atrium, the pre-formed 'J' shape of the atrial pacing wire should reform. Rotate the pacing wire and position the tip in the right atrial appendage.
- Connect the pacing wire(s) to the pacing box and check for stability of the pacing wire(s) by asking the patient to cough, sniff and take some deep breaths. Exclude diaphragmatic pacing.
- Obtain a CXR to exclude a pneumothorax and check the position and integrity of the pacing wire(s). The atrial pacing wire should face anteriorly and loop upwards on a lateral CXR. The ventricular pacing wire should resemble the outline of a 'sock' on a postero-anterior (PA) CXR.

Complications of transvenous pacing

These include pneumothorax, haemothorax, infection, inadvertent arterial puncture, non-sustained VT as the pacing wire is manoeuvred across the tricuspid valve, thromboembolism with pulmonary embolism, and myocardial perforation with cardiac tamponade.

Temporary transoesophageal cardiac pacing

This approach obviates the requirement for central venous access or sterile precautions, and may be considered when fluoroscopy is unavailable. It comprises a transoesophageal pulse generator and gelatine bipolar pill electrodes (for the oral route) or transoesophageal pacing catheters (for the nasal route).

Temporary epicardial cardiac pacing

This involves directly stimulating the epicardium of the atria and/or ventricle using electrodes sutured to the epicardium at the time of cardiac surgery. The pacing wires are pulled through an incision in the skin and secured to the external chest wall. By convention, the atrial wires and the ventricular wire exit from the right and left side of the sternum, respectively. Infection, myocardial damage and/or perforation, tamponade and disruption of coronary anastomoses are the recognized complications.

Setting the pacemaker up

- Check the pacemaker box has a fresh battery and ensure the connections are secure and correct.
- Turn the pacemaker box on and set the pacing rate at 90–110bpm for cardiac surgery, 50bpm for sinus rhythm and 70–90bpm for heart block or bradycardias.

Determine the capture threshold

Capture describes the ability of the electrical impulse to initiate a myocardial depolarization.

- Turn the pacemaker rate to 10bpm above the intrinsic rate and increase the pacemaker output to 3V.
- Slowly decrease the output until loss of capture occurs, then increase it until capture reoccurs after every pacer spike. This is the capture threshold (aim for <1.0 and <1.5V for ventricular and atrial wires, respectively). Set output at 2–3 times the threshold or at 3V, whichever is higher.
- Reset the pacemaker to the prescribed rate.

Determine the sensitivity threshold

Sensitivity refers to the ability of the pacemaker to detect intrinsic myocardial activity. The sensitivity dial indicates the minimum voltage that the pacemaker is able to sense. Therefore, decreasing the sensitivity dial actually increases pacemaker sensitivity, and vice versa.

- Set the pacing rate at 10bpm below the intrinsic rate.
- Lower the pacemaker output to 0.1V to prevent competitive pacing.
- Increase the sensitivity dial until the sense indicator stops flashing and the pace indicator starts flashing.
- Slowly decrease the sensitivity dial until the sense indicator flashes continuously. This value is the sensing threshold. Set the sensitivity dial at half the sensitivity threshold value.
- If there is no underlying rhythm and sensitivity cannot be determined, set the sensitivity dial at 2mV.
- Reset pacemaker to prescribed rate.

Pacemaker mode and variables

- VVI for ventricular pacing only.
- DDD for dual-chamber pacing, allowing AV sequential pacing, which may benefit patients with a low cardiac output state or those patients with a 'stiff' left ventricle.
- The three letter code corresponds to the chamber paced ('V' for ventricle and 'D' for dual chamber), the chamber sensed and the response to sensing ('I' means pacing is inhibited on sensing intrinsic myocardial activity).
- AV interval (~150ms): this is the time interval between a paced or sensed event in the atrium and a paced event in the ventricle.
- Upper rate limit (~135bpm): this is the maximum rate the ventricles will pace at, as determined by tracking the atrial rate.
- PVARP (post-ventricular atrial refractory period, ~300ms): this time interval limits how early after a paced or sensed ventricular beat an atrial event can trigger a ventricular paced event.

Caring for patients with pacemakers

Proper care of the temporary cardiac pacing system includes daily assessment of the patient's haemodynamic status and examination of the insertion site for signs of infection. The underlying heart rhythm, sensitivity and capture thresholds should be determined daily, providing pacing is occurring <90% of the time.

Troubleshooting

The absence of pacing spikes on the ECG

This may be due failure to pace when the intrinsic rate is less than the pacing rate. Or it may be because the intrinsic rate is greater than the set pacemaker rate.

Failure to pace

This describes the failure of the pacemaker box to deliver an electrical impulse, and is indicated by the absence of pacing spikes when the intrinsic heart rate is less than the pacemaker rate. See checklist below.

Failure to capture

This describes the failure of an electrical impulse to initiate a myocardial depolarization, and is revealed by the failure of an appropriately timed pacing spike to be followed by either a 'P' wave or a widened 'QRS' complex. The capture threshold often doubles in the first few days due to endocardial oedema. Therefore, try increasing the output to restore capture.

Failure to sense or undersensing

This describes the failure of the pacemaker to detect intrinsic myocardial activity. It is indicated by regular pacing spikes unrelated to the intrinsic rhythm, which may or may not capture. Try decreasing the sensitivity dial (thereby increasing pacemaker sensitivity).

Inappropriate or oversensing

This describes the situation where the pacemaker is misinterpreting skeletal activity or 'P' and 'T' waves as 'QRS' complexes, and is inhibiting pacemaker activity, causing bradycardic episodes. Try increasing the sensitivity dial (thereby decreasing pacemaker sensitivity).

Causes of failure to pace, capture or sense

- Pacemaker box malfunction or flat battery.
- Insecure or incorrect lead connections.
- Malpositioned, damaged or displaced pacing wire.
- Myocardial infarction/fibrosis adjacent to wire tip.
- Myocardial perforation.
- Certain drugs such as class I antiarrhythmics.
- Electrolyte disturbances which widen the QRS and delay its upstroke, causing undersensing.

Futher reading

Antman EM, Anbe DT, Armstrong PW, *et al.* ACC/AHA guidelines for the management of patients with acute myocardial infarction. *J Am Coll Cardiol* 2004; 44: 671–719.

Francis GS, Williams SV, Achord JL, *et al.* Clinical competence in insertion of temporary transvenous ventricular pacemaker: ACP/ACC/AHA Task Force Statement. *Circulation* 1994; 89: 1913–6.

Gammage MD. Temporary cardiac pacing. Heart 2000; 83: 715–20.

Overbay D, Criddle L. Mastering temporary invasive cardiac pacing. *Crit Care Nurse* 2004; 24: 25–32.

Parker J, Cleland JGF. Choice of route for insertion of temporary pacing wires: recommendations of the medical practice committee and council of the British Cardiac Society. *Br Heart J* 1993; 70: 294–6.

Timothy PR, Rodeman BJ. Temporary pacemakers in critically ill patients: assessment and management strategies. *AACN Clin Issues* 2004; 15: 305–25.

Intra-aortic balloon counterpulsation pump

Intra-aortic balloon pumps were introduced in the 1960s for patients in cardiogenic shock; since then their use has been expanded into other clinical situations to provide earlier haemodynamic support in the management of patients with ischaemia or dysfunctioning myocardium.

The primary aims of intra-aortic counterpulsation are:

1 to increase myocardial oxygen supply
2 to decrease myocardial oxygen demand

The secondary effects are:

1 to improve cardiac output
2 to improve ejection fraction
3 increased coronary perfusion pressure
4 a reduction in heart rate
5 a reduction in systemic vascular resistance.

Physiology

The balloon assists cardiac function by inflating and deflating during the cardiac cycle, using helium gas. Helium is the preferred gas as it has a low density and a rapid diffusion coefficient, therefore allowing rapid inflation and deflation of the balloon.

The balloon inflates at the onset of diastole, augmenting coronary blood flow by the proximal displacement of blood, thereby increasing myocardial oxygen supply. Deflation occurs just prior to systole, lowering systolic blood pressure and afterload, thus reducing myocardial oxygen demand.

For optimal effect, counterpulsation must be timed correctly to the patient's cardiac cycle. This is achieved by either the patient's ECG signal or the arterial waveform.

ECG signal

The most common method used for triggering is the ECG signal, and the R wave is used as the trigger for balloon inflation. Inflation starts at the middle of the T wave and the balloon deflates before the end of the QRS complex. Difficulties in synchronization may arise in cases of tachyarrhythmias, pacemakers and poor ECG signal; in such cases the arterial waveform may be used for triggering instead.

Arterial waveform

The two phases of the cardiac cycle can be identified on the arterial waveform (Fig. 2.3.1). The dichrotic notch represents the closure of the aortic valve and the onset of diastole, it is here where the balloon is inflated, displacing blood towards the openings of the coronary arteries, thus increasing coronary artery perfusion. The start of systole is represented by the arterial upstroke and deflation of the balloon occurs just prior to this point, immediately before the aortic valves open, thus allowing the forward flow of blood.

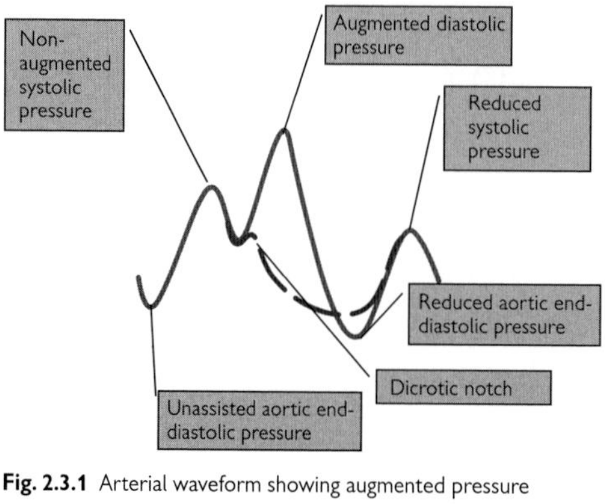

Fig. 2.3.1 Arterial waveform showing augmented pressure

Errors in timing

Errors can occur with the timing of the intra-aortic balloon pump, and this may result in different waveform characteristics and various physiological effects.

Early inflation occurs before the dichrotic notch, and the balloon inflates against a closed aortic valve; this results in a poorly defined dichrotic notch, which lies between the unassisted systole waveform and the augmented diastolic waveform.

Late inflation results in diastolic augmentation occurring after the dichrotic notch, and this results in suboptimal coronary artery perfusion.

Early deflation occurs during diastole, thus an early and sudden drop in diastolic augmentation is seen on the arterial waveform; this results in suboptimal afterload reduction and coronary artery perfusion.

Late deflation is when the balloon remains inflated for too long, thus remaining inflated during systole, resulting in a widened appearance of the diastolic augmentation waveform, reduced assisted aortic end-diastolic pressure and a prolonged rate of rise of assisted systole. Late deflation impedes left ventricular ejection and increases the afterload.

Indications

- Left ventricular failure
- Cardiogenic shock
- Unstable refractory angina
- Mechanical complications of AMI
- Post-myocardial infarction ventricular irritability
- Cardiac support for high risk general surgery patients and percutaneous transluminal coronary angioplasty (PTCA) patients
- Septic shock
- Weaning from cardiopulmonary bypass

Contraindications

- Severe aortic valve dysfunction
- Abdominal aortic aneurysm
- Thoracic aortic aneurysm
- Aortic dissection
- Severe peripheral vascular disease
- Irreversible brain damage

Insertion of the balloon pump

The balloon is inserted percutaneously via either femoral artery. A modified Seldinger technique allows easy and rapid insertion. The balloon catheter is passed into the aorta, over a guide wire, and should lie just distal to the subclavian artery. If not using fluoroscopy, a CXR must be done to confirm the position of the balloon tip. The guide wire can then be removed from the central lumen, which can now be used for arterial pressure monitoring.

If the balloon is placed too proximally, then the left subclavian artery may become occluded, and if the balloon is too distal, then the renal arteries may become occluded.

Once the balloon is secured in place, the patient should not be allowed to sit up, but can be nursed in a 30° head up position. Sitting may result in the balloon migrating inwards, with the risk of perforating the arch of the aorta and occlusion of the subclavian artery. Flexion of the leg in the sitting position may kink the balloon, which will prevent adequate inflation.

Complications

The incidence of complications occurring as a result of balloon pumps has decreased over the years, and balloon pump-induced death has decreased significantly.

All reported complications are listed below, the most common being vascular.

Vascular

- Limb ischaemia
- Femoral artery thrombosis
- Peripheral embolization
- Femoral vein cannulation
- Arterial injury
- AV fistula
- False aneurysm

Balloon related

- Perforation
- Rupture
- Incorrect position
- Gas embolization
- Entrapment

Other

- Haemorrhage
- Visceral ischaemia
- Infection
- Compartment syndrome
- Thrombocytopaenia

The most common vascular complication is limb ischaemia; this may be because many of these patients suffer from co-existing diseases such as diabetes, hypertension and peripheral vascular disease. The patients must therefore have their peripheral pulses, capillary refill and limb temperature checked regularly, and the balloon must be removed immediately if there are any signs of ischaemia.

Other vascular injuries generally require surgical intervention.

Balloon perforation or rupture is indicated by blood in the tubing, low augmentation or gas loss. Treatment is to turn the console off and change the balloon.

Compartment syndrome presents as pain, swelling and hardness of the calf. Treatment is urgent removal of the balloon with or without fasciotomy.

The balloon physically damages platelets during inflation and deflation, and this may result in thrombocytopaenia. All patients on balloon pumps should be anticoagulated using heparin, so beware of heparin-induced thrombocytopaenia as the cause of the low platelets.

Removal of the balloon pump

Patients need to be weaned off the balloon pump by reducing the balloon frequency. 1:1 indicates that inflation and deflation occurs with every cycle, which is the setting most patients are started on. 1:2 indicates inflation and deflation with every other cycle, and 1:3 indicates inflation and deflation for every 3rd cycle. The frequency is gradually weaned from 1:1 to 1:3, or more depending on the console, as the patient requires less support.

Once the patient tolerates less support on the balloon pump, indicated by cardiovascular stability and the absence of myocardial ischaemia, it can then be removed.

To remove the balloon, make sure anticoagulation has been weaned, disconnect the balloon from the pump, then gently pull back and remove. Direct pressure then needs to be applied over the puncture site for at least 30min. Pedal pulses should be confirmed by palpation or Doppler, and the patient should be monitored for bleeding and limb ischaemia.

Further reading

Akyurekli Y, Taichmann JC, Keon WJ. Effectiveness of intraaortic balloon counter pulsation and systolic unloading. *Can J Surg* 1980; 23: 122–6.

Barnett MG, Swartz MT, Peterson GJ *et al.* Vascular complications from intraaortic balloons: risk analysis. *J Vasc Surg* 1994; 71: 328–32.

Eltchaninoff H, Dimas AP, Whitlow PL. Complications associated with percutaneous placement and use of intraaortic balloon counter pulsation. *Am J Cardiol* 1993; 71: 328–32.

Freedman RJ. The intra-aortic balloon pump system: current roles and future directions. *J Appl Cardiol* 1991; 6: 313–8.

Mercer D, Doris P, Salerno TA. Intra-aortic balloon counter pulsation in septic shock. *Can J Surg* 1981; 24: 643–45.

Moulopoulos SD, Topaz S, Koloff WJ, *et al.* Diastolic balloon pumping (with carbon dioxide) in the aorta—a mechanical assistance to the failing circulation. *Am Heart J* 1962; 63: 669–75.

Cardiac assist devices

Over the last few years there have been major developments in cardiac assist device technology for both temporary and longer term haemodynamic support for patients with severe cardiac failure.

General description

Cardiac assist devices are blood pumps that partially support or entirely replace the function of the left or right ventricle.

A left ventricular assist device (LVAD) takes in blood from the left atrium or left ventricle and ejects usually into the ascending or descending aorta, but sometimes more peripherally. As a result, LV preload is decreased and cardiac output increased, restoring organ perfusion. A right ventricular assist device (RVAD) takes blood from the right atrium and ejects into the pulmonary artery. Some patients may require biventricular support using two VADs. Pumps can be extracorporeal or intracorporeal, and cannulation may be direct via thoracotomy or percutaneous. Some pumps produce pulsatile flow and others continuous. Total artificial hearts that replace the heart completely are also available. Recently percutaneously placed devices providing LV support have come into clinical use. Nearly all devices require patients to receive systemic anticoagulation.

Indications for cardiac assist device

Use of a cardiac assist device is indicated in patients with cardiac failure when cardiac output has fallen to a level such that other organ failure secondary to poor perfusion is likely to occur, despite maximal medical therapy. The most common causes of acute cardiac failure requiring circulatory support are acute myocardial ischaemia and following cardiac surgery. In these circumstances, extracorporeal or percutaneous devices for short-term support are used to allow time for cardiac function to recover or for consideration of implantation of a longer term device. Medium-term (extracorporeal pulsatile) devices are usually used as a bridge to recovery or cardiac transplantation.

Patients with slowly deteriorating chronic heart failure are more likely to be managed with long-term intracorporeal (surgically implanted) systems that allow patients to leave hospital, and are implanted either as a bridge to recovery or transplantation or rarely as permanent (destination) therapy. In a randomized clinical trial of LVAD implantation vs medical therapy in 129 patients ineligible for cardiac transplantation, patients receiving an LVAD (Heartmate) survived longer and had better functional status (REMATCH study).

Contraindications to VAD support

- Contraindication to anticoagulation
- Aortic regurgitation—greater than mild (for LVAD)
- Multiple organ failure

Types of pump

Pulsatile

Blood is pumped by pneumatic or electric motor-driven compression of a blood reservoir. Prosthetic valves in the circuit prevent reverse flow. Pumps require adequate preload and afterload—stroke volume (SV) decreases with very high afterload, unless drive line pressure is increased.

Pneumatic

- Thoratec VAD: extracorporeal single chamber (plastic sac) pump used for short and medium-term support. A vacuum is used to enhance filling of the blood sac that is then compressed to produce an SV of 65ml with total flows up to 6.5l/min. Access cannulae contain mechanical one-way valves. Can be used as a long-term VAD.
- Abiomed BVS5000 and AB5000: extracorporeal pumps with two blood chambers—a gravity-filled atrium and a pneumatically compressed ventricle. Two polyurethane valves are positioned within the pump. These pumps have been used extensively for temporary support for left, right or both ventricles. The AB5000 can be used for longer term as a bridge to transplantation or recovery.
- HeartMate LVAS: implantable long-term support for bridge to transplant, recovery or destination therapy. Contains porcine valves and a pump surface that allows a cellular lining to develop, and therefore there is less requirement for anticoagulation. Maximum SV is 85ml.

Electric motor driven

- HeartMate XVE LVAS: similar to HeartMate LVAS but uses an electric motor, rather than air to eject blood.
- Novacor LVAS: intracorporeal device that includes pusher plates to produce flow. Porcine valves are used in the cannulae. This device is only suitable for LV support, but can be used long term.

Non-pulsatile

No valves are included in circuits with these pumps, and filling occurs by suction from the pump. Centrifugal pumps are used for short-term extracorporeal support and axial pumps are placed intracorporeally for longer term ventricular assistance.

Centrifugal

Centrifugal pumps accelerate blood flow from the inlet at the centre of a rotating plate to the outflow at the periphery. These pumps (and axial impellers) are sensitive to changes in preload and afterload, and therefore flow may vary considerably at the same pump revolutions per minute (rpm). They are used to provide temporary cardiac support. Pumps with bearings produce local heat that has been associated with an increased incidence of thrombotic complications.

- Medtronic Bio-pump (BioMedicus): extracorporeal centrifugal pump with bearings.
- Levitronix (Centrimag): a small extracorporeal pump, in which the impeller is rotated by a magnetic field, without bearings. Can be used as an LVAD and/or an RVAD for up to 28 days.

Axial

Axial impeller pumps are smaller than other pumps and have a lower blood-contacting surface area than pulsatile pumps. All models require intracorporeal placement. Blood is pumped by a rotating screw or propeller. There has been considerable interest recently in using this type of pump for long-term ventricular support because of their smaller size and reduced risk of infection.

- Jarvik 2000: small axial pump, rotating at 8000–12000rpm that is implanted into the apex of the left ventricle and ejects into the descending thoracic aorta, providing LV support. Can be implanted using a left thoracotomy.

Used for bridge to transplant, but has also been used for destination therapy.

- Micromed DeBakey and HeartMate II: axial pumps implanted with inflow from the ventricle and outflow in the ascending aorta (LVAD) or pulmonary artery (RVAD).

Complications associated with VADs

Echocardiography (TTE and TOE) is very valuable in diagnosing and managing VAD-associated problems.

Acute

- Haemorrhage
- Air embolus
- Right ventricular failure

RV dysfunction is common after LVAD implantation, and up to 30% of patients may subsequently require RVAD support. Many patients will require inotropic support and pulmonary vasodilators.

- Cannula obstruction
- Haemolysis
- Arrhythmias
- Right to left shunting through patent foramen ovale (LVAD)
- Multiple organ failure

Chronic

- Thrombus formation/haemorrhage
- Stroke
- Infection
- Valve failure
- Device failure

Total artificial hearts

Although total artificial hearts that completely replace both ventricles have been produced, they have not been used widely. Potential advantages over intracorporeal LVADs include absence of arrhythmias and potential RV failure.

Catheter-based temporary assist devices

Recently a number of assist devices that can be used without the need for a thoracotomy have become available. These devices are for short-term support (<10 days) until recovery occurs or longer term support is arranged. Indications for use include cardiogenic shock of any cause, either until cardiac function improves or as a bridge to surgical (long-term) LVAD implantation or to transplantation. A further use being investigated is during high risk revascularization (surgical or medical) in order to decrease myocardial oxygen demand in a large area of ischaemic myocardium. Contraindications to insertion include RV failure (biventricular support will be required) and inadequate peripheral arterial vessels for device placement.

Impella

The Impella (Abiomed Europe, Aachen, Germany) has a catheter-mounted axial flow pump that is passed from the femoral artery retrogradely through the aortic valve into the left ventricle. Blood enters the pump in the left ventricle and is ejected into the aorta.

Two sizes are available. The LP2.5, size 12F, is inserted percutaneously via the femoral artery and can pump up to 2.5l/min. The larger LP5.0 requires insertion via femoral artery cut down, and can pump up to 5l/min.

Versions of the pump that can be placed during cardiac surgery are available. The LD5.0 is placed through the ascending aorta into the left ventricle. Right ventricular assist is also possible using the RD device. With an inflow suction port placed surgically in the right atrium and outflow cannula in the pulmonary artery the system can pump up to 5.5l/min.

The Impella devices can be used for up to 10 days.

Tandem Heart

The Tandem Heart (CardiacAssist Inc., Pittsburgh, PA, USA) is an extracorporeal centrifugal pump. The inflow cannula is passed from the femoral vein into the left atrium via a transeptal puncture. The outflow cannula is placed via the femoral artery into the iliac artery. The system can pump up to 5l/min and be used for up to 14 days. This makes it suitable for temporary support post-myocardial infarction or post-cardiac surgery.

Percutaneous short-term LVAD support is appealing because of the potential wider applicability of pumped circulatory support. Clinical outcome studies of percutaneous LVAD support are awaited.

Venoarterial extracorporeal membrane oxygenation

ECMO for respiratory failure can usually be provided without the need for circulatory support (VV ECMO) and is described in Chapter 1.14.

Some patients may require combined circulatory and pulmonary support, e.g. patients with ARDS combined with acute right ventricular failure, for example post-pneumonectomy. In these circumstances, temporary combined cardiac and pulmonary support can be achieved using venoarterial extracorporeal membrane oxygenation (VA ECMO). Blood is withdrawn from a right atrial cannula, pumped by an extracorporeal pump through an oxygenator and returned into the aorta. Cannulae can usually be placed percutaneously. A centrifugal pump, e.g. Levitronics/ Centrimag, is often used in this situation.

Uses of VA ECMO

- Neonatal respiratory distress syndrome (VV ECMO is also used)
- Failure to wean from cardiopulmonary bypass
- Short-term support of left or both ventricles when combined with acute pulmonary failure
- ARDS with acute right ventricular failure.

Further reading

Boehmer JP, Popjes E Cardiac failure: mechanical support strategies. *Crit Care Med* 2006; 34: 268–77.

Rose EA, Gelijns AC, Moskowitz AJ, *et al.* Long-term mechanical left ventricular assistance for end-stage heart failure (REMATCH Study). *N Engl J Med* 2001; 345: 1435–43.

Therapeutic cooling

Therapeutic hypothermia is being used with increasing frequency to prevent or mitigate various types of neurological injury. Currently, its most frequent usage is in patients who remain comatose following witnessed cardiac arrest with restoration of spontaneous circulation (ROSC). Two randomized controlled trials and 15 non-randomized studies have shown that neurological outcome in this category of patients can be improved by mild (32–34°C) hypothermia. Preliminary findings suggest that patients with other initial rhythms, such as asystole and pulseless electrical activity, may also benefit from therapeutic cooling. Guidelines from the European Resuscitation Council and the American Heart Association formally recommend the use of hypothermia for selected patients who remain comatose following a witnessed cardiac arrest.

Hypothermia can also be used for numerous other indications including severe traumatic brain injury, stroke, hepatic failure, ischaemic spinal cord injury, myocardial infarction and numerous others. Some of these indications require longer treatment periods, with a concomitant increase in the risk of side effects.

Definitions

Induced hypothermia: an intentional reduction of a patient's core temperature below 36.0°C.

Therapeutic hypothermia: controlled induced hypothermia, i.e. induced hypothermia with potentially harmful effects such as shivering being controlled or suppressed. Temperature range usually 32–35.9°C.

A separate but closely related issue is the use of controlled normothermia (therapeutic fever management). Several studies have demonstrated a link between fever (irrespective of its cause) and a worsening of neurological outcome in many types of neurological injury, including post-ischaemic injury following cardiac arrest. This correlation persists after multivariate analysis, and observations from animal studies strongly suggest that the link is causal. Therefore, symptomatic control of fever is becoming an increasingly accepted goal of therapy in patients with neurocritical illness.

Therapeutic normothermia: bringing down and maintaining core temperature within a range of 36.0–37.5°C in a patient with fever, with the potentially deleterious effects such as shivering being controlled or suppressed.

Temperature management in critically ill patients poses special challenges for attending physicians and nurses, as the induction strategy and proper management of side effects can have a substantial impact on outcome. The hypothermia treatment period can be divided into three distinct phases:

Induction phase

Aim: to achieve temperatures ≤34°C and then target temperature as quickly as possible. In this phase, a small overshoot (≤1°C) should be regarded as acceptable provided core temperature remains >30°C.

Maintenance phase

Aim: to control core temperatures tightly within a narrow range, with no or minor fluctuations (maximum 0.2–0.5°C).

Re-warming phase

Aim: slow and controlled rise in temperature, target rate 0.2–0.3°C/h, maximum acceptable rate 0.5°C/h. Reason: rapid re-warming after therapeutic hypothermia can re-trigger harmful processes and adversely affect outcome. The rate of re-warming should be even slower (0.05–0.1°C/hr) when hypothermia has been used in patients with TBI.

Practical aspects

Induction of hypothermia will lead to the activation of counter-regulatory mechanisms to decrease heat loss, including an increase in sympathetic tone, vasoconstriction of skin vessels and shivering. Shivering increases oxygen consumption by 40–100% and has been linked to increased risk of morbid cardiac events; however, these observations have been made in the post-operative setting, where hypothermic patients are awake and have a high rate of metabolism, increased oxygen consumption, excess work of breathing, a high heart rate and a general stress-like response. These adverse events are linked to the haemodynamic and respiratory responses rather than to shivering *per se*, and the side effects are largely absent in controlled hypothermia where patients are sedated, ventilated and have low heart rates. However, shivering can generate significant amounts of heat and can significantly decrease cooling rates; for this and other reasons it should be aggressively treated (especially in the induction phase of cooling). Shivering responses decrease markedly when the temperature decreases below 33.5–34.0°C.

Cardiovascular effects of cooling include bradycardia and a rise in blood pressure. Hypothermia's effect on myocardial contractility is variable (depending on heart rate and filling pressure); in most patients, myocardial contractility will increase, although mild diastolic dysfunction may develop in some patients. Clinically significant arrhythmias may occur, but only if core temperature decreases below 30°C. The most important long-term side effect of hypothermia is an increased risk of infections (especially of the respiratory tract and/or wounds) and bedsores.

The most important potential side effects of cooling are:

- Hypovolemia through hypothermia-induced cold diuresis. If uncorrected this can cause hypotension. Hypothermia *per se* does not decrease blood pressure.
- Electrolyte disorders (cooling causes urinary loss of K, Mg, P as well as intracellular shift; rapid re-warming can cause hyperkalaemia).
- Hyperglycaemia (cooling can cause insulin resistance and decreased insulin secretion).
- Shivering (can be controlled with magnesium, meperidine, quick-acting opiates, propofol or benzodiazepines; additional therapeutic options include ketanserin, clonidine, tramadol, urapidil and doxapram).
- Skin injuries/bedsores (prolonged direct exposure of the skin to ice or ice-packs can cause burns; cooling causes vasoconstriction in the skin; and wound infections can develop more easily due to the immunosuppressive effects of hypothermia).
- Infections, especially airway and wound infections.

Precautions

- Treat infections early and aggressively; consider antibiotic prophylaxis; perform frequent cultures of blood and other sites.

- Use appropriate sedation and analgesia (animal data suggest loss of protective effects if sedation is insufficient; sedation also facilitates cooling by preventing shivering and causing vasodilation).
- Adjust ventilator settings (cooling causes ↓O_2 consumption and ↓CO_2 production); adjust feeding rate (cooling decreases metabolism by 7–10% per °C decrease below 37°C).
- Blood gas analysis and clotting parameters are affected by temperature. Most laboratories warm samples to 37°C before analysis. If blood gas results have not been analysed at the patient's true core temperature, values can be estimated with the following rule of thumb: for pO_2, subtract 5mm Hg for every 1°C below 37°C; for pCO_2, subtract 2mm Hg for every 1°C below 37°C; for pH, add 0.012 points for every 1°C below 37°C.
- Adjust drug dosage (drug clearance, especially by the liver, may change; this includes clearance of sedatives, opiates and paralysing agents. Precaution: use bolus doses during induction phase, avoid high maintenance doses).
- Avoid core temperature ≤30°C (risk of arrhythmias arises at temperatures ≤28–30°C). Hypothermia does not cause arrhythmias at temperatures ≥30°C.
- Avoid 'overtreating'. Bradycardia, mild metabolic acidosis and a slight rise in lactate levels, liver enzymes and amylase are normal consequences of hypothermia, and usually do not require treatment.
- Avoid long-term paralysis. Paralysis can mask inadequate sedation and seizures, and can have adverse consequences such as increased risk of critical illness polyneuromyopathy. Treat shivering with one of the other agents listed above.
- Consider platelet administration before surgery or invasive procedures during cooling.
- General measures: provide good basic intensive care (many of the side effects of cooling can be prevented or controlled with proper intensive care treatment).

Cooling methods

A number of cooling devices have reached the market in recent years that enable reliable maintenance and slow and controlled re-warming. There are invasive systems (cooling catheters for direct cooling of the blood) and non-invasive methods (water-circulating blankets and adhesive pads for surface cooling); 371;1955–69. Air-circulating cooling blankets are ineffective for cooling purposes, and should not be used for induction of hypothermia. In the induction phase, rapid cooling rates can be achieved by combining an invasive or surface cooling device with rapid infusion of cold fluids (1500–3000ml of 4°C saline or Ringers lactate using a pressure bag). Rapid cooling reduces the severity and duration of shivering, and decreases the risk of hypothermia-induced electrolyte disorders.

Controlled normothermia

Most of the side effects listed above do not occur during controlled normothermia. However, shivering does occur because the hypothalamic temperature setpoint is elevated in patients with fever; thus, if core temperature is lowered by external cooling, the patient's normal counter-regulatory mechanisms will be activated. Indeed shivering may be more pronounced than in hypothermic patients, because whereas at 33°C the shivering response is absent or significantly blunted, at 36–37°C the counter-regulatory mechanisms are working at maximum capacity. Therefore, maintaining controlled normothermia is often more difficult than maintaining controlled hypothermia, and extra efforts may be required to combat shivering. This is a problem especially in non-ventilated patients, because the doses of sedatives required to control shivering may be so large that they can induce respiratory failure.

Antipyretic drugs such as paracetamol (acetaminophen) or aspirin can be used as adjunctive treatment to lower temperature. A major advantage is that these drugs do not activate the shivering response. However, their efficacy (especially in non-infectious ('central') fever is relatively low; the average temperature decrease in patients treated with high doses of paracetamol or aspirin is 0.1–0.7.

Conclusions

There is an increasing awareness that temperature can significantly affect outcome in critically ill patients, especially those with neurological injuries. Therapeutic temperature management is therefore likely to gain importance, not just in ICU patients but (certainly in the case of controlled normothermia) also in patients admitted to general wards. Mild hypothermia appears to be well tolerated provided that the side effects are prevented or strictly controlled. Temperature control should be regarded as an important goal of therapy in critically ill patients, especially those with neurological injuries.

Further reading

Diringer MN, Reaven NL, Funk SE, et al. Elevated body temperature independently contributes to increased length of stay in neurologic intensive care unit patients. *Crit Care Med* 2004; 32: 1611–2.

Nolan JP, Deakin CD, Soar J, *et al.* European Resuscitation Council. European Resuscitation Council guidelines for resuscitation 2005. Section 4. Adult advanced life support. *Resuscitation* 2005; 67 Suppl 1: S39–86.

Polderman KH. Therapeutic hypothermia in the Intensive Care unit: problems, pitfalls and opportunities (review). Part 1: indications and evidence. *Intensive Care Med* 2004; 30: 556–75.

Polderman KH: Application of therapeutic hypothermia in the intensive care unit. Opportunities and pitfalls of a promising treatment modality. Part 2: practical aspects and side effects. *Intensive Care Med* 2004; 30: 757-69.

Polderman KH. Induced hypothermia and fever control for prevention and treatment of neurological injuries. Lancet 2008; in press.

Polderman KH. Therapeutic hypothermia and controlled normothermia in the ICU: practical considerations, side effects and cooling methods. *Crit Care Med* 2008 (in press).

Chapter 3

Renal therapy techniques

Chapter contents

Haemodialysis

The first human haemodialysis was performed in 1943 by Willem Kolff in The Netherlands for the treatment of acute renal failure. Following this, haemodialysis was adopted for the treatment of acute renal failure in the immediate post-war years and then for chronic renal failure from the 1960s. Currently haemodialysis is the most common form of replacement treatment for end-stage renal disease (ESRD). Haemodialysis is one method used for treatment of acute renal failure, and ESRD patients will develop critical illness. An understanding of the principles of haemodialysis and how it is carried out is therefore essential.

In haemodialysis, waste solute removal occurs primarily via the principle of diffusion. This is defined as a type of solute movement across a semi-permeable membrane driven by a concentration gradient (Fig. 3.1.1). This principle is employed by separating an extracorporeal blood circuit from a flow of specially prepared warmed fluid called dialysate by a semi-permeable membrane within a specially designed dialyser (Fig. 3.1.2). The dialysate is a solution with a solute composition that will minimize the loss of essential solutes such as sodium, calcium, magnesium, chloride, bicarbonate, etc. Fluid loss is achieved by applying a hydrostatic pressure gradient to the blood compartment. Modern dialysis machines generate the prescribed dialysate composition from a solute concentrate with purified water, and control fluid removal by volumetric measurement according to the treatment prescription.

Extracorporeal circuit

Access

- The success of any extracorporeal treatment is 90% dependent upon the quality of the access.
- Patients with ESRD ideally will have an established surgically created arteriovenous (AV) fistula which allows easy access to the circulation.
- A permanent AV fistula is extremely precious and must be protected particularly from prolonged hypotension. It must not be used for any other purpose.
- In acute renal failure, temporary access to the circulation is normally achieved by the insertion of a large bore dual-lumen catheter sufficient to allow a blood flow of 200ml/min.
- A design that minimizes recirculation of treated blood should be used, e.g. shotgun.
- Temporary large bore arterial access is now rarely used.

Anticoagulation

- Unfractionated heparin remains the most common agent used for anticoagulation; however, fractionated heparin is now being used more commonly.
- In chronic ESRD dialysis there is usually no call for regional anticoagulation of the circuit with little systemic anticoagulation, but this is often necessary in the critically ill. Under these circumstances, protamine can be infused into the venous limb of the circuit to reverse the heparin effect.
- Citrate anticoagulation with calcium reversal has now gained favour and reduces the risk of bleeding to a minimal level. All forms of regional anticoagulation need careful protocols to run properly.
- In the most severely ill, it may be possible to run the circuit without anticoagulant at a high blood flow.

Dialysers, membranes and biocompatibility

Membrane technology has resulted in the hollow fibre dialyser becoming the standard design. This helps minimize the priming volume of the circuit. Membranes are now available in a range of materials compared with the original cuprophane, e.g. polysulphone, polycarbonate, polyacrylonitrile. They can be manufactured with a wide variety of diffusive and hydraulic conductance properties. The only truly biocompatible surface is normal endothelium, but the modern membranes are less likely to activate the alternative complement pathway than the older cellulose-based versions. In general, haemodialysis membranes restrict the passage of solute particles with a molecular weight of >500Da.

Factors that influence solute clearance in dialysis

- *Blood flow.* Solute clearance increases as blood flow increases, but normally the rise in clearance drops off once 250–300ml/min has been achieved. Poor circuit blood flow has a major limiting effect on dialysis efficiency

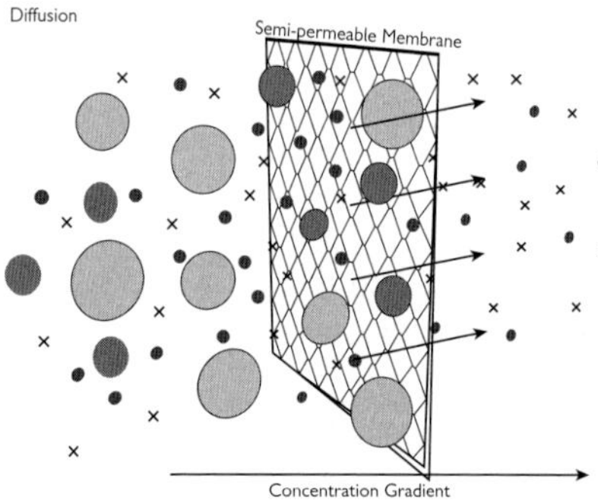

Fig. 3.1.1 Diffusive transport.

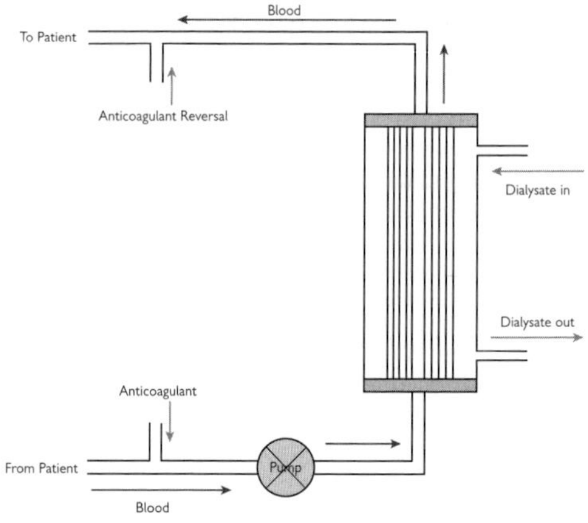

Fig. 3.1.2 Haemodialysis circuit.

- *Dialysate flow.* Solute clearance is affected by the maintenance of the highest solute concentration gradient across the membrane. A high dialysate flow of 500ml/min is the norm in ESRD. Above this level there is little gain in clearance
- *Membrane.* The properties of the membrane will determine the hydraulic conductivity and the rate of transfer of solute of any given size. If a high filtration fraction is generated, protein deposition upon the membrane will reduce hydraulic and solute conductance. Increasing the surface area will raise clearance.

Adequacy of dialysis

For patients with ESRD on chronic dialysis there is a significant body of data on the adequacy of dialysis and calculation of the dialysis dose using the Kt/V_{urea} or urea reduction ratio (URR = 1 – post-dialysis urea/pre-dialysis urea). Kt/V represents the fractional clearance of urea. This relates the dialyser clearance (K) and the time on treatment to the distribution volume of urea. It can be expressed according to a single or, more accurately, a double pool kinetic model. The difference between prescribed and achieved clearance is often significant and is influenced by factors such as recirculation, lower than expected blood flow and lower efficiency of the dialyser than anticipated, e.g. protein adsorption. In ESRD, a KtV value of >1.2 and URR >65% is normally accepted to improve long-term outcome. Even in chronic dialysis practice, it is important to take into account factors other than these calculations alone. There is evidence that the clearance of molecules greater in size than urea and less than albumin, the so-called middle molecules, is important in the prevention of the uraemic syndrome although there is still debate over the identity of the 'uraemic' toxin(s). In acute renal failure there are far fewer data on the best way to estimate the dose for renal replacement therapy (RRT). The patients are seldom in steady state, it is difficult to establish a lean body mass and there is commonly increased protein catabolism following trauma/surgery/bleeding. Most will attempt to keep the blood urea below 30mmol/l prior to commencing the next treatment for an intermittent regime and below 20 mmol/l for a continuous regime.

Buffer

Originally acetate was used as the buffer in the dialysate for reasons of chemical stability, but acetate must be metabolized to bicarbonate and causes vasodilatation, which makes it unsuitable for the critically ill. With changes in dialysate preparations and the use of modern machines, bicarbonate is now the buffer of choice for the critically ill and is also now used in >75% of European chronic dialysis patients.

Performing haemodialysis in the critically ill

The ESRD patient who develops critical illness

With the increasing number and age of patients receiving long-term dialysis support, the number presenting for planned or unplanned critical care support is rising. The ESRD patient will normally require a longer time on dialysis to cope with the increased catabolic load in order to prevent complications such as uraemic pericarditis. Preservation of their access is important, and their treatment must be managed in conjunction with staff experienced in ESRD care. The method of RRT may need to be changed depending upon the acute problem, and it may be necessary to use the methods normally preserved for acute renal failure. Sometimes this may be necessary because the critical care staff may not be familiar with ESRD haemodialysis techniques.

- The technique used should be adapted to both the patient's needs and the unit's expertise.

When should dialysis be started in acute renal failure?

The decision of the timing of the start of RRT has to be tailored to the needs of the individual patient. Much will depend upon the cause of the renal failure and whether this has occurred with single organ disease as opposed to multi-organ failure. In the situation of a simple nephrotoxic insult causing no other major organ failure, such as an excess of gentamicin, RRT can be delayed until the urea is approaching 30mmol/l. Intermittent haemodialysis treatment will allow adequate control and adequate patient mobilization. In the situation of renal failure secondary to sepsis or post-ruptured abdominal aortic aneurysm repair, treatment should be started early and a continuous RRT strategy should be pursued.

Continuous or intermittent, fast or slow?

Dialysis is highly efficient at removing low molecular weight solutes. Short intermittent dialysis regimes have been developed over the years for ESRD, and these are probably only suitable for critically ill patients who are stable, normotensive, non-catabolic and recovering from the illness precipitating their admission to the ICU. This allows them to mobilize and minimizes exposure to anticoagulation. There are also patients in whom rapid solute exchange may be specifically indicated

- Life-threatening hyperkalaemia
- Highly water-soluble low molecular weight poisons with a low volume of distribution, e.g. lithium, ethylene glycol.

Contraindications for short duration high efficiency dialysis would include

- Cerebral injury/oedema
- Hepatic failure
- Severe azotaemia (dysequilibration syndrome)
- Cardiovascular instability.

In these circumstances, the rapid solute change due to the maximum concentration gradient at the start of high efficiency dialysis will cause major water shifts into the brain with the generation of cerebral oedema. Continuous or semi-continuous methods (e.g. sustained low efficiency dialysis; SLED) should be used in these circumstances with a much slower solute transfer to minimize the rate of loss of solute from the blood compartment. In SLED the blood flow and dialysate flow are reduced, which prevents major solute gradients developing between the intra- and extracellular fluid compartments. This minimizes large water shifts across cell membranes. In reality, with the new dialysers that allow selection of the pore size, surface area and hydraulic conductivity, pure diffusive continuous therapies are becoming less common and convective (filtration) and diffusive (dialysis) are now combined as haemodiafiltration

Complications of haemodialysis

- Haemorrhage from access, line disconnection, anticoagulation
- Thrombosis of the extracorporeal circuit
- Air embolism, although this is minimized by modern machines having sophisticated air detectors for the venous side of the circuit

- Dysequilibration syndrome
- Electrolyte abnormalities and haemolysis, although these are very rare with modern machinery unless the dialysate composition is set incorrectly
- Anaphylactoid bradykinin reactions (AN69 membranes in patients receiving angiotensin-converting enzyme inhibitors)
- Pyrogen reactions due to the use of non-pure water
- Hypovolaemia
- Fluid overload This may be from limited ability to remove fluid on haemodialysis compared with haemofiltration
- Hypothermia from heat loss from the circuit and/or the use of unheated dialysate.

Further reading

http://www.adqi.net/

Ronco C, Bellomo R, Kellum J, eds. Critical care nephrology. Saunders, 2008. *ISBN*: 978-1416042525.

Haemo(dia)filtration

Introduction

Despite advances in the understanding, diagnosis and treatment of acute kidney injury (AKI), many aspects remain unresolved. Modern technology has provided different modalities to perform extracorporeal renal support, but it is not clear which is superior in terms of efficacy and outcome.

Indications to start renal replacement therapy (RRT)

RRT is indicated when renal dysfunction leads to one or more of the following:

- Oligo/anuria
- Severe fluid overload
- Pulmonary oedema
- Hyperkalaemia
- Metabolic acidosis

However, recent greater ease of use and a low associated morbidity has led to RRT being considered early in the disease process. This may be related to the perception that maintenance of homeostasis and prevention of complications is increasingly important. There is also some evidence that RRT has some role to play in the management of sepsis and multi-organ dysfunction syndrome (MODS).

Indications to stop RRT

There is no hard evidence on how and when RRT should be stopped. It is generally accepted, however, that increasing urine output during RRT is a signal that the kidneys are improving. Removal of RRT should also be considered if the patient demonstrates haemodynamic stability with decreased requirement for vasopressors and improving condition overall.

Principles of renal replacement

The kidneys filter the blood to remove excess water and waste products. Renal replacement essentially uses semi-permeable membranes to achieve the same result. The membrane may be artificial, as in a filter, or autologous, as in the peritoneum. Many molecules, including water, urea and solutes of various molecular weights, are transported across the membrane by variable combinations of the processes of diffusion (dialysis) and convection (ultrafiltration (UF)).

During diffusion, the movement of solutes depends on their tendency to reach the same concentration on each side of the membrane; this results in the passage of solutes from the compartment with the higher concentration to the compartment with the lower concentration. Diffusion is affected by characteristics of the semi-permeable membrane including thickness, surface area, temperature and diffusion coefficient. Diffusion is provided by dialysis, in which a solution (the dialysate) flows on the other side of the membrane, countercurrent to blood flow, in order to maintain a solute gradient.

In convection, the movement of solute across a semi-permeable membrane is a result of transfer of water across the membrane. In other words, as the solvent (plasma water) crosses the membrane, solutes are carried with it if the pore size of the membrane allows. Convection can be achieved by UF, which creates a transmembrane pressure (TMP) gradient. UF depends on the rate of flow (Qf), the membrane coefficient (K_m) and the TMP gradient between the pressures on both sides of the membrane:

$$\text{Qf} = K_m \times \text{TMP}$$

The TMP gradient is the difference between the pressure in the blood compartment and filtrate compartment. The blood compartment pressure is directly related to blood flow (Qb). The filtrate compartment pressure is modulated by suction in modern RRT machines. The machines are designed to maintain a constant rate (Qf): when the filter is 'fresh' and highly permeable, the pumps retard UF production, generating a positive pressure on the filtrate compartment (TMP is initially dependent only on blood flow). As the membrane fibres become degraded, a negative pressure on the filtrate side is necessary to achieve a constant Qf. With time, TMP progressively increases up to a maximum level at which solute clearance is compromised, and clotting of the filter or membrane rupture is possible.

The size of molecules cleared during convection and UF exceeds that during diffusion, because they are physically dragged to the UF side; however, this gradually becomes limited by the protein layer that progressively closes filter pores during convective treatments. In addition, the membrane itself can adsorb molecules, and this is important for higher molecular weight toxins. The membrane adsorptive capacity is generally saturated in the first few hours of filter use and has a relatively minor impact on mass separation processes. During UF, plasma water and solutes are filtered from the blood, leading to a decrease in blood hydrostatic pressure and increase in blood oncotic pressure. The fraction of plasma water that is removed from the blood during UF is called the filtration fraction and should be kept in the range of 20–25% to prevent excessive haemoconcentration within the filtering membrane. Otherwise, the oncotic pressure gradient could neutralize the TMP gradient, resulting in equilibrium.

Replacing plasma water with a substitute solution completes the *haemofiltration* (HF) process. The replacement fluid can be administered after the filter (post-filter dilution HF), before (pre-filter dilution HF) or both. Post-filter dilution leads to a higher urea clearance (~2000ml/h), but pre-filter dilution prolongs the circuit lifespan by reducing haemoconcentration and protein build-up in the filter fibres. Conventional HF is performed with a highly permeable, steam-sterilized membrane with a surface area of ~1m^2. The addition of convection to the diffusion process allows *haemodiafiltration*: dialysis and replacement solutions run simultaneously within the same filter to obtain additional solute removal.

Choice of mode

RRT may be intermittent or continuous. In general, intermittent RRT is reserved for haemodynamically stable patients. How effectively RRT is applied may be more important than the method chosen. It is difficult to use biochemical or clinical markers to monitor RRT. Urea concentration should be <30mg/dl and creatinine <221µmol/l. Nonetheless, urea and creatinine clearance do not necessarily represent the clearance of other toxins and solutes.

The ideal RRT would include:

- efficient solute removal
- minimum solute disequilibrium
- low UF rate
- haemodynamic stability
- low anticoagulant needs
- minimal interference with patient mobility

Continuous RRT schedule may be adjusted to fulfil the patients needs and the illness.

Practical RRT prescription

During RRT, clearance (K) depends on circuit blood flow (Qb), haemofiltration flow (Qf) or dialysis flow (Qd), the molecular weight of the solutes, and th efilter type and size. Circuit blood flow is mainly dependent on vascular access and operational characteristics of the machines.

In haemofiltration, Qf is strictly linked to Qb by the filtration fraction. In dialysis, however, Qd is not limited by the filtration fraction, but when the Qd/Qb ratio exceeds 0.3 dialysis will be less efficient. Urea and creatinine are generally used as reference solutes in order to measure the effectiveness of the RRT prescription, but their clearance is not directly correlated with outcome of AKI.

Membrane sieving coefficient (SC)

During UF, the driving pressure jams solutes, such as urea and creatinine, against the membrane. The SC determines the amount of solute that passes through the pores of the membrane. The SC is calculated by the ratio of the concentration of the solutes in the filtrate to that in the plasma. An SC of 1.0, as is the case for urea and creatinine, demonstrates complete permeability and a value of 0 total impermeability. Molecular size (<12Da) and filter porosity are the major determinants of SC. During continuous treatments, a minimum urea clearance of 30ml/h/kg (2.8l/h in a 70kg patient) is required.

Techniques

Slow continuous ultrafiltration (SCUF)

Blood is driven by a pump through a highly permeable filter via an extracorporeal circuit, using venovenous access. The ultrafiltrate produced during membrane transit is not replaced and it corresponds to weight loss. It is used only for fluid control in overloaded patients

Circuit blood flow: 100–250ml/min.

Ultrafiltrate flow: 5–15ml/min.

Continuous venovenous haemofiltration (CVVH)

CVVH is similar to SCUF above except that the ultrafiltrate produced during membrane transit is partly or completely replaced to maintain intravascular volume control. Replacement fluid may be delivered before, after or on both sides of the filter (pre- or post-dilution). Clearance for all solutes is convective and equals the UF rate.

Circuit blood flow: 100–250ml/min.

Ultrafiltrate rate: 15–60ml/min.

Continuous venovenous haemodialysis (CVVHD)

In CVVHD, blood is driven through a low permeability dialyser via an extracorporeal circuit in venovenous mode and a counter-current flow of dialysate is delivered on the dialysate compartment. The ultrafiltrate produced during membrane transit corresponds to the patient's weight loss. Solute clearance is mainly diffusive, and efficiency is limited to small solutes only.

Circuit blood flow: 100–250 ml/min.

Dialysis flow: 15-60 ml/min.

Continuous venovenous haemodiafiltration (CVVHDF)

This is a technique where blood is driven through a highly permeable dialyser via an extracorporeal circuit in venovenous mode and a counter-current flow of dialysate is delivered on the dialysate compartment. The ultrafiltrate produced during membrane transit is in excess of the patient's desired weight loss, and replacement solution is needed to maintain fluid balance. Solute clearance is both convective and diffusive.

Circuit blood flow: 100–250ml/min

Dialysis flow: 15–60ml/min

Ultrafiltrate rate: 15–60ml/min.

High volume haemofiltration (HVHF)

This treatment uses highly permeable membranes and haemofiltration with a high volume setting: Qb >200ml/min and Qf >45ml/kg/h in order to increase removal of high molecular weight solutes (such as sepsis and systemic inflammatory mediators).

Anticoagulation

In many RRT modalities blood comes into contact with the artificial surfaces and some form of anticoagulation is needed. To reduce the risk of the filter clotting, vascular access should be of adequate size, kinked tubing should be avoided and the blood flow rate should exceed 100ml/min. Pump flow fluctuations must be prevented (in modern machines this is mainly due to circuit increased resistances rather than flow rate inaccuracies). Venous bubble traps, where air–blood contact occurs, are used to prevent systemic air emboli, and the machine will alarm if bubbles are detected.

There is evidence that when the set-up is perfectly optimized, anticoagulants contribute little to the maintenance of circuit patency. When anticoagulants are relatively contraindicated (risk of bleeding, pre-existing coagulopathy, thrombocytopenia) RRT can still be safely performed and filter life may not be compromised.

Unfractionated heparin is the most commonly used anticoagulant. The dose ranges from 5 to 10IU/kg/h. In some patients, heparin can also be used in combination with protamine administration post-filter (regional heparinization) with a 1:1 ratio (150IU of unfractionated heparin per mg of protamine) and monitoring of prothrombin time (aPTT). Problems with heparin are relatively unpredictable bioavailability, antithrombin III depletion and the risk of heparin-induced thrombocytopenia (HIT).

Low molecular weight heparins are used in some units, but prospective studies have not yet shown them to be superior in prolonging circuit life. Bioavailability is more reliable than unfractionated heparin, and the risk of HIT is lower. However, the anticoagulant effect cannot be reversed and there may be a higher risk of haemorrhage.

Prostacyclin is potentially useful for RRT anticoagulation, being a potent inhibitor of platelet aggregation with a short half-life. It is infused at a dose of 4–8ng/kg/h with or without the adjunct of low dose heparin. Hypotension may be induced by higher doses. High cost and the risk of hypotension limit the use of this agent to short-term treatment.

Citrate chelates calcium to prevent clot formation and can produce regional anticoagulation. Administration of calcium chloride may be required to maintain normocalcaemia. This approach is effective in maintaining filter patency and compares favourably with heparin. It also avoids the risk of HIT and does not lead to systemic anticoagulation. However, the risk of hypocalcaemia, metabolic alkalosis and the cumbersome replacement and dialysate fluid preparation limit its use.

Peritoneal dialysis (PD)

There are reports of the first PD being performed in the mid 18th century; however, it was not until the 1920–1930s that the treatment was re-introduced experimentally for acute renal failure. It began to find some favour in the late 1940s, but was dogged by the problem of peritonitis and access problems. Since the 1970s, continuous ambulatory peritoneal dialysis (CAPD) has been a common form of ESRD therapy, particularly for those with some residual renal function for whom it can be used for many years or where there are contraindications to anticoagulation. Many patients ultimately have to move to haemodialysis in order to achieve adequate control of azotaemia. However, prior to this, intermittent PD was a relatively common method used for the management of acute renal failure or as a (less than ideal) bridge until a place was found on a chronic haemodialysis programme. Other than the lack of need for anticoagulation, the main advantages of PD is that the peritoneum is a natural semi-permeable membrane and that the process can be continuous. CAPD allows near normal patient mobility

Peritoneal membrane structure and solute transfer

The three-pore model of the peritoneal membrane accounts for

- the measurable, but low, rate of transfer of proteins through a small number of large pores >15nm
- some convection with solvent drag (osmotic gradient) through water channels, 0.5nm (aquaporins)
- diffusive solute movement (concentration gradient) through the large number of 4nm pores allowing small solute and water passage.

Solute transport is closely linked to the capillary supply to the visceral and parietal peritoneal membranes, and the effective surface area for solute and fluid exchange is less than the anatomical area of the peritoneal membrane. The rate-limiting steps for solute transfer are therefore the permeability of both the peritoneal capillaries and the permeability and size selectivity of the peritoneal membrane. There is considerable variation between individuals for these factors, which is further significantly affected by inflammation.

Access

A catheter is used to provide access to the peritoneal cavity. Originally these were relatively rigid and introduced blindly over a stylet directly through the abdominal wall. These frequently caused leakage, infection was common and the risk of visceral damage high, but nowadays silastic catheters based upon the design of Tenckhoff and Schechter are used which are tunnelled subcutaneously and have Dacron cuffs placed subcutaneously.

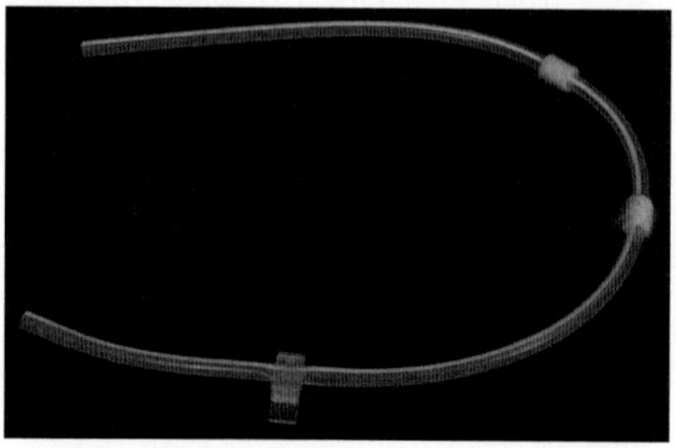

Fig. 3.3.1 Photograph of a peritoneal dialysis catheter.

These may be inserted via a trochar and cannula, minilaparotomy or minilaparoscope even at the bedside. The proper positioning of the catheter is essential to ensure efficient drainage and function of the catheter. Simple issues such as constipation may significantly affect catheter function. Previous abdominal surgery with the likelihood of multiple adhesions is a relative contraindication for PD

Techniques

PD is carried out by filling the peritoneal cavity with sterile pre-prepared dialysate fluid. The peritoneal fluid will achieve solute equilibration with the plasma water in 4–5h, although the optimum dwell time for maximum fluid removal using dextrose as the osmotic agent is 2–3h. The fluid is then drained and replaced with fresh dialysate. A single filling and draining of the peritoneal cavity is called a cycle.

The commonly used CAPD popularized in the late 1970s for ESRD management uses long dwell times and 4–5 cycles per day, 7 days per week. The patient drains and refills the peritoneal cavity, taking 30–40min, at intervals throughout the day. The effluent bags are weighed to determine the volume of fluid removed and the concentration of osmotic agent adjusted to keep the patient's fluid balance neutral. Some patients use machines that cycle on a shorter time basis through the night. These remove the need for inconvenient bag changes, warm the dialysate and can be programmed for targeted fluid removal. The abdomen can be left empty or full throughout the day. The method used will depend upon the method availability, individual circumstances and the wishes of the patient.

Dialysate

General composition

PD fluid contains sodium, chloride, calcium and magnesium. The concentration of these can be adjusted, although this is primarily used for calcium.

Buffer

Lactate has been the standard for many years, but is being replaced by or combined with bicarbonate.

Osmotic agent

Traditionally dextrose has been used in different concentrations—standard, 1.36% (350mosm/kg), or high osmolarity, 3.86%, depending upon the quantity of fluid removal required. The glucose used in CAPD may make a significant contribution to calorie intake. An alternative is glucose polymer (icodextrin) present in a 7.5% concentration. This operates by colloid osmosis as icodextrin has an average molecular weight of 20 000Da.

Biocompatibility

The pH of most commercial fluids is <5.5 and contains high lactate and glucose degradation product concentrations. These factors are felt to damage peritoneal lining cells, and newer fluids use bicarbonate as the buffer with a more neutral pH and fewer glucose degradation products. Patients have much less pain on infusion of these more biocompatible products, and these fluids will hopefully protect the integrity of the peritoneal membrane and prolong the efficiency of the peritoneal membrane to clear solute and water.

PD as renal replacement therapy

Adequacy of PD and assessment of peritoneal function

As mentioned previously there is a wide variation in effective peritoneal surface area, and this can be assessed for long-term PD by measuring the peritoneal solute clearance. The used dialysate is collected for 24h and a plasma sample taken. The urea and creatinine are measured in both the fluid and plasma. With the dialysate volume, a 24h clearance can be calculated, and conventionally this is expressed as weekly clearance by multiplying by 7 and standardized by the body surface area. For the patient's total clearance, the effect of residual renal function must be added to this result. A creatinine clearance of >50l/1.73m^2 is regarded as satisfactory.

Formal testing of the peritoneal membrane can be performed by the peritoneal equilibration test (PET) which gives a value for the rate of transport of water and low molecular weight solute. Patients can then be allocated a category of high to low transporters.

Complications

- *Infection*: this may be of the peritoneum or the tunnel site. Peritonitis is easily detected by the development of cloudiness of the effluent dialysate often associated with pain. Samples are sent for microbiology, and antibiotic treatment is given intraperitoneally according to the centre's regime. Occasionally the cause will be due to a gastrointestinal or gynaecological source rather than external contamination of the dialysate fluid. Prevention of infection has improved greatly over the years, with specific systems introduced to minimize the risk of contamination during bag changes. Many patients now have years between episodes of cloudy fluid/infection,
- Leaks: dialysate may leak through the catheter track, into the pleural space, soft tissues or into a hernial sac
- Catheter insertion complications: bleeding, organ damage, etc.
- Catheter malposition or malfunction, e.g. fibrin blockage.
- Constipation.
- Membrane failure: for solute transport, UF or both.
- Sclerosing peritonitis.
- Pain.
- Hernia development,

Management of acute renal failure by PD

Advantages of PD

- Natural membrane
- Peritoneum impermeable to bacteria
- No necessity for extracorporeal circuit or anticoagulation
- Continuous therapy
- Controllable UF and solute clearance
- No requirement for expensive, sophisticated machinery
- Minimal effects on cardiovascular stability
- Less potential for further vascular insult to the damaged kidney.

What is the place of PD in the critically ill?

Formerly PD was a relatively common form of treatment for acute renal failure but, as the technology of haemodialysis and then continuous RRT developed, it has fallen out of favour other than for paediatric practice where vascular access and extracorporeal circuit management can be extremely difficult. In situations where the sophisticated resources required to apply modern continuous RRT is not available, PD has a continuing place in situations where the peritoneal cavity is not compromised, for example by intra-abdominal surgery. The original method where repeated rigid catheter insertion was used probably has no place, but the modern methods of insertion of Tenckhoff catheters allow relatively simple catheter placement. Ash has recently argued the case for the place of PD in the critically ill and the potential for high frequency cycling allowing the high solute clearances felt necessary for the critically ill.

Management of the CAPD patient with critical illness

There are a large number of ESRD patients receiving PD as their replacement therapy and, on occasion, they will require critical care. Depending upon the problem, management of their renal failure can usually be continued using PD, the one obvious exception being major intra-abdominal surgery. This will need to be supervised by staff fully trained in this treatment to avoid the common complications and ensure good catheter function. The dialysis regime will need to be adapted by increasing the solute clearance, as is normally necessary in the critically ill, and to adjust UF as indicated by the patient's condition.

If there is no-one with CAPD experience present in the critical care unit, then the catheter can be locked and the RRT method with which the unit is familiar instituted until the patient can be transferred to a centre familiar with PD or recovers to be able to supervise their own treatment.

Further reading

Ash SR. Peritoneal dialysis in acute renal failure: the under-utilised modality. *Contrib Nephrol* 2004; 144: 239–54.

Jacobs C, Kjellstrand CM, Koch KM, Winchester JF, eds. Replacement of renal function by dialysis, 4th edn. *Kluwer Academic Publishers, Dordrecht*, 1996.

Johnson RJ, Feehally J, eds. Comprehensive clinical nephrology, 2nd edn. *Mosby, St Louis, MO*, 2003.

Chapter 4

Gastrointestinal therapy techniques

Chapter contents

Insertion of a Sengstaken–Blakemore tube in critical care

The Sengstaken–Blakemore tube is very effective at controlling torrential bleeding from oesophago-gastric varices. Its use is associated with serious complications such as oesophageal ulceration, oesophageal perforation and aspiration pneumonia in 15–20% of cases. Up to 50% of patients will re-bleed once the balloon is deflated. so its primary function is to control bleeding initially prior to further definitive treatment.

Indication

Consider inserting a Sengstaken–Blakemore tube where bleeding from oesophago-gastric varices is not controlled endoscopically, where access to endoscopy is not readily available, if the patient is unable to tolerate endoscopic procedures or if the patient does not consent to an endoscopy. The Sengstaken–Blakemore tube will control bleeding in up to 90% of patients but has to be viewed as a temporary solution, as re-bleeding occurs in ~50% of patients on deflation of the balloon. It is essential to plan the next therapeutic step within 12–24h. This will usually be a further attempt at endoscopic therapy, but other options such as a transjugular intrahepatic portosystemic shunt (TIPSS) and even liver transplantation may be considered.

Equipment

The Sengstaken–Blakemore tube (Fig. 4.1.1.) is a triple lumen tube, and differs slightly from the Minnesota tube, a variant used in the same way, in that the Minnesota has a fourth port to enable aspiration of oesophageal contents and so reduce the risk of aspiration pneumonia. The tubes are usually stored in the fridge of the emergency department, endoscopy, admissions unit or theatres.

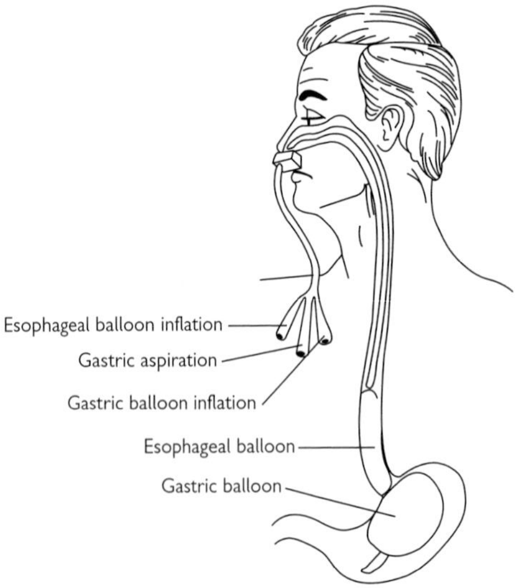

Fig. 4.1.1 A pictorial representation of a Sengstaken–Blakemore tube.

Preparation

It is ideal, though not essential, for the patient to be sedated with an endotracheal tube *in situ* as this reduces the risk of aspiration pneumonia, enables insertion of the tube down the oesophagus rather than trachea, and is more comfortable for the patient. The Sengstaken–Blakemore tube should be removed from the fridge immediately prior to insertion. Colder, stiffer tubes are thought to aid insertion, although they probably warm up and soften in a relatively short time. The balloons and channels are then checked for leaks by insufflating with a 50ml bladder syringe. Deflate completely and clamp off the two balloons, and lubricate the tube with some water-based lubricating jelly to aid insertion. The insertion can be done with the patient lying on their back or side (typically left side). An assistant with suction is always required as variceal bleeds may produce large volumes of blood.

Insertion

The lubricated Sengstaken–Blakemore tube is inserted via the nose or the mouth. The nasal route allows easier nursing and is said to be more comfortable for the patient. Oral insertion can be considered if there is a nasal obstruction or the patient does not tolerate nasal insertion. Lidocaine spray can be used in those who are not intubated. Once the insertion point is anaesthetized, pass the tube through the nostril into the pharynx and gently push down into the oesophagus. There may be a slight resistance as the tube passes the larynx and, on entering the oesophagus, there is then a slight 'give'. Check that the tube has not curled up in the back of the pharynx. Continue passing the tube down the oesophagus to the 55cm mark from the incisors; indicating a position well below the gastro-oesophageal junction (GOJ). Inflate the gastric balloon with water or air and check the position with a chest radiograph: using a mixture of water-soluble contrast material and water may help to visualize the balloon. Once the tube is correctly sited, fill with a maximum volume of 300ml of water (or air). Some clinicians favour filling the balloon completely with 300ml initially, as a tube positioned at 55cm below the GOJ has little risk of complications. Novel techniques are being developed such as using ultrasound to ensure correct placement. Once the balloon is filled, gently pull the tube back until resistance is felt. Apply traction (see below).

Post-insertion

1. Traction on the tube is maintained by applying tape ('Sleek' or red tape is best) to the skin of the nose only. Weighted traction using bags of saline causes necrosis at the GOJ and at the angle of the mouth (if using the oral route). The angle of the mouth can be further protected using a tennis ball, with a unilateral longitudinal slice from one pole to the other, as this will dissipate the pressure over the skin of the face.
2. Aspirate from all the available portals.
3. Chest radiograph to ensure there is no oesophageal perforation (subcutaneous emphysema, pneumonitis) and no evidence of aspiration pneumonia.
4. Check the portals, length of the Sengstaken–Blakemore tube and angle of mouth at regular intervals.
5. Rarely does the oesophageal balloon need insufflating. If it is needed to control bleeding then insufflate to no more than 40mm Hg and deflate every 4h for 15min to prevent oesophageal necrosis; some advocate deflating for 2min every hour.

6 Regularly suction (15min intervals) or put on continuous low-pressure suction to remove secretions via the oesophageal tube as this reduces the aspiration risk.
7 Aspirate the gastric port every 15min for 4h then hourly to check the bleeding rate. Place on free drainage into a bile bag.
8 Release traction at 10h and deflate to prevent necrosis. If no bleeding occurs in 1h, deflate completely, and if no further bleeding occurs in the following hour then remove the Sengstaken–Blakemore tube.
9 The tube must be removed within 36–48h.
10 Clear written instructions on the monitoring and care needed must be available for both nursing and medical staff.

Pharmacological measures

In any bleeding patient, good resuscitation, with blood and fluids (colloids and crystalloids), and close monitoring of fluid balance are most important to ensure a good outcome for the patient.

Diversion of blood flow to the oesophago-gastric varices is caused by portal hypertension, and diversion away from the varices is achieved pharmacologically with terlipressin (Glypressin) 2mg initially then 1–2mg 4–6 hourly up to 72h. The terlipressin constricts the splanchnic vessels and reduces the venous blood flow through the upper gastrointestinal (GI) tract. This results in a reduction in the pressure in the collateral circulation and therefore reduces the risk of bleeding. Glypressin therapy should be initiated in all patients thought to be bleeding from oesophago-gastric varices unless contraindicated (such as coronary heart disease, cardiac failure and polydipsia).

In an encephalopathic patient, lactulose may be given down the gastric port of the tube to encourage bowel action and reduce the risk of encephalopathy. Broad spectrum antibiotics have been proven to reduce both the risk of re-bleeding from varices and the mortality from sepsis in cirrhotic patients admitted with an upper GI bleed.

Follow-up therapy

Following insertion of the Sengstaken–Blakemore tube, plans should be made for further definitive treatment. Once the patient is stable with the Sengstaken–Blakemore tube in place, subsequent endoscopy needs to be performed within the following 24h to allow further attempts at endoscopic therapy. Band ligation of the varix or insertion of the sclerosant ethanolamine are used to achieve haemostasis and to eradicate the varices. A 'second look' endoscopy may be needed after 24–48h to assess for re-bleeding. Discussion with the local Liver Unit will cover potential candidates for TIPSS or liver transplant.

Further reading

Bernard B, Grange JD, Khac EN, *et al.* Antibiotic prophylaxis for the prevention of bacterial infections in cirrhotic patients with gastrointestinal bleeding: a meta-analysis. *Hepatology* 1999; 32: 142–53.

Dearden JC, Hellawell GO, Pilling J, *et al.* Does cooling Sengstaken–Blakemore tubes aid insertion? An evidence based approach. *Eur J Gastronenterol Hepatol* 2004; 1611: 1229–32.

Douglass A, Bramble MG, Barrison I. National survey of UK emergency endoscopy units. *BMJ* 2005; 330: 1000–1.

Kupfer Y, Cappell MS, Tessler S. Acute gastrointestinal bleeding in the intensive care unit. The intensivist's perspective. *Gastroenterol Clin North Am* 2000; 29: 275–307.

Lin AC-M, Hsu Y-H, Wang T-L, *et al.* Placement confirmation of Sengstaken–Blakemore tube by ultrasound. *Emerg Med J* 2006; 25: 487.

Panes J, Teres J, Bosch J, *et al.* Efficacy of balloon tamponade in treatment of bleeding gastric and esophageal varices. Results in 151 consecutive episodes. *Dig Dis Sci* 1988; 334: 454–9.

Vlavianos P, Gimson AES, Westaby D, *et al.* Balloon tamponade in variceal bleeding: use and misuse. *BMJ* 1989; 298: 1158.

Upper gastrointestinal endoscopy

Acute GI haemorrhage is the main indication for endoscopy in the critical care setting. Endoscopy is the primary diagnostic and therapeutic technique used in patients with GI bleeding. Acute upper GI bleeding has an incidence ranging from 50 to 150 per 100 000 of the population each year. The hospital mortality has remained steady at ~10% for patients admitted for GI bleeding but is 30% for patients who develop GI bleeding while in hospital for other reasons. Many of these patients are older or have significant cardiovascular, respiratory or cerebrovascular co-morbidity.

Presentation

Patients may present with vomiting fresh blood or 'coffee ground' altered blood. Patients may also present with melaena (black tarry stools), and ~10% of lower GI bleeds (haemochezia) will have an upper GI cause. The majority of patients require admission, although a small proportion of young/fit patients with self-limiting bleeding may not. Re-bleeding is defined as fresh haematemesis and/or melaena with the development of shock (pulse >100bpm, systolic pressure <100mm Hg) or a reduction in Hb concentration >20g/l over 24h.

Causes

A cause for upper GI bleeding is found in ~80% of cases (Table 4.2.1)

Table 4.2.1 Causes of acute upper gastrointestinal haemorrhage

Diagnosis	Approximate %
Peptic ulcer	35–50
Gastroduodenal erosions	8–15
Oesophagitis	5–15
Varices	5–10
Mallory–Weiss tear	15
Upper gastrointestinal malignancy	1
Vascular malformations	5
Other	5

Hospital management

Patients with significant upper GI bleeding should be looked after by specialist gastroenterologists (physicians or surgeons) in a safe environment. This may be an acute medical ward where the medical and nursing staff have experience of the problem or critical care units for severely ill patients. The management of these patients in specialized units has been shown to reduce the mortality from 11 to 5%. There must be round the clock expertise including access to emergency endoscopy, surgery and indeed blood transfusion. There should be agreed protocols available to all for the management of upper GI haemorrhage. Details of admission and subsequent events must be clearly recorded.

Clinical approach

The management depends on a number of factors including the assessment of severity and cause of bleeding, along with the age and presence of co-morbid factors.

Assessment of severity

It is important to stratify patients into those with a high or low risk of death. The Rockall score has now become the standard scoring score used in most acute centres (see Chapter 20.4).

Resuscitation

The initial management is to establish an adequate airway and to ensure adequate venous access with a least a 14 or 16 gauge IV cannula. A central venous catheter should be considered in patients with signs of major haemorrhage. Initial fluid replacement can be with crystalloid but, if there are signs of shock (pulse >100bpm), then 500ml of colloid should be administered immediately. Blood should be transfused when bleeding is extreme and/or when the Hb is <10g/l. The initial (pre-transfusion) Hb should be interpreted with caution as this is a poor indicator of the severity of bleeding.

Initial investigations

A full set of baseline blood tests should be taken including electrolytes and clotting (particularly when liver disease is suspected). Four units of blood should be cross-matched, although O negative blood can be given in dire situations. ECG, CXR and blood gases are advisable in those with cardiorespiratory disease.

Endoscopy

Most patients can be endoscoped on the next available list, usually within 12–24h. Emergency endoscopy should be considered in:

- patients with chronic liver disease
- patients presenting with shock with significant concurrent illnesses
- patients with clinical evidence of re-bleeding following a primary intervention.

In most cases, endoscopy is best performed in an endoscopy unit but severely bleeding patients may be best managed with an endotracheal tube in place in a critical care setting. Endoscopy must be performed by experienced operators able to achieve haemostasis in patients with bleeding from ulcers and varices. It is equally important that assistants have been adequately trained and are familiar with the endoscopic equipment and their accessories.

Endoscopy will usually reveal the source of bleeding, give some indication of prognosis and enable endoscopic therapy.

The prognosis is partly dependent on identification of stigmata of recent haemorrhage (SRH) as revealed in the Rockall score. It is therefore important to take appropriate steps to identify clearly the source of bleeding. This may involve the use of washing catheters, change of position of the patient and, in experienced hands, any clot should be removed (washed/snared) to expose the bleeding point so that endoscopic therapy can be targeted.

Endoscopic therapy

Patients without SRH have a low risk of re-bleeding and should not be treated endoscopically as their prognosis is good. A variety of techniques have been developed to treat patients with major SRH.

In patients found to have bleeding due to oesophagogastric varices, both sclerotherapy with ethanolamine and band ligation can be used. Sclerotherapy involves the injection of the sclerosant ethanolamine through a needle injection catheter both para- and intravariceally. More recently, band ligators that attach to the distal end of the endoscope have been developed to allow suction of the varix and then release of a tight band around the base of the varix. Often patients will be initially treated with sclerosant, but then bands should be applied as quickly as possible as this technique is better at controlling bleeding and, importantly, reducing the risk of re-bleeding.

If endoscopy fails to stop the bleeding then a Sengstaken–Blakemore tube may be used, and occasionally TIPSS or rarely surgery may be indicated. All patients with variceal bleeds should be started on IV antibiotics.

Patients with bleeding from ulcers can be treated with injection, application of heat or with mechanical clips. Local expertise will determine which techniques are used, but recent studies suggest that dual therapy with two of the above techniques will reduce the risk of re-bleeding by 30%.

Injection therapy involves injecting 1:10 000 adrenaline solution in quadrants around the bleeding point, then direct injection into the bleeding vessel. 95% patients will stop bleeding, but re-bleeding will occur in up to 20% of these. Thermal haemostasis is achieved with heater probes or argon beam plasma coagulators. The heater probe uses both pressure and heat to achieve haemostasis with success equal to injection therapy. A variety of mechanical clips have been developed to apply to bleeding points, and are particularly useful for visible larger vessels.

These techniques can be used to treat other causes of bleeding such as Mallory–Weiss tear, vascular malformations (argon beam particularly useful) and the tricky Dieulafoy lesion.

Medical therapy

A neutral gastric pH is required to improve the stability of clots over bleeding arteries. Whilst there is little evidence to support H_2 antagonists in the acute setting, there is increasing evidence that using proton pump inhibitors (PPIs) early leads to improvements in outcome. In one study from Nepal, high dose oral omeprazole was shown to reduce blood transfusion requirements and the risk of bleeding when compared with placebo. In more recent studies, high dose intravenous PPIs led to reductions in the rate of re-bleeding, blood transfusion requirement, duration of hospital stay and the need for endoscopic therapy. There was a non-statistical trend to reduced mortality in the treated group. A high dose PPI is therefore recommended (80mg bolus followed by an infusion of 8mg hourly for 72h) as part of the initial management of patients with significant upper GI bleeding (see Chapter 20.4).

There is little evidence to support the use of other agents, although there is some evidence that tranexamic acid may reduce the need for surgical intervention.

Follow-up

Patients should resume drinking 4–6h after endoscopy. Repeat endoscopy is required if there is evidence of fresh bleeding or if there if there is concern that optimal treatment was not possible at the initial endoscopy (poor views, etc.).

A surgical opinion is required in bleeding that cannot be stopped by endoscopic intervention and in the following circumstances:

- any patient requiring early endoscopy
- patients >65 who remain unstable after ≥4 units of blood
- patients <65 who remain unstable after ≥8 units of blood
- patients with significant re-bleeding.

Patients who have bled from ulcers should receive standard ulcer healing therapy, which often includes *Helicobacter* eradication. Patients taking non-steroidal anti-inflammatory drugs (NSAIDs) or aspirin should stop these drugs. Patients who bled from gastric ulcers should undergo repeat endoscopy 6 weeks after discharge to ensure ulcer healing and to exclude malignancy. Repeat endoscopy is usually not necessary in the duodenal ulcer group.

Further reading

Holman RA, Davis M, Gough KR. Value of centralised approach in the management of haematemesis and melaena; experience in a district general hospital. *Gut* 1990; 31: 504–8.

Khuroo MS, Yattoo GN, Javid G. A comparison of omeprazole and placebo for bleeding peptic ulcer. *N Engl J Med* 1997; 336: 1054–8.

Lau JYW, Leung WK, Wu JC, *et al.* Omeprazole before endoscopy in patients with gastrointestinal bleeding. *N Engl J Med* 2007; 356: 1631–40.

Lau JYW, Sung JJY, Lee KKC, *et al.* Effect of intravenous omeprazole on recurrent bleeding after endoscopic treatment of bleeding peptic ulcers. *N Engl J Med* 2000; 343: 310–6.

Rockall TA, Logan RFA, Devlin HB, *et al.* Incidence of and mortality from acute upper gastrointestinal haemmorrhage in the United Kingdom. *BMJ* 1995; 311: 222–6.

Stiegmann GV, Goff JS, Michaletz Onody PA, *et al.* Endoscopic sclerotherapy as compared with endoscopic ligation for bleeding oesophageal varices. *N Engl J Med* 1992; 326: 1527–32.

Nasojejunal feeding in critical care patients

Critical care patients are often malnourished, due to either poor nutritional status prior to admission, inadequate calorie intake for nutritional needs or a combination of both. Enteral nutrition (EN) helps the gut function normally and keeps the integrity of the mucosal barrier, and so decreases gut permeability, reducing the risk of bacteraemia and endotoxaemia.

Bacterial and toxin translocation is prevented by the barrier function of the small bowel mucosa, but this is compromised early in the disease process of critically ill patients, as demonstrated by increased gut permeability to polyethylene glycol. Studies of trauma, burns and major surgery patients have shown improved outcome with EN compared with total parenteral nutrition (TPN), and this has been replicated with those with severe acute pancreatitis. Furthermore, EN caused a reduced incidence of systemic inflammatory response syndrome (SIRS), a reduced APACHE II score, C-reactive protein (CRP) and serum IgM antiendotoxin antibodies, but an increased total antioxidant capacity.

Gastroduodenal dysmotility is a common problem in critical care and may result from the underlying illness, but also from medication such as sedatives or analgesics. Dysmotility prevents or reduces efficacy of nasogastric (NG) feeding, and large gastric residual volumes place a patient at risk of reflux, vomiting and aspiration. Nasojejunal (NJ) feeding can overcome these difficulties, and enable the patient to receive sufficient calorie intake.

Nutritional assessment and treatment

General malnutrition (protein-calorie) can be assessed from the history (anorexia, dietary history, calorie intake) and examination (muscle wasting, oedema, angular stomatitis). Objective bedside measurements can include weight loss >10% in the preceding 3 months, blood tests (albumin <35g/l, lymphocytes <1.5×10^9, transferrin <2g/l), skin fold tests (mid-triceps skin fold thickness <8mm in men and 17mm in women, and mid-arm muscle circumference <30cm on men and 26cm in women) and a BMI <$19kg/m_2$. Obese patients should receive nutritional treatment according to their ideal body weight for their height, with a 30% supplement for increased metabolic requirements in critical care settings.

There are several factors to consider for nutritional treatment:

1 Fluid balance
2 Energy from fat and carbohydrates (30–60 kcal/kg/24h)
3 Nitrogen requirements (0.16–0.35g/kg/24h)
4 Electrolytes
5 Trace elements and vitamins

Typical feeding regimes will need working out with hospital dieticians, but typical polymeric feeds are Jevity (Abbott) and Osmolite (Abbott), which comprise protein, carbohydrate, fat, vitamins and minerals. Continuous drip feeding reduces the complications of reflux, aspiration or diarrhoea. Starting rates should be in the order of 30ml/h and increased as the patient tolerates. Additional fluid needs should be provided with water. Feed containers and giving sets should be changed every 24h to prevent bacterial contamination.

Who needs NJ feeding?

Due to difficulties placing and maintaining an NJ feeding system, the NG route should be used routinely, with NJ reserved for particular cases. The main indications for a NJ feeding tube are post-gastric/oesophageal surgery and acute severe pancreatitis, but patients with gastric atony or gastoparesis, who are at risk of aspiration, may also benefit. The risk of aspiration due to NG feeding is 6.5% , whilst the risk of aspiration in NJ feeding is 2.4%. Consider percutaneous endoscopic gastrostomy (PEG) or percutaneous endoscopic jejunostomy (PEJ) in patients requiring long-term feeding (>4–6 weeks). Combining NJ feeding with a gastric aspiration port helps to reduce gastric volumes and so reduces the risk of aspiration.

Methods

1. Bedside NJ insertion

A simple NJ tube can be placed at the bedside by laying the patient at 30–45°. A motility stimulant (e.g. metoclopramide or erythromycin) can be given 30min prior to insertion for improved insertion rates. Mark off the NJ tube at the level of the stomach (40–45cm) and measure off another 25–30cm to allow insertion into the jejunum. Pass the lubricated tube down the nose into the stomach and at the first marked point blow in air to confirm placement. Roll the patient into the right lateral oblique position at the same angle for the head and continue advancing into the duodenum. Blowing in air now should produce fine rather than harsh crackles. Placement in the left lower lung in patients with pulmonary oedema or pneumonia can mimic that of air blown in the stomach. Aspirates of fluid from the duodenum and beyond should be alkaline. Push to the second mark and confirm the position using an abdominal radiograph with or without contrast.

2. Fluoroscopic insertion

Move the patient to a suitable area for radiological screening. Pass an NJ tube using a guide wire and fluoroscopic screening into the jejunum. Position can be checked at the same time.

3. Endoscopic insertion

In the critical care or endoscopy unit pass the gastroscope into the duodenum. A nasobiliary guide wire (ERCP guide wire) is passed down the biopsy channel and, once in the duodenum, pushed as far as possible past the second part into the jejunum. Remove the endoscope and maintain the wire in position either using screening or by inserting it in a stepwise fashion by as much as the endoscope is removed. Once the endoscope is removed, convert the orojejunal guide wire to an NJ wire by a naso-oral exchange. Pass a plastic tube over the guide wire in a Seldinger method into the jejunum. Check the position with a contrast abdominal radiograph or by screening, and remove the guide wire.

Evidence, disadvantages and alternative techniques

Success rates for jejunal placement remains low at 14%, so techniques to make the insertion more reliable have been developed: weighted ends, balloons and spiral corkscrews. ECG monitoring with a change in the polarity as the tube passes the pylorus gives fast placement within 15min (range 7–75) with 65% placed the first time, and a further

30% the second time. The rather expensive Cortrak system uses an external sensor to plot diagrammatically the position of the NJ tube, and an initial study found it correctly placed an NJ tube in 57/57 patients in a faster time, with reduced radiographic costs and shorter time delay to starting EN.

Fluoroscopy can help correct placement of NJ tubes but is often not feasible in the critical care setting, with the need for radiological support, a lead-lined room, being expensive and time consuming.

Endoscopy is useful as it can visualize the upper GI tract, ensuring there are no contraindications to NJ feeding. An alternative technique to the one described passes the NJ tube into the stomach, the endoscope finds it in the stomach and with forceps or a snare brings the tube through the pylorus into the duodenum and beyond towards the jejunum. Unfortunately the tube is easily dislodged on removing the endoscope so this limits its usefulness.

Troubleshooting

1 NJ tube keeps slipping
   - Try a different ended tube such as weight/ balloon/ corkscrew to keep in the jejunum with peristalsis.
   - Use a prokinetic.

2 NJ tube blocked
   - Change tube for a new one.
   - In future, flush tube after each feed, after medications and when not in use. (Unblock with water, soda water or 5% sodium bicarbonate.)
   - Do not use for non-liquid medications or use an NG tube.

3 NJ not positioning correctly
   - Check indication.
   - Seek specialist help—endoscopic or radiological.

4 Abdominal pain and distension
   - Consider slowing feed or stopping for a short period
   - Try pro-kinetics.
   - Would an NG tube satisfy feeding requirements?
   - Should patient be considered for PEG/PEJ?

Summary

- NJ tubes rarely used, but a good way of achieving nutritional goals.
- NJ tubes are difficult to place consistently and easily, though new techniques are increasingly available.
- If emergency feeding needed consider NG feeding in the short term unless vomiting or risk of aspiration.
- Enteric feeding protects gut barrier integrity, is better, cheaper and safer than TPN; but TPN may bridge the gap until enteric feeding is possible.

References

Cohen LD, Alexander DJ, Catto J, *et al.* Spontaeous transpyloric migration of a ballooned nasojejunal tube: a randomised controlled trial. *J Parenter Enteral Nutr* 2000; 24: 240–3.

Davies AR, Froomes PR, French CJ, *et al.* Randomized comparison of nasojejunal and nasogastric feeding in critically ill patients. *Crit Care Med* 2002; 30: 586–90.

Lai CW, Barlow R, Barnes M, Hawthorne AB. Bedside placement of nasojejunal tubes: a randomised-controlled trial of spiral- vs straight-ended tubes. *Clin Nutr* 2003; 22: 267–70.

Marik PE, Zaloga GP. Gastic versus post pyloric feeding: a systematic review. Crit Care 2003; 7: R46–51.

Patrick PG, Marulendra S, Kirby DF, *et al.* Endoscopic nasogastric–jejunal feeding tube placement in critically ill patients. *Gastrointest Endosc* 1997; 45: 72–6.

Pearce CB, Duncan HD. Enteral feeding. Nasogastric, nasojejunal, percutaneous endoscopic gastrostomy and jejunostomy: its indication and limitations. *Postgrad Med J* 2002; 78: 198–204.

Chapter 5

Nutrition

Chapter contents

Enteral nutrition

Is there a rationale for nutrition in the ICU?

Nutrition is an important part of intensive care medicine. This may seem self-evident, but the lack of randomized controlled clinical trials to document the usefulness of nutrition in the ICU has been pointed out. The fact that nutrition may be associated with adverse effects has led to some authors to the point where they question the use of nutrition as such in the ICU. However, the majority of intensivists are in favour of providing nutrition for their patients, basically relating to the fact that sooner or later any individual will starve to death without nutrition. The controversy will then be when and how to provide nutrition for the patients. As for many different routines in the ICU, nutrition should also be protocolized, and exceptions from protocol should be rare and well motivated. The nutritional routines should be well known by everybody working in the unit, and everybody should be well informed and hopefully unanimous behind the rationale for the particular routines used.

Who is responsible for the nutrition?

The decision when to initiate nutrition is a responsibility of the intensivist. If the individual intensivist lacks the appropriate competence, it is advisable to get in contact with a nutritional team, a dietician or any other expert, just like in other cases when the intensivist may be in need of external advice. It is important to integrate the feeding decision in the general medical strategy, taking the fluid balance, possible over- or underhydration and possible interferences with medications or other types of treatment given into account. Furthermore, the decision whether or not to use the GI tract for nutrition is another responsibility of the intensivist.

Access to the GI tract

To assess the GI function is difficult, and there is no generally accepted definition of the functionality of the GI tract. One suggestion is to evaluate the GI function in terms of whether or not enteral feeding is possible. It has been suggested that successful enteral feeding on the level of 80% of the measured energy expenditure may be a proper definition of normal GI tract function. ICU patients are most often fed by nasogastric (NG) or nasojejujunal (NJ) tubes. There are several studies comparing the two techniques, but there is no convincing evidence that one technique is superior to the other. In conjunction with surgical procedures, it is sometimes possible to insert a percutaneous feeding jejunostomy, which might be helpful post-operatively in cases of upper GI tract surgery. There is reasonably good evidence that an early start of enteral feeding is associated with a high success rate. This observation is true regardless of feeding technique or placement of feeding tube.

Energy deficit

Recently there is accumulating evidence that a cumulated energy deficit in long-staying ICU patients is a predictor of morbidity and even mortality. Energy deficit is the difference between measured or estimated energy expenditure and the provided calories. A cumulated energy deficit of >10 000kcal has in several studies been shown to be associated with a high level of morbidity, even when adjusting for underlying pathology. Unfortunately an energy deficit cannot be compensated for later on, and very often the major part of an energy deficit is built up during the initial 2 weeks of ICU stay. This is unfortunate because during the initial period of ICU stay, it is usually quite difficult to predict which patients are going to be the real long-stayers. If this could be predicted with a high accuracy, this would not be a problem, but unfortunately it is difficult and, once the accumulated energy deficit is developed, it will stay as a burden of depletion for the patients. Overfeeding later on will worsen the problem rather than help.

When to start nutrition

Whenever the decision is taken to feed the intensive care patient, the feeding should be with a complete formula containing all macronutrients regardless of whether the feeding is by the enteral or parenteral route. There are several standard formulas enriched with the proper vitamins and trace elements available on the market, usually with a high content of fibres. Similarly there are several all-in-one combinations for parenteral nutrition (PN) to which there are supplements available containing water- and fat-soluble vitamins as well as trace elements. For most patients, these standard formulations are the most appropriate nutrition. For patients with excessive losses from fistulas as well as in burn injuries, there might be an elevated need for trace elements as well as for antioxidants. When patients are fed by the enteral route only, the success rate of enteral feeding is usually on the level 60–70%. This may not be a big problem if the ICU stay will be less than a week with a perspective of resuming ordinary food intake within a short time. However, if 100% of energy expenditure cannot be reached before the energy deficit gets out of hand, it is difficult not to give complementary parenteral feeding to meet the nutritional target. The length of stay is here the crucial factor. There presently is not sufficient documentation to show that a combination of enteral and parenteral feeding to meet the nutritional target will decrease morbidity and mortality. The reason for this is that no such studies are at hand. Still, this is an often advocated strategy for nutritional support in the long-staying ICU patient.

How to estimate the caloric need

The best way to estimate the caloric needs is to perform indirect calorimetry. If such readings are available, dosage of nutrition is no problem. However, in many institutions, this is not possible. Second best then is to have a measurement of carbon dioxide production, which under stable circumstances can give a good estimate. However, overfeeding may give erroneously high values of energy expenditure based on carbon dioxide production, which it is not possible to discover without access to a calculated respiratory quotient. In most cases it is advisable to start up with 20kcal/kg in elderly people >65 years old and 25kcal/kg for younger people. Later on during ICU stay, some patients may develop an extreme hypermetabolism, which sometimes can be difficult to detect. If this hypermetabolism is not recognised and appropriately treated, an extreme accumulated energy deficit may develop, which has a high risk to be detrimental to the patient. Consequently for extreme long-stayers with multiple organ failure access to indirect calorimetry or at least a carbon dioxide production measurement may be crucial.

A nutritional protocol

In general terms, a robust feeding algorithm is to be preferred over a diversified feeding regimen for different underlying disorders. The advantage of specific feeding routines for specific patient groups is not impressive. Still in addition to standard feeds for enteral or parenteral use, there are specific nutrients. Best documented in terms of morbidity and mortality is supplementation with glutamine. For patients needing PN, supplementation with IV glutamine containing dipeptides is demonstrated to give a survival advantage. This is therefore recommended in most guidelines for patients on PN. Glutamine supplementation for patients on enteral nutrition (EN) is more controversial.

Specific nutritional formulations

On the European market there are today a number of different fat emulsions. All of them are demonstrated to be well tolerated, and several offer considerable theoretical advantages. Unfortunately there are presently no clinical studies with clinically relevant end-points that show a preference for any specific IV fat emulsion.

For enteral use there are omega-3 fatty acid-enriched formulas, which in a few recent single-centre studies have been demonstrated to provide advantages in terms of both morbidity and mortality in ICU patients who tolerate enteral feeding. The underlying mechanism is claimed to be that omega-3 fatty acids have anti-inflammatory properties. Although the documentation for these new products has been criticized, the dramatic effect shown cannot be ignored. Available studies are not conclusive as the control formula used has a very high lipid content. More conclusive studies will be needed before a general recommendation can be made concerning the omega-3-enriched formulas.

Further reading

Heidegger CP, Romand JA, Treggiari MM, *et al.* Is it now time to promote mixed enteral and parenteral nutrition for the critically ill patient? *Intensive Care Med* 2007; 33: 963–9.

Simpson F, Doig GS. Parenteral vs. enteral nutrition in the critically ill patient: a meta-analysis of trials using the intention to treat principle. *Intensive Care Med* 2005; 31: 12–23.

Villet S, Chiolero RL, Bollmann MD, et al. Negative impact of hypocaloric feeding and energy balance on clinical outcome in ICU patients. *Clin Nutr* 2005; 24: 502–9.

Wernerman J. Intensive care unit nutrition—nonsense or neglect? *Crit Care* 2005; 9: 251–2.

Wernerman J. Guidelines for nutritional support in intensive care unit patients: a critical analysis. *Curr Opin Clin Nutr Metab Care* 2005; 8: 171–5.

Parenteral nutrition

Nutrition is an essential component of the supportive therapies offered by intensive therapy units (ITUs). Nutritional support improves wound healing, decreases the catabolic response to injury and improves clinical outcomes, including a reduction in complication rates and length of stay.

Enteral nutrition (EN) is preferred over parenteral nutrition (PN) because EN has lower infectious complications, is easier to use and cheaper. However, not all patients are suitable for EN.

Indications

- Gastrointestinal failure of any cause (e.g. major abdominal surgery, trauma or sepsis with a consequent prolonged ileus, short bowel syndrome, enteral fistulae).
- PN may be required in acute pancreatitis (although EN via a jejunal feeding tube has a significantly lower risk of infectious complications, and shorter duration of hospitalization, consequently EN is preferred).
- Inability to absorb EN.

Commencement

There is some evidence that early nutrition has a mortality benefit over delayed nutrition. Consequently PN should be commenced during the first 24–48h of an ITU admission if EN is contraindicated. If EN is not absorbed (including after a trial of promotility agents) then PN should be commenced as soon as possible because PN may have survival advantages over delayed EN (>7 days).

Cessation

Daily review of PN continuation is required. There may be a period where EN and PN are co-administered while establishing EN. Once GI function has recovered, PN is best withdrawn over a period of 24–48h to avoid rebound hypoglycaemia. If rapid cessation of PN is required, frequent blood glucose monitoring is required and a 5% dextrose infusion should be used to maintain normoglycaemia.

Dose

The daily calorie requirement of patients in ITU is difficult to assess. Important in the assessment is a nutritional history, underlying medical conditions and presenting problems to the ITU. Anthropomorphic measurements can be used; however, they can be difficult and unreliable in ITU patients. Measurements of serum albumin, prealbumin, ferritin and lymphocytes are all unreliable as they are independently impacted upon by acute illness. Other methods to assess caloric requirements include predictive equations such as the Harris–Benedict equation and indirect calorimetry. Urinary nitrogen can be measured to assess protein losses; however, given that protein loss varies on a day-to-day basis, the delay in measurement and altering the make-up of the PN bag makes this impractical.

Burns, major trauma and sepsis are all hypermetabolic and catabolic states. Major burns may increase the caloric requirement by up to 150% of baseline and increase protein catabolism.

Given the difficulties in estimating an individual's caloric requirements, many practitioners give 25–30kcal/kg/day and alter the dose depending on individual patient circumstances as this has been shown to be as accurate as more complex approaches.

Requirements

Electrolytes (/kg/day)

Water	30ml
Sodium	1–2mmol
Potassium	0.7–1mmol
Calcium	0.1mmol
Magnesium	0.1mmol
Phosphorus	0.4mmol

Carbohydrate

3–4g/kg/day

Glucose is the optimal carbohydrate in PN and should provide ~60% of non-protein calories.

Lipid

Approximately 40% of non-protein calories should derive from lipid. Lipids are essential for cellular homeostasis and immune function. Lipids are available as long chain triglycerides or medium chain triglycerides, and mixtures of the two. There is insufficient evidence at present to suggest that any single lipid formulation provides a clinically significant benefit over others.

Protein

1–1.5g/kg/day, 1.5–2g/kg/day for patients with catabolic illnesses including burns.

Protein should be a mixture of essential and non-essential amino acids. A recent meta-analysis suggests that glutamine as part of a PN regime may give a survival benefit, although it will not decrease infectious complications. As yet no clinically significant benefit has been demonstrated with branched chain amino acids.

Vitamins and essential elements (daily requirement)

The optimal requirement for vitamins and essential elements in the critically ill or in PN is unclear. The recommended daily allowance of vitamins and essential elements is (Food and Drug Administration):

Vitamin A	700–900mcg
Vitamin D	5mcg
Vitamin E	15mcg
Vitamin C	75–90mg
Vitamin K	90–120mcg
Folic acid	400mcg
Nicotinamide	40mg
Riboflavin	1.3mg
Niacin	16mg
Thiamine	1.2mg
Pyridoxine	1.3mg
Cobalamin	2.4mcg
Pantothenic acid	5mg
Biotin	30mcg
Chromium	20–35mcg
Copper	900mcg
Fluoride	3–4mg
Iodine	150mcg

Iron	8–18mg
Manganese	1.8–2.3mg
Molybdenum	45mcg
Selenium	55mcg
Zinc	8–11mg

There is evidence that the use of selenium and antioxidants to supplement PN improves mortality without decreasing infection rates, ITU length of stay or length of ventilator dependence. Consequently supplementation of PN with selenium and antioxidants may be considered. Supplementation with zinc above baseline requirements has not been shown to improve mortality.

Formulations

Standard formulations of PN are available in combination bags that require thorough mixing before infusion. Most formulations contain ~40% of non-protein calories as lipid, and 60% as carbohydrate with added amino acids, vitamins and trace elements. Most formulations can have the electrolyte concentration altered depending on clinical circumstances, and additional trace elements and vitamins may be added.

Investigation

Daily

- Blood glucose estimation 1–4 hourly as indicated by blood glucose stability
- Electrolytes (including calcium, magnesium, phosphate, sodium, potassium, urea)
- Liver function tests
- Full blood count
- Coagulation screen

Monthly

- Trace elements (selenium, zinc, molybdenum, manganese, copper, iron)

Complications

Relating to access

- Complications of insertion
- Catheter-related bloodstream infection
- Central vein thrombosis

Relating to infusions

- Infection rates are increased in PN compared with EN.
- Liver abnormalities: incudes hepatic steatosis and cholestasis, and hepatic failure may rarely occur. The incidence of hepatic problems varies with duration of PN. Steatosis and cholestasis may relate to excessive caloric provision, but there is evidence that choline deficiency may be important. Both hepatic steatosis and cholestasis usually follow a benign course, although they may require reduction in PN rate.
- Hyperglycaemia: there is increasing evidence that strict glucose control in critical illness leads to reduced morbidity and mortality (from 8 to 4.6%) in surgical patients with blood glucose maintained from 4.4 to6.1mmol/l.
- Rebound hypoglycaemia with sudden cessation of PN infusions.
- Refeeding syndrome: monitor potassium, magnesium, phosphate and calcium levels, especially in patients who are malnourished
- Lipaemia: if lipaemia is a significant problem the rate of PN can be reduced or the lipid component reduced or removed.

Relating to deficiencies

Common deficiencies are thiamine (wet or dry beri-beri or lactic acidosis) or vitamin K (hypocoagulable states); however, all vitamins and trace element deficiencies may develop. Patients on RRT are particularly at risk of deficiencies of water-soluble vitamins.

Further reading

Atkinson M, Worthley LIG. Nutrition in the critically ill patient: Part I. Essential physiology and pathophysiology. *Crit Care Resus* 2003; 5: 109–20.

Buchman A. Total parenteral nutrition-associated liver disease. *J Parenter Enteral Nutr* 2002; 26: S43–8.

Heyland DK, Dhaliwal R, Drover J, *et al.* Canadian clinical practice guidelines for nutrition support in mechanically ventilated, critically ill adult patients. *J Parenter Enteral Nutr* 2003; 27: 355–73.

Heyland DK, Dhaliwal R, Suchner U, *et al.* Antioxidant nutrients: a systematic review of trace elements and vitamins in the critically ill patient. *Intensive Care Med* 2005; 31: 327–37.

Marik PE, Zaloga GP. Meta-analysis of parenteral nutrition versus enteral nutrition in patients with acute pancreatitis. *BMJ* 2004; 328: 1407–12.

Simpson F, Doig GS. Parenteral vs. enteral nutrition in the critically ill patient: a meta-analysis of trials using the intention to treat principle. *Intensive Care Med* 2005; 31: 12–23.

Immune-enhancing nutrition

Immune-enhancing nutrition (IEN) describes feeds that are enriched with specific 'functional' nutrients thought to augment or modify beneficially immune function and the inflammatory response in order to improve clinical outcome. This is particularly pertinent in the ICU patient where the relationship between malnutrition, immune deficiency and nosocomial infection has long been recognized. Nutrients considered 'immune-enhancing' include the amino acids arginine and glutamine, omega-3 (ω3) fatty acids, dietary nucleotides and antioxidant vitamins and minerals, usually combined within IEN.

Their immune-modifying effects appear to be dose dependent, confounding clinical outcome measures generated from intention-to-treat (ITT) results vs subgroup analysis based on delivery of an arbitrary 'threshold' of feed delivery. Research on IEN includes formulated immune-enhancing feeds or the *ad hoc* addition of one or more nutrients to an enteral formula. Such heterogeneity of IEN makes global recommendations for use difficult.

Standard feeds and immune effect

A confounding factor of IEN is that standard feeds *per se* attenuate injury-related catabolism, maintain structural and functional integrity of the GI tract, reduce infectious complications and improve wound healing rates. Early enteral feeding (i.e. within 24h of ICU admission) is associated with a significant reduction in infectious complications. Feeding within 48h of ICU admission significantly reduces ICU mortality by 20% and hospital mortality by 25% in ventilated medical patients despite being independently associated with risk of ventilator-associated pneumonia. This beneficial reduction in mortality exceeds that currently achieved by the use of IEN.

Immune-modifying nutrients

L-Arginine

L-Arginine is a 'conditionally essential' amino acid during metabolic stress and sepsis. Low circulating L-arginine levels give rise to the views of sepsis as an L-arginine-deficient state or a syndrome of excess nitric oxide, a vasoactive product of L-arginine metabolism.

Arginine upregulates macrophage phagocytic activity and neutrophil production of reactive oxygen species (such as peroxynitrite). High level supplementation (above 12g/l) reduces infectious complications and enhances wound healing in elective surgery, but conversely can augment rather than subdue the inflammatory response.

Glutamine

The most abundant circulating amino acid in the extracellular and intracellular compartments becomes 'conditionally essential' during critical illness as plasma glutamine levels fall.

Several controlled studies and a meta-analysis have confirmed glutamine's beneficial influence on the inflammatory response, oxidative stress and gut integrity. The preferred energy substrate for rapidly dividing enterocytes and immune cells, it may also improve glucose metabolism by reducing insulin resistance, and is also a precursor of glutathione.

Supplementary enteral glutamine fails to demonstrate clear clinical benefit, except in the trauma or burns patient where it is a recommended addition.

Omega-3 polyunsaturates

The omega-3 (ω3) long chain polyunsaturated fatty acids (PUFAs) eicosopentanoic acid (EPA) and docosohexanoic acid (DHA) generate potent immunomodulatory activities via direct competition with arachidonic acid—an ω6 PUFA—in the production of eicosanoids. Eicosanoids derived from ω3 PUFAs such as prostacyclin PGI_3 and leukotriene B_5 (LTB_5) downregulate inflammatory processes, in contrast to the proinflammatory eicosanoids derived from ω6 PUFAs, such as LTB_4. Competitive suppression of LTB_4 reduces monocyte generation of key inflammatory mediators such as cytokines IL-1β, IL-6 and tumour necrosis factor (TNF), ameliorating inflammatory eicosanoid production. ω3 PUFAs offset the proinflammatory effects of high-dose arginine-supplemented IEN.

GLA (γ-linolenic acid)

Metabolism of GLA (an ω6 PUFA) to di-homo-γ-linolenic acid (DGLA) blocks formation of proinflammatory leukotrienes from arachidonic acid metabolites. DGLA is the precursor of the less inflammatory prostaglandin E_1 and thromboxane A_1, and augments the effect of long-chain ω3 PUFAs.

Nucleotides

Required by rapidly dividing cells, nucleotides improve immune parameters in experimental animal models and supplemented neonatal feeds. There is no evidence that nucleotides alone confer benefit to the critically ill patient except when included within IEN formula.

Antioxidant micronutrients

Emerging evidence suggests a reduction in 28 day mortality in surgical ICU patients given continuous EN with supplementary infusions of vitamins C and E. Selenium infusions may reduce the mortality rate in patients with septic shock and severe sepsis.

Patient groups

Medical patients

Patients with primary lung failure from chest infection or smoke inhalation injury have an increased mortality with IEN. IEN does not appear to benefit this group.

Pre-surgical patient

Pre-operative IEN given to upper GI cancer patients reduces post-operative infectious complications, but not mortality. ITT evidence is currently less than compelling and there are significant flaws in the design of recent studies.

Post-surgical patient

The incidence of acquired infection and hospital length of stay (LOS) are significantly reduced in elective surgery patients given IEN, although reduction in septic complication rates are non-significant and overall mortality rates similar. Patients requiring ICU whilst being fed IEN demonstrated a trend for increased mortality.

Trauma

Trauma patients are likely to be the most well nourished of critical care patients. IEN lowers the incidence of bacteraemias and intra-abdominal infections, but other infectious complications remain unchanged.

Sepsis

The potential benefit of L-arginine-enriched IEN is limited to mild sepsis (APACHE II score 10–20) rather than those with a pre-existing enhanced inflammatory response present (i.e. severe sepsis or SIRS). Subgroup analysis confirms a significantly higher mortality in septic patients receiving IEN compared with control feed. Comparing IEN with parenteral nutrition, subgroup analysis of severely septic patients demonstrated a 3-fold increase in mortality compared with controls.

ARDS

High-fat respiratory feeds reduce $PaCO_2$ and VCO_2 in ALI and ARDS by altering the respiratory quotient and metabolic load of the feed. Use of an IEN respiratory feed (rich in ω3 EPA and ω6 GLA plus antioxidant vitamins) vs a 'standard' respiratory formula to address the underlying inflammatory pathogenesis of ARDS significantly reduced ventilator days, incidence of organ failure and ICU LOS, with a trend towards reduced mortality, despite significant patient heterogeneity.

Summary

Globally, IEN reduces the risk of infection complications, time on mechanical ventilation, ICU LOS and hospital LOS in selected patient groups, but has no appreciable effect on mortality. Variations in the nutrient profile of IEN feeds (particularly with regard to the level of arginine supplementation), errors in trial design, underpowered studies and *post hoc* interpretation of trial results all create difficulties in recommending IEN to the heterogenous ICU population. The influence of early and appropriate enteral feeding *per se* may be of greater clinical relevance than IEN on positive outcomes in the critically ill patient.

Further reading

Angstwurm MW, Engelmann L, Zimmermann T, *et al.* Selenium in Intensive Care (SIC): results of a prospective randomized, placebo-controlled, multiple-center study in patients with severe systemic inflammatory response syndrome, sepsis, and septic shock. *Crit Care Med* 2007; 35: 118–26.

Coëffier M, Déchelotte P. The role of glutamine in intensive care unit patients: mechanisms of action and clinical outcome. *Nutr Rev* 2005; 63: 65–9.

Crimi E, Liguori A, Condorelli M, *et al.* The beneficial effects of antioxidant supplementation in enteral feeding in critically ill patients: a prospective, randomized, double-blind, placebo-controlled trial. *Anesth Analg* 2004; 99: 857–63.

Kalil AC, Danner RL. L-Arginine supplementation in sepsis: beneficial or harmful? *Curr Opin Crit Care* 2006; 12: 303–8.

Kieft H, Roos AN, van Drunen JD, *et al.* Clinical outcome of immunonutrition in a heterogeneous intensive care population. *Intens Care Med* 2005; 31: 524–32.

Kreymann KG, Berger MM, Deutz NE, *et al.* ESPEN guidelines on enteral nutrition: intensive care. *Clin Nutr* 2006; 25: 210–23.

McCowen KC, Bistrian BR. Immunonutrition: problematic or problem solving? *Am J Clin Nutr* 2003; 77: 764–70.

Montejo JC, Zarazaga A, Lopez-Martinez J, *et al.* Immunonutrition in the intensive care unit. A systematic review and consensus statement. *Clin Nutr* 2003; 22: 221–33.

Sakr Y, Reinhart K, Bloos F, *et al.* Time course and relationship between plasma selenium concentrations, systemic inflammatory response, sepsis, and multiorgan failure. *Br J Anaesth* 2007; 98: 775-84.

Chapter 6

Respiratory monitoring

Chapter contents

Pulmonary function tests in critical illness

Introduction

Pulmonary function test results in critically ill patients can be important prognostically and guide ventilatory and weaning strategies. However, they are not straightforward to measure in mechanically ventilated patients and remain limited to dynamic volumes. Fortunately, most modern mechanical ventilators are able to calculate and display static and dynamic lung volumes, together with derived values for airway resistance, compliance and flow/volume/time curves. The ability to monitor these changes after altering ventilatory parameters has enabled more sophisticated adjustments of ventilation, to prevent potentially damaging mechanical ventilation.

Spirometry measures dynamic lung volumes. This is most useful when assessing the severity of obstructive lung diseases (especially asthma, COPD and obliterative bronchiolitis).

Lung volume measurements by body box plethysmography (gold standard) or helium dilution (prone to under-representation in bullous lung disease or significant gas trapping) detect hyperexpansion or restrictive lung diseases (i.e. small lungs, inflammation or fibrotic lung disease, or abnormalities of the muscles or skeleton of the chest wall).

Lung function tests on mechanically ventilated patients

A number of factors should be considered when performing lung function on the ICU. Such patients are invariably sedated, excluding volitional tests. They are not easily moved, and may not be in an ideal upright position. Their high oxygen requirements may also affect accurate gas exchange measurements. However, the presence of an artificial airway simplifies the measurement of lung volumes and pressure–volume relationships. Those on mandatory modes of mechanical ventilation may be unable to perform a vital capacity (VC) manoeuvre, although a passive complete pressure–volume (P–V) loop will be possible.

Measuring pulmonary mechanics

Lung volumes and VC

Portable spirometers allow bedside measures of VC and forced expiratory volume (FEV) in spontaneously breathing extubated patients. For intubated patients, a pneumotachograph (which measures VC through an accurate flow sensor) is preferred. These values usually will be effort dependent, and may be underestimates possibly due to inadequate effort, underlying lung disease or muscle weakness. A VC of >10ml/kg is a reasonable indicator of the need for assisted ventilatory support in those with neuromuscular disease such as Guillian–Barre syndrome. However, trend monitoring of declining VC, with symptomatic hypercapnic acidosis, is often a more practical marker of the need for intervention in these situations. VC monitoring is less useful for predicting need for ventilatory assistance or successful weaning in other conditions.

Functional residual capacity (FRC) has been measured using a number of different techniques such as simple helium dilution (rebreathing 6 breaths from a 1litre 'bag-in bottle' system), nitrogen washout or prolonged inert gas dilution. FRC (normally 2–3l) is frequently reduced in ventilated patients, for such reasons as supine position, sedatives, neuromuscular blocking agents, abdominal distension and underlying lung disease (e.g. atelectasis, consolidation, pulmonary oedema). Monitoring such measurements (if practical) can help assess the effectiveness of therapeutic strategies such as chest physiotherapy and lung expansion manoeuvres (i.e. recruitment and PEEP).

Compliance and resistance

In a well sedated patient with an indwelling endotracheal tube (ETT), measurements of total respiratory compliance (Crs), airway resistance (Raw) and respiratory resistance (Rrs) can be made during constant flow ventilation. Airway pressure at the proximal end of the ETT (termed pressure at airway opening, Pao), during a brief post-inspiratory pause at varying volumes (between FRC and total lung capacity (TLC)) through the inspiratory cycle, enables plots of volume against Pao, and pressure change against flow to calculate Crs, Raw and Rrs, respectively.

Normal values for Crs are >100ml/cm H_2O. In ALI and ARDS, Crs is often <25ml/H_2O. Monitoring these measurements may allow optimization of ventilatory manoeuvres such as recruitment, and applying PEEP. For example, at the onset of inspiration, as airway pressure is increased, the slope on the V–P curve suddenly increases at the lower inflection point. This represents the improved compliance at closing volume. As pressure is increased, an upper inflection point is encountered where compliance tends to fall again, reflecting overinflation. The optimal airway pressures are between these two points, and so Crs measures and V–P loops may be used to adjust mechanically imposed volumes and pressures between these points, so improving gas exchange and reducing ventilator-induced lung injury.

Airway resistance (Raw) measurements are useful for considering the causes of increased Raw. Normal values in spontaneously breathing patients are <2.5 l/s cmH_2O/l/s. In a normally ventilated patient, this may rise to ~4. In cardiogenic pulmonary oedema, this may be>10, ARDS >15 and obstructive airways disease >20 cmH_2O/l/s.

Intrinsic PEEP (PEEPi)

Intrinsic or auto-PEEP describes the increase in end-tidal alveolar pressure whenever the expiratory time is inadequate to allow the lung to deflate to its relaxation volume. PEEPi occurs if expiratory resistance is increased (i.e. airflow obstruction) or if expiratory time is too short. It is measured with the proximal pressure transducer during an end-expiratory occlusion manoeuvre. At no flow, a positive Pao reflects static PEEPi. A dynamic measurement of PEEPi can be recorded by the airway pressure at which inspiratory flow commences in spontaneously breathing or assisted modes. Dynamic hyperinflation can arise, leading to increased work of breathing (in spontaneous ventilation), reduced ability to trigger the ventilator in assisted modes, increased intrathoracic pressures and consequences, and risks of volu-barotrauma.

If the reduction of PEEPi is deemed beneficial, treating the underlying cause, adjusting ventilation or the application of external PEEP (with cautious monitoring of PEEPi and other parameters of dynamic hyperinflation) are warranted.

Respiratory muscle testing

Bedside assessment of respiratory muscle testing in the ICU may allow prediction of prolonged weaning. The ability to sustain spontaneous breathing is governed by respiratory drive, respiratory muscle strength and endurance, and respiratory muscle loading (combination of resistance, compliance and PEEPi). Respiratory muscle weakness is common during prolonged mechanical ventilation. It is commonly due to the consequences of critical illness such as muscle wasting, critical illness myoneuropathy, malnutrition, hypercatabolism, iatrogenic causes (e.g non-depolarizing blocking agents and steroids, or prolonged neuromuscular blockade) and, less commonly, due to primary neuromuscular disorders.

Strategies

Respiratory drive can be assessed by measuring airway pressure 0.1s after occluding the airway against an inspiratory effort (P0.1). Most modern ventilators have this option. This represents neuromuscular activation of the respiratory system and correlates with the work of breathing. A high value P0.1 >6cm H_2O may imply an unsustainable work of breathing, and is used as one of a number of indicators of failure to wean to extubation. Very low values of P0.1 reflect inadequate drive and probaby weaning failure.

Non-volitional techniques for measuring diaphragm strength are now available on the ICU. They utilize a combination of external magnetic stimulators of the phrenic nerves, with oesopheageal and gastric pressure transducers, thus allowing transdiaphragmatic pressure change (PDi) measurements.

Weaning predictors

Tests of respiratory muscle function have greatest application in the prediction of weaning outcome. Predictors, such as maximum inspiratory pressure, VC and minute ventilation, are frequently falsely positive and negative. Although patients failing a weaning trial may have an elevated pressure–time index and P0.1, these tests have not gained popularity in everyday ICU practice.

The ratio of *respiratory frequency to tidal volume (f/V)* is the most reliable simple predictor of weaning outcome. Thus, a value <80 provides a high likelihood ratio (>7.5) of successful weaning. In contrast, values >105 may suggest a further period of weaning.

Assessment of gas exchange

A wide range of indices of gas exchange efficiency have been proposed, such that arterial blood gas tension (PaO_2) can be assessed at differing concentrations of inspired oxygen(FiO_2).

The PaO_2:FiO_2 ratio is one criterion used to define ALI (<40kpa) and ARDS (<27kPa).

The oxygenation index is another measure that is the product of mean airway pressure, FiO_2 divided by PaO_2. The oxygenation index takes into account ventilatory adjustments and is said to predict outcomes better in paediatric acute respiratory failure than PaO_2:FiO_2.

Venous admixture and shunt

In a lung with abnormal gas exchange, regions with little or poor gas exchange act (e.g. consolidation or collapse) as shunts, and the oxygen tension of mixed venous blood, which is added essentially unchanged to arterial blood, governs PaO_2 to a large extent. Mixed venous PaO_2 reflects peripheral oxygen delivery and consumption. An estimate of venous admixture and shunt is possible with simultaneous sampling of mixed venous, pulmonary arterial and arterial blood. However, practical uses are limited.

Pulmonary function as an outcome predictor in the critically ill

Pulmonary function testing is useful for evaluation of different forms of lung disease or for assessing the presence of disease in a patient with known risk factors, such as smoking. Other indications include:

- Evaluation of symptoms such as chronic persistent cough
- Objective assessment of bronchodilator therapy
- Addressing occupational exposures
- Pre-operative risk assessment prior to thoracic or upper abdominal surgery
- Objective assessment of impairment or disability.

Poorer FEV_1 predicts an increased likelihood of post-operative pulmonary complications, particularly in those with COPD.

A lower gas transfer coefficient (TLCO), and greater rate of decline preceding critical illness, predict an increased mortality in patients with diffuse parenchymal lung disease.

Summary

Pulmonary function testing serves as an important tool in critical illness. Prior information and serial decline can predict worse outcomes from intercurrent critical illness, particularly if associated with the underlying chronic lung condition. Measurements and interpretation of static and dynamic lung function in the critically ill can also provide opportunities to recognize deterioration, optimize ventilatory assistance and predict weaning.

Further reading

Overview of pulmonary function testing. www.uptodate.com
http://www.thoracic.org/sections/publications/statements/

End-tidal CO_2 monitoring

End-tidal carbon dioxide monitoring is now advised for all ventilated patients on a critical care unit and is essential monitoring for the transfer of such patients both within and between hospitals. Whilst useful for monitoring of the presence of ventilation, capnography can also offer other important and valuable information to the critical care practitioner.

There are two types of commonly used gaseous carbon dioxide monitoring used in clinical practice.

Capnography

The instantaneous graphical record of carbon dioxide (CO_2) concentration in the respired gases during respiration.

Capnometry

The measurement and display of CO_2 concentrations on a digital or analogue indicator.

Both methods can be employed in the critical care environment. Analysis of the CO_2 concentration and waveform can help in the management of both the respiratory and cardiovascular systems.

Measurement techniques

Capnography

Four main methods are used to measure CO_2 concentration in respiratory gases: mass spectrography, Raman spectrography, photoacoustic spectrography and, most commonly, infrared spectrography. This final method uses the physical principle that polyatomic gases absorb infrared light. CO_2 selectively absorbs light at a specific wavelength of 4.3μm. The absorption of this wavelength of light is proportional to the concentration of CO_2 molecules and, by comparing them with a known standard, the concentration can be displayed—usually as a partial pressure (mmHg or kPa).

Capnometry

A pH-sensitive chemical indicator in a plastic housing placed in the system between the ETT and the method of ventilation. Exposure to CO_2 causes a change in the paper's colour: purple to yellow. The degree of colour change permits approximation of the CO_2 concentration; however, it cannot be used for accurate measurement.

Location of CO_2 monitors

Capnometers are classified as side-stream or main-stream, depending on the position of the sensor relative to the gas delivery system. Both have advantages and disadvantages.

Side-stream

The senor is located distal to the patient. The gas is sampled through capillary tubing attached to the distal end of the ventilation apparatus, as close to the subject's airway as possible. This may be a T-piece inserted into a breathing system, or a luer lock on an HME. The tubing can also be inserted into the nostril of a spontaneously breathing patient. Optimal gas flow is considered to be 50–200ml/min, which needs to be considered if using expired gas flow to measure tidal volume. It also causes a delay in reading of ~150ms.

Main-stream

Mounted on the breathing system, the capnometer consists of an infrared generator and sensor within a cuvette through which the respiratory gases pass. The sensors are heated to 39°C to prevent water condensation that may produce falsely elevated readings. Care is required as the heat can cause facial burns. The additional weight of the apparatus on the breathing system can cause traction on the ETT. Unlike the side-stream method, the main-stream technique provides immediate readings with respiration.

The capnogram waveform

The normal capnogram is usually displayed at 7mm/s. It has a waveform that is divided in to three phases.

- I Carbon dioxide-free phase. Anatomical dead space and that of the breathing system, HME, catheter mount.
- II An S-shaped upswing which denotes mixed dead space and alveolar gases.
- III A plateau phase due to alveolar emptying. The normal plateau often has a slight upward slope; the highest point of this slope is the end-tidal CO_2 partial pressure ($PetCO_2$) and, if the slope has achieved a plateau, is the closest approximation of the partial pressure of arterial CO_2 ($PaCO_2$).

Volumetric capnography

Plotting the partial pressure of expired CO_2 ($PECO_2$) against time does not account for expiratory flow. Whilst giving useful information about the presence of ventilation and an estimate of the $PaCO_2$, the inclusion of flow measurement allows for a greater amount of pulmonary physiology to be detected and applied in management. This leads to the use of volumetric capnography based on the single breath test for CO_2 (SBT-CO_2). It differs from standard capnography by the integration of gas flow to produce a graph of $PECO_2$ against volume rather than time. The SBT-CO_2 gives more information on the ventilation/perfusion (V/Q) status of the lung.

Clinical applications of capnography

The use of capnography has been a standard requirement for monitoring at induction of general anaesthesia. It is now a requirement for monitoring of ventilated patients on the ICU and transport of ventilated patients both intrahospital and interhospital.

Confirmation of endotracheal intubation

The presence of a capnogram aids in the identification of an appropriately placed ETT, and is mandatory for oral or nasal tubes and tracheostomy. Following intubation, six expired CO_2 waves need to be observed to confirm correct placement, as oesophageal and gastric CO_2 may be present from bag and mask ventilation, the presence of carbonated drinks, etc. The use of capnometry for such procedures is acceptable, but caution must be observed as tracheal secretions or gastric contents may contaminate the capnometer, interfering with its chemical reaction and causing it to read positive for CO_2 in error.

Presence and adequacy of ventilation

The presence of a regular capnogram of correct morphology allows continuous monitoring of ventilation. This is in preference to the display of the $PetCO_2$ value alone. Accidental disconnection or extubation, endotracheal obstruction, ETT cuff leak and ventilator malfunction can all be detected due to a change in the morphology of the capnogram.

Capnography can be used to monitor ventilation in the spontaneously ventilating subject. Sampling can be undertaken at the nose, by adaptation of the nasal cannulae, or by placing the sampling line within the face mask. When oxygen is concurrently at low flow rates, the $PetCO_2$ is a good predictor of $PaCO_2$. At high oxygen flow rates, the mixing with the exhaled gases leads to under-reading of the $PetCO_2$. In patients at high risk of apnoea, e.g. type II COPD, neuromuscular disorders, CO_2 monitoring can contribute to a prompt response in the event of hypopnoea or respiratory arrest.

If neuromuscular blockade is being used, then CO_2 monitoring can aid assessment of its adequacy. Breathing by the patient during mandatory ventilation leads to a characteristic dip within phase III; the so-called 'curare cleft'. Titration of paralysing therapy to prevent this phenomenon can be achieved as a goal and can lead to lower dose requirements.

Estimation of $PaCO_2$

In normal individuals, the difference between $PaCO_2$ and $PetCO_2$, the (a-et)PCO_2 is between 2 and 5mm Hg. It increases with age and disorders that may increase anatomical or alveolar dead space, e.g. COPD, pulmonary embolism, low cardiac output and mechanical ventilation itself. It decreases with large tidal volume low frequency ventilation, as well as in pregnancy and in young children.

Because of this potential variability, it is best to have a concurrent assessment of the $PaCO_2$. Ongoing monitoring can then use the $PetCO_2$ as a surrogate. Dynamic changes in the patient's cardiovascular or pulmonary condition may result in a change in the (a-et)PCO_2, so the $PetCO_2$ cannot be ubiquitously relied on as a guide to $PaCO_2$. Though a raised $PetCO_2$ does usually signify a raised $PaCO_2$, the contrary is not always true.

Cardiovascular status

The delivery of CO_2 to the lungs and the regional perfusion of the alveoli are reflected in the partial pressure of CO_2 in the alveoli. If ventilation remains constant (V), then changes in perfusion (Q) will result in a change in $PECO_2$. This has been demonstrated clinically in both dynamic changes in cardiac output and the detection of pulmonary embolism. Changes that occur in hypermetabolic states such as thryotoxicosis or severe sepsis can increase $PECO_2$ as a reflection of the increase in tissue CO_2 production. A novel method of cardiac output monitoring, the partial rebreathing technique (PRCO), uses a variation of the indirect Fick method. Studies suggest that there is good correlation between this method and other standards. This may have a role as a non-invasive alternative in the mechanically ventilated patient.

Capnography also has a role at cardiac arrest. It reflects well the adequacy of resuscitation. $PetCO_2$ values of <10mm Hg at 20min post-resuscitation are associated with significant mortality. Return of a spontaneous circulation can be signified by a sudden increase in $PetCO_2$.

Alveolar recruitment and PEEP

The application of PEEP as a method to recruit and maintain the patency of collapsed alveoli is a strategy that can be used in respiratory failure, particularly ALI. Dead space is initially large in ALI, as reflected by a high (a-et)PCO_2. The application of PEEP has been shown to reduce this gradient. Other studies have demonstrated that titration of PEEP does not improve (a-et)PCO_2 in all cases of ALI/ARDS. However, the gradient reduces in those that have a demonstrable inflection point on the pressure–volume curve, and those patients that improve oxygenation with the application of PEEP.

The shape of the volumetric capnogram

Alterations in the shape of the capnogram can give information regarding pulmonary function. If all the alveoli had the same PCO_2, the phase II time would be short and the plateau of phase III would be horizontal. The lung is not homogenous due to wide ranges of V/Q ratios. Those areas of the lung that have a low V/Q ratio (underventilated, high PCO_2) empty after those with a high V/Q ratio (well ventilated, low PCO_2). This causes an upward slope of phase III. The respiratory units with the lower V/Q tend to be located distally to those with a higher V/Q. Consequently they empty later in the respiratory cycle. The slope of phase III is thus dependent on the emptying patterns of alveoli with differing time constants and PCO_2 concentrations. A lengthening of phase II and an increase in the gradient of phase III due to an increase in the heterogeneity of alveolar ventilation and perfusion is seen in many causes of respiratory failure; notably acute asthma, COPD, ALI/ARDS, pulmonary fibrosis and pneumonia. In pulmonary embolism, the reduction in perfusion leads to a marked increase in the affected V/Q. The absence of CO_2 in the affected units does not alter the morphology of the SBT-CO_2 trace; it just reduces its height.

Pulse oximetry

Introduction

Pulse oximetry is an essential monitoring technique widely used to determine the oxygen saturation of arterial blood. It is a standard monitor in intensive care as well as anaesthesia and other critical care areas.

Principles

The use of the pulse oximeter is based on two main physical principles, i.e. the Beer–Lambert law and the different absorption spectra of oxy- and deoxy-Hb.

Beer's law describes how the intensity of transmitted light decreases exponentially as the concentration of a substance increases. Lambert's law states that the intensity of transmitted light decreases exponentially as the distance travelled through a substance increases.

These laws are applied using two light-emitting diodes in the pulse oximeter probe which is usually placed on a finger, toe, ear or nose. Red light (660nm) and infrared light (940nm) are transmitted in sequence several hundred times per second, with pauses when both diodes are off to enable compensation for ambient light. Red and infrared light are used at these wavelengths because of their widely differing absorption spectra for oxy- and deoxy-Hb (Fig. 6.3.1).

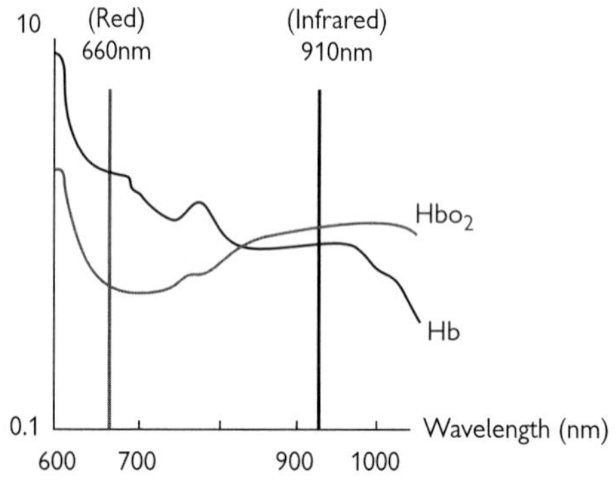

Fig. 6.3.1 Absorption spectra of light as used in the pulse oximeter.

The transmitted light travels through the tissue to a photodetector where the measurements take place.

In the shorter wavelength region (red), oxy-Hb absorbs less light than deoxy-Hb, with the reverse being true in the infrared region (longer wavelength).

At the photodetector, the transmitted light is electronically processed and the relative absorption of the blood at the two wavelengths compared. The isobestic point is the wavelength at which two substances absorb a particular wavelength of light to the same extent and was used in some oximeters to correct for Hb concentration. It can also be used as a reference point where light absorption is independent of saturation.

The pulse oximeter is designed to measure solely arterial oxygen saturation, which requires that the signals from other tissues and capillary and venous blood be filtered out. This is done using the pulsatile nature of arterial blood.

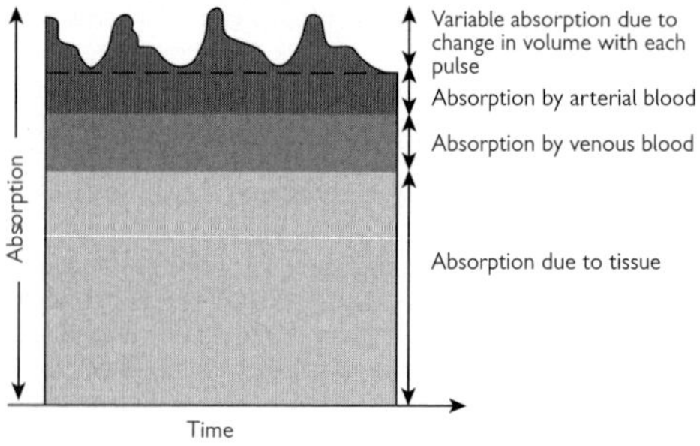

Fig. 6.3.2 Absorption of light transmitted through the finger during pulse oximetry.

The non-pulsatile or constant components of the measurements are discarded, leaving a pulsatile trace from which arterial oxygen saturation can be derived.

Limitations

Calibration

Pulse oximeter calculation of oxygen saturation is based on reference ranges using laboratory measurements from healthy volunteers, and hence cannot include dangerously hypoxaemic levels. It is well established that below saturations of ~70%, pulse oximeters become progressively more inaccurate. Initial set-up, however, on powering up is an automatic process requiring no external calibration procedure.

Perfusion

In hypothermia, hypotension, hypoperfusion, peripheral vasoconstriction (both iatrogenic and primary) and venous congestion, the pulsatile component of the signal can be of insufficient amplitude and quality, such that the reading is inaccurate or absent.

Movement

Movement of the probe or cable by the patient or attending staff can cause artefacts, loss of signal and errors.

The most recent pulse oximetry algorithms have markedly improved performance in low perfusion states and movement.

Arrhythmias

Atrial fibrillation can make the measurement of maximum and minimum absorption more difficult and prone to error.

Electrical interference

Surgical diathermy is a common cause of loss of saturation reading.

Abnormal haemoglobins

Carboxy-Hb has a similar absorption coefficient to oxy-Hb, trending towards a falsely high reading at ~96%. In the case of carbon monoxide (CO) poisoning, e.g. in smoke inhalation, it is essential to remember this point. Where there are suspected high levels of carboxy-Hb, an arterial blood co-oximeter measurement should be taken to confirm the correct carboxy-Hb and O_2 levels as the SpO_2 reading may be misleading. Methaemoglobin (MetHb) has a similar absorption at both emitted wavelengths, giving a saturation reading of ~84%. These readings are the same regardless of the true oxy-Hb saturation. Recently launched multi-wavelength pulse oximeters can now measure carboxy-Hb and MetHb, and consequently have improved accuracy in SpO_2 measurement.

Other intravascular substances

A number of substances can give falsely low saturations when present in tissues and circulating blood, e.g. methylene blue and indocyanin green.

Bilirubin

This has a similar absorption to deoxy-Hb, giving a falsely low reading.

Ambient light

Lights (e.g. in theatre or an anaesthetic room) can affect saturation readings especially if light is bright, direct or flickering (appearing pulsatile).

Nail polish and nicotine

These can absorb infrared light and cause inaccuracies. Nail polish should therefore routinely be removed preoperatively. If this is not possible or if the patient has false nails, the pulse oximeter probe can be placed side to side across the finger, avoiding the nail-bed.

Physical risks

Pressure damage

There have been case reports of pressure necrosis in patients being monitored for long periods, more commonly if poor tissue perfusion is a factor.

Magnetic resonance imaging (MRI)

Burns have been reported due to electrical induction when non-MRI-compatible probes have been used.

Clinical problems

Complacency

SpO_2 readings in the 'normal range' can be falsely reassuring. Because of the sigmoid shape of the Hb dissociation curve, the pulse oximeter can be relatively poor at detecting a significant fall in PaO_2 particularly at the steeper portions of the curve (Fig. 6.3.1).

Time lag

There can be a lag of up to 30s between clinical evidence of cyanosis and pulse oximetry detection of a drop in saturation. This delay is also seen when oxygen saturations improve some seconds after 'pinking up' of a patient following an intervention to treat cyanosis and low saturations. This time lag has been shown to be reduced when an ear probe is used instead of a finger probe.

Despite the expert opinion perception of the advantage of continuous monitoring, there is no published trial evidence of alteration of outcome with pulse oximetry.

Clinical applications

Critical care unit

It is now normal practice to have all patients continuously monitored using a minimum of an ECG and a pulse oximeter.

Anaesthesia

Pulse oximetry has become a mandated standard both during and after general and regional anaesthesia

Ward care, imaging units, endoscopy and patient transport

Continuous oxygen saturation monitoring is becoming more commonplace especially in higher risk patients, and during transport and procedures involving sedation.

Resuscitation

Pulse oximetery can be used during CPR to give a general assessment of adequacy of perfusion.

Investigations

Saturation monitoring can be used during sleep studies to investigate sleep apnoea as well as in cardiac investigations such as exercise tolerance tests.

This simple to use, portable, non-invasive device has become one of the most widely used monitors in hospital medicine. Whilst it has its limitations, it has proved an invaluable addition to clinical observation and other forms of monitoring.

Further reading

Aitkenhead AR, Smith G, eds. Textbook of anaesthesia, 3rd edn. Churchill Livinstone, London 1996.

Yentis, SM, Hirsch, NP, Smith, GB. Anaesthesia and intensive care A–Z, 2nd edn. Elsevier, 2000.

Jubran A. Pulse oximetry. Review article. *Critical Care* 1999; **3**: R11–7.

Chapter 7

Cardiovascular monitoring

Chapter contents

ECG monitoring

ECG monitoring is carried out in order to measure heart rate, rhythm and conduction disturbances, and to monitor pacemaker function. It is essential for the detection of myocardial ischaemia and may also give an indication of electrolyte imbalance.

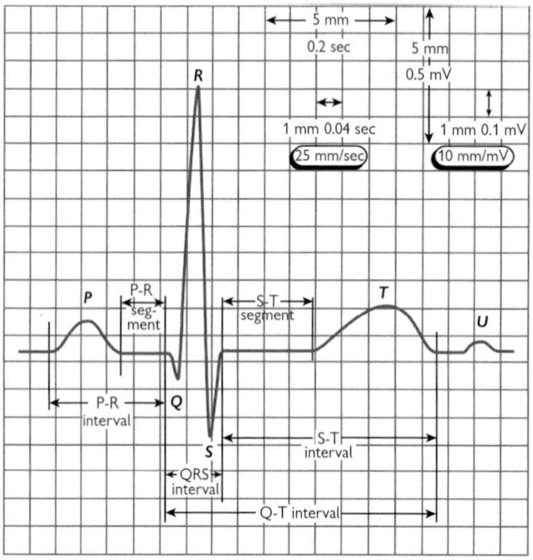

Fig. 7.1.1 Normal ECG configuration.

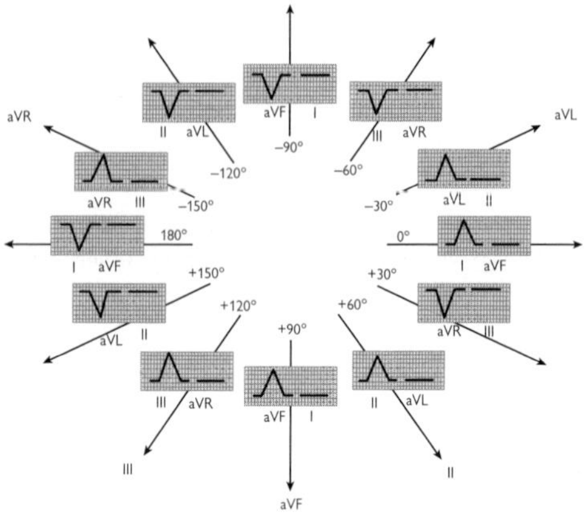

Fig. 7.1.2 ECG leads.

An ECG 'lead' refers to the potential difference recorded between two defined points. The standard calibration for an ECG is 25mm/s and 1mV/cm. If the electrical current is moving towards the positive electrode, then the deflection of the oscilloscope is upwards, if it is away, the deflection is downwards. The frequency range (cycles per second) of an ECG is 0.5–4Hz, i.e. a heart rate of 30–240bpm. The ECG can be broken down into sine waves or harmonics, by Fourier analysis. A minimum of 10 harmonics have to be displayed to produce an ECG waveform, requiring a bandwidth between 0.05 and 40Hz. The bandwidth has to be widened to 0.05–150Hz to enable ST segment analysis. Low and high frequency filters improve the waveform display; the low frequency filter diminishes baseline drift caused by movement and breathing, but exaggerates ST segment changes. The high frequency filter reduces wall power-source noise, but prevents visualization of pacemaker spikes and interferes with QRS and J point recognition. Biological ECG signals are small and require amplification with a differential amplifier to minimize noise. Placing electrodes on bony prominences minimizes interference from muscle activity and the EEG. The signal is then transferred to an oscilloscope for continuous monitoring, or to a printer for interpretation. Adjusting the gain on an ECG monitor may exaggerate or minimize ischaemic changes. It is therefore important to interpret ST elevation or depression when the standard gain of 10mm/mV is selected.

Standard leads

I Between right arm and left arm
II Between left leg and right arm
III Between left leg and left arm

Augmented unipolar leads

The reference electrode is formed by combining leads I, II and III, i.e. the centre of Einthoven's equilateral triangle, where the potential difference is zero.

aVR right arm
aVL left arm
aVF left leg

Unipolar chest leads

The reference electrode is formed by the combined aV leads.

V1 4th intercostals space, right sternal edge
V2 4th intercostals space, left sternal edge
V3 midway between V2 and V4
V4 5th intercostals space, left mid-clavicular line
V5 5th intercostals space, left anterior axillary line
V6 5th intercostals space, left mid-axillary line

Lead selection

In the operating theatre, a single lead ECG display is used, because theatre monitoring employs a three-lead ECG configuration. It is possible to switch between lead I, II and III. During cardiac surgery or on ITU, a five-lead electrode cable is used. This allows the display of seven ECG leads at the same time, including I, II, III, aVR, aVL, aVF and a single unipolar lead, e.g. the lateral chest lead V5.

Three-lead ECG

Lead II or a modified V5 lead should be displayed for detection of arrhythmias, because it monitors down the axis of left ventricular depolarization in patients with a normal cardiac axis. If a pre-operative ECG shows an axis deviation, it is best to display the lead that monitors most closely to the axis of depolarization, i.e. lead I in left axis deviation and lead III in right axis deviation. Coronary ischaemia is best monitored via a lateral chest lead. This is not possible with a three-electrode ECG, but a modified V5 lead can be obtained by placing the right arm lead on the manubrium sterni and the left leg electrode in the standard V5 position. Lead II must be selected on the monitor. This is known as the CM 5 lead and is superior to an individual limb lead for the detection of coronary ischaemia.

Five-lead ECG

Leads II and V4 or V5 should be selected for continuous monitoring. This combination has 90% sensitivity for the detection of inferior or anterior coronary ischaemia

Epicardial ECG monitoring

After cardiac surgery. an atrial ECG can be monitored using the temporary epicardial atrial pacing wires that are placed on the heart. This is useful for the detection of atrial arrhythmias. Similarly, temporary ventricular pacing wires can be used to monitor the ventricular ECG. Epicardial ECG monitoring is also used during off-pump coronary artery surgery, during which the axis and amplitude of a conventional ECG may change due with positioning of the heart. Oesophageal or endotracheal electrodes have also been used during surgery.

ST segment analysis and diagnosis of ischaemia

Subendocardial ischaemia

Subendocardial ischaemia is 'demand ischaemia'. i.e. it produces ST segment depression of >1mm (0.1mV), horizontal or down-sloping. It is measured 60ms after the J point. It is non-localizing to coronary distribution, and leads V5 and V6 are the most sensitive for detection.

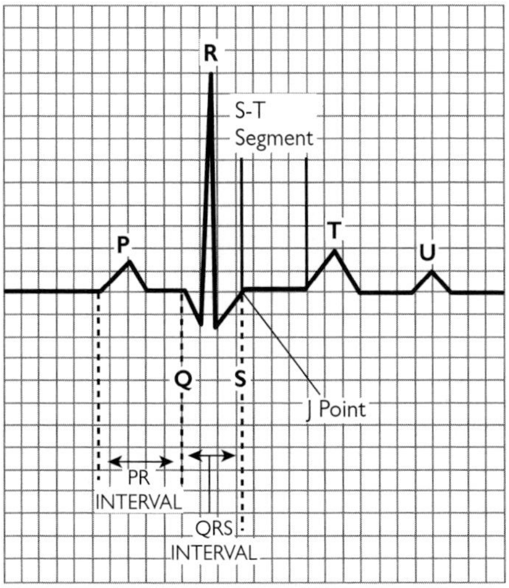

Fig. 7.1.3 J point recognition.

Transmural ischaemia

This is supply ischaemia and produces ST segment elevation. Significant ST elevation is considered to be elevation of 1mm (0.1mV) in two limb leads or 2mm (0.2mV) in two V leads. It is measured at the J point and localizes coronary artery distribution.

It has been shown that ECG monitoring on the ICU has a low sensitivity for detecting myocardial ischaemia, and frequent 12-lead ECGs are superior.

Interpretation and detection of arrythmias

Sinus arrythmia

One P wave per QRS complex, constant PR interval, beat to beat change in RR interval, with respiration in young people.

Sinus bradycardia

Heart rate <40bpm. Often poorly tolerated, resulting in hypotension.

Sinus tachycardia

Heart rate >100bpm. Can precipitate myocardial ischaemia or left ventricular failure.

First degree heart block

The PR interval represents the time for depolarization from the sinoatrial (SA) node to the ventricle. This is usually 0.2s. A prolonged PR interval of >0.2s signifies first degree heart block. This may be a sign of coronary artery disease, rheumatic heart disease, digoxin toxicity or electrolyte imbalance.

Second degree heart block

Mobitz type II

PR interval of conducted beats is constant, but occasionally a P wave is not followed by a QRS complex, because the excitation fails to pass through the AV node and the bundle of His

Wenkebach phenomenon

Progressive lengthening of the PR interval, and then failure of conduction of an atrial beat. The following beat is conducted with a normal PR interval.

2:1 or 3:1 block

Two or three P waves per QRS complex. Normal and constant PR interval in the conducted beats. Wenkebach is usually a benign rhythm, but Mobitz type II, 2:1 or 3:1 block may herald complete heart block in the context of myocardial infarction (MI).

Complete heart block

P waves march through the ECG at a constant rate, whilst the ventricular excitation is a slow ventricular escape rate. There is no relationship between the P waves and the QRS complexes, which are wide due to their ventricular origin. Complete heart block occurs acutely in the context of an MI or may be chronic due to fibrosis around the bundle of His.

Paroxysmal atrial tachycardia

Originates above the ventricles from a site other than the SA node, but including the AV node. The rate is 150–250bpm and is regular. There is one P wave per QRS complex, although the P wave may be hidden in the QRS complex or the T wave. It will compromise the patient if left untreated.

Atrial fibrillation

No P waves, irregularly irregular ventricular rate, with a normal QRS morphology. Is usually associated with significant cardiac disease and can compromise cardiac output, due to inefficient ventricular filling. It is best diagnosed from the arterial waveform, which is irregular, with beat to beat variation in cardiac output.

Atrial flutter

The atrial rate is between 250 and 350bpm, with a 'saw-toothed' P wave appearance. The AV node cannot conduct at this rate so there is a variable block, i.e. 2:1, 3:1 or 4:1, resulting in a ventricular rate of 150, 100 or 75bpm depending on the block. A narrow complex tachycardia with a rate of 150bpm on the ITU is likely to be flutter and is readily treated with a DC shock of 50J.

Junctional tachycardia

This arises from the area around the AV node. The P waves may not be seen, but the QRS complex is a normal shape, because the ventricles are activated normally down the bundle of His.

Ventricular tachycardia

Rapid irregular depolarization from one or more ventricular foci. There are no P waves; the QRS complexes are wide, irregular and vary slightly in shape. It may or may not produce a cardiac output, is life-threatening and requires immediate treatment

Ventricular fibrillation

A rapid irregular rhythm resulting from the discharge of impulses from one or more foci in the ventricles. There are no P waves, no QRS complexes, only bizarre erratic ventricular activity. There is no cardiac output, and immediate cardioversion is required.

Further reading

Hampton J. The ECG in practice, 4th edn. Churchill Livingstone, 2003

Martinez EA, Kim LJ, Faraday N, *et al.* Sensitivity of routine intensive care unit surveillance for detecting myocardial ischaemia. *Critical Care Med* 2003; 31: 2302–8.

Davis PD, Parbrook GD, Kenny G. Basic physics and measurement in anaesthesia, 4th edn. Butterworth–Heinemann, 2002.

Arterial pressure monitoring

Arterial cannulation allows for direct monitoring of the arterial blood pressure and also arterial blood gas sampling. It is essential in intensive care patients with cardiovascular or respiratory failure. It is used during anaesthesia for major surgical cases including cardiac and vascular surgery and situations where major blood loss, cardiovascular instability and pharmacological manipulation of the cardiovascular system is anticipated. It is used in situations where non-invasive blood pressure is unreliable, e.g. arrythmias.

Arterial cannulation

The radial artery is the most commonly used artery for arterial cannulation, as the hand receives collateral blood flow via the ulnar artery. Direct cut-down onto an artery may sometimes be necessary in severely hypovolaemic patients, but this may be more difficult than anticipated. Aortic pressure can be measured post-cardiopulmonary by-pass with a needle placed directly into the aortic root. A non-invasive blood pressure monitor should be available to corroborate the mean arterial pressure.

Allen's test

Allen's test was originally described for assessing arterial blood flow to the hand in thromboangiitis obliterans. The test is now used to assess ulnar arterial blood flow prior to radial arterial cannulation, or harvesting of the radial artery for coronary artery surgery; the ulnar and radial arteries are compressed at the wrist and the patient asked to clench tightly and open the hand. The hand appears white and blanched. Pressure over the ulnar artery is then released and the colour should return to the palm within 5–10s. Delayed return of palmar blood flow, >15s is abnormal and may predict a risk of ischaemic changes if the radial artery is cannulated. The same test can be used prior to ulnar arterial cannulation, but instead collateral circulation via the radial artery is assessed by releasing the pressure over the radial artery. However, overall consensus is that Allen's test is not discriminatory at a particular cut-off time. This does not imply that it never should be performed, but suggests that it should be replaced by more objective tests, such as Doppler ultrasound.

Cannulation

- Awake or asleep: if the patient is awake, explain procedure and infiltrate with local anaesthetic.
- The radial artery can usually be found between the tendon of the flexorcarpi radialis and the head of the radius, but beware aberrant anatomy
- Position the patient's wrist in dorsiflexion, but do not overflex. An assistant can hold the wrist, or a roll of swabs and tape may be used
- Insert the cannula slightly distal to the radial pulse at 45° to the skin. When a flash-back is obtained, advance the needle and the cannula further to compensate for the length of the bevel of the needle. Then carefully slide the cannula off the needle and advance it into the artery. Transfixion can be used especially in babies or small children, and may have a higher success rate. However, the disadvantages include arterial damage and haematoma formation. The radial artery can also be cannulated using a Seldinger technique. This technique involves passing a Seldinger wire into the atery via a needle and then exchanging the needle for a plastic cannula prior to withdrawing the wire.

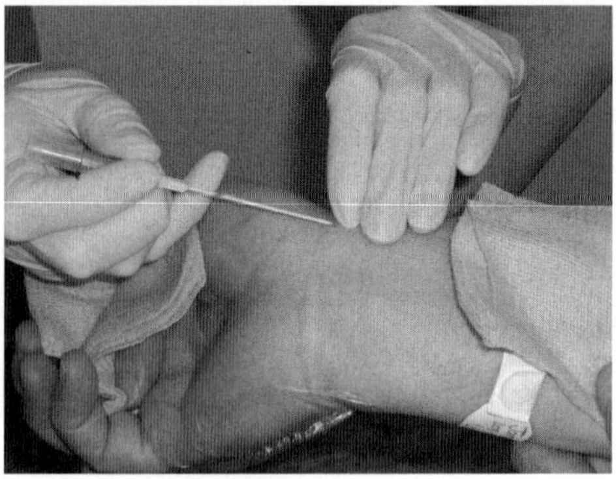

Fig 7.2.1 Arterial cannulation.

Alternative sites for arterial cannulation include:

- Brachial artery

  This is an end artery supplying a large part of the forearm, therefore complications such as thrombosis will have severe consequences.
- Axillary artery

  This is used in neonatal practise.
- Ulnar artery

  The ulnar artery should not be used if the radial artery is occluded or has been damaged by previous cannulation attempts.
- Femoral artery

  This is frequently used in babies and children. A longer catheter is required especially in obese patients. It can easily become occluded if the hip is flexed and is more susceptible to infection.
- Dorsalis pedis artery

  Blood pressure will be 10–20mm Hg higher than in the central circulation.

Complications of arterial cannulation

Ischaemic complications are much more likely in the shocked or hypotensive patient.

- Distal Ischaemia caused by arterial spasm, thrombosis or embolus
- Tissue necrosis
- Bleeding
- Infection
- False aneurysm

Arterial pressure monitoring

In order to monitor arterial pressure, the pressure energy within the arterial cannula has to be transduced to produce an electrical waveform. This requires a system that consists of the following.

A flush system: this consists of a bag of fluid pressurized at 300mm Hg, a drip set and a flow constrictor. This flushes the cannula with heparinized or normal saline at a rate of 3–4ml/h. Excessive flushing of an arterial cannula should be avoided, especially in babies and children, to prevent air or debris entering into the arterial circulation. Flushing with a syringe may cause retrograde cerebral emboli.

Arterial cannula: 20 or 22G parallel-sided stiff Teflon cannula.

Connecting catheter: short and stiff saline-filled to reduce resonance. The number of 3-way taps in the system should be kept to a minimum.

Transducer dome or diaphragm: this detects the small movement of saline to and fro along the catheter. The diaphragm receives this fluctuating pressure energy, and converts it into an electrical signal, the amplitude of which depends on the degree of deformation of the dome. The transducer is placed at the level of the heart and zeroed in this position. Zeroing is carried out by exposing the transducer to atmospheric pressure through an open 3-way tap and pressing 'zero' on the monitor.

Electrical monitor and connections: the input transducer leads to an amplifier and recorder. The frequency range of the arterial pressure waveform is between 0 and 40Hz. The monitor must be able to respond adequately to this range of frequencies.

Normal arterial pressure waveform morphology

Digital readouts of systolic and diastolic blood pressure are displayed as a running average which is updated at frequent intervals. The MAP is a calculated value (diastolic pressure + 1/3 pulse pressure).

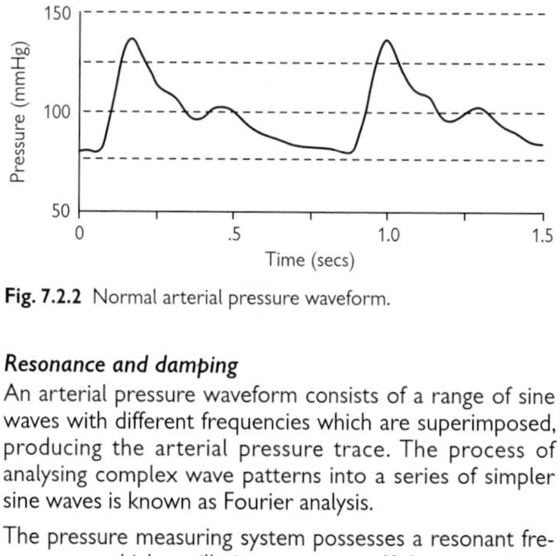

Fig. 7.2.2 Normal arterial pressure waveform.

Resonance and damping

An arterial pressure waveform consists of a range of sine waves with different frequencies which are superimposed, producing the arterial pressure trace. The process of analysing complex wave patterns into a series of simpler sine waves is known as Fourier analysis.

The pressure measuring system possesses a resonant frequency at which oscillations can occur. If this is <40Hz, it falls within the range of the frequencies present in the blood pressure waveform and the sine wave is superimposed on the blood pressure waveform, producing a spiky, distorted, hyper-resonant trace. If the resonant frequency of the system is outside the range of frequencies present in the blood pressure waveform, the problem is avoided. The resonant frequency can be raised by using a shorter stiffer arterial cannula. A hyper- resonant trace will produce elevated systolic pressure readings and decreased diastolic pressure values, but the mean remains accurate. Addition of a rubber bung or an air bubble (caution with air) into the circuit can compensate for underdamping.

A damped trace occurs if there is restriction of transmission of the blood pressure from the artery to the transducer diaphragm. This can be caused by clots, kinks, air bubbles and excessively long or compliant tubing. The systolic pressure will be decreased, whereas the diastolic pressure will be elevated. Again the mean pressure remains relatively accurate.

Difference between central and peripheral arterial pressure

The stiffness of the arterial tree increases with increasing distance from the aortic valve. The blood pressure wave becomes narrower and increases in amplitude in more peripheral arteries. Therefore, even in a supine patient the systolic pressure in the dorsalis pedis artery is higher than in the radial artery, which in turn is higher than in the aorta. The diastolic pressure similarly decreases peripherally and the pulse pressure widens. The effect of temperature and inotropes on the systemic vascular resistance can therefore influence the recording of arterial blood pressure. Non-invasive blood pressure measurements do not always correlate with the invasive blood pressure reading, but the mean pressures should be similar. The nurses will favour the value which suits the target blood pressure!

Using the arterial pressure trace to estimate preload

Systolic pressure variation (SPV) occurs in the mechanically ventilated patient, where changes in intrathoracic pressure and lung volumes produce cyclical variations in blood pressure. An SPV of >10mm Hg is an indicator of hypovolaemia. This 'swing' on the arterial pressure trace can be used to monitor the response to a fluid challenge. Similarly the area under the arterial pressure trace is an indication of cardiac output (see Chapter 7.15).

Further reading

Davis PD, Parbrook GD, Kenny G. Basic physics and measurement in anaesthesia, 4th edn. Butterworth–Heinemann, 2002.

Jarvis A, Jarvis CL, Jones PRM et al. Reliability of Allen's test in selection of patients for radial artery harvest *Ann Thorac Surg* 2000; 70: 1363–5.

Langton JA, Stoker M. Principles of pressuer transducers, resonance, damping and frequency response. *Anaesth Intensive Care Med* 2001; 2: 186–90.

Insertion of central venous catheters

Indications

Central venous access is almost universal in critical care patients.

Indications include:

- monitoring of CVP
- drug administration
- total parenteral nutrition
- fluid resuscitation
- insertion of temporary pacing wires
- insertion of pulmonary artery catheters
- dialysis
- lack of peripheral venous access.

Contraindications

These are relative, but include inability to identify landmarks, limited sites for access, previous difficulties or complications, severe coagulopathy, thrombocytopenia and local sepsis. In addition, if an awake patient is unable to lie flat, central venous cannulation may be impractical without assisted ventilation.

Ultrasound guidance for vascular access

It is now increasingly recommended that ultrasound should be used to guide all central venous access. Ultrasound allows:

- direct visualization of the vessels (artery and vein) and their associated structures
- identification of thrombosis, valve or anatomical abnormalities
- identification of best target vessel
- first-pass cannulation in the midline of a vessel directly avoiding other vital structures
- visualization of guide wire and cannulae entering vein
- reduction of puncture-related complications.

It is likely that the risk of catheter-related sepsis and thrombosis is reduced by limiting the number of needle passes with ultrasound.

Arteries can be distinguished from veins by their round cross-section, their non-compressibility and their pulsatility. Veins, in contrast, show respiratory fluctuation and are easily compressible. In order to maintain sterility during vessel puncture the ultrasound probe should be placed in a sterile plastic sheath. Sterile ultrasound gel is required both inside and outside the sheath. The use of ultrasound requires practice. You should seek instruction before attempting to use it on a patient. You should also be familiar with the landmark approaches to the central veins.

Internal jugular vein

Right internal jugular vein cannulation is associated with a lower incidence of procedural complications and higher incidence of correct tip placement than other approaches. It is especially appropriate for patients with coagulopathy or those patients with lung disease in whom pneumothorax may be disastrous. It may be best avoided in those patients with carotid artery disease or those with raised ICP because of the risks of carotid puncture and of impaired cerebral venous drainage. Internal jugular cannulation is associated with a higher incidence of catheter infection than subclavian cannulation but both have a much lower infection rate than the femoral approach.

The internal jugular vein runs from the jugular foramen at the base of the skull (immediately behind the ear) to its termination behind the posterior border of the sternoclavicular joint where it combines with the subclavian vein to become the brachiocephalic vein. Throughout its length it lies lateral, first to the internal and then to the common carotid arteries, within the carotid sheath, behind the sternomastoid muscle.

Many approaches to the internal jugular vein have been described. Ultrasound will demonstrate the close association of the vein and carotid artery. Choose a site for puncture where the vein does not lie directly over the artery. A typical approach is from the apex of the triangle formed by the two heads of the sternomastoid:

- Slightly extend the neck.
- Turn the head slightly to the opposite side.
- Palpate the carotid artery at the level of the cricoid cartilage.
- Look for the internal jugular vein pulsation. If compressed, the internal jugular can usually be seen to empty and refill.
- To locate the vein, introduce the needle from the apex of the triangle at an angle of 30° and aim towards the ipsilateral nipple. The vein lies typically within 1.5–2cm of the skin surface.
- Often when attempting to puncture the vein it collapses under the pressure of the needle and puncture is not recognized. The vessel may then be located by aspirating as the needle is slowly withdrawn. Blood will be aspirated as the needle tip passes back into the vein, which refills once the pressure has been removed.

External jugular vein

The external jugular vein lies superficially in the neck, running down from the region of the angle of the jaw, across the sternomastoid before passing deep to drain into the subclavian vein. It can be used to provide central venous access, particularly in emergency situations when a simple large-bore cannula can be used for the administration of drugs and resuscitation fluids. Longer central venous catheters can be sited via the external jugular, but the angle of entry to the subclavian vein often leads to inability to pass guide wires centrally and results in a high failure rate.

Subclavian vein

Subclavian vein cannulation is associated with a higher incidence of complications, particularly pneumothorax, and a higher incidence of incorrect line placement than internal jugular cannulation. It is, however, more comfortable for the patient long-term and the site can more easily be kept clean. The subclavian vein is a continuation of the axillary vein. It runs from the apex of the axilla behind the posterior border of the clavicle and across the first rib to join the internal jugular vein, forming the brachiocephalic vein behind the sternoclavicular joint.

- Position the patient supine (some people advocate placing a sandbag between the patient's shoulder blades, which allows the shoulders to drop back out of the way).
- Identify the junction of the medial third and outer two-thirds of the clavicle.
- Introduce the needle just beneath the clavicle at this point, and aim towards the clavicle until contact with bone is made.

- To locate the vein, redirect the needle closely behind the clavicle and towards the suprasternal notch.
- Ultrasound can be used to guide puncture of the vein using a more lateral approach. The axillary vein can be identified under the pectoral muscles at a depth of 3–4cm in the average patient. Longer catheters (20cm left and 25cm right) are required by this approach. Supraclavicular approaches can also be used using both landmark- and ultrasound-guided techniques.

Femoral vein

The femoral vein lies medial to the femoral artery immediately beneath the inguinal ligament. It is particularly useful for obtaining central access in small children and in patients with severe coagulopathy.

- Palpate the femoral artery.
- To locate the vein, introduce the needle 1cm medial to the femoral artery close to the inguinal ligament. It is a common mistake to go too low where the superficial femoral artery overlies the vein.
- Ultrasound should be used to identify the vessels (long saphenous vein, deep and superficial femoral arteries) and ensure that the vein is punctured near the inguinal ligament where the artery and vein lie side by side.

Procedure

Central venous catheterization is almost universally achieved using a catheter over a guide wire (Seldinger) technique. This is associated with a lower incidence of incorrect line placement and complications than cannula over needle techniques.

- For internal jugular, external jugular and subclavian veins, position the patient supine with 10–20° head down tilt. This distends the vein to aid location and helps prevent air embolism.
- Monitor ECG in case of dysrhythmias.
- Universal precautions.
- Use aseptic technique, sterile gown and gloves.
- Prepare sterile field.
- Prepare all equipment.
- Check wire passes through the needle freely. Attach 3-way taps to all open ports of the cannula. Flush the lumens with heparinized saline.
- Inject local anaesthetic to the entry site. Do not forget to anaesthetize suture sites as well.
- Identify the target vessel by ultrasound and/or landmark technique.
- Using a 10ml syringe (partially filled with saline) and needle enter the central vein by the chosen approach, maintaining suction on the syringe at all times.
- Pass the guide wire through the needle. This should pass freely and without any force into the vein. Watch for arrhythmias. Never pull the wire back through the needle once it has passed beyond the end of the bevel: it may shear off.
- Use a scalpel blade to make a small nick in the skin. Hold the blade up and cut away from the wire.
- If provided, pass the dilator over the wire into the vein. Then remove it, leaving the wire in situ.
- Pass the cannula over the wire into the vein. Make sure that before you push the cannula forward the wire is visible at the proximal end. Hold on to the wire at all times, to prevent it being lost inside the patient
- For an average adult patient the central venous cannula via the right internal jugular vein does not need to be inserted more than 12–15cm. Check markings on the cannula. Many are 20cm long and do not need to be inserted up to the hub.
- Draw back blood, check the colour, pulsatility and the pressure of the back flow of blood, flush all the lumens of the line with heparinized saline and lock off the 3-way taps. At this point the patient can be levelled.
- Suture the line into place using the anchorage devices provided and cover with an adhesive sterile dressing.
- If you appear to have missed the vein on the first pass, pull back slowly while maintaining suction on the syringe. You often find you have gone through the vein and can find it on withdrawal.
- Attach a transducer and display the waveform on the monitor.
- Dispose of your sharps and clear away your trolley.
- Obtain CXR to verify central position of the line and check for complications, including pneumothorax and haemothorax.
- Document the procedure in the patient's notes.

Position on chest X-ray

The catheter should lie along the long axis of the vessel and the tip should be in the superior vena cava (SVC) or at the junction of the SVC and right atrium, but ideally outside the pericardial reflection. The pericardium lies below the carina, so ideally catheter tips should be at or above the level of the carina. Catheters below this level may perforate the heart and cause cardiac tamponade. Catheters placed via the subclavian veins or left internal jugular vein must not be allowed to lie with the tip abutting the wall of the SVC. This may cause pain, perforation and accelerated thrombus formation. Either advance the catheter to lie in the long axis of the SVC or pull it back to lie in the brachiocephalic vein. Bear in mind the limitations of CXR; it is useful to confirm central passage and no kinking. The close proximity of the SVC to the pleura, ascending aorta and other structures means that confirmation of the true intravenous position cannot be inferred from a plain CXR.

Common problems with central venous access

Cannot find the vein

Check position (ultrasound and/or landmarks) and try again. If unsuccessful do not persist with repeated passages of the needle in the hope of hitting the vein. You may have misinterpreted the landmarks or the vein may be absent, narrowed or occluded (e.g. with thrombus).

Aspirating blood (needle in vein?) but cannot pass wire

Check needle position by drawing back on the syringe; good flow is essential. Adjust the angle of incidence of the needle to the vein to improve flow. Tip the patient further head down to expand the vein further. Try rotating the needle through 180° and draw back again. Remember the wire must pass easily without force. If this doesn't work, repuncture the vein at a slightly different angle.

Is it arterial?

Occasionally, particularly if using a technique where the wire passes through the barrel of the syringe, it is difficult to know whether you have hit the artery or the vein. In this case it is important to avoid passing a large central venous catheter into the vessel until you are sure. Consider the following:

- Remove the syringe from the needle and observe for pulsatile flow.
- Connect a transducer directly to the needle in the vessel and look at the waveform.
- Pass the wire into the vessel and remove the needle. Pass a 16/18G IV cannula over the wire into the vessel and remove the wire. Attach a transducer or manometer set directly to the cannula. When venous placement is confirmed, pass the wire back through the IV cannula and continue as before.

Arterial puncture

- Needle only, then simply remove and press.
- If large-bore cannula, then action depends on circumstances. If only in situ for a short period then it is usually safe to remove up to 8 French gauge (3mm) and press until bleeding stops. In cases of a larger catheter in situ, carotid puncture in arteriopath, thrombus present, severe coagulopathy or difficulty pressing (subclavian) leave in situ and give platelets and fresh frozen plasma (FFP) before removing. Seek advice and consider the need for surgical exploration and removal under direct vision. Radiological stenting can also be used.

Complications

Complications of central venous cannulation depend in part on the route used but include;

Early	Late
Arrhythmias	Infection
Vascular injury	Thrombosis
Pneumothorax	Embolization
Haemothorax	Erosion/perforation of vessels
Thoracic duct injury (chylothorax)	Cardiac tamponade
Cardiac tamponade	
Neural injury	
Embolization (including guide wire)	

The management of pneumothorax depends upon the size of the pneumothorax and the patient's condition, particularly whether ventilated or not. A small pneumothorax in an unventilated patient with good gas exchange may be observed, or aspirated using a small-bore cannula and syringe with a 3-way tap. Larger pneumothoraces, those that fail to resolve or those that cause any impairment of gas exchange and/or haemodynamics require a formal chest drain. Any significant haemothorax should be formally drained as soon as possible. Once blood has clotted in the chest, drainage is difficult. Seek cardiothoracic/surgical opinion.

Bleeding around the puncture site can occasionally be a persistent problem. If this does not resolve with pressure, use a fine suture (e.g. 5/0 Prolene) to tie a purse string around the puncture site. This usually stops the bleeding.

Line colonization with bacteria and fungi is common, but there is no evidence that changing lines on a regular basis (e.g. every 5–7 days) is of benefit.

Changing catheters over a wire

If new central venous catheters are required, these should usually be placed at a clean site. Occasionally it may be necessary to change a catheter over a guide wire using an existing site. The technique is similar to that described above for placing any central venous catheter.

The main problem is avoiding contamination of the new catheter.

- Cut sutures on the old line before scrubbing.
- Use universal precautions, aseptic technique, gown and gloves.
- Clean and prep the area.
- Pass the wire down the central lumen of the old central venous catheter. (Make sure that the new wire is longer than the old CVP line.)
- Remove the old catheter, leaving the wire in place, and send the tip of the old catheter for culture.
- Clean the puncture site with antiseptic solution.
- Use the wire to site the new line as required.

The problem with this technique is keeping the new line sterile. Wear two pairs of gloves and discard the top pair when you have finished with the old line.

Removing central venous catheters

To remove central lines ensure that all drugs and infusions have been stopped or relocated to other lines. If infection is suspected, send the tip of the line in a dry specimen pot for culture. Removal of central venous catheters can precipitate air embolism, pneumothorax, haemothorax, embolization of thrombus and bacteraemia/sepsis. Make sure the puncture site is below the heart and apply pressure for at least 5min; thereafter apply an occlusive waterproof dressing before sitting the patient up.

Choice of catheter

There are numerous devices on the market, including catheter through needle, catheter over needle, catheter through cannula and catheter over wire. The choice of which to use should depend on the indication for its use, availability of equipment and the skill of the operator.

Other choices include single or multi-lumen catheters, catheter material and long- or short-term use.

Antimicrobial-impregnated devices are also available, but their overall efficacy is still debated.

Catheter-related infections

Intravascular catheter-related infections are a major cause of morbidity and mortality. Coagulase-negative staphylococci, *Staphylococcus aureus*, aerobic Gram-negative bacilli and *Candida albicans* most commonly cause catheter-related bloodstream infection. Management of catheter-related infection varies according to the type of catheter involved. After appropriate cultures of blood and catheter samples, empirical IV antimicrobial therapy should be initiated on the basis of clinical clues, the severity of the patient's acute illness, underlying disease and the potential pathogen involved. In most cases of non-tunnelled central venous catheter-related bacteraemia and fungaemia, the central venous catheter should be removed.

For management of bacteraemia and fungaemia from a tunnelled catheter or implantable device, such as a port, the decision to remove the catheter or device should be based on the severity of the patient's illness, documentation that the vascular access device is infected, assessment of the specific pathogen involved and the ence of complications, such as endocarditis, septic thrombosis, tunnel infection or metastatic seeding.

When a catheter-related infection is documented and a specific pathogen is identified, systemic antimicrobial therapy should be narrowed and consideration given for antibiotic lock therapy, if the central venous catheter or implantable device is not removed.

Further reading

Stonelake P, Bodenham A. The carina as a radiological landmark for central venous catheter tip position. *Br J Anaesthesia* 2006; **96**: 335–0.

Maecken T, Grau T. Ultrasound imaging in vascular access. *Critical Care Med* 2007: 35: S178–85.

Pulmonary artery catheter: indications and use

Introduction

The use of the balloon-tipped, flow-guided catheter to measure the filling pressure of the left side of the heart was first described in 1970 by Swan. The use of the device to measure the cardiac output by a thermodilution method was described in the same paper by Ganz. In the intervening 30 years various other devices have been developed to measure the cardiac output, but the pulmonary artery (Swan–Ganz) catheter has remained the standard against which the other devices have been judged.

Indications

Despite >30 years of international experience with the pulmonary artery catheter, its use has never been validated in an adequately powered RCT. Indications for use are therefore based on expert opinion and consensus statements from a variety of international societies. Potential indications for use of the pulmonary artery catheter as described by Swan and Ganz include:

- Establishing the aetiology of shock states (i.e. cardiogenic vs hypovolaemic vs septic vs obstructive shock)
- Diagnosis of pulmonary hypertension and assessment of the response to treatment
- Differentiation between cardiac and non-cardiac causes of pulmonary oedema
- Monitoring and management of AMI
- Monitoring and management of cardiac performance when restoring spontaneous circulation after cardiopulmonary bypass.
- Monitoring of fluid balance in patients where this is difficult clinically, e.g. burns patients, sepsis with capillary leak
- Assessment of response to inotropic drugs or vasopressors
- Peri-operative optimization of oxygen delivery in high-risk surgical patients

Modifications of the classic Swan–Ganz pulmonary artery catheter also allow:

- Continuous measurement of cardiac output
- Temporary cardiac pacing
- Continuous monitoring of mixed venous oxygen saturation to monitor adequacy of global oxygen delivery.

Use of the pulmonary artery catheter

Use of the pulmonary artery catheter allows the direct measurement of a variety of haemodynamic parameters:

- Right atrial pressure
- Pressures within the right ventricle
- Pulmonary artery pressures
- Pulmonary artery wedge pressure (reflecting the left atrial pressure—see Chapter 7.5)
- The cardiac output

From these data, various other haemodynamic parameters can be derived (see Table 7.5.1)

The measurement of right heart pressures including the pulmonary artery occlusion pressure is described in Chapter 7.5 together with a table of normal values.

Table 7.5.1 Derived haemodynamic parameters

$$\text{Cardiac index} = \frac{\text{Cardiac output}}{\text{Body surface area}}$$

Systemic vascular resistance = MAP – RAP/CO
Systemic vascular resistance index = MAP – RAP/CI
Pulmonary vascular resistance = MPP – PAoP/CO
Oxygen delivery (DO_2) – CO × CaO_2 × 10
Oxygen delivery index (DO_2I) = CI × CaO_2 × 10
Oxygen uptake (VO_2) = (CaO_2 – CvO_2) × CO × 10
Where:
CO = cardiac output (l/min)
CI = cardiac index (l/min/m^2)
MAP = systemic mean arterial pressure
RAP = right atrial pressure
MPP = pulmonary mean arterial pressure
PAoP = pulmonary artery occlusion pressure
CaO_2 = arterial oxygen content (ml/100ml)
CvO_2 = venous oxygen content (ml/100ml)

The cardiac output is measured by the thermodilution method described below

Thermodilution method for the measurement of cardiac output

Cardiac output can be calculated by using the Stewart–Hamilton equation (see Table 7.5.2). A bolus of cold fluid of known volume and temperature is injected through the proximal port of the pulmonary artery catheter into the superior vena cava. This fluid then mixes with the blood in the right ventricle and causes a decrease in the temperature of the blood which is detected by a thermistor at the distal end of the pulmonary artery catheter, i.e. in the pulmonary artery.

Table 7.5.2 The Stewart–Hamilton equation

$$Q = \frac{V(T_B - T_I)K_1K_2}{T_B(t)dt}$$

Where:
Q = cardiac output
V = volume of injectate
T_B = temperature of blood
T_I = temperature of injectate
K_1K_2 = computational constants
$T_B(t)dt$ = integral of blood temperature change

The change in blood temperature detected by the thermistor is plotted against time. The area under the curve is inversely proportional to the cardiac output. If the cardiac output is high, there is a large initial change in the blood temperature, which is short lived. If the cardiac output is poor, the initial change in blood temperature is smaller but the change is more prolonged. Usual practice is to perform three measurements in quick succession and to take the mean value of the measured cardiac outputs; this compensates for the small variations in cardiac output which are seen due to ectopic beats or the respiratory cycle.

A modification of this technique can be used for the 'continuous' cardiac output measurement using a modified pulmonary artery catheter. A heating coil is incorporated into the pulmonary artery catheter to lie within the right atrium and right ventricle. Every 30–60s this heats a bolus of blood; this temperature change is again monitored by a thermistor at the distal end of the catheter, and the cardiac output is calculated from the temperature/time curve. This technique allows a more rapid assessment of the effects of treatment on cardiac output than the intermittent thermodilution technique.

There are several potential sources of error when using the thermodilution method to measure cardiac output:

- Intracardiac shunts
- Too slow injection of cold injectate
- Impairment of thermistor function by impingement against blood vessel wall
- Tricuspid valve regurgitation

Even if the absolute readings of cardiac output are rendered inaccurate by the presence of one of the above factors the trends of the readings may still be useful in guiding treatment.

The thermodilution technique directly measures the cardiac output of the right side of the heart. At equilibrium it is assumed that the output of the right side of the heart is equal to that of the left side.

Pulmonary artery catheter: controversy

Despite 30 years of worldwide experience with the pulmonary artery catheter there is little evidence that it is beneficial to patient outcomes and some suggestion that it may even be harmful. In 1996, Connors *et al.* published a prospective observational study of 5735 patients, 2184 of whom had had their treatment guided by the use of a pulmonary artery catheter. The investigators found that the use of the pulmonary artery catheter was associated with higher mortality rates and increased use of resources, and called for an RCT to assess the effectiveness of the pulmonary artery catheter.

Since the publication of the Connors study, two randomized controlled trials involving the use of the pulmonary artery catheter have been published. The FACTT trial from the ARDSnet group randomly assigned patients with ARDS to management with either a pulmonary artery catheter or a central venous catheter. Use of the pulmonary artery catheter did not improve survival or organ function and was associated with more complications than the use of the central venous catheter alone. The PAC-MAN trial was a multi-centre British study, which randomly assigned 1041 critically ill patients to management with or without a pulmonary artery catheter. Alternative cardiac output monitors could be used at the discretion of the treating units. There was found to be no clear evidence of benefit or harm associated with the use of the pulmonary artery catheter.

Summary

The pulmonary artery catheter can be used to measure and derive a variety of cardiovascular parameters. The clinical value of measuring and manipulating these parameters either by the pulmonary artery catheter or by newer cardiac output monitors such as the oesophageal Doppler remains controversial.

Further reading

Boyd O, Grounds MR, Bennett ED. A randomized clinical trial of the effect of deliberate perioperative increase of oxygen delivery on mortality in high-risk surgical patients. *J Am Med Assoc* 1993; 270: 2699–707.

Connors AF, Speroff T, Dawson NV, *et al.* The effectiveness of right heart catheterisation in the initial care of critically ill patients. *JAMA* 1996; 276: 889–97.

Swan HJ, Ganz W, Forrester J, *et al.* Catheterization of the heart in man with the use of a flow-directed balloon-tipped catheter. *N Engl J Med* 1970; 283: 447–51.

Pulmonary artery catheter: insertion

Introduction

The pulmonary artery catheter has a small (1.5ml) balloon at the tip, just proximal to the distal lumen (Fig. 7.6.1). When inserted into the right atrium this balloon is filled with air and carried by the flow of blood into the pulmonary vasculature, thus guiding the placement of the catheter. The insertion technique can be divided into two stages: (i) cannulation of a large vein with an introducer sheath utilizing the techniques described in Chapter 7.3 and (ii) the passage of the catheter itself. Strict sterile technique should be maintained for the duration of the procedure.

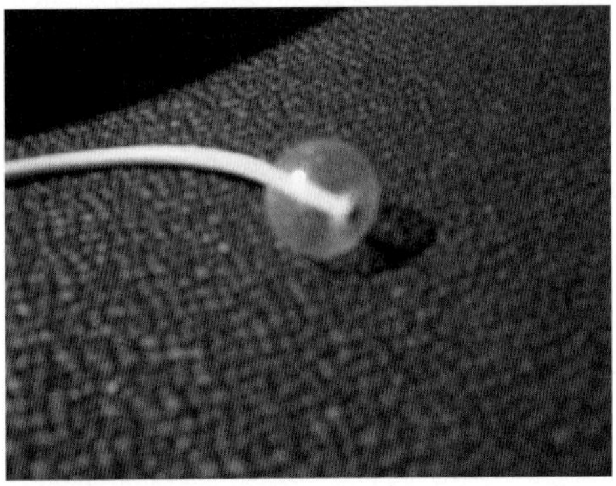

Fig. 7.6.1 The balloon at the tip of the pulmonary artery catheter.

Cannulation of a large vein

Selection of which vein to cannulate will be determined by operator familiarity, the presence of other indwelling vascular devices and patient factors such as the necessity for cervical immobilization. As a general guide:

- **Right internal jugular vein** allows the shortest and straightest route to the right side of the heart
- **Left subclavian** vein offers relatively unrestricted access to the heart
- **Right subclavian and left internal jugular veins** require the catheter to navigate an acute angle to enter the heart
- **Femoral veins** can be used if the other sites are unavailable, but passage of the catheter to the heart is technically difficult.

Most commercially available introducer sheaths are inserted by the modified Seldinger technique. Where appropriate, the insertion of the introducer sheath can be guided by ultrasound. It must be remembered that an introducer sheath is of large diameter (up to 8.5 French) and that the consequences of accidental arterial cannulation are likely to be more severe than would be the case with a standard central venous catheter.

A sterile sleeve is affixed to the introducer sheath through which the pulmonary artery catheter will be passed. This will allow aseptic manipulation of the catheter once it is *in situ*.

Passage of the pulmonary artery catheter

Before starting the insertion procedure, the pulmonary artery catheter should be visually inspected for any obvious faults. The balloon should be inflated to test for integrity. Each of the lumens of the catheter should be flushed with saline to eliminate air bubbles. The markings on the catheter should be inspected to confirm understanding of the distance marking system used (Fig. 7.6.2)

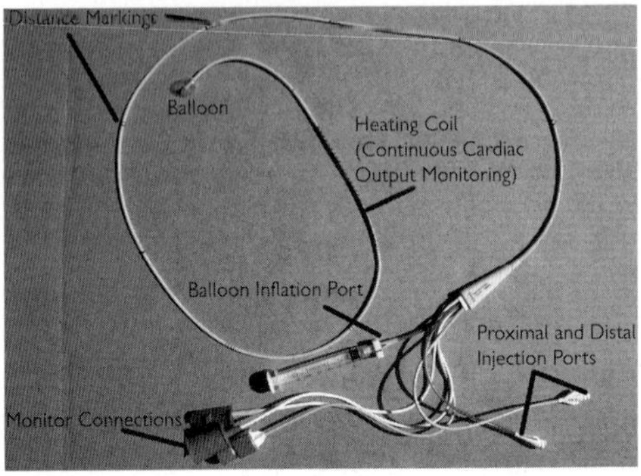

Fig. 7.6.2 Pulmonary artery catheter, markings and features.

The passage of the pulmonary artery catheter through the right side of the heart and into the correct position is monitored by observing the characteristic real-time pressure traces on a monitor. Thus the distal lumen of the catheter should be attached to a pressure transducer system which allows continuous monitoring of the pressure waveform.

Knowledge of the normal pressures on the right side of the heart is invaluable when placing the pulmonary artery catheter (see Table 7.6.1)

Table 7.6.1 Normal right heart pressures (mm Hg)

	Systolic	Diastolic	Mean
Right atrium			0–7
Right ventricle	15–25	0–8	
Pulmonary artery	15–25	8–15	10–20
Wedge pressure			6–12

The pulmonary artery catheter is inserted through the introducer sheath and advanced until a right atrial pressure trace is identified on the monitor. The distance to the right atrium varies depending on the insertion point of the introducer sheath. Typically the right atrial trace will be found at an insertion depth of 15–20cm from the internal jugular veins, 10–15cm from the subclavian veins and 30–40cm if the femoral route is used.

At this point the balloon is inflated with 1.0–1.5ml of air and the inflation port locked. The distance marking on the catheter should be noted. The catheter is now slowly advanced whilst monitoring the pressure trace. The typical right ventricle pressure waveform should be seen after advancing the catheter approximately a further 10cm, and this should change to the pulmonary artery waveform between 10 and 20cm beyond that (Fig. 7.6.3).

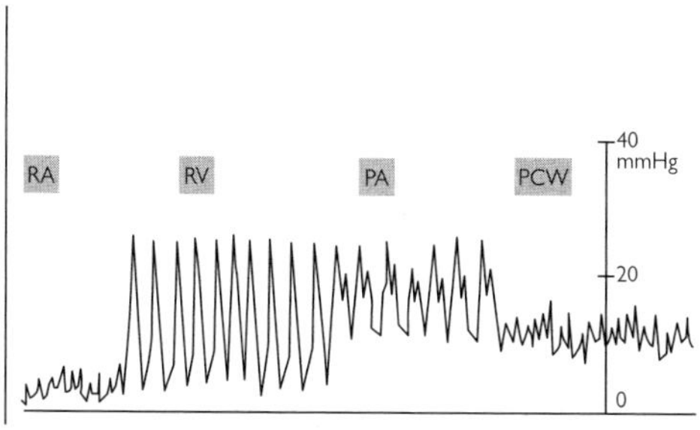

Fig. 7.6.3 Pressure trace during insertion of a pulmonary artery catheter.

Note that the principle differences between the right ventricle and pulmonary artery waveforms are the higher diastolic pressures and the presence of a dicrotic notch in the pulmonary artery waveform. Both of these observations are due to the presence of elastic tissue in the walls of the pulmonary artery.

If the expected pressure changes are not seen after advancing the catheter the appropriate distance, it is possible that the catheter is coiling within the chamber and there is a risk of knotting. The balloon should be deflated and the catheter withdrawn slowly to the starting depth before inflating the balloon and trying again. The balloon should always be deflated before withdrawing the catheter to prevent damage to surrounding structures and minimize the risk of knotting.

Once in the pulmonary artery, the catheter should be advanced a further 10cm or so until the typical wedge pressure trace is seen (Fig. 7.6.3). This is the pulmonary artery occlusion pressure (PAoP). Once the PAoP has been measured (see below) the balloon should be deflated; if the typical pulmonary arterial waveform does not reappear then the catheter should be slowly pulled back until it does. The balloon should never be left inflated or the catheter in the wedged position because this can lead to erosion of the artery wall and subsequent artery rupture or to pulmonary infarction.

When the insertion procedure is complete, a CXR should be performed to confirm the correct position of the catheter and to identify complications of central venous access.

Pulmonary artery occlusion (wedge) pressure

When the pulmonary artery catheter is in the wedged position there is an uninterrupted column of blood between the distal lumen of the catheter and the left atrium. At the end of diastole, when the mitral valve is open, this column of blood extends to the left ventricle, thus the pressure in the left ventricle at end diastole is transmitted to the transducer system along an uninterrupted column of fluid. The PAoP can therefore be used as a marker of left ventricular preload at the end of expiration when artificial intrathoracic pressure manipulations can be discounted.

There are certain circumstances in which the PAoP will not accurately reflect the left ventricular end-diastolic pressure. These include:

- Mitral valve stenosis
- Mitral valve incompetence
- Pulmonary venous obstruction, e.g. from pulmonary fibrosis
- Tip of the catheter lying outside of Wests' zone 3, i.e. the pulmonary capillary bed is compressed by the pressure within the alveoli at some point during the respiratory cycle.

Contraindications

Absolute contraindications to placement of a pulmonary artery catheter include the presence of prosthetic tricuspid or pulmonary valves, endocarditis of tricuspid or pulmonary valves and the presence of right heart thrombus. Caution is advised in patients with recent cardiac arrhythmias and those with coagulopathy.

Complications

The complications of pulmonary artery catheter placement can be divided into those caused by the initial venepuncture which are common to all such procedures (see Chapter 7.3), and those due to the passage or presence of the pulmonary artery catheter itself.

Complications due to the passage of the pulmonary artery catheter include:

- Cardiac arrhythmias.
- Right bundle branch block occurs in up to 5% of insertions. Patients with pre-existing left bundle branch block are at risk of complete heart block
- Cardiac perforation
- Damage to the tricuspid and pulmonary valves
- The catheter may knot if allowed to coil in one of the heart chambers during insertion.

Complications due to the presence of the pulmonary artery catheter include:

- Pulmonary artery rupture. A large observational study suggested that the incidence of pulmonary artery rupture was 0.031%.
- Pulmonary infarction may occur if the balloon is left inflated for prolonged periods of time or if the catheter migrates distally and occludes a small branch artery.
- Infection.
- Venous air.

Further reading

Harvey S, Harrison DA, Singer M. Assessment of the clinical effectiveness of pulmonary artery catheters in managementof patients in intensive care (PAC-Man): a randomised controlled trial. *Lancet* 2005; 366: 472–7.

Kearney TJ, Shabot MM. Pulmonary artery rupture associated with the Swan–Ganz catheter. *Chest* 1995; 108: 1349–52.

Mermel LA, Maki DG. Infectious complications of Swan–Ganz pulmonary artery catheters. Pathogenesis, epidemiology, prevention, and management. *Am J Respir Crit Care Med* 1994; 149: 1020–36.

Echocardiography

Echocardiography provides invaluable and prompt information about systolic and diastolic function, filling status and the function of the intracardiac valves and the great vessels. This has a significant influence on decision making and management in the ICU.

Physics of ultrasound

- Sound is an example of a longitudinal wave oscillating back and forth through a transmitting medium at a fixed velocity, resulting in zones of compression and rarefaction.
- Ultrasound includes that proportion of the sound spectrum above 20kHz. Echo machines use frequencies of 2–10MHz.
- The wavelength (λ) is inversely related to the frequency (f) by the sound velocity (c) so that $c = \lambda f$.
- Sound velocity in a given material is constant but varies in different materials. Ultrasound propagates poorly in air.
- c in blood is 1570m/s, soft tissue 1540m/s and air 330m/s.

Imaging by ultrasound

- Ultrasound waves are generated by piezoelectric crystals in a transducer that vibrate when an alternating current is applied.
- Imaging is achieved by emitting ultrasound pulses from the transducer which are reflected by a boundary between two tissue structures and received by the same transducer, generating a current which is processed to generate an image.
- Wavelength is a determinant of image quality as the spatial resolution is limited to approximately one λ. Therefore, shorter λs (obtained with higher *f*s as *c* is constant) produce better resolution. However, higher *f*s give reduced tissue penetration and thus a reduced image depth.
- The pulsed ultrasound signal is described by the pulse repetition frequency (PRF). This must be set so that there is sufficient time for the pulsed wave to be transmitted, reflected and received in order to display all objects uniquely within a typical 10cm viewing window. There must only be a single pulse present between the transducer and the reflected object at any point in time in order to avoid range ambiguity. With a *c* in tissue of 1540m/s this means that at a depth of 10cm the PRF must be no more than 7.7kHz .
- The strength of reflection at an interface depends on the difference in acoustic impedance (AI) between two media. AI is the product of density and the *c* within the medium. There is a large AI mismatch between tissue and air, preventing imaging within the lung. This also occurs between the transducer and tissue, necessitating a layer of gel between tissue and transducer.

Doppler

- Doppler is used in echocardiography principally to look at aspects of blood flow.
- The Doppler effect is the apparent change in *f* in waves that occurs when the source and observer are in motion relative to each other, with the *f* increasing when the source and observer approach and decreasing when they move apart. This shift in *f* from the transmitted to the received *f* is referred to as the Doppler shift (*fd*) and is given by the Doppler equation;

$$fd = 2.fo.v.\cos\theta/c$$

- Where: *v* is the velocity of blood flow; θ is the angle between the ultrasound beam and blood flow; c is the ultrasound velocity in that medium; *fo* is the transmitting frequency.
- The Doppler shift can therefore be used to measure the velocity of blood flow.

$$v = fd.c/2fo.\cos\theta$$

- v is most accurately measured when ø is zero and the ultrasound beam is in line with the blood flow. Doppler calculations cannot be made when the ultrasound beam is perpendicular to the flow of blood as the cosine of 90° is zero. As long as ø is <20° then the measurement error is <6%.
- Doppler calculated velocities are displayed graphically on the echo machine with *v* on the *x*-axis and time on the *y*-axis. This process requires a formidable amount of electronic processing.
- Colour Doppler is a real-time colourized display of blood flow superimposed on a 2D image. This also requires an enormous amount of computation and is used to identify turbulent flow within the heart that may occur, for example, with valvular pathology.

Indications for echocardiography in the ICU

- Haemodynamic instability: ventricular failure, hypovolaemia, vasodilation, acute valvular dysfunction, cardiac tamponade, pulmonary embolism
- Aortic dissection
- Infective endocarditis
- Source of systemic embolus
- Unexplained hypoxaemia

Indications for transthoracic echo (TTE)

- Imaging of the ascending aorta which is not visualized by transoesophageal echo (TOE) due to interposition of the left main bronchus.
- Imaging of the left ventricular (LV) apex which is frequently foreshortened by TOE.
- Accurate measurement of the pressure gradient across the aortic valve which is frequently underestimated with TOE where alignment of the Doppler beam can be suboptimal.
- When TOE is contraindicated.

Indications for TOE

- Conditions that prevent image acquisition with TTE such as in the presence of hyperinflated lungs, surgical dressings, wounds, drains, prone position or excess fat tissue.
- Examination of posterior structures which are better visualized with TOE such as thoracic aorta, pulmonary veins, left atrium, mitral valve.
- Pathologies where TOE is more sensitive than TTE, e.g. left atrial thrombus, interatrial septal defects, cardiac tamponade.
- In conditions where diagnosis and treatment require more detailed information such as in suspected aortic dissection, infective endocarditis, complex mitral valve pathology.

Contraindications to TOE

Absolute	Relative
Peforated viscus	Atlantoaxial joint disease
Oesophageal stricture	Prior chest irradiation
Oesophageal tumours	Hiatus hernia
Active upper GI bleeding	
Oesophageal diverticula	
Oesophageal scleroderma	
Recent upper GI surgery	

Indications in the ICU

Pulmonary embolism (PE)

- Echo can provide bedside diagnosis in the unstable ICU patient with massive PE when transport outside the ICU for angiography or CT may be unsafe.
- TOE has a sensitivity of 80–92% and a specificity of almost 100%. Echocardiographic features of massive PE are;
  - **(i)** *Acute cor pulmonale*; specifically mid-cavity hypokinesia with preserved function at the apex in contrast to RV dysfunction due to other causes in which wall motion is abnormal in all regions.
  - **(ii)** *Central emboli in the proximal pulmonary arteries;* particularly the main and the right pulmonary artery (detection of left-sided emboli is limited by the poor propagation of ultrasound through air in the left bronchus).

Valvular dysfunction

Echo can be used to assess valvular lesions using 2D imaging, Doppler and colour flow mapping (CFM).

Stenotic lesions

Two-dimensional imaging

- To assess valvular appearance, whether bi- or trileaflet, leaflet, calcification and thickening (rheumatic).
- To assess secondary changes such as spontaneous echo contrast due to obstructed flow (± presence of thrombus), atrial dilatation and ventricular impairment.
- Planimetry can be used to trace a valve area. This is particularly useful with aortic stenosis (AS), with severe AS being a valve area of 0.6–0.8cm^2 .

CFM

- Detects turbulent flow through the restricted lesion and beyond, and gives an indication of its direction and extent.

Doppler

- Measures the velocity(V) across a lesion which can be used to calculate the pressure gradient.
- Severe AS is a mean ΔP 40–50mm Hg, and severe mitral stenosis (MS) is a mean ΔP >12mm Hg. Note that ΔP is flow dependent and therefore underestimates stenotic severity when there is poor LV function.

Regurgitant lesions

Two-dimensional imaging

- To assess leaflet function (inclubing cordal rupture and prolapse) and annular dilatation.
- To look for evidence of endocarditis (see below).

CFM

- To assess the size of the regurgitant jet. For mitral regurgitation (MR) a jet area >50% of the left atrial area is severe and for aortic regurgitation (AR) a jet width >40% of the LV outflow tract. Note that this method tends to underestimate the severity of eccentric (wall hugging) jets of MR.

Doppler

- To assess systolic flow reversal in the pulmonary veins (MR) or the descending thoracic aorta (AR).

Systemic embolization

- TOE is the most sensitive and specific technique for determining the source and potential mechanism of systemic embolization for patients with cerebral ischaemic events or peripheral infarction.
- TOE can identify cardiac sources of embolism including atrial and ventricular thrombi, vegetations, tumours, atrial septal defects or aneurysms, and atheromatous disease of the aorta.
- In critically ill patients with AF, TOE is necessary to exclude the presence of thrombus before cardioversion when a long period of anticoagulation is not possible.

Infective endocarditis (IE)

- The major criteria for the diagnosis of IE are persistent bacteraemia with typical organisms with echocardiographic evidence of endocardial involvement.
- Echocardiographic features of IE are:
  - **(i)** an oscillating intracardiac mass which may be on a valve and/or supporting structure, or in the path of a regurgitant jet or iatrogenic device
  - **(ii)** intracardiac abscess
  - **(iii)** new dehiscence of a prosthetic valve
  - **(iv)** new valvular regurgitation
- TOE is more sensitive and specific than TTE for the detection of vegetations. The sensitivity of TOE for the detection of vegetations on native valves is 82–100% and on prosthetic valves is 77–94%.
- False-positive findings may occur from lesions that resemble vegetations such as: papillary fibroma, ruptured or redundant chordae, non-specific valve thickening or calcification, non-bacterial thrombotic endocarditis, systemic lupus erythematosus (SLE) with cardiac involvement, thrombus, aortic valve Lambl's excrescence or nodule of Arantius.
- In patients with prosthetic valves, vegetations can be mistaken for a sewing ring, surgically severed or retained chordae tendinae, fibrin strands or periprosthetic material.

Unexplained hypoxaemia

TOE can diagnose or rule out cardiac causes of hypoxaemia such as poor ventricular function, MR, pulmonary emboli, intracardiac shunts (patent foramen ovale or atrial septal defect (ASD)) or even to detect pleural effusions.

Estimating pulmonary artery pressure

- Systolic pulmonary artery pressures can be measured in patients with tricuspid regurgitation(TR).
- The ΔP of the TR jet can be measured using Doppler and, if the CVP is known,

  systolic RVP = CVP + TR jet ΔP

  systolic RVP = systolic PAP (if no PV pathology)

Aortic dissection

- TOE provides high resolution real-time imaging of the aorta, resulting in high sensitivity (99%) for identifying dissection.
- The unique advantage of bedside echo over CT or aortography lies in its portability which is of particular value in unstable patients.
- TOE can also identify complications of dissection such as extension of dissection into the coronaries, the presence of pericardial or mediastinal haematoma, the presence, mechanism and severity of AR, the point of entry and exit between the true and false lumen, the presence of thrombus and LV function.
- In suspected aortic dissection when TOE findings are equivocal or negative, aortography, CT or MRI should be performed in addition to TOE.

Clinical application of echocardiography in the ICU

Assessment of LV function

Systolic function/ejection fraction (EF)

- LV systolic function can be quantified by calculating an EF using (1) linear, (2) area and (3) volume measurements.
- Measurements are made in systole and diastole, and machine-integrated software computes diameters, areas and volumes, and provides a value for EF.

(1) Fractional shortening

$$FS = \frac{EDD - ESD}{EDD} \times 100\% \ (30\text{–}40\%)$$

Where EDD = end-diastolic diameter and ESD = end-systolic diameter.

- Measurements are made in the parasternal long axis view using TTE or the transgastric mid short axis view with TOE.
- Fractional shortening may be inaccurate in the presence of regional wall motion abnormalities and must be interpreted taking into account 2D images of the LV.

(2) Fractional area change

$$FAC = \frac{EDA - ESA}{EDA} \times 100\% \ (36\text{–}64\%)$$

Where EDA = end-diastolic area and ESA = end-systolic area.

- Measurements are made by tracing the endocardial border in the parasternal LV short axis view with TTE or the transgastric mid short axis view with TOE.

(3) Ejection fraction (Simpson's discs method)

$$EF = \frac{EDV - ESV}{EDV} \times 100\% \ (55\text{–}75\%)$$

Where EDV = end-diastolic volume and ESV = end-systolic volume.

- In Simpson's disc method ventricular volumes are obtained by tracing endocardial borders and approximating the ventricular cavity with a series of discs of uniform thickness.
- Views used in this method are the apical LV four- or two-chamber view using TTE or the mid-oesophageal four- or two-chamber views using TOE. Simpson's EF method is more accurate than fractional shortening and fractional area change in patients with significant wall motion abnormalities.

Other indices of LV systolic function

- dP/dt of the mitral regurgitant velocity measured with Doppler from the mid-oesophageal ventricular view.
- Mitral annular displacement in systole from the mid-oesophageal ventricular view. A descent of <0.8cm is indicative of significant systolic dysfunction.
- Myocardial movement measured with tissue Doppler imaging.

Regional wall motion abnormality (RWMA)

- In the ICU this may occur in patients on increasing inotropic support, while attempting weaning from ventilation or with severe left ventricular hypertrophy (LVH).
- Wall motion can be graded as follows: (i) normokinesia; (ii) hypokinesia; (iii) akinesia; (iv) dyskinesia; and (v) aneurysmal.
- The parasternal short axis view of the LV (TTE) and the transgastric short axis view (TOE) show areas of myocardium supplied by all three coronaries and as such are ideally suited for looking for ischaemic RWMAs.
- Other causes of altered contractility include: ventricular pacing, ventricular conduction delay, old MI, marked hypovolaemia, severe mitral stenosis and post-cardiopulmonary bypass (Interventricular septum).
- New RWMAs associated with haemodynamic instability are highly indicative of acute myocardial ischaemia.

Cardiac output (CO)

Two echocardiographic methods can be used:

1. Based on measuring LV volumes (EDV and ESV) using Simpson's disc method (see above) and using the patient's heart rate (HR) in the equation:

$$CO = (EDV - ESV) \times HR$$

2. Based on 2D and Doppler echocardiography; SV is given by the equation:

$$SV = VTI_{LVOT} \times CSA_{LVOT}$$

- VTILVOT is the velocity time integral through the left ventricular outflow tract (LVOT).
- CSALVOT is the cross-sectional area of the LVOT.
- VTI LVOT is derived from Doppler analysis of the LVOT. This is obtained from the apical five-chamber view using TTE or from the deep transgastric view using TOE.
- LVOT diameter is measured from the parasternal long axis view with TTE or the mid-oesophageal aortic valve long axis view using TOE. The CSA LVOT is then given by the equation;

$$CSA_{LVOT} = (\pi/4) \times LVOTdiameter^2$$

- The heart rate is then used with the measured SV to calculate cardiac output as with the Simpson's method.

Assessment of preload

2D imaging

- Qualitative estimation of LV volume is often adequate, particularly at the extremes of volumes. Systolic obliteration of the LV cavity is a sign of severe hypovolaemia. However, a large LV EDA may not indicate adequate preload with LV dysfunction.
- Quantitative measurements of LV preload; LV EDA (normal range 9.5–22cm^2) can be obtained by endocardial border tracing. LV EDV (normal range 80–130ml) can be obtained with Simpson's method (see above).
- Studies have demonstrated that changes in LV EDA measured with TOE are related to changes in cardiac output. and were found to be more reliable than the pulmonary artery catheter in determining the cause of hypotension.
- Right atrial (RA) pressure can be estimated from evaluation of the inferior vena cava (IVC) during respiration
- Normal RA pressure (5–10mm Hg) corresponds to normal IVC diameter(1.2–2.3cm) and >50% collapse with respiration. Increased RA pressure leads to a dilated IVC and a failure to collapse with respiration.

Doppler flow

- Transmitral and pulmonary venous flow patterns provide additional loading information.

- Indicators of decreased preload:
  - (i) Decreased early diastolic filling velocity (mitral E wave) and decreased E/A ratio (A is the velocity of late mitral LV inflow due to atrial systole).
  - (ii) Decreased mitral E wave velocity together with decreased pulmonary flow during systole (S wave).
- Indicators of LA pressure:
  - (i) Normal pulmonary flow pattern with predominant S wave is indicative of an LA pressure <8mm Hg.
  - (ii) Dominance of the D wave (pulmonary flow during diastole) occurs with elevated LA pressure.
- AV Doppler flow velocity variation with respiration of >12% in mechanically ventilated patients is indicative of fluid responsiveness (cf. pulse pressure variation seen with LiDCO).

Cardiac tamponade

- Tamponade is suggested by a combination of clinical and echocardiographic features which depend upon the rate of accumulation of pericardial fluid and the presence or absence of cardiac disease.
- Unclotted blood in the pericardium appears as a circumferential echolucent space. Pericardial effusions can be classified into small (<0.5cm), moderate (0.5–2cm) and large (>2cm).
- Tamponade occurs when pressure in the pericardium exceeds the pressure in the cardiac chambers, resulting in impaired cardiac filling. Even relatively small amount of fluid can produce a tamponade effect if accumulated acutely or loculated behind the atria.
- Classical echocardiographic signs of tamponade include: moderate to large pericardial effusion, right atrial collapse (duration >1/3 systole), RV collapse, reciprocal changes in right and left ventricular volumes with respiration, IVC plethora (with elevated right side pressures), respiratory variation in RV and LV diastolic filling, increased RV filling on first beat after inspiration, decreased LV filling on the first beat after inspiration.
- Post-sternotomy tamponade requires TOE as blood is frequently clotted and loculated posteriorly, and may not be visible with TTE.

Assessment of RV function

- RV dysfunction is frequently seen in critical care. RV function is altered by factors increasing RV afterload, such as high levels of peak expiratory pressure and increased pulmonary vascular resistance (from vascular, metabolic and respiratory causes).
- The most common causes of acute cor pulmonale are massive PE and ARDS. Other causes of RV dysfunction include RV infarct, acute sickle cell crisis, air, fat embolism and myocardial contusion.
- RV assessment may alter treatment (fluid loading, vasopressors, thrombolytics) and is of prognostic value.
- Echocardiographicaly, the RV cavity is flat in the four-chamber view or crescent shaped in the short axis view.
- RV walls are thinner than those of the LV, and the interventricular septum acts as part of the LV, moving towards it in systole.
- In RV failure its cavity enlarges, resulting in apical dilatation (in the four-chamber view) and round shape (in the short axis view). RV enlargement is usually associated with IVC dilatation and loss of respiratory collapse, and TR with a jet velocity >2.5m/s).
- The LV and RV interact due to pericardial constraint. The sum of the diastolic ventricular dimensions has to remain constant. Any acute LV or RV dilatation is associated with proportional reduction in LV or RV diastolic dimension. RV dilatation can be quantified by measuring the ratio between the RV EDA and LV EDA. Moderate RV dilatation corresponds to a diastolic ventricular ratio >0.6 and severe RV dilatation to a ratio >1.
- Acute RV failure can lead to distortion of LV size and geometry, and as the RV enlarges the septum is pushed towards the LV, resulting in a small, 'D-shaped' LV cavity with compromised LV filling and function.
- Longitudinal RV function (RV LAX) can be measured by tricuspid annular motion. <1cm = severe RV impairment (compare with mitral annular motion above).

Further reading

American Society of Echocardiography `www.asecho.org` contains comprehensive information regarding guidelines and standards of echopractice.

British Society of Echocardiography `www.bseecho.org` provides information about the accreditation process, learning and courses.

Cheitlin MD, Armstrong WF, Aurigemma GP, *et al.* American College of Cardiology; American Heart Association; American Society of Echocardiography. ACC/AHA/ASE 2003 guidline update for the clinical application of echocardiography: summary article: a report of the American College of Cardiology/American Heart Association Task Force on Practice Guidelines (ACC/AHA/ASE Committee to Update the 1997 Guidelines for the Clinical application of Echocardiography). *Circulation* 2003;108: 1146–62.

Doppler

Introduction

The Doppler effect was first described in 1842 by Christian Doppler, and describes the change in frequency as sound or light waves are reflected off a moving object. This relationship is described by the equation shown in Figure 7.9.1. The Doppler effect can be utilized clinically to measure the velocity of blood flow. An ultrasound beam of known frequency is directed at an angle to intersect the path of the blood flow and reflected back by the red blood cells to an ultrasound detector. The change in the frequency of the reflected ultrasound waves is directly proportional to the velocity of the blood towards or away from the Doppler probe. Measurement of blood flow using the Doppler effect has a variety of clinical applications including the measurement of flow across heart valves and in the assessment of peripheral vascular disease. One of the most common applications of the Doppler effect in the intensive care setting is in the measurement of cardiac output.

The Doppler equation is given as.

$$fd = 2.fo.v.\cos\theta/c$$

Where: v is the velocity of blood flow; θ is the angle between the ultrasound beam and blood flow; c is the ultrasound velocity in that medium; fo is the transmitting frequency.

Doppler measurement of cardiac output

The cardiac output can be calculated by measuring the velocity of blood through the descending aorta with a Doppler probe placed in the oesophagus, or the velocity of blood in the ascending aorta with a probe in the suprasternal notch. The difficulties inherent in maintaining the position of the probe in the suprasternal notch have led to the dominance of oesophageal placement. Two commercially available oesophageal Doppler systems are the CardioQ™ from Deltex Medical and the Hemosonic™ from Arrow International Inc.

Measurement of the velocity of blood (cm/s) in the descending aorta allows the flow of blood (ml/s) to be calculated provided that the cross-sectional area of the aorta is known. The CardioQ™ calculates the aortic cross-sectional area from a nomogram based upon the patient's age, height and weight. The Hemosonic™ directly measures the diameter of the aorta by incorporating M-mode ultrasound capability into the Doppler probe.

Calculation of the cardiac output using the oesophageal Doppler method is dependent on five assumptions:

1. The distribution of blood caudally to the descending aorta and rostrally to the great vessels and coronary arteries maintains is a constant ratio of 70% to 30%
2. That a flat velocity profile exists within the aorta
3. The estimated cross-sectional area is close to the mean systolic diameter
4. There is negligible diastolic blood flow
5. The velocity of blood flow in the aorta is measured accurately

Practical considerations

The descending aorta runs parallel and immediately adjacent to the oesophagus at a depth of ~35–40cm from the teeth. This allows uninterrupted passage of ultrasound waves between the probe and the aortic blood stream. The Doppler probe is most commonly introduced orally in sedated or anaesthetized patients, but may also be introduced nasally in awake patients with mild sedation and topical anaesthesia. The probe should be well lubricated prior to insertion to prevent air between the probe and the oesophageal wall from attenuating the signal. When the probe is at the appropriate depth, it is rotated slowly so that the tip of the probe is facing posteriorly (towards the aorta). Once in position, the probe is manipulated to achieve the optimal Doppler waveform; this will be the clearest signal with the highest peak velocity. The characteristic waveform should be a dark/hollow centre surrounded by red and then white in the trailing edge of the waveform. The waveform should be discrete and well contrasted with respect to the background (Fig. 7.9.2). The gain control alters the contrast between the Doppler waveform and background noise and should be adjusted to give a black background and sharply contrasted Doppler waveform.

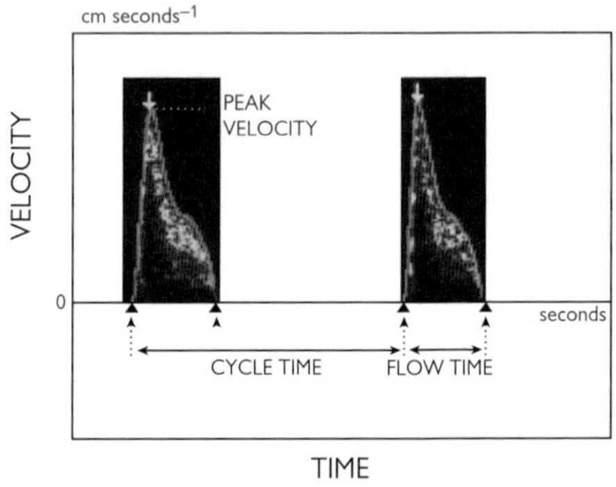

Fig. 7.9.1 Typical Doppler waveform

The positioning technique and waveform recognition require a degree of operator training; however, it has been shown that an acceptable degree of competence can be achieved after the insertion of only 12 probes. Once inserted, Doppler probes have been used in unconscious patients for up to 14 days without complication. The use of an oesophageal Doppler probe is safe in most patients; however, contraindications include the presence of clotting abnormalities, oesophageal varices and recent oesophageal surgery. Readings obtained from an oesophageal Doppler probe may be inaccurate in the following circumstances:

- Coarctation of the aorta
- Thoracic aortic aneurysm (especially if aortic cross-section is calculated from nomogram)
- Presence of a working epidural/intrathecal anaesthetic with subsequent vasodilatation

In these circumstances, whilst the absolute figures from the Doppler probe may be inaccurate, trends in the readings can still be used to guide therapy.

Interpretation of waveform and variables

Transoesophageal Doppler probes are capable of measuring a number of haemodynamic variables, the interpretation of which can then be used to guide treatment.

Peak velocity

The peak velocity of blood in the aorta gives a good estimate of the contractility of the myocardium. Normal peak velocity varies with age; at the age of 20 normal peak velocity is 90–120cm/s, falling to 50–80cm/s by the age of 70.

Stroke volume/cardiac output

Stroke distance is the area under the velocity–time waveform; when multiplied by the aortic diameter this gives a good estimate of the stroke volume. Due to slight beat-to-beat variability in stroke volume, the reading is usually averaged over several beats. The number of beats used for this calculation is the *cycle length*. A cycle length of five beats is usual, but can be increased to improve the accuracy of stroke volume estimation when there is marked beat-to-beat variability, e.g. atrial fibrillation. The cardiac output is calculated from the stroke volume multiplied by the heart rate.

Corrected flow time (FTc)

The flow time is the duration of forward flow of blood in the aorta, i.e. the width of the base of the velocity–time waveform. The flow time varies with heart rate and can be corrected to a heart rate of 60bpm by dividing the flow time by the square root of the cardiac cycle time (analogous to correcting the Q-T interval in ECG interpretation); this value is the corrected flow time (FTc). The normal FTc is 330–360ms. Anything that impedes filling or emptying of the LV will cause a reduction in FTc. Most commonly this is seen in hypovolaemia, but may also be seen with mitral stenosis, PE and excessive use of vasopressors. A prolonged FTc is seen in the vasodilated circulation, e.g. in sepsis. A prolonged FTc of up to 400ms may be regarded as normal in an anaesthetized patient, especially in the presence of a working epidural

In addition to the variables described, the appearance of the velocity–time waveform itself may be diagnostic. as described in Figure 7.9.3.

Clinical application

To date there has been no reported mortality associated with the use of oesophageal Doppler. Morbidity rates are also low; there are case reports of inadvertent insertion into the lower respiratory tract and of epistaxis after nasal insertion.

Single readings may be diagnostic, but observation of dynamic changes with therapy are often more useful.

- *Low stroke volume*. Fluid is best given as boluses, e.g. 200ml, to construct a Starling curve for that patient. If there is less than a 5–10% increase in stroke volume with each bolus it suggests that the plateau point has been reached.
- *Low FTc*. Most commonly represents hypovolaemia. Fluid challenge as above to achieve an FTc of 330–360ms. Other causes, e.g. PE, will not improve with fluids.
- *Low peak velocity*. Consider positive inotropes.
- *Low peak velocity and low FTc*. Consider moves to reduce afterload, e.g. peripheral warming, reduction of vasopressors, glyceryl trinitrate (GTN).

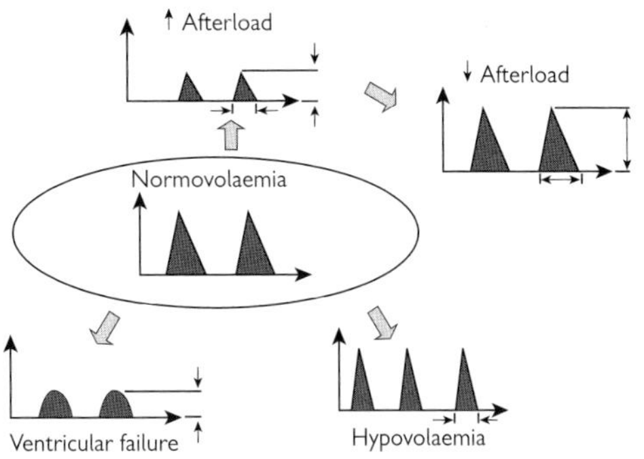

Fig. 7.9.2 Characteristic waveforms.

The use of oesophageal Doppler to measure cardiac output in critically ill patients compares favourably with the use of the thermodilution method using a pulmonary artery catheter.

There is an increasing body of evidence that intraoperative fluid therapy guided by oesophageal Doppler monitoring can result in a lower rate of perioperative complications and a shorter length of hospital stay. A systematic review and meta-analysis of studies using oesophageal Doppler perioperatively found a reduction in hospital stay of nearly 3 days in the Doppler groups.

The ease of use and the data provided by oesophageal Doppler lends itself to use in protocol-driven fluid resuscitation. McKendry *et al.* reported the successful use of a nurse-led, Doppler-guided protocol for fluid optimization post-cardiac surgery. The advent of more flexible probes for nasal insertion in awake patients has allowed for the development of nurse-led early fluid optimization in the setting of critical care outreach teams.

Further reading

Dark PM, Singer M. The validity of trans-esophageal Doppler ultrasonography as a measure of cardiac output in critically ill adults. *Intensive Care Med* 2004; 30: 2060–6.

McKendry M, McGloin H, Saberi D, *et al.* Randomised controlled trial assessing the impact of a nurse delivered, flow monitored protocol for optimisation of circulatory status after cardiac surgery. *BMJ* 2004; 329: 258–62.

Walker D, Usher S, Hartin J, *et al.* Early experiences with the new awake oesophageal Doppler probe. *Br J Anaesth* 2004; 93 : 471.

Pulse pressure algorithms

Cardiac output can be monitored continuously by different devices that analyse the arterial waveform to track changes in stroke volume and cardiac output. The analysis of the arterial pressure wave to determine cardiac output is classified as pulse contour analysis or pulse pressure analysis. Starting from a similar principle three main devices are now available on the market, with different algorithms and features:

- PiCCO system (Pulsion, Munich, Germany)
- LiDCO™plus system (LidCO, Cambridge, UK)
- Flotrac technology and Vigileo Monitor (Edwards Lifesciences, Irvine, CA, USA)

Physiological background

Compliance

Compliance describes the relationship between pressure and volume in the arterial vessels. Knowing the compliance is essential to estimate the changes in volume (stroke volume) from changes

$$C = \Delta V/\Delta P.$$

Where C = compliance, ΔV = changes in volume, ΔP = changes in pressure.

Without knowing the compliance of the arterial tree, more precisely the compliance of the proximal aorta, it is not possible to understand the change in volume that corresponds to a change in pressure. Compliance in the arterial tree is not a linear relationship, and so the same change in pressure does not always reflect the same change in volume. As a general rule, compliance is higher for lower pressures and lower for higher pressures. Another peculiarity of compliance is that it is not constant. The same arterial tree can behave differently in different situations and be characterized by different compliance. For example, vasoconstriction during vasopressor therapy decreases compliance, vice versa vasodilation during vasodilator therapy or sepsis increases compliance.

The aorta is the main arterial vessel of interest, as it is the part of the arterial tree that directly receives the stroke volume. There are three forces that contribute to how the proximal aorta is filled with blood during every heart beat:

- The force of injection of the blood by the pumping of the heart
- The opposing force dependent on the pulsatile inflow (impedance)
- The opposing force dependent on the change in volume that we described as compliance

When blood leaves the aorta there is also another force that opposes the blood flowing peripherally. This is the peripheral resistance.

Reflected waves

A further problem that has to be overcome is the accurate measurement of pressure in the periphery. The arterial pressure recorded is not only dependent on the aortic arterial pressure, but is also the result of the reflection of waves generated peripherally and returning back up the arterial system.

Non-pulsatile flow

Although the flow wave and the pressure wave in the proximal aorta occur almost simultaneously, more peripherally this is not the case as the pressure wave is transmitted ~20 times faster than the flow wave. Moreover, even if it is true that in the proximal aorta the flow is almost pulsatile, blood flows peripherally in both systole and diastole. A pulse pressure algorithm needs to take into consideration all these forces when transforming a pressure to a volume in order to track stroke volume.

Summarizing, an ideal algorithm should:

- Work independently of the arterial site from where pressure is monitored despite changes in waveform shape and pressure through the arterial tree from the centre to the periphery.
- Correct for non-linear compliance and take account of individual variations in aortic characteristics, thus giving an absolute cardiac output.
- Not be affected by changes in vascular resistance causing changes in reflected wave augmentation of the arterial pressure.
- Not rely on identifying details of wave morphology.
- Be only minimally affected by the damping often seen in arterial lines.

History

The first algorithm used in clinical practice was the Wesseling algorithm in 1983. This algorithm is based on the hypothesis that the contour of the arterial pressure waveform is dependent on stroke volume, and that this can be estimated from the integral of the change in pressure over time, considering the interval between the end of diastole to tyhe end of systole (Asys). This is the first algorithm of pulse contour analysis used to determine cardiac output. From this point, new algorithms have been developed.

Devices

PiCCO system

In clinical practice the first pulse contour method using a Wesseling-based algorithm was the PiCCO system (Pulsion Munich, Germany). PiCCO is a cardiac monitor that measures cardiac output and several volumes (intrathoracic blood volume (ITBV), global end-diastolic volume (GEDV), extravascular lung water (EVLW)) via transpulmonary thermodilution. This thermodilution is used to calibrate the pulse pressure algorithm. The pulse pressure algorithm analyses both the systolic and the diastolic part of the arterial pressure to study and determine the non-linear compliance, and the relationship flow/pressure. This part of the process is called calibration and should be repeated every time there is a significant haemodynamic change. In order to perform a thermodilutionm a central venous catheter needs to be in place. 15ml of cold saline is injected through a sensor that detects the temperature and time of the injection. A specialized arterial catheter (usually a femoral artery) detects the changes in blood temperature, producing a thermodilution curve. The same arterial catheter is used to monitor blood pressure, and the arterial waveform is analysed by the pulse pressure algorithm.

PiCCO continuous cardiac output had been studied and validated against the pulmonary artery catheter in several conditions and has proven to be a reliable device, requiring calibration more often only in cases of major haemodynamic changes.

The algorithm also provides the user with the analysis of the variation in either stroke volume (SVV) or pulse pressure (PPV). SVV and PPV represent the variation of stroke volume and of the pulse pressure during the respiratory cycle. In sedated ventilated patients, these indexes have proven to predict the response to a fluid challenge. A large variation (>10–12%) identifies responders and non-responders with good sensitivity and specificity.

LiDCO

The LiDCO™plus system is a cardiac output monitor that measures cardiac output via lithium transpulmonary thermodilution. The LiDCO algorithm for continuous cardiac output monitoring is based on the hypothesis that the change in power in the system (arterial tree) during systole is proportional to the difference in the amount of blood entering the system (stroke volume) minus the amount of blood flowing out peripherally. It is based on the principle of conservation of mass/power and an assumption that following correction for compliance and calibration there is a linear relationship between net power and net flow. This algorithm defines which part of the 'change in power' is determined by the stroke volume. When this is identified, then cardiac output is derived. The calibration is obtained via a lithium dilution technique. In order to perform the calibration, a dose of 0.3mmol of lithium is injected using either central or peripheral venous access. A sensor connected to an arterial line (there is no need for a specialized catheter) which makes it possible to generate a concentration–time curve, and the cardiac output is then calculated. This value is then used to calibrate the pulse pressure algorithm. Further calibrations should be performed in the case of major haemodynamic changes.

Continuous cardiac output of LiDCO has already been validated in several studies. This new algorithm has so far proven to be reliable in both surgical and intensive care patients. The LiDCO algorithm also allows the analysis of the SVV or PPV and of the systolic pressure variation (SPV). As discussed for PiCCO, these indexes are useful predictors of fluid responsiveness.

FloTrac and Vigileo

Flotrac (Edwards Lifescience, Irvine, CA, USA) is the name of the specific transducer incorporated into the Vigileo monitor. The most interesting characteristic of this device is that it does not need to be calibrated and it needs just an arterial line to work. Compliance and resistance are derived from the analysis of the arterial waveform. The hypothesis is that in order to calculate the effects of compliance and peripheral resistance on flow, all the necessary information can be obtained by the analysis of the arterial pressure waveform. Age, weight and sex of the patient are the only variables that the clinician needs to input into the Vigileo monitor. The transducer (Flotrac) can be connected to any functioning arterial access. The algorithm recalculates the compliance continuously, thus bypassing the need for calibration. The Vigileo algorithm also allows the analysis SVV and PPV to be performed. This algorithm is now under validation.

Clinical use of pulse pressure-based algorithms

The most interesting feature of all these devices is that they are able to track changes in cardiac output in real time. Intermittent techniques are not appropriate to measure changes when these occur in a very short time (seconds, minutes). This is particularly useful when evaluating the effect of a fluid challenge or inotrope administration on haemodynamics. When performing a fluid challenge, recognizing an increase in SV (>10%) identifies patients that benefit from fluids. All the devices discussed have features that make them suitable to monitor changes in cardiac output in real time when a therapeutic intervention is applied.

Further reading

Della Rocca G, Costa MG, Pompei L, *et al.* Continuous and intermittent cardiac output measurement: pulmonary artery catheter versus aortic transpulmonary technique. *Br J Anaesth* 2002; **88**: 350–6.

Hamilton TT, Huber LM, Jessen ME. PulseCO: a less-invasive method to monitor cardiac output from arterial pressure after cardiac surgery. *Ann Thorac Surg* 2002; **74**: S1408–12.

Jansen JRC, Wesseling KH, Settels JJ. Continuous cardiac output monitoring by pulse contour during cardiac surgery. *Eur Heart* 1990; 11: 26–32.

Michard F, Teboul JL. Using heart–lung interactions to assess fluid responsiveness during mechanical ventilation. *Crit Care* 2000; **4**: 282–9.

Non-invasive methods

The major criticism to the pulmonary artery catheter is that its level of invasiveness is not supported by an improvement in the patient's outcome. Monitoring cardiac output is essential in haemodynamic patients, so new devices have been developed with the aim of monitoring the circulation, avoiding the invasiveness of pulmonary artery catheterization. Some of these methods, such as pulse pressure analysis, are less invasive but still require the catheterization of blood vessels (arteries, veins or both). Methods that do not need the catheterization of blood vessels are called 'non-invasive methods'. These include:

- Oesophageal Doppler
- Echocardiography
- Electric impedance
- Partial carbon dioxide re-breathing

Doppler ultrasound

The Doppler effect describes why a moving object creates a shift in frequency when referred to an observer. The shift in frequency (emitted or reflected) is proportional to the relative velocity between the object and observer and can be used to estimate the velocity.

Several devices able to measure the flow velocity in the aorta are available. Flow can be measured in the ascending part of the aorta (with a suprasternal notch probe) or in the descending part of the aorta (with an intraoesophageal probe). This method is most widely used. The two most popular oesophageal Doppler devices are CardioQ (Deltex Medical Ltd, Chichester, UK) and Hemosonic 100 (Arrow, Reading, PA, USA).

In order to know the flow, it is necessary to understand the diameter of the descending aorta. The main difference between CardioQ and Hemosonic is that CardioQ uses a normogram to obtain information about the diameter of the aorta. This normogram incorporates age, height and weight. Hemosonic, in order to obtain the information about the diameter of the aorta, uses an M-mode determination. Both CardioQ and Hemosonic cardiac output have been validated against thermodilution.

The accuracy and the precision of Doppler devices have shown good, but not excellent, agreement. Despite this, there are several studies proving that oesophageal Doppler can accurately track changes in cardiac output and guide fluid therapy. Indeed protocols that have used Oesophageal Doppler in the perioperative period to guide fluid therapy have produced an improved outcome.

Doppler ultrasound summary

- Requirements: an intraoesophageal probe (suprasternal notch probe available)
- Easy to use, good level of accuracy and precision
- Disadvantage: difficult to manage in non-intubated patients.

Echocardiography

Cardiac output can be measured with echocardiography with the use of Doppler, looking at flow across the aortic or pulmonary outflow tract. This technique is reliable and accurate although it is user dependent. Studies examining cardiac output by transoesophageal echocardiography have shown acceptable precision and accuracy when compared with pulmonary artery catheterization. Echocardiography also allow a more global overview of cardiac dimensions and function (see Chapter 7.7).

Echiocardiography summary

- Requirements: a trained operator
- Complete vision of cardiovascular dynamics in expert hands
- Disadvantage: operator dependent; long learning curve.

Electric impedance

Electric impedance uses stimulation with a constant electric current with the aim of identifying the electrical impedance variations induced by vascular blood flow. The theory is that the cardiac output is responsible for the variation of the electric impedance. This variation is analysed by an algorithm that estimates the changes in cardiac output. The electrodes can be placed either on the thorax (thoracic electric bioimpedance (TEB)) or on the limbs (whole body electrical bioimpedance (WBEB)).

There are several devices using this principle to track changes in cardiac output, such as BioZ (Cardiodynamics International, San Diego, CA, USA) or Cardioscreen (Messtechnik, Illmenau, Germany).

Validation studies so far have shown the accuracy and precision of this technique. The main advantage is that it is a totally non-invasive technique, while the main disadvantages are that severe fluid shifts (severe oedema, pleural effusions, etc.), arrhythmias, ventilation, etc. affect the reliability of these techniques, making them difficult to trust in critically ill patients.

Electric impedance summary

- Requirements: none.
- Disadvantage: affected by many clinical situations.

Partial carbon dioxide re-breathing

This method is usually classified as non-invasive because it does not require any invasive access, though it can be done only in mechanically ventilated patients. This method is based on a modification of Fick's principle. Fick's principle says that if oxygen uptake happens in the lungs, the cardiac output can be estimated as the ratio between oxygen consumption and the oxygen difference between arteries and veins is known. There is one device that uses this principle (applied to CO_2): the NICO System (Novametrix Medical System, Wallingford, CT, USA). The main advantage of this system is that it can be connected to any mechanical ventilator. The NICO System creates a partial CO_2 re-breathing circuit and analyses the CO_2 concentrations from the end-tidal CO_2 sensor. The shunt percentage is estimated from the analysis of the O_2 utilization (O_2 saturation is obtained via a pulse oximeter connected to the machine). The main disadvantages are that shunts are often present in critically ill patients and NICO compensation is not accurate enough. Indeed not all the studies have proved that NICO is a reliable CO_2 monitor when compared with pulmonary artery catheterization. If implemented, ideally it could be used for every patient on a ventilator.

Partial carbon dioxide concentration summary

- Requirements: a mechanically ventilated patient
- Disadvantages: the shunt fraction is difficult to measure; a low level of precision when high levels of shunt are present.

Further reading

Gan TJ, Soppitt A, Maroof M, *et al.* Goal-directed intraoperative fluid administration reduces length of hospital stay after major surgery. *Anesthesiology* 2002; 97: 820–6.

Moshkovitz Y, Kalushi E, Milo O, *et al.* Recent developments in cardiac output determination by bioimpedance: comparison with invasive cardiac output and potential cardiovascular applications. *Curr Opin Cardiol* 2004; 19: 229–37.

Rocco M, Spadetta G, Morelli A, Dell'Utri *et al. Intensive Care Med* 2004; 30: 82–7.

Vignon P. Hemodynamic assessment of critically ill patients using echocardiography Doppler. *Curr Opin Crit Care* 2005; 11: 227–34.

Measurement of preload status

Preload is the initial stretching of the myocyte before contraction. Unfortunately this stretching cannot be measured *in vivo* and therefore other methods have been developed to estimate preload in clinical practice. Preload can be considered to be the volume of blood at the end of diastole (after atrial contraction) in the ventricles. Knowledge of the preload is important when treating haemodynamically unstable patients to identify which patients will require volume expansion and how much they will need.

Preload indexes

A preload index is an indirect measure of preload that gives us an estimation of the preload itself. A good preload index should correlate with stroke volume in the preload as shown in the Frank–Starling curve (Fig. 7.12.1). The most studied preload indexes are the following:

1 Filling Pressures (CVP, PAoP)
2 Left ventricular end-diastolic area
3 Volumetric indexes (RVEDV, ITBV, GEDV)

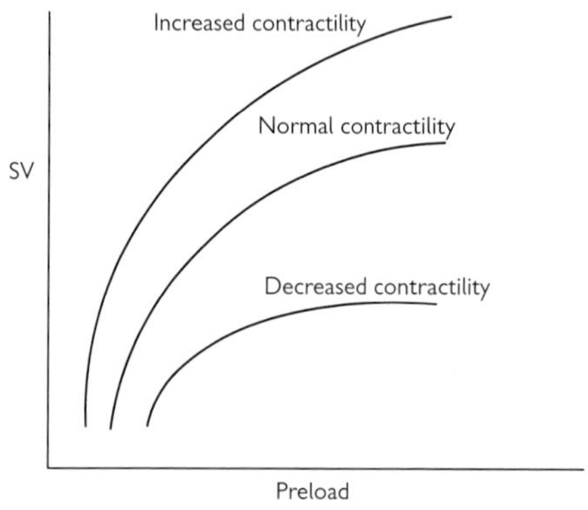

Fig. 7.12.1 Frank–Starling curve.

Filling pressures

Physiological background

Historically pressures such as CVP and PAoP have been used to estimate preload. CVP is a pressure proportional to the volume of blood in the right side of the heart; PAoP is proportional to the volume of blood in the left side of the heart. The assumption behind their use as preload indexes revolves around the belief that myocyte stretching is proportional to the filling pressure of the heart. Unfortunately both CVP and PAoP are intravascular pressures while the pressure that is proportional to the cardiac chamber dilatation is a transmural pressure. A transmural pressure is the result of the difference between an intravascular pressure (that we can measure) and an extravascular pressure, i.e. the intrathoracic pressure. The intrathoracic pressure can be affected by various factors such as mechanical ventilation and PEEP. If changes in intrathoracic pressure were fully transmitted to the intravascular pressure, then the transmural pressure would be the same. This is unfortunately unpredictable. One way of minimizing this problem during mechanical ventilation is by measuring the CVP or the PAoP at the end of the expiratory cycle and without PEEP. This is not always easy nor possible to carry out at the bedside.

A further problem with this relationship is that the compliance of the heart is not linearly related to pressure. If compliance was linear then for every increase or decrease in venous pressure there would be a constant increase or decrease in stroke volume. Unfortunately, this is not the case and even in the preload-dependent part of the Frank–Starling curve changes in volume cannot be accurately predicted by changes in pressure.

Central venous pressure (CVP)

Many studies have failed to prove that CVP is a good preload index. Not even the changes in CVP can predict precisely the changes in stroke volume. Despite this, there is some evidence and good sense that in some situations maintaining a CVP above a minimal level is necessary to avoid hypovolaemia. For example, in a ventilated patient a CVP <10 correlates with a bigger decrease in cardiac output when PEEP is applied. Despite a lack of proof that CVP is a reliable preload index, CVP is still used as a surrogate of preload in many study protocols. For example, a CVP of 8–12mm Hg is often used to define 'normovolaemia' arbitrarily. This is probably guided by common sense and also some evidence that very low and very high values of CVP may be detrimental to the patient.

Pulmonary artery occlusion pressure (PAoP)

No study has ever proven that the PAoP is a reliable preload index. The PAoP cannot reliably guide fluid resuscitation. Despite the fact that the absolute values of PAoP show a poor or no correlation with stroke volume, there is some evidence that a very low or very high PAoP would have some clinical impact. Values <8mm Hg are generally accepted to identify patients who may benefit from volume expansion, while values >18mm Hg may identify patients who probably will not respond to volume expansion and may instead be at risk of developing pulmonary oedema.

Filling pressures key points

- Poor preload indexes
- A wedge pressure >18mm Hg is associated with a higher incidence of hydrostatic pulmonary oedema.
- A wedge pressure <8mm Hg in a mechanically ventilated patient identifies a patient who is more likely to respond to a fluid challenge.

Left ventricular end-diastolic area (LVEDA)

Echocardiography is a valuable tool, but requires training to use it and even then it is an operator-dependent tool. In expert hands echocardiography probably represents the most complete tool to assess the cardiovascular system. A 'quick view' in expert hands can be useful if hypovolaemia is suspected. The area measured in bidimensional mode at the end of diastole is a well accepted measurement of preload and it is considered by many intensivists to be the gold standard. Its role in guiding fluid therapy in the operating theatre is well recognized. In the critically ill patient, LVEDA is more reliable than either CVP or PAoP as a preload index.

Volumetric indexes

With the development of new technologies, new preload indexes have been studied. The most studied volumetric indexes are:

- Right ventricular end-diastolic volume (RVEDV) by a modified pulmonary artery catheter.
- Intrathoracic blood volume index (ITBVI) and global end-diastolic volume index (GEDVI) by the PiCCO system (Pulsion, Munich, Germany)

Right ventricular end-diastolic volume index (RV EDVI)

RVEDVI is a parameter available in some rapid response sensor pulmonary artery catheters. The RVEDV represents the volume of blood in the right ventricle at the end of diastole. It has shown to be a better preload index than filling pressures. Knowledge of the RV EF is important to evaluate the RVEDVI and to identify RV dysfunction. Knowledge of the RV EF allows the Frank–Starling curve to be drawn for the individual patient. The lower the RV EF, the higher will be the value of the RVEDVI. Due to the fact that it requires the placement of a pulmonary artery catheter and because it is not possible to estimate the LVEDV accurately from the RVEDV, the variable has not gained widespread acceptability.

RVEDVI key points

- Better preload Index than filling pressures
- EDV target 80–120ml/m2 (may be adapted according to the RV EF)
- Disadvantage: requires placement of a pulmonary artery catheter.

Intrathoracic blood volume index (ITBVI) and global end-diastolic index (GEDVI)

History: the double indicator technique

The original transpulmonary indicator technique used two indicators to determine cardiac output and volumes. The principle was simple: one indicator would stay only within the vascular system (indocyanin green dye) and a second indicator would spread extravascularly (thermal indicator). From the analysis of the dilution curves of the two indicators, the system (COLD System, Pulsion Medical System, Munich, Germany) was able to measure cardiac output and intravascular and extravascular volumes. The ITBVI represents the volume of blood in the chest; The GEDVI represents the volume of blood in all the heart chambers at the end of diastole. Because of these physiological properties, they have been proposed and validated as preload indexes. These indexes have been studied and validated in many clinical scenarios, proving to be better preload indexes than filling pressures. The COLD system is no longer available; however, a simplified technology has been developed to obtain the same volumetric information with just a single indicator: the PiCCO system.

Single indicator ITBVI and GEDVI

The ITBVI and GEDVI are some of the volumes that the PiCCO system can measure using the transpulmonary thermodilution technique. Analysis of the thermodilution slope allows the PiCCO system to estimate different thermal volumes (such as pulmonary blood volume (PBV), EVLW and the ITBVI and GEDVI). The ITBVI and GEDVI are strictly correlated in their calculation. GEDVI is measured directly and ITVBI is extrapolated using the following formula:

$$ITBVI = GEDVI \times 1.25$$

These measurements have been validated against the double indicator technique (COLD system, Pulsion). Due to the linear relationship between the GEDVI and ITBVI, it is acceptable to extrapolate results from the GEDVI to the ITBVI and vice versa.

Investigators have studied both the ITBVI and GEDVI, demonstrating that they are better indicators of preload than filling pressures (CVP and PAoP). These clinical settings involve both the operating theatre and the ICU. The accuracy of these indicators in terms of measuring preload has been studied even during fluid loading. Volume loading is reflected in increased values of the GEDVI. Whereas the changes in CVP do not reflect changes in stroke volume, changes in GEDVI reflect the changes well.

Clinical use of the ITBVI and GEDVI

In the majority of studies, the ITBVI and GEDVI were targeted to values of 800–1000ml/m^2 and 650–1000ml/m^2, respectively. In critically ill patients, optimizing the preload is challenging. Capillary leak is often present, with the risk of overloading patients and increasing oedema. A way of solving this problem is to guide fluid therapy not by the ITBVI and GEDVI alone, but integrated into protocols that assess all other haemodynamic data such as cardiac output and venous saturation.

Key points of ITBVI and GEDVI

- Good preload index
- ITBVI target 800–1000ml/m2
- GEDVI 650–1000ml/m2.

Further reading

Della Rocca G, Costa MG, Pietropaoli P. How to measure and interpret volumetric measures of preload. *Curr Opin Crit Care* 2007; 13: 297–302.

Ganter CG, Jacob SM, Takala J. Min Anestesiol 2006; 72: 21–36.

Magder S. Central venous pressure: a useful but not so simple measurement. *Crit Care Med* 2006; 34: 2224–7.

Wiesenack C, Fiegl C, Keyser A, et al. Continuously assessed right ventricular end-diastolic volume as a marker of cardiac preload and fluid responsiveness in mechanically ventilated cardiac surgical patients. *Crit Care* 2005; 9: R226–33.

Detection of fluid responsiveness

How to define fluid responsiveness?

Fluid responsiveness is defined as the ability of the heart to increase its stroke volume significantly in response to volume expansion because of the presence of biventricular preload reserve.

Why and when to predict fluid responsiveness

Three different scenarios must be distinguished.

1 *Patients admitted with evidence of acute body fluid losses*: the diagnosis of hypovolaemia is almost certain and the presence of clinical signs of haemodynamic instability (hypotension, tachycardia, oliguria, mottled skin, altered mental status, etc.) strongly suggests that a positive haemodynamic response to volume resuscitation will occur.

2 *Patients admitted with early severe sepsis or septic shock*: large volume resuscitation is necessary, and there is no need for sophisticated parameters to predict volume responsiveness since a positive haemodynamic response is always expected at this early stage.

3 *Patients who have been in the ICU for several hours or days and who experience haemodynamic instability that requires urgent therapy*: only half of these patients still have some preload reserve since they have frequently already been resuscitated. Further fluid infusion has the potential to promote pulmonary oedema in cases of increased pulmonary permeability. Therefore, predictors of volume responsiveness are needed in order to distinguish between patients who can benefit from fluid resuscitation and those in whom fluid loading can be useless and even deleterious.

How to detect fluid responsiveness?

Because clinical evaluation is of poor value for detecting fluid responsiveness, sophisticated parameters have been proposed to help the clinician in the therapeutic decision-making process.

Static markers of cardiac preload

Considering the Frank–Starling relationship (stroke volume vs ventricular preload; Fig. 7.13.1), the response to volume infusion is more likely to occur when the ventricular preload is low than when it is high.

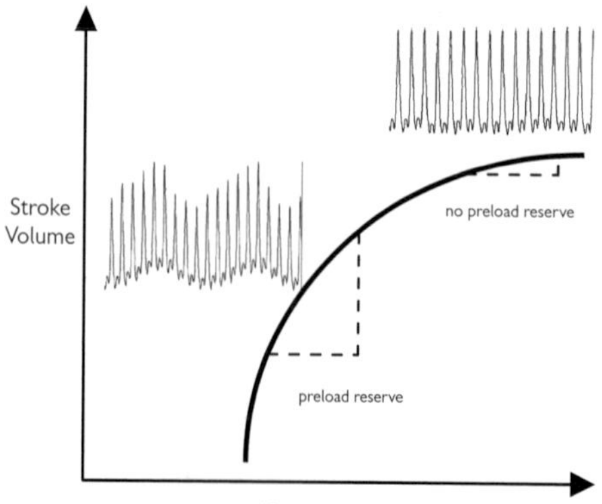

Fig. 7.13.1 Ventricular function curve demonstrating relationship between stroke volume and ventricular preload.

However, except for their lowest and highest ranges, static markers of ventricular preload such as filling pressures (CVPs and PAoP) or cardiac chamber dimensions (LVEDA) fail to predict volume responsiveness reliably. Indeed, there is not one single curve but several relating stroke volume to cardiac preload, depending on the ventricular contractile function. Thus a given value of cardiac preload can be associated with the presence of preload reserve in the case of normal cardiac function or with the absence of preload reserve in the case of decreased contractility.

Dynamic markers of preload responsiveness

Heart–lung interaction indexes

Mechanical insufflation may decrease RV filling through a decrease in venous return. This results in decreased RV stroke volume when the right ventricle has some preload reserve. Because of the long pulmonary transit time, the filling of the left ventricle senses the decrease in RV stroke volume two or three heart beats later and thus generally during expiration. This results in decreased LV stroke volume during expiration if the left ventricle also has some preload reserve. Thus, cyclical changes in LV stroke volume occur in cases of biventricular preload reserve. Since volume responsiveness occurs only in cases of biventricular preload reserve, it has been postulated that the magnitude of the cyclical changes in stroke volume or of its surrogates such as arterial pulse pressure should correlate with the degree of fluid responsiveness. Thus numerous dynamic indices using heart–lung interactions are proposed to assess volume responsiveness in patients receiving controlled mechanical ventilation.

- Respiratory variation of arterial pulse pressure (ΔPP)

Since the arterial pulse pressure (systolic minus diastolic pressure) is directly proportional to LV stroke volume, the magnitude of ΔPP has been proposed as a predictor of fluid responsiveness in patients equipped with an arterial catheter. The ΔPP is calculated as the difference between the maximal (PPmax) and the minimal (PPmin) value of pulse pressure over a single respiratory cycle divided by the average of the two values, and expressed as a percentage:

$$\Delta PP\ (\%) = (PPmax - PPmin)/((PPmax + PPmin)/2) \times 100.$$

In numerous categories of mechanically ventilated patients (septic shock, acute respiratory distress syndrome, cardiac surgery, liver transplantation, etc.), ΔPP was demonstrated to be an accurate marker of fluid responsiveness. Threshold values of ΔPP ranging from 10 to 17% have been reported. Moreover, the fluid-induced decrease in ΔPP correlates well with the percentage changes in cardiac output induced by 500ml fluid infusion. Thus, the ΔPP can be used not only to predict fluid responsiveness but also to assess the actual haemodynamic response to volume infusion. Finally, ΔPP better predicts fluid responsiveness than the systolic pressure variation or its Δ_{down} component.

- Pulse contour-derived stroke volume variation

Pulse contour cardiac output monitoring devices can continuously measure and display stroke volume variation (SVV) which represents the variation of pulse contour stroke volume over a floating period of a few seconds. In patients fully adapted to their ventilator, SVV accurately predicts fluid responsiveness. Threshold values of SVV range between 9.5 and 12.5%.

- Respiratory variation of the peak Doppler aortic blood velocity (ΔVpeak)

Doppler echocardiography allows aortic blood velocity to be measured at the level of aortic annulus (left ventricle outflow track). A value of ΔV_{peak} >12% is predictive of fluid responsiveness.

- Respiratory variation of descending aorta blood velocity (ΔABV) or blood flow (ΔABF)

Oesophageal Doppler monitoring devices allow for the measurement of descending aorta blood velocity or blood flow on a beat to beat basis. A value of Δ_{ABF} >18% is predictive of fluid responsiveness. Since the aortic diameter also varies over the ventilatory cycle, Δ_{ABF} is a better predictor of fluid responsiveness than Δ_{ABV}.

- Respiratory changes in inferior vena cava diameter (ΔDIVC)

The IVC diameter can be measured using echocardiography from short axis or long axis subcostal views. A value of ΔD_{IVC} ((maximal diameter – minimal diameter))/mean of the two values) >12% is predictive of fluid responsiveness.

- Superior vena cava (SVC) collapsibility

The diameter of the SVC can be measured using transoesophageal echocardiography. A value of SVC collapsibility (difference between maximal and minimal diameter divided by maximal diameter) >36% allowed excellent prediction of fluid responsiveness.

- Respiratory changes in pulse oxymetry plethysmographic waveform amplitude (ΔPpleth)

A value of ΔP_{pleth} >14–15% is predictive of fluid responsiveness in mechanically ventilated patients.

Limitations of using heart–lung interaction indexes

- Volume responsiveness is a physiological phenomenon related to a normal preload reserve. Thus, detecting volume responsiveness must not systematically lead to the decision of infusing fluid, in particular in the absence of clinical or biological signs of tissue hypoperfusion.
- The respiratory variation of surrogates of stroke volume cannot be used to assess fluid responsiveness in patients receiving a tidal volume <7ml/kg, in patients with spontaneous breathing activity and in patients with arrhythmias (except for respiratory variation of vena cava diameter).

Passive leg raising

In the cases where the dynamic indices using heart–lung interaction cannot be used (see above), the passive leg raising (PLR) manoeuvre can be used as a test to detect fluid responsiveness. Indeed, lifting the legs by 45° from the horizontal position induces a gravitational transfer of blood from the lower limbs toward the intrathoracic compartment and thus increases cardiac preload. An increase in cardiac output or stroke volume in response to PLR is suggestive of the presence of cardiac preload reserve and hence predictive of fluid responsiveness. Because of the short duration of this test (~1min), a real-time cardiac output or stroke volume measurement method is mandatory. In patients with spontaneous breathing activity and/or cardiac arrhythmias, a PLR-induced increase (>10%) in descending aorta blood flow (oesophageal Doppler) or a PLR-induced increase (>12.5%) in pulsed Doppler stroke volume (echocardiography) can accurately predict fluid responsiveness.

Conclusion

Minimally invasive (ΔPP, SVV) as well as non-invasive dynamic parameters (ΔV_{peak}, Δ_{ABV}, Δ_{ABF}, ΔD_{IVC}, ΔP_{pleth}) testing the sensitivity of the heart to changes in intrathoracic pressure during a mechanical breath can accurately discriminate between responders and non-responders to fluid infusion. In the cases where these indexes are not interpretable (inspiratory efforts, cardiac arrhythmias, low tidal volume), the response of stroke volume (or its surrogates) to PLR is helpful to predict fluid responsiveness.

Further reading

Feissel M, Michard F, Mangin I, *et al.* Respiratory changes in aortic blood velocity as an indicator of fluid responsiveness in ventilated patients with septic shock. *Chest* 2001; 119: 867–73.

Feissel M, Michard F, Faller JP, *et al.* The respiratory variation in inferior vena cava diameter as a guide to fluid therapy. *Intensive Care Med* 2004; 30: 1834–7.

Feissel M, Teboul JL, Merlani P, *et al.* Plethysmographic dynamic indices predict fluid responsiveness in septic ventilated patients. *Intensive Care Med* 2007; 33: 993–9.

Michard F, Teboul JL. Predicting fluid responsiveness in ICU patients: a critical analysis of the evidence. *Chest* 2002; 121: 2000–8.

Monnet X, Rienzo M, Osman D, et *al.* Esophageal Doppler monitoring predicts fluid responsiveness in critically ill ventilated patients. *Intensive Care Med* 2005; 11: 1195–201.

Monnet X, Rienzo M, Osman D, *et al.* Passive leg raising predicts fluid responsiveness in the critically ill. *Crit Care Med* 2006; 34: 1402–7.

Natalini G, Rosano A, Taranto M, *et al.* Arterial versus plethysmographic dynamic indices to test responsiveness for testing fluid administration in hypotensive patients: a clinical trial. *Anesth Analg* 2006; 103: 478–84.

Preisman S, Kogan S, Berkenstadt H, *et al.* Predicting fluid responsiveness in patients undergoing cardiac surgery: functional haemodynamic parameters including the respiratory variation test and static preload indicators. *B J Anaesth* 2005; 95: 746-55.

Vieillard-Baron A, Chergui K, Rabiller A, *et al.* Superior vena caval collapsibility as a gauge of volume status in ventilated septic patients. *Intensive Care Med* 2004; 30: 1734–9.

Chapter 8

Neurological monitoring

Chapter contents

Intracranial pressure monitoring

Introduction

In adults, the normal resting intracranial pressure (ICP) is 0–10mm Hg. ICP may rise to 50mm Hg or so during straining or sneezing, with no impairment in function. It is not, therefore, ICP alone that is important but rather the interpretation of the measurement in pathological conditions. Many of the clinicopathological changes associated with brain injury are the result of pressure differences between the intracranial compartments, with consequent shift of brain structures, rather than the absolute level of ICP.

The deterioration in conscious level accompanying elevation in ICP is probably caused by downward displacement of the diencephalon and midbrain structures. Herniation of the temporal lobe between the brainstem and the tentorial edge into the posterior fossa (tentorial or uncal herniation) causes pupillary dilatation, ptosis, limitation of upgaze and extensor posturing. Tonsillar herniation occurs when the tonsils of the cerebellum herniate through the foramen magnum into the spinal canal. This causes compression of the midbrain with changes in blood pressure, pulse rate and respiratory pattern. Cushing's response, the combination of hypertension and bradycardia, is seen in roughly 1/3 of cases of tonsillar herniation.

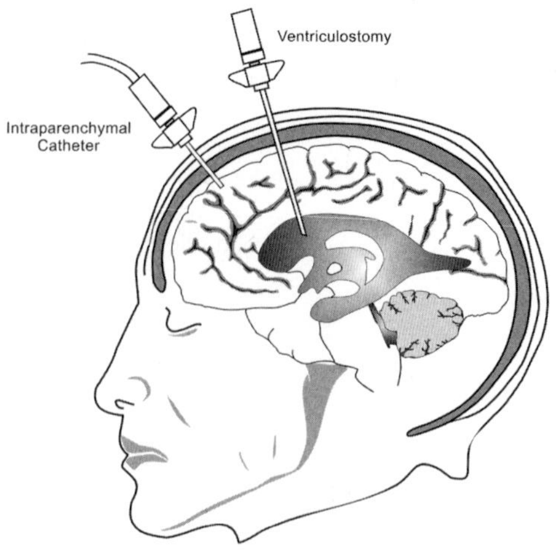

Fig. 8.1.1 Common techniques for measuring ICP.

Indications for ICP monitoring

The Brain Trauma Foundation recommends ICP monitoring in all patients with a closed head injury and a Glasgow Coma Score (GCS) of ≤8 and either (1) an abnormal CT scan or (2) a normal scan and the presence of two of the following three risk factors: age >40 years, unilateral or bilateral motor posturing or a systolic blood pressure <90mm Hg. These patients have a roughly 60% chance of having raised ICP. Both an elevated ICP and an inadequate cerebral perfusion pressure (CPP; see Chapter 8.2) have been shown to correlate with poorer outcome following traumatic brain injury. The optimal levels for the maintenance of ICP and CPP are still debated, but most recommend keeping ICP <20–25mm Hg and CPP >60mm Hg.

Monitoring of ICP may be useful in other conditions. Mortality is improved if ICP is measured in patients who are comatose following intracerebral haemorrhage, and an elevated ICP is a poor prognostic factor in patients with aneurysmal subarachnoid haemorrhage. ICP monitoring in anoxic injury following cardiac arrest or near drowning may be useful in guiding prognosis. ICP measurement may also be of use in hepatic encephalopathy, bacterial meningitis, encephalitis and in conditions such as hydrocephalus or benign intracranial hypertension. ICP monitoring in acute stroke is of little benefit over clinical monitoring alone.

Methods of measuring ICP

The two most commonly used techniques for measuring ICP are intraparenchymal monitors and intraventricular catheters (Fig. 8.1.1).

Intraparenchymal monitors

These are placed via a small incision in the scalp. A hollow bolt is then screwed into the skull such that it penetrates both tables. A 20G spinal needle is passed down the lumen of the bolt to puncture the dura. The transducer is then placed through the lumen of the bolt, 5mm into the brain parenchyma. The monitor should be zeroed to atmospheric pressure prior to insertion. Intraparenchymal monitors are usually inserted into the non-dominant frontal lobe, or the dominant frontal lobe if the non-dominant lobe is the primary site of injury.

Intraventricular catheters

These allow measurement of ICP as well as drainage of cerebrospinal fluid (CSF) to help relieve raised ICP. Placement can be done at craniotomy or through a burr hole. Simple ventriculostomies are tunnelled subcutaneously to reduce the risk of infection and are connected to an external pressure transducer placed at the level of the foramen of Munro or, for clinical purposes, the external auditory meatus. Bolt-drains are larger in diameter and have a pressure transducer within their lumen. They are placed through a hole drilled in the skull vault and secured using a bolt screwed into the skull. Ultrasound or stereotactic guidance is used to direct the catheter if the ventricles are small, whereas normal or large ventricles can usually be found 'free-hand'. ICP is measured by a strain gauge and the trace is generally of better quality and undamped compared with a ventriculostomy with an external transducer.

Complications of ICP monitoring

The transducer drift of modern intraparenchymal monitors is small, infection rates are low and there is no need to change them routinely if prolonged monitoring is required. The risk of significant intracranial bleeding requiring drainage is <1%. Tunnelling of simple ventriculostomies helps to reduce bacterial colonization and ventriculitis. The use of antibiotic-coated or silver-impregnated catheters may also help to reduce infection rates. With bolt-drains, the ICP should not be measured if the drain is open. This leads to a pressure gradient from one end of the drain to the other that is not always uniform. If drainage holes are partially blocked, a pressure gradient develops between the outside and the inside. Catheters with a transducer within them may then underestimate ICP.

ICP in normal and pathological conditions

The normal ICP trace looks similar to an arterial trace (Fig. 8.1.2A). The three peaks are: P1—the percussion wave caused by the arterial pressure being transmitted from the choroid plexus to the ventricle; P2—the tidal wave thought to be due brain compliance; and P3—the dicrotic wave due to aortic valve closure.

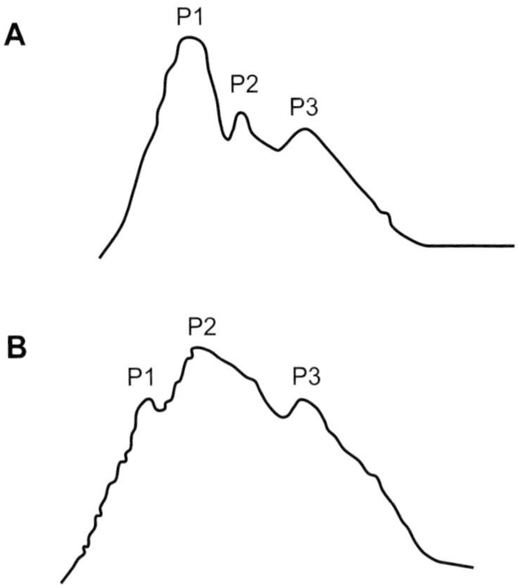

Fig. 8.1.2 Intracranial pressure waveforms.

If intracranial volume increases, the ICP wave shows an initial increase in amplitude although the mean ICP remains little changed. As brain compliance reduces, the P2 component of the pressure wave exceeds P1, with the wave becoming broader (Fig. 8.1.2B).

Lundberg described fluctuations in ventricular pressure in humans in 1960. Lundberg A waves or plateau waves are slow vasogenic waves seen in patients with critical perfusion (Fig. 8.1.3). They may reach 50–100mm Hg high and last 5–20min. Plateau waves can cause critical cerebral ischaemia within minutes and are thought to result from spontaneous reductions in arterial blood pressure resulting in cerebral vasodilatation. This increases ICP, leading to further reductions in cerebral perfusion until maximal cerebral vasodilatation occurs and the wave plateaus. Termination of these waves may occur if arterial blood pressure is increased. Plateau waves are always pathological and indicate greatly reduced cerebral compliance. B waves occur at cycles of 0.5–2/min and can be seen in normal individuals (Fig. 8.1.3). ICP rises to levels 20–30mm Hg above baseline and then falls sharply. Absence of B waves following head injury is a poor sign and may indicate poor autoregulation. C waves are of little clinical importance. They occur with a frequency of 4–8/min and are synchronous with Traub–Hering–Meyer variations in blood pressure.

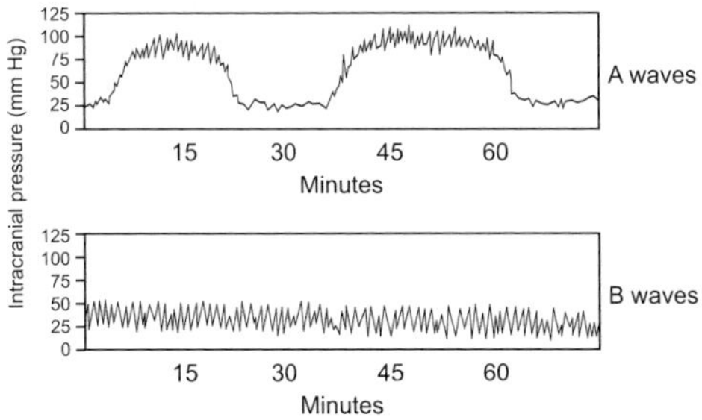

Fig. 8.1.3 Lundberg pressure waves.

Although ICP monitoring can be safely performed in non-neurosurgical centres, outcome from severe brain injury is better if patients are managed on specialized units rather than in a district general hospital. NICE guidance states that all patients with a severe head injury should be managed in specialized centres even if the patient does not require immediate neurosurgery. Protocols to manage severe head injuries have resulted in reduced mortality and improved functional outcome. Rapid access to specialist neurosurgical and non-surgical therapies such as induced hypertension, hypothermia, decompressive craniectomy and barbiturate coma are not generally available outside the specialist centres.

Further reading

Huang SJ, Hong WC, Han YY, *et al.* Clinical outcome of severe head injury using three different ICP and CPP protocol-driven therapies. *J Clin Neurosci* 2006; 13: 818–22.

National Institute of Health and Clinical Excellence. Head injury: triage, assessment, investigation and early management of head injury in infants, children and adults (partial update). 2007. `http://www.nice.org.uk`

The Brain Trauma Foundation. The American Association of Neurological Surgeons. Management and prognosis of severe traumatic head injury. *J Neurotrauma* 2000; 17: 449–27.

Intracranial perfusion

Introduction

The brain receives ~15% of the cardiac output (50ml/100g/min) and consumes 20% of total body oxygen supply. The grey matter of the brain, which consists primarily of the neuronal cell bodies and synapses, has a higher blood flow compared with the white matter, which consists largely of fibre tracts. Critical cerebral blood flow (CBF) is around 20ml/100g/min, with the EEG becoming isolelectric at 15ml/100g/min.

Brain perfusion depends on the difference between MAP and cerebral venous pressure (cerebral perfusion pressure or CPP). As the latter is difficult to measure, ICP is used as a surrogate.

$$CPP = MAP - ICP$$

Regulation of cerebral perfusion

Autoregulation (myogenic regulation)

Autoregulation ensures that CBF remains constant between MAPs from 60 to 160mm Hg (Fig. 8.2.1). The trigger for autoregulation is CPP, with reflex vasoconstriction occurring in response to increases in CPP, and vasodilatation occurring in response to decreases in CPP.

Above and below the values where autoregulation is effective, the relationship between CBF and MAP is linear such that flow is pressure dependent. Autoregulation may be impaired by hypoxia, ischaemia, hypercapnia, trauma and certain anaesthetic agents. How it is impaired is likely to vary between conditions, between patients and even in the same patient at different times in the pathological process.

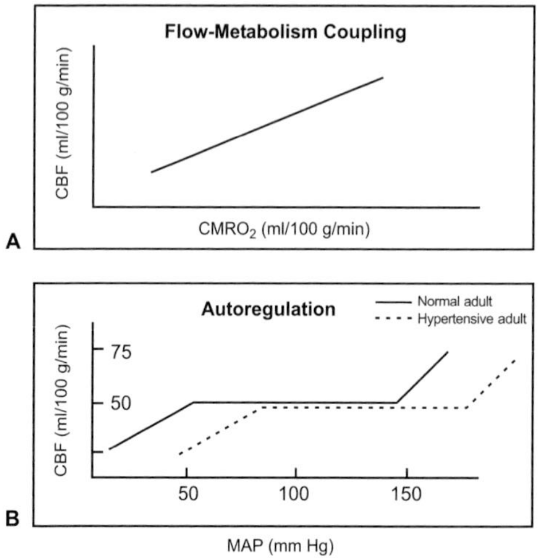

Fig. 8.2.1 Regulation of cerebral perfusion. (A) Flow–metabolism coupling. (B) Autoregulation in the normal adult and in a hypertensive adult.

Flow–metabolism coupling

Flow–metabolism coupling is the direct relationship of the metabolic activity of the brain to CBF (Fig. 8.2.1). The precise mechanisms that control flow–metabolism coupling are unknown but may involve a variety of mediators such as acetylcholine, serotonin, nitric oxide and substance P.

Systemic factors

Carbon dioxide

CBF increases by 3–4% for each mm Hg increase in pCO_2. The responses to changes in pCO_2 occur rapidly, within 30s, and are thought to relate to changes in extracellular or interstitial H^+ concentrations. Tight control of pCO_2 is essential if CPP is critical; increases in CO_2 cause vasodilatation and increased ICP, whereas decreases in pCO_2 below 4kPa have been shown to result in vasoconstriction sufficient to precipitate cerebral ischaemia.

Oxygen

CBF is not affected by changes in paO_2 within the normal range but levels <50mm Hg (6.65kPa) result in cerebral vasodilatation and increases in CBF. Below 30mm Hg (4kPa), CBF is roughly doubled. Again, this will result in an increase in ICP.

Temperature

Brain $cCMRO_2$ is increased by 8% for each degree Celsius increase in temperature. Outcome from brain injury has been inversely correlated with elevation in body temperature. Cooling allows the brain to tolerate periods of low blood flow. Although application of cooling to an unselected group of patients with head injury has been shown to be ineffective, its use is widespread for the control of elevated ICP. Similarly, cooling has been shown to improve neurological outcome following resuscitation from out-of-hospital cardiac arrest (from pulseless VT or VF).

Anaesthetic agents

Thiopentone is a potent cerebrovasoconstrictor and reduces both CBF and ICP. It has been used as a cerebral protection agent for patients with resistant elevations in ICP, and is currently being compared against decompressive craniectomy as a rescue treatment (www.RESCUEicp.com). Propofol is similar to barbiturates with regard to its cerebrovascular effects but causes greater systemic haemodynamic depression. Ketamine causes significant vasodilatation with increases in both CBF and ICP. $CMRO_2$ is little changed and there is a theoretical risk of seizures. Volatile agents are all cerebrovasodilators, thus increasing CBF and ICP to varying degrees. They also decrease $CMRO_2$.

Measurement of CBF

Because of the difficulties in measuring CBF at the bedside, it is not routinely monitored for the majority of brain-injured patients. CPP is used as a simpler measure with the recommendation that it be maintained above 60mm Hg. A number of other techniques allow estimation of either regional CGF or cerebral metabolism.

Transcranial Doppler sonography

Transcranial Doppler sonography (TCDs) allows calculation of the flow velocity of red cells in the major vessels of the circle of Willis. The technique may be applied continuously or intermittently. Most commonly, the middle cerebral artery is studied as this carries 75–80% of the carotid blood flow. TCD measures velocity rather than flow. Although absolute CBF cannot be measured, relative changes in CBF can be measured. Widespread use of the technique is limited by the technical expertise required.

TCD measurements are most commonly used to detect vasospasm following subarachnoid haemorrhage. Clinically significant vasospasm occurs in 20% of cases. Vasospasm is generally considered present when either the flow velocity exceeds 120cm/s or the Lindegaard ratio (the ratio between the velocity in the middle cerebral artery and that in the ipsilateral carotid artery) exceeds 3. The technique can also be used to determine cerebral autoregulation and CO_2 reactivity following head injury. Loss of autoregulation and CO_2 reactivity are poor prognostic indicators. TCD can also be used to measure the pulsatility index which correlates with ICP.

Jugular venous bulb oximetry

Jugular venous oximetry ($SjvO_2$) provides a way of intermittently or continuously measuring cerebral oxygenation and metabolism. As CBF and $CMRO_2$ are closely coupled, CBF can be determined using the difference in arteriovenous oxygen content ($AVDO_2$) between the arterial system and the jugular vein. Both $SjvO_2$ and $AVDO_2$ are global measures and cannot be used to detect regional ischaemia. Evidence from PET scanning suggests that 13% of the brain must become ischaemic before $SjvO_2$ levels fall below 50%.

$AVDO_2 = Hb \times 1.39\ (SaO_2 - SjvO_2)$ (ignoring the amount of dissolved O_2)

Normal values of $SjvO_2$ range from 60 to 75% and for $AVDO_2$ from 2.2 to 3.3μmol/ml. A catheter is inserted into the internal jugular vein in a cephalad direction using the Seldinger technique. The tip of the catheter should be level with the mastoid air cells on a lateral skull X-ray. The accuracy of jugular venous sampling can be affected by contamination of the sample with extracerebral blood, speed of sampling, malpositioning of the catheter and the position of the patient's head. Up to half of desaturations <50% may represent false-positive readings.

$SjvO_2$ monitoring allows detection of episodes of desaturation associated with increases in ICP. A high frequency of desaturations has been correlated with a poor outcome. Monitoring of $SjvO_2$ allows guidance of hyperventilation strategies and helps to distinguish between hyperaemia (when the $SjvO_2$ is high) and vasospasm (when the $SjvO_2$ is low) in patients following subarachnoid haemorrhage. Jugular venous catheters may also be used to measure CBF using thermodilution.

Radiological techniques

Various radiological techniques can be used to assess cerebral perfusion and physiology. Although their use is not widespread, they are helping to define the physiological changes that occur in disease and can be used to direct therapy.

Further reading

Bhatia A, Gupta AK, Neuromonitoring in the intensive care unit. 1. Intracranial pressure and cerebral blood flow monitoring. *Intensive Care Med* 2007; 33: 1263–71.

Bhatia A, Gupta AK. Neuromonitoring in the intensive care unit. 2. Cerebral oxygenation monitoring and microdialysis. *Intensive Care Med* 2007; 33: 1322–8.

Coles JP. Imaging after brain injury. *Br J Anaes* 2007; 99: 49–60.

EEG and CFAM monitoring

Electroencephalogram

The electroencephalogram (EEG) represents the summation of the electrical activity of the brain as recorded from the scalp. Most of the recorded activity arises from the pyramidal neurons of the cerebral cortex. The electrodes are placed according to an internationally recognized system (the 10–20 electrode system). The pattern of electrodes is called a montage.

CFM/CFAM

Cerebral function monitors (CFMs) and cerebral function analysing monitors (CFAMs) are automated EEG processors. The CFM produces a single trace of total power varying with both amplitude and frequency of raw EEG data. The CFAM produces displays of both amplitude and frequency. Both are commonly used as simpler measures of brain electrical activity compared with the EEG.

EEG terminology

The EEG is interpreted according to four main criteria:

1. *Frequency*

   The component waves of the EEG are classified according to their respective frequencies (Table 8.3.1).
2. *Amplitude*

   Most EEG activity is between 20 and 200μV.
3. *Location*

   Multi-channel EEG allows determination of whether activity is localized or generalized. Most CFM/CFAM devices are two channels only.
4. *Paradoxical activity*

   This refers to bursts of abnormal activity.

Table 8.3.1 Clinical interpretation of EEG waves

Wave	Frequency (Hz)	Clinical situation
beta	13–30	Found mainly in the frontotemporal regions. Beta is the dominant frequency when awake and the main frequency in drug-induced coma.
alpha	9–12	Seen in the occipital cortex when awake but with eyes closed. Wanes when eyes opened. Hypoxia or brainstem lesions can produce generalized alpha waves that are unchanged with stimulation.
theta	4–8	Equally dominant with alpha in children but reduces as ageing occurs. 10–15% of adults have theta activity in the temperoparietal regions.
delta	0–4	Occasional delta waves are seen in the awake adult. High voltage delta waves are seen in metabolic encephalopathies of any cause.

Clinical use in ICU

Continuous EEG monitoring is difficult in the ICU. High frequency electrical noise is generated by an array of equipment. Ventilators, nursing procedures and physiotherapy produce mechanical noise.

Seizures and pseudoseizures

Staus epilepticus (SE) is a medical emergency. Mortality is ~10%, with deaths directly attributable to SE, rather than the underlying condition that provoked the seizures, being ~2%. 20–30% of SE is refractory to first-line measures and it is these that more commonly require general anaesthesia to control the seizures and transfer to ICU for management of the airway and ventilation. The EEG is an important tool in the management of both SE and pseudostatus. With seizures, the EEG shows rhythmic spike and wave activity that may be focal or generalized.

Once general anaesthesia is induced for refractory SE, EEG monitoring is desirable as the patient may enter a drug-induced coma with little evidence of convulsions but continue to have repeated seizures (non-convulsive status epilepticus, NCSE). A number of EEG patterns have been described in NCSE. The EEG allows titration of anaesthetic drugs and the use of alternative agents if seizure control is not obtained. NCSE should be considered in patients with unexplained coma or alteration in their mental state, with or without motor signs such as facial myoclonus or nystagmus.

Myoclonic SE is well recognized following anoxic injury, especially in patients resuscitated from cardiac arrest. The EEG usually shows the myoclonic jerking to be associated with generalized, repetitive spikes, sharp waves or triphasic waves occurring at roughly 1s intervals. The prognosis of patients with myoclonic epilepsy associated with anoxic injury is extremely poor.

Pseudostatus due to psychogenic problems is surprisingly common, with up to 25% of patients referred to ICU for the management of refractory seizures having pseudostatus rather than SE. Patients may have received a previous diagnosis of epilepsy and the condition is often refractory to first-line therapy (indeed they often show little response to very high doses of benzodiazepines), resulting in the need for general anaesthesia and ventilation. The EEG allows rapid diagnosis and withdrawal of inappropriate therapy; patients with pseudostatus may have a well-developed alpha rhythm, which can be assessed by passive opening and closing of the eyes. It is essential that the request for EEG details concerns regarding the diagnosis, as <15% of the normal population may have non-specific abnormalities and there is a danger that the EEG is overinterpreted. Such patients must be handled sensitively and referred for appropriate support.

Diagnosis of specific neurological conditions

- Creutzfeldt–Jakob disease

  This is characterized by periodic sharp wave complexes.
- Herpes simplex encephalitis

  Commonly, patients exhibit periodic, lateralized epileptiform discharges in the temporal lobe area.
- Subacute sclerosing panencephalitis

  Patients show paroxysmal bursts of activity in the 2–3Hz region.

Raised ICP

Increases in ICP are commonly associated with both partial and generalized seizures. Prophylactic anticonvulsants are commonly used in cases of severe brain injury with anticipated seizure potential. The optimum duration of

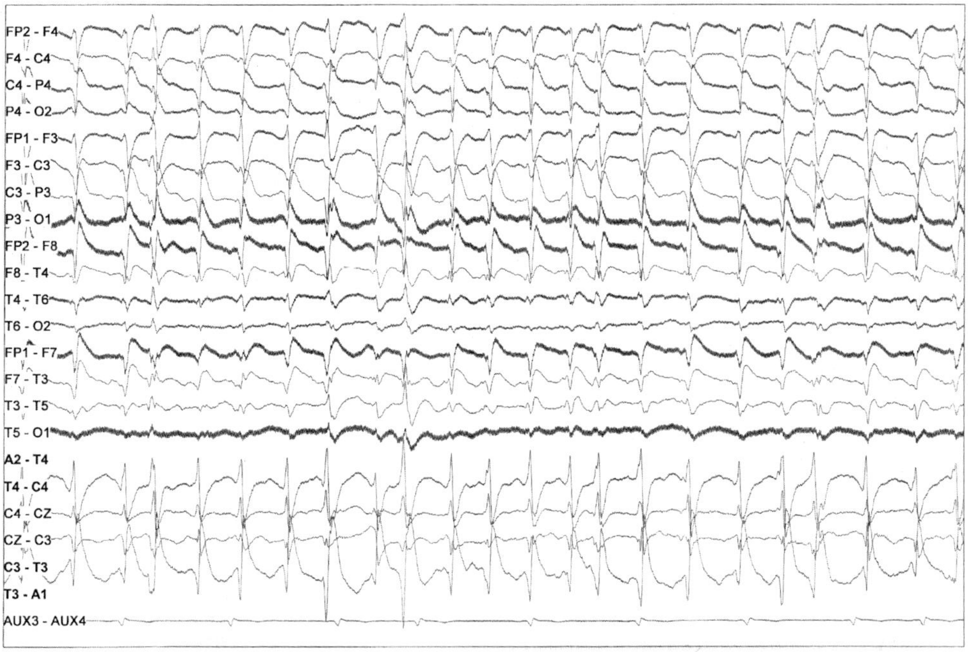

Fig. 8.3.1 EEG frequencies of patients suffering status epilepticus following out-of-hospital cardiac arrest.

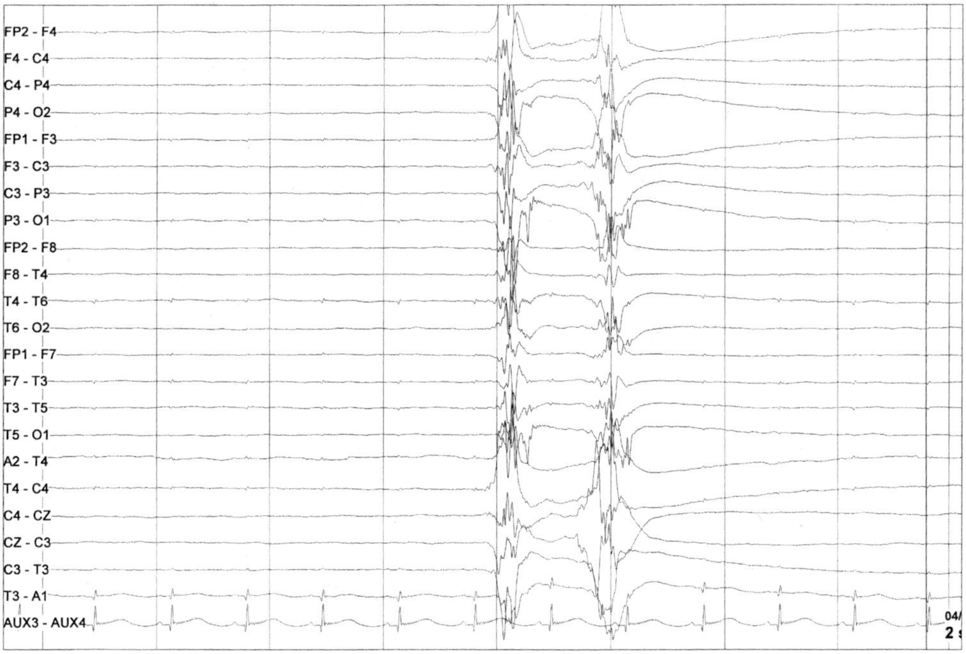

Fig. 8.3.2 EEG frequencies of a patient undergoing burst suppression with thiopentone.

anticonvulsant use and the incidence of seizure activity in unconscious patients are still unclear.

Barbiturate coma is one of the rescue treatments available for intractable, raised ICP when other therapies have failed. The patient is fully loaded with IV barbiturate to produce an isoelectric EEG. A maintenance infusion of barbiturate is then continued and titrated to allow only one or two bursts of activity per screen on the EEG (burst suppression) (Fig. 8.3.2). Therapy is usually continued for a number of days before gradual withdrawal. The use of barbiturate coma is currently being compared with decompressive craniectomy in a phase III clinical trial (www.RESCUEicp.com).

Prognosis

An isoelectric EEG is one of the additional tests suggested in the USA for confirmation of brain death. The EEG has also been used as a prognostic indicator in patients who remain comatose following injury. Burst suppression, low voltage delta activity and a generally low voltage EEG are all poor prognostic indicators. However, EEG patterns that appear more benign do not necessarily correlate with a good outcome.

Further reading

Brenner RP. EEG in convulsive and non-convulsive status epilepticus. *J Clin Neurophysiol* 2004; 21: 319–31.

Other forms of neurological monitoring

Tissue metabolism

Brain tissue oxygenation

The Licox monitor (GMS, Kiel-Mielkendorf, Germany) allows measurement of brain tissue oxygenation that can be used in conjunction with other monitoring modalities to measure the adequacy of cerebral perfusion. The probe is inserted either via a single-lumen bolt, or via a triple-lumen bolt with both an ICP monitor and a microdialysis catheter. Oxygen diffuses from the tissue into an inner electrolyte chamber in the catheter which generates an electric current using a polarographic electrochemical sensor. The probe measures tissue oxygenation from an area of ~15mm^3 around the tip. The risks of infection and significant haemorrhage associated with the technique are low.

Normal brain tissue oxygen values range from 25 to 30mm Hg. Levels <20mm Hg have been reported following head injury and levels <5mm Hg are associated with increased mortality. Improvements in mortality and functional outcome have been reported in patients treated with therapy aimed at maintaining a brain tissue oxygen level >25mm Hg compared with patients treated with a traditional ICP/CPP-guided therapy.

Microdialysis

Microdialysis involves placement of a fine catheter into the brain parenchyma. Dialysis fluid is continuously perfused through the catheterm which is lined with a dialysis membrane, typically with a molecular weight cut-off of ~20kDa. Low molecular weight substances cross the membrane and their concentrations can be measured in the dialysate. Unless there is total equilibration, the concentration of molecules in the dialysate will be lower than that in the extracellular fluid. The proportion of molecule recovered depends on the membrane size, membrane area, diffusion speed of the molecule and the rate of flow of the dialysate.

Glucose, lactate, glutamate, glycerol and the lactate/pyruvate ratio have all been used as markers of cerebral metabolism. Larger membrane sizes allow measurement of polypeptides and cytokines that may be implicated in the damage or repair processes. A recent consensus statement suggests that catheters should be placed in the right frontal region in patients with diffuse head injury, in the area of brain at risk in patients with subarachnoid haemorrhage, and in the penumbral area and a second catheter in normal brain in patients with focal lesions.

The lactate/pyruvate and lactate/glucose ratios are sensitive markers of tissue hypoxia/ischaemia. A high lactate/pyruvate ratio correlates with the severity of injury and outcome in head injury. Alterations in these levels may precede elevations in ICP in acute brain injury, allowing earlier intervention. Similar changes have been seen before development of delayed ischaemic deficits due to cerebral vasospasm in subarachnoid haemorrhage. High levels of the excitatory amino acids glutamate and aspartate have been found in areas of contusion or secondary ischaemic injury.

Cerebral blood flow and metabolism

NIRS

Near-infrared spectroscopy (NIRS) measures regional cerebral oxygen saturation by measuring near-infrared light reflected from the chromophobes in the brain (primarily iron in oxyhaemoglobin and deoxyhaemoglobin, and copper in cytochrome AA_3). Changes in the concentration of near-infrared light as it passes through these compounds can be measured, and this allows calculation of the oxidation status.

Generally, optodes are placed 4–7cm apart on the scalp. Light waves of 700–1000nm can penetrate the scalp, skull and brain to a depth of a few centimetres, allowing illumination of a volume of ~10ml of brain. Normal values of oxygenated haemoglobin are 60–80%. NIRS has been used to monitor patients with brain injury or intracranial haemorrhage, and patients undergoing carotid endarterectomy. The major limitation to its use is the difficulty in distinguishing intracerebral and extracerebral tissues. NIRS is able to follow trends in oxygenation in individual patients.

Laser Doppler flowmetry

Doppler change of laser light can be used to measure movement of red cells within the brain microcirculation. A small Doppler probe is placed within the brain tissue itself. It can obviously only measure CBF within a small area of brain tissue. It has been used experimentally to assess therapeutic interventions, to detect ischaemia and to assess CO_2 reactivity and autoregulation following head injury.

Thermal diffusion flowmetry

The thermal conductivity of brain tissue varies in proportion to CBF. Two thermistors can be placed on the brain surface, and blood flow calculated by means of heating one plate and measuring the thermal difference between plates. Again only a small amount of brain tissue can be assessed.

Peripheral nerve and muscle electrophysiology

Sensory evoked potentials (SEPs)

These are the electrical response of the cortex, brainstem and spinal cord to a peripheral sensory stimulus. They can be recorded in response to stimulation of any sensory nerve, whether cranial or peripheral. The most commonly evoked SEPs are somatosensory (SSEP), visual (VEP) and brainstem auditory (BAEPs).

SSEPs are recorded commonly from the median, ulnar and posterior tibial nerves. SSEPs are a useful method of predicting outcome in post-traumatic and anoxic coma patients. Bilaterally absent SSEPs are strongly associated with poor outcome. SSEPs may also be used in surgery on the spinal column, carotid endarterectomy and cerebral aneurysm surgery.

VEPs are measured in response to a visual stimulus (usually a flashing light or reversing chequerboard). VEPs are profoundly affected by anaesthesia and are occasionally used to assess optic nerve function in pituitary surgery of surgery on the anterior cranial fossa.

BAEPs are used in acoustic neuroma surgery where they have been shown to be useful in preserving the function of the auditory nerve. They may also be used for monitoring during posterior fossa surgery.

Nerve conduction studies

These can be used to diagnose and classify generalized neuropathies that may be seen on the ICU. A stimulus is applied to a nerve at two points along its course, and the response recorded. In axonal neuropathies, the amplitude

Table 8.4.1 Nerve conduction studiy patterns in common clinical conditions

	Motor nerve conduction	Sensory nerve conduction	EMG
Guillain–Barré syndrome	Slowed or blocked	Reduced or absent	Later denervation
Motor neuron disease	Reduced amplitude	Normal	Denervation widespread
Myasthenia gravis	Reduced and falls further with repetition	Normal	Increased jitter on single fibre testing
Critical care polyneuropathy	Reduced	Reduced	Fibrillations

of the response will fall but conduction velocity is well preserved. In contrast, in demyelinating neuropathies, although the amplitude may fall, the conduction velocity is also reduced (Table 8.4.1). Critical illness polyneuropathy is a diffuse axonal neuropathy usually seen in patients with severe sepsis and multi-organ failure. It is usually considered when the patient fails to wean from ventilation and remains profoundly weak. Patients have muscle wasting that often spares the face (although there may be evidence of facial involvement on electrophysiological testing).

Electromyography (EMG)

This examines the electrical activity of a specific muscle. A needle electrode is placed into the muscle, and the spontaneous activity of the muscle is recorded. EMG may help in the diagnosis of motor neuron disease, peripheral nerve root and plexus injuries, and myopathies (Table 8.4.1).

Further reading

Bhatia A, Gupta AK. Neuromonitoring in the intensive care unit. **1**. Intracranial pressure and cerebral blood flow monitoring. *Intensive Care Med* 2007; 33: 1263–71.

Bhatia A, Gupta AK. Neuromonitoring in the intensive care unit. **2**. Cerebral oxygenation monitoring and microdialysis. *Intensive Care Med* 2007; 33: 1322–8.

Stieffel MF, Spiotta A, Gracias VH, *et al.* Reduced mortality rate in patients with severe traumatic brain injury treated with brain tissue oxygen monitoring. *J Neurosurg* 2005; 103: 805–11.

Chapter 9

Fluids

Chapter contents

Crystalloids

Definition

A substance with properties of a crystal; aqueous fluids containing dissolved sugars or salts (Table 9.1.1).

Classification

- Isotonic crystalloids
  - 'Normal saline'
  - Hartmann's (Ringer's lactate)
- Hypotonic crystalloids
  - 'Half-normal saline'
  - 'Dextrosaline'
  - 5% Dextrose
  - 50% Dextrose
- Hypertonic crystalloids.
  - Hypertonic saline

Isotonic crystalloids

In the 1880s Ringer found that a 'balanced' fluid more like plasma retained isolated organ function better than 'normal' saline. Hartmann added lactate in the 1930s.

Pharmacokinetics

- Isotonic so do not lose or gain water by osmosis
- Distribute through the extracellular volume, because sodium is confined extracellularly by cell membrane NaKATPase activity
- Intravascular retention is greater in hypovolaemia
- The plasma volume of 3l is one-fifth of the extracellular volume of 15l, so by 1h ~20% remains intravascularly, i.e. 200ml/l
- *Normal saline*: after rapid infusion of 2l, 24% remains intravascularly at 1h, 22% by 6h (56% remains in the body)
- *Hartmanns*: 18% remains intravascularly at 1h, 14% by 6h (30% remains in the body). More rapid diuresis may be due to mild hypotonicity, inhibiting antidiurectic hormone (ADH), or to lower chloride, reducing renal vasoconstriction,

Pros

- No anaphylactoid reactions
- Saline produces a more sustained volume effect than Hartmann's
- Lactate in Hartmann's is metabolized via pyruvate, to glucose in the liver, or to carbon dioxide and water in peripheral tissues. One litre provides 9kcal.
- Both are cheap,

Cons

Rapid administration of large volumes can cause:

- Dilutional procoagulant effect
- Saline produces a hyperchloraemic metabolic acidosis, of uncertain clinical significance; caused either by decreased strong ion difference due to hyperchloraemia or by dilution of bicarbonate
- Saline (but not Hartmann's) produced abdominal discomfort and subtle cognitive deficits,

Roles

- Appropriate for both fluid resuscitation and maintenance fluid administration
- Outcome in critical care patients resuscitated with saline is as good as with albumin
- Hartmann's avoids hyperchloraemic metabolic acidosis, due to lower chloride and because lactate metabolism consumes hydrogen ions. However outcome benefit not yet demonstrated,

Hypotonic crystalloids

Although initially iso- or hyperosmolar, glucose-containing solutions are rendered hypotonic by cellular uptake and metabolism of glucose.

Pharmacokinetics

- Tonicity is the effective osmolality with respect to the cell membrane. Hypotonic solutions behave like a water load and distribute through the intravascular, interstitial and intracellular volumes
- Half-normal saline distributes half extracellularly like saline and half through the body water.

Pros

- Allow glucose provision, in diabetics and critical care patients not established on nutrition
- Allow supply of IV hydration since intravenous water is hypoosmolar so causes haemolysis.

Cons

- Hypotonic so inappropriate for resuscitation of fluid deficits
- ADH secretion increases in response to non-osmotic factors including surgery, infection and pain. The resulting retention of water over sodium, in conjunction with 'maintenance' hypotonic IV fluid, can cause severe hyponatraemia leading to seizures and death
- 10% dextrose needs a large free flowing vein, and continuous infusion of 50% dextrose needs central access to avoid thrombophlebitis
- Rapid infusion causes hyperglycaemia, glycosuria and osmotic diuresis
- Concurrent 'sliding scale' insulin administration is often necessary to maintain glycaemic control.

Role

- Dextrosaline usage recently restricted in children because of deaths due to hyponatraemia
- Half-normal saline considered safe for fluid maintenance in stable children, although isotonic solutions were recommended if potential water retention, e.g. hypotension, hypovolaemia, perioperative care, sepsis, diarrhoea
- 50% dextrose is used in the emergency treatment of hypoglycaemia and is given with insulin in acute management of dangerous hyperkalaemia
- To supply water over and above saline, e.g. given a supranormal serum sodium. However, in children, correct significant hypernatraemia >160mmol/l slowly with isotonic crystalloid
- More concentrated dextrose solutions reduce the associated water load and are useful for administration alongside isotonic crystalloid maintenance. For instance, 10–20ml/h of 50% dextrose provides 17–34kcal/h. However, central venous access is required to avoid thrombophlebitis.

Table 9.1.1 Crystalloid composition

Fluid	Other names	Na^+ mEql/l	K^+ mEql/l	Cl^- mEql/l	Ca^{2+} mEql/l	Glucose mEql/l	kcal/l	Lactate mEql/l	Calculated osmolarity mOsm/l	Tonicity
Sodium chloride 0.9%	Normal saline	154	–	154	–	–	–	–	308	Isotonic
Ringer's solution	–	147	4		2.2	–	–	–		
Ringer's lactate	Hartmann's solution	130	4	110	2	–	–	28	275	Isotonic
Sodium chloride 0.45% + Dextrose 2%	Half-normal saline + dextrose	77	–	77	–	111	85	–	265	Hypotonic
Sodium chloride 0.18% + dextrose 4%	Dextrose saline	31	–	31	–	222	136	–	262	Hypotonic
5% Dextrose	–	–	–	–	–	278	170	–	278	Hypotonic
10% Dextrose	–	–	–	–	–	556	340	–	556	Hypotonic
50% Dextrose	–	–	–	–	–	2778	1700	–	2778	Hypotonic
Sodium chloride 7.5%	Hypertonic saline	1283	–	1283	–	–	–	–	2567	Hypertonic
Plasma	–	144	5	107	2.3	5	–	<1	290	Isotonic

Hypertonic crystalloids

Hypertonic saline

Hypertonic solutions from 1.8 to 7.5% saline have been employed, either alone or with colloid. Hypertonic 7.5% saline acutely increases intravascular volume by 4–10 times the infused volume, by drawing interstitial and intracellular water into the intravascular space. The salt and water then redistribute through the extracellular volume, over about an hour. Combination of 7.5% saline with either dextran 70 or hetastarch prolongs intravascular retention.

Pros

- Increased intravascular volume
- Haemodilution with reduced viscosity cf starches
- Vasodilation, with reduced afterload and cardiac work, and perhaps improved regional blood flow
- Endothelial 'deswelling' due to osmotic effect may improve capillary blood flow
- Small resuscitation volumes; 250ml of 7.5% hypertonic saline is an effective initial resuscitation fluid.
- Improved microcirculation with splanchnic vasodilatation.

Cons

- Severe hypernatraemia
- Hyperoncotic plasma
- Theoretical risk of central pontine myelinosis
- Potential for rebound intracranial hypertension
- Potential for coagulopathy.

Role

- Amall volumes, so advocated for battlefield resuscitation
- In burns, produce less rise in intra-abdominal pressure than Hartmann's
- Improved outcome in penetrating trauma
- Reduce cerebral swelling and ICP in traumatic brain injury, but no outcome benefit found.

Further reading

Finfer S, Bellomo R, Boyce N, *et al.* A comparison of albumin and saline for fluid resuscitation in the intensive care unit. *N Engl J Med* 2004; 350: 2247–56.

Kuper M, Soni N. Fluids and electrolytes. In: Webster NR, Galley NF, eds. Anaesthesia science. Oxford: *Blackwell*, 2006: 198–200.

National Patient Safety Agency. Patient Safety Alert No 22. Reducing the risk of hyponatraemia when administering intravenous infusions to children. 2007.

Oda J, Yamashita, K, Inoue T, *et al.* Hypertonic lactated saline resuscitation reduces the risk of abdominal compartment syndrome in severely burned patients. *J Trauma* 2006; 60: 64–71.

Wilkes NJ. Hartmann's solution and Ringer's lactate: targeting the fourth space. *Clin Sci (Lond)* 2003; 104: 25–6.

Colloids

Definition

A colloidal fluid is a dispersion of small particles in a continuous fluid phase, which exert an osmotic effect because the endothelium is relatively impermeable to the colloid particles.

- Human plasma derivatives
  - Human albumin solution
- Semi-synthetic colloids
  - Gelatins
  - Dextrans
  - Starches

The ideal colloid has yet to be found, e.g. all colloids can cause anaphylactoid reactions, of which 20% are severe. Consult manufacturer's data sheets for maximum doses. Hypertonic electrolyte carrier solutions are discussed in the previous chapter.

Human plasma derivatives

Human albumin solution (HAS)

Constituents and volume effect

- Derived from plasma from thousands of donors.
- 4.5% HAS is iso-oncotic, whereas 20% HAS is hyperoncotic but 'salt-poor' so mildly hypotonic, so will draw fluid intravascularly
- Initial volume effect is the intravascular volume expansion as a percentage of the fluid volume given.
  - Four hours after administration of 20% HAS:
- 20% leaves the plasma in health
- 32% leaves in sepsis, due to leaky capillaries.

Pros

- Anaphylactoid reactions are very rare
- +ve charge binds drugs, toxins and free radicals
- Antioxidant capacity, clinical relevance unclear
- No itch
- No renal dysfunction.

Cons

- Expensive
- Cannot exclude transmission of infections, e.g. new variant Creutzfeld–Jacob disease (nv-CJD).

Role

- A suggestion from meta-analysis of increased mortality was refuted, but no outcome benefit compared with saline was found in the SAFE study, even in patients with a low plasma albumin
- Possible benefit in sepsis, following paracentesis and in diuretic-induced hepatic encephalopathy
- Possibly harmful in traumatic brain injury
- 'Salt-poor' 20% albumin requires less volume for a given increase in oncotic pressure; benefit suggested when given with furosemide in acute lung injury, though oxygenation does not improve acutely.

Semi-synthetic colloids

Gelatins

Constituents and volume effect

- Gelatins are derived from bovine collagen.
- Gelofusin is 4% succinylated gelatin.
- Haemaccel is urea-linked gelatin.
- Initial 80% volume effect.
- –ve charge of gelofusin repels the endothelium, extending plasma half-life.

Pros

- Initially effective volume expansion
- Near complete renal clearance
- Cheap
- Minimal coagulopathy
- No renal impairment
- Rapid near complete excretion
- No itch.

Cons

- Only 20% remains intravascularly at 90 min
- Highest rate of anaphylactoid reactions
- Bovine origin so possible religious objections, and risk of nv-CJD transmission cannot be excluded
- Calcium in Haemaccel can coagulate transfused blood.

Role

- Most commonly used colloid in the UK
- Good side effect profile except anaphylactoid reactions
- Suitable for short-lived plasma expansion, e.g. during regional or general anaesthesia.

Dextrans

Constituents and volume effect

- Glucose polymers produced by *Leuconostac* bacteria grown in sucrose.
- Iso-oncotic dextran 70 has less initial volume effect than dextran 40, which is hyperoncotic
- Volume effect is relatively prolonged as there is no intravascular metabolism; large molecules are hydrolysed by tissue dextran-1,6-glucosidase and small molecules are renally filtered.

Pros

- Better intravascular persistence than gelatins.

Cons

- Coagulopathy, with reduced factors VII and VIII and von Willebrand factor
- Intermediate risk of anaphylactoid reactions
- Erythrocyte aggregation with rouleaux formation interferes with cross-match
- Acute renal failure, attributed to increased urine viscosity and osmotic pressure
- Half excreted unchanged, half oxidized over days.

Role

- Out of favour due to coagulopathy.
- Superseded by low molecular weight heparins for prophylaxis against deep vein thrombosis
- Avoid in renal failure.

Starches

Constituents and volume effect

- Derived from hydrolysed maize.

Volume effect

- Initial volume effect depends on number of osmotically active particles, and so on concentration

Table 9.2.1 Characteristics of some starches

Fluid	Colloid	MWw (kDa)	MWn (kDa)	Degree of substitution	Plasma half-life (h)	Initial volume effect (%)	COP (mm Hg)	Calculated osmolarity
Albumin 4.5%	Albumin	69	69	–	16	100	25	300
Albumin 20%	Albumin	69	69	–	16	250	100	300
Dextran 40 10%	Dextran 40	40	25	–	4	200	>100	310
Dextran 70 6%	Dextran 70	70	38	–	6	140	75	309
Haes-steril 6%	Pentastarch	200	60	0.5	12	100	34	310
Haes-steril 10%	Pentastarch	200	60	0.5	12	145	80	308
Hespan 6%	Hetastarch	450	70	0.7	24	100	27	310
Voluven	Tetrastarch	130	60	0.4	3	100	36	309
Gelofusin	Succinylated gelatin	30	22.6	–	2	100	13	279
6% Dextran in 7.5% NaCl	Dextran 70	70	38	–	8	700	75	2567
Haemaccel	polygeline	35	24.5	–	2	100	13	300

MWw = weight average molecular weight; MWn = number average molecular weight; COP = colloid osmotic pressure.

Table 9.2.2 The ideal colloid has yet to be found

Fluid	Volume efficacy	Coagulopathy	Anaphylactoid reaction rate	Itch	Renal impairment	Infectious risk	Cost
Ideal...	++	–	–	–	–	–	+
Albumin	++	+	1 in 1010	–	–	+	+++
Gelatin	+	++	1 in 290	–	–	+	+
HES	++	+++	1 in 1724	++	++	–	++
Dextran	++	++++	1 in 366	–	++	–	++

- Duration depends on metabolism, and on osmotically active metabolites seen, e.g. with Voluven
- Metabolism slower with a high molecular weight, a high degree of hyroxyethyl substitution of glucose side chains and a high ratio of C2 compared with C6 substitution,

Pros

- Lowest risk of anaphylactoid reactions
- Sustained volume effect
- Might reduce inflammation and capillary leak, and improve microcirculatory perfusion.

Cons

- Incomplete clearance from the body (50%)
- Incidence of itch up to 13%
- Coagulopathy, with reduced factor VIII and reduced von Willebrand activity. Increased bleeding in neurosurgery and cardiac surgery, more marked with slowly degradable starches
- Renal impairment has been suggested with various starches, e.g. in the recent 'VISEP' trial
- Hyperamylasaemia due to plasma amylase binding complicates the diagnosis of pancreatitis
- Hepatosplenomegaly and ascites in chronic dialysis patients
- Rapidly degraded starches with low molecular weight and low molar substitution, e.g. Voluven (HES 130/0.4) may avoid side effects.

Role

- Effective and sustained volume effect
- Questions remain over side effects
- Avoid in renal failure,

Balanced colloids

- Starch in a more 'balanced' carrier solution (Hextend) containing glucose, lactate and a lower chloride avoids hyperchloraemic acidosis compared with starch in saline (Hetastarch).
- Less coagulopathy *in vitro*
- No outcome benefit demonstrated yet.

Further reading

Kuper M, Gunning M P, Halder, S, *et al.* The short-term effect of hyperoncotic albumin, given alone or with furosemide, on oxygenation in sepsis-induced acute respiratory distress syndrome. *Anaesthesia* 2007; 62: 259–63.

Kuper M, Soni N. Fluids and electrolytes. In: Webster NR, Galley NF, eds. Anaesthesia science. Oxford: *Blackwell*, 2006: 198–200.

Wilkes N J, Woolf R, Mutch M, et al. The effects of balanced versus saline-based hetastarch and crystalloid solutions on acid–base and electrolyte status and gastric mucosal perfusion in elderly surgical patients. *Anesth Analg* 2001; 93: 811–6.

Sodium bicarbonate

The body has developed an efficient system of buffers to minimize the life-threatening tendency to acidaemia and acidosis which follows normal metabolism. Stable blood pH is essential for efficient enzyme activity, and oxygen and carbon dioxide carriage by Hb.

The body has four buffering conjugate pairs,

Bicarbonate/carbonic acid—the main extracellular buffering system and the most important for fixed acids, while playing a major role in transport of volatile acids to the lung.

Tissue and plasma protein/haemoglobin—main intracellular system accounting for 2/3 total body's buffering capacity.

Phosphate system (HPO_4^{2-} and $H_2PO_4^-$)—has plasma buffering capacity equivalent to 20% that of bicarbonate but also active in the renal tubules.

Ammonia/ammonium (NH_3/NH_4^+)—buffering is confined to the renal tubules.

Classical acid–base teaching is that the buffering systems do not operate in isolation but are in equilibrium with each other, the so-called isohydric state. An acid load results in all buffers changing their equilibrium status. Buffers are immediately effective but, once their capacity is exceeded, acidaemia results and acidosis becomes revealed through clinical signs such as ventilatory stimulation, which increases CO_2 removal in an attempt to restore near normal pH. The kidney further reduces acidaemia by accelerating proton excretion; urine pH will fall to 5.5 in the absence of tubular dysfunction. This response is slower than the ventilatory change and reaches maximum efficacy after several hours. The isohydric behaviour of buffers conveniently allows us to examine just one buffer system in order to assess body acid–base status and predict changes under given loads.

Carbonic acid dissociates poorly into the bicarbonate anion and a proton. However, carbonic acid very readily dissociates into dissolved carbon dioxide and water. While carbonic acid is difficult to measure, dissolved carbon dioxide can be readily estimated and is directly proportional to carbonic acid:

$$H_2O + CO_2 = H_2CO_3 = H^+ + HCO_3^-$$

The relative plasma concentrations of H_2CO_3, dissolved CO_2 and bicarbonate are 1:340:6800, respectively. H_2CO_3 is so small that it can be ignored, and the above equation rewritten as:

$$H_2O + CO_2 = H^+ + HCO_3^-$$

The law of mass action for the CO_2/carbonic acid/bicarbonate buffer system becomes:

$$K = [H^+] \times [HCO_3^-]/[CO_2][H_2O]$$

Where *K* is a constant.

$[H_2O]$ is also relatively constant and, by rearranging the equation, $K[H_2O]$ can be replaced by *K*1

$$K1 = [H^+] \times [HCO_3^-]/[CO_2]$$

When this formula is rewritten in the Henderson–Hasselbalch mode (to convert hydrogen ion concentration to its logarithmic representation pH)

$$pH = pK1 + \log [HCO_3^-]/[CO_2]$$

The dissolved carbon dioxide at body temperature can be calculated from the product of CO_2 tension in plasma (40mm Hg (5.3kPa)) and the solubility coefficient (0.03mmol/l/mm Hg). Dissolved plasma CO_2 is 1.2mmol/l (40 x 0.03). Normal plasma $[HCO_3^-]$ is 24mmol/l, so the ratio $[HCO_3^-]/[CO_2]$ is 24/1.2 or 20.

The p*K* of the CO_2/bicarbonate system is 6.1. If these values are substituted in the Henderson–Hasselbalch equation

$$pH = 6.1 + \log 20$$

or

$$pH = 6.1 + 1.3 = 7.4 \text{ (normal plasma pH)}$$

The relationship between the components of the Henderson–Hasselbalch equation is the basis of bicarbonate estimation from measured dissolved CO_2 and pH from blood gas analysis.

Although the p*K* of carbonic acid is rather low at 6.1, resulting in a 20:1 ratio between bicarbonate and carbon dioxide at physiological pH, thus making it seemingly less efficient than a buffer with p*K* 7.4 at normal pH, the carbonic acid system becomes more efficient as pH falls. This is fortunate, since acidosis is the most common acid–base disorder. Furthermore, since it is the only system in which both the numerator, $[HCO_3^-]$, and denominator, $[CO_2]$, can be regulated by independent mechanisms, increased fixed acid loads are not only buffered by bicarbonate but also result in ventilatory stimulation which reduces plasma CO_2, facilitating the return towards normal pH.

An alternative quantitative analysis of carbon dioxide and bicarbonate behaviour has been proposed by Stewart.

Acid–base derangements and restoration by resuscitation, ventilation and/or exogenous buffer administration is readily monitored through central venous or arterial blood sampling.

Persistent acid load from any cause may result in metabolic acidosis. If the cause is due to excess organic acids such as lactate or ketoacids, successful management of the cause progressively reduces production of acids, and the anions (lactate, acetoacetate, β-hydroxybutyrate) associated with the excess protons become metabolized to bicarbonate, therefore correcting acidosis without need for bicarbonate. However, if the cause is excess inorganic acids such as renal failure or renal tubular acidosis, or if reversibility of an organic cause is delayed by institutional processes (wrong diagnosis, delayed ischaemic bowel surgery), buffer base will become exhausted and supplementation required to increase stores or buy time while they are being regenerated.

The homeostatic response to metabolic acidosis results in increased ventilation and CO_2 removal in an attempt to maintain near normal pH. Failure to increase ventilation spontaneously or inadequate mechanical ventilation to mimic hyperventilation will allow acidosis to deteriorate more rapidly. This is apparent from the Henderson–Hasselbalch equation. If pCO_2 remains unchanged, hydrogen ion concentration will double for a 50% fall in bicarbonate concentration. The normal pCO_2 response is a fall of 1.2mm Hg (0.16kPa) for a 1mmol/l fall in bicarbonate concentration.

Common indications for sodium bicarbonate administration

- **Severe inorganic metabolic acidosis**, pH <7.1 and when the precipitating pathophysiology is unlikely to reverse spontaneously, e.g. renal failure or sudden ischaemia of a major organ.
- **Forced alkaline diuresis**. Patients who develop metabolic acidosis following salicylate overdose can benefit from accelerated renal salicylate excretion by promoting an alkaline diuresis. Typically 1l of isotonic (1.26%) sodium bicarbonate is given in the first hour, followed by 500ml of 5% dextrose, 500ml of saline and 500ml of 1.26% sodium bicarbonate at hourly intervals. Efficacy of alkalinization is monitored by measuring urine pH, and dosing is altered to achieve values ≥7 and relating this to the need by observing the fall in blood salicylate.
- **Organic metabolic acidosis** associated with hypopefusion whether cardiogenic or hypovolaemic (blood loss or sepsis) in origin should be corrected with specific resuscitative measures prior to consideration of bicarbonate. Diabetic ketoacidosis usually does not need bicarbonate unless pH is <7.0.
- Management of **hyperkalaemia** or **tricyclic antidepressant overdosage** in the context of cardiac arrest.
- Sodium bicarbonate helps reduce the sensation of dyspneoa and restores plasma $[H_+]$ towards concentrations at which enzyme activity is usually most efficient.

Potential and theoretical dangers of sodium bicarbonate administration

- Hypokalaemia through acid–base changes and precipitation of dysrhythmias.
- Sodium load/hyperosmolar load.
- Overtreatment decreases ionized calcium, causing impaired myocardial contractility and possible dysrhythmias and hypotension.
- Leftward shift oxygen dissociation and decreased tissue oxygen release.
- Intracellular acidosis due to dissolved CO_2 moving across the cellular membrane (relatively impermeable to bicarbonate anion) potentially impairing myocardial contractility. The effect of bicarbonate administration on haemodynamic function has been debated vigorously. The evidence would suggest no detrimental effect on haemodynamics if given at a rate which does not rapidly change ionized calcium. Doses of 100mmol over 40 min appear to be clinically safe.
- Hypercarbia in ventilated patients if ventilation is not temporarily increased during administration.

Quantification of dosage

Various formulations for correcting base deficit have been proposed. The bicarbonate concentration in extracellular fluid is twice that in intracellular fluid. Replacement in the first instance should match the extracellular base deficit. This is calcaulated on the basis that extracellular fluid is 20% body weight.

Therefore

body weight kg x 1/5 x base deficit = sodium bicarbonate (mmol) dose

should significantly correct metabolic acidosis. In practice the dose is about twice this because although bicarbonate is an extracellular buffer, it also facilitates the intracellular buffers to take up protons in accordance with the isohydric behaviour of buffers. The facilitation of intracellular buffer activity effectively results in buffering capacity lost from the extracellular space for a given dose of bicarbonate. This in pharmacokinetic terms is an increase in bicarbonate volume of distribution, although bicarbonate remains predominantly in the extracellular space. It is therefore common to see formulae suggesting doses calculated on the basis of 1/3 to 1/2 body weight. However, in view of the potential for adverse effects on potassium and calcium concentrations if a full corrective dose is given, it is safer to give half the corrective dose to achieve pH 7.2 and reassess whether there is a clinical need for more.

Sodium bicarbonate preparations

Sodium bicarbonate can be given as an oral preparation; this is common for patients with chronic acidotic states such as chronic renal failure or renal tubular acidosis. It is available as a 600mg tablet providing ~7mmol Na and bicarbonate, or 500mg capsules providing 6mmol. Daily dosage depends on the degree of acidosis.

IV solutions are commonly available as the iso-osmolar 1.26% (150mmol Na^+ and 150mmol HCO_3^-/l) or the hyperosmolar 8.4% preparation (1000mmol Na^+ and HCO_3^-/l or 1mmol/ml. The latter is corrosive to veins and should be administered through a central line.

Isotonic bicarbonate is a convenient solution for restoring buffer base when hypovolaemia is significant.

Sodium bicarbonate in dialysate fluids

Bicarbonate-containing dialysate fluids have now replaced acetate for intermittent dialysis. Acetate, together with lactate and citrate, are buffers which with a normal functioning liver are converted to bicarbonate. However, acetate dialysate proved to be problematic with respect to haemodynamic stability and biocompatibility. Lactate, hitherto the most common buffer for continuous dialysis systems, has been replaced by bicarbonate solutions. This is primarily because hyperlactataemia which is commonly observed with lactate dialysate confuses management even though there is effective buffering of acids. However, in those with hepatic dysfunction, it is not metabolized to bicarbonate sufficiently to be an effective buffer.

Buffers are needed in dialysis fluid to deal with the 100mmol of fixed acid protons generated by metabolism each day by normal adults. Kidney failure results in progressive depletion of buffers because protons are instantaneously buffered. Consequently, proton concentrations are extremely low and are not effectively removed by dialysis. However, to avoid development of acidosis, buffers need repletion. Modern bicarbonate dialysate solutions contain between 30 and 40mmol/l, and not 25mmol/l as might be expected. This is in order that bicarbonate not only moves efficiently down a concentration gradient but also replenishes buffer deficit. If lower concentrations were used, the plasma bicarbonate concentration 25mmol/l would be achieved slowly. This would be a problem with the time limits imposed by intermittent dialysis or prove to be less effective with the slower flow of continuous dialysis techniques. It is notable that dialysis often leaves patient very slightly alkalotic.

It should also be noted that convection during haemofiltration removes buffer base; therefore, the replacement buffer solutions have to not only replace the corrected buffer removed but also provide additional buffer to replenish the original buffer deficit more rapidly.

Further reading

Bersin RM, Chatterjee K, Arieff AI. Metabolic and hemodynamic consequences of sodium bicarbonate administration in patients with heart disease. *Am J Med* 1989; 87: 7–14.

Cooper DJ, Walley KR, Wiggs BR, *et al.* Bicarbonate does not improve hemodynamics in critically ill patients who have lactic acidosis. A prospective, controlled clinical study. *Ann Intern Med* 1990; 112: 492–8.

Kaehny WD, Anderson RJ. Bicarbonate therapy of metabolic acidosis. *Crit Care Med* 1994; 22: 1525–7.

Kellum JA. Determinants of blood pH in health and disease. *Crit Care* 2000; 4: 6–14.

Mathieu D, Neviere R, Billard V, *et al.* Effects of bicarbonate therapy on hemodynamics and tissue oxygenation in patients with lactic acidosis: a prospective, controlled clinical study. *Crit Care Med* 1991; 19: 1352–6.

Stewart PA. Modern quantitative acid–base chemistry. *Can J Physiol Pharmacol* 1983; 61: 1444–61.

Blood

Whole blood transfusion is rare, and usually blood components are given, targeted to the specific requirements of patients. The recognition of virally transmitted infection, the apparent detrimental effect of transfusion of stored blood and supply problems have led to a far more objective use of blood products.

1 Red blood cells are usually recommended when there is a percived need to correct haemoglobin/oxygen delivery.
2 Component use should be limited to correction of known deficiencies as highlighted by either laboratory or near patient testing.
3 In an unstable patient with suspected massive haemorrhage, clinical assessment and empirical transfusion therapy is justified, but a process of repeated coagulation testing needs to be used to confirm diagnosis and guide further treatment.
4 In the long-stay ICU patient, strategies to minimize transfusion should be employed. Blood sampling can be minimized and will decrease the volume of blood discarded. Iron supplements, oral or IV (non-septic patient), and potentially the use of recombinant erythropoietin can reduce transfusion need.

Current practice

Red blood cells

Transfusion should be decided on an individual basis taking into consideration the stability of the patient, co-morbidities and age, as well as current physiological status. The study by Herbert suggested withholding transfusion in stable patients, resulted in a better outcome, although this was with non-leucoreduced blood. All blood in the UK now undergoes a 4-log reduction in white cells (99.99% white blood cells (WBCs) removed) before storage.

There are two categories of ICU patient: stable and unstable.

Unstable patients who have overt or covert haemorrhage need to be aggressively resuscitated. Massively bleeding patients can bleed to death, and prompt resuscitation and transfusion can save life.

Uncontrolled bleeding usually needs surgical correction or at least local control, i.e. simple pressure. Resuscitation is targeted at maintaining an adequate circulating volume, but with lower blood pressure than normal. This prevents dislodging clots on bleeding, severed vessels after vasospasm, and platelet plugging. Overenthusiastic resuscitation will promote bleeding, increase the size of haematoma, increase the need for more fluid and blood components, and eventually lead to dilutional coagulation problems in addition to the coagulopathy caused by the initial haemorrhage.

Coagulation tests may alter unexpectedly in such dynamic situations, with non-linear changes in test results. Platelet counts may decline rapidly, for example, therefore early and anticipated transfusion of platelets and FFP is made on an empirical clinical basis.

Caution is also needed in withholding red cell transfusion in those patients who have suffered obvious severe trauma and who may be hypovolaemic but still have misleading normal or high haemoglobin values. Stable non-acute patients do not justify empirical transfusion therapy, and transfusion may be minimized using laboratory or near patient testing results. As a general rule, a Hb level of 7–9g/dl would be deemed adequate in all stable ICU patients. Patients with severe chronic cardiorespratory disease may benefit from a haematocrit of between 28 and 33%, equivalent to a Hb of between 9 and 10g/dl.

In younger patients without cardiorespiratory disease, a level of 70g/l would be sufficient.

Platelet count

In bleeding patients, maintain platelets at 75×10^9/l, while in brain injury of traumatic of haemorrhagic origin this will need to be 100×10^9/l.

In stable non-bleeding ICU patients, 10×10^9/l would seem to be an adequate level, unless some invasive procedure is planned which may then trigger the need for platelet transfusion.

Folate and iron deficiency

Folate replacement has become routine on most ICUs, whereas there is an increasing trend to test iron status in long-stay patients. The interpretation of such tests is fraught with difficulty in such patients as ferritin is an acute phase protein. The use of oral and IV iron supplementation and the use of recombinant erythropoietin can be considered.

Laboratory testing for coagulopathy

FBC and platelet count

The Coulter counter measures platelet counts and corpuscular size, which may hint at other deficiencies leading to abnormal red cell shape. This is a count, and provides no information about red cell or platelet function.

Near patient testing is extremely useful in dynamic unstable situations, but such machines need similar quality control and maintenance to the laboratory machines in use. Spurious results are dangerous, but may occur if sampling procedures have not been followed accurately, e.g. the testing of dilute samples giving falsely low readings, etc.

Tests of coagulation

A problem in assessing coagulation abnormalities is the non-specific nature of the tests and the time to obtain results in clinical practice. Most decisions will need to be made on the more basic available tests conducted by your coagulation and haematology laboratory, these include:

- *Prothrombin time (PT)*. A normal result would be 10–14s and is a measure of extrinsic and common coagulation pathways. Factor VII and factors common to both pathways are evaluated. The test is conducted by adding tissue thromboplastin and calcium ions to plasma.
- *Activated partial thromboplastin time (aPTT)*. A time of 30–40s would be considered normal. It is a measure of the intrinsic pathway. The test involves adding Kaolin, a surface activator, phospholipids and calcium ions to plasma. Failure to correct both PT and aPTT with normal plasma when tested in the laboratory would indicate the presence of inhibitors, e.g. heparinoids or fibrinogen degradation products (FDPs).
- *Thrombin time*. If prolonged, normal being 10–12s, fibrinolyis due to reduced fibrinogen (which may also be measured and needs to be >1g/dl) is suspected. Thrombin time is assayed by adding thrombin to plasma and observing the time to fibrin formation

Treatment

If these tests are abnormal for the patient tested, correction towards a normal value can be obtained by treating with normal plasma usually provided in the form of thawed FFP. It is recommended that thawed plasma can be kept at 4°C for 24h, and so should always be immediately available in large hospitals with a busy laboratory. Otherwise it can be thawed within 20–30min from frozen in a water bath.

A low fibrinogen is treated with reconstituted cryoprecipitate providing no more FFP is indicated, as 3 packs of FFP contains similar amounts of fibrinogen to 10 packs of cryoprecipitate.

Thromboelastogram (TEG)

Not all ICUs will have access to a TEG machine, but many hospitals with a cardiovascular or liver transplant unit or a vascular surgical unit may well be using such machines routinely.

The information obtained from such machines is displayed graphically and can give useful information detecting subtle changes between coagulation fibrinolysis and related haemostatic parameters.

Blood components commonly available in the UK

Red blood cells

All red blood cell concentrates supplied are leucoreduced with 99.99% of the leucocytes removed before storage (4-log reduction). The concentrated red cells are resuspended in 50–80ml of saline adenine glucose with mannitol (SAG-M), with a resultant haematocrit of 0.5–0.7. They are stored for up to 35 days at 4°C.

Cost: ~£135 per bag

Platelets

These are administered in adult bag equivalents. Each adult therapeutic bag can be expected to raise the platelet count by 20 x 10^9/l.

Cost: ~£200 per adult dose

FFP

Provided as packs of 300ml of plasma produced by centrifugation of whole blood from a previously tested donor and frozen to achieve factor VIII concentration of >0.7IU/ml. Three packs of FFP will provide 1.5–3.0g of fibrinogen (VIIa needs fibrinogen to work). Usually given as a 4-pack dose

Cost: $400 per 4-pack dose

Cryoprecipitate

This is provided as 20-40ml of cryoprecipitate rich in factor VIII, von Willebrand factor, factor XIII, fibronectin and fibrinogen. Packs contain at least 150–300mg of fibrinogen and 70IU of factor VIII.

Cost of one unit £33 and of a 10-unit dose £330.

Further reading

BCSH. Guidelines for the use of fresh frozen plasma, cryoprecipitate and cryosupernatant. 2003.

BCSH. Guidelines for the use of platelet transfusions. 2003.

BCSH. Guidelines on the management of massive blood loss. 2006. www.bcshguidelines.co.uk

Blood Transfusion and the Anaesthetist. Red cell transfusion 2001. www.aagbi.org.uk

Blood Transfusion and the Anaesthetist. Blood component therapy. 2005. www.aagbi.org.uk

Corwin HL. Erythropoietin and transfusions among critically ill patients. *JAMA* 2003; 289: 1512.

Hebert PC, Wells G, Blajchman MA, *et al.* A multicenter randomized controlled trial of transfusion requirements in critical care. *N Engl J Med* 1999; 340: 409–17.

Chapter 10

Respiratory drugs

Chapter contents

Bronchodilators

Bronchodilators, as the name suggests, are used in airways disease, particularly in asthma and COPD, to produce a reversal of airway obstruction. An overview of the three main categories is provided here:

β_2 Agonists

β_2 agonists give the greatest bronchodilation amongst the bronchodilators in asthma. They are classified by length of action:

- short–intermediate acting, e.g. salbutamol, terbutaline, fenoterol
- long-acting, e.g. formoterol, salmeterol.

Mode of action

β_2 Agonists directly stimulate the β_2-adrenergic receptor which is found in virtually all types of cells. The receptor is subclassified as β_1, β_2 and β_3. Although both β_1 and β_2 receptors are found in the lungs, bronchodilatory effects are predominantly a function of the β_2 receptor. The receptor consists of a protein folded across the plasma membrane, and is linked to the stimulatory guanine nucleotide-binding protein (G_s). Occupation of the receptor activates the enzyme adenylate cyclase via the G_s protein, and this converts ATP to cAMP, which is responsible for the physiological response, in this case, relaxation of airway smooth muscle.

In addition, β_2 agonists have non-direct bronchodilator actions which may contribute to their therapeutic function:

- enhancement of mucociliary clearance
- inhibition of cholinergic neurotransmission
- inhibiting the release of bronchoconstrictor mediators (e.g. leukotrienes, histamine, prostaglandins) from inflammatory cells (e.g. mast cells)
- reducing microvascular leakage.

There is no evidence however that β_2 agonists have a significant inhibitory effect on chronic inflammation in asthma, hence they must not be used as alternative to inhaled steroids as anti-inflammatory therapy.

Therapeutic use

β_2 agonists are most commonly administered via the inhalation route; other routes include IV, subcutaneous (SC) and oral. β_2 agonists may be inhaled in nebulized form, or as metered-dose inhalation (MDI) in the form of propellant-generated aerosol or as a breath-propelled dry powder (e.g. 'turbohaler', 'accuhaler'). Using the MDI optimally, ~12% of the drug is delivered to the respiratory airways; the remainder is deposited in the mouth, pharynx and larynx. Nebulized doses need to be ~6–10 times that used in MDIs to produce the same level of bronchodilation.

- **Short-acting β_2 agonists** act rapidly and their duration of action lasts 3–4h. In acute asthma, they are the bronchodilators of choice. In this setting, it is common practice to use nebulized β_2 agonists, although studies have shown that supervised administration of β_2 agonists by MDI with a spacer device in the emergency setting appears to be as effective as nebulizers in both adults and children. Short-acting β_2 agonists are also useful in prevention of exercise-induced asthma, or other triggers including cold air and allergens.
- In mild or stable asthma, short-acting β_2 agonists should be used as required by symptoms, and not on a regular basis. Increased usage signals the need for step-up of anti-inflammatory therapy.
- **Long-acting β_2 agonists (LABAs)** were developed later and marked an important milestone in asthma management. The bronchodilator effect lasts >12h. This is particularly important in addressing nocturnal asthma symptoms. LABAs are considered in Step 3 of the BTS/SIGN chronic asthma guidelines. Formoterol is a full agonist compared with salmeterol, and so has a more rapid onset of action. This may make formoterol suitable for symptom relief, as well as symptom prevention in combination with an inhaled corticosteroid. LABAs have been shown to improve asthma symptoms and the need for additional bronchodilator therapy, peak expiratory flow and asthma-specific measures of quality of life.

Side effects

These are due to pharmacological actions on extrapulmonary β_2 receptors. Side effects are uncommon with inhalation therapy, and more significant in oral or IV therapy.

- Muscle tremor—direct stimulation of skeletal muscle β_2 receptors
- Tachycardia—direct effect on heart β_2 receptors, and reflex response to peripheral vasodilatation
- Metabolic—hypokalaemia, hypomagnesaemia, hyperglycaemia
- Transient decrease in PaO_2—increase of ventilation–perfusion mismatch by relaxation of compensatory vasoconstriction in underventilated areas of lung
- Tolerance/subsensitivity/desensitization—occurs with regular use of β_2 agonists and is clearly demonstrated for the non-bronchodilatory responses (tremor, tachycardia and metabolic effects). The mechanism is thought to be due to uncoupling, internalization and/or downregulation of β_2 receptors. Tolerance is not progressive and has not shown to be of clinical importance.

Anticholinergic agents

Anticholinergics are one of the mainstays of treatment in COPD; they are also useful in the treatment of acute asthma exacerbation by nebulization, but are less effective than β_2 agonists.

Mode of action

Anticholinergics are antagonists of muscarinic receptors and inhibit cholinergic nerve reflexes which give airway smooth muscle its tone. As the airways in COPD are structurally narrowed, the bronchodilator effects of anticholinergics are more significantly marked compared with normal airways.

Therapeutic use

Anticholinergics are most commonly administered in MDI. Short-acting agents (e.g. ipratropium bromide) have a maximum effect 30–60min after use, and last from 4 to 6h, hence they are prescribed 4 times daily. The newer long-acting anticholinergica (e.g. tiotropium) last up to 24h, and hence are used once a day. They have been shown to improve patient symptoms and spirometric parameters, and to reduce theexacerbation rate in COPD.

Side effects

Inhaled anticholinergics are minimally absorbed, so have relatively few side effects. Nebulized anticholinergics may rarely precipitate glaucoma in elderly patients by a direct effect on the eyes, hence a mouthpiece should be used as an alternative to a mask. Other potential effects include dry mouth, blurred vision and urinary retention.

Theophyllines

Theophylline has been used in asthma treatment for >60yrs; it has seen its role change gradually with developments in other classes of bronchodilators and anti-inflammatory agents. Further developments included slow-release formulations which countered the rapid absorption and elimination of theophylline, and rapid assays which made therapeutic drug monitoring readily possible.

Mode of action

Although theophylline has traditionally been classified as a bronchodilator, its therapeutic effect in controlling asthma has always been disproportionately greater than is explained by its relatively small degree of bronchodilator ability. There is recognition that theophylline has, in addition, anti-inflammatory, immunomodulatory and bronchoprotective effects that may contribute to its efficacy as preventive treatment for chronic asthma:

- downregulation of the function of immune and inflammatory cells (e.g. T lymphocytes, macrophages, mast cells)
- decrease of fatigue in diaphragmatic muscles
- decrease of airway microvascular leakage
- increasing mucociliary clearance
- central action to block decrease in ventilation which occurs with sustained hypoxia.

These findings suggest, but do not establish, its non-bronchodilator efficacy, and some of these actions give a rationale for added therapy in acute asthma unresponsive to β_2 agonists and systemic steroids, as well as its use in stable COPD.

On a molecular level, two modes of action are known to occur at clinically relevant drug concentrations:

- Inhibition of phosphodiesterases—intracellular cAMP, essential for relaxation of airway smooth muscle, is hydrolysed by phosphodiesterase. Thus its inhibition by theophylline increases cAMP concentration, leading to bronchodilation. Anti-inflammatory effects may be due to action on the isoenzyme via cAMP in inflammatory cells.
- Antagonism of adenosine receptors—this appears to be the mechanism by which theophylline stimulates ventilation in hypoxia, decreases fatigue in diaphragmatic muscles and inhibits release of certain mediators from mast cells.

Therapeutic use

Theophylline is considered in Step 4 of the BTS/SIGN chronic asthma treatment guidelines, if asthma is still uncontrolled with inhaled corticosteroids and LABAs. Theophylline can also be useful in stable COPD as an additional bronchodilator, improving dyspnoea and reducing hyperinflation. The drug is usually given in 2 divided doses at 12h intervals. In acute asthma, evidence for the efficacy of IV theophylline is conflicting; hence it should only be considered for patients with severe acute symptoms unresponsive to other measures. Similarly, the benefits of adding theophylline in acute exacerbation of COPD remain unclear, with a few randomized controlled trials showing no benefit but with increased adverse effects. Doses giving peak serum concentrations between 10 and 20mcg/ml are most effective in symptom prevention and reducing the need for rescue therapy in chronic asthma.

Theophylline is predominantly eliminated by hepatic cytochrome *P450* isoenzymes. Many factors affect plasma clearance and hence plasma concentration:

- Increased plasma clearance—enzyme induction by drugs (e/g. rifamipicin, antiepileptics); cigarette and marijuana smoking, even passive; high-protein, low carbohydrate diet; in children
- Decreased plasma clearance—enzyme inhibition (e.g. ciprofloxacin, macrolides, methotrexate, allopurinol, cimetidine, alcohol); liver disease; cardiac decompensation; septic shock; prolonged pyrexia; in the elderly.

Side effects

Efficacy and toxicity of theophylline are closely associated with serum drug concentration. Side effects include nausea and vomiting, diarrhoea, headaches, irritability and insomnia. Even higher serum concentrations can cause seizures, toxic encephalopathy, hyperthermia, cardiac arrhythmias and death.

Further reading

Barnes PJ. Drugs for airway diseases. Medicine 1999; 27: 37–45.

Barnes PJ. Asthma and COPD: basic mechanisms and clinical management. *Academic Press*, 2002.

British Guideline to the Management of Asthma Update. BTS/SIGN 2007. http://www.brit-thoracic.org.uk.

COPD guidelines. National Institute of Clinical Excellence (NICE) 2004. http://www.nice.org.uk.

Global Strategy for Asthma Management and Prevention. Global Initiative for Asthma (GINA) 2007. http://www.ginasthma.org.

Nelson HS. Beta-adrenergic bronchodilators. *N Engl J Med* 1995; 333: 499–506.

O'Byrne P, Bisgaard H, Godard PP, *et al.* Budesonide/formoterol combination therapy as both maintenance and reliever medication in asthma. *Am J Respir Crit Care Med* 2005; 171: 129–36.

Turner MO, Patel A, Ginsburg S, *et al.* Bronchodilator delivery in acute airflow obstruction. A meta-analysis. *Arch Intern Med* 1997; 157: 1736–44.

Weinberger M, Hendeles L. Theophylline in asthma. *N Engl J Med* 1996; 334: 1380–8.

Nitric oxide

History

Nitric oxide (NO) was identified as an endogenous vasodilator (endothelial-derived relaxing factor) in 1987. It is now known to be a mediator of intracellular signalling and numerous physiological functions, including: neurotransmission, inhibition of platelet and leucocyte adhesion, gastrointestinal motility and host defence. The physiological role of endogenous NO was first demonstrated in healthy volunteers by evaluating the systemic and pulmonary pressor response to an infusion of an unselective inhibitor of NO synthase (NOS). It is a colourless, odourless gas, which is relatively insoluble in water. Environmental NO arises from fossil fuel combustion, cigarette smoke and lightning. Atmospheric concentrations usually range between 10 and 500 parts per billion (ppb), but can be higher in heavy traffic.

Biochemistry

NO is synthesized from L-arginine by NOS. There are three isoforms: one is inducible (NOS II), and two are constitutively expressed, neuronal (NOS I) and endothelial (NOS III). The inducible form NOS II is expressed in response to various stimuli, including proinflammatory cytokines. Relatively large quantities of NO are produced continuously by inducible NOS II in blood vessel walls during an inflammatory response, suggesting that this pathway contributes to the vasculopathy of sepsis. Under physiological conditions, NO is produced in a highly regulated manner by NOS III, and controls local vascular tone by diffusing from the vascular endothelium to act on smooth muscle cells. NO has a high affinity for iron–sulfur groups and haem, which accounts for its very short half-life in blood. In combination with oxyhaemoglobin, NO forms methaemoglobin and nitrate. Nitrate is excreted in urine, whilst most of the methaemoglobin is reduced to ferrous haemoglobin. NO also reacts very rapidly with superoxide species to produce peroxynitrite anions, which may form highly reactive and toxic hydroxyl radicals. These so-called reactive nitrogen species are beneficial when used by leucocytes to kill microbes, but can also cause local tissue damage.

NOS inhibitors were proposed as adjuncts to cardiovascular support in patients with septic shock. Despite reports of successful cases, larger trials demonstrated increased mortality in patients with sepsis associated with the use of non-selective NOS inhibitors, and these agents are not currently used.

Clinical use of inhaled nitric oxide (iNO)

NO donors, including sodium nitroprusside and nitrates, have an established role in treating patients with hypertensive crises, angina and acute heart failure. The objectives of using iNO are: reducing pulmonary vascular resistance, reducing ventilation–perfusion mismatch or replacing circulating NO stores. Endogenous NO activity is decreased after lung transplantation and in patients with sickle cell disease. iNO has been used effectively to support patients with ALI after lung transplantation. However, despite encouraging initial reports, its prophylactic use is of no benefit. High dose iNO may be beneficial in treating sickle crises, but has not been assessed in a randomized trial.

The most common clinical scenarios in which iNO is used are:

Acute lung injury (ALI)

Severe hypoxaemia caused by extensive ventilation–perfusion mismatching is characteristic of ALI. iNO augments hypoxic pulmonary vasoconstriction by selectively vasodilating vessels associated with ventilated alveoli; because the gas is delivered by inhalation the blood supply to unventilated lung units is unaffected. iNO improves indexes of oxygenation in ~2/3 of patients with ALI; however, there is no evidence from multiple randomized placebo-controlled trials that NO improves mortality or shortens the duration of mechanical ventilation. Therefore, the role of iNO is as a rescue treatment in cases where oxygenation is dangerously low despite optimal ventilation.

Right ventricular failure

The right ventricle is exquisitely sensitive to increased afterload. Therefore, iNO can markedly improve RV function, cardiac output and oxygen delivery by reducing pulmonary vascular resistance. The advantages of iNO over other vasodilators are that oxygenation tends to be improved and systemic pressures are maintained. However, in patients with left heart failure, iNO may increase pulmonary blood flow and left atrial pressure, causing an exacerbation of pulmonary oedema. Despite a lack of evidence from randomized trials, iNO is most commonly used in this context to support patients after cardiac surgery. There are also reports of haemodynamic benefit in cases of acute massive PE.

Neonatal hypoxic respiratory failure

In hypoxaemic infants born after 35 weeks of gestation, iNO reduces the need for ECMO, but mortality is not reduced. Oxygenation improves in ~50% of infants. Whether infants have evidence of persistent pulmonary hypertension of the newborn (PPHN) does not affect outcome.

Administration of iNO

NO is most commonly administered to mechanically ventilated patients through an ETT, although it may also be given through a face mask or nasal cannulae. Intermittent flow, co-incident with inspiration, reduces the production of nitrogen dioxide by minimizing the mixing time of oxygen and NO. iNO should be administered at the lowest effective dose for the shortest possible time because the toxic effects of iNO are largely unknown, the physiological benefit of continuous inhalation lasts no longer than 48h and it is very expensive. Dose–response studies in patients with ARDS have demonstrated that over 1 day of continuous inhalation the pulmonary vasculature becomes 10 times more sensitive to its effects. Before starting iNO, all other appropriate strategies to optimize pulmonary vascular resistance or oxygenation should have been deployed. The means of assessing effectiveness, PaO_2:FiO_2 ratio or cardiac output monitoring should also be available before iNO is administered. Reasonable starting doses are 5 and 10ppm to modify oxygenation and pulmonary haemodynamics, respectively. Gradual up-titration every 30min to 20ppm should be tried before concluding that there is no physiological response. Daily dose titration against the relevant physiological parameter should be performed with the expectation of a 10-fold decrease in dose each day and withdrawal after 48h or sooner if there is no longer physiological benefit.

If iNO has been administered for >12h, acute rebound pulmonary hypertension may develop on withdrawal, particularly in children. Incremental withdrawal with close haemodynamic monitoring is advised.

Adverse effects of iNO

Most of the adverse effects of iNO can be predicted from the physiological effects and biochemical reactions of NO. There is a negligible risk of methaemoglobinaemia in adults receiving up to 40ppm iNO, although administration is contraindicated by methaemoglobin reductase deficiency. Potentially damaging reactive nitrogen species are formed in patients with sepsis and ALI, but the contribution of iNO to any pathological effects of these radicals is unknown. The effects of NO inhalation on bleeding time and other indexes of platelet function in healthy volunteers and patients are variable. However, there is an increased risk of intraventricular haemorrhage in preterm infants.

Adjunctive therapies

Phosphodiesterase (PDE) hydrolyses cGMP the secondary messenger of NO signalling in smooth muscle. Orally administered PDE5 inhibitors are selective pulmonary vasodilators, partially because PDE5 is highly expressed in the lung. For example, sildenafil augmented pulmonary vasodilation induced by iNO, although the route of administration of these agents removes their beneficial effects on oxygenation, making them suitable only for the treatment of pulmonary hypertension and right ventricular failure.

Further reading

Adhikari NK, Burns KE, Friedrich JO, *et al.* Effect of nitric oxide on oxygenation and mortality in acute lung injury: systematic review and meta-analysis. *BMJ* 2007; 334 7597: 779.

Atz AM, Lefler AK, Fairbrother DL, *et al.* Sildenafil augments the effect of inhaled nitric oxide for postoperative pulmonary hypertensive crises. *J Thorac Cardiovasc Surg* 2002; 124: 628–9.

Finer NN, Barrington KJ. Nitric oxide for respiratory failure in infants born at or near term. *Cochrane Database Syst Rev* 2006; (4): CD000399.

Gerlach H, Keh D, Semmerow A, *et al.* Dose–response characteristics during long-term inhalation of nitric oxide in patients with severe acute respiratory distress syndrome: a prospective, randomized, controlled study. *Am J Respir Crit Care Med* 2003; 167: 1008–15.

Griffiths MJ, Evans TW. Inhaled nitric oxide therapy in adults. *N Engl J Med* 2005; 353: 2683–95.

Meade MO, Granton JT, Matte-Martyn A, *et al.* A randomized trial of inhaled nitric oxide to prevent ischemia–reperfusion injury after lung transplantation. *Am J Respir Crit Care Med* 2003; 167: 1483–9.

Moncada S, Palmer RM, Higgs EA. Nitric oxide: physiology, pathophysiology, and pharmacology. *Pharmacol Rev* 1991; 43: 109–42.

Stamler JS, Loh E, Roddy MA, *et al.* Nitric oxide regulates basal systemic and pulmonary vascular resistance in healthy humans. *Circulation* 1994; 89: 2035–40.

Mucolytics

Introduction

Mucolytic agents increase expectoration by reducing sputum viscosity or facilitating hypersecretion. Most of the drugs used as mucolytics have been developed to reduce mucus viscosity. This often helps relieve respiratory difficulties. The viscosity of mucus secretions in the lungs is dependent upon the concentrations of mucoprotein, and the presence of disulfide bonds between these macromolecules and DNA.

Mucoactive drugs are defined as being able to modify mucus production, secretion, its nature and composition, and/or its interactions with the mucociliary epithelium. Mucolytic drugs are a type of mucoactive drug, but both terms are used interchangeably .

Expectorants may be confused with mucolytics. Expectorants increase mucus production, without alteration of its chemical properties. Guaifenesin is a widely used expectorant in over-the-counter antitussive agents. It increases volume and thereby decreases viscosity of respiratory tract secretions.

Bronchodilators given via the nebulized route improve expectoration through increasing ciliary beat frequency of the mucociliary escalator.

Properties of mucus

The mucus layer and a periciliary watery layer surround the respiratory airway cilia. Mucus consists of a mixture of transudate and secretions from surface epithelial lining cells and submucosal glands of the conducting airways. It is mainly water (95%) with glycoproteins (2–3%), proteoglycans (0.1–0.5%), lipids (0.3–0.5%), proteins and DNA. The composition changes in disease states, with a reduction in the water component .

Types of mucolytics

Naturally occurring mucolytics include Mugwort, Bromelain, Papain and Clerodendrum.

Pharmacological mucolytics include *N*-acetylcysteine (NAC), Carbocysteine (Mucodyne®), Mecysteine (Visiclair®), and Erdosteine (Erdotin®). These agents hydrolyse glycosaminoglycans—they break down/lower the viscosity of mucin-containing body secretions. They are also antioxidants through the thiol groups being able to reduce free radicals.

NAC is the most widely studied mucolytic. It is a *N*-acetyl derivative of the amino acid l-cysteine, and is a precursor in the formation of the antioxidant glutathione within the body. NAC acts to split the sulfide bonds in the macromolecules, thereby decreasing viscosity, allowing for removal by normal physiological clearance mechanisms. The action of NAC is pH dependent. Mucolytic action is significant at ranges of pH 7–9.

Recombinant DNase (Pulmyzme®) breaks down DNA as the mechanism for its mucolyic action, and has been studied extensively in cystic fibrosis .

Clinical application

Strategies

Mucolytics can be given via the inhaled route or orally.

- Hydration. Traditionally steam inhalation and nebulized saline has been used to facilitate expectoration. There is no evidence of it changing the properties of mucus.
- Hypertonic saline increases expectoration when delivered as an aerosol. It reduces mucus viscoelasticity but can induce bronchospasm. It is effective in cystic fibrosis long term, but this has not been shown in COPD.
- Other agents such as saturated potassium iodide, in liquid form for several weeks, have been studied. However, the metallic taste, rashes and hyperkalaemia prevent its clinical use.
- Surfactant. A surfactant layer separates layers of mucus and periciliary fluid, so facilitating mucus spreading. It also acts to lubricate the cilia. Several observations suggest a potential role for surfactant as a mucoactive substance, but further studies are required.

Indications

Inhaled acetylcysteine is indicated for mucolytic therapy as an adjuvant in respiratory conditions with excessive and/or thick mucus production. Such conditions include: COPD, bronchiectasis, cystic fibrosis and pneumonia.

It is also used post-operatively, as a diagnostic aid, and in tracheostomy care.

Its use in other situations, such as burns-associated inhalational injury, is unclear.

Due to its potential for bronchospasm when given nebulized, it is often mixed with a bronchodilator. This has prevented accurate and robust assessment of its true value, as compared with the oral route.

Mucolytic therapy in specific clinical practice

In COPD

The volume of mucus secretion is ~15ml/day. However, mucus secretion can increase 3-fold in COPD. A number of oral mucolytics have been studied in the short term.

The first reports of aerosolized mucolytics (NAC) in chronic bronchitis in 1968/9 suggested potential benefits.

Carbocysteine can improve exacerbation rates and interval in COPD exacerbators. This has been corroborated in an elderly cohort .

A Cochrane review (n = 6,415, 23 randomized controlled trials, duration 2–24 months) of 10 different oral mucolytics in mild COPD showed a modest reduction in exacerbations, with an number needed-to-treat of 6 to prevent 1 exacerbation .

NAC used over at least 24 weeks can produce clinically relevant improvements in symptoms and exacerbation rates, which extend to a year, without notable side effects. NICE recomends a trial of oral mucolytics in chronic productive cough associated with COPD.

In bronchiectasis

As part of bronchial hygiene, hydration, physiotherapy and mucolytic agents are important considerations in the management of bronchiectasis.

Nebulized NAC is beneficial in some patients, but has not demonstrated clinical improvement in the randomized controlled trial setting.

There are conflicting results on the efficacy of aerosolized recombinant DNase, which breaks down DNA, a major gelatinous product of neutrophils. DNase improves pulmonary function (FEV_1) and reduces hospitalizations in cystic fibrosis, but is not effective in non-cystic fibrosis bronchiectasis.

In mechanically ventilated patients

The delivery of inhaled drugs to the lower respiratory tract of mechanically ventilated patients is complicated by deposition of the aerosol particles in the ventilator circuit and ETT, and the factors governing pulmonary deposition in mechanically ventilated patients are different from those in ambulatory patients.

Systematic reviews of pharmacological therapies for ARDS have shown no benefit on outcomes with the use of NAC (n = 235, 5 studies, relative risk 0.89; 95% confidence interval 0.65–1.21) .

There are reports of resolution of mucus plugging exacerbating status asthmaticus through endotracheal instillation of recombinant DNase .

The use of inhaled agents such as NAC and in mechanically ventilated patients has not demonstrated outcome benefits in larger studies. Furthermore, the possibility of increased airways resistance due to bronchospasm has been reported and, if considered as a rescue therapy, it should only be used with a bronchodilator.

Summary

- There are a number of pharmacological and non-pharmacological methods for altering the composition of mucus in respiratory disease.
- There has not been any evidence for the benefit of inhaled mucolytics in mechanically ventilated patients except reports of rescue therapy in status asthmaticus. Furthermore, they may cause short-lived bronchospasm, and increased airway resistance. Thus, they are not recommended for general use.
- There is evidence for clinically practical improvements in mild and moderate COPD through oral mucolytics such as Carbocysteine and NAC.

Further reading

Adhikari N, Burns KE, Meade MO. Pharmacologic treatments for acute respiratory distress syndrome and acute lung injury: systematic review and meta-analysis. *Treat Respir Med* 2004; 3: 307–2.

Allegra L, Cardaro Cl, Grassi A. Prevention of acute exacerbations of chronic obstructive bronchitis with carbocysteine lysine salt monohydrate: a multicenter double blind placebo-controlled trial. *Respiration* 1996; 63: 174–80.

Clarke, SW, Pavia, D. Mucociliary clearance. In: Scientific Foundations, Crystal, RG, West, *JB, eds. The lung. New York: Raven Press*, 1991.

Durward A, Forte V, Shemie SD. Resolution of mucus plugging and atelectasis after intratracheal rhDNase therapy in a mechanically ventilated child with refractory status asthmaticus. *Crit Care Med*. 2000;28: 560–2.

Elkins, MR, Robinson, M, Rose, RR, *et al*. A controlled trial of long-term inhaled hypertonic saline in patients with cystic fibrosis. *N Engl J Med* 2006; 354: 229.

Fuchs, HJ, Borowitz, DS, Christiansen, DH, *et al*. Effect of aerosolized recombinant human DNase on exacerbations of respiratory symptoms and on pulmonary function in patients with cystic fibrosis. The Pulmozyme Study Group. *N Engl J Med* 1994; 331: 637.

Grandjean EM, Berthet P, Ruffmann R, *et al*. Efficacy of oral long-term N-acetylcysteine in chronic bronchopulmonary disease: a meta analysis of published double blind, placebo-controlled clinical trials. *Clin Ther* 2000; 22: 209–21.

Kory RC, Hirsch SR, Giraldo J. Nebulization of N-acetylcysteine combined with a bronchodilator in patients with chronic bronchitis. A controlled study. *Dis Chest* 1968; 54: 504–9.

Poole, PJ, Black, PN. Oral mucolytic drugs for exacerbations of chronic obstructive pulmonary disease: systematic review. *BMJ* 2001; 322: 1271.

Poole, PJ, Black, PN. Mucolytic agents for chronic bronchitis or chronic obstructive pulmonary disease (Cochrane review). The Cochrane library, issue 3, 2004, Chicester, UK: John Wiley & Sons Ltd.

Richardson PS, Phipps RJ. The anatomy, physiology, pharmacology and pathology of tracheobronchial mucus secretion and the use of expectorant drugs in human disease. *Pharmacol Ther* [B] 1978; 3: 441–79.

Task Group on Mucoactive Drugs. Recommendations for guidelines on clinical trials of mucoactive drugs in chronic bronchitis and chronic obstructive pulmonary disease. Task Group on Mucoactive Drugs. *Chest* 1994; 106: 1532.

Yasuda H, Yamaya M, Sasaki T, *et al*. Carbocisteine reduces frequency of common colds and exacerbations in patients with chronic obstructive pulmonary disease. *J Am Geriatr Soc* 2006; 54: 378–80.

Surfactant

A substance in lung oedema fluid and lung extracts was found in the mid-1950s by Pattle and Clements which lowered surface tension dramatically. It was termed surfactant, i.e. surface active agent. In 1959, Avery and Mead clarified the role played by a lack of surfactant in hyaline membrane disease of premature infants, now called respiratory distress syndrome (RDS) of the newborn.

Surfactant therapy has since been used as routine life-saving therapy in infant RDS, and extension of its use to ALI/ARDS is being currently studied. Furthermore, elucidation of functions outside of surface tension reduction, importantly lung defence and immunomodulation, are being uncovered, leading to studies of its role and possible therapeutic uses in other lung diseases.

Composition

Pulmonary surfactant forms a thin layer at the surface of the lining fluid layer on the alveolar epithelial surface. It is a complex biological mixture of lipids and proteins, with lipids making up to 90% of the total by weight. Of the lipids, ~90% are a mixture of phospholipids, with the remaining 10% being mainly cholesterol. Dipalmitoylphosphatidylcholine (DPPC) is the phospholipid predominantly responsible for the surface tension reduction properties of surfactant. The protein composition includes four unique surfactant proteins (SP)-A, -B -C and -D, in addition to the remaining 80% which are contaminating serum and lung tissue proteins.

SP-A is the most abundant surfactant protein and, along with SP-D, is the more hydrophilic protein, playing a role both in pulmonary host defence and in the recycling of surfactant. SP-B and SP-C are hydrophobic surfactant proteins which are critical in the formation of the surfactant monolayer with its surface tension-lowering properties.

Metabolism

Surfactant metabolism involves a continuous process of synthesis and degradation. The protein and lipid components are both synthesized by type II alveolar epithelial cells. The surfactant phospholipids, which are synthesized from blood-derived phospholipid precursors and from recycled products from the alveoli, are stored in lamellar bodies which are secretory granules found in the cytoplasm of alveolar type II cells. These are released into the alveolar lumen by exocytosis.

After secretion and combination with the surfactant proteins, surfactant is initially transformed into tubular myelin, a transitory large aggregate structure that is then transformed into the final functional layer. The lipid and protein components are separated as the lipid is inserted into a monolayer at the air–liquid interface.

As part of a recycling process, most of the surfactant is taken back up by the type II cells. Additional degradation involves alveolar macrophage phagocytosis, local intra-alveolar catabolism and mucociliary clearance. Certain components are recycled directly back into the new surfactant. Surfactant half-lives of between 15 and 30h have been demonstrated in phospholipid turnover studies.

Normal function

Surface tension reduction and alveolar size regulation

The combination of elasticity of lung parenchyma and surface tension of the fluid at the air–alveolar interface causes the lung to decrease in size. The surface tension plays a much more significant role in this balance, and without surfactant would completely collapse the lung alveoli.

Pulmonary surfactant adsorbs to the alveolar air–water interface and causes dynamic reduction in the surface tension with changes in alveolar size, i.e. surface tension reduces with decrease in alveolar size during expiration until near zero, hence stopping collapse and atelectasis, then rises again with inspiration. This means that alveolar pressure is kept near constant throughout a ventilatory cycle and the respiratory workload is reduced.

This surface tension reduction is achieved by the hydrophobic ends of the phospholipids aligning in parallel and lifting out of the liquid alveolar lining into the air space. The surfactant proteins, particularly SP-B and SP-C, enhance this activity. This structure remains dynamically stable throughout the ventilatory cycle.

Pulmonary defence

Surfactant forms part of the alveolar and bronchial epithelial lining fluid which acts as a non-specific barrier against foreign particles and microorganisms.

There are antibacterial properties of surfactant itself. SP-A and SP-D are collectins, a family of collagenous lectins believed to play an important in first-line innate defence by binding to viruses and by opsonizing yeasts and bacteria.

Additionally, both have been shown to have immunomodulatory roles and have been shown to be involved in modulating the functions of cells of the adaptive immune system, including dendritic cells and T cells.

Lung fluid balance

The presence of the high surface pressure of surfactant within the alveolar space counteracts fluid movement into the alveoli and contributes to preventing alveolar oedema.

Surfactant products

Currently there are several types of surfactant preparations available. The majority of them in clinical use are animal-derived products, of either bovine or porcine origin, which contain some of the surfactant proteins. These products are obtained either by animal lung lavage or lung mincing in saline, with extraction of the active phospholipids and proteins with organic solvents.

The synthetic surfactants available contain DPPC with a synthetic emulsifier to facilitate surface adsorption. The synthetic preparations available for clinical use do not contain surfactant proteins.

ALI/ARDS

ALI and the more severe ARDS are defined as syndromes of inflammation and increased permeability associated with a constellation of radiological and physiological abnormalities that cannot be explained by left atrial or pulmonary capillary hypertension. They are characterized by diffuse injury to the alveolar–capillary barrier, resulting in severe impairment in gas exchange. The aetiology is diverse but can be broadly divided into direct and indirect lung injury. There is an associated mortality of up to 40% for ARDS.

Surfactant dysfunction within ALI/ARDS is thought to contribute significantly to the disease's morbidity and mortality.

The initial exudative phase is characterized histologically by diffuse alveolar damage. There is a combination of defective surfactant and a reduction in the synthesis and recycling of surfactant due to damage and loss of type II alveolar cells. The presence of a protein-rich oedema contaminates the surfactant present, leading to a reduced functional capacity through both a dilutional effect and inactivation by proteolytic effects of the oedema. Furthermore, lung injury leads to an increase in the ratio of minor phospholipids to phosphatidylcholine, thought to be due to the damage and release of cell membrane lipids, thus leading to reduced surface tension-lowering properties.

The administration of exogenous surfactant would seem a logical approach in addressing some of the deleterious effects within ALI/ARDS. There have been several preclinical and small clinical trials using a variety of surfactant preparations, dosing regimes and modes of drug delivery. These have suggested that the use of exogenous surfactant may be beneficial in ALI/ARDS in terms of improving physiological outcomes and potential survival benefits.

However, a large multi-centred, double-blind, placebo-controlled trial in adults showed no benefits; but the surfactant was administered using by nebulizer (with only 5% deposition) and employed a preparation of surfactant without surfactant-specific proteins. Following on from this, there have been 3 recent large multi-centre phase III trials employing direct intratracheal instillation. One of these was with HL 10, a preparation of natural surfactant isolated from pig lungs and containing a mixture of SP-B and SP-C. This trial was concluded for futility. Two further trials using surfactant containing a recombinant protein C with treatment up to 24h including up to four doses have recently been reported. These have shown an improvement of oxygenation but no survival benefit or reduction in the need for mechanical ventilation.

A *post hoc* analysis of these two trials, however, suggested that those patients with a direct pulmonary insult causing ARDS tended towards a reduced mortality. To address this issue, a further trial looking into surfactant use in patients with severe respiratory insufficiency due to direct pulmonary insult is ongoing.

RDS of newborn

RDS is the main cause of respiratory distress in newborn infants, particularly preterm infants. There is a significant reduction in the amount of surfactant present secondary to the immaturity in the development of the type II alveolar cells. This leads to increased surface tension within the terminal respiratory units, resulting in atelectasis and subsequent respiratory failure.

Clinical trials have shown that surfactant therapy (synthetic and animal derived) led to improvements in oxygenation, decreased ventilatory support, decreased risk of pneumothorax and decreased mortality.

When possible, antenatal corticosteroid administration is given to those women at risk of having preterm deliveries. This is believed to speed maturation of fetal lungs and to increase surfactant synthesis and release. There are several strategies of surfactant treatment: immediate preventative treatment in those at high risk of developing RDS, early treatment given within the first 2h of being born and rescue treatment to those with established RDS. All have been shown to lead to improved clinical outcomes.

The prophylactic and early strategies have been demonstrated to be superior to rescue therapy in 2 separate Cochrane meta-analyses. No specific trials have as yet been done comparing early vs prophylactic therapy though there is suggestive indirect evidence that prophylactic is better.

Other uses of exogenous surfactant

One recent study suggested a protective effect of exogenous surfactant instilled to donor lungs before retrieval on post-lung transplantation surfactant function and on early clinical outcome. This was done as post-transplant graft rejection was often found to be related to post-reperfusion surfactant dysfunction. This may provide a further avenue of use for surfactant.

Surfactant dysfunction or deficiency may also play a role in the pathophysiology of other respiratory disorders affecting newborn infants. Hence there may be a role for its use in babies with meconium aspiration syndrome, pneumonia and possibly bronchopulmonary dysplasia.

Conclusion

Current evidence does not support the use of exogenous surfactant in adult patients with ALI/ARDS, although there may be a role for it in certain subgroups, i.e. those with direct lung injury. Further studies looking into different doses, delivery modes (nebulized, intratracheal or bronchoscopic instillation) and duration of treatments are required, and the range of side effects from the drug and delivery need to be clearly understood.

However, for RDS in infants, both synthetic and natural products have been shown to be effective, though natural preparations containing surfactant proteins (specifically SP-B and SP-C) have been found to be superior. With the development of new synthetic products containing surfactant proteins, it remains to be seen whether these will prove to be more effective in this group of patients.

Ongoing research into surfactant pathophysiology may reveal other potential lung diseases that may benefit from therapeutic intervention.

Further reading

Anzueto A, Baughman RP, Guntapalli KK, *et al.* Aerosolized surfactants in adults with sepsis-induced acute respiratory distress syndrome. *N Engl J Med* 1996; 334: 1417–21.

Hohlfeld JM. Pulmonary surfactant and lung fluid balance. In: Gibson GJ, Geddes DM, Costable U, *et al.* Respiratory medicine, 3rd edn, Philadelphia: Saunders, 2003: 93–104.

Horbar JD, Wright EC, Onstad L. Decreasing mortality associated with the introduction of surfactant therapy: an observational study of neonates weighing 601 to 1300 grams at birth. The Members of the National Institute of Child Health and Human Development Neonatal Research Network. Pediatrics 1993; 92: 191–6.

Schwarts RM, Luby AM, Scanlon JW, *et al.* Effect of surfactant on morbidity, mortality, and resource use in newborn infants weighing 500 to 1500 g. *N Engl J Med* 1994; **330**: 1476–80.

Spragg RG, Lewis JR, Walmrath H *et al.* (2004). Effect of Recombinant Surfactant Protein C-Based Surfactant on the Acute Respiratory Distress Syndrome. *N Engl J Med* 351: 884-892.

Struber M, Fischer S, Niedermeyer J, *et al.* Effects of exogenous surfactant instillation in clinical lung transplantation: a prospective, randomized trial. *J Thorac Cardiovasc Surg* 2007; 133: 1620–5.

Helium–oxygen gas mixtures

Nomenclature

Helium–oxygen mixtures are sometimes referred to as heliox, whilst nitrogen–oxygen mixtures are referred to as nitrox. However, heliox is sometimes used to refer specifically to helium 79%–oxygen 21%. In this chapter, heliox will refer to any mixture of helium and oxygen, whilst heliox21 refers to helium 79%–oxygen 21%.

Rationale

The efficiency of gas flow is dependent upon, amongst other things, the physical properties of the gas, specifically its density and viscosity. Reducing the density increases the efficiency of gas flow. Helium is a colourless, odourless gas, is chemically and biologically inert, and its density is 7 times less than nitrogen and 8 times less than oxygen, with a comparable viscosity. Thus, substituting helium for nitrogen in inspired gas mixtures increases the efficiency of convectional and diffusional gas transport.

Indications

Helium–oxygen mixtures should be considered as a rescue therapy in the immediate management of upper and/or lower airway obstruction due to such conditions as: croup, epiglottitis, laryngitis, tracheitis, foreign body aspiration, post-extubation or peribronchoscopy stridor, tumour (upper airway or proximal tracheobronchial tree), tracheomalacia, tracheal stenosis, acute severe asthma and acute severe (hypercapnic) exacerbation of COPD.

Treatment with a helium–oxygen mixture should be initiated in a patient with any of these conditions who despite first-line therapy develops severe respiratory distress, specifically: reports severe dyspnoea, has a very high respiratory rate, is making excessive respiratory effort, is tiring, becomes drowsy or agitated, or is becoming hypoxic and/or hypercapnic. It may prevent the need to intubate or at least create a time window to allow this to be done urgently rather than as an emergency.

Expected effects

Administering helium–oxygen should improve the efficiency of ventilation and thereby reduce respiratory distress. However, it is only a temporizing intervention, i.e. it extends the period of time available for definite treatment for the underlying condition to be delivered; it is not in itself therapeutic.

Presentation

Helium should only be available as heliox21 (79% helium–21% oxygen). This is because you will never want to deliver a gas mixture with <21% oxygen.

Face mask administration

Helium–oxygen gas mixtures can be delivered through any tight-fitting mask. The mask should preferably have a reservoir bag into which the heliox is delivered, and one or more one-way expiratory valves. Every effort should be made to minimize air entrainment. Specialist masks and mixing/nebulizing circuits are available commercially. Supplemental oxygen can be provided either through a Y-piece mixing circuit or via nasal specs worn underneath the tight-fitting mask.

Nebulization

Generating a respirable aerosol using heliox21 through a standard, gas-driven, updraft nebulization chamber requires flow rates of ≥15l/min as compared with air or oxygen which run at 6–8l/min. Thus the efficiency and reliability of respirable particle generation using heliox21 are suboptimal. As a carrier gas for respirable particles, however, heliox21 demonstrates significantly higher delivery than more dense gas mixtures. Ideally, therefore, an alternative particle generation technique should be employed, such as ultrasound or vibrating mesh. Unfortunately, these techniques are not widely available. The choice in an individual circumstance will usually be decided by practicalities such as the need for supplemental oxygen or heliox21 availability. It may be difficult to run a reservoir bag and a nebulizer simultaneously off the same cylinder.

Caution: managing hypoxia (SpO_2 <88%)

In hypoxic patients, a balance needs to be struck between improving ventilation (by minimizing gas density and hence minimizing the FiO_2) and achieving adequate oxygenation (by diluting heliox21 with supplemental oxygen). As a starting guide, aim to achieve an SpO_2 of 88–92%.

Patient monitoring during therapy

Routine respiratory monitoring is all that is required (airway patency, respiratory rate, clinical evaluation of the adequacy of ventilation, SpO_2 and blood gas analysis). Continuous oxygen saturation monitoring should be used in all hypoxic patients. Always assess and optimize face mask position as any air entrainment will reduce the effectiveness of this intervention.

Safety

Standard safety precautions for compressed gases are all that is required. Helium is inert and insoluble in human tissues at atmospheric pressure. Helium does have a high thermal conductivity but does not cause significant airway or whole patient cooling, even in neonates.

Stopping helium–oxygen therapy

Helium–oxygen therapy can be withdrawn as soon as definitive therapy has taken sufficient effect to reduce respiratory distress. It may be useful as an intermittent therapy in such conditions as acute severe asthma where periodic reductions in the work of breathing can prevent decompensation and thereby prevent the need for intubation and mechanical ventilation.

Indications for helium–oxygen mask ventilation (CPAP, BiPAP, PSV)

Heliox may reduce the work of breathing to a similar extent to positive pressure mask ventilation. The effect of these two interventions is additive such that a patient failing one, may benefit from the addition of the other. Delivering heliox mixtures through positive pressure mask ventilation devices is problematic, as none is currently designed for this. Some clinicians have tried entraining heliox21 at 15l/min into the mask, or as near to it in the circuit as practical. However, the efficacy of this technique, in particular the actual gas mixture delivered to the patient, is uncertain.

Indications for helium–oxygen IPPV via endotracheal or tracheostomy tube

Severe inspiratory and/or expiratory flow limitation necessitates the use of dangerously high airway pressures

(≥35cm H_2O) and/or high levels of intrinsic PEEP. The effectiveness of instituting helium–oxygen will be limited by the degree to which oxygen supplementation is required. A reversible pathology should have been identified and a treatment plan instituted. Patients may respond to relatively small reductions in gas density such that even an FiO_2 of 0.7 should not necessarily preclude a therapeutic trial. It is sometimes possible to decrease the FiO_2 gradually as ventilation improves, thus decreasing the gas density further.

Patient monitoring during IPPV therapy

Routine respiratory/ventilator monitoring is all that is required. There are currently only two commercially available ventilators designed for use with heliox. Of note, both of these can be used to deliver mask ventilation. Some other ventilators can be connected to heliox in place of air. Heliox may interfere with both internal performance and patient monitoring. Extreme care needs to employed to avoid the delivery of excessive or inadequate tidal volumes. Always use a pressure control mode and measure the FiO_2. Switching gas mixtures between heliox and nitrox usually requires recalibration of the pneumotachograph, which in most ventilators cannot be performed whilst delivering ventilation to a patient. Capnography is also affected by substituting helium for nitrogen. The efficacy of heliox over nitrox should be evident almost immediately, with a maximal effect seen within 15min.

Stopping helium–oxygen therapy

Assuming that helium–oxygen has proven to be efficacious and that a sufficient time interval has elapsed to allow definitive therapy to have taken effect, then institute a trial of switching the inspiratory gas mixture back to nitrogen oxygen. If this results in a significant deterioration in respiratory mechanics, then re-institute helium–oxygen and set a time interval at which a re-trial of nitrogen–oxygen will be undertaken. Intermittent use of a helium–oxygen mixture may be considered as part of a weaning strategy.

Published trials

There are a significant number of published trials of heliox in a variety of settings. These have been extensively reviewed However, there is currently insufficient evidence to justify its routine use.

Further reading

Ball JA, Grounds RM. Calibration of three capnographs for use with helium and oxygen gas mixtures. Anaesthesia 2003; 58: 156–60.

Chatmongkolchart S, Kacmarek RM, Hess DR Heliox delivery with noninvasive positive pressure ventilation: a laboratory study. *Respir Care* 2001; 46: 248–54.

Colebourn CL, Barber V, Young YD. Use of helium–oxygen mixture in adult patients presenting with exacerbations of asthma and chronic obstructive pulmonary disease: a systematic review. Anaesthesia 2007; 62: 34–42.

Fink JB. Opportunities and risks of using heliox in your clinical practice. *Respir Care* 2006; 51: 651–60.

Hess DR. Heliox and noninvasive positive-pressure ventilation: a role for heliox in exacerbations of chronic obstructive pulmonary disease? *Respir Care* 2006; 51: 640–50.

Hess DR, Fink JB, Venkatamaran ST, *et al.* The history and physics of heliox. *Respir Care* 2006; 51: 608–12.

Hurford WE, Cheifetz IM. Should heliox be used for mechanically ventilated patients? *Respir Care* 2007; 52: 582–94.

Kim IK, Saville AL, Sikes KL. *et al.* Heliox-driven albuterol nebulization for asthma exacerbations: an overview. *Respir Care* 2006; 51: 613–8.

Myers TR. Use of heliox in children. Respir Care 2006; 51: 619–31.

Oppenheim-Eden A, Cohen Y, Weissman C, *et al.* The effect of helium on ventilator performance: study of five ventilators and a bedside pitot tube spirometer. *Chest* 2001; 120: 582–8.

Smith SW, Biros M. Relief of imminent respiratory failure from upper airway obstruction by use of helium–oxygen: a case series and brief review. *Acad Emerg Med* 1999; 6: 953–-6.

Tassaux D, Jolliet P, Thouret JM, *et al.* Calibration of seven ICU ventilators for mechanical ventilation with helium–oxygen mixtures. *Am J Respir Crit Care Med* 1999; 160: 22–32.

Wigmore T, Stachowski E. A review of the use of heliox in the critically ill. *Crit Care Resusc* 2006; 8: 64–72.

Cardiovascular drugs

Chapter contents

β-Adrenergic agonists

β-Adrenergic agents are used commonly for cardiovascular support in critical care to increase cardiac output via β_1 receptor-mediated inotropic and chronotropic effects (see Chapter 11.6) in order to maintain adequate organ perfusion.

Non-cardiovascular indications for β_2 agonists include bronchodilatation (Chapter 10.1) and uterine relaxation. Research is ongoing into the potential benefits of β_2 agonists in reducing EVLW in patients with ARDS.

Effects of β-adrenergic agonists

Most β-adrenergic agonists in clinical use are active at more than one type of adrenergic receptor (β_1, β_2, β_3, α_1 and α_2).

- Cardiac—β_1 (and to a much lesser degree β_2) effects include increased heart rate, increased conduction velocity throughout the heart and increased rate of idioventricular pacemakers. All β-adrenergic agonists increase myocardial oxygen consumption and may precipitate myocardial ischaemia in susceptible patients (dobutamine is used to carry out myocardial stress testing). Beta agonists increase the incidence of cardiac arrhythymias.
- Blood vessels— β_2 agonists induce vasodilatation in coronary muscle, skeletal muscle, and pulmonary, splanchnic and renal arterioles and arteries. α_2 agonists cause vasoconstriction in splanchnic, renal and skin vessels, and to a lesser degree in coronary and pulmonary arterioles and arteries.
- Metabolic effects— β_2 agonists cause increased glycogenolysis, gluconeogenesis in liver and skeletal muscle, increased potassium uptake in skeletal muscle, and increased lipolysis.

The clinical effects of a specific agent result from the sum of actions at different receptors and may alter as dose increases. In addition, effects may vary with alterations in intravascular volume.

As with vasoconstrictor drugs, it is important to optimize circulating volume for a particular patient before initiating β agonist therapy. This may include the use of cardiac output monitoring.

The half-lives of all the β agonists listed in this chapter are very short (a few minutes) with the exception of ephedrine. Caution should be used in patients already receiving monoamine oxidase inhibitors (MAOIs).

In some patients, particularly with sepsis, increasing doses of β agonists may be required to achieve the same clinical effects.

Drugs

Epinephrine (adrenaline)

Epinephrine is a naturally occurring catecholamine in the adrenal medulla. It is a mixed α-, and $\beta_1$and β_2-adrenergic agonist. At low doses, β_2-mediated vasodilatation predominates, but at higher non-physiological doses increasing vasoconstriction (skin, mucosa, GI tract, kidneys and systemic veins) occurs as a result of α_1-adrenergic receptor agonism.

Epinephrine is used most commonly as an inotrope in patients with low cardiac output despite optimal fluid resuscitation and unresponsiveness to other inotropes.

Epinephrine infusion has been associated with increased arterial blood lactate concentration, metabolic acidosis and worsening markers of splanchnic perfusion. As with all β agonists, epinephrine increases the incidence of arrhythmias. In general, it is used to manage patients with low cardiac output unresponsive to other inotropic agents.

Epinephrine is given as a IV bolus during cardiac arrest (as part of resuscitation algorithms) because of its vasoconstrictor action.

Epinephrine is the drug of choice for the management of anaphylactic shock both because of α_1-mediated vasoconstriction and β_2-mediated inhibition of mast cell release of inflammatory mediators including histamine.

- Dose—IV bolus (during cardiac arrest): 1mg. IM (anaphylaxis): 0.5mg. IV infusion: 0.01–1mcg/kg/min; usually started at dose in the range 0.02–0.05mcg/kg/min.
- Adverse effects—tachycardia, arrhythmias, vasoconstriction with potential organ dysfunction and necrosis, metabolic acidosis, hyokalaemia, increased blood glucose and lactate concentrations, increased metabolic rate.

Norepinephrine (noradrenaline)

Norepinephrine is the neurotransmitter found in sympathetic post-ganglionic nerve fibres and is a mixed β_1 and α_1 agonist. Infusion results in increased blood pressure and usually no change or an increase in cardiac output. Care must be taken to ensure that patients are not or do not become hypovolaemic, as in these circumstances cardiac output may decrease and peripheral perfusion become severely impaired.

Norepinephrine is generally used to maintain adequate MAP following volume resuscitation and after adequate cardiac output has been restored. Norepinephrine is therefore commonly used in combination with another β agonist or PDE3 inhibitors in patients with cardiogenic shock.

In patients with volume-resuscitated septic shock, norepinephrine infusion has been reported to improve urine output and glomerular filtration rate (GFR).

- Dose—IV infusion: 0.01–1mcg/kg/min. Normal starting dose: 0.02–0.05mcg/kg/min.
- Adverse effects—vasoconstriction with potential organ dysfunction and necrosis, metabolic acidosis, arrhythmias.

Isoprenaline

Isoprenaline is a synthetic agonist at β receptors and has no α-adrenergic effects. Infusion results in increased heart rate and cardiac output, but decreased MAP because of β_2-mediated vasodilatation. Its main use is as a chronotrope for the temporary management of bradycardias. It is also occasionally used as an inotrope in patients with pulmonary hypertension because of its pulmonary vasodilator effects.

- Dose—IV infusion: 0.5–10mcg/min.
- Adverse effects—tachycardia, arrhythmias.

Dopamine

Dopamine is the natural metabolic precursor of epinephrine and norepinehrine, and is an agonist at dopamine, α and β receptors.

Effects vary according to infusion rate. At doses of 0–5mcg/kg/min, dopamine receptor effects predominate, resulting in renal and splanchnic vasodilatation. Urine output may increase as a result of a proximal tubular diuretic effect. At doses of 5–10mcg/kg/min, β_1 effects result in increased heart rate and contractility. At doses of 10–20mcg/kg/min, α_1 receptor-mediated effects are more marked, leading to vasoconstriction.

Dopamine has been used to maintain blood pressure in patients with septic shock, but norepinephrine is more likely to be effective.

Addition of low-dose dopamine infusion to other cardiovascular support in critically ill patients does not decrease the requirement for acute RRT.

In patients post-cardiac surgery, use of dopamine is associated with an increased incidence of atrial fibrillation.

- Dose—IV infusion: 1–10mcg/kg/min. Normal starting dose is 2–5mcg/kg/min.
- Adverse effects—tachycardia, arrhythmias, vasoconstriction, nausea and vomiting.

Dobutamine

Dobutamine is a synthetic agonist at mainly β_1 but also β_2 and α_1 receptors. IV infusion causes increased heart rate and stroke volume, and vasodilatation. The effect on blood pressure is variable, and often concurrent norepinephrine infusion is required to prevent hypotension. It is used primarily for the management of low cardiac output, despite adequate fluid resuscitation, in patients with cardiogenic shock, usually post-MI or following cardiac surgery. Dobutamine has been recommended as the first-choice agent to increase cardiac output, when required, in patients with septic shock.

- Dose—IV infusion: 0–20mcg/kg/min. Usual starting dose is 2–5mcg/kg/min, and it is rarely required to use >10mcg/kg/min.
- Adverse effects—tachycardia, arrhythmias, hypotension.

Dopexamine

Dopexamine is a synthetic dopamine receptor and β_2 receptor agonist. Dopexamine infusion causes increased heart rate, stroke volume and systemic vasodilatation (including renal and splanchnic), resulting in increased cardiac output. Its inotropic effects are mild.

- Dose—IV infusion: 0.5–6mcg/kg/min.
- Adverse effects—tachycardia, hypotension.

Ephedrine

Ephedrine is a direct α and β agonist, but also increases norepinephrine release from sympathetic nerves. Administration results in increased heart rate, cardiac output and blood pressure. Although it is active if given orally, it is usually administered as an IV bolus. Tachyphylaxis occurs, making it unsuitable for IV infusion. Its main use is as treatment of temporary hypotension associated with epidural or spinal anaesthesia.

- Dose—IV bolus: 3–6mg every 3min, maximum 30mg.
- Adverse effects—tachycardia, arrhythmias, CNS stimulation.

Salbutamol

Salbutamol is a selective β_2 agonist primarily used for its bronchodilator effect. It is rarely used for cardiovascular support for patients with pulmonary hypertension.

- Dose—IV infusion: initially 3–20mcg/min.
- Adverse effects—tachycardia, arrhythmias, hypokalaemia.

Role of β agonist drugs

High-risk surgical patient

A number of studies have reported improved survival of high-risk surgical patients when cardiac index or oxygen delivery are optimized to above normal levels during the perioperative period using fluids and β agonists. This does not appear to be agent specific and has been reported in various studies using dobutamine, epinephrine and dopexamine.

Post-cardiac surgery

Low cardiac output post-cardiac surgery is relatively common. Patients requiring a low degree of inotropic support are often managed with dopamine as this can usually be managed in level 2 critical care areas. For patients requiring more support, epinephrine, dobutamine or a PDE3 inhibitor are commonly used.

Cardiogenic shock

Agents with both inotropic and vasodilator properties such as dobutamine or PDE3 inhibitors are common choices. Low dose epinephrine may be added if required. Tachycardia may limit doses of β agonists.

Septic shock

In patients with septic shock and low cardiac output unresponsive to optimization of intravascular volume, dobutamine has been recommended as the inotrope of choice. Cardiovascular optimization needs to be carried out as early as possible in order to decrease the incidence of multi-organ failure. Norepinephrine is the first-line drug to increase MAP.

Multi-organ failure

Several meta-analyses have consistently reported that attempting to target supranormal values of cardiac index or oxygen delivery in patients with established multi-organ failure does not improve survival.

Further reading

Brunton L, ed. Goodman and Gilman's pharmacological basis of therapeutics, 11th en. New York: McGraw Hill.

Dellinger RP, Levy MM, Carlet JM, *et al.* Surviving Sepsis Campaign; international guidelines for management of severe sepsis and septic shock: 2008. *Crit Care Med* 2008; 36: 296–327.

Rhodes A, Bennett ED. Early goal-directed therapy: an evidence-based review. *Crit Care Med* 2004; 32: S448–50.

Rivers E, Nguyen B, Havstad S, *et al.* Early goal-directed therapy in the treatment of severe sepsis and septic shock. *N Engl J Med* 2001; 345: 1368–1377.

Phosphodiesterase inhibitors

Phosphodiesterases (PDEs) are a family of enzymes that inactivate cAMP. PDE inhibitors increase cAMP levels, leading to increased contractility in myocardial cells and relaxation in smooth muscle. To date, 11 PDE subtypes have been identified in mammals, although only 5 subtypes have been found to have clinical relevance in humans. PDE inhibitors relevant to critical care will be discussed in this section and are classified into non-selective and selective inhibitors.

Non-selective PDE inhibitors

Methylxanthines

Theophylline and aminophylline (water-soluble complex of theophylline and ethylenediamine) act through non-specific PDE3 and 4 inhibition, resulting in increased intracellular cAMP levels. In addition, theophyllines are competitive antagonists of adenosine receptors. The main effects are increased heart rate, bronchodilatation, diuresis and anti-inflammatory effects. Adverse effects include tachyarrythmias, tremor, electrolyte and glucose abnormalities, and nausea, vomiting and diarrhoea.

The clinical utility of theophylline in the critical care setting is controversial. Meta-analyses have not found benefit for the use of IV theophylline for acute severe asthma. However, international consensus guidelines recommend its use as rescue therapy for patient's refractory to standard asthma treatment.

No RCTs have demonstrated a benefit for theophylline in COPD patients suffering acute exacerbations. However, it may have a role in patient's refractory to standard therapy.

Small studies have shown increased diaphragmatic strength and mucociliary clearance in patients in ICUs. Due to risk–benefit considerations, theophylline is not routinely used for these indications in critically ill patients.

IV theophylline is administered as aminophylline slowly over 20min; it is extremely irritant. The initial loading dose is 250–500mg (5mg/kg), followed by an infusion at 500mcg/kg/h. Extreme caution should be used in patients already on chronic theophylline therapy because of the risk of adverse effects.

Theophylline undergoes hepatic metabolism, and this is impaired in hepatic and cardiac failure. Plasma theophylline levels should be measured 4–6 hourly, aiming for a target concentration of 10–20mg/l. Adverse effects may be seen in the therapeutic range and are more likely with theophylline levels >20mg/l. Arrhythmias and convulsions may pre-date other signs of toxicity. An important side effect of theophylline is hypokalaemia, the incidence of which is increased when it is used in combination with β agonists.

Selective PDE inhibitors

Phosphodiesterase type 3 Inhibitors

PDE3 isoforms (A and B) are localized to numerous tissues, notably cardiac tissue, vascular smooth muscle and platelets. PDE3 inhibitors cause increased intracellular calcium accumulation (via inhibition of cAMP breakdown), resulting in improved contractility in cardiac myocytes.

In addition, there is increased lusitropy (diastolic relaxation), as the re-uptake of calcium is also a cAMP-dependent activity. There is evidence that the rate of re-uptake of calcium by the sarcoplasmic reticulum of the cardiac myocyte is increased with the use of PDE3 inhibitors. This diastolic relaxation is of particular benefit in neonates, children, and adults with poorly compliant ventricles.

The inhibition of PDE 3 in vascular smooth muscle results in the potentiation of cGMP, causing vasodilatation. As a consequence, these agents result in reductions in systemic vascular resistance, pulmonary vascular resistance and venous pressures.

There is some evidence for synergistic action between PDE3 inhibitors and β agonists such as dobutamine in the setting of low cardiac output states. This effect has been well described in neonatal cardiac surgery.

PDE3 inhibitors may also be useful as first-line inotropic agents in patients who have either been on long-term β-blockers, or who have a clinical indication for β-blockade in the setting of a low cardiac output state.

As with all potent vasodilators, caution should be exercised in their use in the presence of left or right cardiac outflow tract obstruction of any cause.

PDE3 inhibitors are usually given by IV infusion and it is important to consider that their half-lives are considerably longer than those of cathecholamines. Dose reduction may be necessary in the presence of renal impairment and particularly in elderly patients. Acute tolerance does not appear to be a feature of these agents.

There is concern about a potential increase in mortality with the long-term use of PDE3 inhibitors in patients with chronic heart failure. The reasons for this are unclear, but may be related to hypotension and an increase in both ventricular and atrial arrhythmias. There is no evidence of increased mortality with PDE3 inhibitors used short-term in the intensive care setting.

The main role for PDE3 inhibitors is in cardiac surgical intensive care patients. There appears to be little difference between agents in terms of effect. Due to the marked reduction in systemic vascular resistance, there is currently no role for these agents in patients with septic shock.

Milrinone

- Milrinone is administered IV as a loading dose of 20–50mcg/kg over 10min (diluted), followed by infusion at a rate of 0.1–0.75mcg/kg/min. The loading dose is often omitted if hypotension is anticipated. It is usually continued for at least 12h post-cardiac surgery or for 48–72h in congestive cardiac failure. It has a half-life of 30–60min, but this may be significantly prolonged in patients with renal dysfunction. In this scenario, dose reduction is necessary to prevent severe vasodilatation.
- Milrinone has been studied extensively in cardiac surgical and heart failure patients. There is evidence that it facilitates weaning from cardiopulmonary bypass. In the cardiac intensive care setting, milrinone increases cardiac index without a marked increase in heart rate, but at the expense of reduced systemic vascular resistance.
- In a comparison study with dobutamine, both drugs increased cardiac index significantly, but there was a greater achievement in MAP in patients receiving dobutamine. Milrinone had a slightly better safety profile,

with the dobutamine group suffering a higher incidence of hypotension and new AF.

- Milrinone has been found to be as effective as 20ppm NO in reducing pulmonary artery pressures in patients with pulmonary hypertension.
- Milrinone is generally preferred to other PDE3 inhibitors because of better PDE3 selectivity and its shorter half-life.

Enoximone

- Enoximone causes an increase in cardiac index, and reduction in systemic vascular resistance when compared with both placebo and dobutamine. As with milrinone, enoximone has been found to facilitate weaning from cardiopulmonary bypass.
- Enoximone is administered as a bolus of 0.5–1.5mg/kg, followed by an infusion at 5–10mcg/kg/min. It has a half-life of 2h.

Amrinone

- Amrinone has similar effects to the other PDE3 inhibitors.
- Impaired coagulation has been reported in some patients recieving amrinone due to a reduction in platelet count and/or platelet function.
- Amrinone is administered as a loading dose of 0.75–1.5mg/kg, followed by an infusion of 10mcg/kg/min. It has an elimination half-life of 3.5h.

Dipyridamole

This antiplatelet agent owes part of its mechanism of action to PDE3 inhibition. It also has a role in the management of pulmonary hypertension through PDE5 inhibition.

Phosphodiesterase type 4 inhibitors

Two experimental agents are currently being evaluated in phase III trials in patients suffering from asthma and COPD. Selective PDE4 inhibition has anti-inflammatory and immune-modulating functions in the respiratory mucosa, resulting in clinical improvement in bronchoconstriction, mucous hypersecretion and airway remodelling.

Phosphodiesterase type 5 inhibitors

PDE5 inhibitors prevent the breakdown of cGMP in pulmonary vascular smooth muscle, increasing intracellular levels, resulting in vasorelaxation in the pulmonary vascular bed and, to a lesser extent, the systemic circulation. PDE5 receptors are also found in the lower oesophageal sphincter, visceral smooth muscle and corpus cavernosum.

Sildenafil

- Sildenafil is licensed for use in erectile dysfunction and pulmonary hypertension.
- The dose is 12.5–50mg tds orally, and an IV formulation is available. In the context of pulmonary hypertension, the long-term use of sildenafil has been associated in improvements in RV mass and functional status.
- In intensive care patients, it is often used as a step-down therapy from iNO in patients with severe pulmonary hypertension. In this setting its use seems logical, but no outcome studies have been reported. Systemic hypotension may occur.
- Recent evidence has suggested a role for sildenafil in the management of myocardial ischaemia reperfusion injury. Thus it may find clinical application in the management of cardiac arrest and myocardial stunning post-cardiac surgery

Further reading

Amsallem E, Kasparian C,; Haddour G, *et al.* Phosphodiesterase III inhibitors for heart failure. *Cochrane Database Syst Rev* 2005; (1): CD002230.

Feneck RO, Sherry KM, Withington PS, *et al.* European Milrinone Multicenter Trial Group: comparison of the haemodynamic effects of milrinone with dobutamine in patients after cardiac surgery. *J Cardiothorac Vasc Anesth* 2001; 15: 306–15.

Gillies M, Bellomo R, Doolan L, *et al.* Bench-to-bedside review: inotropic drug therapy after adult cardiac surgery—a systematic literature review. *Crit Care* 2005; 9: 266–79.

Kroegel C, Foerster. M. Phosphodiesterase-4 inhibitors as a novel approach for the treatment of respiratory disease: cilomilast. *Expert Opin Invest Drugs* 2007; 16: 109–24.

Mitra A, Bassler D, Watts K, *et al.* Intravenous aminophylline for acute severe asthma in children over two years receiving inhaled bronchodilators. *Cochrane Database Syst Rev* 2005, Issue 2.

Parameswaran K, Belda J, Rowe BH. Addition of intravenous aminophylline to beta2-agonists in adults with acute asthma. *Cochrane Database Syst Rev* 2000, Issue 4.

Vasodilators

In critically ill patients, vasodilators may be indicated for treatment of systemic or pulmonary hypertension, reduction of cardiac preload or treatment of vasospasm in specific arterial systems.

Caution is required if administering vasodilators to patients with low fixed cardiac output, e.g. severe aortic stenosis, because of the risk of inducing severe hypotension.

Nitrates

Nitrates act directly on smooth muscle by release of NO from the parent molecule. Tolerance to nitrates can be reduced by the use of nitrate-free periods.

Glyceryl trinitrate (GTN)

GTN acts primarily on venous capacitance vessels, reducing venous return (preload). It has some arteriolar effect, decreasing afterload, and is a coronary vasodilator.

Onset of action is 2–5min with a half-life of 3min. GTN undergoes hepatic and extrahepatic metabolism via red cells and vascular endothelium. Tachyphylaxis is common, with tolerance occurring within 24–48h.

- Indications: congestive cardiac failure, cardiac ischaemia.
- Contraindications: aortic stenosis, hypertrophic obstructive cardiomyopathy (HOCM), hypotension, tamponade, severe anaemia, hypertensive encephalopathy.
- Dose and route: available sublingually, orally, transdermally and IV. Start IV infusion 10mcg/min and titrate by 10mcg/min to a maximum 200mcg/min.

Isosorbide mononitrate (ISMN)

ISMN is an orally administered nitrate used for angina prophylaxis and treatment of heart failure.

Isosorbide dinitrate (ISDN)

ISDN has slower onset and is longer acting than GTN and can be administered sublingually, orally or by IV infusion.

Directly acting vasodilators

Sodium nitroprusside (SNP)

The main action of SNP is relaxation of vascular smooth muscle in both arteries and veins that occurs via NO-stimulated increase in cGMP. At low doses, arterial vasodilatation predominates.

The hypotensive effect of SNP is seen within 1–2 min and may cause reflex tachycardia. Myocardial ischaemia can occur via a coronary steal syndrome.

Circulatory half-life is ~2min. Nitroprusside metabolism can lead to methaemoglobin formation and metabolic acidosis. Specific therapy for overdose includes administration of sodium nitrite followed by sodium thiocyanate. Tachyphylaxis may occur.

- Indications: immediate reduction of blood pressure in hypertensive crises, acute congestive cardiac failure, controlled hypotension intraoperatively.
- Contraindications: aortic coarctation, congenital optic atrophy, high output cardiac failure, severe B_{12} deficiency.
- Dose: start 0.3–0.5/mcg/kg/min and titrate to maximum 8mcg/kg/min.

Hydralazine

Hydralazine preferentially dilates arterioles via stimulation of cGMP. It is associated with reflex sympathetic activity, resulting in tachycardia. Hydralazine causes renin to be released by the juxtaglomerular apparatus, with subsequent angiotensin production, aldosterone release and sodium retention; thus β-blockers or diuretics are often administered concurrently.

Onset of action is within 5–10m IV, 20–30min orally. The half-life is 2–4h, but in patients with renal disease the half-life may increase up to 16h.

- Indications: hypertension, hypertensive crisis.
- Contraindications: SLE, severe tachycardia, high output heart failure, myocardial insufficiency due to mechanical obstruction, porphyria.
- Dose and route: orally, 10–25mg bd–qds for hypertension. Increase to 50–75mg qds in cardiac failure. By slow IV injection, 5–10 mg, may be repeated after 20–30min. By IV infusion, initially 200–300mcg/min, maintenance usually 50–150mcg/min.

Diazoxide

Diazoxide is an arteriolar vasodilator and antihypertensive. It inhibits insulin release, and hyperglycaemia may occur.

Onset of action is 5–10min with duration of action of 4–12h. Diazoxide is extensively protein bound, partly hepatically metabolized and partly excreted unchanged.

Difficult to use to control blood pressure over short time periods because of long half-life.

- Indications: hypertensive emergencies.
- Contraindications: ischaemic heart disease.
- Dose: by rapid IV injection, 1–3mg/kg with a maximum single dose of 150mg. Can be repeated after 5–15min as required.

Calcium antagonists

Calcium channel blockers have antianginal, antiarrythmic and vasodilatory effects. In cardiac muscle, calcium antagonism reduces myocardial contractility and cardiac output in a dose-dependent fashion. Impulse generation at the sinoatrial node and conduction via the atrioventricular node are calcium dependent, and blockade decreases sinus node pacemaker rate and atrioventricular node conduction velocity.

There are three classes of calcium channel antagonists:

- Dihydropyridines (nifedipine, amlodipine, nimodipine)
- Diphenylalkylamines (verapamil)
- Benzothiazepines (diltiazem)

Nifedipine is an arteriolar vasodilator. It can be administered orally, sublingually or IV. Sublingual administration may cause rapid severe hypotension.

Onset of action is 2–5min. It is hepatically metabolized with a plasma half-life of 4h.

- Indications: angina, hypertension, Raynaud's syndrome.
- Contraindications: aortic stenosis, porphyria, cardiogenic shock.
- Dose: 5–20mg tds.

Nimodipine has selective cerebral vasodilatory effects. It is indicated in the prevention and treatment of ischaemic neurological deficit following subarachnoid haemorrhage.

Peak plasma concentrations are reached within 1h, orally or IV. Half-life is 1–2h. Nimodipine undergoes hepatic metabolism; the dose should be halved in liver failure.

- Contraindications: severely raised ICP.
- Dose: orally, 60mg 4 hourly; IV, 500mcg–1mg/h initially, increased to 2mg/h as blood pressure tolerates.

Verapamil and *diltiazem* are used as antiarrythmic and antianginal agents, and have limited vasodilatory actions. They should be used carefully in the presence of accessory conducting pathwaysm e.g. Wolf–Parkinson–White syndrome, as VF may be precipitated.

α-Adrenergic receptor antagonists

Adrenergic receptors are subdivided into α_1 and α_2, and β_1, β_2 and β_3 subtypes.

- α_1 receptors are responsible for vasoconstriction, gut smooth muscle relaxation, increased salivation and gluconeogenesis.
- α_2 receptor agonists inhibit noradrenaline and acetylcholine release and stimulate platelet aggregation.

α-Blockade causes reduced systemic vascular resistance. There may be reflex sympathetic stimulation.

Phentolamine is a non-selective reversible competitive antagonist at both α_1 and α_2 receptors Onset of activity is rapid, with duration of action of 10–15min.

- Indications: phaeochromocytoma.
- Dose: 2–5mg (IV), repeat as necessary

Phenoxybenzamine is a non-selective irreversible α_1 and α_2 receptor antagonist. Noradrenaline re-uptake is blocked, potentiating the action of β agonists. Duration of action is 3–4 days.

- Indications: phaeochromocytoma.
- Dose: orally, initially 10mg bd, increased to 1–2mg/kg in divided doses; IV, 1mg/kg daily, slow injection over 2h daily.

Prazosin is a competitive α_1 receptor antagonist.

- Indications: essential and renovascular hypertension, Raynaud's disease, benign prostatic hypertrophy.
- Dose: initially 500mcg bd/tds at night, increased to 20mg/day in divided doses.

Other α receptor antagonists

Phenothiazines (chlorpromazine) and butyrophenones (haloperidol, droperidol) are competitive α antagonists.

Mized α and β antagonists

Labetolol is a competitive antagonist at both α_1 and β receptors, although β-blockade is predominant.

- Indications: hypertensive emergencies.
- Dose: orally, initially 100mg bd, titrate to maximum 2.4g/day in divided doses; IV bolus, 10–20mg over 1min, repeated every 5min to maximum dose of 200mg; IV infusion, 2mg/min, increased as needed. Dose range 50–160mg/h.

Carvedilol is a non-selective β-blocker with α_1 antagonistic actions that cause vasodilatation. It is used in the treatment of hypertension and in congestive cardiac failure.

Centrally acting vasodilators

Clonidine is a centrally acting partial α_2 agonist. There is a risk of rebound hypertension if stopped suddenly.

Onset of action is 30–60min, peak action at 2–4h, and half-life is 8–12h. 50% is excreted renally unchanged.

- Indication: post-operative blood pressure control.
- Contraindication: (relative) depression.
- Dose: orally, 50–100mcg tds, increased to maximum 1.2mg/day; IV bolus, 10mcg repeated until desired effect; IV infusion, 0.5–1.0mcg/kg/h.

Methyldopa, an analogue of L-dopa, causes decreased blood pressure by reduction in peripheral vascular resistance. It is hepatically metabolised and is renally excreted. Onset of action is 4–6h, half-life is 2h. Peak effect occurs at 3–6 h.

Side effects include sedation, lactation, extrapyramidal signs and neuropsychiatric sequelae. Coombs test may become positive; may cause problems with X-matching blood.

- Dose: orally, 250–300mg bd/tds, increase to maximum 3g/day.

Angiotensin inhibitors

Angiotensin-converting enzyme (ACE) inhibitors

ACE inhibitors act by binding irreversibly to the angiotensin I binding site in the lung and preventing conversion to angiotensin II. Peripheral vascular resistance is decreased; cardiac output and heart rate are unchanged.

ACE inhibitors are used post-MI for their ventricular remodelling properties, and have been shown to improve long-term survival.

Oral administration is usual, although enalaprilat is available as an IV agent for use in patients who are unable to take oral therapy.

ACE inhibitors are renally excreted. Half-life is dependent on the preparation.

- Indications: hypertension, post-MI, cardiac failure, ischaemic heart disease.
- Contraindications: hyperkalaemia, acute renal dysfunction, renovascular disease, pregnancy, hereditary angioedema.
- Dose: captopril 12.5–50mg 8 hourly. Onset of action 20–30min, duration of activity 4h. Peak effect 90min post-dose. May cause profound hypotension in critically ill; usual to start with test dose of 6.25mg.

Pulmonary vasodilators

In critically ill patients, pulmonary vasodilators are used to prevent and treat acute RV failure. In addition, inhaled pulmonary vasodilators are often used to improve oxygenation in patients with ARDS, although RCTs have not demonstrated improved survival.

Pulmonary hypertension in the critically ill

Vasodilators used in this setting include GTN, SNP, isoprenaline (Chapter 11.1), phentolamine, prostacyclin, and PDE inhibitors types 3 and 5 (see Chapter 11.2).

Vasodilators administered by inhalation are NO (Chapter 10.2) and iloprost.

Chronic pulmonary vasodilator therapy

Treatment options have expanded over the last few years and now include oral agents, inhaled and IV therapies.

- Prostanoids (epoprostenol (IV), iloprost (inhalation), treprostanil (SC), beraprost (oral)).
- Endothelin receptor antagonists (bosentan, ambrisentan, sitaxentan).

Further reading

Bersten AD, Soni N, eds., Oh's intensive care manual, 5th edition, Butterworth-Heinemann, 2003.

Galie N, Manes A, Branzi A. Prostanoids for pulmonary hypertension, *Am J Respir Med* 2003; 2: 123–37.

Joint Formulary Committee. British National Formulary. 53rd edn. London: British Medical Association and Royal Pharmaceutical Society of Great Britain, 2007.

Katzung BG. Basic and clinical pharmacology, 6th edn. Appleton & Lange, 1995.

LaRaia A, Waxman A. Pulmonary arterial hypertension: evaluation and management, *South Med J* 2007; 100: 393–9.

www.merck.com The Merck Manual, 18th edn. Merck & Co, 2006–2007.

Vasopressors

There are few good quality clinical trials to guide use in specific clinical situations.

Classes of vasopressors

1 α_1-Adrenergic receptor agonists: norepinephrine, metaraminol, phenylephrine and ephedrine. α_1 Agonists, used primarily for their inotropic action, including adrenaline and dopamine, are described in Chapter 11.1.
2 Vasopressin receptor agonists: vasopressin, terlipressin.
3 Nitric oxide synthase (NOS) inhibitors: L-NMMA, L-NAME. In a clinical RCT, L-NMMA was found to increase mortality
4 Guanylate cyclase inhibitors: methylene blue.

Corticosteroids may be used as an adjunct to vasopressors in septic shock, and are considered in Chapter 27.9.

Indications

1 Vasodilation, such as that caused by SIRS, spinal cord injury, vasodilator and sedative drugs.
2 Cardiogenic shock, to improve coronary perfusion pressure (second-line treatment after an intra-aortic balloon pump).
3 Maintenance of CPP in brain-injured patients with raised ICP.
4 Cardiopulmonary resuscitation.

Contraindications and cautions

1 Hypovolaemia, for which the primary treatment is fluid resuscitation, with or without a procedure to control haemorrhage. In reality, bolus doses of vasopressors may be required to defend blood pressure whilst resuscitation is taking place.
2 Low cardiac output states: studies of norepinephrine have demonstrated that cardiac output may increase by 10–20%. Phenylephrine has been shown to increase cardiac output in septic shock, and vasopressin either decreases or does not alter cardiac output.
    - A fall in cardiac output is less likely if the patient has been adequately fluid resuscitated.
    - Measurement of cardiac output and markers such as lactate, base deficit and mixed or central venous oxygen saturation may be invaluable in assessing the effect of vasopressors.
    - It may seem logical to titrate vasopressors to the systemic vascular resistance (SVR). However,it is preferable to titrate vasopressors to the MAP that is clinically relevant and measured directly.

Effects and sideeffects

Cardiovascular effects

- Increased systolic and diastolic blood pressure, LV stroke work, myocardial oxygen demand and coronary perfusion pressure. Epinephrine may increase MAP in patients who do not respond adequately to other vasopressors, due to its greater inotropic activity.
- Venoconstriction and increased preload.
- Pulmonary vascular resistance may increase (e.g. norepinephrine) or decrease (e.g. vasopressin).
- Coronary artery dilation (e.g. norepinephrine) or constriction (e.g. vasopressin).
- Tachycardia, particularly with drugs which have significant β_1 activity, e.g. epinephrine, dopamine, ephedrine. Reflex bradycardia may occur with vasopressors that have little or no chronotropic activity. Norepinephrine usually causes either no change or a small decrease in heart rate.
- All vasopressors are potentially arrhythmogenic (particularly epinephrine and dopamine) and may cause myocardial ischaemia.

Effects on the splanchnic circulation

- Norepinephrine usually has little effect on splanchnic blood flow, but a reduction in flow may occur, particularly if the patient is hypovolaemic. In combination with dobutamine, norepinephrine usually increases blood flow to the gut.
- Dopamine increases mesenteric blood flow.
- Epinephrine, phenylephrine and vasopressin all decrease splanchnic blood flow and may cause clinically important ischaemia, manifest as ileus, malabsorption, stress ulceration or bowel infarction.

Effects on renal function

- Norepinephrine increases urine output and creatinine clearance in patients with volume-resuscitated septic shock, used alone or when combined with dobutamine.
- Similar improvements have been noted with vasopressin and phenylephrine.

Effects on the skin

- Ischaemic extremities and skin lesions may occur with any vasopressor, but particularly with vasopressin.

Metabolic effects

- Adrenaline causes increased glucose production and suppression of insulin release, leading to hyperglycaemia. Hepatic clearance of lactate is impaired, and therefore lactate is a less useful marker of tissue perfusion.

Pharmacology of specific agents

α_1-Adrenoceptor agonists

α_1 Receptors are present throughout the peripheral arterial and venous systems. Stimulation of the receptor leads to G-protein-mediated activation of phospholipase C, and a cascade of intracellular signals leading to calcium-mediated vasoconstriction.

Norepinephrine is the amine neurotransmitter at post-ganglionic sympathetic nerve terminals, and is an agonist at all adrenergic receptors. However, when exogenous norepinephrine is administered as an IV infusion the α_1 effects predominate.

- Dose: 0.01–1.5 mcg/kg/min by IV infusion
- Half-life: 2min, leading to a steady-state plasma concentration within 10min of starting or changing a constant rate infusion.
- Metabolism: primarily in the liver, kidneys, brain and lungs by monoamine oxidase (MAO) and catechol-o-methyltransferase (COMT), to inactive metabolites.
- Interactions: effects may be exaggerated and prolonged in patients taking MAOIs, even though this interaction is associated more often with indirect acting sympathomimetics.

Metaraminol is a synthetic amine with both direct and indirect sympathomimetic actions. The direct action is mainly on α_1 receptors, although it has some β receptor activity. The indirect action involves stimulation of the release of norepinephrine from nerve terminals.

- Use: short-term treatment of hypotension, e.g. in the initial resuscitation of the shocked patient, at the start of haemofiltration, during anaesthesia for procedures on ITU.
- Dose: 0.2–1.0mg by IV bolus.

Phenylephrine is a direct acting synthetic sympathomimetic amine, with potent α_1 agonist activity and no β receptor activity.

- Dose: 50–100mcg by IV bolus, 0.5–8mcg/kg/min by IV infusion.
- Duration of action: 5–10min.
- Metabolism: in the liver by MAO.

Ephedrine has both direct and indirect sympathomimetic actions.

- Dose: 3–6mg by IV bolus.
- Duration of action: the elimination half-life is 4h. However, the duration of clinical activity is often just a few minutes. This may be due to tachyphylaxis, as norepinephrine stores in nerve terminals become depleted. For the same reason, repeated boluses may be ineffective after the first 12–15mg.
- Not metabolized by COMT or MAO. Some is metabolized in the liver, but 65% is excreted in the urine unchanged.

Vasopressin receptor agonists

Vasopressin is released from the posterior pituitary gland in response to increased plasma osmolality, decreased arterial blood pressure or decreased intravascular volume.

It acts on three subtypes of vasopressin receptor:

- V1 receptors mediate vasoconstriction, both directly and by increasing vascular responsiveness to catecholamines.
- V2 receptors are found in the renal collecting ducts. Stimulation leads to increased water reabsorption.
- V3 receptors are found mainly in the CNS system, where they modulate secretion of adrenocorticotrophic hormone (ACTH).

Arginine vasopressin (AVP) also known as antidiuretic hormone (ADH). It is an agonist at V1, V2 and V3 receptors.

- The plasma concentration of endogenous AVP usually increases in early septic shock. In more prolonged shock, a state of vasopressin deficiency develops. Infusion of vasopressin may allow reduction or withdrawal of other vasopressors. At doses >0.05U/min complications including cardiac arrest and regional ischaemia become more likely. These limit its use, and mean that it cannot generally be titrated as a sole vasopressor.
- Dose in septic shock: 0.01–0.04U/min by IV infusion.
- Dose in cardiac arrest: 40U IV bolus
- Half-life: 6min, duration of action 30–60min.
- Metabolism: primarily in the liver and kidneys

Terlipressin is a selective V1 receptor agonist. Terlipressin has a longer duration of action than vasopressin, and can therefore be give by IV bolus. It is primarily used to treat variceal bleeding in a dose of 2mg IV four times daily. In refractory septic shock, can be used when AVP not available.

- Dose in septic shock: initial bolus of 0.5mg, repeated every 30min to a maximum of 2mg. Then 0.5–1mg four times daily.
- Half-life: 6h, duration of action 2–10h.

Desmopressin is a synthetic selective V2 receptor agonist, used to treat neurogenic diabetes insipidus and bleeding disorders. It is not used as a vasopressor.

Guanylate cyclase inhibitors

Methylene blue inhibits the activity of NOS as well as guanylate cyclase.

In vasoplegic shock caused by cardiopulmonary bypass, one trial has shown a reduction in mortality and duration of shock with methylene blue compared to conventional vasopressors.

- Dose: an initial bolus of 1–2mg/kg over 15–30min then a continuous infusion of 0.25–1mg/kg/h for 3h to 3 days.

Use of vasopressors in specific situations

Septic shock

- Current guidelines recommend either dopamine or norepinephrine as the first-line vasopressor in septic shock. An observational study demonstrated increased mortality in patients treated with dopamine rather than other catecholamines.
- The target MAP of 65mm Hg may be adequate for most patients, depending on their pre-morbid blood pressure.
- A recent trial in patients with septic shock compared treatment with adrenaline vs the combination of norepinephrine and dobutamine. No significant difference was found in either mortality or serious adverse events.
- Phenylephrine by IV infusion may be useful when tachycardia limits treatment with norepinephrine, and adrenaline.
- Initial reports of the VASST study show no overall mortality benefit in patients with septic shock treated with vasopressin rather than norepinephrine alone.

Cardiac arrest

- Current international guidelines recommend epinephrine 1mg by IV bolus as the first-line vasopressor in cardiac arrest. Vasopressin may have a role in refractory ventricular fibrillation or out-of-hospital arrest in asystole.

Brain injury

- There are no good trials comparing different vasopressors for augmentation of CPP. However, it is common practice to use norepinephrine or dopamine to maintain a CPP of 60–70mm Hg.

Further reading

Annane D, Vignon P, Renault A, *et al.* Norepinephrine plus dobutamine versus epinephrine alone for management of septic shock : a randomised trial. *Lancet* 2007; 370: 676–84.

Beale RJ, Hollenberg SM, Vincent JL, *et al.* Vasopressor and inotropic support in septic shock: and evidence-based review. *Crit Care Med* 2004; 32: S455–65.

Faber P, Ronald A, Millar BW. Methylthioninium chloride: pharmacology and clinical applications with special emphasis on nitric oxide mediated vasodilatory shock during cardiopulmonary bypass. *Anaesthesia* 2005; 60: 575–87.

Hollenberg SM, Ahrens TS, Annane D, *et al.* Practice parameters for hemodynamic support of sepsis in adult patients. *Crit Care Med* 2004; 32: 1928–48.

LeDoux D, Astiz ME, Carpati CM, *et al.* Effects of perfusion pressure on tissue perfusion in septic shock. *Crit Care Med* 2000; 28: 2729–32.

Levin RL, Degrange MA, Bruno GF, *et al.* Methylene blue reduces mortality and morbidity in vasoplegic patients after cardiac surgery. *Ann Thoracic Surg* 2004; 77: 496–9.

Mullner M, Urbanek B, Havel C, *et al.* Vasopressors for shock. *Cochrane Database Syst Rev* 2004; (3): CD003709.

Russell JA. Vasopressin in septic shock. *Crit Care Med* 2007; 35: S609–15.

Sakr Y, Reinhart K, Vincent JL, *et al.* Does dopamine administration in shock influence outcome? Results of the sepsis occurrence in acutely ill patients (SOAP) study. *Crit Care Med* 2006; 43: 589–97.

Antiarrhythmic agents

Arrhythmias represent disturbances in normal sinus rhythm, occurring as a result of disordered impulse formation or conduction, or action potential disorders.

Arrhythmias are common in intensive care patientsm and have been shown to prolong ICU stay, with a trend towards increased mortality. Atrial arrhythmias, in particular AF, predominate in post-surgical patients especially following cardiac and thoracic surgery. In contrast, ventricular arrhythmias are more common in the mixed ICU patient population.

Antiarrhythmic agents are traditionally classified according to their primary electrophysiological effect in the Vaughn Williams classification (Table 11.5.1). Although many agents have multiple modes of action and do not fit easily into any one class, other classification systems have proved complex and are not routinely used. Other commonly used drugs such as adenosine and digoxin are not included in this classification.

Table 11.5.1 Vaughn Williams classification

Class	Action	Drugs
Class I	Na channel blockers	
Ia	ADP prolonged	Procainamide
Ib	ADP shortened	Lignocaine
Ic	ADP unchanged	Flecanide
		Propafenone
Class II	β-Blockers	Esmolol
		Metoprolol
Class III	K channel blockers	Amiodorone
		Sotalol
Class IV	Ca channel blockers	Verapamil
		Diltiazem

Clinical classification

It is more useful clinically to divide antiarrhythmic agents according to their use in the treatment of tachyarrhythmias.

- Supraventricular tachycardias (SVTs)
  - Verapmil
  - Adenosine
  - β-Blockers
  - Digoxin
- Ventricular tachycardias (VTs)
  - Lignocaine
- Both SVTs and VTs
  - Amiodorone
  - Procainamide
  - Sotalol
  - Flecanide

It is important to note that most have a narrow therapeutic index and all are potentially proarrhythmic. In the majority of patients with haemodynamic instability secondary to an arrhythmia, the initial treatment of choice will be direct current cardioversion (DCCV). Exceptions to this include treatment of torsade de pointes and arrhythmias secondary to drug toxicity, in particular digoxin toxicity.

Commonly used antiarrhythmic agents

Verapamil

Competitive calcium channel blocker (class IV antiarrhythmic agent).

Use: treatment of SVT, AF and atrial flutter.

Dose: initially 5–10mg IV over 2–3 min. A further 5mg every 20min if no response (maximum 20mg). Orally 40–120mg tds.

As effective as adenosine in terminating SVT, but potential for hypotension as has significant negative inotropic effects. Use with caution in patients with poor ventricular function. Avoid IV use if recently treated with β-blockers as may result in severe hypotension and asystole. Avoid in Wolff–Parkinson-White as VT or VF may be precipitated.

Adenosine

Endogenous nucleoside with rapid onset and ultrashort duration of action. Termination of SVT mediated via α_1 receptors, depressing SA and AV nodal activity.

Use: diagnosis and treatment of cardiovascularly stable SVT.

Dose: initial 3mg followed by further 6mg then 12mg after 1–2min if not effective. Administer as a fast IV bolus.

As effective as verapamil in terminating SVT, but associated with increased incidence of minor side effects including dyspnoea, chest discomfort and facial flushing.

Digoxin

A cardiac glycoside with multiple mechanisms of action including inhibition of Na-K-ATPase (which results in slowed AV node and pacemaker cell conduction) and increased efferent vagal activity.

Use: rate control in AF and atrial flutter if monotherapy with a β-blocker or calcium channel blocker unsuccessful.

Dose: 10–15mcg/kg (usually 500mcg) IV over 30min 6 hourly until effective (max 20mcg/kg).

Digoxin has a narrow therapeutic range, and side effects are common, exacerbated by hypokalaemia and hypomagnesaemia. Toxicity may precipitate any form of arrhythmia, most commonly junctional bradycardia, bigeminy and heart block. Treatment of arrhythmias resulting from toxicity includes correction of electrolyte imbalance and digoxin antibodies. Temporary pacing may be required. The use of DCCV remains controversial as severe ventricular arrhythmias may be precipitated.

Digoxin is no longer indicated as montherapy for rate control in AF and has no role in AF prophylaxis for cardiac surgery or in the treatment of post-operative AF.

β-Blockers

A group of drugs which act by the reversible blockade of β_1 cardiac adrenoreceptors (class II).

β-Blockers are used for rate control in acute SVT including AF and atrial flutter. Longer acting β-blockers are the treatment of choice for rhythm control in persistent AF and rate control in permanent AF and symptomatic paroxysmal AF. β-Blockers are also indicated for AF prophylaxis post-cardiac surgery.

Esmolol

Use: rate control in acute SVT in theatre and on ICU.

Dose: 0.25mg/kg IV bolus or 50–150mcg/kg/min infusion.

Esmolol has a rapid onset (<2min) and offset (<20min) of action and is available for IV use only. Hypotension and bradycardia may occur, but side effects are limited due to the short duration of action.

Amiodorone

A broad-spectrum class III antiarrhythmic agent that also demonstrates class I, II and IV activity.

Use: multiple uses in almost all arrhythmias, especially when other antiarrhythmics have proved ineffective or are contraindicated. It can be used for rate control or cardioversion in AF and atrial flutter, as AF prophylaxis post-cardiac surgery, in haemodynamically stable VT and SVT, and in cardiac arrest with persistent VT or VF. It should be used as first-line treatment for pharmacological cardioversion in persistent AF with structural heart disease and for non-life-threatening cardiovascularly unstable AF if delay in DCCV.

Dose: initially IV 5mg/kg (300mg) over 30–60min followed by 15mg/kg over 23h (maximum 1.2g in 24h). Dilute in dextrose 5%. Further maintenance is usually by oral route. Following cardiac arrest 300mg IV.

Although bradycardia and hypotension can occur after bolus injection, amiodorone tends to be a cardiovascularly stable drug with low proarrhythmic potential.

Hypothyroidism and thyrotoxicosis are common side effects and can present within 48h of treatment. Thyrotoxicosis can be refractory to treatment, with amiodorone therapy needing to be withdrawn to gain control. Several patterns of amiodorone-induced pulmonary toxicity have been reported. Of particular concern in ICU patients is a reported incidence of ARDS in 10–50% of patients treated with amiodorone.

Procainamide

A class Ia antiarrythmic agent.

Use: first-line treatment of sustained monomorphic VT in stable patients. Also used for repetitive zoomorphic VT. It can also be used in the treatment of SVT.

Dose: 100mg by slow IV infusion not exceeding 50mg/min. Repeated every 5min up to a maximum of 1g. Can be given orally, 50mg/kg daily in divided doses.

The use of procainamide has been limited by a number of cardiac and non-cardiac side effects. Rapid administration may result in hypotension, reduced cardiac output, prolongation of the Q-T interval and torsades de pointes. Chronic use may cause a lupus-like syndrome in up to 20% of patients.

Sotalol

A β-blocker classified as a class III antiarrhythmic agent possessing additional class I activity.

Use: has been used to treat both ventricular and supraventricular arrhythmias, although recently limited to treatment of ventricular arrhythmias. May be useful in repetitive polymorphic VT. Recommended for the prevention of postoperative AF in cardiac surgery.

Dose: 1–1.5mg/kg over 20min IV infusion. Orally 80–160mg bd. Not commonly used as an acute treatment given need for slow IV infusion administration.

There is a small risk of precipitating torsades de pointes especially with hypokalaemia. Bradycardia and hypotension may be a problem in patients with poor LV function.

Lignocaine

A class Ib antiarrhythmic agent.

Use: essentially limited to patients with sustained polymorphic VT associated with myocardial ischaemia unresponsive to procainamide or amiodorne.

Dose: initial bolus of 1mg/kg IV followed by an infusion.

Lignocaine is no longer recommended in the ALS algorithm for the treatment of ventricular tachyarrhythmias.

Magnesium

Although not classed as an antiarrhythmic agent, magnesium is often used in the treatment of ventricular arrhythmias.

Use: drug of choice in the treatment of torsade de pointes. Also used for polymorphic VT, particularly in the setting of acute MI and in digoxin overdose. May be used as an adjunct for rate control in AF.

Dose: 5–10mmol over 10–15min IV.

Key points

- DCCV is the treatment of choice in patients with haemodynamic instability secondary to a tachyarrhythmia.
- Correct underlying electrolyte imbalances.
- All antiarrhythmic drugs are potentially proarrhythmic.

Further reading

Blomström-Lundqvist C, Scheinman MM, Aliot EM, *et al.* ACC/AHA/ESC guidelines for the management of patients with supraventircular arrhythmias executive summary: a report of the American College of Cardiology/American Heart Association Task Force on Practice Guidelines, and the European Society of Cardiology Committee for Practice Guidelines (Writing Committee to Develop Guidelines for the Management of Patients with Supraventricular Arrhythmias). *J Am Coll Cardiol* 2003; 42: 1493–531.

Holdgate A, Foo A. Adenosine versus intravenous calcium channel antagonists for the treatment of supraventricular tachycardia in adults. *Cochrane Database Syst Rev* 2006; (4): CD005154.

National Clinical Guideline for the Management of Atrial Fibrillation. NICE Guideline 36. 2006.

Reinelt P, Karth GD, Gepert A, *et al.* Incidence and type of cardiac arrhythmias in critically ill patients: a single centre experience in a medical–cardiological ICU. *Intensive Care Med* 2001; 27: 1466–73.

Zipes DP, Camm AJ, Borggrefe M, *et al.* ACC/AHA/ESC 2006 guidelines for management of patients with ventricular arrhythmias and the prevention of sudden cardiac death executive summary: a report of the American College of Cardiology/American Heart Association Task Force on Practice Guidelines, and the European Society of Cardiology Committee for Practice Guidelines (Writing Committee to Develop Guidelines for the Management of Patients With Ventricular Arrhythmias and the Prevention of Sudden Cardiac Death). *J Am Coll Cardiol* 2006; 48: 1064–108.

Chronotropes

Chronotropes (from the Greek khronos, meaning time) are drugs that alter the heart rate.

Positive chronotropes:

1 β_1 agonists: isoprenaline, dobutamine, adrenaline.
2 Antimuscarinic agents: atropine, glycopyrrolate.
3 Glucagon
4 Triiodothyronine(T_3)

Negative chronotropes:

1 β_1 antagonists: propranolol, esmolol, metoprolol
2 Calcium channel antagonists: verapamil, diltiazem.
3 Digoxin
4 Amiodarone
5 Magnesium (high dose IV)

Isoprenaline

Isoprenaline is a synthetic catecholamine and acts as a β_1 and β_2 agonist. There are no α effects. Because of this, it increases heart rate, contractility and cardiac output. Systemic and pulmonary vascular resistance is decreased.

Half-life: 2min.

Pharmacokinetics: 60% is excreted unchanged and the remaining is conjugated in the liver or metabolized by MAO and COMT.

Dose: IV 0.02–0.5mcg/kg/min. It can be administered safely through a peripheral line.

Indications

1 Bradycardia unresponsive to atropine, when electrical pacing is not available.
2 Use as a temporary therapy in AV block either to reduce the block or to increase rate of idioventricular foci.

Contraindications

1 Do not use in resuscitation of asystole because isoprenaline-induced vasodilatation results in reduced carotid and coronary blood flow.

Adverse effects

1 Hypotension
2 Proarrhythmogenic
3 Coronary steal
4 Tachycardia
5 May unmask pre-excitation in patients with an accessory conduction pathway.

Dobutamine

Dobutamine is a synthetic catecholamine distributed as a racemic mixture. Dobutamine is a direct β_1 agonist, with limited β_2 and α effects, and has no $\alpha 2$ or dopaminergic activity. It increases the heart rate, contractility, cardiac output and decreases both SVR and pulmonary vascular resistance (PVR). The blood pressure either increases or remains unchanged.

Half-life: 2min.

Pharmacokinetics: It is metabolized by COMT and conjugation in the liver. It produces an active metabolite.

Dose: 2–20mcg/kg/min. It is supplied in 20ml vials containing 250mg. It is diluted at least up to 50ml in 5% dextrose before infusion.

Adrenaline

Adrenaline is a natural catecholamine produced by the adrenal medulla. It is direct agonist at α_1-, α_2-, $\beta_1$and β_2-adrenergic receptors. At doses <0.03mcg/kg/min β receptors are preferentially activated. At higher doses, even α receptors are activated. Heart rate and contractility are increased at all doses. At low doses, SVR decreases, but increases at higher doses due to α-mediated vasoconstriction.

Pharmacokinetics: rapidly taken up by neurons and tissues, and metaboliaed by MAO and COMT.

Administration: IV, SC, via ETT and IM.

Dose: 0.5–1.0mg bolus for resuscitation. 0.02–0.2mcg/kg/min for both inotropic and chronotropic effects.

Availability: epinephrine is available in vials at concentrations of 1:1000 and 1:10 000m and pre-filled syringes at a concentration of 1:10 000. A 1:100 000 concentration is available for paediatric use.

Atropine

Atropine is a tertiary amine consisting of tropic acid and tropine. The levorotatory form is active, but is commercially available as the racemic mixture. It antagonizes acetylcholine at muscarinic receptors, resulting in vagolysis and tachycardia. Atropine is included in the bradyarrhythmia and asystole resuscitation algorithms.

Dose: IV bolus of 0.4–1.0 mg in adults up to 3mg. In children, use 20mcg/kg (minimum 0.1mg and maximum 0.4mg, may be repeated).

Pharmacokinetics: the heart rate effects are seen within seconds of IV administration and last up to 15–30min. If given IM, PO or SC, offset occurs in ~4h. The drug is minimally metabolized and undergoes renal elimination.

Adverse effects

1 Tachycardia
2 Bradycardia at low doses
3 Sedation
4 Central anticholinergic syndrome at higher doses
5 Urinary retention
6 Increases intraocular pressure in narrow-angle glaucoma.

Glycopyrrolate

Glycopyrrolate is a synthetic quaternary amine containing mandelic acid. It does not cross the blood–brain barrier and is devoid of central effects. It causes less tachycardia when compared with atropine. Its use is in mild bradycardia and to counter muscarinic effects of neostigmine. Atropine remains the drug of choice in life-threatening bradyarrhythmias.

Dose: IV bolus of 0.1–0.2mg repeated every 2–3min. Use 5–10mcg/kg in children.

Glucagon

Glucagon is a peptide hormone produced by the α cells of the pancreas. It increases intracellular cAMP, acting via a specific receptor. It increases heart rate, contractility, atrioventricular conduction and cardiac output. This effect is seen even in the presence of β-blockade.

Pharmacokinetics: termination of action is by redistribution and proteolysis in liver, kidney and plasma. Duration of action is 20–30min.

Dose: 1–5 mg IV slowly; 0.5–2.0 mg IM/SC. It is infused at 25–75mcg/min.

Adverse effects

1 Hyperglycaemia
2 Hypokalaemia
3 Nausea and vomiting
4 Tachycardia
5 Allergic reactions.

Triiodothyronine (T_3)

T_3 and thyroxine are thyroid hormones, of which T_3 is the active form. It enters the cell and acts via receptors on the nucleus and mitochondria. It stimulates gene transcription and accelerates oxidative phosphorylation. T_3 increases heart rate and contractility.

Dose: IV 0.4mcg/kg as bolus followed by 0.4mcg/kg infused over 6h.

It is rarely used to increase the heart rate alone. It may be of use post-bypass when conventional therapies have failed, but is not recommended routinely. One has to be careful not to induce cardiac ischaemia.

Esmolol

Esmolol is an ultrashort-acting selective β_1 antagonist that reduces heart rate. It is used to prevent tachycardia and hypertension in response to laryngoscopy, intubation and other perioperative stimuli.

Dose: 0.25–0.5mg/kg boluses followed by an infusion of 50–200mcg/kg/min. Transient hypotension can occur during loading dose. It is available in 10ml (10mg/ml) vials for bolus administration and in ampoules containing 2.5g in 10ml for continuous infusion.

Pharmacokinetics: it is rapidly eliminated by red cell esterases. Its distribution half-life is 2min and its elimination half-life is 9min. The side effects are therefore quickly reversible.

Contraindications

1 Sinus bradycardia
2 Heart block
3 Cardiogenic shock
4 Overt heart failure
5 Asthma.

Propanolol

Propranolol is a non-selective β_1 and β_2 antagonist. It decreases the heart rate, reduces myocardial contractility and suppresses renin release. Cardiac output and myocardial oxygen demand are reduced.

Pharmacokinetics: it is highly lipid soluble and crosses the blood–brain barrier. It has a greater volume of distribution, and half-life is ~4–6h. It is metabolized in the liver.

Dose: administration of propranolol is titrated to desired effect, beginning with 0.5mg and progressing by 0.5mg increments every 3–5min. It is administered at the rate of 1mg/min. Total dose is <10 mg. It is supplied as 1mg/ml ampoule.

Adverse effects

1 Marked bradycardia
2 Bronchospasm
3 Congestive heart failure
4 Atrioventricular heart block
5 Withdrawal syndrome following discontinuation.
6 Raynaud's phenomenon.

Metoprolol

Metoprolol is a selective β_1 antagonist. Mechanism of action and effects are similar to propranolol.

Dose: by IV injection, up to 5mg at rate of 1–2mg/min, repeated after 5min if necessary, up to a total dose of 10–15mg.

Verapamil

Verapamil is a calcium channel antagonist belonging to the phenylalkylamine group. It preferentially binds to L-type calcium channels in its depolarized inactivated state (use-dependent blockade). These channels are present in both the myocardial and vascular smooth muscle cells. Verapamil causes vasodilatation, reduces the heart rate andcontractility, and may cause hypotension.

Pharmacokinetics: elimination occurs by hepatic metabolism and the plasma half-life is 3–10h.

Dose: IV loading dose of 5–10mg. Dose may be repeated after 30min. Maintenance: 5–15mg/h. PO: 40–80 mg 3–4 times a day. Paediatric doses: 75–200mcg/kg IV.

Adverse effects

1 Hypotension
2 Severe bradycardia especially in combination with β-blockers
3 Reduces digoxin elimination and can precipitate digoxin toxicity.

Diltiazem

Diltiazem is a calcium channel antagonist belonging to the benzothiazepine group. It blocks the L-type calcium channels similar to verapamil, but to a lesser extent. It reduces SVR, reduces the heart rate and contractility, but to a lesser extent than verapamil. It is thus less likely to compromise the cardiac output.

Pharmacokinetics: eliminated by both hepatic metabolism (60%) and renal excretion (35%). Plasma elimination half-life is 3–5h. The active metabolite is desacetyldiltiazem.

Dose: IV loading dose of 20mg over 2min. It may be repeated after 15min. Maintenance dose of 5–15mg/h infusion, depending on heart rate control. PO: 120–360mg/day.

Adverse effects

1 Hypotension
2 Bradycardia
3 Used with caution in combination with β-blockers and digoxin.

Magnesium

Magnesium is the second most abundant intracellular cation. It stabilizes the excitable cell membrane.

Dose: 5ml of 50% over 30min. May be repeated.

Caution

1 Monitoring of serum magnesium levels is required.
2 It should be avoided in patients with renal insufficiency.
3 May cause AV nodal blockade.

Digoxin

Digoxin is a cardiac glycoside, $C_{41}H_{64}O_{14}$, derived from leaves of the foxglove plant. It increases the force of contraction

Chamber paced	Chamber sensed	Response	Rate response	Antitachycardia
O-none	O-none	O-none	O-none	O-none
A-atrium	A-atrium	I-inhibit	R-adapt	P-ATP
V-ventricle	V-ventricle	T-triggered		S-shock
D-dual	D-dual	D-dual		D-dual
S-single	S-single			

due to increases in intracellular calcium concentration resulting from inhibition of Na^+/K^+ ATPase. It has vagotonic action on the AV node, so it is useful for rate control in SVT.

Dose: IV loading of 0.25–0.5mg increments up to 1.0mg. Maintenance of 0.125–0.250mg/day.

Onset: gradual onset over 15–30min. Peak effect occurs 1–5h after IV administration.

Offset: it has a long half-life of 1.7 days. The main route of elimination is through the kidneys.

Disadvantages

1 Long half-life
2 Low therapeutic index.
3 Interindividual variations in therapeutic and toxic serum levels and dosages.

Adverse effects

1 Can precipitate any arrhythmia.
2 Loss of appetite, nausea, vomiting and diarrhoea
3 Blurred vision, visual disturbances, confusion, drowsiness, dizziness, nightmares, agitation and/or depression
4 Acute psychosis, delirium, amnesia.

Amiodarone

Amiodarone is a class III antiarrhythmic agent. It blocks potassium channels, and is an α and β receptor non-competitive antagonist.

Pharmacokinetics: has very high lipid solubility resulting in marked tissue accumulation. It is metabolized hepatically and the elimination half-life is 20–100 days.

Dose: loading dose of 300mg (5mg/kg) over 30–60min. Maintenance: 900mg (15mg/kg) over 23h.

Adverse effects

1 Haemodynamic instability due to myocardial depression and α blockade.
2 Prolongation of QT interval
3 Multiple drug interactions
4 Long-term: hypo/hyperthyroidism, corneal deposits, hepatitis, pulmonary fibrosis and photosensitivity.

Electrical methods

Electrical pacing of the heart is a reliable method of rate support.

Pacing can be either temporary or permanent.

Advantages

1 Immediate effect
2 Reliable
3 Ability to synchronize atrial and biventricular contractions
4 Reduced risk of untoward effects and proarrhythmia
5 Ability to incorporate cardiovertor-defibrillator.

Pacemakers are coded using five letters and used as shorthand to designate pacing modes.

Indications for temporary cardiac pacing:

1 Sinus bradycardia/escape rhythm causing haemodynamic compromise
2 Bridge to permanent pacing
3 Following cardiopulmonary bypass
4 During AMI: asystole, AV block
5. Bradycardia dependent tachyarrhythmias

Indications for permanent pacing:

1 AV heart block—type II second degree or third degree block
2 Bifascicular/trifascicular block
3 Sinus node dysfunction
4 Hypersensitive carotid sinus syndrome
5 Bradyarrhythmias following heart transplant
6 Prophylaxis for tachyarrhythmias—with β-blockers—paroxysmal SVT, paroxysmal AF and long QT syndrome.

Adaptive rate pacing is used in patients with chronotropic incompetence. The heart rate is increased according to the physiological need. This need is detected by various methods:

- activity-based sensors
- QT-based sensors
- minute ventilation sensors

Overdrive pacing and cardioversion–defibrillation are methods used to stop tachyarrhythmias. Modern pacemakers can be incorporated with an ICD (internal cardiovertor–defibrillator).

Further reading

Ali-Melkkila T, Kaila T, Antila K, *et al.* Effects of glycopyrrolate and atropine on heart rate variability. *Acta Anaesthesiol Scand* 1991; 35: 436–41.

Carruthers SG, McCall B, Cordell BA, *et al.* Relationships between heart rate and PR interval during physiological and pharmacological interventions. *Br J Clin Pharmacol* 1987; 23: 259–65.

Clemo HF, Wood MA, Gilligan DM, *et al.* Intravenous amiodarone for acute heart rate control in the critically ill patients with atrial tachyarrhythmias. *Am J Cardiol* 1998; 81: 594–8.

Gray RJ, Bateman TM, Czer LS, *et al.* Esmolol: a new ultrashort-acting beta-adrenergic blocking agent for rapid control of heart rate in postoperative supraventricular tachyarrhythmias. *J Am Coll Cardiol* 1985; 5: 1451–6.

Hays JV, Gilman JK, Rubal BJ. Effect of magnesium sulphate on ventricular rate control in atrial fibrillation. *Ann Emerg Med* 1994; 24: 61–4.

Joradaens L, Trouerbach J, Calle P, *et al.* Conversion of atrial fibrillation to sinus rhythm and rate control by digoxin in comparison to placebo. *Eur Heart J* 1997; 18: 643–8.

Miller MR, Kim N, Goodman SN, *et al.* The evidence regarding the drugs used for ventricular rate control. *J Fam Pract* 2000; 49: 47–59.

Resuscitation Council UK. Advanced life support provider manual, 5th edn. Resuscitation Council UK.

Antianginal agents

Antianginal agents are of key importance to the critical care physician. Patients may develop ischaemia and require treatment while under our care and, with increasing numbers of patients with significant co-morbidities, many patients are taking these agents when they become sick and require intensive care

Pathophysiology

Unstable angina or acute coronary syndrome and stable angina have different pathophysiology and treatment. The best way to prevent angina in a critically ill patient with stable angina is to ensure they are well oxygenated, that their blood pressure (especially the diastolic and therefore coronary perfusion) is well maintained and that tachycardia is prevented. Antianginal agents should be used with great caution in patients who are unstable as you will block many of the receptors you might well be trying to stimulate in a few hours time to maintain that blood pressure.

β-Blockers

These are first-line antianginal agents in stable patients. Think about this as you pile in adrenergic drugs to a patient with a past history of angina. They have negative inotropic and negative chronotropic actions and limit myocardial oxygen demand. They are also effective antihypertensives. These combined actions reduce LV wall tension and thus further improve blood supply and oxygen delivery to the myocardium. By preferentially prolonging diastole they further increase coronary perfusion. They have been extensively investigated for pre-optimization of high risk surgical patients and are recommended by the American Heart Association for continuation in patients already taking these drugs and for initiation in high risk (and possibly intermediate risk) patients undergoing vascular and high risk surgery.

Other beneficial actions

β-Blockers inhibit platelet aggregation, reduce the risk of ventricular arrhythmias in acute ischaemia, slow conduction and have actions on cardiac remodelling that make them beneficial in chronic heart failure.

Cardiac and circulatory adverse actions

Heart failure: due to inhibition of the sympathetic drive, β-blockers carry the risk of worsening LV dysfunction. In the setting of critical illness, this is a significant concern; it occurs in <6% of patients who are stable before initiation of β-blockade.

Cardiac conduction abnormalities: β-blockers should be avoided in patients with sick sinus syndrome, and there is a risk of precipitating heart block in those with conduction abnormalities. This can be exacerbated by drug interactions (e.g. calcium channel blockers, digoxin).

Peripheral vascular disease: symptomatic worsening has been observed in those with severe arterial disease, and most surgeons will prefer to stop them in the context of peripheral vascular surgery, however this is probably overstated and the evidence is poor.

Inhibition of coronary vasodilatation: is overcome by the beneficial effects of β-blockade on myocardial oxygen demand in stable patients. In the critically ill patient with acute circulatory insufficiency this may become clinically significant, especially as diastolic blood pressure falls. The relative potency of pressors at β_1 and β_2 receptors in increasing myocardial contractility without necessarily overcoming existing β-blockade of coronary vasodilatation to the same extent may worsen ischaemia.

Abrupt withdrawal can precipitate acute hypertensive crises, crescendo angina and heart failure. Beware the unexplained post-operative crisis following accidental omission!

Extracirculatory adverse actions

Bronchoconstriction is worsened by β-blockade, especially with non-selective agents, and high doses of selective agents.

Hyperkalaemia: catecholamines cause uptake of potassium into cells and β-blockers inhibit this, it is rarely of clinical relevance.

Hypoglycaemia is worsened and recovery slowed in those on β-blockers. The symptoms of hypoglycaemia, sweating, tachycardia, anxiety are masked by β-blockade. These effects are less or absent if cardioselective agents are used.

Pharmacokinetics and drug specifics

The intensivist must be aware of the metabolism and elimination of common drugs. **Atenolol** is excreted 50% in the faeces and 50% in the urine, mostly as unchanged drug; there is ~10% liver metabolism and the half-life is 6–9h in healthy individuals; accumulation in renal failure is common and presents frequently to acute medicine. **Metoprolol** (also bisoprolol, propranolol, oxprenolol) is extensively metabolized in the liver by the CYP2D6 enzyme complex. The half-life is bimodally distributed in the population and is either ~3h or 8h (hence some patients need tds administration and others bd). The hepatic metabolism makes this drug particularly useful in the recovering critical care patient. **Carvedilol** is hepatically metabolized, but one metabolite is 13 times more potent at β-blockade and is then excreted in the faeces. **Sotalol** is entirely excreted unchanged in the urine; this drug also has class III antiarrhythmic activity at higher doses (>80mg bd). **Labetalol** is hepatically metabolized, and also has α-blocking activity. **Esmolol** is degraded by red cell esterases, with a half-life of 9min; it is used for acute hypertension and supraventricular arrhythmias, and not for angina.

β-Blocker overdose

These patients will present with hypotension and bradycardia. The PR interval may be prolonged, and QRS complexes may be broadened. Hypoglycaemia and mild hyperkalaemia may be noted (if accumulation has resulted in renal failure this may be marked).

Treatment should be according to ABC principles (see Chapter 25.1); specific therapy includes **atropine** (0.5mg IV repeated every 5min to 3mg), **glucagon** 5mg IV bolus (increases intracellular cAMP and therefore calcium independently from β adrenoreceptors) repeated if no response after 5min and followed by infusion of 1–5mg/h. **Calcium** (10ml of 10% calcium chloride centrally or 30ml of 10% calcium gluconate peripherally). **Insulin and glucose** have also been used in β-blocker overdose titrating up to 50U in 50g glucose over 1h. **Catecholamines** will often be necessary, but may result in myocardial ischaemia for the reasons postulated above. **PDE inhibitors** are attractive as the increase in cAMP will be independent of β-blockade. Other therapies that can be added in desperation include sodium bicarbonate for arrhythmia, magnesium (especially if QT prolonged with sotalol), aminophylline, transvenous pacing, aortic balloon pump, haemodialysis, and even methylene blue to inhibit NO production and increase vascular tone.

Calcium channel blockers

These drugs are frequently used for angina and blood pressure control in patients who cannot tolerate β-blockade. There are two pharmacological (and functional) groups. The dihydropyridines (nifedipine, amlodipine, felodipine) reduce afterload and cause coronary vasodilatation, whereas the non-dihydropyridines (diltiazem, verapamil) are also rate controlling. Systematic analysis does not show any benefit for these drugs in preventing MI or mortality; therefore, β-blockers remain first line unless contraindicated. In the recovering critically ill, amlodipine has become commonly used as an antihypertensive due to its lack of effect on heart rate and conduction, and avoidance of β-blockade 'in case' the patient deteriorates and requires catecholamine support; there is, however, no evidence that this is any safer than cautious β-blockade with an appropriate agent.

Pharmacokinetics and drug specifics

Amlodipine is hepatically metabolized, has a peak effect at 6–12h and an elimination half-life of 30–50h if hepatic function is normal. **Diltiazem** has a half-life of 4h and is hepatically metabolized, but has active metabolites and these are partially excreted in the urine. **Nifedipine** is hepatically metabolized to inactive metabolites; the half-life is 2–5h, but slow release preparations are usually used and these must not be crushed for NG tube administration; its use is best avoided in critically ill patients. **Verapamil** is hepatically metabolized; its use in the critically ill is best avoided due to the risk of heart failure.

Calcium channel blocker overdose

These patients will be hypotensive and may or may not be bradycardic depending on the agent. An ABC approach plus specific therapy with **calcium** (10ml of 10% calcium chloride, repeated as necessary or followed by infusion at 0.5mEq calcium/kg/h). **Glucagon** can also be used (see above). **Vasopressors** (noradrenaline) may be necessary and also PDE inhibitors (only once pressors are initiated and can be titrated to counter hypotension). **Insulin** and glucose treatment has been used successfully (see above). Transvenous pacing and aortic balloon pump may be necessary.

Nitrates

These are used for their arterial and venous dilatation, reducing pre- and afterload and myocardial work. GTN infusion (50mg in 50ml titrated from to 15ml/h) provides rapid relief of unstable angina in in-patients. Rapid reversibility makes GTN especially useful in critically ill patients for angina and hypertensive crises. Prolonged administration (>24h) results in tolerance to the nitrate and reduced efficacy. Headache and tachycardia are common side effects, and nitrates should be avoided in those with RV infarction and HOCM. Prolonged administration of IV nitrates can result in methaemoglobinaemia and possibly resistance to heparin. Look for transdermal nitrate patches in hypotensive obtunded patients with a past history of ischaemic heart disease and remove (especially before defibrillation). Sublingual nitrates are normally avoided in critically ill patients due to the unpredictable degree of hypotension.

Other antianginal drugs

Opiates provide important symptomatic relief and should always be used to ameliorate the sympathetic drive in acute ischaemia. They do not provide outcome benefit.

Potassium channel sensitizers such as **nicorandil** have an arterial and venous vasodilatory action but may also have a role in ischaemic pre-conditioning and myocardial protection. Its use in the critically ill patient remains experimental.

Ranolazine is a fatty acid oxidase inhibitor which also prevents calcium overload in myocytes. Intensivists should be aware that it causes prolongation of the QT interval.

Ivabridine has a specific action on the sinus node pacemaker current, reducing heart rate. Its use in those intolerant of β-blockade is increasing.

Further reading

Fleisher LA, Beckman JA, Brown KA, *et al.* ACC/AHA 2006 Guideline update on perioperative cardiovascular evaluation for noncardiac surgery: focused update on perioperative beta-blocker therapy. Circulation 2006; 113: 2662–74. `http://circ.ahajournals.org/cgi/content/full/113/22/2662`

Held PH, Yusuf S, Furberg CD. Calcium channel blockers in acute myocardial infarction and unstable angina: an overview. *BMJ* 1989; 299: 1187–92.

Antiplatelet agents

Platelets interact with a range of clotting factors, endothelial surfaces and tissue components, as well as with each other to form a blood clot. Most of the time they are inactive awaiting stimulation, until there is vessel injury when they are appropriately activated to form a component of the blood clot plugging the gap. There are a variety of situations where there is inappropriate activation or where we do things to the patient that result in undesirable platelet activation. There are a series of drugs that can be used to prevent this.

Aspirin

Acts by irreversibly acetylating cyclo-oxygenase type 1 (COX-1) found in platelets. This is achieved at low doses (usually 75mg daily) and prevents COX-1 from producing prostaglandin H_2 which would otherwise be used in production of thromboxane A_2 which is stored in platelets and acts as a local amplifier of platelet activation.

Clinical use

Coronary disease: aspirin is used in stable coronary disease for primary and secondary prevention, and in unstable disease for treatment of MI.

The second international study on infarct survival (ISIS-2) demonstrated that 160mg aspirin daily reduced 5 week mortality by 23% in acute ST elevation myocardial infarction (STEMI). This was the same as the reduction achieved by streptokinase (25%) and, used together, an odds reduction of 42% is achieved (from 13.2 to 8.0% mortality). Aspirin is an important therapy!

GI bleeding: a past history of GI bleeding should not prevent the administration of aspirin acutely in STEMI.

Cerebrovascular disease: aspirin is also used for secondary prevention of cerebrovascular disease, giving ~22% odds reduction (from 21.4 to 17.8% in a pooled analysis of 21 trials).

Issues in intensive care

GI bleeding is a major side effect of aspirin. This risk should be put in perspective. In a meta-analysis of 22 randomized trials of aspirin therapy, the increased risk of major bleeding from aspirin was 70%, but this translates to an absolute annual increase of only 0.13% in stable patients (769 patients need to be treated with aspirin to cause one major bleed). Clearly these absolute risks will be greater in the intensive care population.

Bronchospasm is seen in up to 10% of new users.

Perioperative: in general, aspirin should not be suspended for operations, as this significantly increases the risk of perioperative coronary events, unless bleeding would be catastrophic, e.g. intracranial surgery.

Reversal of aspirin: requires platelet transfusion.

Dipyridamole

Inhibits adenosine deaminase and phosphodiesterase (PDE), resulting in accumulation of adenosine and cAMP. It is used as a second-line agent in stroke prevention in conjunction with aspirin or in those intolerant of aspirin. It is also used in cardiac stress testing due to its vasodilatory action. There are few reports of overdose, but hypotension and MI are reported. Dipyridamole has a half-life of 10h; more rapid reversal requires platelet transfusion.

Clopidogrel

Clopidogrel and ticlopidine are thienopyridines that block binding of ADP to the type II low affinity purine receptor (P2Y12) on the platelet surface and interrupt platelet activation. Ticlopidine has a higher incidence of adverse effects (neutropenia and thrombotic thrombocytopenic syndrome) than clopidogrel and consequently is less commonly used.

Clinical use

Acute coronary syndrome

Clopidogrel is a key drug in the management of unstable angina and non-ST elevation MI (NSTEMI), and studies have demonstrated a reduction in vascular events when clopidogrel is added to aspirin therapy for up to 12 months (MI reduced from 6.7 to 5.2% in the CURE study at 1yr). There is an increase in bleeding, and individual patient risks should be considered when starting this treatment (major bleeding increased from 2.7 to 3.7% in CURE). Clopidogrel is frequently used as first-line therapy in patients intolerant of or allergic to aspirin.

Post-coronary stenting

Clopidogrel reduced the relative risk of in-stent thrombosis by 26.9% at 1yr (absolute reduction of 3%) following percutaneous coronary intervention (PCI) in the CREDO study (the control group was given clopidogrel for 3 months post-PCI and both groups continued aspirin). Evidence suggests that pre-treatment with thienopyridines further reduces instent thrombosis provided the loading dose (300mg clopidogrel) is at least 6h before the procedure (it may be possible to improve the outcomes when loading in advance is impossible by giving a larger loading dose, 600mg).

Issues in intensive care

Cardiothoracics: there is evidence that clopidogrel therapy may significantly increase bleeding post-operatively, incidence of return to theatre and transfusion requirements in cardiothoracic surgery. If possible it should be suspended 5 days before bypass surgery. This effect is mitigated if clopidogrel is started at least 4h post-operatively in those with low drain outputs, where there may be an outcome benefit to starting clopidogrel. An assessment on an individual patient basis and their likelihood of having an unstable coronary event during drug suspension should be made.

Non-cardiac surgery and medical patients: there are very few data. Individual assessment of coronary risk vs bleeding risk should be made. If the patient has had coronary stent implantation within **1 month** (bare metal stents) or **3 months** (coated or drug-eluting stents) then only severe or life-threatening bleeding should prompt cessation of clopidogrel as the risk of stent occlusion is significant.

Perioperative: platelet transfusion should only be used in the context of overt haemorrhage and not pre-emptively even if a decision to stop clopidogrel is made pre-operatively (neurosurgery may be an exception).

There is only one reported case of clopidogrel overdose and that was without symptoms.

Reversal: requires platelet transfusion.

GpIIb/IIIa receptor antagonists

There are two classes of agent:

- Antibody to the receptor (abciximab, ReoPro®)
- Small molecule inhibitors (tirofiban, Aggrastat®; and eptifibatide, Integrilin®)

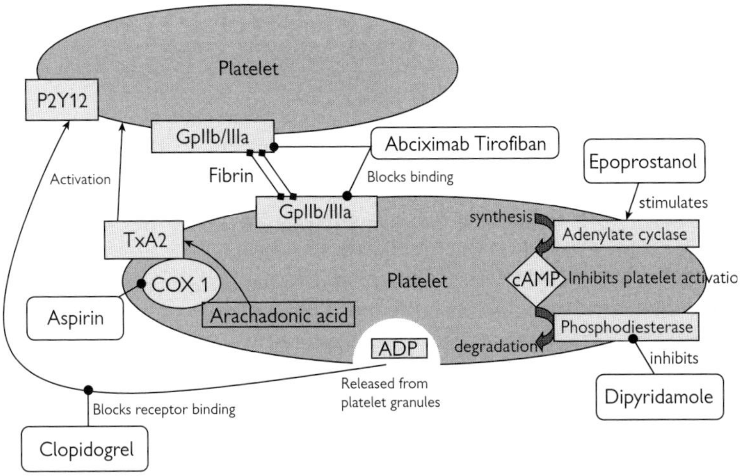

Fig. 11.8.1 Mechansim of action of antiplatelet drugs.

These agents act by blocking the GpIIb/IIIa receptor on the platelet surface. This receptor binds fibrin so is key to creating the meshwork of fibrin and activated platelets that forms the platelet plug of a clot.

Abciximab has complex pharmacokinetics, but the key point is that the molecule takes days to clear from the plasma completely, and clinically platelet function takes ~48h to recover from cessation of an infusion. Recovery of platelet function is much more rapid from the small molecule inhibitors (within a few hours).

Abciximab can cause a unique form of thrombocytopenia occurring between 30min and 24h of administration that results in a profound drop in platelets, believed to be due to the presence of 'pre-formed' antibodies to 'hidden' epitopes on platelets. Confusingly pseudothrombocytopenia can also be seen, but this recovers within 4h, and different platelet counts are seen with different anticoagulants in the sampling tube, e.g. EDTA vs citrate. Both these are much less common with tirofiban or eptifibatide.

Clinical use

STEMI: should not be used in STEMI, where primary therapy is thrombolysis, unless used prior to angiography and primary angioplasty ± stent. They are frequently used in the context of failed thrombolysis or re-infarction whilst awaiting transfer for rescue PCI.

NSTEMI: meta-analysis shows that if the serum troponin is elevated and if PCI is planned, there is mortality and MI benefit to using these drugs, and this benefit is still seen with concurrent clopidogrel therapy.

Bleeding risk: is elevated especially with concurrent use of other agents. All the GpIIb/IIIa inhibitors require dose adjustment in patients with renal failure, and use with caution in the elderly and with weight adjustment in smaller patients.

Reversal: platelet transfusion, but tirofiban and eptifibatide reverse within a few hours anyway.

Epoprostenol (prostacyclin, PGI_2, Flolan®)

This is used in intensive care as a method of anticoagulation for extracorporeal circuits. It acts by stimulating adenylate cyclase and increasing cAMP levels, which inhibits platelet activation. It is useful for its very rapid reversibility within a few minutes of stopping the infusion (half-life is 6min). Its use is limited by cost and profound vasodilatation (it is also used for pulmonary vasodilatation in idiopathic pulmonary hypertension).

Summary of indications

Aspirin

- Primary prevention in high risk patients (coronary and cerebrovascular)
- Secondary prevention all patients
- Pre- and post-coronary stenting

Dipyridamole

- Second-line therapy in cerebrovascular disease in combination with aspirin

Clopidogrel

- Second-line therapy in high risk coronary disease in combination with aspirin
- Pre- and post-coronary stenting
- Alternative to aspirin in those intolerant

GpIIb/IIIa inhibitors

- STEMI: failed thrombolysis pending rescue PCI or pending primary PCI
- NSTEMI: positive troponin, only if proceeding to PCI
- Caution in renal failure, elderly, small patients.

Further reading

Bosch X, Marrugat J. Platelet glycoprotein IIb/IIIa blockers for percutaneous coronary revascularization, and unstable angina and non-ST-segment elevation myocardial infarction. *Cochrane Database Syst Rev* 2001; (4): CD002130.

ISIS-2 Collaborative Group. Randomised trial of intravenous streptokinase, oral aspirin, both, or neither among 17,187 cases of suspected acute myocardial infarction: ISIS-2. Lancet 1988; 2: 349–60.

Yusuf S, Zhao F, Mehta SR, *et al.* Effects of clopidogrel in addition to aspirin in patients with acute coronary syndromes without ST-segment elevation. *N Engl J Med* 2001; 345: 494–502.

Diuretics and the critically ill

Introduction

Diuretics are frequently used in the critically ill, although the rationale for their use is not always logical.

The most common reasons are for reduction of tissue or pulmonary oedema, to promote urine output for oliguric states, to control ascites and occasionally to change blood acid–base balance to help weaning, such as with acetazolamide.

Tissue oedema, pulmonary oedema and ascites

- Tissue oedema is the accumulation of fluid in the interstitial space. It results in circulating hydrostatic forces overwhelming the protective safety factors described by Guyton. These relate lymphatic flow, interstitial oncotic pressure and capillary hydrostatic pressure assuming normal endothelial permeability in a given tissue. In health, tissues have remarkably different capillary permeabilities from each other. For example, brain has non-fenestrated capillaries while muscle, subcutaneous tissue, intestines, kidneys and liver are progressively more permeable. The variability between these components explains why it is considerably easier to develop skin oedema than pulmonary oedema for a given hypervolaemic state.
- In the critically ill, the tendency for greater capillary permeability with systemic inflammatory states exacerbates the tendency to oedema. Tissue and pulmonary leakiness result in oedema with modest capillary hydrostatic pressure rises.
- Pulmonary oedema may be hydrostatic, as it is with iatrogenic circulating hypervolaemia. This is more likely in those with unheralded cardiac dysfunction and uncommon in fluid-deficient septic or haemorrhagic patients. It also follows the hypervolaemic state associated with the hyperaldosteronism of cardiac dysfunction or the mechanical perturbation associated with valvular incompetence or pericardial constriction. Equally, a significant reduction in cardiac performance through abnormal rhythms or deteriorating contractility may acutely or insidiously precipitate pulmonary oedema through left atrial pressure rises.
- Ascites is a hallmark of patients with severe cirrhosis. Mechanical obstruction by slow portal vein flow or thrombosis results in peritoneal cavity fluid accumulation. This is the result of hepatic sinusoidal outflow obstruction due to fibrosis. Continuing fluid accumulation is halted by the dynamic balance between peritoneal hydrostatic pressure and the forces of transudation. Reduction of the former by aspiration leads to a rapid re-accumulation of ascites. Cirrhotics also retain sodium, which promotes ascites and peripheral oedema. Two theories for salt retention have been proposed although both result in increased aldosterone activity

1. Underfill theory which suggests that splanchnic pooling and peripheral vasodilatation reduce the effective intravascular volume and stimulate secondary sodium retention.
2. Overflow theory suggests primary sodium retention through intrahepatic hypertension and an ill-defined hepatorenal reflex. The latter stimulates renal sympathetics, which promote sodium retention.

The decompensated cirrhotic is characterized by vasodilatation, arteriovenous fistulae, and fluid and albumin loss through ascites, which all lead to reduced effective intravascular volume. The latter stimulates compensatory secondary sodium retention, oliguria and impaired water excretion.

Appropriateness of diuretics for oedema

- While diuretics may be an appropriate treatment for patients with hydrostatic pulmonary oedema due to circulating hypervolaemia, they are less appropriate for the hyperpermeable pulmonary congestion or oedema of inflammatory states.
- Where oedema is largely driven by sodium retention and hyperaldosteronism, diuretics are appropriate and of value, although control of the driving mechanism such as myocardial dysfunction is likely to be more successful for oedema control.
- Diuretic therapy for hyperpermeability, pulmonary oedema of chest infection or aspiration pneumonitis may modestly improve oxygenation particularly if there is alveolar rather than interstitial oedema; however, the improvement is short lived because defective permeability is not resolved. Large oxygenation improvement suggest a significant hydrostatic component
- Diuretic therapy to achieve negative balance may in hyperpermeability states result in circulating hypovolaemia, renal dysfunction, a fall in cardiac output and greater inotrope need, which are associated with poor outcomes. Paradoxically these patients may still continue to have peripheral oedema if the underlying inflammation persists.
- There is a common belief that peripheral oedema is a marker for pulmonary or internal organ oedema, and that 'dry' states improve tissue oxygenation. The improvement in survival rates associated with more aggressive resuscitation and fluid maintenance techniques suggests that the latter is a better overall haemodynamic package.
- In critical illness, increased capillary permeability is common. Oedema formation, particularly in subcutaneous and muscle tissue where the safety factors are not as well developed, is expected. Unresolved systemic inflammation will result in consecutive days of positive balances struggling to achieve an appropriate circulating volume to maintain multi-organ function in the face of permeability losses. The more rapidly the specific therapies of timely surgery or antibiotics are instituted to halt the inflammatory process, the less likely are oedema formation and multi-organ failure.
- It is notable that in the recovery phase of systemic inflammation, when permeability tends back to normal, spontaneous diuresis occurs without haemodynamic perturbations and indeed diuretics may be used to accelerate losses of excess total body saline with little further haemodynamic impact other than through unheralded rhythm changes consequent to large potassium and magnesium losses.

Indications for diuretic therapy

- Hydrostatic pulmonary oedema
- Congestive cardiac failure

- Hypertension
- Cerebral oedema
- Hyperaldosteronism-mediated oedema, nephrosis, cirrhosis, cor pulmonale
- Peripheral oedema to promote mobility
- Promote urine output for renal function
- Change arterial blood chemistry to aid weaning
- Help manage poor oxygenation in permeability pulmonary oedema

Commonly used diuretics in the critically ill

Thiazides

Bendrofluazide

This is a weak diuretic which produces a sustained daily diuresis by inhibiting sodium uptake in the cortical thick ascending limb of the loop of Henle and in early distal tubules. It has to gain tubular access by glomerular filtration to be active. It is used for long-term hypertension management and uncommonly used in the acute phase of critical illness.

Metolazone

Metolazone is a powerful thiazide given in doses 5–10mg twice daily, but only available in oral preparations. It can provide significant diuresis when loop diuretics are becoming ineffective. It can be used for resistant peripheral oedema, and in the critically ill can help provide a diuresis in those with non-oliguric chronic renal failure.

Loop diuretics

Frusemide

Frusemide is a powerful short-acting agent very commonly used either to improve pulmonary function consequent to cardiac failure or less effectively to 'dry out lungs' in those with pulmonary congestion or oedema related to systemic or localized pulmonary inflammation.

Frusemide is also use to accelerate oedema clearance in those in the recovery phase of critical illness. In addition, it is increasingly used as an infusion to drive a diuresis to maintain renal function. Infusions can be effective in low doses, starting in diuretic-naive kidneys from 1mg/h.

It acts by enzymatic inhibition of cortical and medullary thick ascending loop of Henle Na^+ K^+ $2Cl^-$ co-transporter. This tubular cell brush border-sited enzyme facilitates the movement of sodium into the tubular cell; sodium is then is pumped out of the cell into the interstitium by energy-dependent Na^+ K^+ ATPase. Consequently, frusemide reduces tubular energy requirements.

Like thiazides, frusemide increases delivery of sodium- and chloride-rich filtrate to distal tubular potassium and hydrogen ion-secreting sites. The diuretic-driven plasma volume contraction causes an increase in aldosterone secretion which promotes sodium exchange for K^+ and H^+ ions at these sites. The loss of chloride and the cation exchanges result in hypokalaemia and a mild metabolic alkalosis. Magnesium losses are also substantial.

A further consequence of large quantities of chloride and sodium reaching distal tubules is stimulation of the juxtaglomerular apparatus which results in renin- and adenosine-mediated afferent glomerular arteriolar vasoconstriction.

Aldosterone antagonists

Spironolactone

This is available only as an oral preparation; it is a competitive antagonist of aldosterone with a linear diuretic response in doses between 25 and 100mg. It has a long duration of action and its active elements are spironolactone and its metabolite canrenone. It is commonly combined with loop diuretics for its synergistic diuretic effect while sparing potassium losses. Its main use is to control hyperaldosteronism-driven oedematous states, typically cardiac, cirrhotic or nephrotic. It has been shown to reduce mortality associated with severe cardiac failure (EFs <35%)

Amiloride

Amiloride also acts at the collecting tubule, but prevents sodium uptake by the sodium pump and not by aldosterone inhibition.

Potassium canrenoate

Potassium canrenoate is an IV aldosterone antagonist. It is a prodrug metabolized to the active canrenone. It is given in an equivalent dose range to spironolactone. The above drugs alone are not very powerful, but with loop diuretics they minimise the tendency to hypokalaemia.

Carbonic anhydrase inhibitors

Acetazolamide

This is available as either IV or oral preparations. 250–500mg 6 hourly is a modestly effective diuretic. By inhibition of carbonic anhydrase in the proximal tubule it facilitates bicarbonate and sodium loss. The resulting high sodium tubular content leads to greater potassium–sodium exchanges in the distal collecting tubules and results in hypokalaemia.

Consequently acetazolamide is one of the few causes of hypokalaemic, hyperchloraemic metabolic acidosis.

Acetazolamide can be used to provide a mild hyperchloraemic metabolic acidosis to correct metabolic alkalosis which is impeding weaning. Typically patients receiving loop diuretics develop a mild metabolic alkalosis (chloride and K losses). They may also have a secondary metabolic alkalosis that accompanies hypercarbia of hypoventilation. Such patients have apneoic episodes during attempts at weaning if the pH > 7.45.

Impaired weaning can be managed with a few days course of acetazolamide until pH is mildly acidotic. It should be noted that CSF pH might take a further 48h to correct; therefore, apneoa episodes on a ventilator may continue. Potassium and magnesium losses will be large, and plasma concentrations should be kept at the high end of the normal range.

The diuretic effect of acetazolamide tends to tail off after a few days.

Osmotic diuretics

Mannitol

Mannitol is commonly used as pulse therapy to reduce cerebral oedema and improve ICP control. It does not cross the blood–brain barrier and provides an osmotic gradient for cerebral cellular and extracellular water movement to the vascular space. Theoretically it would be expected that mannitol is more effective for management of cytotoxic cerebral oedema (white and grey matter cellular swelling due to ischaemia) than vasogenic (capillary permeability, interstitial) oedema, which affects mainly white matter.

Mannitol promotes diuresis by gaining access to the renal tubule. It has a molecular weight of 182Da and is readily filtered. It inhibits sodium and water uptake in all parts of the tubule by it osmotic effect.

Hypovolaemia and renal impairment may follow continuous aggressive therapy (>6 pulses/day) in the absence of urine loss replenishment.

Further reading

Better OS, Schrier RW. Disturbed volume homeostasis in patients with cirrhosis of the liver. *Kidney Int* 1983; 23: 303–11.

Guyton A. Textbook of medical physiology, 8th edn. New York: Elsevier, 1991.

Kaufmann AM, Cardoso ER. Aggravation of vasogenic cerebral edema by multiple-dose mannitol. *J Neurosurg* 1992; 77: 584–9.

Pitt B, Zannad F, Remme WJ, *et al.* The effect of spironolactone on morbidity and mortality in patients with severe heart failure. Randomized Aldactone Evaluation Study Investigators. *N Engl J Med* 1999; 341: 709–17.

Rocco VK, Ware AJ. Cirrhotic ascites. Pathophysiology, diagnosis and management. *Ann Intern Med* 1986; 105: 572–85.

Levosimendan

The most studied calcium sensitizer, levosimendan, has recently been introduced in many countries for the treatment of acutely decompensated chronic heart failure (HF) and has both positive inotropic and vasodilatatory effects. It differs from classic inodilators because of its ability to improve myocardial efficiency, enhancing myofilament response to calcium (Ca^{2+}) and leading to increased myocardial contraction without increasing intracellular calcium concentration.

Levosimendan displays Ca^{2+} dependent binding to the N-terminal domain of cardiac troponin C with higher affinity at high Ca^{2+} concentration and lower affinity at low Ca^{2+} concentration. By stabilizing the Ca^{2+}-troponin C (TnC) complex, levosimendan inhibits troponin I (TnI) effect and prolongs the actin-myosin cross-bridge association rate. Thus, the positive inotropic effect is obtained without an increase of intracellular calcium concentration or a significant increase of myocardial oxygen demand, usually seen with other inotropes.

Levosimendan also increases cyclic Adenosine Monophosphate (cAMP) due to phosphodiesterase inhibition but the contribution of the cAMP system to its action appears to be rather small.

Levosimendan is associated with an increased rate of relaxation and reduced relaxation time, thus improving diastolic performance.

The beneficial effects of levosimendan are also related to its vasodilatatory effect mediated by a Potassium-ATP-channel opening effect in cardiac and smooth muscle cells in an ATP-dependent manner and levosimendan-induced decrease in right and left ventricular afterload seems to be beneficial in failing hearts.

Levosimendan improves coronary blood flow, decreases myocardial oxygen extraction, and improves ischaemic myocardium performance. This was first shown in animals and healthy humans, but was later shown in patients with congestive HF, acute myocardial infarction (AMI), after PCI of AMI patients with LV dysfunction and after coronary artery bypass grafting (CABG) where, despite improved cardiac performance, it did not increase myocardial oxygen consumption or change myocardial substrate utilization.

Levosimendan has a half-life of approximately 1.3 hours. The drug is metabolized by the liver and has two active metabolites, OR-1855 and OR-1896, with long half-lives (75-78 hours), that are excreted by the kidney and prolong the duration of the hemodynamic effects of their parent compound. This long half-life is markedly increased in patients with severe chronic renal failure or end-stage renal disease undergoing haemodialysis as compared with healthy subjects.

Clinical Studies

Several clinical trials have shown the beneficial effect of levosimendan on short-term hemodynamic and clinical signs in patients with AHF. Kivikko *et al* (**DATE**) reported a 30% increase in CO and a 50% decrease in PCWP after 24 hours infusion in class III-IV heart failure patients. The Levosimendan Infusion versus DObutamine (LIDO) study enrolled 203 patients with severe low-output heart failure and compared the effects of levosimendan with those of dobutamine in a double blind fashion over 24 hours. The primary end point of hemodynamic improvement (an increase of 30% or more in cardiac output, and a decrease of 25% or more in PCWP) was achieved by 28% of the levosimendan patients and 15% of the dobutamine patients (P = .022). Interestingly, a subgroup analysis demonstrated that the use of β-blockers enhanced the hemodynamic effects of levosimendan but reduced the hemodynamic effects of dobutamine. In the LIDO study, levosimendan treatment was also associated with a significant decrease in mortality. At 31 days, all-cause mortality was significantly lower with levosimendan compared with dobutamine (hazard ratio 0.43 [95% CI 0.18-1.00] P = .049). The patients were also followed retrospectively for 180 days and this analysis revealed that 26% of the levosimendan patients had died, compared with 38% in the dobutamine group (hazard ratio 0.57 [95% CI 0.34-0.95] P = .029).

In addition, levosimendan is safe in patients with acute coronary syndromes and it improves the function of stunned myocardium in patients who undergo percutaneous coronary intervention. Importantly, the inodilatory effects of levosimendan are accentuated by concomitant use of beta blocking agents in the LIDO trial. In the Randomized Multicenter Evaluation of Intravenous Levosimendan Efficacy (REVIVE) trial, levosemindan significantly improved a composite of clinical signs and symptoms of acute decompensated heart failure over five days as assessed by patients and their physicians. In the Survival Of Patients With Acute Heart Failure In Need Of Intravenous Inotropic Support (SURVIVE) study a statistically significant difference was seen early, especially in patients chronically treated with a beta blocker, but it was not evident in 180-day survival.

Drug Use

Treatment with Levosimendan is usually initiated with a 10 minute loading bolus of 3 to 6 mcg/kg followed by a 24h continuous infusion of 0.05 to 0.2 mcg/kg/min. If the patient has hypotension, one should either skip the loading dose or associate Norepinephrine in low dose. Most patients show improvement in hemodynamic function during the next 24h, usually heralded by a significant increase in urine output and a significant decrease in the PCWP. This diuretic effect is often the cause of electrolyte imbalance that has been associated with arrhythmia. Magnesium and potassium should be pre-emptively administrated in order to prevent arrhythmia unless there is a contra-indication such as renal failure.

As a powerful vasodilator, levosimendan may be a harmful drug. Although this drug has a minor influence on myocardial oxygen demand *per se*, in patients with active ischemia or obstructive CAD, levosimendan induced hypotension, especially in the hypovolemic patient, may precipitate tachycardia, aggravate ischemia, and increase myocardial damage, worsening long term prognosis. Hypotensive patients or patients with active ischemia are not good candidates for levosimendan administration and should have these problems addressed first.

In countries where it is available, early levosimendan infusion can be considered for patients who remain symptomatic with dyspnea at rest despite initial therapy, particularly those with a history of chronic heart failure, chronically treated with beta-blockers. It has also been used to restore right or left ventricular function in patients after cardiac surgery, in unresponsive cardiogenic shock after heart transplantation primary graft failure, and RV dysfunction in acute respiratory distress syndrome patients.

References

Gheorghiade M, Teerlink JR, Mebazaa A. Pharmacology of new agents for acute heart failure syndromes. *Am J Cardiol*. 2005; **96(6A)**: 68G-73G.

De Luca L, Colucci WS, Nieminen MS, *et al.* Evidence-based use of levosimendan in different clinical settings. *Eur Heart J*. 2006; **27**(16): 1908-20.

Kass DA, Solaro RJ. Mechanisms and use of calcium-sensitizing agents in the failing heart. Circulation 2006; **113**(2): 305-15.

Givertz MM, Andreou C, Conrad CH, Colucci WS. Direct myocardial effects of levosimendan in humans with left ventricular dysfunction: alteration of force-frequency and relaxation-frequency relationships. *Circulation* 2007; **115**(10): 1218-24.

Morelli A, Teboul JL, Maggiore SM, *et al.* Effects of levosimendan on right ventricular afterload in patients with acute respiratory distress syndrome: a pilot study. *Crit Care Med* 2006; **34**(9): 2287-93.

Toller WG, Stranz C. Levosimendan, a new inotropic and vasodilator agent. *Anesthesiology* 2006; **104**(3): 556-69.

Michaels AD, McKeown B, Kostal M, *et al.* Effects of intravenous levosimendan on human coronary vasomotor regulation, left ventricular wall stress, and myocardial oxygen uptake. *Circulation* 2005; **111**(12): 1504-9.

De Luca L, Proietti P, Celotto A, *et al.* Levosimendan improves hemodynamics and coronary flow reserve after percutaneous coronary intervention in patients with acute myocardial infarction and left ventricular dysfunction. *Am Heart J* 2005; **150**(3): 563-8.

Follath F, Cleland JG, Just H, *et al.* (2002) Efficacy and safety of intravenous levosimendan compared with dobutamine in severe low-output heart failure (the LIDO study): a randomised double-blind trial. *Lancet* 2002; **360**(9328): 196-202.

Mebazaa A, Nieminen MS, Packer M, *et al.* Levosimendan vs dobutamine for patients with acute decompensated heart failure: the SURVIVE Randomized Trial. *Jama* 2007; **297**(17): 1883-91.

Gastrointestinal drugs

Chapter contents

H2 blockers and proton pump inhibitors

Physiology of acid secretion

There is continual basal acid secretion and an increase after meals, from the parietal cells in the body and fundus of the stomach. The dominant mechanism for acid secretion is mediated by histamine from enterochromaffin cells, in turn stimulated by gastrin, released from antral G cells in response to amino acids. Other stimuli acting on parietal cells include acetylcholine, gastrin, calcium and pituitary adenylate cyclase-activating polypeptide.

Pharmacology

Histamine receptor-2 blockers (H2Bs)

- can cause bradycardia on rapid injection
- have a short half-life, resulting in an elevated pH for 4–8h after an intravenous bolus
- possess a degree of renal elimination and therefore require dose adjustment with renal impairment
- cimetidine is known to be an enzyme inhibitor increasing the plasma levels of many drugs, e.g theophylline, metronidazole, diazepam and phenytoin
- exhibit tachyphylaxis or tolerance.

This feature of tolerance is demonstrated in a trial where healthy volunteers were exposed to two drugs in a crossover fashion. Results are shown in Table 12.1.1 from continuous infusions, but similar results were obtained for intermittent dosing. pH during days 1, 2 and 3 is displayed as a median value, and the percentage time spent above a pH value of 4 and 6.

Table 12.1.1 Effects of ranitidine and omeprazole on intragastric pH

	Day 1	Day 2	Day 3
Ranitidine median pH	5	3	2.7
Omeprazole median pH	>6	>6	>6
Ranitidine % time pH >4	70%	38%	26%
Omeprazole % time pH >4	95%	>99%	>99%
Ranitidine % time pH >6	30%	<11%	<11%
Omeprazole % time pH >6	59%	>70%	>70%

Ranitidine—50mg loading dose + 0.25mg/kg/h infusion or 100mg qds.

Omeprazole—80mg loading dose + 8mg/h infusion or 80mg loading dose + 40mg qds.

Proton pump inhibtiors (PPIs)

- do not exhibit tachyphylaxis
- have an elimination half-life of ~1h
- bind irreversibly to the H^+/K^+ ATPase proton pump and thus require the synthesis of new pump enzyme to terminate their effect—a process that can take up to 48h
- do not require dose adjustment in the elderly or those with renal impairment
- may need dose adjustment in hepatic impairment
- do exhibit drug interactions.

Omeprazole reduces the clearance of carbamazepine, diazepam and phenytoin.

Lansoprazole is a weak inducer of cytochrome P450, affecting the metabolism of phenytoin, theophylline and warfarin.

Pantoprazole does not inhibit or induce the cytochrome P450 system.

Pathophysiology of stress ulcers

Factors contributing to mucosal disease

- Defects in gastric glycoprotein mucus. This is contributed to by refluxed bile salts and uraemic toxins.
- Gastric acid hypersecretion. Although acid secretion in most critically ill patients is normal or subnormal, in patients with *head injuries* and *extensive burns* there can be hypersecretion.
- Ischaemia. Even with apparently normal systemic circulation, visceral perfusion can be decreased, decreasing secretion of mucus and bicarbonate.
- *Helicobacter pylori* infection. This has not been well studied in the critically ill.

Coagulation effects

In vitro studies have shown at a pH of 6.4 the effectiveness of coagulation and platelet aggregation is halved. A further drop in pH to 5.4 results in practical cessation of coagulation and platelet aggregation activity. Clot lysis by pepsin is inhibited if pH is >4. The literature has suggested aims of treatment are:

- A *pH >4* to prevent stress ulceration
- A *pH >6* to prevent clot lysis with an acute GI bleed

Stress ulcer prophylaxis

The significant study in this area that gives us both definitions and risk factors for stress ulcers is by the Canadian Critical Care Trials Groups, led by Cook, and published in 1994. It was a prospective, multi-centre, cohort study involving 2252 patients in four university-affiliated, medical–surgical ICUs.

Definitions

- Occult bleeding: guaiac +ve gastric aspirate or stool
- Overt bleeding: haematemesis, haematochezia or malaena
- Clinically significant bleeding: haemodynamic change or need for transfusion

Risk factors

Mechanical ventilation >48h

There is a 16-fold increase risk of bleeding; odds ratio 15.6 (P <0.001)

Coagulopathy

There is a 4-fold increase in the risk of bleeding; odds ratio 4.3 (P <0.001)

Of 847 patients with one of these two risk factors, 3.7% had clinically significant bleeding, and of 1405 patients without risk factors, 0.1% had clinically significant bleeding.

Benefits of prophylaxis

H2Bs

In Cook's meta-analysis of 1996 which included 7218 patients, it was shown that in patients given H2Bs the prevalence of clinically significant bleeding has an odds ratio of 0.44 (95% confidence interval (CI), 0.212–0.88) vs placebo/no therapy, and an odds ratio of 0.86 (95% CI, 0.46–1.59) vs antacids.

However, in the more recent meta-analysis by Messori, which excluded studies using cimetidine and only used placebo-controlled trials and therefore only had 398 patients, ranitidine was not shown to have a treatment effect on clinically important bleeding. This paper discussed the need for an RCT, but there was difficulty in the ethics in using a placebo control. It also asked the question of whether it realistic to expect cimetidine to be effective and ranitidine ineffective as their results seemed to show.

PPIs

There have been few studies evaluating PPIs specifically for stress ulcer prophylaxis, resulting in insufficient evidence of superiority. Their use is, however, becoming more popular. Studies have shown that enteral or IV administration of a PPI does maintain a pH of at least 4.

Risks of prophylaxis

Ventilator-associated pneumonia

There remains concern over a possible increased rate of VAP in those treated with prophylaxis. The proposed mechanism is through aspiration of colonized secretions. A large randomized study comparing the use of sulcralfate (no pH effect) and ranitidine found no difference in the rate of VAP. However, this area remains controversial.

In addition, the use of PPIs and H2Bs has been associated with decreased neutrophil function and lower production of reactive oxygen intermediates. This has uncertain clinical significance; interpreted as deleterious for control of infection or beneficial in aiding ulcer healing and preventing systemic inflammation.

Infectious gastroenteritis

Increased rates of infection are proposed due to loss of the protective role of gastric acid as a bactericidal barrier. Patients treated with PPIs and achlorhydric patients have been shown to be at risk of upper GI colonization and infections, including *Clostridium difficile* disease.

Outcomes

Patients who develop clinically important GI bleeding have a higher mortality. This equates to a 20–30% increase in absolute risk of mortality and an increase of 1–4 in relative risk. Length of ICU stay is also extended by ~4–8 days. It is disappointing that prophylaxis has not demonstrated a statistically significant reduction in mortality despite >50 randomized trials and several meta-analyses. HR2Bs do reduce the rate of clinically significant GI bleeding by 50%, and hence the associated costs of endoscopic treatment. The evidence supports a broad range of practice patterns.

Treatment of acute bleeding after endoscopy

Up to 20% of patients rebleed after endoscopic treatment, particularly those noted to have a visible non-bleeding vessel, adherent clot or ulcer size >1cm.

H2Bs are unlikely to be effective in active bleeding, or preventing rebleeding after haemostasis from endoscopic injection or thermo/electro-coagulation.

PPIs are effective in preventing rebleeding after haemostasis as they raise pH close to neutrality and allow the formation of stable clots. This topic has been the subject of a Cochrane Review in 2007. The rate of rebleeding was decreased from 17.3 to 10.6%. Use of PPIs decreased the need for surgery (odds ratio 0.61, 95% CI 0.48–0.78). Overall they found no difference in all-cause mortality, apart from the Asian studies in which mortality was reduced.

One regimen used is omeprazole 80mg bolus + 8mg/h for 3 days and 20mg/day for 2 months. This decreased transfusion requirements, decreased the rate of rebleeding from 20 to 4% in the first 3 days (number needced to treat of 5–6). In addition, studies have shown the use of PPIs in preventing rebleeding to be cost-effective.

Further reading

Abpi Compendium of Data Sheets and Summaries of Product Characteristics. Datapharm Publications Ltd, 2000.

Conrad S. Acute upper gastrointestinal bleeding in critically ill patients: causes and treatment modalities. *Crit Care Med* 2002; **30**: S365–8.

Cook DJ, Fuller HD, Guyatt GH, *et al.* Risk factors for gastrointestinal bleeding in critically ill patients: Canadian Critical Care Trials Groups. *N Eng J Med* 1994; **330**: 397–81.

Cook DJ, Griffith LE, Walter SD, *et al.* The attributable mortality and length of intensive care unit stay of clinically important gastrointestinal bleeding in critically ill patients. *Crit Care* 2001; 5: 368–75.

Cook D, Guyatt G, Marshall J, *et al.* A comparision of sucralfate and ranitidine for the prevention of upper gastrointestinal bleeding in patients requiring mechanical ventilation. Canadian Critical Care Trials Group. *N Engl J Med* 1998; 338: 791–7.

Cook DJ, Reeve BK, Guyatt GH, *et al.* Stress ulcer prophylaxis in critically ill patients: resolving discordant meta-analyses. *JAMA* 1996; 275: 308–14.

Fennerty MB. Pathophysiology of the upper gastrointestinal tract in the critically ill patient: rationale for the therapeutic benefits of acid suppression. *Crit Care Med* 2002; **30**: S351–5.

Messori A, Trippoli , Vaiani M, *et al.* Bleeding and pneumonia in intensive care patients given ranitidine and sucralfate for prevention of stress ulcer: meta-analysis of randomised controlled trials. *BMJ* 2000; 321: 1103.

Netzer P, Gaia C, Sandoz M, *et al.* Effect of repeated injection and continuous infusion of omeprazole and ranitidine on intragastric pH over 72 hours. *Am J Gastroenterol* 1999; 94: 351–7.

Antiemetics

Nausea and vomiting are protective reflexes designed to prevent the body from ingesting noxious substances. Vomiting is the forceful expulsion of the contents of the upper GI tract through the mouth and associated with contraction of the abdominal muscles. Nausea is the unpleasant sensation that precedes vomiting. The genesis of nausea and vomiting in critically ill patients has myriad causes. Included in these is post-operative nausea and vomiting (PONV), ileus and gastroparesis, use of opiate analgesia and sepsis. Symptoms of nausea and emesis may be overlooked when dealing with a complex patient with multiple problems. Prolonged recovery times in post-surgical patients and risk of aspiration pneumonitis are clear reasons why nausea and vomiting should be adequately treated in critically ill patients. To understand the principle actions of antiemetic drugs it is useful to know the mechanisms underlying nausea and vomiting.

Mechanisms of nausea and vomiting

Vomiting centre

The vomiting reflex is initiated by the vomiting nucleus situated in the medulla oblongata. Afferent impulses from numerous other areas of the nervous system synapse in the vomiting centre:

- Cortical input from pain, memory, anticipation or fear
- Sensory inputs from smell and taste
- Direct vagal afferents from the GI tract
- Impulses coordinated in the chemoreceptor trigger zone via the nucleus tractus solitarius

Chemoreceptor trigger zone (CTZ)

The CTZ is a collection of cells found on the Area Postrema on the surface of the brain. It lacks an effective blood–brain barrier and so is sensitive to input of noxious stimuli within both the CSF and the blood. As such, opiates, chemotherapy and anaesthetics all act via the CTZ. Vagal afferents from the GI tract synapse in the CTZ in addition to direct stimulation of the vomiting centre.

Neurotransmitters

Many neurotransmitters are implicated in the process of nausea and vomiting, but only six have been involved in pharmacological attempts to treat nausea and vomiting:

- Serotonin receptors (5-HT) are found on vagal afferents and in high concentrations within the CTZ. The 5-HT_3 subgroup is especially prominent.
- Histamine is implicated in the transmission of impulses from the vestibular system, but is also involved in gut neural output. The H_1 receptor subtype predominates.
- Dopamine is found in high concentrations in the CTZ especially the D_2 subgroup.
- Acetylcholine is involved in vestibular transmission of impulses.
- Substance P acts upon neurokinin-1 (NK-1) receptors which are involved in multiple pathways.
- Cannabinoid receptors (CB_1) are found in the vomiting centre and again are involved in multiple pathways. Agonism of these receptors allays emesis.

Motor outputs

Once the inputs have been processed in the vomiting centre, there is a combination of neural outputs:

- Vagal afferents to the oesophagus, stomach and small intestine (giant retrograde contraction).
- Somatomotor neurons supplying the diaphragm and muscles of the anterior abdominal wall.
- Autonomic and somatic output to the anal and bladder sphincters to prevent expulsion in response to large increases in intra-abdominal pressure.
- Parasympathetic output to the heart and salivary glands leading to bradycardia and salivation.
- Sympathetic output to skin constrictors resulting in skin pallor.

Antiemetic drugs

Anticholinergics

These drugs act by direct effects on the vestibular pathway but also have effects on modulation of impulses from the gut. *Scopolamine* can be used transdermally and is effective when applied preoperatively.

Scopolamine

- Indication: motion sickness or pre-medication.
- Dose: 1mg patch applied 5–6h before journey/operation. Lasts 72h.
- Side effects: drowsiness, dry mouth, dizziness, blurred vision and difficulty micturating.
- Caution in renal or hepatic dysfunction.

Antihistamines

Predominant effects are on the vestibular pathways so especially useful in motion sickness disorders and middle ear surgery. Drugs include *cinnarizine, cyclizine* and *promethazine*. Drowsiness is a common side effect.

Cyclizine

- Indication: nausea and vomiting; motion sickness
- Dose: 50mg tds IV/PO/IM.
- Side effects: drowsiness, dry mouth, blurred vision, difficulty micturating.
- Avoid in liver disease, safe in renal impairment.

Antidopaminergics

Non-specific antagonism of dopamine receptors, but antiemetic effects are modulated by the D_2 subtype. These drug types are useful where the main mechanism of emesis is in the CTZ (e.g. opiate side effect). Three classes: benzamides (*domperidone, metoclopramide*) are both prokinetics and antiemetics; phenothiazines (*prochlorperazine and chlorpromazine*) have weak antimuscarinic effects in addition; butyrophenones (*droperidol, haloperidol*) are similar in effects to phenothiazines.

Metoclopramide

- Indication: nausea and vomiting due to GI disorders.
- Dose: 10mg tds IV/PO/IM.
- Side effects: extrapyramidal disorders, drowsiness, neuroleptic malignant syndrome, arrhythmias.
- Reduce dose in hepatic or renal impairment (increased risk of extapyramidal side effects).

Chlorpromazine

- Indication: nausea and vomiting.
- Dose: 25–50mg qds IV/PO/IM.
- Side effects: extrapyramidal, drowsiness, neuroleptic malignant syndrome, arrhythmias, hypotension.
- Reduce dose and use with caution in hepatic or renal failure.

5-HT$_3$ receptor antagonists

The advent of 5-HT$_3$ receptor antagonists in the mid-1980s revolutionized the treatment of chemotherapy-induced emesis. Since then, they have been found to be useful in many other clinical contexts. Drugs in this class include *ondansetron, granisetron and tropisetron.*

Granisetron

- Indication: chemotherapy-induced nausea and vomiting; prophylaxis and treatment of PONV.
- Dose: 1mg bd IV.
- Side effects: diarrhoea, abdominal pain, QT prolongation.
- Avoid in cardiac conduction disorders. Safe in hepatic and renal impairment.

Corticosteroids

The mechanism of steroids acting as antiemetics is not clear. In humans undergoing chemotherapy, the rate of *cisplatin*-induced emesis is inversely related to the serum cortisol level, suggesting a link. The presumed mechanism is by effects on eicasonoid metabolism. *Dexamethasone* is the most commonly used drug in this class, and appears to be especially efficacious in PONV.

Dexamethasone

- Indication: nausea and vomiting from chemotherapy or in the prophylaxis of PONV.
- Dose: 4–8mg od IV/PO.
- Side effects: peptic ulceration, proximal myopathy, dysphoria, hyperglycaemia, immunosuppression.
- Care in infection and reduce dose in renal or hepatic impairment. Adrenal suppression on withdrawal after prolonged treatment.

Neurokinin-1 (NK$_1$) receptor antagonists

Substance P is the endogenous stimulant at this receptor, and antagonism of its effects provides antiemetic actions against a large array of stimuli. In view of this, they are assumed to work at the level of the brainstem, although this has not been clarified yet. *Aprepitant* is the only drug in this class licensed at present and has a narrow indication in delayed phase chemotherapy-induced emesis.

Aprepitant

- Indication: adjunct to dexamethasone and 5-HT$_3$ antagonists in emetic chemotherapy.
- Dose: 125mg IV pre-chemotherapy, Then 80mg od for 2 days.
- Side effects: hiccoughs, diarrhoea, constipation.
- Reduce dose in hepatic impairment.

Cannabinoid CB$_1$ receptor agonist

The proposed area of activity is in the vomiting centre and so are broad-spectrum antiemetics. In clinical practice, they tend to be used in chemotherapy-induced emesis. *Nabilone* is the best known of this class of drugs.

Nabilone

- Indication: adjunct in emetic chemotherapy.
- Dose: 1–2mg bd po.
- Side effects: drowsiness, euphoria, dry mouth, sleep disturbance.
- Avoid if history of psychiatric disturbance; contraindicated in severe hepatic impairment.

Miscellaneous agents

Specific 5-HT$_{1A}$ agonists such as *buspirone* have been shown in humans to reduce emesis following *cisplatin* chemotherapy, but they are not licensed as antiemetics. GABA$_B$ receptor agonists such as *baclofen* have also shown some antiemetic activity in neurologically impaired children.

Clinical approach

PONV

Scoring systems for PONV have been well validated, with the risk of it rising from 10% with no risk factors up to 80% with 4 risk factors. This makes stratifying patients simple and the administration of prophylactic antiemetics appropriate. *Metoclopramide, dexamethasone* and 5-HT$_3$ receptor antagonists in combination are commonly used.

On the ICU

Clearly the use of different agents in critically ill patients will depend on the clinical scenario and the side effect profile. Simple measures such as the insertion of NG tubes to decompress the stomach and adequate pain relief help to reduce the incidence of nausea and vomiting. Prokinetics such as *metoclopramide* have a role as first-line agents, but some care must be taken in prescribing phenothiazines and butyrophenones in view of their risk of cardiac side effects.

Dexamethasone will have effects on the glycaemic control of a patient, which remains integral to intensive care practice, so they are not commonly used. The 5-HT$_3$ receptor antagonists have a reasonable side effect profile and, while more expensive than some other agents, can be used with relative safety.

The role of more novel agents such as *aprepitant* and *cannabinoids* is unclear.

Further reading

Andrews PLR, Rudd JA. The role of tachykinins and the tachykinin NK$_1$ receptor in nausea and emesis. In: Holzer P, ed. Handbook of experimental pharmacology. Berlin: *Springer*, 2004: 359–440.

Hornby PJ. Central neurocircuitry associated with emesis. *Am J Med* 2001; 111: 106S–12S.

Hursti TJ, Fredrikson M, Steinbeck G, *et al.* Endogenous cortisol exerts antiemetic effects similar to that of endogenous corticosteroids. *Br J Cancer* 1993; 68: 112–4.

Kreis ME. Postoperative nausea and vomiting. *Auton Neurosci* 2006; 129: 86–91.

Miner WJ, Sanger GJ. Inhibition of cisplatin induced vomiting by selective 5-hydroxytriptamine M-receptor antagonism. *Br J Pharmacol* 1986; 88: 497–9.

Sanger GJ, Andrews PLR. Treatment of nausea and vomiting: gaps in our knowledge. *Auton Neurosci* 2006; 129: 3–16.

Gut motility agents

Introduction

Delayed gastric emptying (also referred to as gastric stasis and gastroparesis) is common in critical illness. Critical care management should include

- supportive measures (hydration, nutrition, placement of gastric tube for decompression)
- minimizing use of opioids
- optimizing glycaemic control and medications.

Normal gastric emptying reflects a coordinated effort between different regions of the stomach and the duodenum, as well as complex extrinsic modulation by the CNS and distal gut factors: normal gastric emptying consists of fundic relaxation to accommodate food, antral contractions to break up large food particles, pyloric relaxation to allow food to exit the stomach, and antropyloroduodenal coordination of motor events. Gastric dysmotility includes delayed gastric emptying (gastroparesis), rapid gastric emptying (as seen in dumping syndrome) and other motor dysfunctions such as impaired fundic distension most commonly found in functional dyspepsia. The importance of these gastric dysrhythmias is uncertain. Critically ill patients (without diabetes mellitus) are thought to have disturbed motility of the proximal stomach and loss of fundic wave activity. There is enhanced pyloric pressure and reduced antral pressure. The feedback loop of bulky duodenal nutrients leading to pyloric relaxation is absent, further contributing to delayed gastric emptying.

Indications

Gut motility agents are indicated in patients with large nasogastric aspirates, vomiting and paralytic ileus.

The following factors should be considered before prescribing gut motility agents.

- Patients on critical care units are frequently prescribed PPIs, which can delay gastric emptying. Consider using H_2 antagonists as an alternative agent.
- Tachyphylaxis occurs with conventional prokinetics after only a few days of treatment. Consider switching or combining gut motility agents.
- Enteral nutrition is always desirable, and clinicians should persevere in establishing enteral feeding (oral, NG and NJ) according to local protocols.
- Enteral feeding is best established with low fat feed without non-digestible fibre; continuous feed or frequent small meals.

Erythromycin

IV erythromycin is the treatment of choice during acute episodes of delayed gastric emptying. Infusions produce high amplitude gastric propulsive contractions, which then dump food residue into the duodenum. Erythromycin also stimulates fundic contractility and inhibits the accommodation response of the stomach after food. An RCT with small numbers showed that IV erythromycin improves gastric motility and early nutritional intake in critically injured patients. Within the dosage range of 70–200mg this is a dose-independent effect. A single bolus dose of IV erythromycin facilitates active bedside placement of post-pyloric feeding tubes in critically ill adult patients.

Evidence supporting the use of oral erythromycin remains generally weak. A dose of up to 250mg qds can be used.

The main limitations for the use of erythromycin are its side effects: gastrointestinal toxicity, ototoxicity, pseudomembranous colitis and prolongation of the QTc interval. Therefore, erythromycin should only be used in the short term and with caution if administered simultaneously with the enzyme inhibitors CYP3A4.

The potential epidemiological impact of the increased macrolide use and evidence of the spread of resistance should be borne in mind when using erythromycin as a prokinetic agent in critically ill patients. Erythromycin can be recommended, if patients have failed other treatments for impaired gastrointestinal dysmotility and are intolerant of metoclopramide.

Erythromycin vs metoclopramide

A small RCT comparing IV administration of erythromycin and metoclopramide concluded that erythromycin is more effective than metoclopramide in treating feed intolerance. The effectiveness of both treatments declined rapidly over time, but combination therapy of both medications proved more successful in reducing gastric aspirates (day 1 = 92% and day 6 = 67%).

Metoclopramide

Metoclopramide has antiemetic and prokinetic properties. It is a useful alternative for those who cannot take erythromycin or as an adjunct to erythromycin therapy.

Metoclopramide acts by blocking D_2 receptors in the GI tract. Its side effects are due to its central phenothiazine-like action on dopaminergic pathways, which has made the drug less popular in recent years. However, during short-term use, the risk of tardive dyskinesia is minimal. Injection of an antiparkinsonian drug, such as procyclidine, will control dystonic attacks.

The advantage of the drug is that it can be given enterally in tablet or liquid form or by slow IV injection at a dose of 10mg tds (up to 40mg per day can be tolerated by adults).

Domperidone

Oral metoclopramide and domperidone are equally effective in alleviating the symptoms of gastroparesis in diabetes, but no evidence for IV use/ICU available to date. Domperidone acts on the CTZ and has the advantage over metoclopramide that it is less likely to cause sedation and dystonias, because it does not readily cross the blood–brain barrier.

Cisapride

Stimulates 5-HT_4 receptors, resulting in acetylcholine release from the myenteric plexus.

Effects are abolished by atropine. This leads to increased antral and duodenal contractility, which is maintained over long-term treatment (1yr), in healthy subjects and in various gastric stasis syndromes. Cisapride may be more potent and better tolerated than equivalent doses of metoclopramide Dose-dependent side effects include abdominal discomfort and increased bowel frequency. The main drawback of cisapride is the significant drug interactions with medications that are metabolized by cytochrome P450-3A4 which have led to arrhythmias and death. Its use is therefore restricted.

The dose is 10mg qds, usually in liquid form.

Gastroparesis and diabetes

Critical illness and diabetes melllitus are both associated with delayed gastric emptying. Furthermore, 1/3 of ICU patients have diabetes mellitus. It has therefore been thought that critically ill diabetic patients are at increased risk of gastroparesis. Studies comparing NG feeding of diabetic and non-diabetic patients have shown no difference in gastric motility during critical illness. However, NG feeds are liquid meals and their absorption has been shown to be variable, whereas gastric emptying after a solid or semi-solid meal is consistently slow in diabetic patients.

Diabetic patients in critical care should therefore receive the same treatment as their non-diabetic counterparts.

Acute hyperglycaemia is thought to result in reduced antral motility, in increased pyloric pressures and in decreased compliance of the gastric fundus, leading to slow gastric emptying. It is also thought that delayed gastric emptying itself leads to poor glycaemic control. Hyperglycaemia attenuates the effects of prokinetic drugs. Therefore, hyperglycaemia needs to be treated diligently and without delay.

Treatment

A pilot study of injecting **botulinum toxin** into the pylorus of oesophagectomy patients has shown promising results: no patient who received the injection developed delayed gastric emptying or aspiration pneumonia in the postoperative period. After a median follow-up time of 5.3 months, only 1 out of 12 patients had required intervention for symptoms of gastric stasis.

Patients not responding to supportive measures and medical treatment need to be considered for early jejunal (postpyloric) feeding tube placement. Other surgical treatments are not suitable for ICUs, including the pioneered technique from the USA where gastric motility is achieved by enteric electrical stimulation with an implantable gastric pacing device.

Summary

- Supportive measures—gastric decompression, hydration, minimizing use of opioids
- Optimizing glycaemic control
- Medications—erythromycin and metoclopramide
- Placement of jejunostomy feeding tubes.

Further reading

Abell T, Lou J, Tabbaa M, *et al.* Gastric electrical stimulation for gastroparesis improves nutritional parameters at short, intermediate, and long-term follow-up. *J Parenter Enteral Nutr* 2003; 27: 277–81.

Berne JD, Norwood SH, McAuley CE, *et al.* Erythromycin reduces delayed gastric emptying in critically ill trauma patients: a randomised, controlled trial. *J Trauma* 2002; 53: 422–5.

Chapman M, Fraser R, Vozzo R, *et al.* Antor-pyloro-duodenal motor responses to gastric and duodenal nutrient in critically ill patients. *Gut* 2005; 54: 1384–90.

Feldman M, Smith HJ. Effect of cisapride on gastric emptying of indigestible solids in patients with gastroparesis diabeticorum. A comparison with metoclopramide and placebo. *Gastroenterology* 1987; 92: 171.

Griffith, D, McNally A, Therese RN, *et al.* Intravenous erythromycin facilitates bedside placement of postpyloric feeding tubes in critically ill adults: a double-blind, randomized, placebo-controlled study. *Crit Care Med* 2003; 31: 39–44.

Horowitz M, Wishart JM, Jones LK, *et al.* Gastric emptying in diabetes: an overview. *Diabet Med* 1996; 13(9 Suppl 5): 16–22.

Maganti K, Onyemere K, Jones MP. Oral erythromycin and symptomatic relief of gastroparesis. A systematic review. *Am J Gastroenterol* 2003; 98: 259

Mutlu GM, Mutlu EA, Factor P. GI complications in patients receiving mechanical ventilation. *Chest* 2001; 119: 1222–41.

Schmidt HB, Werdan K, Muller-Werdan U. Autonomic dysfunction in the ICU patient. *Curr Opin Crit Care* 2001; 7: 314–22.

Umperrriez GE, Isaacs SD, Bazargan N, *et al.* Hyperglycaeamia: an independent marker of in-hospital mortality in patients with undiagnosed diabetes. *J Clin Endocrinol Metab* 2002; 87: 978–82.

Wehrmann T, Lembcke B, Caspary WF. Influence of cisapride on antroduodenal motor function in healthy subjects and diabetics with autonomic neuropathy. *Aliment Pharmacol Ther* 1991; 5: 599.

Antidiarrhoeals

Diarrhoea is a common problem in critically ill patients. Incidences vary from 14.7 to 38%. Diarrhoea in this setting can lead to excess fluid shifts, resulting in haemodynamic instability and electrolyte disturbances. In addition, skin care problems related to the buttocks and perineum are an issue. As a general rule, diarrhoea due to infective causes should be passed without any attempt to reduce the frequency or consistency of the stool. In the situation where infective causes are excluded and where other measures such as changing the feeding regimen have been attempted, then resort to antidiarrhoeal drugs may be appropriate.

Risk factors and causes of diarrhoea

A broad differentiation of diarrhoea into infective and non-infective causes is a useful starting point for deciding on the role of antidiarrhoeals. Where infectious agents are identified, then appropriate antibiotic treatment should lead to resolution of the symptoms. *Clostridium difficile* is the main cause of antibiotic-induced diarrhoea in the UK, and treatment with metronidazole or vancomycin is indicated.

Where infection is excluded, then drug=induced causes should be sought:

- Laxatives
- Antibiotics
- Magnesium-containing oral medications
- H_2 receptor antagonists
- Proton pump inhibitors.

Where possible, these medications should be discontinued. Other risk factors, where modifiable, should be addressed. These include:

- Hypothermia/fever
- Hypoalbuminaemia
- Re-use of previously suspended oral feed
- Malnutrition
- Sepsis syndrome.

Once all these factors have been addressed, then by a diagnosis of exclusion it can be assumed that the diarrhoea is related to enteral feeding. Enteral feeding-associated diarrhoea remains the most common cause of diarrhoea in critically ill patients. Treatment involves cessation of feed or antidiarrhoeal drugs

Antidiarrhoeal drugs

These can be roughly divided into antimotility drugs, anantispasmodics and bulk-forming drugs.

Antimotility drugs

These drugs act to slow down peristalsis in the gut and thus increase the transit time in the colon, allowing for more absorption of water and solute. Commonly used opiates include *loperamide* and *codeine* phosphate. The side effects of opiates include dependence, and nausea and vomiting. *Co-phenotrope* (Lomotil®) is a combination of *diphenoxylate*, an opioid derivative, and *atropine* sulfate in proportions of 100 parts to 1 part, respectively. Side effects of this drug mainly relate to the opioid.

Loperamide

- Indication: symptomatic treatment of acute diarrhoea and chronic diarrhoea.
- Dose: 4mg PO initially then 2mg following each loose stool, max 16mg daily.
- Side effects: dizziness, drowsiness, urticaria, paralytic ileus.
- Reduce dose in hepatic impairment.

Codeine phosphate

- Indication: symptomatic treatment of acute diarrhoea and chronic diarrhoea.
- Dose: 30mg qds PO.
- Side effects: nausea, drowsiness, respiratory depression, hypotension.
- Caution in respiratory disease; reduce dose in renal failure; may precipitate coma in liver disease.

Co-phenotrope

- Indication: adjunct to rehydration in acute diarrhoea.
- Dose: 2.5mg/25mcg PO, initially 4 tablets then 2 tablets every 6h.
- Side effects: see codeine phosphate and atropine.
- Cautions: see codeine phosphate.

Antispasmodics

These are antimuscarinics (see also diphenoxylate above) and help to reduce gut motility, but are especially useful at alleviating the spasms associated with both acute and chronic diarrhoea. Tertiary amines such as *atropine* tend to be better absorbed than the quarternary amines such as *propanthiline* and *hyoscine*; however, the latter agents tend to cross the blood–brain barrier less due to their reduced lipid solubility. Oral absorption is poor for all these agents, but *hyoscine* is used IV to good effect during endoscopy. Side effects are as for all muscarinics, and include bradycardia, dry mouth, photophobia and urinary retention.

Atropine

- Indication: symptomatic relief of GI disorders associated with muscle spasm.
- Dose: 600–1200mcg od PO.
- Side effects: bradycardia, urinary retention, nausea, vomiting, giddiness. May precipitate angle-closure glaucoma.
- Caution in Down syndrome or tachycardia.

Hyoscine butylbromide (Buscopan®)

- Indication: symptomatic relief of GI disorders associated with muscle spasm.
- Dose: 20mg qds PO/IV.
- Side effects: see atropine.
- Cautions: see atropine.

Bulk-forming agents

These agents are essentially fibre replacements and act by increasing faecal mass. They can act as laxatives in patients with small, hard stools but are also useful in the diarrhoea associated with diverticular disease. Included in this class are *ispaghula husk* and *methylcellulose*. The main concern with these drugs is that adequate oral hydration is maintained, as there is a risk of intestinal obstruction

Ispaghula husk (Fybogel®)

- Indication: diarrhoea associated with diverticular disease.
- Dose: 3.5g od PO,

- Side effects: flatulence, abdominal distension, intestinal obstruction.
- Ensure adequate fluid intake orally.

Methylcellulose

- Indication: diarrhoea associated with diverticular disease.
- Dose: 4mg PO initially then 2mg following each loose stool, max 16mg daily.
- Side effects: see *Ispaghula*.
- Cautions: see *Ispaghula*.

Enteral supplements

Recent research into the role of fibre and into live microbial feed supplements has shown promise in the treatment of enteral feeding induced diarrhoea.

Soluble fibre

The physiological effects of fibre on the gut include:

- Prolongation of intestinal transit time.
- Generation of short chain fatty acids.
- Reduction in *C. difficile* toxin production.
- Binding of bile salts.

It is therefore not surprising that they may be beneficial in enteral feeding-associated diarrhoea. Indeed in a randomized, double-blinded study, they have been shown to reduce the severity and time of diarrhoea. This was only in sepsis related patients and only in a small number (25 patients).

Probiotics

A probiotic is a live microbial feed supplement that improves intestinal microbial balance. They are found in enriched commercial products such as cheeses and yoghurts. *Saccharomyces boulardii* has been shown to reduce the incidence of enteral feeding-associated diarrhoea in a series of 128 critical care patients. These were patients with sepsis, so it is not certain whether this can be extrapolated to the general adult ICU population.

Prebiotics

Prebiotics are food ingredients that are non-digestible and benefit the host by stimulating the growth of certain bacteria in the colon. Commonly used prebiotics include:

- Inulin
- Fructo-oligosaccharides
- Galacto-oligosaccharides
- Soya-oligosaccharides
- Xylo-oligosaccharides
- Isomalto-oligosaccharides
- Pyrodextrins

They clearly have a place in the treatment of recurrent *C. difficile* diarrhoea, but no large studies to date have been performed in critically ill patients to examine their role in these patients.

Synbiotics

Combinations of probiotics with prebiotics are termed synbiotics. The principles are the same as for prebiotics and probiotics. One study examined the administration of an infusion of *Bifidobacterium lactis, Lactobacillus acidophilus, Lactobacillus bulgaricus, Streptococcus thermophilus* and oligofructose to critically ill patients and found they favourably altered the upper GI bacterial milieu, but there was no clear clinical benefit.

Further reading

Bleichner G, Blehaut H, Mentac H *et al. Sacchromyces boulardii* prevents diarrhoea in critically ill tube fed patients. *Intensive Care Med* 1997; 23: 517–23.

Elpern EH, Stutz L, Peterson S, *et al.* Outcomes associated with enteral tube feedings in a medical intensive care unit. *Am J Crit Care* 2004; 13: 221–7.

Jain PK, McNaught CE, Anderson AD, *et al.* Influence of symbiotic containing *Lactobacillus acidophilus* La5, *Bifidobacterium lactis* Bb12, *Streptococcus thermophilus, Lactobacillus bulgaricus* and oligofructose on gut barrier function and sepsis in critically ill patients: a randomised, controlled trial. *Clin Nutr* 2004; 23: 467–75.

Montejo JC. Enteral nutrition-related gastrointestinal complications in critically ill patients: a multicentre study. The Nutritional and Metabolic Working Group of the Spanish Society of Intensive Care Medicine. *Intens Care Med* 1999; 25: 95–101.

Spapen H, Diltoer M, Van Malderen C, *et al.* Soluble fiber reduces the incidence of diarrhea in septic patients receiving total enteral nutrition: a prospective, double blind, randomized, and controlled trial. *Clin Nutr* 2001; 20: 301–5.

Wiesen P, Van Gossum A, Preiser J-C. Diarrhoea in the critically ill. *Curr Opin Crit Care* 2006; 12: 149–54.

Constipation in critical care

Constipation is a common problem, affecting 20% of the general population. Constipation is more prevalent in ICU patients, often due to medication but also due to lack of normal physiological function, such as balanced diet, exercise and biofeedback. This aspect of critical care management can be overlooked when management of life-threatening conditions takes precedence. Constipation is unpleasant for the patient: common symptoms are flatulence, bloating, abdominal pain and feeling of incomplete emptying, overflow diarrhoea, nausea and vomiting. Ventilatory weaning and urinary function can also be affected.

Constipation may be due to colonic 'inertia', due to a primary disease of the colon (stricture, cancer, anal fissure), or a secondary phenomenon due to metabolic disturbances (hypercalcaemia, hypothyroidism, diabetes mellitus) or neurological disorders (Parkinsonism and spinal cord lesions). Constipation as a disorder of pelvic floor dysfunction occurs when colonic transit time is normal, but stool is stored in the rectum for prolonged periods of time.

It is imperative to confirm the diagnosis of constipation, and to exclude an underlying condition, before starting medical treatment. Where possible, any underlying cause should also be treated.

In the critical care environment, medications are often responsible for constipation, see Table 12.5.1 for examples.

Table 12.5.1 Types of medications causing constipation

Anticholinergics	Antihistamines
	Anticholinergics
	Antidepressants
	Anticholinergics
Cation-containing agents	Iron supplements
	Aluminium (antacids, sucralfate)
Neurally active agents	Opiates
	Antihypertensives
	Ganglion blockers
	Vinca alkaloids Calcium channel blockers
	5-HT_3 antagonists

Treatments

Some ICUs have developed treatment protocols for the management of constipation. Bowel protocols may be useful in special situations (e.g. liver disease and spinal cord injury). The main advantage of a bowel protocol is regular assessment of bowel function.

Stimulant laxatives

Stimulant laxatives act by increasing peristalsis and by increasing the amounts of water in the stool, either by reducing the absorption of the water in the colon or by causing active secretion of water in the small intestine. The most commonly used stimulant laxatives are anthraquinones, i.e. **senna** and **danthron**; bisacodyl and docusate sodium are also stimulant laxatives. Stimulant laxatives are very effective, but they can cause diarrhoea with resulting dehydration and loss of potassium and other electrolytes. They also are more likely than other types of laxatives to cause intestinal cramping. **Parasypathomimetics** (neostigmine and pyridostigmine) enhance parasympathetic activity in the gut and increase GI motility. They are rarely used for this effect, as **bowel obstruction needs to be excluded** before use. They should not be used shortly after bowel anastomosis.

Osmotic laxatives

These increase the amount of water in the large bowel either by drawing fluid into to bowel or by retaining the fluid they were administered with.

Hyperosmolar laxatives

The semi-synthetic substance **lactulose** is the most commonly used substance in this category. The result is osmotic diarrhoea with low faecal pH, which discourages the proliferation of ammonia-forming organisms. Marcrogols (e.g. **Movicol**) are inert polymers of ethylene glycol, which sequester fluid in the bowel. Lactulose is used in the treatment of hepatic encephalopathy.

Saline laxatives

These contain non-absorbable ions such as magnesium, sulfate, phosphate and citrate (e.g**. magnesium hydroxide, magnesium sulfate**, sodium phosphate, sodium citrate, phosphate enema). Saline laxatives act within a few hours and are therefore useful in critical care. The magnesium in magnesium-containing laxatives is partially absorbed from the intestine and into the circulation, hence caution in chronic renal failure with long-term use of magnesium-containing laxatives.

Bulk-forming laxatives

Fibre is defined as material made by plants that is not digested by the human GI tract. Fibre is one of the mainstays in the treatment of constipation. Dietary intake of fibre in the form of fruit and vegetable is impractical for most ICU patients. Many types of fibre within the intestine bind to water and keep the water within the intestine. The fibre adds bulk (volume) to the stool and the water softens the stool. Increased bulk leads to increased peristalsis. The effect of bulk-forming laxatives may take some time to develop. Adequate fluid intake must be maintained during treatment to avoid bowel obstruction. Commonly used agents contain **ispagula husk** (Fybogel, Fibrelief, Isogel, Regulan).

Emollient laxatives

Emollient laxatives are generally known as stool softeners. They are used rarely in the current management of acute constipation. They contain **docusate** (e.g. Colace), which is a wetting agent that enhances the mixing of water with stool within the colon. Although docusate generally is safe, it may allow the absorption of mineral oil and some medications from the intestine. The use of emollient laxatives is not recommended together with mineral oil or with some prescription medications. Emollient laxatives are commonly used when there is a need to soften the stool temporarily and make defecation easier (e.g. after surgery, childbirth or heart attacks). They are also used for individuals with haemorrhoids or anal fissures. Other examples of stool softeners are the following

Enemas

There are many different types of enemas. By distending the rectum, all enemas (even the simplest type, the tap water enema) stimulate the colon to contract and eliminate stool. Other types of enemas have additional mechanisms of action. For example, saline enemas cause water to be drawn into the colon. Phosphate enemas (e.g. Fleet) stimulate the muscles of the colon. Mineral oil enemas lubricate and soften hard stool. Emollient enemas (e.g. Colace Microenema) contain agents that soften the stool. Enemas are particularly useful when there is faecal impaction, which is hardening of stool in the rectum. The frequent use of enemas can cause disturbances of the fluids and electrolytes in the body. This is especially true of tap water enemas.

Suppositories

As is the case with enemas, different types of suppositories have different mechanisms of action. There are stimulant suppositories containing **bisacodyl** (e.g. Dulcolax). **Glycerin** suppositories are believed to have their effect by irritating the rectum

Special situations

Palliative care

in this setting, it is important to consider differential diagnoses, such as malignant bowel obstruction, epidural cord compression, hypercalcaemia and medications as the cause of constipation. Symptom relief is paramount. Protocols for management of constipation have been developed locally in the UK and by the hospice movement and are freely available online, e.g. http://www.cancerhelp.org.uk/help/default.asp?page=1436

Spinal cord injury

Bowel dysfunction is common and disabling after spinal cord injury. The goal of treatment is to establish predictable and timely bowel evacuation as soon as possible, preventing constipation, faecal impaction or incontinence.

Liver failure

In patients with hepatic encephalopathy, plasma ammonia levels are high and treatment with lactulose is aimed at reducing or inhibiting GI ammonia production and by removal of ammonia from the gut.

Miscellaneous drugs

Several prescribed drugs that are used to treat medical diseases consistently cause (as a side effect) loose stools, even diarrhoea. There are several small studies that have examined these drugs for the treatment of constipation. **Colchicine** is a drug that has been used for decades to treat gout. Colchicine has also been demonstrated to relieve constipation effectively in patients without gout. **Misoprostil (Cytotec)** is a drug used primarily for preventing stomach ulcers caused by NSAIDs such as ibuprofen. Diarrhoea is one of its consistent side effects. Several studies have shown that misoprostil is effective in the short-term treatment of constipation. Misoprostil is expensive, and it is not clear if it will remain effective and safe with long-term use. Orlistat **(Xenical)** is a drug that is used primarily for reducing weight. It works by blocking the enzymes within the intestine that digest fat. In studies, orlistat has been shown to be effective in treating constipation. Orlistat has few significant side effects as very small amounts of the drug are absorbed from the intestine.

Conclusion

For the treatment of constipation arising due an intensive care admission, stimulant and osmotic laxatives should be used as first-line treatment as soon as the problem is identified. For patients with pre-existing constipation, treatment should be restarted as soon as possible. This may be more urgent in special circumstances such as spinal cord injury or liver failure.

Further reading

AGA guideline: constipation. *Gastroenterology* 2000; 119: 1761.

Als-Nielsen, B Gluud L, Gluud C. Nonabsorbable dissacharides for hepatic encephalopathy. *Cochrane Database Syst Rev* 2004; (2): CD003044.

BNF section 1.6 http://www.bnf.org/bnf/bnf/current/1001.htm

Locke GR III. AGA technical review on constipation. *Gastroenterology* 2000; 119: 1766.

Chapter 13

Neurological drugs

Chapter contents

Opioid and non-opioid analgesics in the ICU

Opioid analgesics

Opioid analgesic drugs remain the mainstay of pain relief in the Critical Care Unit. Abnormal GI function in the critically sick consequently makes enteral administration undesirable. IV administration remains the mainstay. Pharmacokinetic considerations consequent upon organ dysfunction leading to altered absorption, distribution and metabolism usually play the most important role in the choice of agent.

Most analgesics used on the ICU are metabolized via phase I or II pathways, and they are generally effectively metabolized in all but those with severe liver dysfunction. Metabolism is generally affected by liver blood flow rather than hepatocyte function. Opioids exert their analgesic action by binding to the opioid receptors at both spinal and supraspinal sites. Unwanted effects include bradycardia, miosis, hypothermia, nausea, urinary retention, respiratory depression and constipation.

Route of administration

The IV route is the most reliable way of delivering opioids in the critically ill. Extradural opioids have been used, often in combination with local anaesthetics; inhalational and transmucosal opioids are only rarely used. Patient-controlled modes of administration require a fully conscious and orientated patient, and are therefore only of limited value in the CCU.

Choice of drug

The most commonly used opioids are morphine, fentanyl, alfentanil and remifentanil

Morphine

Morphine is the most often prescribed agent because of its low cost, excellent analgesic efficacy and euphoric effects. It has a peak effect within 20min, and duration of action between 2 and 7h. It has low lipid solubility and volume of distribution, and its duration of action is determined by hepatic metabolism. It is metabolized by the liver to the water-soluble morphine-6-glucuronide and morphine-3-glucuronide, which are then renally excreted. Morphine-6-glucuronide is 2–800 times analgesically more potent than morphine and accumulates in renal dysfunction. This can lead to unwanted prolonged sedation and respiratory depression Morphine-3-glucuronide is not analgesically active.

Fentanyl, alfentanil and remifentanil

Fentanyl is a synthetic opioid; it is the preferred analgesic agent for critically ill patients with haemodynamic instability and for patients manifesting symptoms of histamine release with morphine or morphine allergy. Fentanyl is 50–100 times more potent than morphine; it has extremely low bioavailability and therefore can be given by any route other than the GI tract. It is extremely lipid soluble and has an onset of action within 30s, with a peak effect in 5–15min. It has a short half-life of 30–60min following redistribution, but accumulation in peripheral compartments can increase the half-life to 9–16h.

Fentanyl is metabolized in the liver to pharmacologically inactive metabolites, which are renally excreted. In critically ill patients with renal failure there is an increase in the volume of distribution and half-life of fentanyl. Fentanyl has minimal cardiovascular effects compared with morphine. Following a long infusion of fentanyl, accumulation may cause prolonged respiratory depression.

Alfentanil is a phenylpiperidine synthetic opioid. It has similar pharmacodynamic properties to the other newer opioids, but it shows considerable variability in its pharmacokinetic profile from patient to patient. Interindividual variability in alfentanil clearance is likely to result from differences in hepatic P450-3A4 expression and to P450-3A4-related drug interactions.

Remifentanil has an extremely short context-sensitive half-life and is independent of hepatic and renal function . In the cardiac- and neuro-ICU setting, remifentanil's short half-life is especially desirable. It allows good neurological assessment when required, profound haemodynamic stability and early extubation after bypass surgery. One study suggests that the intraoperative use might even reduce the need for a post-operative ICU stay after major abdominal surgery.

Table 13.1.1 outlines commonly use regimes for opioid infusion in Critical Care Units.

Table 13.1.1 Infusion rates for commonly used opioids in critical care

Drug	MEAC ng/ml	$t_{1/2}$ terminal (min)	Dose mcg/kg/h
Alfentanil	50–100	90	30–60
Fentanyl	1–3	185	1–5
Sufentanil	0.2–0.5	160–210	0.2–1.0
Remifentanil	n/a	10–20	30–60
Morphine	10–30	100–180	50–100

MEAC = minimally effective analgesic concentration.

Non-opioid analgesics

Non-steroidal anti-inflammatory drugs (NSAIDs)

NSAIDs have opioid-sparing effects and have both central and peripheral sites of analgesic activity. The use in the critically ill is however controversial. Their metabolism and excretion is dependent on liver and kidney function, both of which pathways are frequently impaired in the ICU patient. NSAIDs decrease the prostaglandin-dependent renal blood flow and are associated with an increased gastric ulceration risk. It seems prudent to avoid this class in the critically ill in the absence of any definite gain to be had.

A new class of agents has been developed that selectively inhibit the inducible cyclo-oxygenase enzyme, COX-2. By sparing physiological tissue prostaglandin production while inhibiting the COX-2-related inflammatory processes, these agents are thought to offer the potential of effective analgesia with fewer side effects than previous NSAIDs. They have been shown to be as effective as NSAIDs in the management of post-operative analgesia. Adverse effects on renal blood flow, which are similar those of to conventional NSAIDs, and concerns regarding potential prothrombotic effects of at least some of the COX-2 agents, will limit their use in the critically ill patient.

Ketamine

This IV anaesthetic agent has intense analgesic properties even at subanaesthetic levels, maintaining the airway, and has stimulatory effects on the respiratory and cardiovascular system. It is used in specific painful procedures, particularly in burn patients for dressing changes.

Hallucinations and emergence phenomena can be attenuated by the co-administration of benzodiazepines.

There is furthermore some evidence, that ketamine can be useful in chronic pain states such as central pain, complex regional pain syndrome, fibromyalgia and neuropathic pain. Either alone or in combination with opioids it provides rapid, effective and prolonged analgesia .

Neuropathic pain agents

Some patients may be suffering from or develop neuropathic pain. This sort of pain may be difficult to manage with standard analgesics, and consideration should be given to adding in specific drugs for neuropathic pain as outlined in Table 13.1.2. Patients may also have pre-existing neuropathic pain problems; medication should be continued where possible.

Table 13.1.2 Adjuvant therapies for pain in critical care.

Drug	Dose mg	Neuropathic pain	Sleep	PTSD
Tricyclic antidepressants	20–100 nocte	+	++	+
Gabapentin	100–900	++	+	+?
Pregabalin	25–300	++	+	+?

PTSD = post-traumatic stress disorder.

Adjuvant therapies

Especially in patients with features of chronic pain or altered sleep patterns, tricyclic antidepressants have been used extensively. There might be a rationale for using these drugs in the medium- to long-stay patient where a constellation of pain, anxiety and depression co-exists, possibly along with a disturbed sleep pattern. There is evidence that the usage of tricyclics, and possibly some of the drugs used to treat neuropathic pain, may reduce the development of post-traumatic stress disorder (PTSD) in ICU survivors.

Alternative therapies

No evidence exits to support the use of alternative therapies in the critically ill. In the absence of any untoward effects, however, the use of transcutaneous electrical nerve stimulation (TENS), acupuncture, aromatherapy, etc., should not be withheld. Anecdotal evidence suggests a benefit from acupuncture in neuropathic pain, and reduced sedative and analgesic requirements following aromatherapy.

Summary

Opioids are the most commonly used analgesic agents, often giving in combination with sedative drugs. There is no doubt that this method is effective and cheap, and staff have a wealth of experience in its use. However, such regimes do not provide satisfactory pain relief in all patients.

What is needed to avoid patients experiencing pain while in Ithe CU is individualized, goal-directed analgesic regimes in their own right, not as a side effect of sedation. In concert with analgesia, anxiety, the physical environment and the patient's sleeping pattern need to be considered. Adherence to a clear protocol may be as important as choice of medication.

Further reading

Barr J, Donner A. Optimal intravenous dosing strategies for sedatives and analgesics in the intensive care unit. *Crit Care Clin* 1995; 11: 827–47.

Breen D, Karabinis A, Malbrain M, *et al*. Decreased duration of mechanical ventilation when comparing analgesia-based sedation using remifentanil with standard hypnotic-based sedation for up to 10 days in intensive care unit patients: a randomised trial. *Crit Care*. 2005; 9: R200–10.

Curtis SP, Ng J, Yu Q, *et al*. Renal effects of etoricoxib and comparator nonsteroidal anti-inflammatory drugs in controlled clinical trials. *Clin Ther* 2004; 26: 70–83.

Kuhlen R, Putensen C. Remifentanil for analgesia-based sedation in the intensive care unit. *Crit Care* 2004; 8: 13–4.

Muellejans B, Matthey T, Scholpp J, *et al*. Sedation in the intensive care unit with remifentanil/propofol versus midazolam/fentanyl: a randomised, open-label, pharmacoeconomic trial. *Crit Care* 2006; 10: R91.

Roemsing J, Moeniche S. A systematic review of COX-2 inhibitors compared with traditional NSAIDs, or different COX-2 inhibitors for post-opereative pain. *Acta Anaesthesiol Scand* 2004; 48: 525–46.

Wilson W, Smedira N, Fink C, *et al*. Ordering and administration of sedatives and analgesics during the withholding and withdrawal of life support from critically ill patients. *JAMA* 1992; 267: 949–53.

http://www.anzca.edu.au/publications/acutepain.htm

Sedation management in ICU

Drugs with sedative, analgesic and neuromuscular blocking activity are used in different combinations to facilitate care of the critically ill. Sedative agents alleviate anxiety, reduce the stress response and improve tolerance of ICU interventions.

Indications for use of sedation

1. To maintain patient comfort while being managed within critical care areas.
2. To facilitate compliance with mechanical ventilation.
3. To help control raised ICP.
4. To manage anxiety, agitation and delirium.
5. To augment analgesia through the opiate-sparing effect of some sedative agents.

Prior to starting sedation, any underlying cause of discomfort or agitation should be treated. Furthermore, the undesirable effects of sedative infusions should be considered, as sedative use can complicate neurological assessment, prolong the duration of mechanical ventilation and increase length of stay in the ICU and the hospital .

The amnesic properties of some sedatives may modify post-traumatic stress (PTSD) by reducing recollection of unpleasant or frightening memories. Unfortunately, oversedation and withdrawal can contribute to PTSD symptoms.

Sedative agents

A number of drug classes with distinct features are available. Sedation can be administered by intermittent bolus dose or continuous infusion. IV infusions provide constant levels of sedation to increase patient comfort. However, their use is an independent predictor of increased length of stay in the ICU and the hospital .

Determining appropriate dosing of drugs can be difficult. The decreased protein binding and the impaired renal and hepatic function that occur in critical illness lead to changes in half-life and volume of distribution.

Benzodiazepines

Benzodiazepines are the most commonly used sedatives. They act on benzodiazepine receptors, which enhance the effect of γ-aminobutyric acid (GABA) on chloride channels, causing intracellular influx of chloride ions. This increases resting membrane potential, inhibiting excitation.

They have anxiolytic, anticonvulsant, amnesic and centrally mediated muscle relaxant properties.

- *Diazepam* has a rapid onset of action, and patients generally will awaken rapidly after a bolus dose. With continuous infusions, the half-life and active diazepam metabolites lead to a prolonged sedative effect.
- *Lorazepam* is eliminated by conjugation to inactive glucuronides. It has a slower onset of action, making it less useful for acute agitation, and a prolonged half-life, making it difficult to titrate.
- *Midazolam* has a rapid onset of action and a short half-life, making it ideal for the critically ill. Accumulation and prolonged sedative effects are reported in critically ill patients who are obese, in renal failure or have low serum albumin.. Prolonged sedative effects may also be caused by the accumulation of the active metabolite, α-hydroxymidazolam, or its conjugated salt.

Tolerance to benzodiazepines may occur within hours to several days of therapy, and escalating doses of midazolam have been reported. Benzodiazepines can also cause delirium (both hypo- and hyperactive forms).

Propofol

Propofol is a non-water-soluble propylphenol formulated as an aqueous emulsion in intralipid solution. It is a short-acting GABA agonist with sedative and hypnotic effects but no analgesic properties. The plasma level of propofol rapidly falls after discontinuation, and recovery time is short compared with other sedatives. This is due to redistribution from plasma to the tissues. With prolonged infusions, the tissues become saturated and recovery is longer. No changes in kinetic parameters have been reported in patients with renal or hepatic dysfunction.

Propofol improves control of ICP and decreases CBF and metabolism. Rapid awakening from propofol makes it useful for patients in whom frequent neurological assessment is needed.

Propofol causes a dose-dependent drop in blood pressure through reduced SVR and bradycardia. Also, the lipid base of propofol can function as a medium for bacterial growth, and long-term or high dose infusions may result in hypertriglyceridaemia, and some cases of pancreatitis have been reported.

Propofol infusion syndrome is a rare but lethal complication. It is reported in paediatric and occasionally in adult critical care. There is a severe metabolic acidosis, rhabdomyolysis, haemodynamic collapse and bradycardia progressing to asystole. This may be due to impaired fatty acid oxidation or inhibition of phosphorylation in the mitochondria. Risk factors include hypoxia, sepsis, cerebral injury and high propofol dose.

Whilst propofol has experimental evidence of anticonvulsant activity in animal models, abnormal epileptiform movement has been reported in clinical anaesthetic practice.

Etomidate

Etomidate is now rarely used in the ICU because it is associated with adrenocortical insufficiency and has been shown to increase mortality in critically ill patients.

Butyrophenones

Haloperidol has sedative effects, and boluses are used to alleviate delirium. Haloperidol infusions have been used successfully in the management of agitated patients in critical care. There is a risk of complete heart block, ventricular tachycardia and QTc prolongation—with the accompanying possibility of torsades de pointes.

Phenothiazines

Phenothiazines block muscarinic, α_1-adrenergic, H_1 histaminic, DA_1 and DA_2 receptors. They have antipsychotic properties that are mainly due to their DA_2 receptor blocking activity in the limbic system. Chlorpromazine 50–100mg can be administered IM, but IV bolus doses (2.5–10mg) cause severe hypotension. An infusion of 10–20mg/h is less likely to compromise blood pressure.

Central α_2 agonists

These include clonidine and dexmedetomidine.

Dexmedetomidine is a selective α_2 agonist. It has sedative and analgesic-sparing properties, and produces anxiolysis comparable with benzodiazepines. Rapid administration of dexmedetomidine leads to transient elevation of blood pressure, whilst dexmedetomidine infusions cause bradycardia or hypotension.

Volatile anaesthetic agents

Inhaled anaesthetic agents such as the halogenated hydrocarbon isofluorane can be administered via the breathing circuit, and these may be used when intolerance of other sedatives occurs or to help treat refractory bronchospasm. A concentration of 0.3–0.6% isofluorane should provide satisfactory sedation. A common problem on the ICU has been the requirement for an anaesthetic machine and scavenging of exhaled gases. The development of anaesthetic-conserving devices can allow the use of an ICU ventilator which does not need a gas-scavenging system.

Opioids

Whilst primarily used as analgesic agents, the sedative and antitussive properties of opioids enhance the effects of other sedatives. Whilst opioids have sedative effects, they do not diminish awareness or produce any sort of amnesia for stressful events.

Sedation monitoring

Ideally sedation should attain the goal of a calm ICU patient, easily aroused, with maintenance of the normal sleep–wake cycle. Some patients may require deeper levels of sedation to facilitate mechanical ventilation. Daily interruption of sedative infusions leads to reduction of duration of ventilation and length of stay. Subjective sedation scales as part of a protocol improve outcome and are recommended by international guidelines. Sedation and delirium scales such as the Richmond Agitation and Sedation Scale (RASS) and the Confusion Assessment Method (CAM-ICU) should provide accurate, reliable data that are simple to collect. A defined sedation goal, using sedation scales, can reduce length of stay.

Summary

- Sedation may facilitate invasive treatments for critically ill patients.
- Long-acting sedative drugs contribute to confusion and prolonged length of stay.
- Sedation monitoring should be routine in critical care.
- Sedation protocols incorporating monitoring and daily hold reduce length of stay.
- Short-acting drugs and non-benzodiazepine hypnotics look promising and need further evaluation

Further reading

Bailie GR, Cockshott ID, Douglas EJ, *et al.* Pharmacokinetics of propofol during and after long-term continuous infusion for maintenance of sedation in ICU patients. *Br J Anaesth* 1992; 68: 486–91.

Kam PC, Cardone D. Propofol infusion syndrome. Anaesthesia 2007; 62: 690–701.

Kelly DF, Goodale DB, Williams J, *et al.* Propofol in the treatment of moderate and severe head injury: A randomized, prospective double-blinded pilot trial. *J Neurosurg* 1999; 90: 1042–52.

Kollef MH, Levy NT, Ahrens TS, *et al.* The use of continuous i.v. sedation is associated with prolongation of mechanical ventilation. *Chest* 1998; 114: 541–8.

Sackey PV, Martling CR, Granath F, *et al.* Prolonged isoflurane sedation of intensive care unit patients with the Anesthetic Conserving Device. *Crit Care Med* 2004; 32: 2241–6.

Jacobi J, Fraser GL, Coursin DB, *et al.* Clinical practice guidelines for the sustained use of sedatives and analgesics in the critically ill adult. *Crit Care Med* 2002; 30: 119–41.

Kress JP, Pohlman AS, O'Connor MF, *et al.* Daily interruption of sedative infusions in critically ill patients undergoing mechanical ventilation. *N Engl J Med* 2000; 342: 1471–7.

Agent	Receptor	Dose (bolus)	Dose (infusion/ maintenance)	Plasma protein binding	Half-life (h)	Active metabolites	Elimination
Diazepam	BZ	0.03–0.1mg/kg q 0.5–6h		98%	20–120	Active metabolites desmethyldiazepam; 3-hydroxydiazepam; oxazepam	Desmethylation and hydroxylation produces active metabolites Conjugation of active metabolites to inactive glucuronides
Lorazepam	BZ	0.02–0.06mg/kg q 2–6 h	0.01–0.1mg/kg/h	90%	8–15	None	Conjugation to inactive glucuronides
Midazolam	BZ	0.02–0.08 mg/kg q 0.5–2h	0.04–0.2mg/kg/h	96%	3–11	α-Hydroxymidazolam	Hydroxylated by hepatic cytochrome P-450 to α-hydroxymidazolam and excreted by the kidney
Propofol	GABA		2–12mg/kg/h	98%	26–32		Conjugates of 2, 6-di-idopropyl-1, 4-quinol
Haloperidol		0.03–0.15mg/kg q 0.5–6h	0.04–0.15mg/kg/h		18–54		

BZ = benzodiazepine; GABA = γ-aminobutyric acid.

Muscle relaxants

Neuromuscular blockade is used in as an aid to intubation and as an adjunctive treatment for particular situations in the already ventilated and adequately sedated patient.

Physiology

Depolarization of the motor neuron results in the fusion of vesicles containing acetylcholine with the neuronal membrane, each releasing ~10 000 molecules of acetylcholine into the synaptic cleft. The acetylcholine receptors are grouped together on the postsynaptic membrane at the motor end plate by a complex series of steps during synapse formation that depend upon the action of agrin released from the nerve and rapsyn within the muscle fibre. The synaptic cleft is only 20nm, enabling rapid association of acetylcholine with the receptor, opening non-selective ion channels and resulting in membrane depolarization and calcium influx into the muscle fibre. The available pharmaceutical agents act on the nicotinic acetylcholine receptor (nAChR) on the postsynaptic membrane.

Depolarizing blockers

Suxamethonium is the only available depolarizing blocker, it acts by binding the nAChR, resulting in ion channel opening and muscle depolarization; it then occupies the receptor for far longer than acetylcholine, preventing further depolarization until it has dissociated from the receptor and diffused away to be metabolized by plasma cholinesterase.

Use

Suxamethonium is used in rapid sequence induction and intubation at a dose of 1.0–1.5mg/kg. Its onset of action is <1min and duration is usually 7–8min.

Cautions

Potassium is released from muscles during depolarization and serum levels rise by 0.5–1.0mmol/l following suxamethonium. Avoid in hyperkalaemia.

Any cause of severe immobility or dennervation results in a decrease in acetycholine release, and this in turn causes upregulation of acetylcholine receptors. The receptors produced are also of a 'fetal' type, resulting in an increased sensitivity to suxamethonium, failure to aggregate at the muscle end plate and increased ion flux when activated.

Under these conditions, suxamethonium can cause a dramatic rise in potassium, leading to cardiac arrest, and must be **avoided**.

> Avoid suxamethonium in:
> - Hyperkalaemia
> - Burns (if >24h after injury)
> - Crush injuries (if >2 days after injury)
> - Guillain–Barré syndrome
> - Spinal cord injury
> - Stroke
> - Prolonged immobilization or neuromuscular blockade (i.e. do not use or use with great caution for the re-intubation of intensive care patients).

One in 3200 patients are homozygous for plasma cholinesterase deficiency and will remain paralysed for 3–8h.

Suxamethonium can cause malignant hyperthermia (see Chapter 22.13) and should also be avoided in those with a family history of myotonia and those with muscular dystrophy. Suxamethonium is less effective in conditions reducing the number of acetylcholine receptors, such as myasthenia gravis. Due to the tonic contraction, its use is often avoided in patients with penetrating ocular injury and raised ICP, although this is an area of debate.

Non-depolarizing blockers

There are two classes of acetylcholine receptor competitive antagonists, aminosteroids and benzylisoquinolinium compounds; however, the differences in the functional properties of each agent are more important clinically.

Aminosteroids

Pancuronium is long acting with a half-life of 100–130min, a time of onset of 1–3min and is 60–80% eliminated by the kidneys, the remainder being hepatic. Its duration is therefore increased in renal and hepatic failure. It is vagolytic, and use can result in tachycardia which may be undesirable in the critically unwell.

Vecuronium is shorter acting (half-life 80–90min) with a time of onset of 1.5–3min and is only 10–20% eliminated by the kidneys, the remainder being hepatic metabolism; however, one of its highly active metabolites is eliminated by the kidney and it has been associated with prolonged blockade following infusion. It is not vagolytic.

Rocuronium has a very rapid onset of 1.0–1.5min, and this has led to its use in modified rapid sequence induction in those patients in whom suxamethonium is contraindicated. If propofol is used as an induction agent, the incidence of 'acceptable' intubating conditions is the same as for suxamethonium; however, if the more stringent 'excellent' intubating conditions are applied, suxamethonium is better (RR 0.87)

Rocuronium has a half-life of 60–100min and is <10% eliminated by the kidney, the remainder being hepatically metabolized; its duration of action increases in hepatic failure and in the elderly.

Benzylisoquinolinium compounds

Atracurium has an intermediate duration of action, with a half-life of 21min and an onset of 2.0–2.5min. It has the great advantage of being metabolized by Hofmann degradation and ester hydrolysis, making it ideal for patients with renal or hepatic dysfunction (although degradation is slowed in acidosis and hypothermia). It can cause histamine release and hypotension. An inactive metabolite, laudanosine, causes seizures in dogs, but even in very prolonged administration in humans this does not appear to reach toxic concentrations or cause problems.

Cisatracurium is a potent isomer of atracurium with very similar properties, except dosing is 70% lower and therefore there is less histamine release, hypotension and laudanosine production.

Mivacurium is metabolized by plasma cholinesterases, has an onset of 1.5–2.5min and a duration of action of only 2–5min. Its use in the critically ill has not been extensively investigated.

Clinical use of prolonged muscular blockade

There is a distinct lack of good evidence from trials for the use of prolonged neuromuscular blockade in intensive care. The following are areas where neuromuscular blockade is used when conventional therapies are failing and/or adequate sedation and analgesia alone fail to produce the desired effect.

Facilitating mechanical ventilation

Whilst it is becoming more unusual with modern ventilators, there are occasions when patient–ventilator asynchrony impacts negatively on gas exchange despite prolonged attempts to adjust ventilator settings and increasing sedation. Evidence for benefit in the literature is lacking, and the use of muscular blockade must be approached on a case by case basis. Beware that some patients suffer clinically significant worsening of ventilation–perfusion mismatching on paralysis; if this happens don't do it again to that patient! Whilst there is no particular reason why it is necessary if sedation is adequate, some ICUs paralyse patients who are being turned prone to improve their ventilation.

Reduction of oxygen consumption

This is often cited as a reason for paralysing difficult to oxygenate patients. However, the literature does not support the efficacy of this. Again, in the most difficult patients, it is often attempted and should be done so on a case by case basis.

Shivering when actively cooling

When actively cooling patients for therapeutic reasons shivering can limit the cooling process and potentially result in a harmful increase in metabolic demand. In this context, the use of muscular blockade to allow further cooling may be necessary.

Muscle spasm and hyperpyrexia

Rarely, conditions such as tetanus can lead to dangerous and intractable muscle spasms, and muscular blockade may be necessary to allow adequate ventilation. In the specific case of malignant hyperpyrexia, dantrolene is used as it acts directly on the muscle to prevent release of calcium from the sarcoplasmic reticulum and therefore uncouples myocyte contraction. The dose of dantrolene is 1mg/kg repeated as necessary to a maximum of 10mg/kg. It has also been used in severe neuroleptic malignant syndrome.

Management of raised ICP

Once again the evidence for doing this is rather limited; however, there are situations when everything else has been done and the pressure is still high. Most ICUs will have a protocol for managing raised ICP, and neuromuscular blockade will feature somewhere, usually before barbiturate coma or craniectomy.

There is no particular reason to use paralysis for transfer of patients with raised ICP if adequate sedation can be achieved; however, we all know that despite very high doses of sedation and analgesia some patients still gain additional relaxation and a fall in ICP following neuromuscular blockade, particularly during transfers and procedures. Use it in conjunction with ICP monitoring on a case by case basis.

Monitoring

Is essential when using prolonged neuromuscular blockade. The first monitor is clinical assessment:

Is the blockade adequate?

This will depend on the indication; to achieve ventilator synchrony a very small degree of block may be enough, whereas to abolish a cough reflex in a patient with critically raised ICP a much higher degree of block is required.

Is the blockade too much?

The best clinical assessment is to have frequent 'block breaks'. If bolus blockade is being used, wait until movement starts to cause problems again before giving more; if an infusion is used a daily hold is an absolute minimum, and 12 hourly may be more appropriate. This answers two questions: first, do they still need muscular blockade as well as sedation; and, secondly, are they receiving an appropriately titrated dose.

Electrical stimulation 'twitch testing'

Should always be used as an objective adjunct to clinical assessment. There are various guidelines used; however, in general, the presence of clinically adequate block but with at least two out of four contractions on a 'train of four' test still present can be regarded as an appropriately titrated dose.

Essential care

Patients who are paralysed must have special attention paid to:

- Pressure areas (including peripheral nerve compression)
- Physiotherapy and joint mobility
- Deep vein thrombosis prophylaxis
- Eye care and closure

⚠ Problems and complications

Prolonged paralysis and neuropathy

This is the most significant complication of using neuromuscular blockers. Prolonged recovery from neuromuscular blockade may be a simple pharmacodynamic phenomenon in the critically ill patient failing to metabolize the drugs as predicted. Many drugs can potentiate the duration of neuromuscular blockade; rather than learning lists, just stick to regular suspension of the infusion and be aware of your individual patient's clinical response and recovery.

More severely, neuromuscular blockade is a major risk factor for critical care myopathy, or acute quadriplegic myopathy syndrome (AQMS). It is not possible to screen for AQMS, and only 50% of patients have a measured rise in serum creatine phosphokinase concentration. Concomitant steroids are especially high risk for severe myopathy. There may also be an increased risk with aminoglycoside antibiotics or cyclosporin.

Further reading

Murray MJ, Cowen J, DeBlock H, *et al.* Clinical practice guidelines for sustained neuromuscular blockade in the adult critically ill patient. *Crit Care Med* 2002; 30: 142–56.

Perry J, Lee J, Wells G. Rocuronium versus succinylcholine for rapid sequence induction intubation. *Cochrane Database of Syst Rev* 2003; (1): CD002788.

Anticonvulsant drugs

Anticonvulsant drugs are commonly used in intensive care patients, most often in patients with established epilepsy or in patients being treated specifically for status epilepticus (SE). This chapter discusses in detail the anticonvulsant drugs commonly used to treat SE.

First-line drugs: benzodiazepines

Diazepam

Diazepam is very effective in SE, and has been extensively studied. As with all benzodiazepines, its mechanism of action is via potentiation of the inhibitory neurotransmitter GABA. It can be administered by IV bolus injections or rectally, and has a rapid onset of action. Good brain levels are attained within 1min of a standard IV dose. Rectal administration produces a peak level after 20min. It is highly lipid soluble, is rapidly redistributed and therefore has a short duration of action. Sedation and hypotension may occur, and after repeat dosing, diazepam accumulates, resulting in persisting high peak levels. This may result in sudden and unexpected CNS depression and cardiorespiratory collapse. Diazepam is metabolized by hepatic enzymes.

Bolus IV diazepam should be given undiluted at a rate not exceeding 2–5mg/min, with standard adult bolus dose being 10–20mg, with additional 10mg doses being given at 15min intervals to a maximum of 40mg. It should not be mixed with other drugs.

Lorazepam

Lorazepam has a smaller volume of distribution and is less lipid soluble than diazepam. It has a slower onset but a longer duration of action. It has significant advantages over diazepam. It does not accumulate in lipid stores, and has strong cerebral binding and a long duration of action due to its distribution half-life. Lorazepam is extremely effective in status, and it is effective for up to 12h after a single dose (longer than diazepam). Its main disadvantage is the rapid development of tolerance, with repeated doses being much less effective. It shares the sedating side effects of all benzodiazpeines, but sudden cardiorespiratory collapse is much less likely because of its relative lipid insolubility and the lack of accumulation after a single dose.

It is administered by IV bolus, and, as distribution is slow, the rate of injection is not critical. In adults, a bolus dose of 0.07mg/kg to a maximum of 4mg is given, which can be repeated once after 20min if required. It is usually available as a 1ml ampoule of 4mg/ml.

Midazolam

Unlike other benzodiazepines, midazolam is water soluble but becomes lipophilic at physiological pH, allowing rapid transfer across the blood–brain barrier. It may therefore be used buccally, intranasally and IM, as well as via the IV route. Buccal midazolam (10mg in 2ml) has been shown to be as effective as rectal diazepam (10mg) in the management of acute seizures in children. Because it is water soluble, midazolam takes 3 times longer than diazepam to peak EEG effects, and therefore repeat dosing should be delayed by several minutes to assess sedative effects fully. Its action is short lived because of a short half-life, and therefore the relapse rate is high after a single bolus injection. It is more suited as the benzodiazepine of choice for use as an infusion, as it is less likely to accumulate because of its smaller volume of distribution and kinetic characteristics. As with other benzodiazepines, it causes sedation, hypotension, respiratory depression and occasional respiratory arrest.

Midazolam bolus can be used in early status at a dose of 5–10mg IV, which can be repeated once after 15min. If used as an infusion in intensive care, a loading dose of 0.15mg/kg should be administered, followed by an infusion of 0.05–0.4mg/kg/h. It is available in 5ml ampoules containing 2mg/ml, or a 2ml ampoule containing 5mg.

Second-line drugs

Phenytoin

This is a drug of first choice in established SE. It is highly effective and has a long duration of action. It can also be continued as long-term treatment. It causes minimal respiratory or cerebral depression, although hypotension is more common. Initial infusion takes 20–30min in adults, and the onset is slow. It therefore needs to be given in conjunction with a short-acting rapid onset benzodiazepine. It is well known that phenytoin has easily saturable pharmacokinetics, but this is less of a problem in the acute setting. However, careful monitoring of level is required. It must be given in normal saline to prevent precipitation, and must not be mixed with other drugs for the same reason. It should not be given IM because of erratic absorption, and can cause thrombophlebitis. Other CNS effects can occur in the acute setting, particularly at high doses, such as nystagmus and ataxia. Other adverse effects include nausea and vomiting, rash and hepatic blood dyscrasias.

If the drug is then continued in the longer term via the oral route once the status has been abolished, then its interaction with other drugs may become problematic. This is because it is highly protein bound and because it is metabolized via the P450 enzyme system and is therefore a powerful inducer of hepatic enzymes. Phenobarbitone and carbemazepine have variable and unpredictable effects (either increase or decrease) on phenytoin levels since they both induce and compete for hepatic enzymes. Sodium valproate may elevate phenytoin levels by displacing it from its protein-binding site and also by inhibiting its metabolism. It decreases levels of many other drugs, including phenobarbitone. It inhibits carbemazepine, warfarin, oestrogens, benzodiazepines and corticosteroids. Other drugs whose levels are reduced by phenytoin and require monitoring and adjustment include frusemide and cyclosporin. Drugs that significantly increase phenytoin levels include isoniazid, omeprazole, cimetidine and sulfonamides. Drugs that lower phenytoin levels include amiodarone.

Adult loading does is 15–18mg/kg, and the rate of administration should not exceed 50mg/min, with a lower infusion rate (<20mg/min) in the elderly. Phenytoin is usually available as 5ml ampoules containing 250mg of phenytoin sodium.

Fosphenytoin

This is an inactive water-soluble phenytoin prodrug, which is metabolized to phenytoin. The equimolar equivalent of 1mg of phenytoin is 1.5mg of fosphenytoin, and is supplied in a ready mixed solution of 50mg phenytoin equivalents (PE) per ml (i.e. 75mg/ml). This is to standardize the solution to that of parenteral phenytoin. Fosphenytoin can be given at three times the rate of phenytoin, and should be given at 150mg/min. Fosphenytoin is completely bioavailable following IM administration, although it is not routinely recommended in the treatment of SE as this route has not been well studied in this particular circumstance. Peak concentration occurs at 30min after administration. The half-life is 15min. Although more expensive, it causes less thrombophlebitis, less hypotension and is better tolerated and easier to administer. Hepatic or haemopoietic adverse reactions, like those seen with phenytoin, also may occur.

Phenobarbitone

This is also a drug of choice in the treatment of established status. It is highly effective, has a rapid onset of action, has prolonged anticonvulsant effect and may also have a cerebral protective effect. Tolerance is unusual, and once seizures are controlled they usually do not recur. There is also some evidence that if given with barbiturate anaesthesia it can reduce the risk of relapse following anaesthetic withdrawal. The disadvantages are excessive sedation, hypotension and respiratory depression. Skin reactions are rare. With more prolonged therapy after the initial treatment of status, there is a risk of accumulation, and therefore blood level monitoring is essential. Although it is a very stable drug, it should not be given via the IV infusion with other agents (e.g. phenytoin) as precipitation may occur.

Similarly to phenytoin, it is a powerful hepatic enzyme inducer, and therefore also may increases the metabolism of oestrogen, steroids, warfarin, benzodiazepines and carbemazepine. Its effect on phenytoin is unpredictable.

Loading adult dose in adults is 10mg/kg (doses up to 20mg/kg have been used), at a rate of 100mg/min, followed by maintenance of 1–4mg/kg/day (either IV or orally). Phenobarbitone is usually available in 1ml ampoules containing 200mg.

Sodium valproate

Sodium valproate is available in IV form and, although it is not recommended as first-line treatment for established SE, it may be a useful third-line agent, which some units administer before using general anaesthetic agents. It is certainly useful for administration to patients who for any reason cannot take their usual dose of valproate by mouth, or whose serum level of valproate is low and must be increased quickly. In general, it is well tolerated, but patients with known liver dysfunction or mitochondrial disease may not be good candidates for this drug. Cases of pancreatitis have been reported after IV valproate.

Valproic acid is given as an IV loading dose of 20mg/kg dissolved in normal saline and infused at a rate of 20–50mg/min.

Third-line drugs: anaesthetic agents

Thiopentone

Thiopentone is used for barbiturate anaesthesia in SE. It is a very effective anticonvulsant drug, and may have cerebral-protective effects. The most significant side effect is hypotension, and many patients require pressor therapy. It also has saturable pharmacokinetics and a strong tendency to accumulate. If high doses are given, blood levels may remain high despite discontinuation, and days may pass before recovery of consciousness. Blood monitoring is essential, of both thiopentone and its metabolite pentonbarbitone. Other toxic effects include hepatic and pancreatic disturbance, and rarely acute hypersensitivity. It should be used with caution in the elderly, and in those with hepatic, renal or cardiac dysfunction. Thiopentone should be made up in normal saline and should not be administered with other drugs.

The following regime is recommended in SE: a 100–250mg bolus over 20s, with further 50mg boluses every 2–3min until seizures are abolished, with intubation and ventilation. An infusion of 3–5mg/kg/h should continue to attain a blood level of ~40mg/l. After 24h, metabolism may be at saturation, and blood levels should be measured once or twice daily to ensure they are not excessive. Thiopentone should continue until seizure activity has ceased as monitored by burst suppression on EEG for 12–24h. The usual preparation is a vial containing 2.5g with 100ml of dilutant to produce a 2.5% solution.

Propofol

This non-barbiturate anaesthetic agent is also used in the treatment of resistant SE. Although it has significantly less inherent antiepileptic properties compared with thiopentone, there is growing evidence of its usefulness in the management of status, and its ease of use offers some advantages. It also has neuroexcitatory effects, which can cause muscle rigidity or abnormal movements including myoclonus, which can be mistaken for seizures. Seizures have, however, been reported to occur occasionally with propofol withdrawal. It is extremely lipid soluble and has a high volume of distribution, and thus acts rapidly in SE. It remains effective during continuous infusion, and a major advantage is that recovery of consciousness following discontinuation is very quick. It causes profound respiratory and cerebral depression, but hypotension is uncommon and cardiac side effects are few. Long-term use (e.g. in patients with prolonged intractable status) causes lipaemia, acidosis and rhabdomyolysis.

The dose may need to be reduced when administered with ongoing use of benzodiazepines, opiates and phenothiazines. It may potentiate neuromuscular blockade of vecuronium. Higher doses may be required with concomitant theophylline administration.

In SE, a bolus of 1–2mg/kg is administered, followed by an infusion of 1–5mg/kg/h, as guided by the EEG burst suppression pattern. After the patient has been seizure free for 12–24h, the dose can be gradually reduced over 24h to minimize the risk of rebound seizures. It is available as 20ml ampoules containing 10mg/ml as an emulsion.

Further reading

Kumar A, Bleck TP. Intravenous midazolam for the treatment of refractory status epilepticus. *Crit Care Med* 1992; 20: 483–8.

Limdi NA, Shimpi AV, Faught E, *et al.* Efficacy of rapid IV administration of valproic acid for status epilepticus. *Neurology* 2005; 64: 353–5.

Lowenstein DH, Alldredge BK. Status epilepticus, *N Engl J Med* 1998; 338: 970–6

Shorvon SD. Status epilepticus: its clinical features and treatment in children and adults. Cambridge: Cambridge University Press, 1994.

Shorvon S, Dreifuss F, Fish D, *et al.* The treatment of epilepsy. Oxford: Blackwell Science Ltd, 1996.

Cerebroprotective agents

Cerebroprotection is the prevention or reduction of brain injury from an ischaemic or hypoxic insult before or during the time of insult. **Neuroresuscitation** refers to prevention or reduction of injury after the injury has occurred.

Understanding the pathophysiology of ischaemia is essential as this points to which agents might work. The ischaemic cascade involves release of excitatory neurotransmitters (such as glutamate), opening of cell membrane channels to allow calcium and sodium influx, generation of free radicals and ultimately membrane depolarization. Cell death occurs via two processes:

- Necrosis: early, via process of inflammation.
- Apoptosis: delayed, via mitochondrial and DNA damage.

Cerebroprotective agents inhibit one or more points along the path of cell death. Ideal agents would also enhance repair.

Clinical models requiring cerebroprotection generally involve either focal or global cerebral ischaemia. These include stroke, traumatic brain injury (TBI), vasospasm following aneurysmal subarachnoid haemorrhage (aSAH), cardiac arrest and cardiopulmonary bypass.

Despite extensive preclinical evidence, most clinical trials have so far failed to demonstrate clear cerebroprotective efficacy. Much of this is a reflection of the limitations of preclinical and clinical trials. The timing of therapy appears critical, i.e. early institution or even initiation prior to the insult. It is likely that multitherapy is the most effective strategy.

The following list is by no means exhaustive. Focus is on those agents which currently show promise.

Pharmacological cerebroprotection

N-methyl-D-aspartate (NMDA) antagonists

Proposed mechanism of action: blockade of excitotoxic activity. Many have dose-limiting side effects in humans. Multiple clinical trials in stroke and TBI have failed to prove efficacy. An RCT of 171 patients undergoing coronary artery bypass graft (CABG) demonstrated a reduction in neuropsychological deficit at 2 months in patients receiving *remacemide* pre- and post-operatively .

Anaesthetic agents

Proposed mechanisms of action: reduction in CMR and reduction in ICP, both of which may limit secondary damage, sodium channel blockade, inhibition of lipid peroxidation, free radical scavenging and potentiation of GABA-mediated inhibition. Clinical trials are small and inconclusive. The Brain Trauma Foundation guidelines for the management of severe traumatic brain injury include thiopentone as 2nd tier therapy for severe refractory intracranial hypertension. Although cerebroprotection has not been conclusively demonstrated, thiopentone, propofol and volatile agents may extend the window of ischaemic tolerance.

Magnesium

Proposed mechanism of action: inhibition of glutamate release, NMDA receptor blockade, calcium channel blockade, vasodilation. Large clinical trials in stroke and TBI have failed to demonstrate clear benefit. The MAGPIE trial demonstrated a significant reduction in the incidence of eclampsia in women with pre-eclampsia, which may be relevant to the discussion of cerebroprotection. The FAST-MAG trial is designed to evaluate the effect of early administration of magnesium on outcome in acute stroke patients. Magnesium loading dose is delivered in the field by paramedics within 2h of symptom onset. A phase III trial in aSAH patients is currently underway The aSAH clinical model has the advantage that the cerebroprotective intervention can be in place *before* the insult (vasospasm) occurs.

Erythropoietin

Erythropoietin (EPO) secretory sites and receptors have been identified within the brain. Hypoxia and other stressors may result in increased production of EPO and expression of EPO receptors (*hypoxic cerebral pre-conditioning*).

Proposed mechanisms of action: blockade of apoptosis pathway at multiple steps (both neuronal and endothelial cells), enhancement of neurogenesis and angiogenesis. A phase II clinical trial has shown safety in stroke patients. A phase II trial in aSAH patients is currently underway.

HMG CoA reductase inhibitors (statins)

Proposed mechanisms of action: anti-inflammatory (reduced thrombogenesis and platelet activation), improved vasomotor reactivity (upregulation of endothelial NOS), reduced generation of reactive oxygen species. Two large clinical trials have demonstrated the role of statins in the prevention of stroke. There is some evidence that statins may reduce the ischaemic deficit following vasospasm in aSAH patients . A phase III clinical trial is currently underway.

Progesterone

Proposed mechanism of action: reduced excitotoxicity through GABA-mediated inhibition, alteration of blood–brain barrier to reduce oedema formation, inhibition of apoptosis, anti-inflammatory. A phase II clinical trial has demonstrated safety in TBI patients .

Hypothermia

A wealth of preclinical trials point to hypothermia as a cerebroprotectant. This is likely to be due to more than reduction of the CMR, as even mild hypothermia (T = 34°C) appears beneficial. Proposed mechanisms of action include reduction in excitoxicity, lipid peroxidation and free radical damage. Promising phase II trials in TBI did not translate into a positive phase III study. Clifton *et al.* investigated the effect of hypothermia (target T 33°C within 8h of injury) on outcome at 6 months following TBI. The study was halted after enrolment of 392 of planned 500 patients because the treatment was not effective. Patients >45yrs had poorer outcomes. The current NABIS:H IIR trial by the same investigators examines the effect of hypothermia (target T 33°C within 4h of injury) in patients <45yrs.

Two trials published simultaneously demonstrated that mild to moderate therapeutic hypothermia improves neurological outcome after cardiac arrest. Although the studies were relatively small (77 patients and 273 patients, respectively), their conclusion has been incorporated into ILCOR recommendations for advanced life support of unconscious patients with spontaneous circulation after out-of-hospital cardiac arrest . Importantly, the need for avoidance of hyperthermia is stressed.

Other strategies

Decompressive craniectomy

Wide decompressive craniectomy to reduce raised ICP makes good sense in terms of prevention of secondary brain injury. It has been well described in the setting of TBI and stroke. Two large multi-centre trials involving TBI patients are currently underway.

Maintenance of cerebral blood flow and oxygenation

Whilst the search for definitive cerebroprotective agents continues, preventative and supportive strategies must not be forgotten. Careful attention to maintenance of CBF is paramount. Targets should be set to achieve adequate CPP, appropriate arterial carbon dioxide tension, promotion of cerebral venous drainage and early control of raised ICP. Cerebral oxygen delivery needs to meet cerebral oxygen requirements. Early airway protection, controlled ventilation, appropriate sedation, control of seizures and prevention of hyperthermia will all promote cerebral oxygen demand vs supply balance. These fundamental strategies remain the mainstay of cerebral protection.

Further reading

Amarenco P, Bogousslavsky J, Callahan A 3rd, *et al*, Stroke Prevention by Aggressive Reduction in Cholesterol Levels (SPARCL) Investigators. High-dose artorvostatin after stroke or transient ischemic attack. *N Engl J Med* 2006; 355: 549–59.

Arrowsmith JE, Harrison MJ, Newman SP, *et al.* Neuroprotection of the brain during cardiopulmonary bypass: a randomised trial of remacemide during coronary artery bypass in 171 patients. *Stroke* 1998; 29: 2357–62.

Clifton GL, Miller ER, Choi SC, *et al.* Lack of effect of induction of hypothermia after acute brain injury. *N Engl J Med* 2001; 344: 556–63.

http://www.clinicaltrials.gov/ct/show/NCT00178711

http://www.braintrauma.org/guidelines

http://www.fastmag.info

http://www.rescueicp.com

http://www.stashtrial.com

http://www.surgery.cuhk.edu.hk/imash-trial

Lynch JR, Wang H, McGirt MJ, *et al.* Simvastatin reduces vasospasm after aneurysmal subarachnoid hemorrhage: results of a pilot randomized clinical trial. *Stroke* 2005; 36: 2024–6.

Muir KW, Lees KR, Ford I, *et al.* Magnesium for acute stroke (Intravenous Magnesium Efficacy in Stroke trial): randomised controlled trial. *Lancet* 2004; 363: 439–45.

Temkin NR, Anderson GD, Winn HR, *et al.* Magnesium sulphate for neuroprotection after traumatic brain injury: a randomised controlled trial. Lancet *Neurol* 2007; 6: 29–38.

The Hypothermia after Cardiac Arrest Group. Mild therapeutic hypothermia to improve the neurologic outcome after cardiac arrest. *N Engl J Med* 2002; 346: 549–56.

Tseng MY, Czosnyka M, Richards H, *et al.* Effects of acute treatment with pravastatin on cerebral autoregulation, and delayed ischemic deficits after aneurysmal subarachnoid haemorrhage: a phase II randomized placebo-controlled trial. *Stroke* 2005; 36: 1627–32.

Wright DW, Kellermann AL, Hertzberg VS, *et al.* ProTECT: a randomised clinical trial of progesterone for acute traumatic brain injury. *Ann Emerg Med* 2007; 49: 391–402.

Mannitol and hypertonic saline

Introduction

The capillary endothelial cells within the brain are connected via tight junctions forming a blood–brain barrier (BBB). The BBB is a semi-permeable membrane that limits bulk movement of fluid from the brain capillaries into the parenchyma. The BBB is moderately permeable to water but relatively impermeable to small solutes and proteins. Glucose and certain amino acids are actively transported across the BBB. The BBB is not present in the choroid plexus or in certain areas of the hypothalamus.

The BBB may be disrupted by pathology, especially in head injuries and anoxic insults. When this occurs, there is flow of proteins and electrolytes into the brain parenchyma creating a hydrostatic pressure that results in fluid movement into the tissue. This is known as vasogenic oedema. Cytotoxic oedema is due to swelling of the neuronal and/or glial cells, frequently results from hypoxic injury and is the predominant process in the very acute stages following brain injury.

Mannitol

Mannitol is a low molecular weight solute (182Da) that can be added to crystalloid solution to make it hyperosmolar. It is commonly used as a 20% solution (1098mosm/kg). The European Brain Injury Consortium and the Brain Trauma Foundation recommended mannitol as the osmotic drug of choice in brain-injured patients. The Brain Trauma Foundation recommends 2ml/kg of 20% mannitol, infused over 20min, for patients with clinical signs of raised ICP or deteriorating neurological function, before ICP monitoring is instituted. These guidelines are based on studies that show better ICP control and slightly better outcomes in patients given mannitol compared with barbiturate coma. As such, there remains considerable confusion over the optimal treatment regime, the effectiveness of mannitol, especially compared with hypertonic saline solutions, and the timing of its usage.

Actions of mannitol

Mannitol reduces ICP within a few minutes. Distribution is rapid, with a half-life of ~10min. Its diuretic action occurs within 1–4h, such that its beneficial effects cannot result from it being an osmotic diuretic. Serum osmolarity is increased following mannitol administration. This draws water into the vascular compartment from all tissues (including the brain), resulting in a temporary increase in blood pressure. If autoregulation is intact, the increase in CPP will cause cerebral vasoconstriction and consequent reduction in ICP. The haematocrit is reduced following mannitol administration. This may also increase CBF and oxygen delivery. Mannitol also decreases CSF production, which leads to a reduction in cerebral volume and consequently a reduction in ICP. It is also a free radical scavenger.

Mannitol does accumulate in the interstitium following repeated doses. If this rises significantly, there is a theoretical risk that the normal gradient between brain and blood is reversed and cerebral oedema is worsened. If repeated doses are given, it is prudent to measure serum osmolality. The concern that toxicity is induced if the serum osmolality exceeds 320mosm/kg is largely theoretical. It is important to ensure that patients do not become dehydrated through repeated mannitol usage as that may worsen cerebral injury and increase the risk of renal impairment. There is no evidence that administration of mannitol results in reduction of cerebral water content from normal brain alone, causing a worsening of midline shift in the presence of a mass lesion.

Practical administration

The priorities in the management of a patient with acute intracranial hypertension, from whatever cause, are the same as for all critically ill patients, namely ABC (control of airway, breathing and circulation). The airway must be protected, 100% oxygen applied and the pCO_2 controlled between 4 and 5kPa. These may require intubation and ventilation. ICP should be presumed to be at least 20mm Hg in a patient who is comatose, and the cerebral perfusion pressure (CPP = MAP – ICP) should be maintained above 60mm Hg, with the use of inotropes as necessary. If the patient shows signs of coning at any stage (pupillary dilatation and/or contralateral hemiparesis), 2ml/kg of 20% mannitol should be administered. This dose can be repeated if there is no response or if signs of coning recur. As detailed above, this is not a treatment but rather a holding measure until other therapies can be employed. Hypotension, secondary to the diuretic effects of mannitol, should be avoided, as this may cause secondary brain injury. The use of high doses of mannitol as a rescue therapy for patients with a GCS of 3 and pupillary abnormalities has been discredited.

Hypertonic saline

Hypertonic saline (HTS) is an attractive alternative to mannitol as an osmotic agent. The BBB permeability to sodium is low, thus producing an osmotic gradient where the BBB is intact. Administration of HTS produces an increase in circulating blood volume and consequent rise in CPP. HTS may also modulate the inflammatory response by reducing leucocyte adhesion to the endothelium. HTS does not have the diuretic properties of mannitol, thus reducing the risk of hypotension and volume depletion following its usage. A variety of concentrations of HTS are available ranging from 3% (1026mosm/kg) to 23.4% (8008mosm/kg).

Animal studies have suggested that HTS may be more effective than mannitol in reducing raised ICP, and with a longer duration of action. In adult patients with raised ICP, HTS has been shown to produce a significant decrease in ICP that correlates with increasing serum osmolarity. Interestingly, the effects of HTS seem to extend long after the osmotic effects have disappeared and to be poorly correlated with serum sodium concentration. HTS may produce decreases in ICP in patients who are refractory to the action of mannitol, suggesting that the two agents have differing mechanisms of action. Outcome studies in the adult population are limited. A number of trials have reported the beneficial effects of HTS in paediatric populations where it has been used largely as an infusion rather than as bolus, rescue therapy. Osmolalities have been allowed to rise as high as 371mOsm/kg.

HTS may cause a number of systemic side effects. These include coagulopathies, fluid overload and electrolyte disturbances. In particular, HTS may cause a non-anion gap metabolic acidosis, hypokalaemia and hypocalcaemia. Concerns regarding renal impairment, central pontine myelinolysis and rebound increases in ICP have not been confirmed. HTS of >2% concentration should be given via a central venous catheter due to the risk of thrombophlebitis, thus limiting its usage in the pre-hospital setting.

Rebound oedema may occur if hyperosmolar therapy has been prolonged, leading to equilization of the osmolar gradient across the BBB. Within a few hours of hyperosmolar therapy, levels of intracellular electrolytes and organic osmoles increase. These restore cell size to normal despite the hyperosmolar state. When hyperosmolar therapy is discontinued, a reverse gradient may be established, leading to an increase in brain water content. It is therefore, important to wean hyperosmolar solutions slowly.

Further reading

Ogden AT, Mayer SA, Connolly ES Jr. Hyperosmolar agents in neurosurgical practice: the evolving role of hypertonic saline. *Neurosurgery* 2005; 57: 207–15.

Task Force of the American Association of Neurological Surgeons and Joint Section in Neurotrauma and Critical Care. Guidelines for the management of severe head injury. *Brain Trauma Foundation,* 1995.

Wakai A, Roberts I, Schierhout G. Mannitol for acute traumatic brain injury. *Cochrane Database Syst Rev* 2007; (1): CD001049.

Chapter 14

Haematological drugs

Chapter contents

Anticoagulants and heparin-induced thrombocytopenia

Introduction

For >50 years, the options for therapeutic anticoagulation were limited to unfractionated heparin (UFH) and oral vitamin K antagonists. While highly effective, both drugs have major safety problems. Both have narrow therapeutic ranges, substantial interindividual dose variability, major side effects and require regular therapeutic drug monitoring, with a narrow therapeutic window and high incidence of bleeding complications.

Low molecular weight heparins (LMWHs; 1980s) represented a substantial advance in therapeutic anticoagulation. Predictable pharmacokinetics with thus no requirement for monitoring, as well as a longer half-life and thus less frequent dosing, and a lower frequency of heparin-induced thrombocytopenia (HIT). In the 1990s several new parenteral anticoagulants appeared, including the synthetic heparin derivatives fondaparinux and the direct thrombin inhibitors argatroban, hirudin and bivalirudin. The present decade sees the emergence of an exciting new generation of oral anticoagulants, which do not require routine therapeutic monitoring. These are mainly oral direct thrombin inhibitors such as Dabagatran and oral antiXa agents such as Rivaroxaban.

Unfractionated heparin

Composition

UFH is a naturally occurring glycosaminoglycan produced by mast cells and basophils derived from tissues rich in mast cells, such as porcine intestine or bovine lung. The heparin molecule is a polymer of repeating disaccharide units, primarily comprising sulfated glucosamine and uronic acid. Heparin is a heterogeneous mixture of differing chain lengths, but most preparations have a mean molecular weight of 13 000–15000Da.

Mechanism of action and pharmacology

The anticoagulant activity of heparin is mediated by endogenous antithrombin, a physiological inhibitor of coagulation. A specific pentasaccharide sequence of the heparin molecule binds to antithrombin inducing a conformational change and a 1000-fold increase in antithrombin activity. In turn, antithrombin inhibits thrombin and factor Xa, both essential factors for normal coagulation. Only the pentasaccharide sequence is required for the inhibition of factor Xa (anti-Xa activity), whereas a longer sequence of 18 saccharides, including the pentasaccharide, is necessary for thrombin inhibition.

Anticoagulant activity in different heparins depends on the distribution of heparin chain molecular weights. The activity of heparins is standardized in either International Units (IU) as determined by the World Health Organization international standard, or United States Pharmacopoeial (USP) units. Heparins are only active when administered parenterally; IM administration should be avoided as it can result in large haematomas. The half-life of IV UFH is 45–60min, demanding continuous IV infusion for effective anticoagulation. UFH given SC has a lower bioavailability than IV heparin. By the SC route, UFH activity starts at 2h and lasts ~10h, necessitating twice daily administration.

Dosing

Treatment with IV UFH is usually initiated with an IV bolus over 5min (5000IU for a 70kg adult) followed by continuous IV infusion (15–25IU/kg/h, or 1400IU/h for a 70kg adult). The aPTT ratio (aPTT-R) is measured 4–6h after commencing the infusion, and the rate of infusion adjusted accordingly. Thereafter, the APTT-R should be monitored at least once every 24h, as heparin requirements can change rapidly over time. The platelet count should be checked before starting UFH and repeated at least every other day between days 4 and 14 of UFH treatment. If the patient has received heparin within the last 100 days, platelet count monitoring should begin within 24h of starting heparin to monitor for HIT.

Prophylactic doses of SC UFH range from 5000 to 7500IU bd. aPTT monitoring is not required when prophylactic doses are used, but the platelet count should be monitored as HIT can occur.

The aPTT is sensitive to both thrombin and factor Xa inhibition. The aPTT can be expressed in seconds or as a ratio to a control aPTT time (aPTT-R). An aPTT-R of 1.5–2.5 is usually associated with therapeutic anticoagulation, but because aPTT reagents have differing heparin sensitivity, local reference ranges should be used. Clinical use of the activated clotting time is now restricted to monitoring the very high heparin doses used for anticoagulation in extracorporeal circuits.

Reversal

As IV UHF has a short half-life, cessation of the infusion is usually sufficient for the management of mild bleeding symptoms. For more severe bleeding, rapid reversal of the anticoagulant activity of UFH can be with 1mg protamine for every 100IU of heparin given within the previous hour up to a maximum of 40–50mg protamine. The dose can be repeated if necessary. Protamine is a protein derived from fish milt, and can lead to allergic reactions.

Indications and contraindications

The main indication in UK hospitals is perioperative bridging of warfarin in patients with mechanical heart valves, during vascular surgery and extracorporeal circuits, and in renal failure. Otherwise for the treatment of venous thromboembolism and thromboprophylaxis, UFH has been largely superseded by LMWH except in renal failure. The only absolute contraindications to all types of heparin are current major bleeding or confirmed history of HIT, especially if in the last 100 days.

Adverse effects

A slight fall in platelet count (of <30% compared with baseline) occurs in up to 1/3 of patients within the first 4 days of starting heparin. This is a reversible dose-dependent phenomenon, not associated with bleeding or thrombosis, and does not require cessation of heparin.

Falls in platelet count of >50% compared with baseline should raise the possibility of HIT. HIT is a life-threatening complication of heparin treatment and occurs in 0.3–6.5% of those receiving UFH. The onset is typically between 5 and 10 days after starting UFH, unless heparin has previously been administered, in which case it may begin earlier. The cause is development of an IgG antibody to heparin and platelet factor 4, which forms a complex capable of activating and depleting platelets. Because the thrombocytopenia is due to platelet activation, patients with HIT are paradoxically at high risk of both venous and arterial thrombosis; bleeding is rare. Other features may include necrotizing skin changes at heparin injection sites or a history of anaphylactic reactions to heparin injection. A clinical scoring system for suspected HIT has been developed, and can be useful in determining the need for further investigation.

The diagnosis of HIT may be confirmed by specific enzyme-linked immunosorbent assay (ELISA) or by functional platelet studies. The treatment is immediate cessation of all heparins (including line flushes and including LMWH), and initiation of an alternative anticoagulant such as danaparoid, hirudin or fondaparinux at therapeutic doses. Platelet transfusion is contraindicated, and warfarin should not be started until the platelet count has recovered, as it may cause microvascular necrosis.

Low molecular weight heparins

LMWHs are produced by the depolymerization of UFH.

Mechanism of action and pharmacology

The anticoagulant activity of LMWHs is mediated by antithrombin. An antithrombin-binding pentasaccharide sequence alone is required for the inhibition of factor Xa (anti-Xa activity), whereas a longer sequence of 18 saccharides, including the pentasaccharide, is required for the bridging function necessary to inhibit thrombin. This explains the higher ratio of anti-Xa to anti-IIa activity of smaller LMWH molecules.

In contrast to UFH, which is rapidly cleared by the reticuloendothelial system, LMWHs are cleared slowly by a renal mechanism. In those with normal renal function, the bioavailability and clearance of SC LMWHs are sufficiently predictable to allow dosing without monitoring.

Dosage and monitoring

LMWHs should be dosed according to the manufacturer's instructions.

Given the renal clearance of LMWHs, bleeding complications are more common; with renal failure, dose adjustment is necessary and should be guided by monitoring of the anti-Xa level or UFH should be used.

One of the advantages of LMWHs is that routine monitoring is not necessary unless there is renal failure or in morbidly obese patients.

If monitoring is required, the aPTT is not sufficiently sensitive to anti-Xa activity so direct measurement of plasma anti-Xa activity is required. As anti-Xa activity declines rapidly *in vitro*, analytic samples must be rapidly transported to the laboratory on ice, centrifuged at 4°C, separated and either assayed immediately or frozen at –70°C for subsequent analysis. Target anti-Xa ranges vary by LMWH product and indication; manufacturers' data should be consulted. Because of the risk of HIT, patients receiving LMWHs should have a baseline platelet count on the day of starting treatment, and platelet counts every 2–4 days between days 4 and 14 of treatment.

Reversal

Most bleeding complications can be managed by dose reduction or cessation of LMWH. For severe bleeding, partial reversal of the anticoagulant activity of LMWH can be achieved with 1mg protamine for every 100IU of LMWH given within the previous 8h (maximum 40–50mg protamine); this can reverse up to 90% of anti-IIa and 60% of anti-Xa activity. A partial return of LMWH anticoagulant activity may be seen 3h after reversal due to continued LMWH absorption from the SC injection site. Protamine can be re-administered if necessary.

Adverse effects

HIT is rare when compared with the rate with UFH. Patients with cutaneous reactions to LMWHs may tolerate other LMWH formulations or danaparoid, but cross-reactivity rates are high. Fondaparinux is a useful alternative in this scenario.

Danaparoid

Danaparoid sodium is a low molecular weight heparinoid derived from animal intestinal mucosa. It is a mixture of heparan, dermatan and chondroitin sulfates, and, like LMWHs, inhibits factor Xa via antithrombin, with little anti-IIa activity. Danaparoid is administered parenterally, either IV or SC, and has an elimination half-life of 24h. It is used primarily for the treatment of HIT. Clearance of danaparoid is partially renal, so dose reduction and therapeutic monitoring is required in patients with renal failure. There is no specific reversal agent for danaparoid—it is not neutralized by protamine sulfate.

Coumarins

The coagulation factors II, VII, IX and X, as well as the naturally occurring anticoagulants protein C and S, are dependent upon vitamin K. In each case, synthesis of the functional protein requires the post-translational γ-carboxylation of N-terminal glutamine residues, and warfarin antagonizes the effect of vitamin K.

Peak serum concentrations are reached at ~3h of oral administration, and the half-life is 36–42h. Warfarin is highly protein bound, mainly to albumin. Despite rapid absorption of warfarin and other coumarins, the onset of the anticoagulant effect is delayed as it requires the gradual depletion of functional coagulation factors. Metabolism is hepatic, requiring the cytochrome P450-2C9 hepatic microsomal enzyme.

A number of genetic and environmental factors affect the absorption, pharmacokinetics and pharmacodynamics of coumarins. Genetic polymorphisms of the CYP2C9 enzyme are primarily responsible for differences in warfarin metabolism. The most common polymorphisms, CYP2C9*2 and CYP2C9*3, are each seen in ~10% of Caucasians, and are associated with a reduced warfarin requirement. A small proportion of individuals (<1%) have a hereditary resistance to coumarins mediated by reduced affinity of the coumarin receptor and require very large doses of coumarins (e.g. ≥30mg warfarin daily) to achieve an anticoagulant effect.

Interactions

Foods rich in vitamin K1 (phytonadione) reduce the efficacy of coumarins by overcoming its inhibition of vitamin K recycling. Numerous drugs and herbal remedies are known to interact with coumarins and alter the anticoagulant effect. In addition, antiplatelet agents, including NSAIDs, can lead to an increase in bleeding risk.

Monitoring

Because of the considerable interindividual variability in dose requirements, and the myriad food and drug interactions, coumarins require routine therapeutic monitoring of the INR.

Reversal

Administration of vitamin K1 can reverse the anticoagulant effects of coumarins, but takes at least 6h, as it necessitates the *de novo* production of active γ-carboxylated coagulation factors by the liver.

A dose of 10mg vitamin K will make anticoagulation with coumarins difficult during the following 2 weeks, so 1mg vitamin K may therefore be preferable in patients without life-threatening bleeding.

FFP contains all the vitamin K-dependent coagulation factors, and can reverse warfarin when given at a dose of 15–20ml/kg. As the half-life of factor VII is short, vitamin K replacement should be given concomitantly.

Prothrombin complex concentrates (PCCs) are plasma-derived products containing the vitamin K-dependent coagulation factors in a concentrated form. The activity of PCCs is usually expressed in terms of units of factor IX, the typical dose required for warfarin reversal being 20IU/kg in a slow IV push over several minutes. Although more expensive than FFP, PCCs have the advantage of a small volume of administration, rapid preparation (no thawing required) and more complete reversal of warfarin activity. They are the treatment of choice when fast reversal is required. As with FFP, vitamin K replacement should be given in conjunction with PCCs.

Adverse effects

The principal adverse effect of coumarins is bleeding, with a risk of fatal haemorrhage of 0.25%/yr in unselected patients, the risk being much higer in critical care patients. In individuals with hereditary protein C deficiency, coumarin-induced skin necrosis due to microvascular thrombosis can occur. This complication can be avoided by using an alternative anticoagulant (e.g. a LMWH) during coumarin loading.

Synthetic pentasaccharides

Fondaparinux

Fondaparinux is a synthetic pentasaccharide—consisting of the antithrombin-binding pentasaccharide sequence found in the heparin molecule. Like LMWHs, fondaparinux binds the antithrombin molecule causing a conformational change, which enhances its activity against factor Xa. Because there are no additional saccharides to provide the necessary bridging function for thrombin binding, fondaparinux has no anti-thrombin activity.

Fondaparinux is given as an SC injection and has a half-life of 17h, making it suitable for once-daily dosing. Clearance is exclusively renal, so it is not recommended in those with a creatinine clearance of <30ml/min. Fondaparinux does not bind to platelet factor 4, so has no capacity to cause HIT. The dose is 2.5mg SC once daily for thromboprophylaxis and acute coronary syndrome, or 7.5mg SC once daily for treatment of venous thromboembolism.

There is no specific reversal agent for fondaparinux—protamine sulfate is ineffective. Experimental data indicate that recombinant activated factor VII may partially reverse the anticoagulant effect of fondaparinux.

Parenteral direct thrombin inhibitors

Unlike heparins, direct thrombin inhibitors are not dependent on endogenous antithrombin for their anticoagulant effects.

Hirudin

Hirudin is a 65 amino acid polypeptide, originally discovered in the saliva of the medicinal leech, *Hirudo medicinalis*. Two recombinant derivatives are available: lepirudin and desirudin. Hirudin is an irreversible direct thrombin inhibitor, binding to both the active and substrate recognition sites of the thrombin molecule. Hirudin is given either as an IV infusion or by twice-daily SC injection. It is not active orally.

As the clearance of hirudin is exclusively renal, the half-life is highly dependent on renal function. With normal renal function, hirudin has a half-life of 60min after IV administration, but in those with end-stage renal failure the half-life can be as long as 300h.

Hirudin requires therapeutic monitoring. The aPTT is usually used, with a typical target aPTT-R of 2.0–2.5. The ecarin clotting time may be a better alternative for hirudin monitoring, but is less widely available.

Hirudin is licensed for the treatment of thrombosis associated with HIT. Its major adverse effect is bleeding. 40–70% of patients develop hirudin antibodies after a week of treatment. The antibodies are rarely inhibitory, but may bind to hirudin and reduce renal clearance, resulting in a prolongation of half-life.

There is no specific reversal agent for hirudin. Options in bleeding patients include blood product support, activated prothrombin complex concentrates or recombinant activated factor VII. Hirudin is not cleared by haemodialysis.

Bivalirudin

Bivalirudin is a recombinant 20 amino acid polypeptide analogue of hirudin. It binds to the substrate-binding site of thrombin, but, unlike hirudin, can be cleaved by thrombin itself, making bivalirudin a reversible thrombin inhibitor. Bivalirudin has a half-life of 25min following IV injection. Because only a proportion of excretion is renal, clearance is less dependent upon renal function than for hirudin. Bivalirudin is monitored using the aPTT or ecarin clotting time. Because of its short half-life, the clinical use of bivalirudin is usually restricted to the management of acute coronary symptoms and to anticoagulation during PCI.

There is no specific reversal agent for bivalirudin. Because of the short half-life, bleeding can be managed with blood product support alone until the anticoagulant activity declines.

Argatroban

Argatroban is a small molecule reversible thrombin inhibitor derived from the amino acid arginine. It is only active parenterally. The half-life is ~40min, and clearance is primarily hepatic. Dose adjustment is recommended in those with moderate liver failure. Argatroban is monitored using the aPTT. As with hirudin and bivalirudin, there is no specific reversal agent. Argatroban has been used principally in the management of HIT and during percutaneous coronary procedures in patients at risk of HIT.

Thromboprophylaxis in critical care patients

Such is the risk of venous thromboembolism in patients admitted for critical care, that thromboprophylaxis should be administered unless there is a bleeding risk. Each ICU should have a policy for using thromboprophylaxis. The reader is referred to the gold standard of thromboprophylaxis, the American College of Chest Physicians guidelines.

Further reading

Avling BM. How I treat heparin-induced thrombocytopenia and thrombosis. *Blood* 2003; 31: 31–7.

Baglin T, Barrowcliffe TW, Cohen A, *et al.* Guidelines on the use and monitoring of heparin. *Br J Haematol* 2006; 133: 19–34.

Baglin T, Keeling DM, Watson HG *et al.* Guidelines on oral anticoagulation (warfarin): third edition—2005 update. *Br J Haematol* 2005; 132: 277–85.

Geerts WH, Bergqvist D, Pineo GF, Heit JA, Samama CM, Lassen MR, Colwell CW. Prevention of venous thromboembolism: American College of Chest Physicians Evidence-Based Clinical Practice Guidelines (8th Edition). *Chest.* 2008; 133(6 Suppl):381S–453S.

Keeling D, Davidson S, Watson H, *et al.* The management of heparin-induced thrombocytopenia. *Br J Haematol* 2006; 133: 259–69.

Lo GK, Juhl D, Warkentin TE, *et al.* Evaluation of pretest clinical score (4 T's) for the diagnosis of heparin-induced thrombocytopenia in two clinical settings. *J Thromb Haemostasis* 2006; 4: 759–65.

Mueller RL, Scheidt S. History of drugs for thrombotic disease. Discovery, development, and directions for the future. *Circulation* 1994; 89: 432–49.

Thrombolysis

The thrombotic and fibrinolytic systems are exquisitely balanced. This ensures the rapid generation of thrombus and its localization at the site of vessel injury. Fibrinolysis prevents the excess deposition of fibrin and enables its rapid removal. This minimizes the potential disruption to the blood supply. Fibrinolysis is a surface-bound phenomenon, with most of the events being catalysed by fibrin itself. It is frequently stated that fibrin is the architect of its own destruction.

Definition of thrombolysis

Thrombolysis is the infusion of thrombolytic agents to dissolve or directly destroy thrombi in blood vessels. Thrombolysis uses integral parts of the fibrinolytic pathway to achieve thrombus destruction. It is used in the management of AMI, acute ischaemic stroke, PE and aterial occlusion involving thrombus. The key to the successful use of thrombolysis is identifying those patients who are most likely to benefit from treatment and to initiate treatment as promptly as possible. Close observation is required because of the inherent increased risk of bleeding associated with these agents.

Physiology of fibrinolyis

The major components of the fibrinolytic system are plasminogen, plasmin and tissue plasminogen activator (tPA). Plasminogen is produced in the liver and is incorporated into thromboses as they are formed. The generation of fibrin and its binding to tPA leads to an increased affinity of tPA for plasminogen. This leads to the generation of plasmin at the site of the fibrin clot. Plasmin proceeds to digest the fibrin chains in an asymmetrical pattern, producing fibrin degradation products and dissolving the thrombus. Fibrinolysis is inhibited by the actions of plasminogen activator 1 (PAI-1) and α_2-antiplasmin (α_2-AP). PAI-1 acts directly on tPA to antagonize its action. This process is summariaed in Figure 14.2.1. The decreased level of fibrinogen causes an increase in the INR and aPTT; the thrombin time is prolonged.

Three agents are used in clinical practice for thrombolysis: streptokinase, urokinase and alteplase (recombinant tPA).

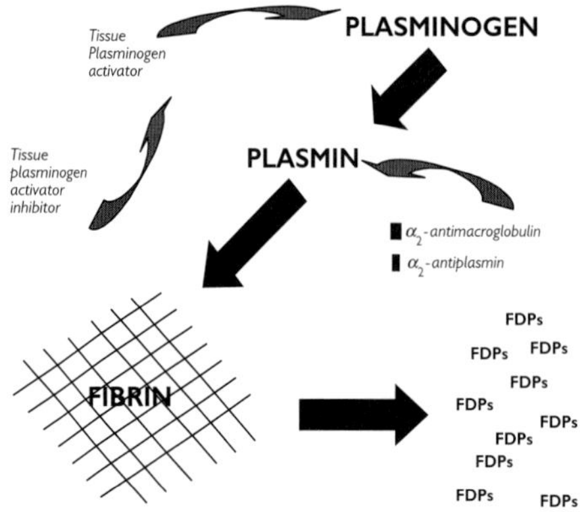

Fig. 14.2.1 Overview of thrombolysis.

Streptokinase

Streptokinase is a produced by β-haemolytic *Streptococcus*, and was the first agent to be used for thrombolysis on a large scale. The benefits of streptokinase were confirmed in the Second International Study of Infarct Survival. In this study, the addition of streptokinase led to a significant reduction in mortality in patients who had suffered an AMI. Streptokinase works by binding to and activating plasminogen. Streptokinase has a short half-life of ~20min. Streptokinase stimulates an antibody response. This limits the ability to give a repeat dose. When antibody titres to streptokinase are high, treatment with streptokinase is unlikely to produce satisfactory thrombolysis.

Urokinase

Urokinase directly activates plasminogen; it is also known as urokinase-type plasminaogen activator (u-PA). It was initially isolated from human urine. When compared with streptokinase, it does not induce an antigenic response. Urokinase is mainly used for clearing thrombosed indwelling central venous catheters.

Tissue plasminogen activator

tPA plays a central role in limiting and localizing the normal haemostatic response. tPA is a serine protease and is produced by the endothelium. It is the major naturally occurring physiological enzyme responsible for converting plasminogen to plasmin. Recombinant tPA has now been synthesized. It does not produce an antigenic response. It is also moderately more effective than streptokinase at clot lysis. It is currently the first-line choice in the UK for thrombolysis when urgent percutaneous coronary angiography is not available. tPA has a half-life of ~5min and is rapidly cleared from plasma by the liver.

Contraindications to thrombolysis

The major contraindications to thrombolysis are a recent stroke, the presence of a cerebral malignancy or metastases, and pregnancy. The risk of haemorrhagic complications is significantly increased in patients who have undergone recent surgery, or those with significant retinopathy or a profound coagulopathy. The clinical decision to use it must be made after a careful assessment of the potential risks and benefits.

Factors influencing a successful outcome

The age and nature of the thrombus are key factors influencing the speed of lysis. The younger the thrombus, the greater the chance of success. Arterial thrombi tend to resolve more promptly than venous thrombi, and continuous catheter-directed infusion is preferable to bolus infusion.

Myocardial infarction

All the currently available trials show that thrombolytic agents reduce the mortality in acute STEMI. The GUSTO-1 trial showed that recombinant tPA was superior to streptokinase. Thrombolysis has resulted in a 30% reduction in the mortality from MI.

Acute limb ischaemia

The most important treatment for acute limb ischaemia to try to prevent limb loss is the rapid initiation of anticoagulation with heparin. This prevents further propagation of the thrombus and stimulates tPA release. Thrombolysis in these patients can help to buy time before a definitive procedure can be undertaken. It can open up vessels to allow a graft or enable a subsequent angioplasty.

Pulmonary embolism

Thrombolyis for PE remains a controversial issue. In view of the potentially life-threatening consequences of thrombolytic therapy, it should be reserved only for cases where the diagnosis has been confirmed and there is evidence that the PE is causing haemodynamic compromise or RV failure (i.e. a massive PE). It is worth considering that hypotension requiring vasopressor support is an independent risk factor for massive haemorrhage post-thrombolysis. Studies suggest that thrombolysis produces a short-term improvement in oxygenation and haemodynamic function. Specifically there is evidence to suggest that it leads to a lower pulmonary artery pressure and PVR. However, there is no overall impact on mortality, even in those patients who have suffered a massive PE. It is reasonable to continue to have PE as a specific indication for thrombolysis as it can be life saving for individual patients. Doses vary considerably, but a dose of tPA of 100mg infused over 2h has been recommended in the ACCP guidelines. The patient should also receive anticoagulation with heparin.

Further reading

Buller HR, Agnelli G, Hull RD, *et al.* Antithrombotic therapy for venous thromboembolic disease: the Seventh ACCP Conference on Antithrombotic therapy for venous thromboembolic disease. *Chest* 2004; 126: 401s.

ISIS-2. ISIS-2 (Second International Study of Infarct Survival) randomised trial of intravenous streptokinase, oral aspirin, both or neither among 17,187 cases of suspected myocardial infarction: Lancet 1988; 2: 349–60.

Thabut G, Thabut D, Myers RP, *et al.* Thrombolytic therapy of pulmonary embolism: ameta-analysis. *J Am Coll Cardiol* 2002: 40: 1660–7.

The GUSTO Investigators. An international randomized trial comparing four thrombolytic strategies for acute myocardial infarction. *N Engl J Med* 1993: 329: 673–82.

Antifibrinolytics

Tranexamic acid (*trans*-4-aminomethylcyclohexane-1-carboxylic acid) is a synthetic lysine analogue that is a competitive inhibitor of plasmin and plasminogen. There is large variation in dose used. *In vitro* studies have suggested a dose of 10mcg/ml is required to inhibit fibrininolysis. Tranexamic acid is distributed throughout all tissues, and the plasma half-life is 120min, with most of it being renally excreted. Studies of plasma levels confirmed that the Horrow regime, which has been shown to reduce blood loss in cardiac surgery, of 10mcg/kg followed by 1mg/kg/h, attained theses levels. Other studies have used up to 5g per patient with no ill-effect. A Cochrane review has shown no increased thrombotic risk with tranexamic acid or EACA.

EACA (ε-aminoncaproic acid) is also a synthetic lysine analogue that has a potency that is 10 times weaker than tranexamic acid. It is therefore administered in a loading dose of 150mg/kg followed by a continuous infusion of 15mg/h. The initial elimination half-life is 1–1.15h and therefore must be administered by continuous infusion in order to maintain therapeutic drug levels.

Aprotinin is a broad-spectrum serine protease inhibitor isolated from bovine lung, which forms irreversible inhibitory complexes with a number of serine proteases. In particular, it is a powerful antiplasmin agent. The initial elimination of aprotinin is 1.5–2h and, like the synthetic antifibrinolytics, it is renally excreted. In cardiac surgery, the 'high-dose' or Hammersmith regime, i.e. 2million KIU to the patient and cardiopulmonary bypass prime, and an infusion of 500 000 KIU/h) has been shown to reduce perioperative bleeding in open cardiac surgery. Lower doses do produce adequate antiplasmin effects. It is licensed in a dose of 2million units to treat hyerfibrinolysis.

A recent Food and Drug Administration (FDA) warning was issued to cover the use of aprotinin. This was based on two studies in cardiac surgery. An open study by Manago *et al.* suggested that aprotinin usage in cardiac surgery was associated with an increased risk of MI, stroke and renal failure, and another study by Karkonti *et al.* cited an increased risk of renal problems in those receiving aprotinin when compared with tranexamic acid. However, Manago's study was open and it remains unclear whether the perhaps sicker patients received aprotinin. A randomized triple blinded study of aprotinin vs tranexamic acid vs EACA (BART), has shown that there is an increased morbidity & mortality in the aprotinin-treated group. At the current time, due to the current FDA warning on aprotinin, its greater costs and need to give a test dose, which is often impractical in an emergency situation, tranexamic acid and EACA are to be preferred. A dose of tranexamic acid 1–2gm is recommended by the authors in emergency situations where hyperfibrinolysis is suspected.

Further Reading

Fergussion DA, Hébert PC, Mazer CD, *et al.* BART Investigators. A comparison of aprotinin and lysine analogues in high-risk cardiac surgery. *N Engl J Med.* 2008;358(22):2319–31. Epub 2008 May.

Henry DA, Carless PA, Moxey AJ, *et al.* Antifibrinolytic use for minimising perioperative allogeneic blood transfusion. *Cochrane Database Syst Rev.* 2007 Oct 17;(4):CD001886. Review.

Chapter 15

Miscellaneous drugs

Chapter contents

Antibiotics

Introduction

Infection is a common reason for admission to an ICU and a common complication of stay in an ICU. The presence of infection in patients in ICU is an important risk factor for increased mortality and morbidity.

Antimicrobial chemotherapy remains the cornerstone of therapy of patients with infection, and antibiotics are one of the most common therapies administered in the intensive care setting. Often antibiotic use in ICUs is for (empirical) treatment of infections, for prophylaxis such as in selective digestive decontamination of the digestive system (SDD), for prevention of ventilator-associated pneumonia (VAP) or for non-antimicrobial use such as the use of erythromycin as a prokinetic agent for gut motility.

The effective management of infection in ICU requires an integrated multi-disciplinary approach involving intensivist(s), infectious disease (ID) physician/microbiologist and pharmacists, systematic and comprehensive diagnostic measures, use of appropriate antimicrobial therapy and supportive care.

Important issues in antimicrobial management of infection in ICU patients

Severity of infection

('Severe') sepsis is the most common reason for admission to ICU. The reported incidence of sepsis in ICU is as high as 35%, with mortality rates from 27 to 54% in sepsis and septic shock, respectively. Patients developing nosocomial sepsis in ICU generally have significant co-morbidities and risk factors for complex, difficult to treat drug-resistant infections, associated with high mortality.

Whist fever in an ICU patient is the most common trigger for treatment with broad-spectrum antibiotics, it is a non-specific sign of infection. At the same time, its importance as an important early warning signal of sepsis must be appreciated.

Early appropriate antimicrobial therapy

The key to ensuring survival in severe sepsis is the combination of antibiotic therapy and rapid removal of infected tissue or devices.

Two very important aspects of 'early appropriate antimicrobial therapy' are:

1 ***'Time-to-first dose'*** of antibiotic': intensive monitoring, close supervision and expertise generally, of staff in the ICU, means that sepsis is more rapidly diagnosed compared with most emergency departments and, other hospital wards/units. Yet, sepsis in ICU carries a very high mortality.

   The international guidelines for the management of patients with severe sepsis; recommend initiation of antibiotic therapy within 1h of presentation (recommendation grade E, i.e. level of evidence IV or V). Rather alarmingly, only 50% of septic shock patients receive antibiotics within 6h of onset of hypotension!

   This necessitates a concerted effort in ICU and pharmacy staff to ensure that the first dose is ordered stat, it is readily available as a supply of pre-mixed antibiotics and is administered concomitantly with other resuscitative measures without waiting until after the blood pressure is normalized.

2 ***The new treatment paradigm:*** *'getting therapy right first time'.*

'Appropriate (empirical) antimicrobial therapy' is comprises of 4 Rs:

1 **Right drug–bug match**; in other words, using the 'best guess antibiotic' targeting the 'most likely pathogens'.
2 **Right regimen**: Dose, route, frequency, duration.
3 **Right tissue concentration** for effective eradication,
4 **Right cost**, i.e. cost-effectiveness.

Factors influencing choice of initial (empirical) therapy

Epidemiology of infection

Nearly half of the infections in ICU patients are acquired before admission to ICU and usually before admission to hospital, in the community (community-acquired); and, approximately half of infections are acquired following admission to ICU (hospital/ICU-acquired). The community-acquired pneumonias and intra-abdominal sepsis are the most common community-acquired infections treated in ICU, and VAP and central intravascular catheter-related bacteraemia are the most common nosocomial infections seen in the ICU.

Antibiotic resistance

ICUs are usually the 'hot zone' of antibiotic resistance, and pathogens such as methicillin-resistant *Staphylococcus aureus* (MRSA) have become endemic in many ICUs. There are several risk factors for emergence of antimicrobial resistance such as:

- Selective pressure from use of broad-spectrum antibiotics for empirical therapy of septic patients.
- Crowding of patients with complex medical problems into a small area.
- Use of invasive devices, e.g. central lines, catheters, etc., for monitoring or therapeutic purposes.
- Immunocompromised status of critically ill patients.
- High intensity of care required by ICU patients providing greater opportunities for cross-transmission of infection between patients and from the contaminated environment by the healthcare workers from lapses in infection control.

Current challenges of antibiotic-resistant bacteria in ICU are:

MRSA: MRSA strains are all resistant to: β-lactams; penicillins (oxacillin, flucloxacillin, amoxicillin/co-amoxiclav, etc.), cephalosporins and carbapenems (meropenem/imipenem/ertapenem). **Hospital/healthcare-acquired MRSA** (HA/HACI MRSA) strains are multi-drug resistant (MDR), i.e. in addition to β-lactams, they are resistant to other multiple classes of antibiotic such as macrolides (erythromycin, clarithromycin) and quinolones (ciprofloxacin, moxifloxacin, levofloxacin), and are distinct from **community-associated MRSA** (CA-MRSA) strains. CA-MRSA is an emerging pathogen in patients without traditional risk factors for HA/HCAI MRSA (e.g. recent hospitalization, prior antibiotic therapy, recent surgery, nursing home residence, etc.), carries a distinctive virulence factor (the **panton-valentine leucocidin, PVL**), causes mainly skin and soft tissue infection and, less frequently, necrotizing pneumonia, involves predominantly children and young adults and is usually susceptible to multiple classes of antimicrobials such as erythromycin, co-trimoxazole, chloramphenicol and fluroquinolones. **Anti-MRSA treatment options** are mainly IV vancomycin and IV teicoplanin. Clinical isolates of vancomyin intermediate, and vancomycin-resistant *Staphylococcus aureus* (VISA and VRSA) have also been reported.

Newer agents include:

Linezolid (IV/PO 600mg every 12h) is a member of a new class of antibiotics, the oxazolidinones, with a novel mechanism of inhibition of microbial protein synthesis without risk of cross-resistance with other protein synthesis inhibitor antibiotics such as macrolides, clindamycin, etc. It is 100% bioavailabile by the IV and oral route, is a suitable alternative to vancomycin, particularly in MRSA pneumonia, but can cause reversible myelosuppression and optic neuropathy on prolonged therapy.

Daptomycin (IV 4–6mg/kg once daily) is a cyclic lipopeptide with a unique mechanism of action, its clinical use is limited to skin infections, and possibly MRSA bacteraemia and/or endocarditis.

Tigecycline (IV 100mg loading dose followed by 50mg twice daily) is a glycylcycline antibiotic with activity against MRSA and Gram-negative bacteria (except *Pseudomonas aeruginosa*) including MDR strains, and *Acinetobacter baumannii.*

MDR Gram-negative bacteria:

Extended-spectrum β-lactamase (ESBL)-positive *Klebsiella pneumoniae,* and other MDR Gram-negative bacilli with inducible β-lactamases such as *Enterobacter, Citrobacter, Serratia* spp. are resistant to 2nd- and 3rd-generation cephalosporins, i.e. cefuroxime, cefotaxime, ceftriaxone, ceftazidime, gentamicin and quinolones, and usually cause urinary tract infections (UTIs), respiratory tract infections or wounds. Localized lower UTIs may be treated with piperacillin–tazobactam (Tazocin®) or ticarcillin–clavulanate (Timentin)

Severe systemic infections such as hospital-acquired pneumonia/VAP, or urosepsis require treatment with carbapenems.

Temocillin Negaban®) (IV 1–2g every 12h), a Ticarcillin derivative; re-launched in the UK in 2006, is active against ESBL *Klebsiella* and *Escherichia coli*, and other MDR *Enterbacter* spp., and is a useful carbapenem-sparing (narrow-spectrum) antibiotic to treat these MDR Gram-negative bacteria infections.

MDR *Acinetobacter baumannii* can occasionally cause epidemics of infection in ICU patients. Epidemic strains are resistant to many broad-spectrum antibiotics such as cephalosporins, piperacillin–tazobactam and ciprofloxacin, and have variable susceptibility to aminoglycosides sensitive only to carbapenems. Carbapenemase-producing strains of *A. baumannii* have been reported and are sensitive to only Colistin and Tigecycline.

Other MDR pathogens in ICUs include MDR *Pseudomonas aeruginosa, Stenotrophomonas maltophilia* treatment choice(s) should be based on antimicrobial susceptibility.

Other risks of antibiotic therapy

'Collateral damage' from antibiotic therapy refers to ecological adverse effects of antibiotic therapy, namely the **selection** of antibiotic-resistant organisms and the unwanted development of **colonization or infection** with such organisms, including *Clostridium difficile*. The following class(es) of antibiotics have been associated with risk of collateral damage:

3rd-generation cephalosporins: VRE, ESBL-producing *Klebsiella, Enterobacter* spp., MDR *Acinetobacter* spp., *Clostridium difficile*-associated disease (CDAD).

Quinolones: MRSA, quinolone-resistant Gram-negative bacilli, ESBLs including *P. aeruginosa*, quinolone-resistant *Acinetobacter* species, CDAD.

Carbapenems: carbapenamase-producing *K. pneumoniae, Enterobacter* spp., MDR *P. aeruginosa, Acinetobacter baumannii, Stenotrophomonas maltophilia.*

While there is no one solution that can be applied to all ICUs, the use of prescribing guidelines which encourage the use of narrow-spectrum antibiotics and limit use of broad-spectrum antibiotics, and use of treatment algorithms involving review of microbiological investigations to de-escalate therapy should be used to delay the emergence of drug resistance and prolong the utility of newer drugs.

Further reading

Cinel I, Dellinger RP. Current treatment of severe sepsis. *Curr Infect Dis Rep* 2006; 8: 358–65.

Dellinger RP, Carlet JM, Masur H, *et al.* Surviving sepsis campaign guidelines for management of severe sepsis and septic shock. *Crit Care Med* 2004; 32: 858–73.

Kumar A, Roberts D, Wood KE, *et al.* Duration of hypotension before initiation of effective antimicrobial therapy is the critical determinant of survival in human septic shock. *Crit Care Med* 2006; 34: 1589–96.

Marik PE. Fever in the ICU. *Chest* 2000; 117: 855–69.

McDonald LC. Trends in antimicrobial resistance in health care–associated pathogens and effect on treatment. *Clin Infect Dis* 2006; 42: S65–71.

Antifungals

In a critical care setting, systemic antifungal agents may be prescribed to treat or prevent infections in two broad categories of patients: those with classic risk factors such as prolonged neutropenia, haematopoietic stem cell transplantation (HSCT) or HIV infection/AIDS, who may be admitted to ICU for advanced supportive care; and a broad group of less severely immunocompromised critically ill patients; who may also be susceptible to these infections.

During the last decade, the landscape of invasive fungal infections has changed significantly with regards to the epidemiology, diagnosis and therapeutic options. Although the incidence of invasive fungal infection has also increased in line with the broadening spectrum of the 'at-risk' population, parallel developments in antifungal chemotherapy have brought optimism of improved outcome for patients.

Systemic antifungal agents used to treat invasive mycoses and mucocutaneous forms of candidiasis are described in this chapter. Although *Pneumocystis jirovecii* (formerly *Pneumocystis carinii*) now is classified among the fungi, traditional therapy has been with trimethoprim–sulfamethoxazole and hence is not described here. The echinocandin class of antifungal drugs (described later) are active against the cyst form of *P. jirovecii* and offer a potential for prophylactic therapy, but they lack activity against the trophozoite form causing pneumonia.

There are **three main families of systemic antifungal agents**:

1. **Polyenes**, e.g. amphotericin B: conventional amphotericin B deoxycholate (cAMB (Fungizone)) and lipid-based preparations such as liposomal amphotericin B (L-AMB (Ambisome)), amphotericin B lipid complex (ABLC (Abelcet)), amphotericin B colloidal dispersion (ABCD (Amphocil, Amphotec))
2. **Azoles**:

   1st-generation triazoles: fluconazole (Diflucan), itraconazole (Sporanox; Janssen-Cilag)

   Newer triazoles: voriconazole (Vfend, Pfizer), posaconazole (Noxafil, Schering-Plough)
3. **Echinocandins**: caspofungin (Cancidas, MSD), micafungin (Mycamine, Astellas) and anidulafungin (Eraxis: Pfizer)
4. **Miscellaneous**: flucytosine

Amphotericin B

1. A polyene antibiotic derived from *Streptomyces nodosus*.
2. Introduced in 1959 (without any randomized trials) for treatment of many invasive fungal infections, it has been the workhorse of antifungals. It is considered to be the 'gold standard' for antifungal therapy and is the only antifungal with an indication for initial therapy of many fungal infections.
3. *Mechanism of action*: it binds ergosterol in the fungal cell (absent in mammalian cells) wall rendering the cell leaky and resulting in cell death.
4. Broad spectrum of activity against most fungi that cause human disease. *Aspergillus terreus*, *Scedosporium* spp., *Trichosporon* spp. and *Candida lusitaniae* are resistant. Its spectrum is not influenced by the choice of formulation.
5. *Adverse effects*: parenteral administration of the conventional amphotericin B is often associated with unpleasant infusion-related reactions such as fever, chills and rigors that can be prevented or reduced either by slowing the rate of infusion or by pre-medication with antihistamines/hydrocortisone and paracetamol. Dose-limiting nephrotoxity; usually reversible on discontinuation of therapy. Monitoring with estimated GFR (eGFR) is recommended.
6. Lipid-based formulations due to their altered pharmacological distributions are less toxic than cAMB.
   - These permit higher doses to be administered without dose-limiting side effects of cAMB.
   - These can be used safely use in patients intolerant of cAMB, particulary those with renal insufficiency or at risk for developing nephrotoxity.
   - None of the lipid fomulations has been proven superior to cAMB in treatment of infections caused by *Candida* or *Aspergillus* spp.
   - There is no difference in efficacy between the three lipid-based formulations, though infusion-related side effects such as fever, rigors and hypotension are more common with ABCD and the toxicity profile of L-AMB has been shown to be better than that of ABLC.
   - However, there is a wide variation in the drug acquisition costs. Lipid formulations are more expensive than cAMD, and L-AMB is the most expensive lipid formulation.
   - The choice of formulation should be individual patient based.
7. Drug interactions. Amphotericin B can augment nephrotoxicity of gentamicin, cyclosporin and certain anticancer drugs.

Azoles

The azoles are a large group of synthetic agents.

Mechanism of action: fungal cell membrane active agents that act by Inhibiting the cytochrome P450- (CYP-450) dependent fungal enzyme lanosterol demethylase, thereby inhibiting ergosterol synthesis and disrupting cell membrane activity.

Fluconazole

- *Spectrum of activity* includes *Candida albicans*, *C. parapsilosis*, *C. tropicalis* and *Cryptococcus neoformans Blastomyces dermatidis*, *Coccidioides immitis*, *Histoplasma capsulatum*, and *Paracoccidioides* spp..
- *C. krusei* and *C. glabrata* tend to be resistant. It has no activity against *Aspergillus* spp.
- Fluconazole has an excellent safety profile and is available in oral and IV formulations; it is 100% bioavailable by the oral route and the generic drug is inexpensive compared with proprietary voriconazole and posaconazole.
- Itraconazole has broader activity against yeasts and is also active against *Aspergillus* spp. Itraconazole has less reliable gastric absorption and greater potential for drug interactions.
- Voriconazole has a broader spectrum of activity against all species of *Candida* including *C. krusei* and *C. glabrata*, and is also active against fluconazole-resistant *C. albicans*. It is the only antifungal drug approved for primary treatment of invasive aspergillosis. It is available in oral and IV formulation. Blood concentrations are highly variable and require monitoring when used to treat invasive mycoses, and has multiple drug interactions.

- Posaconazole is the newest triazole with an extended spectrum of activity against yeasts, moulds and dimorphic fungi. It is licensed by the EC for the treatment of invasive aspergillosis, fusariosis, chromoblastomycosis and coccidiodomycosis in adults who are refractory, or intolerant of other antifungals. It is also indicated for prophylaxis of invasive fungal infections in high-risk haematological malignancy patients and HSCT recipients on high dose immunosuppressive therapy for graft vs host disease. It is available only as an oral suspension and has a lower drug interaction profile compared with other triazoles

Echinocandins

- Echinocandins are naturally occurring and synthetic lipopeptide antifungal agents.
- *Mechanism of action*: inhibit fungal cell wall synthesis through non-competitive inhibition of 1,3-β-D-glucan synthase, an essential component of fungal cell wall, absent in mammalian cells.
- *Spectrum of activity*: echinocandins are fungicidal against *Candida* spp., including fluconazole-resistant isolates, and fungistatic against *Aspergillus* spp. They lack activity against *Cryptococcus neoformans*, *Trichosporon* spp., *Fusarium* spp. and the zygomycetes (*Rhizopus*, *Mucor*, etc.)
- Echinocandins' unique mechanism of action at the fungal cell wall offers a sound theoretic potential for synergy with cell membrane-active polyenes (AMB) and triazoles (fluconazole, voriconazole) in combination therapy for mould infections. Also, absence of cross-resistance with azoles is advantageous in treatment of fluconazole-resistant candidiasis.
- Oral bioavailability is only 3% so IV route of administration is required.
- Their excellent safety profile, very low potential for CYP450-mediated drug interactions and tolerability in critically ill patients with renal and/or hepatic impairment and polypharmacy in units with high rates of triazole-resistant non-albicans *Candida* infections makes this class of drugs the standard of care for ICU patients.
- High drug acquisition costs is the major limiting factor to their wider use in ICUs.

Caspofungin

Caspofungin is indicated for the treatment of invasive candidiasis (candidaemia, oesophageal candidiasis) in adult patients, 'salvage therapy' of invasive aspergillosis in adult patients and empirical therapy for presumed fungal infections (such as *Candida* or *Aspergillus*) in febrile neutropenic adult patients.

A dose regimen of a single 70mg loading dose on day 1, followed by 50mg daily thereafter is recommended. Caspofungin dose should be halved in patients with moderate hepatic insufficiency (Child–Pugh score 7–9). No dose adjustment is required with renal impairment.

Micafungin and Anidulafungin

These are not yet licensed in the EU.

- Micafungin is FDA approved for antifungal prophylaxis in HSCT recipients and in treatment of oesophageal candidiasis. It requires no loading dose,
- Anidulafungin is FDA-approved for the treatment of oesophageal candidiasis, candidaemia and deep-tissue candidiasis. It is unique because it undergoes slow biotransformation in humans rather than being metabolized. In clinical trials it has demonstrated superiority to fluconazole for treatment of oesophageal candidiasis.
- Neither micafungin nor anidulafungin need dose adjustment with hepatic or renal impairment.

Flucytosine

Flucytosine (5-FC) is a synthetic pyrimidine that gets incorporated into RNA, replacing uracil, thereby disrupting protein synthesis in the susceptible fungal cells.

- It has a very limited spectrum of activity that includes *Candida* spp, *Cryptococcus neoformans* and *Cladosporium* spp.
- It is available as oral and IV formulations. The oral drug is almost completely absorbed but it requires blood level monitoring due to risk of bone marrow suppression.
- Mainly used in combination therapy with AMB in treatment of cryptococcal meningitis

Important considerations about use of antifungals in critically ill patients

1. These drugs have been designed, developed and clinically validated for use in patients with haematological malignancies, HSCT or HIV/AIDS patients. Patients with baseline characteristics that are commonly seen in ICU patients were excluded in clinical trial validation studies.
2. Therefore, the pharmacokinetics and pharmacodynamic parameters, drug interactions with other drugs, safety data in renal and/or hepatic impairment must be cautiously extrapolated with these caveats.
3. The role of experts such as haematologists, HIV physicians and antimicrobial stewardship teams including a clinical microbiologist and antimicrobial and ICU specialist pharmacist cannot be overemphasized.

Further reading

Bellman R. Clinical pharmacokinetics of systemically administered antimycotics. *Curr Clin Pharmacol* 2007; 2: 37.

Meersseman W, Lagrou K, et al. Invasive aspergillosis in the ICU: an emerging disease. *Intensive Care Med* 2007; 33: 1679–81.

Metcalf SC, Dockrell DH. Improved outcomes associated with advances in therapy for invasive fungal infections in immunocompromised hosts. *J Infect* 2007; 55: 287–99.

Toya SP, Douskou M. Candiduria in intensive care units: association with heavy colonization and candidaemia. *J Hosp Infect* 2007; 6: 201–6.

Antiviral agents

Antiviral agents target different stages in the life cycle of viral pathogens such as inhibition of viral cell attachment and entry, prevention of viral uncoating, viral genome replication (e.g. scyclovir), and viral assembly and maturation.

In immunocompetent patients, acute virus infections are cleared by the patient's immune system itself; most antiviral agents are used in the management of persistent infections.

However, acute viral meningitis and meningoencephalitis are important causes of admission to hospital. An estimated incidence of 5–15 cases per 100 000/yr of viral meningitis occurs in the UK, enterovirus being the most common pathogen. Herpes simplex virus (HSV) CNS infections affect all ages and cause most fatal cases of encephalitis. The arboviruses, a group of >500 arthropod-transmitted viruses, are the leading cause of encephalitis worldwide.

This chapter addresses antivirals commonly used in the ICU.

Acyclovir

Acyclovir a nucleoside analogue and requires intracellular activation to exert antiviral activity. It is active against herpesviruses.

Acyclovir is a preferred substrate for the viral thymidine kinase (TK) that phosphorylates acyclovir to acyclovir monophosphate within virus-infected cells. Acyclovir monophosphate is then progressively transformed by cellular kinases to acyclovir diphosphate and acyclovir triphosphate, which competitively inhibits the viral DNA polymerase and blocks viral DNA synthesis.

Resistance to acyclovir in herpesviruses is due to the lack of production of viral TK, altered TK substrate specificity and altered viral DNA polymerase. These viral enzyme changes are due to point mutations or base insertions or deletions in the corresponding genes.

Acyclovir has been associated with nausea, diarrhoea, rash, headache, renal insufficiency and neurotoxicity. Acyclovir dose adjustments are needed for renal insufficiency.

Acyclovir is effective in primary and recurrent genital as well as orolabial HSV infections. Systemic acyclovir is used to treat HSV encephalitis (see Table 15.3.1). Acyclovir is also effective for treating varicella and herpes zoster infections in immunocompromised patients.

Ganciclovir

Ganciclovir is a nucleoside derivative that is available for the treatment of cytomegalovirus (CMV) infections. Ganciclovir must be phosphorylated to ganciclovir triphosphate to exert its antiviral activity. In CMV-infected cells, the *UL97* gene of CMV encodes a protein kinase that phosphorylates ganciclovir to ganciclovir monophosphate, with cellular kinase performing futher phosphorylation to the triphosphate which inhibits the CMV DNA polymerase.

Resistance in CMV isolates is due to, reduced intracellular ganciclovir phosphorylation caused by point mutations or deletions in the phosphotransferase encoded by the *UL97* gene and, point mutations in viral DNA polymerase.

Ganciclovir can cause myelosuppression, rash, liver function test abnormalities and CNS side effects, from headache to convulsions and coma.

Ganciclovir is used in life-threatening CMV pneumonia and in CMV retinitis (see Table 15.3.1).

Foscarnet

This is an inorganic pyrophosphate analogue which reversibly and non-competitively inhibits the activity of the viral DNA polymerase. Foscarnet is inhibitory for most ganciclovir-resistant CMV, and acyclovir-resistant HSV and varicella-zoster (VZV) strains.

CMV and HSV can become resistant to foscarnet due to point mutations in DNA polymerase of these viruses.

Nephrotoxicity and metabolic abnormalities such as hypocalcaemia, hypercalcaemia, hypomagnesaemia and hypophosphataemia are common side effects.

Foscarnet has been used to treat gancyclovir-resistant CMV retinitis and acyclovir-resistant mucocutaneous HSV infections (see Table 15.3.3 1).

Cidofovir

Cidofovir is a nucleoside phosphonate analogue that must be phosphorylated to its diphosphoryl derivative by cellular phosphorylating enzymes. Codofovir diphosphate is a competitive inhibitor of the viral DNA polymerase, which leads to cessation of viral DNA chain elongation. It has inhibitory activity against herpes viruses and other DNA viruses such as papilloma, pox and adenoviruses.

Table 15.3.1 Antiviral agents and adult doses

Viral infection	Drug	Adult dosage
Herpes simplex virus		
Genital herpes	Acyclovir	400mg PO tid or 200mg PO 5 times/day for 7–10 days
Encephalitis	Acyclovir	10–15mg/kg/8h IV for 14–21 days
Cytomegalovirus		
Retinitis	Ganciclovir	5mg/kg/12h IV for 14–21 days
	Foscarnet	60mg/kg/8h IV for 14–21 days
	Cidofovir	5mg/kg IV once weekly x2 then every other week
Influenza virus		
Influenza A and B viruses	Oseltamivir	75mg PO bid for 5 days
Varicella-zoster virus		
Varicella in immunocompromised hosts	Acyclovir	10mg/kg/8h IV for 7–10 days
Herpes zoster in normal hosts	Acyclovir	800mg PO 5 times daily for 7–10 days
Herpes zoster in immunocompromised hosts	Acyclovir	10mg/kg/8h IV for 7–10 days

Cidofovir is also inhibitory for acyclovir-resistant HSV strains and ganciclovir-resistant CMV.

Fever, nausea, headache, rash, anterior uveitis, nephrotoxicity and neutropenia are some of the principal side effects of cidofovir. Monitor renal function and neutrophil count within 24h before each dose.

IV cidofovir is approved for the treatment of CMV retinitis in AIDS patients.

Oseltamivir

This is a neuraminidase inhibitor which is effective for prophylaxis and treatment of both influenza A and B.

High level resistance because of histidine to tyrosine mutation in codon 274 of the N1 neuraminidase can emerge during treatment of H1N1 and in some patients treated for H5N1 infections.

Oseltamivir is generally well tolerated. Long-term prophylaxis is associated with headache, rash, hepatic inflammation thrombocytopenia and CNS toxicity, such as hallucination and extrapyramidal signs.

Early treatment of acute influenza reduces time to functional recovery by 1–3 days, and also decreases the risk of lower respiratory tract complications leading to hospitalization.

For treatment of pandemic flu, readers should refer to Health Protection Agency and Department of Health, UK latest pandemic flu guidelines.

Further reading

CDSC. Viral meningitis associated with increase in echovirus type 13. *Commun Dis Rep CDR Wkly* 2000; 10: 277–8.

Chou S, Guentzel S, Michels KR, *et al.* Frequency of *UL97* phosphotransferase mutations related to ganciclovir resistance in clinical cytomegalovirus isolates. *J Infect Dis.* 1995; 172: 239–42.

Coen DM, Richman DDAntiviral agents. In: Knipe DM, Howley PM, eds. Fields virology, 5th edn, Vol. 1. Philadelphia, PA: Lippincott Williams & Wilkins, 2007: 447–85.

Erice A. Antiviral susceptibitily testing. In: Storch GA, ed. Essentials of diagnostic virology, Churchill Livingstone, 2000: 271–89.

Gaudreau A, Hill E, Balfour HH, *et al.* Phenotypic and genotypic characterization of acyclovir-resistant herpes simplex viruses from immunocompromised patients. *J Infect Dis.* 1998; 178: 297–303.

Hayden FG. Antiviral drugs (other than anti-retrovirals). In: Mandell, Douglas and Bennett's, Principles and practice of infectious diseases, 6th edn, Vol 1. Philadelphia, PA: Elsevier Churchill Livingstone, 2005: 514–51.

Ho DD, Hirsch MS. Acute viral encephalitis. *Med Clin North Am* 1985; 69: 415.

Lurain NS, Thompson KD, Holmes EW, *et al.* Point mutations in the DNA polymerase gene of human cytomegalovirus that result in resistance to antiviral agents. *J Virol* 1992; 66: 7146–715.

N-Acetylcysteine

Modes of action

N-Acetylcysteine (NAC) is the acetylated form of the amino acid L-cysteine. It is a sulfhydryl group donor and a precursor for glutathione production. Its primary systemic use is as an antioxidant as it can directly scavenge oxygen radicals, and act indirectly by boosting glutathione levels.

It enhances NO synthesis and cGMP levels, resulting in vasodilation and inhibition of platelet aggregation.

It also cleaves disulfide bonds, converting them to sulfhydryl groups and thereby reducing the chain length of mucoproteins in lung secretions, enabling easier clearance.

Uses

- *Paracetamol poisoning*. Glutathione is a powerful endogenous antioxidant but becomes rapidly depleted in paracetamol poisoning if normal hepatic conjugation pathways become saturated, resulting in a greater proportion of paracetamol being converted to *N*-acetyl-*p*-benzoquinone imine (NAPQI) by the CYP2E1 mixed-function oxidase enzyme. This unstable and toxic metabolite is normally rendered non-toxic by conjugation with glutathione. When glutathione levels are depleted by ~70%, hepatotoxicity is likely as NAPQI is free to cause widespread damage to hepatocytes in a familiar centrilobular pattern. Decision to treat in paracetamol poisoning is based upon the paracetamol blood level and known time of ingestion using a nomogram.
- *COPD*. There is some evidence that oral NAC can prevent or reduce the number of acute exacerbations in COPD.
- *See notes*. The evidence for other uses of NAC is discussed below.

Routes

- IV
- Oral
- Nebulized

Side effects/complications

Anaphylactoid reactions: incidence ~0.2%. Mostly this is limited to urticarial rashes and pruritis, but 10% of those affected can experience hypotension and/or bronchospasm

Nebulized NAC causes bronchorrhoea which may cause problems in those with an inadequate cough. In intubated patients, secretions may increase. Occasionally bronchospasm can occur.

IV co-administration of certain drugs can lead to precipitation, notably erythromycin, tetracyclines and ampicilin.

Notes

- *Paracetamol poisoning:* any patient who might have liver enzyme induction due to concurrent medication or chronic alcohol abuse, or who might have glutathione depletion prior to overdose due to malnutrition, HIV, etc., should be considered for NAC treatment at blood paracetamol levels below the normal treatment line on the nomogram.
- *Non-paracetamol-induced liver failure*. Despite reports of improvements in hepatosplanchnic perfusion and some measures of hepatic function, little good evidence exists to support the use of NAC in this situation, with the exception of liver failure due to amanita phalloides ingestion and carbon tetrachloride, chloroform or potassium permanganate poisoning. Nevertheless, it continues to be recommended as adjunctive therapy in acute liver failure.
- *Radiocontrast-induced nephropathy*. NAC appears to have some benefit in preventing this problem, particularly those patients with pre-existing chronic renal impairment
- *Acute respiratory distress syndrome:* despite initial suggestions that NAC may improve oxygenation and reduce ventilator-dependent days, no convincing benefit has been demonstrated to date
- *Sepsis and multi-organ failure:* many studies have shown an increase in cardiac index with NAC. Initiation of NAC treatment after the initial 24h post-hospital admission is not of any benefit and may be detrimental. Whether there is a reduction in proinflammatory cytokine levels in sepsis is still debated.
- *Myocardial ischaemia*: the combination of oral NAC and transdermal nitroglycerin has been shown to reduce the incidence of refractory angina, MI and death in patients with angina. Unfortunately severe headaches are associated with this combination. In AMI, it may improve cardiac function post-thrombolysis .
- *Other lung diseases*: in cystic fibrosis, NAC use has not shown any improvement in lung function; however, there is some recent evidence it can modulate lung inflammation. NAC may promote some marginal benefits in idiopathic pulmonary fibrosis.
- *Heavy metal poisoning:* NAC has the ability to chelate some heavy metals and improve their excretion rates.
- *HIV/AIDS*: longer term administration of NAC has been shown to improve immune function and serum albumin levels in HIV-infected patients

Drug dosages

Whilst there is consensus regarding the doses required in paracetamol poisoning, clinical studies conducted on the efficacy of NAC for other indications have often used a different dosing regimen. The IV doses given below are for paracetamol poisoning.

- *IV administration:* it is available in ampoules at concentrations of 10 or 20% which can be diluted in 5% dextrose solutions. Initial treatment is 150mg/kg over 15min then 50mg/kg over 4h, followed by 100mg/kg over 16h. This last infusion rate can be continued past 24h of treatment.
- *Oral administration:* 400–1200mg/day.
- *Nebulized:* the 20% solution is highly osmotic and can be too irritant to be delivered undiluted. Dilution should be with saline or water for injection. Regimes can be varied, but 6–10ml of a 10% solution 3–4 times per day is usual.

Further reading

Brok J, Buckley N, Gluud C. Interventions for paracetamol (acetaminophen) overdoses. *Cochrane Database Syst Rev* 2006; (2): CD003328.

Kramer BK, Hoffmann U. Benefit of acetylcysteine for prevention of contrast-induced nephropathy after primary angioplasty. *Nat Clin Pract Nephrol* 2007; 3: 10–11.

Sklar GE, Subramaniam M. Acetylcysteine treatment for non-acetaminophen-induced acute liver failure. *Ann Pharmacother* 2004; 38: 498–500.

Activated protein C

Introduction

The microcirculation in sepsis is characterized by unrestricted and/or inappropriate activation of coagulation and inflammatory pathways, resulting in tissue hypoperfusion. The protein C anticoagulant pathway composed of thrombin, thrombomodulin, endothelial protein C receptor (EPCR), protein C and protein S is essential for the negative control of both coagulation and inflammation. Within this complex system, activated protein C (APC) serves as a key regulator in preserving the internal milieu and restoring the microcirculation, through its potent cytoprotective and anticoagulant properties. Drotrecogin alfa (activated) (DrotAA), a synthetic form of APC, was approved in 2002 for use in patients with severe sepsis and multiple organ failure.

Chemistry

APC is an anticoagulant glycoprotein with serine protease activity and has a molecular mass of 55kDa. DrotAA is a recombinant form of human APC, and is prepared using a human cell line that processes the complimentary DNA for inactive protein C zymogen. Following post-translational modifications, the secreted recombinant protein C is activated by cleavage with thrombin. The activated product—APC—is then purified and presented in a powder form for IV infusion.

Mode of action

The cytoprotective and anticoagulant actions are probably responsible for the clinical benefits observed with DrotAA. There is an ongoing debate as to which of the varied modes of action is most important, but the major clinical benefits are attributed to the cytoprotective actions.

Cytoprotective actions

The cytoprotective effects of APC are mediated through the cellular receptors EPCR and protease-activated receptor 1 (PAR1). Stimulation of these receptors leads to alteration in gene expression profiles, resulting in anti-inflammatory and antiapoptotic activity, and endothelial barrier stabilization.

Antiapoptotic actions

- Alteration in activity of apoptotic inhibitors and apoptotic transcription factors

Endothelial barrier stabilization

- Upregulation of sphingokinase reduces endothelial permeability and stabilizes the cellular cytoskeleton

Anti-inflammatory actions

- Inhibits translocation of nuclear factor-κB

Anticoagulant effects

- Activation of the fibrinolytic pathway by inactivating plasminogen activator inhibitor
- Complexing with protein S and directly inhibiting factor Va and VIIIa preventing thrombin formation
- Inhibiting proinflammatory cytokine-mediated release of tissue factor from monocytes and endothelial cells

Dose

DrotAA is administered IV as a continuous infusion at 24mcg/kg/h for 96h. The currently recommended dose and duration of infusion were selected from a phase II clinical trial in 131 patients with severe sepsis. The dose selected was that which had greatest effect on D-dimer level.

Pharmacokinetics

DrotAA infusion shows linear pharmacokinetics with rapid achievement of steady state and prompt decline in plasma activity with $t_{1/2}$ α and $t_{1/2}$ β of 13min and 1.6h, respectively. Plasma DrotAA activity reduces by ~80% 1h after drug discontinuation.

Indications

The key to appropriate use of DrotAA lies in the early assessment of the risk of death. However, there is still no consensus on a good operational definition of 'high risk' in patients with severe sepsis. In the USA, DrotAA is recommended in patients 'at high risk of death, e.g. those with an APACHE II score of 25' since subset analysis demonstrated that the treatment benefit in the PROWESS trial was in this subgroup. In the EU, DrotAA is licensed for patients with 'severe sepsis and multiple organ dysfunction', irrespective of pre-treatment APACHE II score. The PROWESS trial demonstrated an increased treatment effect as the number of organ dysfunctions increased. DrotAA is indicated in adult patients with severe sepsis who are at high risk for death. Risk for death is currently best determined by clinical judgement and presence of organ dysfunction.

Outcome data

Clinical trials in adults

The PROWESS trial (*n* = 1690), was the first phase III multi-centre RCT of DrotAA in adults. The trial demonstrated a 19.4% relative reduction and 6.1% absolute reduction in 28-day mortality. To obtain additional efficacy and safety data prior to licensing, a single-arm open-label study known as the ENHANCE trial (*n* = 2434) was performed. Using similar entry criteria, the trial showed a mortality rate similar to that in PROWESS (25.3% vs 24.7%) in the DrotAA treatment arm, thereby confirming efficacy. The subsequent ADDRESS trial (*n* = 2613), was a multi-centre RCT enrolling patients with severe sepsis and low risk of death. This trial failed to show a mortality benefit with DrotAA, suggesting that the favourable risk–benefit profile may only be apparent in patients at high risk of death.

Clinical trials in children

The RESOLVE trial (*n* = 477) was a multi-centre RCT in paediatric patients, and could not replicate the mortality benefits observed in the adult studies. Although there was no overall difference in the bleeding events during the 28 day study period, CNS bleeding events were more common with DrotAA treatment compared with placebo. Interestingly, in children with severe sepsis and disseminated intravascular coagulation, there were strong trends towards improvement in mortality.

Registries

Descriptive analyses of national audits and registries have confirmed the mortality benefit reported in the clinical trials. The findings of the Promoting Global Research Excellence in Severe Sepsis (PROGRESS) database of 12 492 patients with severe sepsis from 37 countries showed that the adjusted odds ratio (OR) for hospital

Table 15.5.1 Incidence of serious bleeding and fatal ICH events in the PROWESS, ADDRESS and XPRESS trials

Trial	PROWESS (*n* = 1690)		ADDRESS (*n* = 2613)		XPRESS (*n* = 1994)	
	DrotAA	Placebo	DrotAA	Placebo	Heparin + DrotAA	Placebo + DrotAA
Serious bleeding events						
During infusion	2.4%	1%	2.4%	1.2%	2.3%	2.5%
0–28 days	3.5%	2%	3.9%	2.2%	3.9%	5.2%
Fatal CNS bleeding events						
During infusion	0.2%	0	0	0.1%	0.1%	0.2%
0–28 days	0.2%	0.1%	0.2%	0.1%	0.3%	0.4%

mortality associated with DrotAA was 0.75, and a greater treatment effect was seen for patients with ≥3 organs in failure. The OR of mortality associated with DrotAA treatment has been variously reported from other registries from the UK, Poland, Belgium and Italy as between 0.65 and 0.85.

Exclusion criteria and contraindications

The main exclusion criteria used in the clinical trials are summarized below.

Increased bleeding risk

- Platelet count <30 000/mm^3
- Warfarin use within the preceding 7 days
- Acetylsalicylic acid dose >650mg/day
- Surgery within the preceding 12h
- Head trauma or stroke within 3 months
- GI bleeding within 6 weeks

Expected survival <24h or moribund state

Known hypercoagulable conditions

Altered immune system function

- HIV infection with a last known CD4 count of <50/mm^3
- History of organ transplantation
- Advanced cancer

Severe chronic illness

- Chronic renal failure requiring haemodialysis or peritoneal dialysis
- Known or suspected portosystemic hypertension, chronic jaundice, cirrhosis, or chronic ascites

Acute pancreatitis with no established source of infection

Complications

Bleeding is the most common adverse event observed with DrotAA. 'Serious' bleeding was defined in the trials as any intracranial haemorrhage (ICH), any life-threatening bleeding, any bleeding event classified as serious by the investigator or any bleeding that required the administration of 3 units of packed red cells on two consecutive days. Table 15.5.1 shows the incidence of serious bleeding and fatal ICH events in three of the larger trials involving DrotAA.

Drug interactions

Heparin

The XPRESS trial (*n* = 1994), was a phase IV multi-centre RCT comparing DrotAA with or without concomitant heparin use in patients with severe sepsis. The trial showed preserved efficacy of DrotAA treatment and no harmful interactions between heparin and DrotAA.

Antiplatelet drugs and warfarin

The use of these antiplatelet drugs and anticoagulants does not represent an absolute contraindication to the use of DrotAA provided coagulation abnormalities are corrected prior to starting DrotAA infusion.

Controversy

Over the last few years there has been significant debate as to the reported efficacy and the risk–benefit profile of DrotAA. The questions regarding the perceived efficacy of DrotAA arise from various aspects of the conduct of the PROWESS trial, and the relatively high cost of the drug. The mortality benefit reported in the PROWESS trial has not been replicated in all patient groups with severe sepsis, and consequently some clinicians have ongoing scepticism.

In the light of these issues and an assumption that there is still clinical equipoise among critical care physicians, a second randomized double-blind placebo-controlled trial is planned to be underway by 2009, called the PROWESS Shock trial.

Further reading

Abraham E, Laterre PF, Garg R, *et al.* Drotrecogin alfa (activated) for adults with severe sepsis and a low risk of death. *N Engl J Med* 2005; 353: 1332–41.

Bernard GR, Vincent JL, Laterre PF, *et al.* Efficacy and safety of recombinant human activated protein C for severe sepsis. N Engl J Med 2001; 344: 699–709.

Bernard GR, Wright TJ, Ely EW, *et al.* Safety and dose-relationship of recombinant human activated protein C (rhAPC) on coagulopathy in severe sepsis. *Crit Care Med* 2001; 29: 2051–59.

Eichacker PQ, Natanson C. Increasing evidence that the risks of rhAPC may outweigh its benefits. *Intensive Care Med* 2007; 33: 396–99.

Laurent OM, Berislav VZ, Griffin JH. The cytoprotective protein C pathway. *Blood* 2007; 109: 3161–72.

Levi M, Levy M, Williams MD, *et al.* Prophylactic heparin in patients with severe sepsis treated with drotrecogin alfa (activated). *Am J Respir Crit Care Med* 2007; 176: 483–90.

Nadel S, Goldstein B, Williams MD, *et al.* Drotrecogin alfa (activated) in children with severe sepsis: a multicentre phase III randomised controlled trial. *Lancet* 2007; 369: 836–43.

Vincent JL, Bernard GR, Beale R, *et al.* Drotrecogin alfa (activated) treatment in severe sepsis from the global open-label trial ENHANCE: further evidence for survival and safety and implications for early treatment. *Crit Care Med* 2005; 33: 2266–77.

Chapter 16

Resuscitation

Chapter contents

Basic and advanced resuscitation

Recovery from cardiac arrest depends on an intact 'Chain of Survival', which comprises:
- Early recognition and call for help
- Early CPR
- Early defibrillation
- Post resuscitation care.

Prevention

- In-hospital cardiac arrests are usually not sudden or unpredictable: in ~80% there is deterioration in clinical signs during the preceding few hours.
- The cardiac arrest rhythm is usually pulseless electrical activity (PEA) or asystole, and prognosis is poor.
- Earlier recognition and treatment can prevent some cardiac arrests, deaths and unanticipated ICU admissions.
- Strategies such as critical care outreach and medical emergency teams might reduce the incidence of cardiac arrest, but this has been difficult to prove.
- Earlier recognition also enables a do not attempt resuscitation (DNAR) decision to be applied, if this is appropriate.

In-hospital resuscitation

After in-hospital cardiac arrest, the division between basic life support (BLS) and advanced life support (ALS) is arbitrary; in practice, in-hospital resuscitation is a continuum. For all in-hospital cardiac arrests, ensure that:
- cardiorespiratory arrest is recognized immediately
- help is summoned using a standard telephone number—it should be 2222 in the UK
- CPR is started immediately
- a compression:ventilation (CV) ratio of 30:2 is used.

Risks to the rescuer

There are few reports of harm to rescuers from doing CPR.
- Wear gloves. Eye protection, aprons and face masks, may be necessary.
- Infection risk is lower than perceived. There are reports of infections with tuberculosis (TB), and severe acute respiratory distress syndrome (SARS). HIV transmission has never been reported.

Mechanism for the production of blood flow during chest compressions

- Chest compressions generate blood flow by increasing intrathoracic pressure and compressing the heart directly; however, perfusion of the brain and myocardium is, at best, 25% of normal.
- The CPP achieved during CPR correlates with restoration of spontaneous circulation (ROSC).
- In the presence of VF, chest compressions increase the amplitude and frequency of the VF waveform and the likelihood that attempted defibrillation will be successful.
- Pauses in chest compressions of as little as 10s before shock delivery reduce the chances of successful defibrillation. Frequent interruptions in chest compressions reduce survival from cardiac arrest. Each time chest compressions are stopped the CPP decreases rapidly and takes time to reach previous levels once chest compressions are resumed.

Advanced life support

The ALS algorithm enables a standardized approach to cardiac arrest management (see Appendix 1). Cardiac arrest rhythms are classified as:
- Shockable rhythms—VF/VT. In adults, the most common rhythm at the time of cardiac arrest out of hospital is VF, which may be preceded by a period of VT, by a bradyarrhythmia or, less commonly, supraventricular tachycardia (SVT).
- Non-shockable rhythms—asystole and PEA.

Treatment of shockable rhythms

- Start CPR and assess rhythm. If using an old monophasic defibrillator, consider resuming chest compressions while charging the defibrillator (older equipment is slow to charge). See Chapter 2.1 for more detail on defibrillation.
- Give one shock of 150–200J biphasic (360J monophasic).
- Immediately resume chest compressions (CV ratio 30:2) without reassessing the rhythm or feeling for a pulse.
- Continue CPR for 2min, then pause briefly to check the monitor:
- If VF/VT persists:
  - Give a further (2nd) shock of 150–360J biphasic (360J monophasic).
  - Resume CPR immediately and continue for 2min.
  - Pause briefly to check the monitor; if VF/VT persists, give adrenaline 1mg IV followed immediately by a (3rd) shock of 150–360J biphasic (360J monophasic). Do not delay a shock to wait for adrenaline—if the adrenaline is not ready, give it after delivery of the shock.
  - Resume CPR immediately and continue for 2min.
  - Pause briefly to check the monitor; if VF/VT persists, give amiodarone 300mg IV followed immediately by a (4th) shock of 150–360J biphasic (360J monophasic).
  - Resume CPR immediately and continue for 2min.
  - Give adrenaline 1mg IV immediately before alternate shocks (i.e. approximately every 3–5min).
  - Give further shocks after each 2min period of CPR and after confirming that VF/VT persists.
- If organized electrical activity compatible with a cardiac output is seen, check for a pulse:
  - If a pulse is present, start post-resuscitation care.
  - If no pulse is present, continue CPR and switch to the non-shockable algorithm.
- If asystole is seen, continue CPR and switch to the non-shockable algorithm.

Precordial thump

- If the onset of VF/VT is both witnessed and monitored, give a precordial thump if a defibrillator is not available for immediate delivery of a shock.
- The mechanical energy of the precordial thump is converted to electrical energy, which may be sufficient to achieve cardioversion.
- A precordial thump is most likely to be successful in converting VT to sinus rhythm.
- Successful treatment of VF by precordial thump is much less likely unless the thump is given within the first 10s of VF onset.

Treatment of PEA

- Start CPR 30:2.
- Give adrenaline 1mg IV as soon as intravascular access is achieved.
- Continue CPR 30:2 until the airway is secured—then continue chest compressions without pausing during ventilation.
- Recheck the rhythm every 2min and check for a pulse if organized electrical activity is seen
- Give further adrenaline 1mg IV every 3–5 min (alternate loops) until ROSC is achieved

Treatment of asystole and slow PEA (rate <60/min)

- Treat as for PEA but inject atropine 3mg after the first dose of adrenaline is given.

Airway and ventilation

- Many patients on an ICU will already be intubated at the time of cardiac arrest. Tracheal intubation provides the most reliable airway during CPR but if a tracheal tube is not already in place, attempts at intubation should be made only by trained personnel.
- A supraglottic airway device (e.g. laryngeal mask airway (LMA) or Proseal LMA) is an alternative to tracheal intubation.
- If a supraglottic airway device has been inserted, attempt continuous chest compressions without stopping for ventilations. If gas leakage is excessive, interrupt the chest compressions to enable adequate ventilation.

Drug delivery

- Peak drug concentrations are higher and circulation times are shorter when drugs are injected into a central vein compared with a peripheral vein.
- On the ICU, a central venous catheter (CVC) is often *in situ* at the time of cardiac arrest. If not *in situ*, insertion of a CVC is not an immediate priority—it requires interruption of CPR and is associated with several potential complications.
- Peripheral venous cannulation is quicker, easier and safer. Flush drugs injected peripherally with at least 20ml of fluid and elevate the extremity for 10–20s to facilitate drug delivery to the central circulation.
- Consider the intraosseous route if the IV route is impossible. Giving a drug through the tracheal tube results in highly variable, and usually ineffective, plasma drug concentrations.

Reversible causes

Identify and treat reversible causes during CPR for all cardiac arrests. This is particularly important in the ICU where potentially reversible causes are more common.

- Hypoxia
- Hypovolaemia
- Hyperkalaemia, hypokalaemia, hypocalcaemia, acidaemia and other metabolic disorders
- Hypothermia
- Tension pneumothorax
- Tamponade
- Toxic substances
- Thromboembolism (pulmonary embolism or coronary thrombosis).

Post-resuscitation care

See Chapter 16.2.

Outcome

Despite developments in the emergency services, the outcome from out-of-hospital cardiac arrest (OHCA) remains very poor, with survival to hospital discharge of ~5–10%. After in-hospital cardiac arrest, the survival to hospital discharge is 15–20% (40% after VF and 6% after PEA or asystole). The majority of survivors have a good neurological recovery. The outcome from cardiac arrest in a critical care area is better than in other in-hospital locations.

CPR on the ICU

Many aspects of CPR on the ICU are specific to this environment:

- Most cardiac arrests will be both monitored and witnessed.
- There should be minimal delay before starting CPR.
- Many patients are already receiving positive pressure ventilation at the onset of cardiac arrest.
- Mechanical ventilation can be continued during chest compressions, but the airway pressure alarms will be distracting and, if a pressure mode is being used, inadequate tidal volumes will be given.
- Continuous invasive arterial pressure monitoring is frequently in place—this provides some indication of the effectiveness of chest compressions and is helpful in detecting when ROSC has been achieved.
- The presence of a CVC is helpful— drug delivery by this route is both rapid and reliable.

Further reading

Cook TM, Hommers C. New airways for resuscitation? *Resuscitation* 2006; 69: 371–87.

Edelson DP, Abella BS, Kramer-Johansen J, *et al.* Effects of compression depth and pre-shock pauses predict defibrillation failure during cardiac arrest. *Resuscitation* 2006; 71: 137–45.

Hillman K, Chen J, Cretikos M, *et al.* Introduction of the medical emergency team (MET) system: a cluster-randomised controlled trial. *Lancet* 2005; 365: 2091–7.

Nolan JP, Deakin CD, Soar J, *et al.* European Resuscitation Council guidelines for resuscitation 2005. Section 4. Adult advanced life support. *Resuscitation* 2005; 67 Suppl 1: S39–86.

Nolan J, Soar J, Lockey A, *et al.* Advanced life support, 5th edn. London: *Resuscitation Council (UK)*, 2006.

Sandroni C, Nolan J, Cavallaro F, *et al.* In-hospital cardiac arrest: incidence, prognosis and possible measures to improve survival. *Intensive Care Med* 2007; 33: 237–45.

Post-cardiac arrest management

With the exception of patients resuscitated from a very brief period of cardiac arrest, most of those with ROSC will initially be comatose, and many of these will require admission to an ICU. Unconscious, mechanically ventilated survivors of cardiac arrest account for 5.8% of all admissions to ICUs in the UK. Of these, 43% survive to leave the ICU and ~30% survive to hospital discharge. Two-thirds of patients dying after admission to ICU following out-of-hospital cardiac arrest (OHCA) die from neurological injury and 25% of patients dying after admission to ICU following in-hospital cardiac arrest die from neurological injury.

Airway and ventilation

- There are no data supporting precise indications for intubation, ventilation and sedation after cardiac arrest.
- Although cerebral autoregulation is either absent or right-shifted in a majority of patients in the acute phase after cardiac arrest, cerebrovascular reactivity to changes in arterial carbon dioxide tension seems to be preserved.
- There are no data to support the targeting of a specific arterial PCO_2 after resuscitation from cardiac arrest—aim for normocarbia.

Circulation

Coronary revascularization

- Acute changes in coronary plaque morphology are found in 40–86% of cardiac arrest survivors, and in 15–64% in autopsy studies.
- Primary PCI is the treatment of choice after OHCA and STEMI.
- The safety of thrombolysis after CPR is well established.
- Prior CPR is not a contraindication to thrombolysis—restoration of coronary perfusion is a priority.
- If there is evidence of coronary occlusion, consider immediate revascularization by thrombolysis or PCI.
- The optimal technique for revascularization will depend on local facilities for PCI as well as patient factors.
- Management of the ventilated, haemodynamically unstable post-cardiac arrest patient in the cardiac catheter laboratory is challenging and requires the presence of an experienced ICU clinician.

Myocardial dysfunction after cardiac arrest

- Haemodynamic instability is common after cardiac arrest and manifests as hypotension, low cardiac index, arrhythmias and impaired contractility on echocardiography. This post-resuscitation myocardial dysfunction (or myocardial stunning) is usually transient and often reverses within 24–48h.
- The post-resuscitation period is associated with marked elevations in plasma cytokine concentrations, manifesting as a sepsis-like syndrome and multiple organ dysfunction, which has recently been termed the post-cardiac arrest syndrome.
- Infusion of fluids may be required to increase right heart filling pressures or, conversely, diuretics, vasodilators and inotropes/balloon pump may be needed to treat myocardial dysfunction.
- In the presence of a significant inflammatory response, noradrenaline may be required to maintain an adequate blood pressure.
- Early echocardiography will enable the extent of myocardial dysfunction to be quantified and may guide therapy.

Blood pressure control after cardiac arrest

In the absence of definitive data, target the MAP to achieve an adequate urine output, taking into consideration the patient's normal blood pressure.

Prophylactic antiarrhythmic therapy

There are no data to support or refute the use of prophylactic antiarrhythmics in patients who have survived cardiac arrest. However, it is reasonable to continue an infusion of an antiarrhythmic drug that restored a stable rhythm successfully during resuscitation.

Disability (optimizing neurological recovery)

Cerebral perfusion

- Immediately after ROSC there is a period of cerebral hyperaemia. After 15–30min of reperfusion, however, global cerebral blood flow (CBF) decreases and there is generalized hypoperfusion associated with a decrease in CBF to ~50% or less of normal.
- Normal cerebral autoregulation is lost, leaving cerebral perfusion dependent on MAP.
- Under these circumstances, hypotension will compromise CBF severely and will compound any neurological injury; therefore, maintain MAP at the patient's normal level.

Sedation

- Although it has been common practice to sedate and ventilate patients for up to 24h after ROSC, there are no data to support a defined period of ventilation, sedation and neuromuscular blockade after cardiac arrest.
- The duration of sedation and ventilation may be influenced by the use of therapeutic hypothermia.
- There are no data to indicate whether or not the choice of sedation influences outcome, but short-acting drugs (e.g., propofol, alfentanil, remifentanil) will enable earlier neurological assessment.

Prevention and control of seizures

- Seizures and/or myoclonus occur in 5–15% of adult patients who achieve ROSC, and in 10-40% of those who remain comatose.
- Seizures increase cerebral metabolism by up to 3-fold.
- Seizures and myoclonus *per se* are not related significantly to outcome, but status epilepticus and, in particular, status myoclonus are associated with a poor outcome.
- There are no studies that address directly the use of prophylactic anticonvulsant drugs after cardiac arrest in adults.
- Prolonged seizure activity may cause cerebral injury, and should be treated promptly and effectively with benzodiazepines, phenytoin, sodium valproate, propofol or a barbiturate.
- Clonazepam is the drug of choice for the treatment of myoclonus, but sodium valproate and levetiracetam may also be effective.

Temperature control

Treatment of hyperthermia

A period of hyperthermia is common in the first 48h after cardiac arrest. The risk of a poor neurological outcome increases for each degree of body temperature >37°C. Treat any hyperthermia occurring in the first 72h after cardiac arrest with antipyretics or active cooling.

Therapeutic hypothermia

- Mild hypothermia started after ROSC reduces the neurological injury caused by reperfusion and the post-cardiac arrest syndrome.
- Based on favourable results from two randomized clinical trials, unconscious adult patients with spontaneous circulation after out-of-hospital VF cardiac arrest should be cooled to 32–34°C. Start cooling as soon as possible and continue for at least 24h.
- Induced hypothermia might also benefit unconscious adult patients with spontaneous circulation after OHCA from a non-shockable rhythm, or cardiac arrest in hospital.
- Rapid infusion of ice-cold fluid 30ml/kg is a very effective, simple method for initiating cooling. Treatment can then be continued using either internal (intravascular cooling) or external techniques (e.g. circulating water blankets). Intravascular cooling enables more precise temperature control.
- Treat shivering by ensuring adequate sedation and giving neuromuscular blocking drugs. Bolus doses of neuromuscular blockers are usually adequate, but infusions are necessary occasionally. Use of continuous neuromuscular blockade could mask seizure activity.
- Rewarm the patient slowly (0.25–0.5°C/h) and avoid hyperthermia.
- Complications of mild therapeutic hypothermia include increased infection, cardiovascular instability, coagulopathy, hyperglycaemia and electrolyte abnormalities such as hypophosphataemia and hypomagnesaemia.

Blood glucose control

- There is a strong association between high blood glucose after resuscitation from cardiac arrest and poor neurological outcome.
- Tight control of blood glucose (4.4–6.1mmol/l) has been shown to reduce mortality in critically ill patients, particularly those in ICU for >3 days, but this has not been demonstrated in post-cardiac arrest patients specifically.
- Comatose patients are at particular risk from unrecognized hypoglycaemia, and the risk of this complication occurring increases as the target blood glucose concentration is lowered.
- In common with all critically ill patients, patients admitted to a critical care environment after cardiac arrest should have their blood glucose monitored frequently and hyperglycaemia treated with an insulin infusion. The blood glucose concentration that triggers insulin therapy, and the target range of blood glucose concentrations, should be determined by local policy.

Prediction of outcome in comatose survivors after cardiopulmonary resuscitation

- Predicting the final outcome of individual patients remaining comatose after resuscitation from cardiac arrest is problematic.
- Prognosis cannot be based reliably on the circumstances surrounding cardiac arrest and CPR.
- The decision to admit a comatose post-cardiac arrest patient to ICU should be based predominantly on the patient's status before the cardiac arrest.
- Absent pupil or corneal reflexes within days 1–3 after CPR, or absent or extensor motor responses 3 days after cardiac arrest reliably predict a poor outcome in the normothermic patient.
- Myoclonic status epilepticus within the first day after a primary cardiac arrest reliably predicts a poor outcome.
- Burst suppression or generalized epileptiform discharges on the EEG predict poor outcome, but this is too imprecise for use in individual cases. Timely access to EEG recording and interpretation may be a problem on many ICUs.
- Bilateral absence of the N2O component of the somatosensory evoked potential (SSEP) with median nerve stimulation recorded on days 1–3 or later accurately predicts a poor outcome.
- A serum neuron-specific enolase (NSE) concentration >33mcg/l 1–3 days after CPR accurately predicts a poor outcome.

Further reading

Adrie C, Adib-Conquy M, Laurent I, *et al.* Successful cardiopulmonary resuscitation after cardiac arrest as a 'sepsis-like' syndrome. *Circulation* 2002; 106: 562–8.

Bernard SA, Gray TW, Buist MD, *et al.* Treatment of comatose survivors of out-of-hospital cardiac arrest with induced hypothermia. *N Engl J Med* 2002; 346: 557–63.

Hypothermia After Cardiac Arrest Study Group. Mild therapeutic hypothermia to improve the neurologic outcome after cardiac arrest. *N Engl J Med* 2002; 346: 549–56.

Laurent I, Monchi M, Chiche JD, *et al.* Reversible myocardial dysfunction in survivors of out-of-hospital cardiac arrest. *J Am Coll Cardiol* 2002; 40: 2110–6.

Laver S, Farrow C, Turner D, *et al.* Mode of death after admission to an intensive care unit following cardiac arrest. *Intensive Care Med* 2004; 30: 2126–8.

Wijdicks EF, Hijdra A, Young GB, *et al.* Practice parameter: prediction of outcome in comatose survivors after cardiopulmonary resuscitation (an evidence-based review): report of the Quality Standards Subcommittee of the American Academy of Neurology. *Neurology* 2006; 67: 203-10.

Fluid challenge

Definition

A fluid challenge is a specific volume of fluid given over a specified time period in order to determine whether the cardiac output will respond to further volume.

Rationale

Hypovolaemia may due to bleeding, GI, urinary or skin losses, or may be caused by internal losses such as third spacing. Relative hypovolaemia may result from an increase in venous capacitance secondary to inflammatory processes such as sepsis or pancreatitis, or as a side effect from drugs. Venous return and therefore preload is reduced, leading to a reduced stroke volume and cardiac output. Perfusion to vital organs is lowered and will lead to progressive organ failure if not corrected. Circulatory support with inotropes is inappropriate in the hypovolaemic patient and may increase myocardial oxygen demand

Overt hypovolaemia due to exsanguination is self-evident. However it can be a difficult diagnosis in the critically ill patient as the clinical signs lack sensitivity and specificity.

Clinical indicators of hypovolaemia

- Thirst, dry mouth, reduced skin turgor
- Tachycardia, reduced blood pressure, reduced CVP/pulmonary artery wedge pressure (PAWP)
- Reduced urine output (<0.5ml/kg/h), increased toe–core gap
- Raised urea, raised sodium, raised lactate, reduced urinary sodium (<20mmol/l)

Whilst abnormal values suggest hypovolaemia, normal values do not exclude it. Increased variations in arterial pulse pressure with breathing in sedated mechanically ventilated patients are due to changes in stroke volume that occur with changes in intrathoracic pressure, and may suggest hypovolaemia. Passive leg raising to increase venous return temporarily can be used, but may not be reliable in awake patients.

Unfortunately there is no linear relationship between pressure and volume in a vascular compartment that can change its capacitance 3-fold. Therefore, the response to fluid is not reliably predictable for any given CVP and may even fall with volume repletion (e.g. in conditions with intense peripheral vasoconstriction such as pre-eclampsia). The CVP may be falsely high if the patient has intrinsic heart or lung disease.

A more dynamic measurement of the likely response to fluid can be obtained by administering a specific volume of fluid as a fluid challenge. In order for the fluid challenge to result in an increase in stroke volume and cardiac output, the fluid challenge has to increase cardiac preload significantly and this has to increase stroke volume significantly. Therefore, the patient can be a non-responder because either preload is not increased or one or both of the ventricles is operating on the flat part of the Frank–Starling curve.

Performing a fluid challenge

To test this mechanism requires a variable amount of fluid. Filling pressures represent the net effect of preload, ventricular compliance and afterload. The initial fluid challenge technique proposed by Weil and Henning in 1979 measured CVP at 10min intervals after 100–200ml of fluid. If the change in CVP was <2mm Hg, the fluid was continued. If it was 2–5mm Hg it was stopped and the CVP re-measured after 10min. If it was >5mm Hg, it was stopped. The values were 3–7mmHg if the PAWP was being used.

Vincent has recently modified this technique allowing for the continuous monitoring that is now available. He suggests a larger volume over a longer time period in line with the regime suggested in the surviving sepsis campaign (i.e. 500–1000ml crystalloid or 300–500ml colloid over 30min). Goals should be set at the outset, such as an increase in MAP. Because the most serious adverse effect of a fluid challenge is acute pulmonary oedema secondary to congestive cardiac failure, Vincent suggests setting 'safety limits' such as a set CVP/PAWP which, when reached, alerts the practitioner to stop the infusion. If the MAP is rising along with the CVP, fluid can be infused until the desired MAP is reached. If the CVP is rising without any change in MAP, this indicates the fluid challenge is unsuccessful and other forms of circulatory support are required.

Type of fluid

There is no consensus as to the most suitable fluid. Colloids are widely used, as they are believed to stay in the circulation longer due to their larger molecular weight. This maintains osmotic pressure, and so a smaller volume can be given compared with a crystalloid to achieve the same haemodynamic response. Colloids may be blood products (HAS or FFP) or synthetic (modified gelatins, dextrans or hydroxyethyl starches). They have different molecular weights and therefore remain in the circulation for varying amounts of time. They also differ in their safety profile. Low to medium molecular weight colloids such as gelatins and albumin may leak in to the interstitial space more rapidly than high molecular weight colloids such as hydroxyethyl starches. A number of Cochrane systematic reviews have looked at the difference in mortality when different fluids are used for resuscitation. They found no difference between crystalloids and colloids, no difference between any of the colloids, and no difference between hypertonic and nearly isotonic fluids. In the latter two reviews, the authors noted large confidence intervals and therefore could not exclude significant clinical differences.

The choice of fluid used should be made on the basis of the underlying disease, the type of fluid lost, the severity of circulatory failure, the serum albumin of the patient and the risk of bleeding.

Colloids

Human albumin

Human albumin solution is available as 5 or 20%, the former being used for hypovolaemia, the latter for the treatment of hypoalbuminaemia in the presence of salt and water overload. In the UK, human albumin is expensive and there are concerns over the risk of transmission of infections, as with any blood product. A Cochrane systematic review showed no benefit in terms of mortality when albumin was used for resuscitation. This review was mainly made up of patients from the SAFE trial, which showed no difference in outcome between normal saline and human albumin when given as a bolus in 7500 patients.

Gelatins

Gelatins are produced by the hydrolysis of bovine collagen and then cross-linked with urea to produce Haemaccel or succinylated to produce Gelofusine. They remain in the circulation for ~2h, with renal excretion occurring within 48h. They are isotonic and the amount of chloride is lower than normal saline (145). Haemaccel has a significant amount of calcium (Ca 6.25) and so should not be infused through the same giving set as citrated blood. Gelatins also have the potential to cause allergic reactions.

Dextrans

Dextrans are polysaccharides derived from fermentation of sucrose which is then hydrolysed and fractionated into different molecular weights.

Dextran 40 has a molecular weight of 40 000Da. It is hypertonic and is not used for the treatment of hypovolaemia. It can cause renal tubular obstruction and renal failure.

Dextran 70 is produced as a 6% solution in normal saline or 5% dextrose. Its average molecular weight is 70 000Da. Osmolality is 335mosm/kg and is therefore mildly hypertonic. Plasma half-life is 6h. It can precipitate anaphylactic reactions and interfere with haemostasis.

Hyroxyethyl starches

Hydroxyethyl starches are prepared by hydroxyethyl substitution of amylopectin, a glucose polymer. They are generally presented in solution in normal saline and so may cause a hyperchloraemic acidosis. They vary in molecular weight but remain in the intravascular space for at least 6h. Hydroxyethyl starches may have adverse effects on coagulation and may also cause intractable itching if large volumes are used.

Crystalloids

Normal saline

Normal saline has long been used for resuscitation. However, the high chloride present will result in a hyperchloraemic acidosis when given in large volumes. The hyperchloraemic acidosis is caused by the high chloride content of normal saline (154mmol). This excess of negative chloride ions lead to a decrease in the strong ion difference, which causes a normal anion gap anion gap metabolic acidosis.

Hartmann's solution.

Hartmann's solution has a lower chloride concentration than normal saline but is mildly hypotonic, so may exacerbate cerebral oedema in those with brain injury. However, its main benefit is that its use is not associated with a normal anion gap acidosis.

Hypertonic saline

Hypertonic solutions are considered to expand intravascular volume by causing an osmotic shift of fluid from the extracellular and interstitial compartments to the intravascular space, thereby increasing blood pressure. The perceived advantage is that a small amount can be given over a short period with less risk of interstitial oedema. In particular it may be the fluid of choice in head injuries where the patient is hypovolaemic, as an increased MAP is required to maintain CPP, but not at the expense of a large fluid load that may result in interstitial oedema and brain swelling. The osmotic gradient may even draw water out of the brain tissue, thereby reducing ICP. However, if the blood–brain barrier is interrupted, the hypertonic saline may in fact pass across, drawing excessive amounts of water with it and thereby increasing intracranial pressure.

Hypertonic solutions may also prevent interstitial oedema whenever there is acute lung injury such as after trauma or surgery.

There are data in animals and humans to suggest that hypertonic saline has a favourable effect on haemaodynamic variables, ICP, and gut and respiratory function. However, there are no conclusive RCTs in humans at present.

Further reading

Bunn F, Alderson P, Hawkins V. Colloid solutions for fluid resuscitation. *Cochrane Database Syst Rev* 2003; (1): CD001319.

Bunn F, Roberts I, Tasker R, *et al.*. Hypertonic versus near isotonic crystalloid for fluid resuscitation in critically ill patients. *Cochrane Database Syst Rev* 2004; (3): CD002045.

Finfer S, Bellomo R, Boyce N, *et al.* A comparison of albumin and saline for fluid resuscitation in the intensive care unit. *N Engl J Med* 2004; 350: 2247–56.

Roberts I, Alderson P, Bunn F, *et al.* Colloids versus crystalloids for fluid resuscitation in critically ill patients. *Cochrane Database Syst Rev* 2004; (4): CD000567.

Vincent JL, Weil MH. Fluid challenge revisited. *Crit Care Med* 2006; 34: 1333–7.

Weil MH, Henning RJ. New concepts in the diagnosis and fluid treatment of circulatory shock. Thirteenth annual Becton, Dickinson and Company Oscar Schwidetsky Memorial Lecture. *Anesth Analg* 1979; 58: 124–32.

Chapter 17

Respiratory disorders

Chapter contents

Upper airway obstruction

There are few medical conditions that are as rapidly and predictably lethal as the loss of upper airway patency. Because of the relative infrequency with which upper airway obstruction (UAO) is encountered by most physicians, opportunities to acquire significant clinical experience are limited. This, combined with the frequently subtle presentation of UAO and the clinician's inability to visualize the upper airway in its entire extent through routine physical examination, may hamper diagnosis of this condition until a crisis results.

Pathophysiology

The sites of UAO may be within the airway lumen, in the walls or extrinsic to the airway. Further, sites of UAO maybe can be divided into supraglottic, glottic and infraglottic above the carina. Finally, UAO will behave differently during inspiration and expiration if intrathoracic or extrathoracic. The intrathoracic airway dilates during inspiration as it is exposed to outward force of negative intrapleural pressure. Positive intrapleural pressure during expiration causes compression and narrowing. The compliant extrathoracic airway, not exposed to intrapleural pressure, collapses during inspiration and increases in diameter during expiration. UAO is likely to occur at sites of anatomic narrowing such as the hypopharynx at the base of the tongue, and the false and true vocal cords at the laryngeal opening.

Causes

Functional causes

- CNS depression
- Peripheral nervous system and neuromuscular abnormalities
- Recurrent laryngeal nerve interruption (post-operative, inflammatory, tumour infiltration)
- Obstructive sleep apnoea
- Laryngospasm
- Myasthenia gravis
- Guillain–Barre polyneuritis
- Hypocalcaemia (causing vocal cord spasm)
- Tetanus

Mechanical causes

- Foreign body aspiration

Infections

- Epiglottitis
- Supraglottitis
- Retropharyngeal cellulitis or abscess
- Parapharyngeal abscess
- Ludwig's angina
- Diphtheria
- Bacterial tracheitis
- Laryngotracheobronchitis

Laryngeal oedema

- Allergic
- Hereditary angioedema

Haemorrhage and haematoma

- Post-operative
- Anticoagulation therapy
- Coagulopathy

Trauma

Burns

Neoplasm

- Pharyngeal, laryngeal and tracheobronchial carcinoma
- Vocal cord polyposis

Congenital

- Vascular rings
- Laryngeal webs, laryngocoele

Miscellaneous

- Cricoarytenoid arthritis
- Achalasia of the oesophagus
- Hysterical stridor
- Myxoedema

Clinical presentation and initial evaluation

May be complete or partial.

Complete UAO

- Rapidly progressing series of events. Patient is unable to breathe, speak or cough, and may hold the throat between the thumb and index finger (the universal choking sign). Anxious and agitated. Vigorous attempts at respiration with intercostal and supraclavicular retraction. Heart rate and blood pressure raised. Patient becomes rapidly cyanosed,
- Respiratory efforts diminish, loss of consciousness, bradycardia and hypotension. Cardiac arrest.
- Death is inevitable if the obstruction is not relieved within 2–5min of the onset,

Partial UAO

- Stable, or progressive deterioration,
- Signs and symptoms may be mild but as they worsen they include coughing, inspiratory stridor, crowing or noisy respiration, dysphonia, aphonia, choking, drooling and gagging. Dyspnoea, feeble cough, respiratory distress and signs of hypoxaemia and hypercarbia such as anxiety, confusion, lethargy and cyanosis may be present as the obstruction worsens.
- Powerful inspiratory efforts against an obstruction may produce dermal petechiae and subcutaneous emphysema. Partial airway obstruction that is worsening should be aggressively managed and, if rapidly progressing, immediate preparation for treatment as complete obstruction should be made.
- In stable, non-progressing cases of partial obstruction, specific diagnostic evaluation may be undertaken provided the patient is strictly observed for any signs of deterioration and facilities for skilled airway management are immediately available.

Special investigations

Laryngoscopy and bronchoscopy

Laryngoscopy using flexible naso-endoscopy in a stable, cooperative patient is useful in diagnosing foreign bodies, retropharyngeal or laryngeal masses and other glottic pathology. In skilled hands it is quick, simple and atraumatic.

If laryngoscopy is conducted using a flexible intubating laryngoscope or bronchoscope, definitive airway control can be achieved at conclusion of examination by railroading an ETT into the trachea. Disadvantages are need for a skilled operator, time to achieve local anaesthetic topicalization of the airway and a cooperative patient. It can be very difficult in the presence of blood and secretions. It is a traumatic procedure and may lead to worsened swelling, bleeding and oedema, and catastrophic loss of the airway.

Radiographic imaging

AP and lateral plain neck radiographs can be useful in detecting radiopaque foreign bodies, retropharyngeal masses and epiglottitis. A lateral view should be obtained during inspiration with the neck fully extended.

CT scanning in stable patients enables assessment of the integrity of the thyroid, cricoid and arytenoid cartilages, as well as the status of the airway lumen.

Management

A myriad of techniques using a huge variety of equipment have been described for management of UAO. The key principles are to have agreed a set number of techniques and to provide training and equipment for these for each institution.

General measures

Reverse hypoxia with 100% oxygen. Gain IV access as soon as practicable. Continuous monitoring and observation with the most skilled personnel available. Assess the airway carefully to delineate where and what type of UAO is present. Plan the approach to airway management with Plan A and subsequent back-up plans in the event of failure.

Airway equipment should be readily available, ideally in a movable trolley with an agreed contents list that is maintained regularly. Such a list would include a choice of laryngoscopes, blades and ETTs, fibreoptic bronchoscope or laryngoscope, bougies, a choice of supraglottic airway devices such as LMA™ and intubating laryngeal mask airway (ILMA™) and equipment necessary for a surgical airway (cricothyroidotomy set, tracheostomy tray and equipment for trans tracheal jet ventilation), emergency drugs and good suction,

Principles of airway management techniques

Airway manoeuvres

Try simple manoeuvres to open airway, jaw thrust, insertion of an oropharyngeal or nasopharyngeal airway may be effective in the unconscious or obtunded patient.

Consider the coma position to maintain the airway if the cervical spine is clear.

Endotracheal intubation

If UAO persists, the key principle in gaining formal airway control is not to lose oxygenation during the intubation attempts. Supraglottic airway devices such as the LMA and ILMA can provide a means of oxygenation and a conduit for endotracheal intubation.

If a full stomach is likely and a rapid sequence intubation indicated, then careful head and neck positioning and cricoid pressure with the BURP manoeuvre (Backward, Upward and Rightward Pressure) may improve laryngeal visualization. Pre-loading the ETT onto a bougie will minimize apnoeic time. Use of a CO_2 detector (capnography or single use device) will ensure correct placement of the ETT in the trachea.

If appropriate skills are available then flexible endoscopic techniques (FOI) may be considered. This can be achieved through an LMA, for example, or under local anaesthesia if time permits. Siting of a cricothyroid cannula beforehand can provide oxygenation using transtracheal jet ventilation during the intubation attempt and can remove the sense of extreme urgency from the situation. Care with allowing time for exhalation and not overinflating the lungs will avoid barotrauma, especially in the presence of severe UAO.

In the presence of blood and excessive secretions, FOI may be impossible. Retrograde tracheal intubation over a J-tip guide wire passed cranially via the cricothyroid membrane can be useful in this scenario.

Surgical airway

Indicated when earlier airway plans have failed or at the outset if endotracheal intubation is not possible (e.g. bleeding into an oral surgery microvascular flap with severe UAO) or if an unstable cervical spine is threatened by available airway techniques. The key principle here is to recognize the need for a surgical airway early and not wait till the patient is already severely hypoxic.

Percutaneous transtracheal jet ventilation using one of the proprietary needle cannula/catheters/jet ventilation systems (e.g. VBM Manujet™) inserted through the cricothyroid membrane can be achieved relatively quickly.

Cricothyrotomy with a wide bore cannula or even an ETT with a minimum internal diameter of 5mm will allow adequate gas exchange through a normal breathing circuit. The cricothyroid space is 9mm by 30mm in an adult; therefore, up to a size 8.5mm outer diameter tube should avoid complications such as laryngeal fracture and vocal cord damage. Complications such as subglottic stenosis, thyroid fracture, haemorrhage and pneumothorax are uncommon.

Emergency tracheostomy is rarely required. Formal surgical tracheostomy under local anaesthesia may be a prudent approach under some controlled conditions

Further reading

American Society of Anesthesiologists Task Force on Management of the Difficult Airway. Practice Guidelines for Management of the Difficult Airway: An Updated Report by the American Society of Anesthesiologists Task Force on Management of the Difficult Airway. *Anesthesiology* 2003; 98: 1269–77.

Difficult Airway Society, http://www.das.uk.com/

Henderson JJ, Popat MT, Latto IP, et al (2004). Difficult Airway Society guidelines for management of the unanticipated difficult intubation. *Anaesthesia* 59: 675–94.

Langeron O. Trauma airway management. *Curr Opin Crit Care* 2000; 6: 383–9.

Respiratory failure

Definition

Respiratory failure is a condition in which the respiratory system is unable to maintain adequate gas exchange to satisfy metabolic demands, i.e. oxygenation of and/or elimination of carbon dioxide from mixed venous blood. The respiratory system consists of a gas-exchanging organ (the lungs) and a ventilatory pump (respiratory muscles/thorax) either or both of which can fail and precipitate respiratory failure.

Classification

Respiratory failure is generally classified into:

- ***Hypoxaemic (type I).*** This is the most common form of respiratory failure and is invariably associated with parenchymal lung diseases (Table 17.2.1). It is characterized by a PaO_2 <8.0kPa (60mm Hg) with a normal or low pCO_2.
- ***Ventilatory (type II).*** This is secondary to failure of the ventilatory pump, and characterized by hypoventilation with hypercapnia ($PaCO_2$ >6.0kPa (45mm Hg)), which in the absence of supplemental oxygen is invariably associated with hypoxaemia (Table 17.2.1).

Table 17.2.1 Common causes of respiratory failure

Type I: hypoxaemic	Type II: hypercapnic
Pneumonia	COPD
ARDS/ALI	Severe asthma
Pulmonary fibrosis	Drug overdose (opiates)
Pulmonary oedema	CNS insult (trauma, CVA)
Asthma	Primary muscle disorders
COPD	Myasthenia gravis
Pneumothorax	Poliomyelitis
Pulmonary embolus	Kyphoscoliosis
Obesity	Polyneuropathies
Pulmonary hypertension	Obesity hypoventilation syndrome

Pathophysiology

Hypoxaemic—type I

Type I respiratory failure derives from the effects of one or more of the following four pathophysiological mechanisms: ventilation/perfusion mismatch, true shunt, diffusion impairment or reduced inspired oxygen concentration.

Ventilation/perfusion (V/Q) mismatching occurs when alveolar units are poorly ventilated in relation to their perfusion (low V/Q units). As the degree of V/Q maldistribution increases, hypoxaemia worsens because a greater proportion of the cardiac output will be poorly oxygenated. This effect is amplified because the sigmoid shape of the haemoglobin dissociation curve means that high or normal V/Q alveolar units cannot compensate for the units at low V/Q ratio.

True shunt occurs when deoxygenated mixed venous blood bypasses ventilated alveoli, resulting in 'venous admixture'. The quantity of blood which would be required to reduce the saturation of the pulmonary end-capillary blood to the observed value of PaO_2 is called the shunt fraction (Qs/Qt) and can be calculated as;

$$Qs/Qt= (CcO_2 - CaO_2)/(CcO_2 - CvO_2)$$

or more simply as;

$$Qs/Qt= (1 - SaO_2)/(1 - SvO_2)$$

Where CcO_2 = capillary oxygen content; CaO_2 = arterial oxygen content; CvO_2 = venous oxygen content CcO_2 = capillary oxygen content; SaO_2 = arterial oxygen saturation; SvO_2 = mixed venous oxygen saturation.

In practice, it is difficult to distinguish between true shunt and V/Q mismatch, and they often occur simultaneously. V/Q mismatch results in hypoxaemia because the distribution of alveolar oxygen tension is uneven. However, when breathing FiO_2 1.0, the alveolar oxygen tension becomes uniform with V/Q mismatch, whereas there is no effect in true shunt, and, therefore, it may be possible to distinguish the two processes.

Diffusion impairment occurs when the movement of oxygen from the alveolus to the pulmonary capillary is impaired and there is insufficient time for oxygenation to occur. This is invariably related to extensive and/or destructive lung disease where V/Q mismatch is also a significant factor, and in its pure form occurs rarely in clinical practice.

Reduced inspired oxygen concentration is not a problem in conventional practice (outside of extreme environments), and is easily overcome by increasing the FiO_2.

Initially, the hypoxaemia present in type I respiratory failure is frequently associated with an increase in the ventilation, and therefore decreased $PaCO_2$. However, as the condition persists or progresses, fatigue of the respiratory muscles or CNS impairment can lead an increase in $PaCO_2$.

Another factor that may contribute to hypoxaemia is low mixed venous oxygen saturation (SvO_2). Normally, only 20–30% of the delivered oxygen is extracted by the tissues, and the resulting venous oxygen levels can be measured using a central venous catheter (central venous oxygen saturation, $ScvO_2$) or in the pulmonary artery using a pulmonary artery catheter (mixed venous oxygen saturation, SvO_2). SvO_2 values of ~65–75% represent an optimal balance between global oxygen supply and demand. It is clear that the lower the SvO_2 the greater will be the effect of shunt or low Va/Q ratio on PaO_2. Increasing SvO_2 with early use fluids, blood transfusion and inotropic support to optimize cardiac output, can have a favourable effect on arterial oxygenation and also survival.

Hypercapnic—type II

In normal conditions $PaCO_2$ is maintained within strict limits (4.8–5.9kPa (36–44 mmHg)). Hypercapnic respiratory failure may occur either acutely, insidiously or acutely upon chronic CO_2 retention. The common denominator in type II respiratory failure is reduced effective alveolar ventilation (VA) for a given CO_2 production (VCO_2). The relationship between end-tidal CO_2 and VCO_2 is:

$$[\text{end-tidal } CO_2] = VCO_2/VA;$$

$$[\text{end tidal } CO_2] = VCO_2/(VE(1 - VD/VT)$$

end-tidal concentration in % approximates to end-tidal value in kPa. Partial pressure can be substituted and there is a close but unpredictable relationship between $PaCO_2$ and end-tidal CO_2, so the equation can be rewritten

$$PaCO_2 = VCO_2/(VE(1 - VD/VT)\times f)$$

Where VE is minute ventilation and VD is dead space ventilation, VT is tidal volume and f is respiratory frequency.

Under conditions where VCO_2 remains unchanged, the resulting pCO_2 will depend on the interaction between respiratory rate, tidal volume and the degree of dead space ventilation. Although the latter is often assumed to be fixed, in reality the physiological dead space may vary within a given patient and depends on the interaction between alveolar and pulmonary vascular pressures. This can be particularly important in critically ill patients where the precarious cardiovascular status interacts with the need for positive pressure ventilation. VCO_2 is rarely the limiting factor in normal lungs (see below), but even normal (carbohydrate-based feeds) or slightly increased (increased work of breathing) VCO_2 may be a problem with extensive lung disease.

Clinically, type II (hypercapnic) respiratory failure occurs under four circumstances.

- ***Central CNS depression*** with reduction of the respiratory drive (e.g. drugs, CNS diseases)
- ***Impaired respiratory muscle function*** (e.g. neuromuscular diseases, malnutrition, drugs, skeletal deformities, respiratory muscle dysfunction or fatigue from excessive mechanical load)
- ***V/Q mismatch*** (high V/Q, with increase in dead space ventilation)
- ***Increased*** CO_2 ***production*** in extreme cases (malignant hyperthermia) can be the sole cause

Acute vs chronic respiratory failure

Acute type II respiratory failure develops over minutes to hours and is invariably associated with an acidosis (pH <7.35). In chronic type II respiratory failure, hypercapnia develops over a much longer period, allowing time for renal compensation with an increase in bicarbonate concentration and minimal change in pH. The distinction between acute and chronic hypoxaemic (type I) respiratory failure cannot easily be made on the basis of arterial blood gases, but clinical markers of chronic hypoxaemia, such as polycythaemia or cor pulmonale, suggest a long-standing disorder.

Clinical assessment

The assessment of a patient with suspected respiratory failure requires a thorough clinical history and examination in conjunction with specific investigations, with individual findings dependent on the precipitating cause. The degree to which this is feasible may depend on the severity and rapidity with which the patient is deteriorating, and it is not uncommon for some of this process to occur following the instigation of empirical therapy and sometimes ventilatory support. None the less, this process should be completed as soon as is practicable. Repeated clinical observation, including pulse oximetry monitoring may be necessary.

Essential investigations

- Arterial blood gas analysis
- ECG
- CXR
- FBC
- Septic screen (sputum, blood culture)

Several indices are used in clinical practice to assess and monitor gas exchange in ventilated and non-ventilated patients.

$P(A–a)O_2$ gradient: the alveolar to arterial (A–a) oxygen gradient is calculated by subtracting the PaO_2 from the alveolar PAO_2, calculated using the alveolar gas equation:

$$PAO_2 = PIO_2 - (PaCO_2/R)$$

The normal A–a gradient varies with age and FiO_2. Hypoventilation can be differentiated from other causes of hypoxaemia by the presence of a normal A–a gradient.

$P(a/A)O_2$ ratio or respiratory index: this is calculated by dividing the $P(A–a)O_2$ gradient by PaO_2. Unlike the $P(A–a)O_2$ gradient it is relatively unaffected by the FiO_2. The normal $P(a/A)O_2$ ratio varies from 0.74–0.77 when FiO_2 is 0.21, to 0.80–.82 when FiO_2 is 1.

PaO_2/FiO_2 ratio: this is probably the most widely used index, being easy to calculate and a good estimate of shunt fraction. A PaO_2/FiO_2 ratio of <200mm Hg (26.6kPa) indicates ARDS and relates to a shunt fraction of >20%, and <300mm Hg (40kPa) defines ALI.

Oxygenation index (OI): this index takes into account the mean airway pressure and is calculated as:

$$OI = (FiO_2 \times Paw \times 100/PaO_2)$$

Principles of treatment

Respiratory failure is managed by a combination of specific and supportive measures. General principles are the following.

- Ensure airway patency
- Administer oxygen to maintain SaO_2 >90%
- Correct hypoperfusion and anaemia
- Correct reversible causes (e.g. drain pleural effusion or pneumothorax)
- Pharmacological management to treat infection, bronchoconstriction
- Physiotheraphy to mobilize secretions
- Consider non-invasive ventilatory support (CPAP/bilevel) to improve oxygenation, reduce work of breathing and reduce hypercapnia
- Early assessment for mechanical ventilation if non-invasive respiratory support contraindicated or failed.

Further reading

Hess DR, Kacmarek RM. Indices of oxygenation and ventilation. In: Hess DR, Kacmarek RM, eds. Essentials of mechanical ventilation. New York: McGraw-Hill, 2002: 240–5.

Lumb AB. Nunn's applied respiratory physiology, Elsevier, 2005.

Mellemgaard K. The alveolar-arterial oxygen difference: its size and components in normal man. *Acta Physiol Scand* 1966; 67: 10–20.

Rivers E, Nguyen B, Havstad S, *et al.* Early goal-directed therapy in the treatment of severe sepsis and septic shock. *N Engl J Med* 2001; 345: 1368–77.

West JB Respiratory physiology—the essentials, 7th edn. Baltimore: Williams and Wilkins, 2004.

Wood LD. The pathophysiology and differential diagnosis of acute respiratory failure. In: Hall JB, Schmidt GA, Wood LD, eds. *Principles of critical care.* New York: McGraw-Hill, 2005: 417–26.

Pulmonary collapse and atelectasis

The terms atelectasis and collapse are often used interchangeably. Pulmonary collapse can affect any anatomical division of the lung, i.e. the whole lung, a single lobe or segments or subsegments of a lobe. It occurs due to a reduction or complete cessation of ventilation.

Causes

Obstructuve (resorptive) atelectasis.

Intrinisic obstruction of the airway with distal resorption of air obstruction: inhaled foreign body, aspiration, neoplasms, mucus plugs (asthma, bronchiectasis, **a**llergic bronchopulmonary aspergillosis (ABPA), secretions (pneumonia), endobronchial intubation.

Relaxative (passive) atelectasis

Interruption of the negative pressure holding visceral and parietal pleura in close contact causes the lung to retract: pneumothorax, pleural effusions.

Compressive atelectasis

External compression of the lung by chest wall, pleural or mediastinal structures. Can be localized or regional in nature: neoplasms (primary or secondary), lymphadenopathy (e.g. sarcoid, TB, lymphoma), cardiomegaly (especially affecting left and middle lobe bronchus), loculated pleural collections, abdominal distension (ascites, ileus, abdominal compartment syndrome), obesity, neuromuscular weakness, chest pain (e.g. post-surgical, trauma).

Adhesive atelectasis

Increased surface tension within the alveoli due to decreased production or inactivation of surfactant: ARDS, infant respiratory distress syndrome (IRDS), pulmonary oedema, near drowning.

Cicratrization atelectasis

Loss of lung volume due to parechymal scarring: granulomatous disease, radiation, necrotizing pneumonia.

Rounded atelectasis (folded, trapped lung)

A distinct condition associated with inflammatory pleural disease, usually asbestosis, with minimal volume loss.

Consequences

- Hypoxaemia
  - V/Q mismatching
  - Reduced FRC
- Increased work of breathing
  - Surfactant dysfunction in collapsed region
  - Decreased thoracoabdominal compliance (passive and compressive atelectasis)
  - Increased risk of infection
  - Increased bacterial growth in collapsed region
  - Development of respiratory failure

The severity of the changes seen depends on the degree and rapidity of the developing collapse.

Incidence

Pulmonary collapse is not uncommon, the exact frequency depending on the cause. In patients who have undergone open abdominal surgery the incidence of significant subsegmental collapse approaches 20–25%.

Clinical features

Presenting features will depend on speed of onset, cause and severity of the atelectasis. Many patients may be asymptomatic, but common symptoms include breathlessness, cough and chest pain, and some may report systemic features. A full medical history may help identify the aetiology.

Examination findings

- Fever, tachycardia
- Tachypnoea
- Low SaO_2
- Reduced expansion on the affected side
- Trachea deviated towards the side of the collapse*
- Dull percussion note over affected area*
- Reduced breath sounds over affected area*
- Other signs that the patient is at risk of collapse, i.e. chest and abdominal wounds, abdominal distension, neuromuscular abnormalities.

(*only if significant volume of the lung affected)

Differential diagnosis

It is often difficult clinically to differentiate collapse from consolidation or pleural fluid, and frequently these entities will co-exist (Table 17.3.1).

Investigations

- CXR: ideally a PA film, but a lateral may be useful.
- Markers of infection and inflammation (FBC, CRP, sputum and blood cultures) as indicated
- Arterial blood gases (ABGs) to assess the degree of respiratory compromise
- CT may demonstrate the anatomy and may define causes, e.g. endobronchial lesion, lymphadenopathy
- Chest ultrasound may differentiate collapsed lung from a pleural effusion
- Bronchoscopy: both diagnostic (large airway obstruction, e.g. foreign body, sputum plug, tumour) and therapeutic

Table 17.3.1 Radiographic differences between collapse, consolidation and pleural fluid

	Collapse	Consolidation	Effusion
Volume loss	Marked	Minimal	Variable
Compensatory hyperinflation	Marked	Absent	Absent
Tracheal shift	Towards lesion	Absent	Away from lesion
Mediastinal shift	Towards lesion	Absent	Away from lesion
Diaphragm position	Unilateral elevation	Not elevated	Not elevated
Air bronchogram	Absent	Present	Absent

Radiology

Radiographic signs of collapse may be direct or indirect

Direct

- Displacement of intralobular fissures
- Loss of aeration
- Vascular and bronchial crowding

Indirect

- Elevation of hemidiaphragm
- Mediastinal displacement
- Hilar displacement
- Compensatory hyperinflation of remaining lung
- Crowding of ribs

Lobar collapse is associated with well defined patterns on the chest radiograph. However, CXR signs can be subtle and easily overlooked by the unwary clinician. Total lung collapse results in complete opacification of the effected hemithorax, with indicators of marked volume loss on that side, mediastinal shift and hyperinflation of the contralateral lung. Subsegmental (plate, discoid) atelectasis may appear as peripheral band-like densities perpendicular to the pleural surface.

Generic management

Stabilize the patient

- Oxygen,
- 'ABC'
- Assess the need for ventilatory support (invasive or non-invasive i.e. respiratory rate, ABGs)

Identify causes and treat

It is important to identify the likely causes of collapse as some are amenable to specific therapeutic interventions:

Intrinsic airway obstruction:

- bronchoscopy to remove the source of obstruction
- endobronchial stenting for a neoplastic lesion

Removing external sources of compression:

- Drain pleural effusion
- Treat pneumothorax
- Drain large ascites

Re-expansion of collapsed lung:

- CPAP
- Mechanical ventilation with PEEP

Specific management options

Physiotherapy

There is little evidence for the prophylactic use of physiotherapy for the prevention of atelectasis. However, there is evidence for its efficacy in treatment. Including manual treatments (percussion, vibration and positive pressure assist devices) in conjunction with patient positioning.

Fibreoptic bronchoscopy

Aside from its diagnostic use, bronchoscopy can be used for therapeutic intervention, e.g. to remove a foreign body, or, more commonly, remove retained secretions. It is commonly applied in the ICU, achieving similar results to physiotherapy. Case series demonstrate an improvement in PaO_2, lung compliance and CXR findings. It can be considered in lobar and segmental rather than subsegmental collapse, but may be less effective in patients who demonstrate air bronchograms on the preceding chest film.

Mucolytics (N-acetylcysteine, DNase)

Such therapies aim to reduce the viscosity of secretions, making them easier to clear and reducing mucus plugging. Although DNase has been shown to be effective in cystic fibrosis, definitive evidence in other conditions is scarce.

Mechanical ventilation

The following manoeuvres can be considered in isolation or in concert to re-expand collapsed regions/prevent regional (dependent) lung collapse;

- Higher levels of PEEP/CPAP
- Recruitment manoeuvres: transient application ofhigh levels of PEEP (30–40cm H_2O)
- Positioning the patient with collapsed segments in non-(less) dependent position,

Further reading

Ashizawa K, Hayashi K, Aso N, *et al.* Lobar atelectasis: diagnostic pitfalls on chest radiography. *Br Radiol J* 2001; 74: 89–97.

Hansell DM, Armstrong P, Lynch D, *et al.* Basic patterns of lung disease. In: Imaging of diseases of the chest. Phillidelphia: Elsevier Mosby, 2005: 69–141.

Kreider M, Lipson D. Bronchoscopy for atelectasis in the ICU: a case report and review of the literature, *Chest* 2003; 124: 344–50.

Schindler MB. Treatment of atelectasis: where is the evidence? *Crit Care* 2005; 9: 341–2.

Stiller K. Physiotherapy in intensive care: towards an evidence-based practice. *Chest* 2000; 118; 1801–13.

Chronic obstructive pulmonary disease (COPD)

Definition

COPD is characterized by slowly progressive airflow obstruction that is not fully reversible with treatment. Airflow obstruction is defined as an FEV_1 (forced expiratory volume in 1s) of <80% predicted **and** an FEV_1/FVC (forced vital capacity) ratio of <0.7.

Smoking is by far the most important cause of COPD. Others include air pollution, occupational dust (e.g. coal) and chemical (e.g. cadmium) exposure, and genetic causes (α_1-antitrypsin deficiency).

Severity defined on the basis of FEV_1:

Mild:	FEV_1 50–80% predicted
Moderate:	FEV_1 30–49% predicted
Severe:	FEV_1 <30% predicted

Differential diagnosis

Asthma, bronchiectasis, cardiac failure, lung cancer, bronchiolitis. These conditions may also co-exist with COPD.

Investigations include CXR, pulse oximetry and measurement of acute bronchodilator reversibility plus (where indicated) full lung function testing, peak flow diary, FBC, ABGs, ECG, echocardiogram, sputum culture, α_1-antitrypsin level and thoracic CT scan.

Management of stable COPD

Most treatments for stable COPD aim at controlling symptoms, preventing exacerbations and maintaining or improving exercise capacity and quality of life. Only long-term oxygen therapy (LTOT) in hypoxaemic patients has been shown to reduce mortality. Smoking cessation reduces the rate of decline of lung function while lung transplantation and lung volume reduction surgery can result in improved lung function. However, surgery is only appropriate and available for a small minority of COPD patients.

Current management of stable COPD includes:

- Inhaled bronchodilators: short- and long-acting β_2 agonists and anticholinergics.
- High dose inhaled corticosteroids to prevent exacerbations in moderate and severe COPD.
- Oral modified release theophyllines.
- Oral mucolytics in patients with productive cough.
- Diuretics for oedema due to cor pulmonale.
- Oxygen: short burst for relief of acute dyspnoea. LTOT for patients with PaO_2 <7.3kPa (or <8.0kPa plus polycythaemia or cor pulmonale). Ambulatory oxygen for patients who desaturate on exercise and in whom exercise capacity and/or symptoms improve when oxygen is administered.
- Pulmonary rehabilitation: multi-disciplinary programme comprising physical training and disease education suitable for all patients in whom dyspnoea limits their activity.
- Smoking cessation: nicotine replacement therapy, bupropion or varenicline combined with an appropriate support programme.
- Pneumococcal and annual influenza vaccination.
- Dietetic advice for patients with abnormal BMI.
- Nocturnal NIV may be of value in patients with chronic hypercapnic ventilatory failure with nocturnal hypoventilation and repeated admissions.
- Lung transplantation: single or double lung if FEV_1 is <25% predicted and/or cor pulmonale are present **plus** severe symptoms despite maximal medical therapy. Recipients must be non-smokers, <65 years old.
- Lung volume reduction surgery: consider in patients with upper lobe predominant emphysema where symptoms persist despite maximal medical therapy. Lung function parameters should be at least 20% predicted and $PaCO_2$ <7.3kPa.
- Bullectomy for patients with significant dyspnoea or complications due to a single large bulla.

Acute exacerbations of COPD (AECOPD)

A major cause of morbidity and mortality accounting for 1 in 8 of acute medical admissions. Typically patients present with increased dyspnoea, cough or wheeze, chest tightness, sputum volume and/or purulence.

Causes

Commonly infective (viral and bacterial), but others include air pollution (nitrogen and sulphur dioxide, ozone and particulates) and temperature changes. In some cases the cause is unidentifiable. The most common bacterial pathogens are *Haemophilus influenzae*, *Streptococcus pneumoniae* and *Moraxella catarrhalis*. Viral causes include rhinovirus, influenza, coronavirus and adenovirus.

Differential diagnosis

Pneumonia, pulmonary oedema, PE, pneumothorax, pleural effusion, lung cancer, UAO, recurrent aspiration.

Investigations

CXE, ECG, ABGs, FBC, U&Es, CRP plus blood cultures if pyrexial, and theophylline level if the patient is on oral theophylline therapy.

Assess severity

Signs of a severe exacerbation include severe dyspnoea/tachypnoea, use of accessory muscles and pursed lip breathing, acute confusion, new peripheral oedema, new cyanosis and respiratory acidosis on ABGs. Mortality rises sharply in patients with a pH of <7.25. If none of the above is present, the patient may be suitable for home management of their exacerbation dependent upon other co-morbidities and social circumstances.

Controlled oxygen

Aim to maintain adequate levels of oxygenation without precipitating worsening hypercapnia and acidosis. Ideally SaO_2 should be between 90 and 95%, although in some patients with chronic hypoxia a target of 85–90% is more appropriate. Oxygen should be delivered via face masks that allow accurate determination of FiO_2. SpO_2 should be monitored, and ABGs repeated regularly according to response to treatment.

Hypoxaemia may recover slowly following AECOPD, after other symptoms have improved. This only requires treatment if the patient is symptomatic. For oxygen to be supplied to a patient's home, a Home Oxygen Order Form (HOOF) needs to be completed. In these circumstances, the respiratory team should be contacted so that assessment for LTOT can be arranged ~6 weeks later.

Nebulized bronchodilators

Salbutamol 2–4 hourly plus as required, and ipratropium 6 hourly should be prescribed until the patient has recovered sufficiently to use inhalers. Nebulizers should be driven with compressed air in patients with severe respiratory acidosis, with supplemental oxygen being delivered via nasal cannulae if required.

Systemic steroids

All patients should be prescribed oral prednisolone 30mg/day for 1–2 weeks. IV hydrocortisone should only be used in patients who are unable to take parental medication. There is no proven benefit in continuing steroids beyond 14 days either to promote further recovery or to prevent exacerbations, although a small minority of patients with advanced COPD require maintenance therapy.

Antibiotic therapy

Antibiotics should be reserved for patients with increased sputum purulence unless there is other clinical evidence of infection (e.g. pyrexia, high CRP) or consolidation on CXR. In the absence of pneumonia, a single antibiotic given orally is appropriate for all patients able to take parental medication. Choice of antibiotic will be determined by local policy and is influenced by recent previous antibiotic therapy, previous sputum results and recent hospitalization.

Intravenous aminophylline

Consider only in patients with a severe exacerbation who are not responding adequately to nebulized bronchodilators, particularly those with predominant wheeze. A loading dose should not be given to patients who were on oral theophylline prior to admission. Aminophylline levels should be measured within 24h of starting treatment and daily thereafter.

Treatment of acute respiratory failure

NIV has been shown to reduce mortality and hasten recovery in AECOPD patients presenting with hypercapnic respiratory failure compared with standard medical care. It reduces the need for intubation and has a lower complication rate than treatment with invasive ventilation. It should be used in hypoxaemic patients with a pH of <7.35 **and** a $PaCO_2$ of >6kPa in whom a trial of optimal medical management as described above has been ineffective. It is important to be aware of iatrogenic hypercapnic acidosis caused by the administration of high concentration oxygen. Such patients often improve once the FiO_2 is lowered without the need for NIV.

NIV should be delivered on a dedicated unit with appropriate levels of monitoring and staff training/experience. This usually means ITU/HDU or a high monitoring bay on an admission or respiratory ward. Prior to commencement of NIV, the ceiling of therapy should be agreed, in particular if invasive ventilation on ITU is to be commenced if the patient is deteriorating despite NIV. Patients with a pH of <7.25 are at increased risk of treatment failure with NIV and, if appropriate, should be treated on ITU or considered for invasive ventilation at the outset.

Invasive ventilation

Patients with good pre-exacerbation functional status and no clinically significant co-morbidities should be considered for invasive ventilation if they are deteriorating despite maximal medical therapy including NIV. The mortality rate for this group (~25%) compares favourably with that of patients requiring invasive ventilation for other causes of ARF. However, the prognosis deteriorates in patients requiring >72h of ventilation. NIV has been used to assist weaning patients from invasive ventilation.

Respiratory stimulants

Doxapram is now cheifly used when NIV is unavailable, contraindicated or not tolerated. It can be used along with NIV in patients who are particularly drowsy and CO_2 retaining.

Physiotherapy

There is a lack of good evidence for the benefit of physiotherapy in AECOPD. However, it is probably of value in patients with significant sputum production, particularly when using a positive expiratory pressure mask to assist coughing.

Palliative care

Opioids (initially oramorph 2.5mg up to 4 hourly) should be given to patients with dyspnoea that is not responsive to other therapy. This treatment is also useful for cough. Opioids should not be reserved solely for patients who are in the terminal phase of their illness. Where anxiety is a major factor, benzodiazepines should also be administered (e.g. lorazepam 0.5–1mg up to 8 hourly). The palliative care team should be involved.

Prognosis

Following admission with AECOPD, recovery takes 1–2 weeks, but in 25% of patients is more than a month, with some patients never regaining their previous functional level. The 3 month mortality rate is ~15%. One-quarter of patients are re-admitted within 3 months. For patients requiring either NIV or admission to ITU, the 1yr mortality is ~50%.

Further reading

Breen D, Churches T, Hawker F, *et al.* Acute respiratory failure secondary to COPD treated in the intensive care unit: a long term follow up study. *Thorax* 2002; 57: 29–33.

Burge PS, Calverley PMA, Jones PW, *et al.* Randomised, double-blind, placebo controlled study of fluticasone propionate in patients with moderate to severe COPD: the ISOLDE trial. *BMJ* 2000; 320: 1297–303.

Chu CM, Chan VL, Lin AWN, *et al.* Readmission rates and life threatening events in COPD survivors treated with non-invasive ventilation for acute hypercapnic respiratory failure. *Thorax* 2004; 59: 1020–5.

National Institute of Health and Clinical Excellence, National clinical guideline on management of COPD in adults in primary and secondary care. NICE guideline. *Thorax* 2004; 59 suppl. 1: 1–232.

Plant PK, Owen JL, Elliott MW. Early use of non-invasive ventilation for acute exacerbations of COPD on general respiratory wards: a multicentre randomised controlled trial. *Lancet* 2000; 355: 1931–5.

ARDS: diagnosis

History and definition

The adult respiratory distress syndrome was first described in a case series of only 12 patients from Colorado in 1967. The North American–European Consensus Conference (NAECC) proposed that the syndrome be defined as the acute onset of refractory hypoxaemia in association with bilateral pulmonary infiltrates with no evidence of elevated left atrial pressure (Table 17.5.1). These definitions are now established, but inevitably they lack a pathognomic test, the X-ray criteria are subjective and the oxygenation criteria do not take account of the provision of ventilatory support. The NAECC simultaneously changed the name to acute respiratory distress syndrome (ARDS) recognizing that, whilst the pathological appearances are superficially similar to the respiratory distress syndrome of the newborn, the condition does occur in children and is otherwise distinct The value of dividing the syndrome into ALI and ARDS is questionable as the outcome of patients presenting in either category is similar.

Table 17.5.1 NAECC definition of ALI and ARDS

	Timing	Oxygenation	CXR	Exclusion of cardiogenic pulmonary oedema
ALI	Acute	PaO_2/FiO_2 ≤300mm Hg	Bilateral opacities consistent with pulmonary oedema	PAoP ≤18mm Hg if measured or no clinical evidence of left atrial hypertension
ARDS		PaO_2/FiO_2 ≤200mm Hg		

PaO_2/FiO_2 = arterial partial pressure of oxygen/inspired oxygen fraction; PAoP = pulmonary artery occlusion pressure.

Causes and risk factors

The likelihood of developing ARDS depends on the type and number of predisposing conditions and on patient characteristics. For example, predisposing factors include alcoholism and emerging genetic polymorphisms, whilst diabetes mellitus is protective. Although the causes of ALI/ARDS may be divided into direct and indirect injuries (Table 17.5.2), outcomes are similar if other variables are controlled for.

Epidemiology and incidence

A recent survey in a defined region of the USA reported that the incidence and mortality of ALI/ARDS increases with age from 16 per 100 000 person-years and 24% for teenagers, to 306 per 100 000 person-years and 60% for those >75 years. The majority of patients with ALI/ARDS have either been weaned from ventilatory support or have died within the first 10 days; ~10% of patients require support for >1 month. Mortality rates from most observational studies vary between 35 and 60%, although this will vary depending on the age of the patient and the presence of non-pulmonary organ dysfunctions, particularly shock and hepatic failure. In specialist centres, survival rates have improved over the last 20 years. Most ARDS patients tend to die *with* rather than *from* respiratory failure and, despite severe acute lung damage, chronic respiratory failure afflicts a small proportion of survivors. Chronic weakness and neuropsychiatric problems that may be permanent are the greatest barrier to survivors returning to their normal lives.

Table 17.5.2 Clinical risk factors for ARDS

Direct lung injury	Indirect lung injury
Pneumonia (12%)*	Sepsis syndrome (40%) and shock
Aspiration of gastric contents (20%)	Multiple trauma
Thoracic trauma/pulmonary contusion	Blood product transfusion (35%)**
Inhalation injury (smoke, toxin, near drowning)	Acute pancreatitis
Reperfusion injury (lung transplant, pleural effusion drainage)	Drug overdose/drug reaction
Thoracic irradiation	Cardiopulmonary bypass
Fat embolism syndrome	Pregnancy related (eclampsia, amniotic fluid embolism)
	Tumour lysis syndrome
	Head injury/raised intracranial pressure

Figures in parentheses are the approximate percentage of patients with single risk factors that develop ARDS.
*For patients with pneumonia admitted to an ICU.
**For the transfusion of 15 units of blood in 1 day.

Differential diagnoses

The clinical criteria used to define the syndrome are vague, e.g those used to exclude cardiogenic pulmonary oedema, which is the most important differential. Numerous conditions may present as ARDS despite not sharing the characteristic pathology (diffuse alveolar damage) and pathophysiology:

- acute neutrophilic inflammation
- dysfunction of the alveolar-capillary membrane causing pulmonary oedema
- microvascular dysfunction causing ventilation–perfusion mismatching and hypoxaemia
- fibroproliferation.

Some of these less common conditions, such as acute eosinophilic pneumonia, acute interstitial pneumonitis, cryptogenic organizing pneumonia, diffuse alveolar haemorrhage and bilateral pulmonary embolism, have specific treatments, emphasizing the importance of diagnosing the underlying cause of ARDS. Other conditions may be managed differently because of their relatively poor prognosis, e.g. lymphangitis carcinomatosa.

Clinical features and investigations

The primary aim of the initial clinical assessment is to identify the underlying causes of ARDS and organ system failures that require urgent support. Excluding cardiogenic pulmonary oedema is based on the patient's history, CXR and ECG in the first instance, although further information may be obtained from a pulmonary artery catheter and echocardiogram in selected cases. Thoracic CT demonstrates characteristic appearances in ARDS, with an indirect cause and evidence of the initial insult when the cause of ARDS was pulmonary. Subsequent assessments should focus on detecting the complications of ARDS and critical illness, most notably hospital-acquired infection. Thoracic CT not uncommonly reveals pathology that is not evident on a plain chest film, e.g. pneumothorax, pleural effusion, pneumonia and lung abscess.

Further reading

Acute Respiratory Distress Syndrome Network. Ventilation with lower tidal volumes as compared with traditional tidal volumes for acute lung injury and the acute respiratory distress syndrome. *N Engl J Med* 2000; 342: 1301–8.

Bernard GR, Artigas A, Brigham KL, et al. The American–European Consensus Conference on ARDS. Definitions, mechanisms, relevant outcomes, and clinical trial coordination. *Am J Respir Crit Care Med* 1994; 149: 818–24.

Dakin J, Griffiths M. The pulmonary physician in critical care 1: pulmonary investigations for acute respiratory failure. *Thorax* 2002; 57: 79–85.

Griffiths MJD, Evans TW. Acute respiratory distress syndrome. In: Gibson GJ, Geddes DM, Costabel U, *wt al.*, eds. Respiratory medicine, 3rd edn. London: Saunders, 2003: 736–63.

Montgomery AB, Stager MA, Carrico CJ, *et al.* Causes of mortality in patients with the adult respiratory distress syndrome. *Am Rev Respir Dis* 1985; 132: 485–9.

Rubenfeld GD, Caldwell E, Peabody E, *et al.* Incidence and outcomes of acute lung injury. *N Engl J Med* 2005; 353: 1685–93.

Rubenfeld GD, Herridge MS. Epidemiology and outcomes of acute lung injury. *Chest* 2007; 131: 554–62.

Wheeler AP, Bernard GR. Acute lung injury and the acute respiratory distress syndrome: a clinical review. *Lancet* 2007; 369: 1553–64.

ARDS: general management

Introduction

Despite the large number of studies carried out investigating novel therapies for patients with ARDS, only the use of low tidal volume ventilation has been shown to improve mortality. However, improvements in the survival of these patients in specialist centres have preceded the widespread adoption of protective ventilation and emphasize the importance of optimizing supportive care. Carrying out clinical trials in a highly heterogenous critically ill population of patients is fraught with pitfalls, which are exacerbated by the loose criteria that define the syndrome.

General supportive care

In the absence of specific treatments for ARDS, the management involves aggressive treatment of the underlying causes, and prevention and treatment of the complications of ARDS and critical illness. Accordingly, prophylaxis against stress ulceration, venous thrombosis and pressure ulcers should be administered as indicated. In essence, the objective is to buy time and to optimize conditions for the lungs to recover.

Infection

Non-pulmonary sepsis and pneumonia are amongst the most common causes of ARDS. Conversely, sepsis and VAP are common complications of ARDS. VAP is difficult to diagnose in patients with ARDS because of the frequent co-existence of pulmonary infiltrates and raised indices of inflammation. The importance of preventative measures including oropharyngeal antiseptics and prompt aggressive antibiotic treatment cannot be overemphasized.

Nutrition

All patients with respiratory failure should receive a high fat, low carbohydrate diet to reduce carbon dioxide production and thus ventilatory demand. Enteral nutrition removes the disadvantages of parenteral feeding, such as catheter-related infection and impaired hypoxic pulmonary vasoconstriction. The advantages of enteral feeding include improved gut barrier function (decreasing translocation of bacteria and their toxins) and a decreased incidence of stress ulceration. So-called 'immunonutrition' contains supplements designed to influence specifically inflammatory responses and GI integrity. Small studies have demonstrated benefits in respiratory parameters and the duration of mechanical ventilation, but not on mortality; multi-centre studies will be required to determine the effects on mortality. Similarly, the role of tight glycaemic control in the management of ARDS is uncertain.

Sedation and paralysis

Protocols that include regular interruption of sedative infusions shorten the duration of mechanical ventilation and facilitate weaning. Neuromuscular junction blockers are commonly required to manage patients with ARDS. Their use, particularly when given simultaneously with corticosteroids, is associated with critical illness neuromyopathy, a major cause of morbidity in survivors.

Fluid management

Whilst pulmonary oedema in ARDS is not caused by fluid overload or high left atrial pressure, the high permeability of the pulmonary microvasculature results in leakage of osmotically active molecules into the interstitial space. The formation of oedema, therefore, depends directly on hydrostatic pressure, because osmotic forces are less able to retain fluid in capillaries. Whilst removing lung water improves respiratory function, dehydration of critically ill patients may precipitate multiple organ failure. A recent study compared the effects of liberal and conservative fluid administration strategies in 1000 patients with ALI. Although there was no effect on mortality, the conservative strategy improved lung function and shortened the duration of mechanical ventilation without increasing non-pulmonary organ failures.

Corticosteroids

Corticosteroids may modify the course of lung injury by reducing the activity of a variety of proinflammatory and fibrogenic mediators. However, their administration is not beneficial early in the course of the syndrome. Several small studies suggested clinical benefits of extended moderate- to high-dose methylprednisolone when given to patients with ARDS at least 1 week after diagnosis. A recent randomized, blinded trial involving 180 patients who had acute lung injury for at least 7 days demonstrated no effect on mortality of methylprednisolone vs placebo. However, methylprednisolone increased the number of ventilator-free and shock-free days, with an improvement in oxygenation and compliance. Methylprednisolone did not increase the rate of infectious complications, but was associated with a higher rate of neuromuscular weakness. Unfortunately, these data have not ended the controversy over the role of corticosteroids in the treatment of ARDS.

β-Adrenergic agonists

Besides other effects, β agonists increase fluid clearance from the airspace of the lung. A continuous infusion of salbutamol decreased an index of lung water in patients with ARDS. Larger trials powered to determine the effect of salbutamol on survival in ARDS are planned.

Surfactant replacement

Deficiency and dysfunction of surfactant contributes to the pathogenesis of ARDS by encouraging alveolar collapse and compromising host defence. Despite therapeutic success in neonates with respiratory distress syndrome, multiple trials of synthetic surfactant preparations in adults with ARDS have shown no survival benefit. Possible explanations for this failure include inadequate surfactant delivery to diseased lung units, and poor biological activity of the synthetic preparations.

Further reading

Baudouin SV. Exogenous surfactant replacement in ARDS—one day, someday, or never? *N Engl J Med* 2004; 351: 853–5.

Brun-Buisson C. Preventing ventilator associated pneumonia. *BMJ* 2007; 334: 861–2.

Griffiths MJD, Evans TW. Acute respiratory distress syndrome. In: Gibson GJ, Geddes DM, Costabel U, *et al*, eds. Respiratory medicine, 3rd edn. London: Saunders, 2003: 736–63.

Kress JP, Pohlman AS, O'Connor MF, *et al*. Daily interruption of sedative infusions in critically ill patients undergoing mechanical ventilation. *N Engl J Med* 2000; 342: 1471–7.

Milberg JA, Davis DR, Steinberg KP, *et al*. Improved survival of patients with acute respiratory distress syndrome (ARDS): 1983–1993. *JAMA* 1995; 273: 306–9.

Perkins GD, McAuley DF, Thickett DR, *et al*. The beta-agonist lung injury trial (BALTI): a randomized placebo-controlled clinical trial. *Am J Respir Crit Care Med* 2006; 173: 281–7.

Singer P, Theilla M, Fisher H, *et al.* Benefit of an enteral diet enriched with eicosapentaenoic acid and gamma-linolenic acid in ventilated patients with acute lung injury. *Crit Care Med* 2006; 34: 1033–8.

Steinberg KP, Hudson LD, Goodman RB, *et al.* Efficacy and safety of corticosteroids for persistent acute respiratory distress syndrome. *N Engl J Med* 2006; 354: 1671–84.

Wiedemann HP, Wheeler AP, Bernard GR, *et al.* Comparison of two fluid-management strategies in acute lung injury. *N Engl J Med* 2006; 354: 2564–75.

ARDS: ventilatory management

Introduction

Despite the heterogenous nature of ARDS, the ARMA ARDS network study of 860 patients demonstrated the dramatic effect that ventilatory management has on survival in this syndrome. In essence, invasive mechanical ventilation is a necessary evil that is required in almost all cases, but which further damages the lung and contributes to multiple organ failure.

Ventilator-associated lung injury

Experiments carried out 30–40 years ago demonstrated that high tidal volume and high pressure ventilation caused lung injury in healthy animals, and that previously damaged lung was particularly susceptible to these effects. Similar models implicated the effects of overdistension (volutrauma) as opposed to high airway pressure (barotrauma). and demonstrated the injurious effects of cyclic expansion and collapse of lung units deficient in surfactant activity (atelectotrauma). The 'biotrauma hypothesis' addresses the question of how the effect of injurious mechanical ventilation affects mortality, when only a small minority of patients succumb to respiratory failure. The hypothesis is supported by clinical studies demonstrating that injurious, as opposed to protective, mechanical ventilation was associated with the detection of increased concentrations of inflammatory mediators in bronchoalveolar lavage and plasma. From these studies it can be inferred that injurious mechanical ventilation stimulates the production of inflammatory mediators that overspill from the lung into the systemic circulation and contribute to multiple organ failure.

Ventilation strategy

It is now accepted that mechanical ventilation is inevitably damaging to the injured lung and it is neither necessary nor desirable to strive to achieve normal ABGs in patients with ARDS. The ARMA study demonstrated improved survival by selecting a tidal volume target of 6 as opposed to 12ml/kg predicted body weight (PBW). However, it is not known whether 6ml/kg is the optimal tidal volume and there does not appear to be a threshold, or safe plateau pressure, below which there is no advantage in decreasing tidal volume. PEEP recruits collapsed lung, reduces intrapulmonary shunting and improves oxygenation, making it a central part of the mechanical ventilation strategy in ARDS, because large parts of the lung are collapsed owing to deficient surfactant activity. PEEP also has detrimental effects primarily by overdistending compliant alveoli or by decreasing venous return, RV function and oxygen delivery. In patients being ventilated with a target tidal volume of 6ml/kg, there was no benefit in using high (14mm Hg) against low (8mm Hg) PEEP in the ALVEOLI ARDS network study. Similarly, the application of high airway pressure for a limited period (recruitment manoeuvres) confers short-term physiological benefit only, but may be useful to rescue patients with life-threatening hypoxia.

Alternative modes of respiratory support

There is very little evidence to favour one ventilatory mode over another in adult patients with ARDS. High frequency ventilation aims to minimize tidal volume whilst maintaining recruitment through a high mean airway pressure. This mode improves oxygenation and should theoretically cause less ventilator-associated lung injury: large studies are underway to define its role in adult ARDS. Perhaps the ultimate means of resting the injured lung is to perform Extra Corporeal Oxygenation. This technique requires that the patient's blood passes across a membrane to supplement gas exchange. Because of associated complications, this has traditionally been used as a salvage therapy, which is only of proven benefit in children. However, newer devices such as the Novalung® require a less invasive approach and less anticoagulation, suggesting that this and similar devices may have an increasing role in the future.

Adjuncts to ventilatory support

In many cases of ARDS, especially those with an indirect non-pulmonary cause, there is a predominance of collapse and consolidation in dependent lung regions. Turning patients from supine to prone improves ventilation–perfusion matching and significantly affects gas exchange in ~2/3 cases of ARDS. Furthermore, the weight of the mediastinum is removed from the left lower lobe, secretion clearance may be enhanced and ventilator-associated lung injury may be mitigated. Large studies have failed to demonstrate a benefit in terms of survival or duration of mechanical ventilation with **prone positioning**, whilst the procedure is labour intensive and associated with tube displacement and a higher incidence of pressure sores. **Inhaled vasodilators**, nebulized prostacyclin or Nitric Oxide (NO) also improve oxygenation in ~2/3 cases of lung injury, but have repeatedly failed to improve survival in multi-centre clinical trials.

Recommendations for instituting invasive mechanical ventilation in patients with ARDS

It is not possible to describe ideal ventilator parameters for all patients with ARDS; mechanical ventilation settings need to be individualized and changed with time to suit the patient's condition. This is best achieved with an empirical approach and patience; however, some guidelines may be applied:

- Tidal volume of 6ml/kg predicted body weight (PBW), calculated as follows: for men, PBW = 50.0 + 0.91 (height in cm − 152.4); and for women, PBW = 45.5 + 0.91 (height in cm − 152.4). If the plateau pressure is >30cm H_2O, try to decrease tidal volume further if gas exchange targets can still be met. This may be unnecessary if there is an extrapulmonary cause of restriction, e.g. abdominal distension.
- Respiratory rate of 20/min, which will tend to mitigate respiratory acidosis but ensure that expiration is completed before the subsequent inspiration starts in order to avoid breath stacking.
- Accept a pH >7.2 and do not worry about hypercapnia unless there is concurrent intracranial hypertension or other contraindications. Respiratory acidosis is generally well tolerated unless the rise in carbon dioxide tension is rapid.
- Oxygen saturation target of 88–92% to minimize oxygen toxicity.
- Set PEEP between 14 and 8mm Hg, start at a high level and decrease, until the compliance or oxygenation deteriorates.

- Whilst muscle relaxants and full sedation may be required initially, these should be withdrawn or minimized as soon as possible to avoid neuromuscular sequelae.
- Refractory hypoxaemia may be improved by prone positioning, recruitment manoeuvres and the administration of an inhaled vasodilator such as NO, although none of these interventions can be recommended for routine use.

Further reading

Acute Respiratory Distress Syndrome Network. Ventilation with lower tidal volumes as compared with traditional tidal volumes for acute lung injury and the acute respiratory distress syndrome. *N Engl J Med* 2000; 342: 1301–8.

Brower RG, Lanken PN, MacIntyre N, *et al.* Higher versus lower positive end-expiratory pressures in patients with the acute respiratory distress syndrome. *N Engl J Med* 2004; 351: 327–36.

Ferguson ND, Villar J, *et al.* Understanding high-frequency oscillation: lessons from the animal kingdom. Intensive *Care Med* 2007; 33: 1316–8.

Gattinoni L, Caironi P, Cressoni M, *et al.* Lung recruitment in patients with the acute respiratory distress syndrome. *N Engl J Med* 2006; 354: 1775–86.

Guerin C, Gaillard S, Lemasson S, *et al.* 2004. Effects of systematic prone positioning in hypoxemic acute respiratory failure: a randomized controlled trial. *JAMA* 292: 2379–87.

Hager DN, Krishnan JA, Hayden DL, *et al.* Tidal volume reduction in patients with acute lung injury when plateau pressures are not high. *Am J Respir Crit Care Med* 2005; 172: 1241–5.

Pinhu L, Whitehead T, Evans,T, *et al.* Ventilator-associated lung injury. *Lancet* 2003; 361: 332–40.

Ranieri VM, Giunta F, Suter PM, *et al.* Mechanical ventilation as a mediator of multisystem organ failure in acute respiratory distress syndrome. *JAMA* 2000; 284: 43–4.

Asthma

A chronic inflammatory disorder of the airways in which many cell types play a role, in particular mast cells, eosinophils and T lymphocytes. In susceptible individuals, this inflammation causes recurrent episodes of wheezing, breathlessness, chest tightness and cough, particularly at night and/or in the early morning. These symptoms are usually associated with widespread but variable airflow limitation that is at least partly reversible either spontaneously or with treatment. The inflammation also causes an associated increase in airway responsiveness to a variety of stimuli.

The diagnosis is a clinical one and not always simple. There is no confirmatory blood test, radiographic sign or histopathological feature.

The diagnosis can usually be made by a combination of history (particularly if typical), pulmonary function testing, spirometry, serial measurements of peak expiratory flow rates (PEFR) or bronchial provocation testing by methacholine or exercise. A therapeutic trial of bronchoodilators often aids diagnosis by the above methods.

The differential diagnosis includes respiratory and non-respiratory conditions that may cause similar symptoms, co-exist or worsen asthma severity. Allergic rhinitis (in most allergic asthma and 50% of non-allergic asthma) may present as post-nasal drip syndrome. Gastro-oesophageal reflux can exacerbate asthma symptoms.

Variable airflow obstruction is characteristic of asthma. A non-smoker with cough, shortness of breath and/or wheezing who has expiratory airflow obstruction that reverses to normal with treatment or over time probably has asthma. In contrast, the person with symptoms with consistently normal spirometry probably does not have asthma, and alternative diagnoses (e.g, recurrent bronchitis) should be sought.

Clinical approach

History: key points

- Cough, wheeze, breathlessness (classic triad),
- Chest tightness, chronic cough, recurrent 'infections' (often a misdiagnosis leading to a new diagnosis of asthma),
- Episodic symptoms; time course hours–days, particulary nocturnal symptoms (or early morning wakening).
- Triggers; exercise, cold air, allergen exposure (e.g. animal hairs, housedust mite, moulds, pollens, cockroaches) and non-specific irritants (e.g. cigarette smoke or fumes),
- Atopy; personal or family history, in association with symptoms, favours a diagnosis of asthma,
- Childhood symptoms of asthma, 'wheeziness', recurrent 'bronchitis' or eczema favour diagnosis of asthma,
- Occupational history,
- Drug history; aspirin/NSAIDs/β-adrenergic antagonists may exacerbate asthma.

Features that suggest an alternative diagnosis to asthma include:

- Lack of response to bronchodilators or corticosteroids,
- Onset after 50 years—although late-onset asthma is well recognized,
- Greater than 20 pack year smoking history suggests increasing likelihood of COPD.

Examination: key points

- Widespread, high-pitched, polyphonic wheezes. More commonly in expiration.
- These are distinguishable from monophonic wheezes of fixed airway narrowing or upper airway sounds heard over the neck.
- Nasal polyps, which appear as glistening, grey, mucoid masses within the nasal cavities, should prompt questioning about concomitant aspirin sensitivity and chronic sinusitis.
- Inhaler technique, as part of full assessment.

Classification

- Acute asthma, status asthmaticus
- Chronic asthma; mild, mild intermittent, mild persistent, moderate persistent, severe
- Allergic ('extrinsic') or non-allergic ('intrinsic')
- 'Brittle asthma'
- Corticosteroid-resistant asthma
- Occupational asthma
- Cough variant asthma
- Factitious asthma (paradoxical vocal cord motion)

Investigations

- Pulmonary function testing—FEV1/FVC <0.7; PEFR reduction with bronchodilator reversibility (>15%)
- Total serum IgE and peripheral blood eosinophilia
- Allergy sensitivity testing—to common inhaled allergens by skin testing or specific IgE (RAST).
- Methacholine testing (PC_{20} = concentration causing a 20% fall in FEV_1)
- Chest radiograph – exclude other diagnoses
- Exhaled NO—marker of airway inflammation under evaluation

Management

Chronic asthma

Goals of treatment are freedom from symptoms of asthma, minimizing exacerbations, eliminating impairment of daily activities, reducing pharmacological side effects, optimizing lung function (FEV_1 and/or PEFR >80% predicted or best) and patient/carer education about asthma, its prevention and early treatment. These are achievable through:

- Regular monitoring of symptoms/lung function (PEFR)
- Avoiding and controlling asthma trigger factors
- Appropriate pharmacological therapy
- Patient education (including asthma management plans)

Pharmacological treatments

A *stepwise* approach aims to abolish symptoms and optimize lung function by initiating treatment at the level/dosing most appropriate to achieve this. As symptoms emerge, early control and maintaining it by stepping up treatment as necessary and stepping down when good control established.

'*Relievers*': short-acting β agonists (SABAs) for short-lived relief in all with symptomatic asthma. Anticholinergics can be added in acute excerbations.

'*Preventers*': inhaled corticosteroids (ICS) should be used regularly. Sodium cromoglycate works in some patients. Theophylline or leukotriene receptor antagonists can be used as 'add-on' treatments at ≥step 3 (see below).

Specific therapies: sublingual immunotherapy, monoclonal anti-IgE (e.g, omalizumab); seek specialist advice.

Stepwise approach

Step 1: mild intermittent asthma; SABA as required.

Step 2: regular preventer therapy; ICS 200–800mcg/day beclomethasone dipropionate equivalent.

Step 3: add-on therapy; Add long-acting β agonists (LABAs) or combination ICS–LABA. Increase the ICS dose if required. Consider sequential add-on therapies.

Step 4: persistent poor control; increase ICS up to 2000mcg/day and/or add-on therapies. Stop ineffective add-on therapies. Consider review asthma, and specialist referral.

Step 5: frequent or continuous oral corticosteroids. Consider trials of steroid-sparing agents if long-term oral corticosteroids likely. Specialist monitoring.

Acute severe asthma

Acute severe asthma and status asthmaticus or near-fatal asthma remain important causes of preventable mortality. The predictors of morbidity include underperception of severity, poor asthma management and previous ICU admission. International guidelines for management are published.

	Moderate exacerbation	Acute severe	Life threatening
PEFR	50–75%	33–50%	<33%
Respiratory effort/rate (RR)		RR >25/min	RR >25/min
		Cannot complete sentence in a breath	Feeble effort/silent chest
Heart rate (HR)		HR ≥110/min	HR ≥110/min; arrythmias, bradycardia, hypotension
Arterial blood gas (ABG)		SpO2 >92%	SpO_2 <92%
		PaO_2 >8kPa	PaO_2 <8kPa
		$PaCO_2$ 4.6–6.0kPa	$PaCO_2$ 4.6–6.0kPa
		normal	normal >6.0kPa
Other features			exhaustion, confusion, coma

Clinical features

Management

Immediate treatment: O_2 (high flow), nebulized bronchodilator (salbutamol 5mg ± ipratropium bromide 500mcg (O_2 driven), Hydrocortisone IV 100mg bd–qds (prednisolone 30–40mg PO).

Review: monitor PEFR, O_2 sats, repeat ABG if no improvement, check serum K^+. If no response, further back-to-back nebulized bronchodilators (or every 15min).

Life-threatening: IV magnesium Mg^{2+} (20ml 10% $MgSO_4$) over 20min and/or **SC terbutaline** (5mg in 10ml normal saline) over 24h or **IV salbutamol** (250mcg slow bolus) and/or **IV aminophylline** 500–750mg in normal saline over 24h (monitor levels). Good fluid resuscitation. Discuss with ICU; need for intubation and mechanical ventilation.

Only consider NIV in an ICU setting with senior experts and only if no indication for immediate intubation.

Follow-up

Transfer of care from ICU through to the respiratory ward, and asthma clinic follow-up, with close monitoring, discharge planning and management planning.

Further reading

British Thoracic Society/Scottish Intercollegiate Network. British guideline on the management of Asthma. *Thorax* 2003; 58 Suppl: 1–94.

Global Initiative for Asthma Management and Prevention. NHLBI/WHO Workshop Report, US Department of Health and Human Services. National Institutes of Health, Bethesda, 1995; Pub #95-3659.

http://www.ginasthma.com;www.thoraxjnl.com

Asthma: ventilatory management

Some patients with severe acute asthma/status asthmaticus develop respiratory failure and require supportive care with mechanical ventilation. Approximately 4% of all patients hospitalized for acute asthma require mechanical ventilation. Although life-saving, mechanical ventilation and its associated interventions (e.g, sedatives, paralytics) can also cause morbidity and mortality.

The median duration of mechanical ventilation is ~3 days. The indications for intubation and mechanical ventilation are clinically rather than guideline determined. Thus, a reduced level of consciousness, impending respiratory failure and cardiorespiratory arrest are undisputed indications.

Where possible, intubation should be performed semi-electively, by someone with experience in airway management, and preferably with a large bore ETT (e.g. size 8mm). Manipulation of the airway can cause increased airflow obstruction due to exaggerated bronchial responsiveness. Hence, adequate venous access, non-invasive monitoring, and sedation should be optimized prior to intubation.

Ventilatory strategy

The ventilatory strategy for an asthmatic patient is governed by the need to prevent dynamic hyperinflation and its consequences. Hypotension is a common consequence of pre-existing hypovolaemia, when positive pressure ventilation is applied, in conjunction with the use of anaesthetic agents and sedatives. Bronchospasm, airway inflammation, airway oedema and mucus plugging increase airflow obstruction, decrease expiratory flow and prolong the required complete expiratory time.

Dynamic hyperinflation occurs when increased airway resistance prolongs expiratory flow, so that the next breath interrupts exhalation of the tidal volume, leading to air trapping or 'breath stacking'. The consequences of progressive increases in intra-thoracic pressure, due to intrinsic PEEP and elevated inspiratory plateau pressure (Pplat) are cardiovascular collapse and barotrauma.

Hence, ventilation strategies include: low tidal volumes, slow respiratory rate with prolongation of expiratory time, and pressure limitation. This should minimize dynamic hyperinflation, and consequent hypotension and barotrauma (pneumomediastinum and pneumothorax). The low minute ventilation may lead to relative hypoventilation and resultant hypercapnia (i.e. permissive hypercapnia). Permissive hypercapnia is generally well tolerated so long as adequate oxygenation is achieved and in the absence of contraindications, particularly intracranial pathology, or myocardial ischaemia. Other potential complications include pneumothorax, often the result of excessive 'hand-bagging', and cardiac dysrrythmias.

Ventilatory settings

In general, controlled modes of ventilation are preferred in the immediate post-intubation period, in view of the frequently difficult airway hyper-reactivity, tendency to dynamic hyperinflation and a desire to rest the fatigued respiratory muscles. An example of typical ventilator settings in a pressure-limited mode of ventilation are shown in Table 17.9.1.

Table 17.9.1 Typical ventilator setting for severe asthma

Respiratory rate	10–14 breaths/min
Tidal volume	≤8ml/kg
Inspiratory flow	80–100l/min
Extrinsic positive end-expiratory pressure (extrinsic PEEP)	≤80% of the intrinsic PEEP
Minute ventilation	≤115ml/kg
Inspiratory Pplat	<30cm H_2O

PEEP can be detrimental and should be generally avoided in ventilated and paralysed patients. Intrinsic PEEP increases the magnitude of the drop in airway pressure that the patient must generate to trigger a breath, thereby increasing the patient's workload. Careful application of extrinsic PEEP at levels less than the intrinsic PEEP will reduce this gradient and the work of breathing. Thus, ventilator-set PEEP levels up to 80% of intrinsic PEEP are often helpful in spontaneously breathing patients if set, monitored and adjusted at the bedside. Note that measurements of intrinsic PEEP may be underestimated in severe widespread airway closure, due to impedance of end-expiratory alveolar pressures.

In view of the potential for further dynamic hyperinflation, which may go unrecognized, one should be prepared to decompress manually if necessary (by disconnecting from the ventilator tubing momentarily).

β_2-adrenoceptor agonists are usually delivered to ventilated patients by in-line nebulizer. The amount of drug reaching the airways depends on the nebulizer design, driving gas flow, characteristics of the ventilator tubing and the size of the endotracheal tube.

Sedation and Anaesthesia

Personal experience and local practice account for the variation in agents used. Propofol, with its rapid onset and offset is a good agent for intubation and short-term sedation, although additional fluid resuscitation is necessary to counter its vasodilatory properties. Etomidate is also used, in view of a low risk of cardiovascular side effects. Ketamine, with its bronchodilator and sympathomimetic properties, is useful for induction and sometimes after intubation in persisting severe bronchospasm, as an infusion. Caution is warranted in patients with ischaemic heart disease, hypertension, intracranial pathologies and pre-eclampsia, and the associated dysphoria is often distressing. Thiopentone is generally avoided due to vasodilation and histamine release. Opiates may be used as co-induction agents, although boluses can cause histamine release and worsening bronchoconstriction. Fentanyl, which causes less histamine release than morphine, is more appropriate in the acute setting.

Neuromuscular blocking agents

Suxamethonium may be used in rapid sequence induction. The use of neuromuscular agents is sometimes necessary to achieve control of ventilation, and reduce dynamic hyperinflation. Potential additional benefits include reduction in oxygen consumption, and reduction in carbon dioxide and lactic acid production. The preferred agents are vecuronium and pancuronium. Although all these agents may cause histamine release in large boluses, potentially worsening bronchoconstriction, long-term muscle relaxation with vecuronium is associated with low levels of histamine release as compared with atracurium. The risk of myositis and myopathy, associated with a rise in creatinine kinase (CK), is greater with the concomitant use of corticosteroids than without neuromuscular blockers. Therefore, minimizing the duration of use with monitoring is necessary.

Weaning

Weaning from ventilation is usually commenced following signs of stabilization of ventilation, and reductions in dynamic hyperinflation. There often appears to be a well defined time, specific to patients, at which this occurs, albeit difficult to predict. Sometimes it is heralded by a lack of need for frequent changes in ventilatory parameters, and the production of copious secretions, thought to be related to the loosening of trapped sputum plugs as bronchiolar bronchoconstriction and inflammation settle. Preparation for extubation comes with recognition of a possible sympathetic response-induced bronchoconstriction. Bronchodilators and inhalational anaesthetic agents are often useful in this situation.

Other techniques in severe asthma with mechanical ventilation

Despite use of the treatments mentioned above, some patients continue to demonstrate refractory bronchoconstriction, extreme overinflation and mucus plugging. Various additional methods have been used to alleviate these factors. The routine use of these adjunctive therapies cannot be recommended on the basis of existing clinical studies.

General anaesthesia

Inhalational anaesthetic agents such as isoflurane and sevoflurane are potent bronchodilators and are effective for mask induction in severe asthma. They have been used for maintenance of anaesthesia in refractory cases, although this is limited by the few ICU ventilators which can deliver inhalational anaesthetics, and anaesthetic ventilators, which may not have the capabilities for ventilating patients with very severe airway resistance.

Manual decompression

During expiration, manual compression may reduce hyperinflation. However, it has not been fully evaluated in studies. The use of mucolytics, expectorants or chest physiotherapy has not been shown to provide any direct benefit.

Adrenaline

Adrenaline has both a bronchodilator effect from its β_2-adrenoceptor agonist action, and an α agonist vasoconstrictor effect, thus possibly reducing mucosal oedema formation. However, it is not superior to 'pure' β_2-adrenoceptor agonists and is not recommended for routine use in the treatment of asthma. It may benefit non-responding patients and can be given either nebulized, SC or IV.

Heliox

There have been few studies of its use in acute severe asthma. Heliox, a blend of helium and oxygen with a lower density than nitrogen–oxygen mixtures (helium–oxygen mixture in ratios 80:20 or 70:30), although not recommended for routine use, has been shown to improve airway pressures and gas exchange in intubated patients with asthma. However, it can also cause ventilator malfunction, including inaccurate measurement of tidal volume and oxygen concentration.

Extracorporeal life support

The removal of carbon dioxide and maintenance of oxygenation through an artificial membrane can be used for patients with severe refractory asthma complicated by refractory respiratory acidosis. However, clinical outcome studies are absent.

Follow-up

Patients with status asthmaticus who require mechanical ventilation have increased in-hospital mortality compared with patients who do not require mechanical ventilation (7 vs 0.2%). Patients who survive to hospital discharge remain at high risk of death Transfer of care from ICU through to the respiratory ward, and asthma clinic follow-up, with close monitoring, discharge planning and management planning are thus vital.

Further reading

Abroug F, Nouira S, Bchir A, *et al.* A controlled trial of nebulized salbutamol and adrenaline in acute severe asthma. *Intensive Care Med* 1995; 21: 18–23.

Afessa B. Morales I, Cury JD. Clinical course and outcome of patients admitted to an ICU for status asthmaticus. *Chest* 2001; 120: 1616–21.

Anzueto A, Frutos-Vivar F, Esteban A, *et al.* Incidence, risk factors and outcome of barotrauma in mechanically ventilated patients. *Intensive Care Med* 2004; 30: 612.

Krishnan V, Diette GB, Rand CS, et al. Mortality in patients hospitalized for asthma exacerbations in the United States. *Am J Respir Crit Care Med* 2006; 174: 633.

Mutlu GM. Factor P, Schwarn DE, *et al.* Severe status asthmaticus: management with permissive hypercapnia and inhalation anesthesia. *Crit Care Med* 2002; 30: 477–80.

Scoggin CH, Sahn SA, Petty TL. Status asthmaticus: a nine-year experience. *JAMA* 1977; 238: 1158.

Tassaux D, Jolliet P, Thouret JM, *et al.* Calibration of seven ICU ventilators for mechanical ventilation with helium–oxygen mixtures. *Am J Respir Crit Care Med* 1999; 160: 22.

Pneumothorax

Definition

A pneumothorax is defined as the presence of air in the pleural cavity, and can be classified as either primary or secondary.

Primary pneumothorax

- Patients without *clinically apparent* lung disease. More common in tall thin males (M:F 5:1) with a peak incidence between10 and 30yrs. Most have unrecognized underlying lung disease, with subpleural bullae found in almost all patients who undergo thoracotomy. Cigarette smoking increases the risk by 100 times.

Secondary pneumothorax

- Spontaneous—underlying lung disease (COPD, asthma, cystic fibrosis, interstitial lung disease, TB, lung abscess, PCP).
- Traumatic—penetrating and non-penetrating thoracic and upper abdominal trauma.
- Iatrogenic—pleural biopsy or aspiration, central venous access, mechanical ventilation, percutaneous tracheostomy.

Incidence

Both primary and secondary pneumothoraces are relatively common reasons for medical consultation and hospital admission. In the critical care population overall, the incidence of pneumothorax is ~3%, although in ventilated patients the incidence can be much higher, and predominantly related to ventilator-induced barotrauma, or invasive procedures (Table 7.10.1). In general, morbidity and mortality are determined by the underlying condition. However, in the critically ill, pneumthoraces are associated with increased morbidity and mortality.

Table 17.10.1 Risk factors for pneumothorax in critically ill

High plateau pressures	Interstitial lung disease
Central venous acess	HIV disease (PCP)
ARDS/ALI	Low body weight
Asthma/COPD	

Clinical features

Symptoms and signs

Patients commonly present with ipsilateral pleuritic chest pain and dyspnoea. The severity of the symptoms relates to the size of the pneumothorax (small pneumothoraces may be asymptomatic). Patients with secondary pneumothoraces or any tension pneumothorax may have more dramatic presentations with severe dyspnoea, hypoxia, hypercapnia and cardiovascular instability. This particularly applies to ventilated patients with their underlying lung pathology and increased risk of tensioning.

Physical examination may reveal;

- Tachypnoea (may be missing in ventilated patients)
- Asymmetrical chest wall movement (decreased expansion on affected side)
- Hyper-resonance on percussion
- Tracheal deviation—towards affected side in simple pneumothorax; ***away from affected side in tension pneumothorax.***
- Subcutaneous emphysema
- Tachycardia
- Hypoxia
- Hypercapnia*
- Hypotension*
- Pulsus paradoxus*

(*tension pneumothorax/secondary pneumothrax with severe underlying lung disease)

Additional findings in ventilated patients

- Increased peak airway pressures (volume control)
- Decreased tidal and minute volumes (pressure-'controlled' modes)

Investigations

Chest X-ray

In the absence of life-threatening cardiovascular compromise, it is advisable to confirm a suspected pneumtothorax with a CXR prior to instigating treatment. Classically a pneumothorax appears as a sharp white apicolateral line, beyond which there are no lung markings. In the intensive care patient, however, diagnosis may be more difficult, with anteromedial (38%) or subpulmonic (26%) pneumothoraces being common. In addition, pleural adhesions may result in loculated or encysted pneumothoraces which may be indistinguishable from bullae. Radiological findings associated with pneumothoraces in this population include:

- Increased lucency over diaphragm/upper abdomen
- Deep sulcus sign
- Visualization of the inferior surface of the lung
- Ovoid hypodense regions
- Fluid level
- Temporal changes in line and drain positions
- Mediastinal air and surgical emphysema

In patients with significant surgical emphysema, bullous lung disease or complex chest pathology, CT scanning may be required both for diagnosis and to guide further management.

Radiologocal signs of tension pneumothorax

- Shift of mediastinum to contralateral side
- Flattening or inversion of ipsilateral diaphragm

Conditions mimicking a pneumothorax on CXR

- Bullae
- Visceral gas within the chest
- Skin folds

Arterial blood gas analysis

- Hypoxaemia and mild respiratory alkalosis common
- Hypercapnia and acidosis dictate emergent management

Management (Table 17.10.2)

Primary spontaneous pneumothoraces: usually well tolerated and, if small (<2–3cm) and asymptomatic, can be observed and discharged if there is no deterioration after a period of hours. With larger, symptomatic pneumothoraces, aspiration should be attempted, and can be repeated if not fully effective initially. If aspiration fails, intercostal drain insertion with underwater seal is then recommended.

Secondary pneumothorax: intercostal drainage is agreed first-line management in most symptomatic patients.

Iatrogenic pneumothoraces, in the absence of significant underlying lung disease, may be treated with simple aspiration. Otherwise an intercostal drain should be considered.

Table 17.10.2 Acute management of symptomatic pneumothorax

- High flow oxygen
- If life-threatening cardiovascular compromise consider needle decompression, 2nd intercostals space, mid-clavicular line on the affected side. Leave *in situ* until intercostal drain in place
- Drainage
  Aspiration
    primary pneumothorax >2–3 cm
  Intercostal drain
    primary pneumothorax not responding to aspiration
    secondary pneumothoraces
    mechanically ventilated patients
- Post-drainage CXR

Chest drain management

- In simple pneumtohoraces there is no evidence that large tubes (20–24F) are better than smaller tubes (10–14F). Large bore drains are reserved for those with complex pneumothraces (hydro/haemothoraces), large air leaks, e.g. bullous lung disease, mechanical ventilation.
- For larger bore drains, the use of a trocar is not recommended, and the drain should be placed using blunt dissection.
- Intercostal drains should not be removed unless the air leak has resolved (no bubbling) and there is radiographic resolution.
- There is no place for the routine clamping of chest drains.
- Complications of drain insertion include penetration of major organs or vessels and ultrasound guidance, failure of resolution, pleural infection and surgical emphysema.
- If there is significant surgical emphysema, consider a malpositioned, kinked or blocked tube, or an air leak too large for the capacity of the drain.

In patients with an ongoing air leak despite a larger sized drain, high volume, low pressure (–10 to –20cm H_2O) suction can be considered in the appropriate setting. In the non-mechanically ventilated patient, a persisting air leak beyond 2–5 days should prompt a chest physician/thoracic surgical involvement (Table 17.10.3).

Surgical pleurodhesis (pleurectomy, abrasive) is the most effective approach to resolve persistent leaks and for preventing recurrence. Chemical pleurodhesis with talc slurry is less effective, but may be preferred in those too frail for surgery.

Table 17.10.3 Indications for surgical referral

- Air leak after 2–4 days in secondary and 3–5 days in primary pneumothoraces
- Second ipsilateral pneumothorax
- Contralateral pneumothorax
- Bilateral pneumothoraces
- Spontaneous haemothorax
- High risk activities, e.g. diving, flying

Prevention

In the critically ill, pneumothoraces are associated with increased morbidity and mortality. The following strategies to reduce risks should be considered.

- Adherence to lung protective ventilation strategies
- Ultrasound-guided insertion of CVCs

Special circumstances

Air transport/flying

- A patient with an untreated, closed pneumothorax should not fly due to the risk of gas expansion and worsening clinical condition.
- If air transport is essential, a functioning intercostal drain is essential.
- Current guidelines recommend a period of 6 weeks following either a definitive surgical procedure or a CXR showing complete resolution before flying.
- In patients with underlying lung disease, without definitive surgery, recurrence risk remains significant up to a year later, and alternative transport measures may need to be considered.

The British Thoracic Society recommends specialist referral for anyone with a pneumothorax who takes part in high risk activities such as diving or frequent flying (pilots, flight crew).

Further reading

Baumann MH, Strange C, Heffner JE, *et al.* Management of spontaneous pneumothorax, An American College of Chest Physicians Delphi Consensus Statement. *Chest* 2001; 119 55590–602

British Thoracic Society guidelines for the management of spontanoues pneumothorax. *Thorax* 2003; 58 Suppl 2: 39ii–58ii. (www.brit-thoracic.org.uk/guidelines_since_1997.html)

British Thoracic Society guidelines for the insertion of a chest drain. *Thorax* 2003; 58: 53–59. (www.brit-thoracic.org.uk/guidelines_since_1997.html)

de Lassence A, Timsit JF, Tafflet M, *et al.* Pneumothorax in the intensive care unit: incidence, risk factors and outcome. *Anesthesiology* 2006; 104: 5–13.

Rankine JJ, Thomas AN, Fluetcher D, *et al.* Pneumothorax in critically ill adults. *Postgrad Med J* 2000; 76: 399–404.

Empyema

Empyema is a condition in which purulent fluid accumulates in a body cavity. The name comes from the Greek word *empyein* meaning pus-producing. Empyema in the pleural cavity is sometimes called *empyema thoracis*, or empyema of the chest, to distinguish it from empyema elsewhere in the body. An empyema develops when the fluid in the pleural space is infected and progresses from free-flowing fluid to a complex inflammatory collection.

Empyemas may develop in association with the following:

- Infection of parapneumonic effusion
- Rupture of lung abscess
- Thoracic trauma
- Complicating thoracic surgery
- Complication of chest drains
- Complication of diagnostic pleural fluid aspiration
- Oesophageal rupture
- Spread of infection from mediastinum
- Bronchopleural fistulae (BPFs)

The following aerobic Gram-positive and Gram-negative organisms can cause infection

- Streptococcal (*Streptococcus milleri*)
- *Staphylococcus aureus*
- *Escherichia coli*
- *Pseudomonas* species
- *Haemophilus influenzae*
- *Klebsiella* spp.

More rarely an anerobic or mixed growth can be found

Staphylococcus aureus is most commonly found in association with nosocomial empyemas, post-operative empyemas and in the immunocompromised.

Stages of empyema

In 1962, the American Thoracic Society described three stages of empyema, which continue to be applied in the classification of the disease):

1. Exudative (acute) stage: protein-rich pleural fluid remains free flowing. High neutrophil count, normal glucose and pH levels. This stage lasts for 24–72h. Drainage of the effusion and appropriate antimicrobial therapy are normally sufficient for treatment.
2. Fibrinolytic (transitional) stage: increasing fluid viscosity, activation of coagulation factors and fibroblast activity. Glucose and pH levels start to fall. This stage lasts for 7–10 days.
3. Organizing (chronic) stage: loculated pus in the pleural space with adherence to the visceral and parietal pleura. This may progress with the formation of pleural peels in which the pleural layers are indistinguishable.

Clinical approach

History: key points

- Symptoms are non-specific and include: chest pain, fever, sweating, shortness of breath, malaise, loss of appetite, weight loss.
- Delayed clinical improvement or relapse of pneumonia
- A recent history of chest drain insertion, pleural aspiration, interventional endosocopy, thoracoscopy, cardiac or thoracic surgery

Examination: key points

- Tachycardia
- Percussion note dull
- Absent breath sounds

Special investigations

Imaging of the pleural space is a key element in assessment and management

- CXR to detect effusion
- Ultrasound may detect small effusions not clearly seen on CXR and may also demonstrate the presence or absence of septae within the pleural fluid collection
- Contrast-enhanced CT of the chest provides the most information, and will demonstrate fluid, loculation and thickening of the pleural membranes
- CT and ultrasonography can be used in the placement of drainage catheters
- MRI is rarely used in the imaging of pleural effusion and empyema

Diagnostic pleural sampling:

All patients with a pleural effusion in association with sepsis or a pneumonic illness require pleural fluid aspiration. All patients with unexplained fever or rising CRP should have aspiration or re-aspiration of a pleural effusion. Failed aspiration is an indication for an ultrasound scan. Normally effusions <1cm on X-ray (or ultrasound) can be safely observed but require repeated imaging.

Aspiration should be performed with full sterile technique. Fluid should be sent, before antibiotic therapy is commenced, for the following:

- Microbiology
- Gram stain and culture, acid- and alcohol-fast bacilli (AAFB) staining and culture
- Protein, glucose, lactate dehydrogenase (LDH)
- Cytology
- pH (fluid should be collected in a heparinized syringe avoiding the presence of air and measured in a blood gas analyser)

Frank pus should not be put through a blood gas analyser as pH yields no additional information (drainage is already indicated)

Natural history

If left untreated or with inappropriate or delayed treatment, empyema results in significant morbidity. The presence of purulent fluid and pleural thickening results in restriction of movement and expansion of the lung. Atelectasis of the underlying lung results in ventilation–perfusion mismatch. As a result of the above, gas exchange is severely impaired, resulting in hypoxia and hypercapnia. Even with treatment, the 30-day post-operative mortality after *video-assisted thoracoscopy (VATS)* debridement and open decortication has been reported to range between 1.3 and 6.6%.

Complications of empyema

- Empyema necessitans: A swelling appears over the chest wall, which has a positive cough impulse, in communication with the underlying empyema. Resolves with treatment of the underlying empyema.

- Fibrothorax: Adhesion of the two layers of pleura, so that the lung is covered by a thick layer of non-expansible fibrous tissue
- BPF

Management

The choice of the appropriate treatment depends on the nature of the underlying disease, stage of the empyema and the patient's co-morbidity. The aims of treatment are to control infection, clear infection from and prevent recurrence of infection within the pleural space, and to restore normal pulmonary function. In addition, there is good evidence that optimizing nutrition will improve prognosis. The cornerstones of management are:

- Drainage
- Antibiotics
- Early surgical intervention
- Nutritional supplementation

Indications for drainage

- Pus on aspiration
- Cloudy or turbid fluid
- Organisms seen on Gram stain/culture
- Clear fluid with pH <7.2
- Pleural fluid LDH >1000
- Positive culture and glucose <2.2mmol/l
- Poor clinical progress during treatment with antibiotics alone
- Loculated effusion
- Effusion with pleural thickening

Choice and siting of drain

Stage I and II effusions may be managed by antibiotics and closed drains. Drains can be inserted under ultrasound or CT guidance to improve position.

Small bore 12–16F Seldinger-type chest drains can be used and are well tolerated, but may block and should be flushed regularly. Large bore chest drains block less often but are less well tolerated,

Multiple drains may be needed to manage loculated effusions. Pleural adhesions may form quickly as drainage progresses, leading to the formation of undrained loculations. Frequent cross-sectional imaging is needed to detect such loculae so that additional drainage catheters may be placed if needed.

Intrapleural fibrinolytics

Fibrinolytics may be used in the treatment of pleural infection. Intrapleural urokinase or tissue-type plasminogen activator in combination with careful image-guided placement of chest tubes may be effective However, a double-blind RCT demonstrated that intrapleural administration of streptokinase does not improve mortality, the rate of surgery or the length of the hospital stay among patients with pleural infection.

Antibiotics

All patients should receive antibiotics as soon as pleural infection is identified, and this should cover community-acquired bacterial pathogens, including anaerobes, pending culture and sensitivity results. Patients with suspected nosocomial infection require broader spectrum antibiotic cover, including for MRSA. There are no controlled trial data to address optimal length of treatment with antibiotics; depending on response, most patient are treated for at least 21 days

Medical thoracoscopy

Can be used as a drainage procedure and can be performed early in the course of the disease, under sedation, with local anaesthesia, is less expensive and avoids the need for general anaesthesia. It is useful in patients at high surgical risk.

Surgical intervention

Surgery should be considered in all patients with a loculated effusion, those who are not responding to drainage and once the effusion has become organized (stage III). Primary treatment strategy of VATS is associated with a higher efficacy, shorter hospital duration and less cost than a treatment strategy that utilizes catheter-directed fibrinolytic therapy. VATS debridement is associated with less pain and shorter recovery period than open thoracotomy. The time frame between onset of symptoms and surgery where VATS debridement can be performed with success has been shown to be between 1 and 2 weeks

For pleural empyema in an organizing phase, full thoracotomy with decortication remains the treatment of choice. Perfusion and spirometry improve significantly in patients after the decortication, but the function of the affected lung remains impaired.

Summary of treatment according to stage:

1. Exudative: treat with antibiotics and thoracocentesis or chest tube drainage.
2. Fibrinolytic: treat with fibrinolysis via chest tube or thoracoscopic (VATS) debridement. VATS is preferred in good-risk patients
3. Organizing: requires formal decortication by thoracotomy in order to prevent recurrence and restriction.

Further reading

Davis CW, Gleeson FV, Cavies RJ. BTS guidelines for the management of pleural infection. *Thorax* 2003; 58 Suppl 2: ii18–28.

Evans AL, Gleeson FV. Radiology in pleural disease: state of the art. *Respirology* 2004; 9: 300–12.

Light RW. Parapneumonic effusions and empyema. *Proc Am Thorac Soc* 2006; 3: 75–80.

Maskell NA, Davies CW, Nunn AJ, *et al.* U.K. controlled trial of intrapleural streptokinase for pleural infection. *N Engl J Med.* 2005; 352: 865-74.

Rzyman W, Skokowskia J, Romanowicz G, *et al.* Decortication in chronic pleural empyema—effect on lung function. *Eur J Cardiothorac Surg* 2002; 21: 502–7.

Tassi GF, Davies RJO, Noppen M. Advanced techniques in medical thoracoscopy. *Eur Respir J* 2006; 28: 1051–9.

Wait MA, Sharma S, Hohn J, *et al.* A randomized trial of empyema therapy. *Chest* 1997; 111: 1548–51.

Wurnig PN, Wittmer V, Pridun NS, *et al.* Video-assisted thoracic surgery for pleural empyema. *Ann Thorac Surg* 2006; 81: 309–13.

Haemoptysis

Haemoptysis, the expectoration of blood from the respiratory tract, is potentially life-threatening. It should be distinguished from haematemesis or bleeding from the nasal–pharyngeal compartment. Mortality related to acute haemoptysis is influenced by the quantity and rate of blood loss

Massive haemoptysis is the loss of blood at a rate that poses an immediate threat to life. Quantitatively, this may equate to the expectoration of as little as 200–600ml of blood/24h. This is because the nature of haemoptysis is unpredictable and its severity difficult to ascertain clinically. Sentinel bleeds may be inconspicuous, and the magnitude of bleeding may be underestimated by blood retention within the lower airways.

The bronchial circulation is the most common **source of bleeding** (90%), followed by the pulmonary (5%) and non-bronchial systemic (5%) circulation. In many cases the culprit vessels are fragile anastomoses that link the bronchial and pulmonary circulation. Pulmonary haemorrhage may be complex if bleeding involves the pleurae.

The most common **causes of haemoptysis** in non-Western countries include complications of pulmonary tuberculosis (including bronchiectasis and ruptured Rasmussen's aneurysms), lung abscesses and bronchogenic carcinoma. In Western countries, bronchial neoplasms, inflammatory lung disorders (e.g. chronic bronchitis, infections including fungal lung disease, pulmonary vasculitides, fungal, cystic fibrosis and non-TB bronchiectasis), thromboembolism, coagulopathies as well as iatrogenic causes are encountered. Bleeding pulmonary AV malformations, ruptured aortic aneurysms and unusual disorders (e.g. bronchial Kaposi's sarcoma) make up the rest.

Death due to massive haemoptysis usually results from asphyxiation (loss of gas exchange surface) rather than exsanguination.

Diagnostic evaluation

Key points

- *Plain radiography* is readily available and may reveal pulmonary masses and cavities. However, it has a low overall sensitivity in diagnosing haemoptysis or localizing the site of bleeding.
- *Contrast-enhanced CT* may identify tell-tale aetiological signs (tumour, bronchiectasis, aneurysm) or localize the site of haemorrhage. Even so, it fails to reveal the cause of haemoptysis in up to 10% of cases. CT angiography using multi-detector row helical CT (MDCT) enhances the identification of bleeding arteries over conventional CT. It is believed to achieve comparable sensitivity to conventional angiography for distinguishing bleeding from the bronchial and non-bronchial systems.
- *Laboratory tests.* A full haematology profile, renal and liver biochemistry, inflammatory markers and clotting panel as well as urinalysis comprise the primary laboratory work-up of any patient with haemoptysis. Additional tests may be ordered to narrow specific diagnoses such as vasculitis, infections or pulmonary–renal syndromes.
- *Bronchoscopy* is a widely available and versatile tool. Although its diagnostic accuracy in localizing bleeding sites is reduced by 'normal' chest imaging, it enables a range of endobronchial therapies to be administered.
- *Selective bronchial angiography*, when available, can localize the bleeding site relatively accurately, characterize the nature of the vascular lesion and guide embolotherapy.

Clinical management

Immediate measures

Priorities of clinical management are: (1) securing the upper airway, (2) preserving gas exchange and (3) replacing lost circulating volume. Administer high-flow oxygen and continuously monitor SpO_2, blood pressure and pulse rate. Secure IV access with large-bore peripheral cannulae; don't waste time attempting central venous cannulation. Infuse colloid or crystalloid fluids unless blood, either matched or group O negative, is available.

If immediate tracheal intubation is necessary, use an ETT (size 8–10) large enough to pass a flexible fibreoptic bronchoscope. Positioning the patient with the culprit lung dependent is an intuitive (but unproven) manoeuvre. Enlist anaesthetic or ICU help immediately.

Medical treatment

Aggressively identify and treat any coagulopathy. Beware of the patient with co-existing liver or renal disease, or those on antithrombotic or antiplatelet agents. The empiric use of tranexamic acid to inhibit fibrinolysis is popular in minor haemoptysis but its value remains unproven. The role of antitussive agents in haemoptysis is also controversial; in theory, they may help to decrease cough-related shear forces within the airways. Use desmopressin and related vasoconstrictors cautiously; their systemic haemodynamic effects may be unacceptable to individuals with coronary artery disease or hypertension. Antimicrobial agents should be targeted against the likely pathogen, either bacterial or fungal.

The use of conservative measures alone in significant haemoptysis is associated with very high mortality. Whilst awaiting bronchoscopic or angiographic intervention, judge whether early cardiothoracic input is necessary.

Rigid vs flexible bronchoscopy

Early bronchoscopy, compared with a deferred procedure, is more likely to identify the site of bleeding. A rigid bronchoscope has a larger luminal calibre, providing superior suction, but is more limited in its reach, particularly to the upper lung lobes and peripheral airways. Rigid bronchoscopy also requires general anaesthesia. In contrast, flexible bronchoscopy affords greater manoeuvrability and can be performed on the ward. In cases where iatrogenic haemoptysis has arisen due to bronchoscopic lesional biopsies, the instrument must be kept advanced in the airway but a short distance away from the site of bleeding so as not to disrupt and clot formation and still facilitate suctioning of the airways.

Therapeutic intervention via flexible bronchoscopy

The initial bronchoscopic goal in managing haemoptysis is identification of the bleeding lung segment so that the tip of the bronchoscope can be wedged within it. However, massive haemoptysis often obscures endoscopic visualization of the field. Maintain high-flow suction to remove blood and instill ice-cold saline and epinephrine (1:100 000 dilution) to promote vasoconstriction. Endobronchial application of tranexamic acid and fibrin–thrombin agents has not produced consistent results.

The most established manoeuvre to occlude a bleeding pulmonary segment is to produce tamponade using a Fogarty balloon-tip catheter. A small catheter (size 4–7F) may be passed through the inner channel of the bronchoscope for this purpose. A larger catheter will need to be advanced in parallel to the bronchoscope via an *in situ* ETT. This method frees the endoscopic channel for suctioning and drug instillation. However, catheter-induced bronchial blockade provides only temporary reprieve and carries recognized ischaemic airway complications. We advise occlusion of the segmental or lobar bronchus for ~2–4min at a time. The balloon should be gradually deflated to check if fresh bleeding has ceased, and re-inflated if bleeding persists, and further checks made at 5min intervals.

If a balloon catheter has already been advanced into the airways prior to placement of an ETT, the bronchoscope will have to be removed before the ETT can be placed. Both single-lumen and double-lumen tubes have been used to protect the bronchial tree in life-threatening haemoptysis. The former isolates the contralateral bronchus by shielding access to the bleeding side. With the latter, the higher (tracheal) cuff acts as a proximal blocker while the longer endobronchial arm is positioned 'cuffed' within the contralateral bronchus to ventilate the non-bleeding lung. Secure placement of a double-lumen ETT requires considerable skill.

Additional measures

Successful use of recombinant factor VIIa to promote haemostasis has been described in case reports of patients with significant haemoptysis. However, its efficacy has yet to be confirmed in a controlled trial. Laser photocoagulation and radiotherapy have no role in the emergency treatment of haemoptysis.

Percutaneous angiography and bronchial artery embolization (BAE)

Selective bronchial angiography may provide vital diagnostic information in the pre-operative setting or immediately prior to therapeutic embolotherapy. In skilled hands, BAE is highly successful in controlling life-threatening haemoptysis in patients unsuitable for surgery. Typical angiographic findings in large-volume haemoptysis include vessel tortuosity, hypertrophy, hypervascularity, aneurysmal dilatation and AV shunting. Dye extravasation is an unusual finding. A variety of embolization materials are used, including polyvinyl alcohol foam, absorbable gelatin particles and stainless steel platinum coils.

BAE is not without risk; recognized complications range from transient visceral ischaemia (e.g. chest pain or dysphagia) to catastrophic spinal infarction.

Surgical management of haemoptysis

Emergency surgery for acute massive haemoptysis carries a significant risk of death. Indications for emergency thoracotomy have decreased with advances in bronchoscopic and radiological intervention. However, surgery remains the management of choice for haemoptysis resulting from leaking aortic anerysms, traumatic chest injuries, pulmonary vessel haemorrhage and bleeding from a mycetoma unsuccessfully controlled by other means.

Further reading

Dweik RA, Stoller JK. Role of bronchoscopy in massive hemoptysis. *Clin Chest Med* 1999; 20: 89–105.

Gottlieb LS, Hillberg R. Endobronchial tamponade therapy for intractable hemoptysis. *Chest* 1975; 67: 482–3.

Hirshberg B, Biran I, Glazer M, *et al.* Hemoptysis: etiology, evaluation and outcome in a tertiary referral hospital. *Chest* 1997; 112: 440–4.

Mal H, Rullon I, Mellot F, et al. Immediate and long-term results of bronchial artery embolization for life-threatening hemoptysis. *Chest* 1999; 115: 996–1001.

Meijer K, de Graaff WE, Daenen SM, *et al.* Successful treatment of massive hemoptysis in acute leukemia with recombinant factor VIIa. *Arch Intern Med* 2000; 160: 2216–7.

Naidich DP, Funt S, Etenger NA, *et al.* Hemoptysis: CT–bronchoscopic correlations in 58 cases. *Radiology* 1990; 177: 357–62.

Remy-Jardin M, Bouaziz N, Dumont P, *et al.* Bronchial and non-bronchial systemic arteries at multi-detector row CT angiography: comparison with conventional angiography. *Radiology* 2004; 233: 741–9.

Yoon YC, Lee KS, Jeong YJ, *et al.* Haemoptysis: bronchial and non-bronchial systemic arteries at 16-detector row CT (MDCT). *Radiology* 2005; 234: 292–8.

Yoon W, Kim JK, Kim YH, *et al.* Bronchial and nonbronchial systemic artery embolization for life-threatening hemoptysis: a comprehensive review. *Radiographics* 2002; 22: 1395–409.

Inhalation injury

Smoke inhalation injury occurs in about one-third of patients with major burns, and contributes significantly to their mortality. It is the most frequent cause of death at the scene of a fire. Injury to the airway and tracheobronchial tree may also result from inhalation of chemicals (such as chlorine gas), drugs and biological weapons. Systemic disturbances are common, but depend on the nature and toxicity of the inhaled substance.

Pathophysiology

Discreet pathophysiological phases of lung injury may be seen. An exudative phase is characterized by neutrophil influx, formation of oxygen free radicals, macrophage activation and production of inflammatory mediators with an increase in pulmonary capillary permeability. Injury to type II pneumocytes results in decreased surfactant production. Hyaline membranes may form on the denuded alveolar basement membranes. Transpulmonary fluid flux increases, with an increase in EVLW and increased pulmonary shunt fraction. Upregulation of NO has been implicated in the pathogenesis of associated lung injury.

In some patients the exudative phase may be followed by uncomplicated repair and resolution; however, others may develop a fibrotic phase. During this fibrosing alveolitis, neoangiogenesis and increased collagen deposition is seen.

Overall, injury results from damage due to heat, hypoxia and toxins (local and systemic):

Heat

Exposure to the mucous lining of the airway and tracheobronchial tree results in immediate erythema, oedema and ulceration. Airway compromise due to oedema is a significant risk. Thermal damage is usually limited to the supraglottic region due to the heat exchanging capacity of the upper airway. Dry gases have a lower specific heat capacity than saturated gases with less potential to cause injury. Distal thermal damage is rare, but can result from inhalation of superheated particles or saturated gases.

Oxygen

Environmental hypoxia occurs due to the consumption of oxygen during combustion.

Toxins

Toxins causing direct damage to the epithelium of the airways include sulfur dioxide, nitrogen dioxide, chlorine and ammonia. Their effects result from pH or free radical damage. Distal carriage can occur in the presence of carbon particles. Increased alveolar capillary permeability and lung water contribute to decreased lung compliance. Epithelial cast formation and sloughing, mucociliary dysfunction and oedema result in increased airway resistance, airway obstruction, atelectasis and predisposition to bacterial overgrowth and the development of pneumonia. Ventilation–perfusion mismatch with increased pulmonary shunt results.

Systemic toxins include the asphyxiants carbon monoxide, hydrogen cyanide and hydrogen sulfide. These bind to mitochondrial cytochromes causing disruption of the electron transport chain. Carbon monoxide has a higher affinity for haemoglobin than oxygen, preventing binding of the latter and impairing oxygen carriage. Other systemic toxins include hydrocarbons, organophosphates and metal fumes.

Presentation

Presentation will vary according to the severity and type of injury and presence or absence of cutaneous burn. History (e.g. fire in enclosed space) is essential in identifying the risks of carbon monoxide and cyanide poisoning, significant inhalation injury and airway compromise. Signs and symptoms can develop up to 36h after inhalation injury.

Assessment

Initial assessment should take the form of the trauma primary survey. The presence or absence of cutaneous burns does not predict the potential for airway or respiratory compromise. The specific causes of hypoxia should be sought and treated.

Airway

Obstruction or risk of obstruction must always be considered early while administering high flow humidified oxygen. It is a clinical diagnosis; blood gas analysis and oximetry should not be relied upon. Decreased oxygen saturation is a late and pre-terminal sign of airway and breathing compromise.

Hoarse voice, carbonaceous sputum on deep cough, singed facial and nasal hair, and erythema and oedema of the mucosa in the mouth should raise suspicions of potential airway compromise. Swelling may not reach its maximum until 24h after injury, and may occur rapidly during fluid resuscitation. Paradoxical (abdominal) breathing pattern, tracheal tug and intercostal muscle recession with inability to speak are signs of imminent airway obstruction.

Breathing

Respiratory distress due to inhalation injury usually takes several hours to develop. If evident on presentation, airway compromise must be excluded. Clinical signs include tachypnoea, intercostal recession, accessory muscle use, wheeze and bronchorrhoea. Soot or burn discoloration and the potential presence of carboxyhaemoglobin render cyanosis an unreliable sign.

Circulation/disability/exposure

Cardiovascular, neurological and external signs will vary according to the extent and type of other injuries. Reduced conscious level in the absence of head injury and following resuscitation should prompt investigation for systemic toxins.

Monitoring

Vital signs should be monitored continuously during the assessment and initial management phase. Pulse oximetry can give erroneously high readings in the presence of significant carboxyhaemoglobin.

Specific investigations

Arterial blood gas analysis with co-oximetry is essential to assess carboxyhaemoglobin levels.

Blood should be drawn for cyanide levels; however, the results may take several days to be ascertained. Cyanide toxicity should be suspected and treated in patients with persistent high blood lactate levels, acidaemia, high mixed venous oxygen saturation, low oxygen extraction ratio and deteriorating neurological and cardiac function despite appropriate resuscitation.

Corrected anion gap and osmolar gap should be calculated if acidaemia persists. Toxicology screen should be considered, particularly in patients with reduced or inconsistent neurological levels.

Bronchoscopic examination is useful in assessing the tracheobronchial tree of patients who are stable and have undergone endotracheal intubation. It can be combined with therapeutic lavage

CXR signs may lag behind the clinical course of the patient. A normal chest radiograph does not exclude significant, early inhalation injury.

Management

Initial management

Attention to airway, breathing and circulatory abnormalities forms the central tenet of initial management.

Airway swelling and obstruction is progressive, and may be exacerbated during fluid resuscitation, emphasizing the need for constant reassessment. High flow humidified oxygen should be administered to all patients in the first instance. If airway compromise is anticipated, expert endotracheal intubation should be performed with prior preparation for difficult or failed intubation.

Respiratory management should focus on oxygen delivery. Inhalation injury commonly triggers ALI and ARDS; however, this may develop insidiously over a period of hours or days. If mechanical ventilation is required, standard recruitment and lung protection measures should be employed. High frequency oscillatory ventilation has been associated with improved outcome and reduced incidence of pneumonia. Early bronchoscopy is recommended to record level and degree of injury. Lavage should be performed if pulmonary contamination is present; however, consideration should be given to the fact that excessive saline lavage may induce lung injury.

Regular administration of aerosolized bronchodilators should be considered. Nebulized heparin and NAC have been used to reduce cast formation, distal airway obstruction and atelectasis.

Antibiotic and steroid therapies have no proven prophylactic role but may be required in specific situations. Pneumonia is the most common cause of death in hospitalized patients suffering from inhalation injury.

Carboxy-Hb levels >10% should be treated with 100% inspired oxygen therapy. The half-life of carboxy-Hb is reduced from 240min at an inspired oxygen concentration (FiO_2) of 21% to ~80min at an FiO_2 of 100%. Hyperbaric therapy should be considered in patients with carboxy-Hb >40%, or 20% if pregnant and in patients who have had lowered conscious level from no other cause.

Suspicion of cyanide poisoning (see above) should prompt empiric treatment. Sodium thiosulfate acts slowly by catalysing the metabolism of cyanide. Sodium nitrite reduces cyanide binding by oxidation of haemoglobin to methaemoglobin. Methaemoglobin levels of ~40% should be targeted. Cyanide-binding agents such as dicobalt edetate or hydroxycobalamin may be used, though the former may induce cardiac arrhythmias and instability if used in the absence of cyanide poisoning.

Cardiovascular support primarily involves fluid resuscitation. This can be extremely difficult to assess, particularly if large burns co-exist. Widespread increases in capillary permeability result in fluid redistribution into the interstitium, including that of the lung and airway. Patients with major burns and inhalation injury require far greater fluid resuscitation than those with either injury alone. Limitation of fluid resuscitation in victims of smoke inhalation has not been supported in clinical trials. Crystalloid resuscitation for the first 24h is based on historic evidence, but its use in preference to colloids and blood should be balanced against other injuries. New colloids are available and in development which may alter the recommended fluid resuscitation regimes.

Lung injury is a trigger of SIRS and multiple organ dysfunction. Inotrope and vasopressor therapy may be required. Adrenal insufficiency should be considered in patients refractory to vasopressor therapy, and replacement therapy commenced if appropriate. Improvement in cardiac output and blood pressure may enhance oxygenation through improved lung perfusion and reduced intrapulmonary shunt.

Hypoxic pulmonary vasoconstriction combined with increased thromboxane release following smoke inhalation may result in pulmonary hypertension and RV dysfunction.

Longer term management considerations

Chest physiotherapy remains widely accepted management despite a lack of evidence to support it. Tracheostomy should be considered in patients requiring long-term mechanical ventilation or pulmonary toilet.

ALI and ARDS from any cause is associated with increased resting energy expenditure; dramatically so if burns are also present. Careful attention to nutritional management should be considered at an early stage and reviewed continuously.

Therapies employed in the management of long-term critically ill and mechanically ventilated patients should be considered. Examples include the use of prophylaxis against venous thromboembolism and GI stress ulceration.

Further reading

Enkhbaatar P, Traber DL. Pathophysiology of acute lung injury in combined burn and smoke inhalation injury. *Clin Sci* 2004; 107: 137–43.

Freitag L, Long WM, Kim CS, *et al.* Removal of excessive bronchial secretions by asymmetric high-frequency oscillations. *J Appl Physiol* 1989; 67: 614–9.

Heimbach DM, Waeckerle JF. Inhalation injuries. *Ann Emerg Med* 1988; 17: 1316.

Herndon DN, Barrow RE, Traber DL, *et al.* Extravascular lung water changes following smoke inhalation and massive burn injury. *Surgery* 1987; 102: 341–9.

Herndon DN, Tranber DL, Traber LD. The effect of resuscitation on inhalation injury. *Surgery* 1986; 100: 248–51.

Orzel RA. Toxicological aspects of firesmoke: polymer pyrolysis and combustion. *Occup Med* 1993; 8: 414–29.

Ware LB, Matthay MA. The acute respiratory distress syndrome. *N Engl J Med* 2000; 342: 1334–49.

Pulmonary embolism

Pulmonary thromboembolism embolism (PE) is defined as a migration of a clot to the pulmonary circulation causing compromised or obstructed flow. Hypoxaemia, shock and death are potential results in massive PE.

Pathophysiology

Clinically significant PE comes from deep veins, most commonly from femoral or Iliac veins and less likely from pelvic or the inferior vena cava. CVCs can induce deep venous thrombosis (DVT). Untreated, calf vein thrombi may extend into the popliteal and femoral veins, causing proximal DVT and PE. This is unlikely to occur when asymptomatic popliteal clot is discovered in patients who are progressively ambulating after surgery.

PE causes hypoxaemia by inducing atelectasis (depletion of surfactant), bronchoconstriction secretion and reperfusion injury to the endothelial–epithelial barrier.

Massive PE produces significant dead space with elevation of $PaCO_2$ and the potential for severe pulmonary artery hypertension-induced right to left shunt through a patent foramen ovale. The morbidity and mortality of PE are almost always due to additional emboli following initial diagnosis.

Risk factors

Venous stasis, activation of blood coagulation, and vascular damage (Virchow's triad). The most common clinically identifiable risk factors are: previous history of DVT or PE, prolonged immobilization, underlying malignancy, paralysis and recent surgery or pregnancy.

Diagnosis

Clinical presentation depends upon the size, location, number of emboli and the patient's underlying cardiorespiratory reserve.

The classic triad of chest pain, haemoptysis and dyspnoea is present in <20% of patients. 97% of patients with PE have at least one of the following: pleuritic chest pain, dyspnoea or respiratory rate >20/min. Chest pain can be reproducible.

Table 17.14.1 Well's criteria for pulmonary embolism

Clinical features	Points
Clinical symptoms of DVT	3
Other diagnosis less likely than PE	3
Heart rate >100/min	1.5
Immobilization or surgery within past 4 weeks	1.5
Previous DVT or PE	1.5
Haemoptysis	1
Malignancy	1

Risk score interpretation:

6 points indicates high probability of DVT (87.4%)

2–6 points indicates moderate risk (27.8%)

<2 points indicates low risk (3.4%).

Clinical examination is not reliable in diagnosis of either PE or DVT, but applying a pre-test probability score such as Well's criteria (see Table 17.14.1) may be clinically useful.

Physical findings

Tachycardia and tachypnoea are the most common signs. More specific physical exam findings include right sided S3 sound, wildly split second sound, murmur of tricuspid regurgitation and an accentuated S2 closure sound. Fever of >100.0°F is present in 14% of patients with angiographically proven PE and no source of fever. It is rarely more than 101.0°F.

CXR

CXR usually is normal, but can show enlarged heart, pleural effusion, Westermark sign (dilatation of pulmonary artery proximal to the emboli with sharp cut-off), pulmonary infiltrates, elevated hemidiaphragm and atelectasis. Pulmonary infarction can manifest as wedge- shaped pulmonary infiltrates on chest radiograph.

ECG

ECG findings including tachycardia and non-specific ST-T elevation lack specificity, with more specific findings being signs of RV strain such as P pulmonale, S1Q3T3, right bundle branch block or right axis deviation.

Echocardiogram signs of acute pulmonary artery hypertension include right heart dilation, tricuspid regurgitation, pulmonary artery dilation, loss of respiratory variation in vena cava diameter, and interventricular septum bulge into the LV. Acute RV dilation with hypokinesis sparing the apex is the characteristic finding.

Further investigation

Patients with low pre-testing clinical probability of PE

Normal quantitative D-dimer in the low to intermediate risk patients measured by ELISA probably rules out PE especially in the emergency department.

If D-dimer is positive, multidetector CT angiogram (CTA)/CT venogram (CTV) of femoral and popliteal veins is recommended. If negative, there is no need for further intervention. Based upon location and certainty of the clot, additional testing may be necessary due to increased false-positive results in this group. Across all risk categories, CTA/CTV has a sensitivity of 90% and specificity of 95%.

Patients with intermediate pre-testing clinical probability

29–38% of patients with intermediate clinical probability have PE. PE is present in 8% if CTA is negative. If CTA/CTV is negative, PE is ruled out, but venous ultrasound is needed if only CTA (without CTV) is used.

Patients with high clinical probability

If CTA is negative in a patient with a high probability clinical assessment, PE may still be present in 40%, while if CTA/CTV are negative, PE is present in 18%. With negative CTA/CTV in a high clinical probability setting, a digital subtraction angiogram (DSA) is useful.

V/Q scan

A normal V/Q scan rules out PE, but a high probability V/Q scan rules in PE in most cases. Low or intermediate probability results in V/Q scan in the presence of high clinical probability warrants further investigation.

Diagnostic notes

DSA is the gold standard in evaluation for PE

If the initial testing is V/Q lung scanning, leg ultrasound is recommended when:

- non-diagnostic (low or intermediate probability) lung perfusion scan
- normal perfusion scan in high clinical probability (high risk patients) or high probability scans in low risk patients. CTA/CTV is an option to leg ultrasound in these scenarios
- leg ultrasound may be used in combination with negative CTA to enhance the negative predictive power.

Miscellaneous

The healthy RV cannot generate mean pulmonary artery pressure >40mm Hg in an acute situation like PE. The presence of higher pressure reflects pre-existing pulmonary hypertension. In mechanically ventilated patients, a fall in end-tidal CO_2 ($ETCO_2$) might be useful in raising the clinical suspicion of PE, while the decrease in difference between $PaCO_2$ and $ETCO_2$ probably indicates an effective thrombolysis.

Treatment

LMWH is at least as effective as UFH in treating PE. Therapy with heparin for at least 4–5 days is recommended while the patient is on vitamin K antagonist even if the INR is >2. Intermittent injection of heparin is associated with a higher rate of bleeding than heparin infusion; therefore, it is not recommended. Consider thrombolytics in haemodynamically unstable patients (vasopressor requirement). There are not enough data to support routine use of thrombolytics in PE complicated with RV dysfunction without haemodynamic compromise, although it may be appropriate in some scenarios. Thrombolysis failure, which is defined as persistent RV dysfunction and haemodynamic instability, is expected in 8% of cases. In this case, rescue surgical embolectomy may lead to a better outcome than repeated thrombolysis.

In massive PE, infusion of a large amount of fluids might have a deleterious effect on the LV function as a result of RV dilation and interventricular shift toward LV, causing decreased LV compliance and lowered cardiac output. Blood flow to coronary arteries depends upon the aortic pressure as the upstream pressure. In light of the increased right heart pressures (downstream pressure), it is important to maintain systemic blood pressure to maintain filling of right heart coronary artery. A combined inotrope/vasopressor is preferred to maintain blood pressure in massive PE to increase cardiac output and improve oxygen transportation.

An IVC filter is indicated when anticoagulation is contraindicated or when thrombolysis would be given but is contraindicated.

Further reading

Buller HR, Agnelli G, Hull RD, *et al.* Antithrombotic therapy for venous thromboembolic disease: the Seventh ACCP Conference on Antithrombotic and Thrombolytic Therapy. *Chest* 2004; 126 (3 Suppl): 401S–28S

Davidson B, Karmy-Jones R. When pulmonary embolism treatment isn't working. *Chest* 2006; 129: 839–40.

Dellinger RP. Pulmonary thromboembolism in critical care board review. Northbrook, IL: American College of Chest Physicians, 2007.

Kruip MJ, Leclercq MG, van der JHeul C, *et al.* Diagnostic strategies for excluding pulmonary embolism in clinical outcome studies. A systematic review. *Ann Intern Med* 2003; 138: 941–51.

McConnell MV, Solomon SD, Rayan ME, *et al.* Regional right ventricular dysfunction detected by echocardiography in acute pulmonary embolism. *Am J Cardiol* 1996; 78: 469–73.

PIOPED Investigators. Value of the ventilation/perfusion scan in acute pulmonary embolism: results of the Prospective Investigation of Pulmonary Embolism Diagnosis (PIOPED). *JAMA* 1990; 263: 2753–9.

Stein PD, Afzal A, Henry JW, *et al.* Fever in acute pulmonary embolism. *Chest* 2000; 117: 39–42.

Stein PD, Woodard PK, Weg JG, *et al.* Diagnostic pathways in acute pulmonary embolism: recommendations of the PIOPED II Investigators. *Am J Med* 2006; 119: 1048–55.

Wiegand UK, Kurowski V, Giannitsis E, *et al.* Effectiveness of end-tidal carbon dioxide tension for monitoring thrombolytic therapy in acute pulmonary embolism *Crit Care Med* 2000; 28: 3588–92.

Wood KE. Major pulmonary embolism: review of a pathophysiologic approach to the golden hour of hemodynamically significant pulmonary embolism. *Chest* 2002; 121: 877–905.

Community-acquired pneumonia

Community-acquired pneumonia (CAP) has an overall incidence of 5–11 per 1000 adults. It is characterized by cough, tachypnoea, sputum production, focal chest signs and evidence of systemic sepsis. A CXR will show shadowing in one or more lung segments. About 30% of such patients are admitted to hospital and, of these, 5–10% require ICU admission. This chapter will deal with severe CAP in adults, and will not include patients in hospital >10 days, those with acute exacerbations of COPD or patients with severe immunosuppression.

Aetiology

Of patients admitted to ICU, the most common organisms isolated are:

- *Streptococcus pneumoniae* (22%)
- *Legionella* (18%)
- Viral (10%)
- *Staphylococcus aureus* (9%). May complicate influenza
- *Chlamydia pneumonia*. This can be present as a co-pathogen to *S. pneumonia* or occur in isolation.

In 1/3 of cases no organism is isolated. However, the mortality rate of patients with positive and negative microbiology investigations is similar. Clinical and radiological features are not helpful in distinguishing between different aetiologies. Patients from nursing homes are at risk of aspiration pneumonitis.

Initial management

In severe CAP, initial management should follow standard ABCDE assessment. The airway should be assessed, and high flow oxygen administered to ensure an oxygen saturation (SaO_2) >92%. Signs of respiratory distress, respiratory rate, poor perfusion, shock, focal chest signs and level of consciousness are noted. IV access is established, baseline investigations performed and IV antibiotics commenced (see below). The CURB-65 score should be measured.

CURB-65

The CURB-65 score is a 6-point scale (0–5) for assessing severity and risk of death in CAP. One point is given to each of

- **C**onfusion: new onset confusion (mini-mental test ≤8)
- **U**rea: raised urea >7 mmol/l.
- **R**espiratory rate: ≥30 breaths/min
- **B**lood pressure: systolic blood pressure <90mm Hg and/or diastolic blood pressure ≤60mm Hg
- **65**: age ≥65yrs

Mortality rates are: score 0, 0.7%; score 1, 3.2%; score 2, 13%; score 3, 17%; score 4, 41.5%; score 5, 57%. Patients with a score of ≥3 require urgent hospital admission and assessment for ICU admission.

Investigations

All patients with severe pneumonia require a CXR, FBC, U&Es, liver function tests (LFTs), CRP, blood gas analysis and lactate.

Microbiological investigations required are;

- Blood cultures, ideally before the first dose of antibiotic, although this should not be delayed. They are positive in 10–20%.
- Sputum culture with urgent Gram stain. Intubated patients should have a broncoalveolar lavage sample taken (blind or bronchoscopic), again with urgent Gram stain.
- Urine for pneumococcal C polysaccharide antigen and *Legionella* antigen testing. This is 95% specific and 80% sensitive, and is especially useful if antibiotics have been given prior to cultures being taken.
- Paired serology testing (on admission and 7–10 days later) for *Mycoplasma*, *Chlamydiae* and viruses.

Treatment

CAP which requires ICU is a severe illness with a high mortality. Treatment consists of early administration of appropriate antibiotics, within 8h of admission, and supportive care. Patients may require ICU for the support of the respiratory system, the circulation and other organ systems.

Antibiotic therapy

In all patient groups *S. pneumoniae* is the most common pathogen in severe CAP. Unlike meningitis, penicillin resistance of *S. pneumoniae* is not an issue in the treatment of pneumonia, since tissue levels approximate blood levels. *Legionella* and *C. pneumoniae* are sensitive to clarithromycin.

- Initial antibiotic therapy should consist of co-amoxiclav 1.2g 8 hourly IV, or cefuroxime 1.5g 8 hourly IV, plus a macrolide, usually clarithromycin 500mg 12 hourly IV.
- In patients with anaphylactic reactions to β-lactams discuss with the local microbiology department. Quinolones (e.g. levofloxacin 500mg 12 hourly IV) with enhanced pneumococcal activity are one option.
- In confirmed *Legionella*, treatment is continued with clarithromycin, and rifampicin (600mg 12 hourly IV) can be added.
- Rifampicin can be considered in severe CAP which is failing to improve.
- Treatment with antibiotics should continue for 10 days, extending to 14–21 days in cases of legionella, staphylococci or Gram-negative enteric bacilli.

Note that MRSA and *Pseudomonas* are not covered by this regime

- The incidence of MRSA is rising in the community, particularly in some nursing homes. The local microbiology department should be notified early if MRSA is suspected.
- MRSA pneumonia is treated with linezolid 600mg 12 hourly IV (vancomycin has poor lung penetration)
- *Pseudomonas* is a rare cause of CAP (<4%). The American Thoracic Society recommends cover in patients with the following four risk factors: bronchiectasis; malnutrition; broad-spectrum antibiotics for >7 days within the last month; and chronic steroid therapy (>10mg prednisolone/day).
- Treatment of *Pseudomonas* pneumonia is with ceftazidime 2g 8 hourly IV plus gentamicin

Ventilation

- NIV can produce a transient improvement in oxygen saturation, but >50% of patients subsequently require intubation.
- Patients >40yrs old, and those with a respiratory rate >38 have the highest failure rates. If NIV or CPAP are undertaken for CAP it should be in an intensive care environment, where invasive ventilation can be undertaken rapidly

- Invasive ventilation should aim at ensuring a safe level of oxygenation (PaO_2 >8kPa) whilst minimizing pulmonary barotrauma and volotrauma. Tidal volumes should be set at 6–7ml/kg, with plateau pressures ≤30cm H_2O.
- In severe lobar pneumonia, much of the lung may not be recruitable. High levels of PEEP can damage normal alveoli and worsen shunt. ARDS can complicate severe CAP and may be more PEEP responsive.

Circulation

Septic shock worsens the prognosis in CAP, and should be treated with optimal volume loading and inotropes (noradrenaline ± dobutamine). In the acute stage (ideally within 6h) poor organ perfusion (lactate 4mmol/l) and septic shock should be managed as described by Rivers *et al.*

- CVP >8mm Hg
- MAP >65mm Hg
- Central venous saturation of ≥70%.

Hydrocortisone 50mg qds for 7 days and activated protein C can be considered. After the initial resuscitation, fluid management should be more cautious to avoid worsening gas exchange and increasing lung water.

Complications

Parapneumonic effusions and lung abscess

Up to 50% of patients with bacterial CAP develop parapneumonic effusions.

- Effusions should be tapped under ultrasound control. The appearance is noted, and microscopy and culture requested. The pH is measured anaerobically in a blood gas syringe.
- A complicated parapneumonic effusion is defined as clear fluid with a pH <7.2.
- In empyema, the fluid is cloudy; frank pus, or organisms are present on Gram stain
- Both require effective pulmonary drainage and, in the case of an empyema, a surgical opinion.

Lung abscesses are more common in debilitated patients, alcoholics and following aspiration. A variety of organisms may be responsible. Treatment consists of prolonged antibiotics, and a surgical opinion.

Systemic complications

- Patients with *S. aureus* or *S. pneumoniae* may develop metastatic infections, including meningitis, endocarditis and septic arthritis.
- *Legionella* can produce a variety of complications including encephalitis, pericarditis, pancreatitis, polyarthropathy, hyponatraemia, abnormal liver function, thrombocytopaenia, diarrhoea and renal failure.

Prognosis

The CURB-65 score gives the best early indication of mortality. Mortality is worsened by the presence of significant co-morbidities, septic shock, and in *Pseudomonas* pneumonia.

Further reading

British Thoracic Society Pneumonia Guidelines (2001, updated 2004)
http://www.brit-thoracic.org.uk/bts_guidelines_pneumonia_html

Chiou CCC, Yu VL. Severe pneumococcal pneumonia; new strategies for management. *Curr Opin Crit Care* 2006; 5: 470–6.

Lim WS, Van der Eerden MM, Laing R, *et al.* Defining community acquired pneumonia severity on presentation to hospital; an international derivation and validation study. *Thorax* 2003; 58: 377–82.

Rivers E, Nguye B, Havstad S, *et al.* Early goal-directed therapy in the treatment of severe sepsis and septic shock. *N Engl J Med* 2001; 345: 1368–77.

Wilkinson M, Woodhead MA. Guidelines for community acquired pneumonia in the ICU. *Curr Opin Crit Care* 2004; 1: 59–63.

Hospital-acquired pneumonia

Definition and epidemiology

Hospital-acquired pneumonia (HAP) is defined as a pneumonia beginning >48h after hospital admission. It represents the second most common nosocomial infection, accounting for >25% of all ICU nosocomial infections. Its incidence is between 5 and 15 episodes per 1000 hospital admissions. More than 80% of HAP episodes in ICU are related to mechanical ventilation—VAP. HAP mortality in the ICU may vary from 30 to 70% in different series.

Pathogenesis

For HAP occurrence there must be the entry of pathogens into the lower respiratory tract, followed by colonization, then overwhelming host's defences. The balance among pathogen virulence, host's defence and bacterial burden (related to volume of aspiration) is the most important factor for HAP/VAP development. Important mechanisms associated with pathogenesis are:

- Aspiration of oropharyngeal pathogens and leakage of bacteria around the cuff of tracheal tube (>90% of episodes)
- Colonization of tracheal tube (biofilm)
- Condensate on ventilator circuits, nebulizer and humidifiers
- Inhalation or direct inoculation of pathogens into the lower airway
- Haematogenous spread (uncommon).

Risk factors

The risk factors for HAP include patient characteristics and infection control-related problems. The main risk factor is intubation and mechanical ventilation, increasing the risk of HAP 6- to 21-fold.

Severe acute or chronic illness	Advanced age
Immunocompromise	Coma
Hypotension	Alcoholism
COPD	Respiratory failure

Patient-related risk factors include:

An important issue in HAP is the increasing rates of HAP episodes due to MDR pathogens, especially in ICU. Risk factors associated with MDR HAP are:

- Antimicrobial therapy in last 90 days
- Current hospitalization >5 days
- Immunosuppressive disease or therapy
- Hospitalization for >2 days in the preceding 90 days
- Residence in nursing home
- 'Homecare'
- Chronic dyalisis
- Family member with MDR infection

Aetiology

Most common pathogens include aerobic Gram-negative bacilli (*P. aeruginosa*, *E. coli*, *K. pneumoniae* and *Acinetobacter baumannii*). Gram-positive cocci, *S. aureus*, particularly MRSA, are a very important issue in most ICUs. Polymicrobial episodes are very common.

Several factors such as age, diabetes mellitus, head trauma and coma, local flora and previous exposure to antibiotics may increase the frequency of specific pathogens.

Early-onset pneumonia (<5 days)	**Late-onset pneumonia (>5 days)**
S. pneumoniae	*P. aeruginosa*
H. influenzae	MRSA
MSSA	*Acinetobacter baumannii*

In VAP patients, a very important issue is the time of onset of pneumonia.

Prevention

HAP episodes must be considered preventable until proven otherwise. Prevention of HAP/VAP episodes constitutes a cornerstone of optimal clinical practice on ICU. The application of a bundle of evidence-based interventions (care bundlles) has demonstrated reduction in pneumonia incidence. The main evidence-based interventions are:

- No ventilatory circuit tube changes unless specifically indicated
- Hand hygiene
- Appropriatelly educated and trained staff
- Daily interruption of sedation
- Reduce duration of intubation and of mechanical ventilation through an improvement on sedation management and early weaning
- Oral hygiene with chlorhexidine
- Control endotracheal cuff pressure at least every 24h
- Infection control measures
- Avoid intubation and reintubation as possible
- Semi-recumbent position (30–45°)

Diagnosis

HAP diagnosis should be suspected in every patient with a new or progressive radiographic infiltrate with purulent respiratory secretions plus new onset of fever, leucocytosis or hypoxaemia.

Clinical approach

Initial clinical approach should include:

- Comprehensive medical history, looking for risk factors associated with specific pathogens.
- CXR, evaluating the presence of complications such as pleural effusion.
- Arterial oxygenation/respiratory rate assessment
- Assess presence of organ dysfunction/evaluate severity scores.
- All patients should have blood cultures collected
- Samples of lower respiratory tract secretions should be obtained (see below).

Microbiological fiagnosis

Quantitative cultures should be obtained by non-invasive (endotracheal aspirate) or invasive techniques (bronchoscopy-guided bronchoalveolar lavage or protected specimen brush (PSB)). The choice of method depends on local expertise, availability and cost. A large RCT failed in demonstrating any difference between an invasive and non-invasive approach.

Treatment

The therapeutic approach of HAP/VAP must be patient-based and institution-specific. Empirical treatment choice must be guided by characteristics of patients, local pattern of antimicrobial resistance and direct staining of respiratory samples.

Initial empiric therapy for HAP/VAP according to time to onset and presence of risk factors

Onset	Pathogens	Antibiotic therapy
Early onset without risk factors	*S. pneumoniae* *H. influnzae* MSSA Enterobacteriaceae	Ceftriaxone or Quinolone or Ampi/sulbactam or Ertapenem
Late onset or with risk factors for MDR pathogen	GNB MDR *P. aeruginosa* *K. pneumoniae* *Acinetobacter baumannii*	Antipseudomonal cephalosporin or Antipseudomonal carbapenem or Piperacilin/tazobactam and quinolone or aminoglycoside
	MRSA	Linezolid or vancomycin

Key points

- **Empirical antibiotic choice driven by local microbiological data**
- Data demonstrate an important variability in pathogens in different centres and different ICUs.
- **Prompt initiation of appropriate antimicrobial treatment**
- Appropriate initial antibiotic treatment is associated with better outcomes in HAP/VAP patients. The shorter the delay in starting empirical treatment, the better the impact on prognosis, LOS and cost.
- **Appropriateness of antimicrobial treatment (dose, pharmacokinetics/dynamics considerations, tissue penetration)**
- To achieve optimal antibiotic treatment, appropriate dosage, route of administration and regimen should be employed to ensure tissue penetration (e.g. linezolid has a better tissue penetration than vancomycin when treating VAP due to MRSA).
- **Modification of empirical antimicrobial treatment (de-escalation, rescue therapy)**
- The empiric antibiotic treatment must be reviewed once the culture results are available. De-escalation consists of a broad-spectrum initial antibiotic therapy, followed by a simplification of the regimen based on culture results and clinical evolution. Such a strategy is associated with lower mortality. Rescue therapy is implemented when there is primary resistance on cultures or a poor clinical evolution.
- **Evolution assessment**
- Clinical parameters such as fever and resolution of hypoxaemia (PO_2/FiO_2 ratio) are valuable markers of clinical resolution in VAP. Use of clinical scores, such as CPIS (Clinical Pulmonary Infection Score), may be useful. Use of biomarkers such as CRP or procalcitonin are promising strategies to evaluate resolution, but their use still needs to be evaluated by further studies. Optimal duration of therapy is unknown. A randomized trial concluded that outcomes are similar when treating patients for 8 or 15 days.

Further reading

American Thoracic Society. Guidelines for the management of adults with hospital-acquired, ventilator-associated, and healthcare-associated pneumonia. *Am J Respir Crit Care Med* 2005; 171: 388–416.

Canadian Critical Care Trial Group. A randomized trial of diagnostic techniques for ventilator-associated pneumonia. *N Engl J Med* 2006; 355: 2619–30.

Chastre J, Wolff M, Fagon JY, *et al.* Comparison of 8 vs 15 days of antibiotic therapy for ventilator-associated pneumonia in adults: a randomized trial. *JAMA* 2003; 290: 2588-98.

Rello J, Sá-Borges M, Correa H, *et al.* Variations in etiology of ventilator-associated pneumonia across four treatment sites: implications for antimicrobial prescribing practices. *Am J Respir Crit Care Med* 1999; 160: 608–13.

Rello J, Vidaur L, Sandiumenge A, *et al.* De-escalation therapy in ventilator-associated pneumonia. *Crit Care Med* 2004; 32:2183–90.

Resar R, Pronovost P, Haraden C, *et al.* Using a bundle approach to improve ventilator care processes and reduce ventilator-associated pneumonia. *Jt Comm J Qual Patient Saf* 2005; 31: 243–8.

Pulmonary hypertension

Definition

Pulmonary hypertension is said to occur when the mean pulmonary artery pressure exceeds 25mm Hg at rest or 30mm Hg with exercise. The term pulmonary arterial hypertension (PAH) denotes a series of apparently unrelated disorders which share the histopathological entity of plexogenic pulmonary arteriopathy (PPA). Examples include idiopathic PAH, familial PAH and pulmonary hypertension associated with scleroderma, hepatic cirrhosis, HIV infection and Eisenmenger's syndrome. In addition, pulmonary hypertension can occur in association with cardiac diseases (left heart failure, mitral valve disease), respiratory disorders (emphysema, pulmonary fibrosis), pulmonary thromboembolic disease and various miscellaneous conditions. Although these latter conditions are more common causes of pulmonary hypertension, the severity of pulmonary hypertension is usually less than that seen in PAH and the histopathology is not PPA in nature.

Idiopathic PAH was typically described in young females, although with increasing awareness the condition is now being diagnosed in patients beyond the 4th and 5th decades of life. The incidence and prevalence of the condition is estimated to be 4 per million and 10 per million of the population, respectively. The prevalence of PAH is estimated to be in the region of 100 per million of the population. The incidence and prevalence of pulmonary hypertension in patients with cardiac and respiratory disorders are not precisely known, although they are believed to be considerably higher than for PAH.

Pulmonary h9ypertension

Diagnostic classification (World Congress on Pulmonary Hypertension Venice 2003)

1 Pulmonary arterial hypertension (PAH)
   - Idiopathic PAH
   - Familial PAH
   - Related to
      - Connective tissue diseases
      - HIV
      - Portal hypertension
      - Anorexigens
      - Congenital heart diseases
   - Pulmonary capillary haemangiosis
   - Pulmonary veno-occlusive disease
   - Others (e.g. glycogen storage disease, splenectomy)

2 Associated with left heart disease
   - Atrial or ventricular dysfunction
   - Valvular disease

3 Associated with lung disease/hypoxaemia
   - COPD
   - Interstitial lung diseases
   - Sleep-disordered breathing
   - Developmental abnormalities
   - Chronic exposure to high altitude

4 Associated with chronic thrombotic and/or embolic disease
   - Obstruction of proximal pulmonary artery
   - Obstruction of distal pulmonary artery
   - Non-thrombotic pulmonary emboli

5 Miscellaneous
   - Histiocytosis
   - Lymphangioleiomyomatosis

PAH is associated with a poor survival and a poor quality of life. There is no cure, limited treatment options and incomplete understanding of the disease.

Pathology

PPA occurs in a select group of disorders. The reason why this pathological entity occurs is not clear, although it is possible that the lung only has a finite number of responses to injury which feed into final common pathway mechanisms. This may explain why similarities occur in patients with conditions such as obliterative bronchiolitis following lung transplantation and those with obliterative bronchiolitis associated with rheumatoid disease or respiratory syncytial virus infection in childhood. Likewise, although many conditions have been implicated as causing ARDS, the pathology is similar regardless of aetiology. In PPA there is initial vasoconstriction and subsequent smooth muscle migration from the inner half of the media of muscular pulmonary arterioles into the lumen to become myofibroblasts capable of laying down either smooth muscle or fibrous tissue. The cells proliferate in a concentric fashion and ultimately obliterate the lumen. When sectioned, the vessels have the appearance of a cut onion, hence the term onion skin proliferation. As the radius gets progressively compromised, the resistance to flow increases. At points of weakness in the vessel (proximally at branching areas) the vessel distends and ruptures. Haemorrhage occurs and primitive blood vessels grow into this area in a haphazard or plexiform arrangement. The combination of concentric laminar intimal (onion skin) proliferation and plexiform lesions is referred to as PPA. Some authors believe that plexiform lesions may represent a form of collateral irculation.

Why these particular changes occur in diseases with such diverse aetiology and clinical presentation is not understood. Immunoreactive cells in the lung for gastrin-releasing peptide and calcitonin may be important factors in smooth muscle migration. There is extensive ongoing research into endothelial dysfunction in patients with PAH.

Survival

PAH carries a poor prognosis, and for those patients with class IV New York Heart Association (NYHA) status, the 5-yr actuarial survival is significantly lower than that for patients with lung, breast, prostate, colon and gastric carcinoma. A median survival of 2.8yrs has been reported for untreated patients in class III or IV NYHA. Survival and quality of life have improved for selected patients treated with agents such as endothelin receptor antagonists, prostacyclin analogues and PDE inhibitors.

Prognostic factors

The following factors are useful in predicting mortality in PAH:

1 Aetiology
2 Functional capacity (NYHA or PAH class)
3 Exercise capacity (unencouraged 6min walk test)
4. Haemodynamics (severity of RV dysfunction)
5 Echo parameters (pericardial effusion carries worse prognosis).

Quality of life

Patients with PAH have similar quality of life scores when compared with those for patients with chronic obstructive lung disease and end-stage renal failure.

Natural history

Early on, patients with pulmonary hypertension may be asymptomatic or exhibit dyspnoea with exertion. In the early stages of the disease, the non-specific nature of the symptoms may lead to either failure of diagnosis or incorrect diagnosis. Many patients have had their symptoms attributed to depression. As the condition progresses, the PVR rises and the cardiac output falls. At this stage, patients may change from having relatively few symptoms to experiencing dyspnoea, chest pain, palpitations or syncope with exertion and subsequently at rest. As the condition progresses further, right heart failure and death occur.

Median survival from diagnosis if NYHA functional class III or IV and untreated is 2.8yrs.

Therapeutic targets

Abnormalities in endothelial function with respect to vasoreactivity, intimal proliferation and thrombus formation are believed important in the pathogenesis of this condition. Increasing attention has been given to endothelin 1 (which causes vasoconstriction and cellular proliferation), NO (which via cGMP promotes vasodilatation and is antiproliferative) and prostacyclin (which, acting via cAMP, also potentiates vasodilatation and is antiproliferative). NO or prostacyclin analogues are important in managing patients with this condition, as are endothelin receptor antagonists. Recently attention has focused on PDE type 5 inhibitors.

Therapeutic options

Current drugs available have improved quality of life and prolonged survival for some patients with PAH. Drug therapy can be given orally, e.g. Sildenafil (a PDE type 5 inhibitor) or Bosentan (endothelin A and B receptor antagonist), by inhalation (prostacyclin), SC (prostacyclin analogues) and IV (prostacyclin). Other treatment options include atrial septostomy and lung transplantation. A small number of patients (<10%) will respond to calcium channel blockers. These patients will have demonstrated a positive vascular reactivity test at cardiac catheterization where the pulmonary artery pressure can be reduced to close to normal values following administration of agents such as NO with an increase in or unchanged cardiac output. Other therapeutic agents being considered include lipid-lowering drugs, anti-inflammatory agents, monoclonal antibodies and antiplatelet agents. Further experience with these therapies is awaited.

Patients with NYHA functional class II and IV should be evaluated for bilateral lung transplantation. Some patients with chronic thromboembolic pulmonary hypertension may be candidates for pulmonary thromboendarterectomy. Atrial septostomy has been used to palliate patients with advanced PAH due to its potential to decompress the failing right ventricle and improve cardiac index.

Genetic aspects

Disease-causing mutations in bone morphogenetic protein receptor II (BMPR2) may underlie familial PAH. Mutations have been detected in 55% of families, and show autosomal dominance with incomplete penetrance. Thus far up to 26% of sporadic cases (idiopathic PAH) have BMPR2 mutations. BMPs are a family of secreted growth factors. BMPR2 regulates cell proliferation in response to ligand binding. Mutations lead to a loss of the inhibitory action of BMP on vascular smooth muscle cell growth. As a consequence, inappropriate cellular proliferation can occur.

Current theories on the pathophysiology of pulmonary hypertension

Patients may have a genetic predisposition (e.g BMPR2 mutation) or have a risk factor such as autoimmune disease or HIV, and this facilitates vascular injury. When vascular injury occurs, endothelial cell dysfunction follows and can give rise to inflammation and loss of local vasoreactivity, and facilitate thrombus formation. Smooth muscle cell dysfunction can also occur independently. As a consequence, disease progression and vascular remodelling ensue.

Summary

PAH is a progressive and lethal disease whose initial symptoms can be non-specific. A comprehensive diagnostic approach is required to identify associated conditions and characterize haemodynamics and functional profiles. Although at present there is no cure for PAH, it is hoped that increasing awareness and understanding of disease mechanisms will facilitate the development of effective treatment modalities.

Further reading

ACCP. Evidence-based clinical practice guidelines. Diagnosis and management of pulmonary arterial hypertension. *Chest* 2004; 126: S1–92

Madden BP, Sheth A, Wilde M, *et al.* Does Sildenafil produce a sustained benefit in patients with pulmonary hypertension associated with parenchymal lung and cardiac disease? *Vascul Pharmacol* 2007; 47: 184–8.

Chapter 18

Cardiovascular disorders

Chapter contents

Hypertension

Definition

Hypertension is defined as sustained SBP ≥140mm Hg and/or DBP ≥90mm Hg (Table 18.1.1). In the UK, the prevalence of hypertension is ~32%. Of these, only 22% have controlled BP (<140/90mm Hg). Essential (primary) hypertension accounts for 80–90% of cases. Secondary causes of hypertension include renal and endocrine disorders and drug-induced hypertension (Table 18.1.2).

Table 18.1.1 BHS definitions of hypertension

	SBP	DBP
Optimal BP	<120	<80
Normal BP	<130	<85
High–normal blood pressure	130–139	85–89
Grade 1 hypertension (mild)	140–159	90–99
Grade 2 hypertension (moderate)	160–179	100–109
Grade 3 hypertension (severe)	>180	>110

Table 18.1.2 Causes of secondary hypertension

Renal
Renovascular disease
Atherosclerotic renal artery stenosis
Fibromuscular dysplasia
Renal parenchymal disease
Acute and chronic glomerulonephritis
Polycystic disease
Diabetic nephropathy
Collagen vascular disease
Renal transplantation
Endocrine
Adrenal cortex
Conn's syndrome (primary aldosteronism)
Cushing's syndrome
Congenital adrenal hyperplasia
Dexamethazone-responsive aldosteronism
Adrenal medulla
Pheochromocytoma
Hyperparathyroidism
Acromegaly
Coarctation of aorta
Drug induced
Oral contraceptives
Cyclosporin
Steroids
Carbenoxolone and liquorice
Tyramine and MAOIs
Erythropoetin
NSAIDs
Pregnancy induced hypertension

Treatment of uncomplicated essential hypertension

First-line therapy

Young non-black individuals tend to have higher activity of the renin–angiotensin–aldosterone system (RAAS) as evidenced by higher plasma renin activity (PRA). They respond well to angiotensin-converting enzyme (ACE) inhibitors and angiotensin II receptor blockers (ARBs), whereas those with a low PRA, i.e. the elderly and black individuals, respond better to either calcium channel blockers (CCBs) or diuretics (Fig. 18.1.1).

Drug combinations

BP control on monotherapy is rarely achieved. The most effective way to control BP is to combine 2 or more antihypertensive agents that lower BP by different mechanisms. ACE inhibitors and ARBs (A) combine well with CCB (C) and diuretics (D). This gives rise to the A/CD rule for combining drugs, in which a drug from A group is added to another from either the C or D groups (Fig. 18.1.1). The next step is to add a drug from each group: A + C + D.

Management of hypertension in different patient groups

The elderly

Low-dose thiazide diuretics are the preferred first-line treatment. Dihydropyridine CCBs are suitable alternatives when thiazides are contraindicated or not tolerated.

The very elderly

No firm evidence exists to guide treatment for patients above the age of 80yrs. If antihypertensive treatment has been started before the age of 80, they should be continued.

Diabetes mellitus

Type 2 diabetes

ACE inhibitors and ARBs have an antiproteinuric effect and delay progression from microalbuminuria to overt nephropathy. Combined use of ACE inhibitors and ARBs is more effective in reducing albuminuria and to some extent BP.

Type 1 diabetes

ACE inhibitors have a specific renoprotective action independent of the BP-lowering effect. ACE inhibitor therapy should be titrated to the maximum tolerated recommended dose. The target BP in type 1 diabetes with nephropathy is <130/80mm Hg or lower, <125/75mm Hg, when there is proteinuria ≥1g/24h.

Ethnic groups

Afro-Caribbean hypertensive subjects are more responsive to diuretics and CCBs. ACE inhibitors and ARBs in monotherapy may be less effective in blacks because the RAAS is frequently suppressed but when these drugs are combined with a diuretic or a CCB they are quite effective.

Hypertensive crises

A hypertensive crisis is defined as severe hypertension with ongoing or impending target organ damage (TOD). The rate of the rise in BP in relation to the previous levels of BP is more important than the absolute BP level.

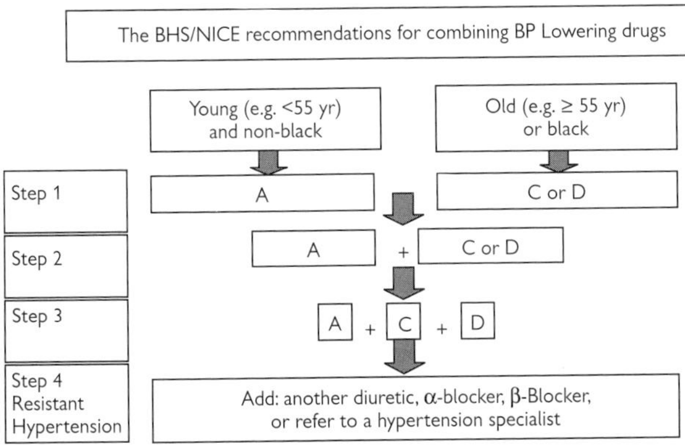

Fig. 18.1.1 The BHS/NICE recommendations for combining BP-lowering drugs.

A **hypertensive emergency** is defined as a situation that requires immediate BP lowering (not necessarily to normal values) to prevent or limit TOD. **Hypertensive urgency** is a situation in which severely elevated BP is not accompanied by any evidence from history, physical examination or laboratory investigation of acute TOD. Individuals under this category could be:

1. Known hypertensive patients who are not compliant with their medication; prior therapy should be restarted (if there are no side effects).
2. For patients taking their medications regularly, therapy should be increased (either by increasing the dose(s) of drugs or by adding new drugs).
3. For patients on no treatment, hypertension therapy should be started with oral agents (e.g. nifedipine SR or LA, or amlodipine) and a follow-up appointment arranged urgently with a hypertension clinic.

Individuals with untreated severe or accelerated hypertension have a dreadful long-term prognosis. The most common causes of death are renal failure, strokes and MI.

Management of hypertensive emergencies

The key to a successful outcome is the prompt recognition and initiation of treatment. Full medical history and physical examination including palpation of all peripheral pulses and a fundoscopic examination is mandatory. Specific points in the patient's past medical history include patient's BP prior to presentation and drug history (including prescription, over-the-counter and recreational drugs).

Initial investigations should include FBC, electrolytes, urea, creatinine, urine dipstick, CXR and ECG. These tests should be performed simultaneously with the initiation of antihypertensive therapy.

The approach in treating hypertensive emergency is initially to reduce BP by ~15–25% with further reductions accomplished more gradually. The initial reduction should be achieved over a period of 2–4h, with less rapid reduction over the next 24h.

Pathophysiology

A sudden increase in PVR (e.g. secondary to non-compliance) triggers an increase in circulating levels of vasoconstrictor substances such as angiotensin II and noradrenaline.

Aortic dissection

Aortic dissection must be excluded in any patient presenting with severe hypertension and chest pain, back pain or abdominal pain. It is life-threatening, with very poor prognosis if not treated (mortality is 1%/h). Aortic dissection is classified as type A if it involves the ascending aorta or type B if it does not. Surgical treatment is usually required for type A dissection, whereas type B responds more favourably to medical treatment. Severe refractory hypertension is nearly omnipresent, especially in the acute phase even in patients without history of hypertension.

Propagation of the dissection is dependent not only on the elevation of the BP itself, but also on the velocity of LV ejection and the rate of increase of the aortic pulse wave. Therefore, the immediate reduction of BP and shear stress is of paramount importance to prevent the extension, haemorrhage and rupture of the dissection. BP should be reduced quickly (within 15–30min) to the lowest tolerated level that preserves adequate organ perfusion. The initial treatment of choice is a combination of IV β-blocker (e.g. esmolol or metoprolol) or a combined α–β blocker (e.g. labetalol) and a vasodilator (e.g. SNP or dihydropyridine CCB). The recent CAFÉ trial, a substudy of the ASCOT trial, has shown that a combination of a dihydropyridine CCB and an ACE inhibitor was more effective in reducing central aortic pressure than a combination of a β-blocker and a diuretic. Therefore, the combination of a CCB and an ACE inhibitor should be considered in the treatment.

Acute pulmonary oedema

More than 90% of patients with heart failure have a history of hypertension. The clinical syndrome of heart failure is usually characterized by signs and symptoms of intravascular and interstitial volume overload. IV GTN is the drug of choice in the initial treatment, together with an IV loop diuretic (e.g. frusemide) and diamorphine. GTN reduces both preload and afterload while improving coronary blood flow. There is very little clinical experience with the use of ACE inhibitors in patients with acute LV failure, but a short-acting ACE inhibitor (e.g. captopril) may be added if necessary.

It is important to stress here that patients with malignant hypertension who present with acute (flash) pulmonary oedema may not have volume overload. In fact, they may have volume depletion secondary to pressure naturesis. Therefore, IV diuresis may exacerbate the hypertension and cause further clinical deterioration. The use of diuretics should be reserved for patients who are clinically fluid overloaded and should not be prescribed routinely.

STEMI and ACS

Hypertension is very common in patients presenting with acute coronary syndrome (ACS). The overall prevalence of hypertension in US patients presenting with NSTEMI is ~50% while in Europe the prevalence is ~34%.

IV GTN is the drug of choice for ACS and STEMI as it reduces PVR while improving coronary perfusion. β-Blockers attenuate the activity of the adrenergic system and the RAAS, and improve survival in post-MI patients. In ACS, β-blockers should be started IV then switched to oral when the patient is stable. When β-blockers are contraindicated, a non-dihydropyridine CCB (diltiazem or verapamil) can be used if the patient does not have severe LV dysfunction. Short-acting dihydropyridine CCB should not be used in the treatment of hypertensive crisis when associated with ACS or acute STEMI. ACE inhibitors could be added if hypertension persists, as they significantly improve survival during STEMI. SNP, unlike GTN, increases heart rate and provokes ST segment elevation, and should not be used alone.

Cocaine overdose

Cocaine overdose is often associated with uncontrolled severe hypertension and coronary artery vasoconstriction leading to angina, MI and sudden death. These effects are mediated through α-adrenergic receptors and therefore β-blockers alone (i.e. without α-blockers) may exacerbate the hypertension and the clinical condition, and are therefore contraindicated. A non-dihydropyridine CCB (e.g. diltiazem or verapamil) or a combined α–β blocker, e.g. labetalol, may be used.

Severe pre-eclampsia and eclampsia

Pre-eclampsia is defined as hypertension (BP ≥140/90mm Hg) in the second half of pregnancy (i.e. after 20 weeks of gestation) associated with proteinuria and oedema. Eclampsia is the occurrence of seizures in a patient with pre-eclampsia. Treatment with antihypertensive drugs is not usually indicated for BP <160/100mm Hg. ACE inhibitors and ARBs are contraindicated in pregnancy because of the increase in foetal and neonatal morbidity and mortality. Methyldopa remains the mainstay of treatment for patients with moderate gestational hypertension because of its foetal and neonatal safety. The drug, however, has many adverse side effects.

For pre-eclamptic patients with severe hypertension, IV hydralazine or labetalol could be given. SNP can cause profound reflex paradoxical bradycardia and hypotension, and should be avoided.

Malignant hypertension

Malignant (accelerated) hypertension is a syndrome characterized by severely elevated BP accompanied by retinopathy including papilloedema, nephropathy, encephalopathy and microangiopathic haemolytic anaemia. Pathologically it is characterized by fibrinoid necrosis in arterioles, myointimal proliferation in small arteries, platelet and fibrin deposition, and breakdown of normal vascular autoregulation function. The resulting vasoconstriction induces severe elevation in BP and widespread endothelial damage. The resulting renal ischaemia prompts massive release of renin and angiotensin II, triggering a vicious cycle. The rapid increase in BP enhances pressure natriuresis, which further stimulates the RAAS, resulting in secondary hyperaldosteronism, hypokalaemia and metabolic alkalosis.

Malignant hypertension rarely occurs *de novo*, and is usually a consequence of untreated essential or secondary hypertension such as renal artery stenosis, phaeochromocytoma or scleroderma. The incidence of malignant hypertension remains stable across the UK and Europe, with ~1–2 cases per 100 000 per year. Malignant hypertension has a very poor prognosis if untreated, with a mortality rate >90% within 1yr, but with proper treatment 5yr survival is 60–75%.

Most patients who present with malignant hypertension have volume depletion secondary to pressure naturesis. Therefore, further diuresis may exacerbate the hypertension and cause further deterioration in kidney function.

Hypertensive encephalopathy

Hypertensive encephalopathy is much less common these days with the use of modern antihypertensive drugs. It is believed to be due to cerebral oedema secondary to failure of CBF autoregulation and rapid elevation of cerebral perfusion. Symptoms and signs include headache, nausea and vomiting, visual disturbances, altered level of consciousness, confusion, disorientation, focal or generalized seizures and retinopathy including papilloedema. Diagnosis may be difficult as it is one of exclusion requiring that stroke, encephalitis, vasculitis, subarachnoid haemorrhage and mass lesions need to be excluded. The definite criterion to confirm the diagnosis is a prompt improvement in the patient's clinical condition with the response to antihypertensive treatment. The goal of treatment is to reduce BP by ~25% within the first hour or to a level of 160/100mm Hg, whichever value is higher. It must be emphasized that cerebral hypoperfusion and neurological deterioration may result if more reductions in BP are achieved quickly. In this case, BP should be allowed to increase and further reductions should be attempted more slowly.

Stroke

Appropriate treatment of hypertension in the setting of acute stroke remains contentious. There is little scientific evidence and no clinically established benefit for rapid lowering of BP among persons with acute ischaemic stroke. Aggressive lowering of BP may cause neurological worsening. However, it is generally agreed that severe hypertension (BP >180/110mm Hg) may be an indication for treatment as higher BP levels is a contraindication to IV thrombolysis. If thrombolysis is not considered, then emergency administration of antihypertensive drugs should be withheld unless the SBP is >220mm Hg and/or DBP is >120mm Hg. Treatment could be started with IV labetalol.

A reasonable goal would be to lower BP by 25% within the first day. Previously hypertensive patients with mild to moderate strokes who are not at high risk for increased ICP may have their usual pre-stroke antihypertensive medications restarted 24h after their stroke.

Drugs for the treatment of hypertensive emergencies

Sodium nitroprusside

SNP dilates arteriolar resistance and venous capacitance vessels and decreases both the afterload and preload. It is a very potent agent with an immediate onset and short duration of action; plasma $t_{1/2}$ is 2–3min. Continuous arterial BP monitoring is recommended to avoid overreduction in BP. The drug is light sensitive and should be shielded from light to prevent degradation. The usual dose is 0.3–10mcg/kg/min. Cyanide poisoning may occur with prolonged or high dose administration, especially in individuals with renal or hepatic insufficiency. Manifestations of poisoning include CNS depression, seizures and lactic acidosis.

GTN

GTN dilates arteriolar resistance and venous capacitance vessels. It reduces preload and afterload, improves LV function and reduces myocardial oxygen demand. GTN dilates both epicardial coronary vessels with stenosis and collaterals, and increases blood supply to ischaemic areas. It is the drug of choice for reducing BP in individuals with STEMI, ACS and acute pulmonary oedema. However, the BP-lowering effect of GTN is not as predictable as with SNP, and higher doses (up to 300mcg/min) may be required to achieve an adequate response. Onset of action is almost immediate, with a very short duration of action ($t_{1/2}$ 3–5min). The starting dose is 5–15mcg/min. Nitrate tolerance is a problem even within the first 24h.

Labetalol

Labetalol is a selective α_1- and non-selective β-adrenergic receptor blocker. Its differential effects on α:β receptors are 1:3 after oral administration and 1:7 after IV administration, respectively. The drug can be given IV as a 20–80mg mini-bolus injection (q 10min) or 2–4mg/min infusion. Labetalol produces a prompt and controlled reduction in BP in patients with hypertensive crises, with onset of action within 5min and duration of action of 3–6h. The drug is contraindicated in patients with acute LV failure, heart block and COPD.

Esmolol

Esmolol is an ultrashort-acting β_1-selective adrenergic blocking agent with an extremely brief $t_{1/2}$ of <10min. This agent is available for IV use both as a bolus and as an infusion. The recommended loading dose is 0.5–1mg followed by an infusion of 50–200mcg/kg/min.

Further reading

Antonios TF, Cappuccio FP, Markandu ND, *et al.* A diuretic is more effective than a beta-blocker in hypertensive patients not controlled on amlodipine and lisinopril. *Hypertension* 1996; 27: 1325–8.

Dahlof B, Sever PS, Poulter NR, *et al.* Prevention of cardiovascular events with an antihypertensive regimen of amlodipine adding perindopril as required versus atenolol adding bendroflumethiazide as required, in the Anglo-Scandinavian Cardiac Outcomes Trial-Blood Pressure Lowering Arm (ASCOT-BPLA): a multicentre randomised controlled trial. *Lancet* 2005; 366: 895–906.

Ravid M, Lang R, Rachmani R, *et al.* Long-term renoprotective effect of angiotensin-converting enzyme inhibition in non-insulin-dependent diabetes mellitus. A 7-year follow- up study. *Arch Intern Med* 1996; 156: 286–9.

Williams B, Lacy PS, Thom SM, *et al.* Differential impact of blood pressure-lowering drugs on central aortic pressure and clinical outcomes: principal results of the Conduit Artery Function Evaluation (CAFE) study. *Circulation* 2006; 113: 1213–25.

Williams B, Poulter NR, Brown MJ, *et al.* Guidelines for management of hypertension: report of the fourth working party of the British Hypertension Society, 2004-BHS IV. *J Hum Hypertens* 2004; 18: 139–85.

Tachyarrhythmias

Excessive rapidity in the action of the heart, usually defined as a heart rate >100bpm, and associated with increased incidence of major cardiac events and length of ICU stay. Tachyarrhythmias may arise from the atria or the ventricles.

Atrial fibrillation (AF)

Characterized by uncoordinated atrial activation. Main features are described in Table 18,2,1.

Management principles

- Correction/removal of potential cause(s)
- Restoration of sinus rhythm if possible (chemical/electrical cardioversion)
- Prevention/exclusion of intracardiac thrombus (TOE)
- Rate control (amiodarone/β-blocker/calcium channel blockade) where cardioversion is not possible
- Anticoagulation may be required and should be tailored to the individual patient situation

Prophylaxis and maintenance of sinus rhythm

- Risk of post-cardiothoracic surgery AF is reduced by amiodarone, β-blockade or dltiazem. Digoxin should not be used.
- In post-operative AF, rhythm control should be the initial option.
- If antiarrhythmics are required to maintain sinus rhythm, β-blockade/amiodarone may be considered

Atrial flutter

Atrial flutter is the expression of rapid and regular atrial excitation. The main features are described in Table 18.2.1.

Management principles

- Generally, as for AF
- Digoxin may convert to AF (rate control easier)
- Overdrive atrial pacing may be used to cardiovert (success rate of approximately <50%)

Multi-focal atrial tachycardia

Multi-focal atrial tachycardia is an irregular cardiac rhythm caused by at least 2 different sites of competing atrial activity with the sinus node. The main features are described in Table 18.2.1.

Management principles

- Frequently transient. May spontaneously convert to sinus rhythm, AF or atrial flutter
- Treat any precipitating cause
- Antiarrhythmics (β-blockers, magnesium or verapamil) may be used
- Electrical cardioversion is not generally effective

Pre-excitation syndromes

Characterized by intermittent tachycardia (narrow or broad complex) associated with an accessory AV connection where a re-entry circuit between atria and ventricles occurs. Includes the Wolf–Parkinson–White (WPW) syndrome. Note that pre-excitation (delta wave) is seen in only 3/1000 ECGs.

Management principles

- AF is potentially life-threatening (may degenerate to VF)
- In 50% of patients with WPW, cardiac arrest is the first manifestation
- Adenosine should be avoided

Table 18.2.1

Rhythm	Substrate	ECG features	Incidence	Risk factors
AF	Following 4–6 re-entry circuit wavelets in the atria near anatomical/functional barriers	Absent P waves; fibrillatory waves and irregular ventricular response (intact AV conduction)	4–5% general ICU; 25–40% cardiac ICU	Age, diabetes, hypertension, structural and ischaemic heart disease, cardiac failure, changes in intravascular volume, increased sympathetic activity, inotropic agents, intracardiac lines, electrolyte imbalance, lung disease, SIRS, hyperthyroidism
AFl	Multiple re-entrant/ ectopic atrial waves	Regular 'saw-tooth' atrial deflexion waves best seen in leads II, III and aVF	5.2% general ICU	As AF, plus pericarditis
MAT	?Triggered activity due to intracellular calcium overload or delayed 'afterdepolarization'	Atrial rate >100bpm and ≥3 morphologically distinct P waves. P–P intervals are irregular and there is an isoelectric baseline between P waves	0.05–0.32% in-patients. ICU incidence not known—probably underdiagnosed	COPD, hypoxaemia, PE, congestive heart failure and electrolyte imbalance.
VT	Originates from one or more ventricular ectopic foci, rate >100bpm	Wide QRS complexes (>140ms), negative precordial, independent atrial activity, capture and fusion beats	41% general ICU	Cardiac disease, electrolyte imbalance, hypoxaemia, acidaemia, drugs
TdP	Cycles of alternating electrical polarity with electrical axis rotating around the baseline.	Characteristic paroxysms of 5–20 beats at heart rate >200bpm and alternating electrical axis in 10–12 beats	Not known	Risk factors: drugs electrolyte imbalance, subarachnoid haemorrhage, QT_c prolongation and insecticide poisoning

AF = atrial fibrillation; Afl, atrial flutter; MAT = multi-focal atrial tachycardia; VT = ventricular tachycardia; TdP = Torsade de pointes.

- Early consultation with an electrophysiologist is advised for the ICU patient with a pre-excitation syndrome
- Electrical cardioversion should be used in emergency

Ventricular tachycardia

Characterized by a regular broad-complex tachycardia. The main features are described in Table 18.2.1.

Management principles

- In all cases: correction/removal of potential cause(s)
- Non-sustained VT with haemodynamic compromise: consider lignocaine/amiodarone infusion or ventricular pacing
- Sustained VT with no haemodynamic compromise: lignocaine/amiodarone and, if no myocardial ischaemia, consider procainamide. If drug treatment fails, cardioversion
- Sustained VT with haemodynamic compromise: cardioversion
- Polymorphic VT with normal QT interval: may be associated with myocardial ischaemia; therefore, electrical cardioversion is recommended with a plan for revascularization where possible
- Torsade de pointes: the main features described in Table 18.2.1. In addition to correction/removal of potential causes, IV magnesium. Consider overdrive pacing or isoproterenol

Key points

- Treatment of all tachyarrhythmias on the ICU should include correction/removal of potential causes.
- Restoration of sinus rhythm is the main goal.
- Where standard pharmacological or electrical therapy fails, expert advice should be sought from an electrophysiologist as specialist intervention may be required.

Further reading

Blomstrom-Lundqvist C, Scheinman MM, Aliot EM, *et al.* ACC/AHA/ESC guidelines for the management of patients with supraventricular arrythmias. *J Am Coll Cardiol* 2003; 42: 1493–531.

Grant AO. Recent advances in the treatment of arrhythmias. *Circ J* 2003; 67: 651–5.

National Collaborating Centre for Chronic Conditions. Atrial fibrillation; national clinical guideline for management in primary and secondary care. London: Royal College of Physicians, 2006.

Trappe HJ, Brandt B, Weismuller P, *et al.* Arrhythmias in the intensive care patient. *Curr Opin Crit Care* 2003; 9: 345–55.

Trohman RG. Supraventricular tachycardia: Implication for the intensivist. *Crit Care Med* 2000; 28 (Suppl.): N129–35.

Bradyarrhythmias

A slow ventricular rate, usually defined as <60bpm, but may be absolute (<40bpm) or relative (excessively slow for the patient's clinical status). Bradyarrhythmias are due to either sinus node dysfunction or AV conduction disturbances.

Causes of bradyarrhythmia

These are divided into intrinsic (degeneration, acquired cardiac diseaseùincluding cardiac surgery, infiltrative diseases, congenital heart disease, infection) and extrinsic (neurological, pharmacological, endocrine, electrolyte disturbance, hypothermia). Bradyarrhythmia is common in intensive care settings. It is usually transient and often related to extrinsic factors such as drugs and airway manipulation.

Factors which increase the likelihood of arrhythmia in ICU include:

1. Pre-existing cardiac disease
2. Treatment with antiarrhythmics
3. Recent macrovascular event
4. Microvascular disease causing ischaemia
5. Altered acid–base balance
6. High CO_2
7. Abnormal electrolyte balance
8. Endogenous catecholamines (pain, anxiety)
9. Exogenous catecholamines (inotropes)
10. Suction/bronchoscopy/airway manoeuvres
11. Deep anaesthesia/sedation
12. Anaesthesia drugs (muscle relaxants, regional)

Sinus node dysfunction (sick sinus syndrome:

- 1:600 patients >65yrs.
- Multiple ECG manifestations including: sinus bradycardia, sinus arrest, sinoatrial block, tachy-brady syndrome, AF.
- Most common manifestation in the ICU is excessive bradycardia upon treatment of tachyarrhythmia.
- Sinus node dysfunction post-anterior MI is relatively common (5–30%). Often associated with concomitant AV node block. Treatment is usually not required unless associated with cardiac failure, hypotension or continuing myocardial ischaemia.
- In tachy-brady syndrome, pharmacological intervention to control the ventricular rate during tachycardia by blocking AV conduction with β-blockers, calcium channel blockers or digitalis may not be possible without pacing due to sinus node depression.

Atrioventricular conduction disturbance

- Abnormalities arise in the AV node or the bundle of His.
- Multiple ECG manifestations including: first/second/third degree AV block, bundle branch block, fascicular block.
- Narrow QRS implies block in the AV node; wide QRS implies infranodal block.
- Most common cause focal injury (MI), but may result from right heart catheter-related trauma.
- Where seen in conjunction with aortic endocarditis, may indicate aortic root abscess with risk of progression to high grade AV block.
- Myocardial ischaemia should be excluded with development of new bundle branch block. Budle branch block in anterior MI may result from large infarct size, LV dysfunction or conduction abnormalities. It is associated with poor prognosis.
- First degree (PR interval >0.2s): does not normally require intervention.
- Second degree (Mobitz type I, Wenckebach): progressive lengthening of PR interval until failed conduction.
- Second degree (Mobitz type II): constant PR interval with intermittent failure of conduction.
- Third degree (complete heart block): independent atrial and ventricular activity.

Risk of progression to high grade AV block

The risk of progression to high grade AV block and to asystole need to be assessed in all patients with AV conduction disturbances. Where indicated, back-up pacing should be considered:

- First degree and Morbitz type I second degree AV block—low risk
- Morbitz type I second degree AV block with wide QRS—high risk especially in the context of anterior MI
- Morbitz type II second degree AV block with wide QRS or associated with anterior MI—high risk

Specific conditions

Infective endocarditis (IE)

Development of new AV block or bundle branch block in IE implies an aortic root abscess, usually in the non-coronary cusp. This complication is associated with significant risk of abrupt development of high grade AV block, and immediate temporary pacing wire insertion is indicated. The case should be discussed with cardiologists and cardiac surgeons.

Lyme disease

AV block is the most common manifestation of myocarditis in this condition. Antibiotic treatment usually resolves the AV block, but temporary pacing may be required.

Clinical approach

Although the clinical approach to the ICU patient with bradycardia does not differ from that in the non-ICU setting, the thresholds at which intervention may be indicated differ, and have to be tailored to each individual patient. Principles of management include exclusion/removal of potential causes, assessment of the haemodynamic impact of the bradycardia and special investigations, whilst rapidly assessing full clinical status of the patients. Further principles of management are outlined below:

1. Immediate intervention may not be required if the patient is haemodynamically stable.
2. Correct electrolytes and ensure adequacy of oxygenation and ventilation. This should be carried out simultaneously with other treatment if haemodynamically compromised. Serum potassium should be maintained at >4.5mmol/l in patients with cardiac disease or post-cardiac surgery (excluding post-cardiac transplantation).
3. Treat all reversible ischaemia. AMI must be considered as a cause of bradyarrhythmia and managed appropriately.
4. If rate is slow and the patient is haemodynamically compromised then consider pacing. Indications for pacing are discussed below.

Pharmacotherapy

Intermittent sinus node dysfunction may respond to a small dose of atropine, but the response is unpredictable. With prolonged bradyarrhythmia and severe, aggravating ventricular irritability not responding to atropine or isoprenaline, temporary pacing should be considered. The following drugs are used to treat bradyarrhythmia:

Glycopyrrolate

Class: muscarininc anticholinergic agent. Synthetic quaternary amine with no central effect.

Indications: treatment of bradycardia, antisialogogue.

Dose: 200–600mcg IV bolus. Peak effect occurs 3min after IV injection.

Interaction: none

Adverse effect: dry mouth, inability to sweat, fever.

Atropine

Class: muscarininc anticholinergic agent. Naturally occurring tertiary amine which penetrates blood–brain barrier

Indications: Treatment of bradycardia when associated with haemodynamic compromise or ventricular ectopy

Dose: 0.02mg/kg. Repeat in 5min if required. 3mg is needed for complete vagal blockade in adult

Interaction: none

Adverse effects: dry mouth, inhibition of sweating, difficulty swallowing, hallucination, blurred vision

Contraindication: glaucoma

Isoprenaline

Class: short-acting synthetic catecholamine with pure β-adrenergic-stimulating properties ($\beta_1 > \beta_2$)

Indications: in emergencies to increase heart rate in bradycardia or in heart block

Dose: 0–10mcg/min

Interactions: none

Adverse effects: reduction in diastolic blood pressure, headache, tremor, palpitations, arrhythmia and sweating

Adrenaline

Class: β- and α-adrenergic receptor agonist

Indication: asystole, inotropic therapy, anaphylactic reaction, acute severe asthma

Dose: for bradyarrhythmia 5–10mcg IV bolus via central vein. Followed if necessary by infusion 0.01–0.2mcg/kg/min

Interaction: exaggerated pressor and tachycardiac response with other sympathomimetics

Adverse effects: tachycardia, hypertension, vasoconstriction, arrhythma, hyperglycaemia, thrombophrebitis/necrosis if given via peripheral vein

Pacing

Pacing is a definitive life-saving treatment for bradyarrhythmia. Various modes of pacing are available, including: mechanical, transcutaneous, transvenous, transoesophageal and transthoracic. Clinical judgement is required for symptomatic bradyarrhythmia secondary to extrinsic causes. Although a change in drug therapy should be considered for drug-induced bradyarrhythmia, pacing may be an acceptable approach if no agent with equivalent efficacy is available. Atrial pacing is preferred in the patients with sinus node dysfunction as it reduces the incidence of AF, pacemaker syndrome and thromboembolism.

Indications for pacing in general ICU:

1 Symptomatic sinus bradycardia (SBP <80) unresponsive to drug therapy
2 Morbitz type II second degree AV block
3 Third degree AV block
4 Bilateral bundle branch block (alternating bundle branch block or right bundle branch block with alternating left anterior fasicular block/left posterior
5 Newly acquired or age-indeterminate bifasicular block with first degree AV block.
6 Newly acquired AV block or bundle branch block in IE

Indications for pacing in AMI

A degree of AV block occurs in 12–25% of AMI, commonly associated with inferoposterior MI causing AV nodal ischaemia with RV impairment. The sinus and AV nodes are relatively resistant to permanent injury by infarction, and normal function should recover over time. However, permanent damage occurs more readily to the bundle of His. Anterior MI often cause AV nodal block in the bundle of His, and it can progress suddenly to complete heart block. Therefore, even transient complete AV block in the His–Purkinje system due to infarction justifies the insertion of a pacemaker.

1 AV block post-anterior MI associated with cardiac failure, hypotension or continuing myocardial ischaemia
2 First degree AV block and bundle branch block associated with anterior MI
3 Newly acquired bifasicular block associated with anterior MI
4 Alternating bundle branch block with anterior MI

Indications for pacing after cardiac surgery

AV block is one significant complication of cardiac surgery particularly post-valve replacement and in surgery for congenital heart disease (1–3%). Epicardial wires are inserted perioperatively for the management of arrhythmias (bradycardia, nodal/junctional arrhythmia, AV block) associated with haemodynamic compromise, and those who are at high risk of post-operative arrhythmia.

Further reading

European Society of Intensive Care Medicine. Patient-centred Acute Care Training (PACT) arrhythmia module, www.esicm.org.

Gregoratos G, Abrams J, Epstein AE, *et al*. ACC/AHA/NASPE 2002 guideline update for implantation of cardiac pacemakers and antiarrhythmia devices: summary article: a report of the American College of Cardiology/American Heart Association Task Force on Practice Guidelines (ACC/AHA/NASPE Committee to Update the 1998 Pacemaker Guidelines). *Circulation* 2002: 106: 2145–61.

Mangrum JM, DiMarco JP. The evaluation and management of bradycardia. *N Engl J Med* 2000; 342: 703–9.

Myocardial infarction: diagnosis

Acute coronary syndromes (ACS) are differentiated into three categories: unstable angina (UA), non-ST-segment elevation myocardial infarction (NSTEMI) and ST-segment elevation myocardial infarction (STEMI). All share a common pathophysiology: plaque rupture with subsequent platelet activation, adhesion and aggregation, thrombin generation and ultimately thrombus formation. Classification by ECG provides a useful framework for management and treatment of ACS, as those with STEMI benefit from early reperfusion therapy (pharmacological or mechanical), vs those patients with NSTEMI or UA for whom catheter-based therapy requires risk stratification.

Due to increased sensitivity of new troponin assays, a joint ACC/ESC committee proposed the following definition of an acute, evolving or recent MI:

Typical rise and gradual fall (troponin) or rapid rise and fall (CK-MB) of biochemical markers of myocardial necrosis with at least one of the following:

- Ischaemic symptoms
- ECG changes indicative of ischaemia (ST-segment elevation or depression)
- Development of pathological Q waves on the ECG
- Coronary artery intervention (e.g. angioplasty)

Clinical approach

Signs and symptoms

The symptoms of angina are described as (1) substernal chest discomfort with characteristic quality and duration that is (2) provoked by exertion or emotional stress and (3) relieved by rest or nitroglycerin. Angina is classified as typical (all 3) or atypical. While typical angina raises the probability of coronary artery disease (CAD), symptoms not characteristic of typical angina (i.e. sharp stabbing pain or pain reproducible by palpation) do not exclude ACS. At least 1/5 of MIs are clinically unrecognized because of atypical symptoms. In one study, 7% of patients with pain fully reproduced with palpation were found to have ACS.

In patients with a history of CAD, assess if chest discomfort is similar to prior episodes of angina.

Physical examination

The bedside examination is important for excluding alternative diagnoses such as aortic dissection or pericarditis, as well as diagnosing certain complications.

- Distended neck veins—elevated RV diastolic pressure
- Pulmonary crackles—elevated LV filling pressure
- Holosystolic murmur at apex—mitral regurgitation from papillary muscle dysfunction
- Holosystolic murmur at left lower sternal border—acute ventricular septal defect due to septal rupture

History

- Assess cardiac risk factors for CAD
- History of CAD/coronary intervention/CABG
- History of peripheral arterial disease
- Diabetes
- Hypertension
- Hyperlipidaemia
- Smoking
- Family history of premature CAD
- Prior stroke/transient ischaemic attack (TIA)

ECG

The findings on ECG will depend on the duration of symptoms, size of myocardium affected, and location and extent of ischaemia/infarction. An initially normal ECG does not exclude ischaemia or even acute infarction. If the initial ECG is normal and symptoms persist, it should be repeated at 5–10min intervals.

The first ECG changes with total coronary occlusion will usually be peaked T waves in the anatomic area of the myocardium in jeopardy followed within minutes by ST-segment elevation.

The diagnosis of STEMI is defined by ≥1mm of ST elevation in two anatomically contiguous leads, new or presumably new left bundle branch block (LBBB), or true posterior MI. The finding of LBBB in the setting of possible ACS is a common cause for delay in reperfusion or treatment due to concern regarding diagnosis and risk of therapy. This is an ideal situation for direct referral to cardiac catheterization when merited.

True posterior infarction is suggested by marked ST-segment depression confined to leads V_1–V_4 and accompanied by tall R waves in the right precordial leads and upright T waves.

Localization of ischaemia/infarction

- I and aVL—high lateral
- V_5 and V_6—lateral
- II, III, aVF—inferior
- V_1, V_2, V_3, V_4—anterior-septal

Patients with inferior STEMI and haemodynamic compromise should be assessed with a right precordial V_4R lead to detect ST-segment elevation (≥1mm) and an echocardiogram to screen for RV infarction.

Biochemical cardiac markers

Biochemical cardiac markers of injury should be measured in all patients who present with chest pain consistent with ACS, for both the diagnosis of myocardial necrosis and the estimation of prognosis. There is a quantitative relationship between the level of marker elevation and the risk for adverse outcome.

CK-MB begins to appear 4–8h after onset of infarction and peaks at 12–24h, with return to baseline at 2-4 days. Levels may be elevated in patients with severe skeletal muscle damage. Cardiac troponins (I and T) have greater sensitivity and specificity than CK-MB. Both convey prognostic information beyond that supplied by the ECG, clinical characteristics at presentation and predischarge exercise test. Although troponins accurately identify myocardial necrosis, necrosis may not necessarily be secondary to atherosclerotic CAD.

Important caveats

Women present more often than men with atypical chest pain and symptoms. Diabetic patients may have atypical symptoms or none at all due to autonomic dysfunction. Elderly persons may have atypical presentations such as generalized weakness, stroke, syncope or a change in mental status.

Traditional risk factors for CAD are only weakly predictive of acute ischaemia, and are less important than symptoms, ECG and cardiac biomarkers.

Echocardiography

Echocardiography can be very useful in patients with suspected ACS, particularly those with equivocal ECG findings. The presence of a regional wall motion abnormality is highly suggestive of acute ischaemia, and its absence suggests that a large ischaemic territory is not present. Echocardiographic findings can also sometimes suggest alternative diagnoses.

Echocardiography provides a good measure of overall LV performance, allows for evaluation of valvular structure and function, and can identify areas of akinesis and thinning suggestive of previous infarction. Echo is also the procedure of choice for rapid identification of complications of MI.

Further reading

Dzau VJ, Antman EM, Black HR, *et al.* The cardiovascular disease continuum validated: clinical evidence of improved patient outcomes: Part I: Pathophysiology and clinical trial evidence (risk factors through stable coronary artery disease). *Circulation* 2006; 114: 2850–70.

European Society of Cardiology
`http://www.escardio.org/knowledge/guidelines/`

GRACE ACS Risk Management Tools
`http://www.outcomes-umassmed.org/grace/acs_risk/acs_risk.swf`

Jaffe AS, Babuin L, Apple FS. Biomarkers in acute cardiac disease: The present and the future. *J Am Coll Cardiol* 2006; 48: 1–11.

Thygesen K, Alpert JS, White HD, *et al.* Universal definition of myocardial infarction. *Circulation* 2007; 116: 2634–53.

Rothwell PM, Coull AJ, Silver LE, *et al.* Population-based study of event-rate, incidence, case fatality, and mortality for all acute vascular events in all arterial territories (Oxford Vascular Study). *Lancet* 2005; 366: 1773–83.

Thygesen K, Alpert JS, White DH; on behalf of the Joint ESC/ACCF/AHA/WHF Task Force for the Redefinition of Myocardial Infarction. Universal definition of myocardial infarction. *Eur Heart J* 2007; 28: 2525–38.

Wang K, Asinger RW, Marriott HJ. ST-segment elevation in conditions other than acute myocardial infarction. *N Engl J Med* 2003; 349: 2128–35.

NSTEMI

General principles

Risk stratification

It is essential to identify those patients at highest risk for future cardiac events who may benefit from a more aggressive or invasive therapeutic approach. Factors predicting high risk:

- Presence and extent of ST-segment depression
- Elevated cardiac biomarkers
- Haemodynamic instability
- Persistent chest pain despite appropriate medical therapy

TIMI rsk score

The TIMI risk score predicts outcome in patients with UA or NSTEMI from 7 variables on presentation:

- Age ≥65yrs
- Presence of at least three risk factors for CAD (hypertension, diabetes, dyslipidaemia, smoking or positive family history of early MI)
- Prior coronary stenosis ≥50%
- Presence of ST-segment deviation on admission ECG
- At least two anginal episodes in prior 24h
- Elevated serum cardiac biomarkers
- Use of aspirin in prior 7 days

Patients are considered to be low risk (score of 0–2), intermediate risk (3–4) or high risk (5–7). The composite endpoint of all-cause mortality, MI and severe recurrent ischaemia at 14 days varies according to the number of TIMI risk factors (score of 0 or 1, 4.7% vs score of 6 or 7, 40.9%).

Initial medical therapy

Antiplatelet therapy

Aspirin

All patients should receive 162–325mg of uncoated aspirin (ASA) as soon as possible after onset of symptoms. The first tablet should be chewed to establish high blood levels rapidly.

Clopidogrel

Clopidogrel can replace ASA in intolerant patients, and leads to significant benefits in NSTEMI when given in addition to ASA. Standard dosing regimen from the CURE trial is a 300mg loading dose followed by a maintenance daily dose of 75mg; higher loading doses are under investigation. One issue with clopidogrel is significantly increased bleeding rates in those persons who undergo emergent or urgent coronary artery bypass surgery in <5 days.

Glycoprotein IIB/IIIA Inhibitors

These should be given to any patients in whom PCI is planned. For those not undergoing PCI, they should be reserved for those at high risk for cardiac events such as a TIMI score ≥4, elevated serum troponin, continuing ischaemia, symptoms of heart failure, impaired systolic function, sustained ventricular tachycardia or haemodynamic instability.

There are three glycoprotein IIB/IIIA inhibitors: tirofiban, eptifibatide and abciximab. The infusion should be started on presentation and continued for 48–72h or until PCI is performed. Abciximab is beneficial in PCI, but was not effective as medical therapy for NSTEMI in the GUSTO IV trial. Eptifibatide and tirofiban have been shown to be effective in patients with high risk features not undergoing PCI, and can also be used in patients undergoing PCI.

Anticoagulation

Heparin

The rationale for use of both heparin and ASA is 2-fold: they interfere with thrombin formation at different sites, and rebound after heparin discontinuation can be blunted by ASA. LMWH is preferred by many physicians because of a lower incidence of HIT, ease of administration without need for monitoring, and a lesser degree of platelet activation.

UFH should be given by bolus (60U/kg IV, maximum 5000U) and infusion (12U/kg/h, maximum 1000U/h) adjusted to maintain aPTT between 50 and 70s.

Direct thrombin inhibitors (DTIs)

DTIs, which include bivalirudin, lepirudin and hirudin, are another alternative to UFH. Bivalirudin compared with UFH has shown significantly less bleeding the ACUITY and REPLACE-2 trials, with similar outcomes in terms of ischaemic events.

Antianginals

Nitrates

Sublingual GTN is administered to patients presenting with chest pain, followed by IV GTN for hypertension, heart failure or if chest pain persists after three sublingual GTN tablets. Caution must be observed in severe RV infarction, severe aortic stenosis or patients who have taken PDE inhibitors for erectile dysfunction within the previous 24h.

β-Blockers

Multiple controlled trials have demonstrated the efficacy of β-blockers in AMI. Although no randomized trials specifically address β-blockers in UA and NSTEMI, they are recommended.

Further medical therapy

Lipid-lowering therapy (statins)

A mortality benefit of atorvastatin 80mg daily was demonstrated in the PROVE-IT TIMI 22 and MIRACL trials. Initial intensive statin therapy, rather than gradual uptitration, is recommended due to the suggestion of benefit in the first 30 days in the PROVE-IT TIMI 22 trial.

Renin–angiotensin–aldosterone inhibition

ACE inhibitors/ARBs

Oral ACE inhibitors should be administered within the first 24h of MI onset in patients with an anterior STEMI, heart failure or LVEF ≤40%. This class of drugs reduces mortality in patients with MI as demonstrated in ISIS-4 (captopril) and GISSI-3 (lisinopril). These drugs should not be administered IV in the 1st 24h or in patients with hypotension (SBP <100mm Hg).

ARBs (valsartan and candesartan) are generally reserved for patients intolerant of ACE inhibitors. ARBs were as effective as ACE inhibitors in the immediate post-MI setting in the VALIANT study, but the combination of the two demonstrated an increased incidence of adverse effects without improving survival.

Aldosterone antagonists

Eplerenone, an aldosterone antagonist, when given to patients an LVEF ≤40%, and symptomatic heart failure or diabetes along with ACE inhibitors and standard therapy in the EPHESUS trial, reduced mortality significantly at 30 days (3.2 vs 4.6% with standard care).

Early invasive vs conservative therapy

Cardiac catheterization may be undertaken in patients presenting with symptoms suggestive of unstable coronary syndromes for one of several reasons: to assist with risk stratification, as a prelude to revascularization and to exclude significant epicardial coronary stenosis as a cause of symptoms when the diagnosis is uncertain.

An early invasive approach has now been compared with a conservative approach in several prospective studies. Two earlier trials, the TIMI IIIb study and the VANQWISH trial, both performed before use of coronary stenting and platelet glycoprotein IIb/IIIa inhibitors was widespread, were negative. More recently, several trials, including a substudy of FRISC II, TACTICS TIMI-18 and RITA-3 found a significant reduction in the combined end-point of death, MI or recurrent angina with invasive management. The most recent comparison, the ICTUS study, found no difference in a composite of death, MI or rehospitalization for angina at 1yr between a group assigned to early invasive management and another assigned to selectively invasive management. As >40% of patients in the selectively invasive group were revascularized in the first month, this trial probably argues not so much against an early invasive strategy as for selection of those patients most likely to benefit. Alternatively (or in parallel), improved adjunctive antiplatelet, antithrombin and lipid-lowering therapy may have narrowed the difference between strategies.

Further reading

ACC guidelines UA/NSTEMI `http://content.onlinejacc.org/cgi/reprint/50/7/e1`

Anderson JL, Adams CD, Antman EM, *et al.* ACC/AHA 2007 guidelines for the management of patients with unstable angina/non-ST-elevation myocardial infarction—executive summary. A Report of the American College of Cardiology/American Heart Association Task Force on Practice Guidelines (Writing Committee to Revise the 2002 Guidelines for the Management of Patients With Unstable Angina/Non-ST-Elevation Myocardial Infarction). *Circulation* 2007; 116: 803–77.

Bavry AA, Kumbhani DJ, Rassi AN, *et al.* Benefit of early invasive therapy in acute coronary syndromes: a meta-analysis of contemporary randomized clinical trials. *J Am Coll Cardiol* 2006; 48: 1319–25.

Cannon CP, Braunwald E, McCabe CH, *et al.* Intensive versus moderate lipid lowering with statins after acute coronary syndromes. *N Engl J Med* 2004; 350: 1495–504.

Dzau VJ, Antman EM, Black HR, *et al.* The cardiovascular disease continuum validated: clinical evidence of improved patient outcomes. Part II: clinical trial evidence (acute coronary syndromes through renal disease) and future directions. *Circulation* 2006; 114: 2871–91.

The TIMI Study Group `http://www.timi.org`

Yusuf S, Zhao F, Mehta SR, *et al.* Effects of clopidogrel in addition to aspirin in patients with acute coronary syndromes without st-segment elevation. *N Engl J Med* 2001; 345: 494–502.

STEMI

Risk stratification—before reperfusion

Risk stratification in STEMI can be based on initial history, physical examination, ECG and CXR. High risk features include advanced age, low blood pressure, tachycardia, heart failure and anterior MI. Killip class (I = no congestive heart failure, II = rales, S3, congestion on CXR, III pulmonary oedema, IV cardiogenic shock) can be used for clinical stratification.

A TIMI risk score for STEMI includes 8 predictors:

- Age ≥75 years—3 points; 65–74 years—2 points
- History of diabetes, hypertension or angina—1 point
- Systolic blood pressure <100mm Hg—3 points
- Heart rate >100 beats/min—2 points
- Killip class II–IV—2 points
- Weight <76kg—1 point
- Anterior ST elevation or LBBB—1 point
- Time to reperfusion therapy >4h—1 point

The TIMI risk score for STEMI has been validated in predicting in-hospital mortality. There is a continuous relationship between the score and 30 day and 1yr mortality regardless of reperfusion strategy.

The location of the MI in STEMI by ECG can predict outcomes. The greater the number of leads with ST elevation, lack of ST resolution at 90–180min after thrombolysis, presence of Q waves, or anterior compared with inferior infarcts.

Therapy

Initial management

The initial goals when the diagnosis of STEMI is made include:

- Relief of ischaemic pain
- Assessment of haemodynamic state
- Initiation of reperfusion therapy (primary PCI or thrombolysis)
- Antithrombotic therapy to prevent rethrombosis or subtotal stenosis at the site of ruptured plaque

In the emergency department, initial management includes oxygen, ASA, β-blockers, analgesia, GTN, and anticoagulation with heparin.

Acute therapy

Reperfusion therapy should be accomplished with either primary PCI or thrombolysis as discussed below.

Antiplatelet therapy should include ASA, clopidogrel and, in patients undergoing PCI, glycoprotein IIb/IIIa inhibitors (tirofiban, eptifibatide or abciximab).

IV GTN should be used in patients with heart failure, hypertension or persistent chest pain after three sublingual GTN tablets.

β-Blockers should be administered to all patients without contraindications who experience STEMI.

β-Blockers

These medications appear to reduce the magnitude of infarction, complications, rate of re-infarction and frequency of ventricular tachyarrhythmias. These benefits are mediated by reducing heart rate, systemic arterial pressure and myocardial contractility, thereby decreasing myocardial oxygen demand. In ISIS-1, >16 000 patients given atenolol had reduced mortality at 7 days (4.3% vs 3.7%, $P < 0.02$).

In conjunction with fibrinolytic therapy, IV β-blockers reduce the incidence of subsequent non-fatal re-infarction and recurrent ischaemia. A key to prevention of recurrent ischaemia is judicious but aggressive titration of β-blockade to achieve both heart rate and blood pressure control (heart rate ≤60 beats/min and blood pressure ≤120/80.

β-Blockers should not be administered acutely to patients with siginificant bradycardia, SBP <100mm Hg, moderate–severe heart failure, AV block or reactive airway disease/active wheezing. Many of these patients will tolerate β-blockers when started later.

Important update regarding IV β-bockers:

Based on results of the COMMIT-CCS2 trial, it seems reasonable to defer IV β-blockers in patients who are haemodynamically compromised, as mortality may be increased in such patients.

Reperfusion therapy

Rapid reperfusion is the most important objective in treatment of patients with STEMI. A decision must be made as soon as possible regarding primary PCI vs thrombolysis. While door to balloon time is the standard of care measurement, with a goal door to needle time (thrombolysis) <30min, and goal door to balloon (primary PCI) <90min, the decision should be make by assessing time and risk.

Reperfusion therapy, particularly fibrinolytics, is most effective when instituted with the first 3h. Unfortunately, patients with STEMI present at a mean of 3–4h after symptom onset. In addition, achieving prompt reperfusion when transfer to another hospital is required is challenging. In the NRMI 4 registry, only 5.3% of patients transferred for primary PCI had a door to balloon time ≤90min.

All patients with cardiogenic shock or Killip class ≥3 should receive primary PCI. In addition, patients with contraindications to fibrinolysis should be reperfused with PCI. Absolute contraindications to fibrinolysis in STEMI include:

- Any prior intracranial haemorrhage (ICH)
- Known structural cerebral vascular lesion (e.g. AV malformation)
- Known malignant intracranial neoplasm
- Ischaemic stroke within 3 months EXCEPT acute ischaemic stroke within 3h
- Suspected aortic dissection
- Active bleeding or bleeding diathesis (excluding menses)
- Significant closed-head or facial trauma within 3 months

Primary PCI vs thrombolytics

Treatment with primary PCI, if timely, high quality at a high volume centre, is the treatment of choice, with multiple randomized trials demonstrating improved survival compared with thrombolysis, with a lower risk of ICH and recurrent MI.

Fibrinolysis is successful in achieving reperfusion in 75–85% of patients. As many as 1/2 to 2/3 of patients presenting with AMI may be ineligible for lytic therapy, however. The major advantages of primary PCI over thrombolytic therapy include a higher rate of normal (TIMI grade 3) flow, lower risk of ICH and the ability to stratify risk based on the severity and distribution of CAD.

A meta-analysis of 23 trials (n = 7739) by Keeley *et al.* demonstrated a 2% absolute mortality reduction at 4–6 weeks (P = 0.0002). However, this analysis has some limitations:

- Time from symptom onset to treatment (<6h in nine of the trials, <12h in 13 of the trials)
- Small size of studies (15/23 trials had <500 patients)
- Variable definition of end-points (e.g. re-infarction)
- Use of both fibrin-specific and non-specific fibrinolytic agents

In both the VIENNA and PRAGUE-2 trials, comparing streptokinase vs transfer for primary PCI, patients who had symptom onset to treatment <3h had no difference in 30 day mortality.

When primary PCI is compared with tPA and the SHOCK trial is excluded, mortality rate is not statistically significantly reduced, P = 0.081.

The Achilles heel of thrombolysis is that 5–15% of patients with successful thrombolysis will reocclude.

Patients who present with STEMI should receive reperfusion based on the time from symptom onset (<3h, either strategy is acceptable), mortality risk (age, heart rate, BP, Killip class and location of MI), risk of bleeding (>75yrs old and female sex have highest risk of ICH) and time for transfer to a skilled PCI laboratory. If the patient presents within 3h, and there is no delay to an invasive strategy, either fibrinolysis or primary PCI is acceptable. If the patient presents within 3h, is not high risk and the expected door to balloon time exceeds the door to needle time by >60min, fibrinolysis is generally preferred. If a skilled PCI lab is available with surgical back-up and a door to balloon time <90min, if the patients is at high risk or if presentation is >3h from symptom onset, an invasive strategy is generally preferred.

Other medical therapy

Patients with STEMI should be treated with ASA, clopidogrel, β-blockers, ACE inhibitors and high dose statins.

Anticoagulation

Heparin

Patients undergoing reperfusion should receive UFH or LMWH. These agents should be used after STEMI in patients who are at high risk for systemic emboli (large or anterior MI, AF, previous embolus, known LV thrombus or cardiogenic shock).

For patients receiving thrombolytic therapy rather than primary PCI, the EXTRACT-TIMI 25 trial demonstrated that enoxaparin administered for the duration of the hospitalization was associated with a 17% relative risk reduction in death or MI at 30 days compared with UFH for 48h.

The OASIS-6 study, compared fondaparinux (2.5mg daily for up to 8 days) vs control (placebo in stratum 1 and UFH in stratum 2). This complicated trial demonstrated a 14% relative risk reduction in death/MI at 30 days compared with control driven mainly by the reduction in stratum 1 (UFH not indicated, 11.2% vs 14 %). There was no difference in stratum 2 (UFH indicated, 8.3% vs 8.7%). There was a concerning increased rate of guiding catheter thrombosis in the primary PCI cohort on fondaparinux (n = 22 vs n = 0, P <0.001). This drug requires further studies before routine use can be recommended.

Glycoprotein IIb/IIIa inhibitors

Studies comparing use of abciximab with half-dose fibrinolytic with full-dose lytic have shown no difference in 30 day mortality, although there is a decrease in non-fatal re-infarction.

ACC guidelines state that it is reasonable to start abciximab in patients undergoing primary PCI (with or without stenting). The data supporting this treatment are limited to smaller studies with composite end-points driven primarily by decreased urgent target vessel revascularization, rather than mortality or re-infarction.

Use of tirofiban or eptifibatide is also considered reasonable, but there are fewer data than with abciximab to support their use in STEMI undergoing primary PCI.

Risk stratification—discharge and beyond

The importance of post-infarct risk stratification is to identify patients at increased risk for arrhythmic and non-arrhythmic cardiac death.

Stress testing

Pre-discharge stress testing is usually performed to detect residual ischaemia in patients with more than one coronary lesion or those who received successful thrombolytic reperfusion.

It is not performed in patients who have been fully revascularized (PCI or CABG) unless as part of a cardiac rehabilitation programme. Low level stress testing appears to be safe in appropriate patients:

- Patient has undergone in-hospital cardiac rehabilitation
- ECG stable for 48–72h
- No symptoms of recurrent angina or heart failure

Complications

Ventricular free wall rupture

Ventricular free wall rupture typically occurs during the first week after infarction. The classic patient is elderly, female and hypertensive. Early use of fibrinolytic therapy reduces the incidence of cardiac rupture, but late use may actually increase the risk. Free wall rupture presents as a catastrophic event with shock and electromechanical dissociation. Salvage is possible with prompt recognition, pericardiocentesis to relieve acute tamponade and thoracotomy with repair. Emergent echocardiography or pulmonary artery catheterization can help make the diagnosis.

Ventricular septal rupture

Septal rupture presents as severe heart failure or cardiogenic shock, with a pansystolic murmur and parasternal thrill. The hallmark finding is a left-to-right intracardiac shunt ('step-up' in oxygen saturation from right atrium to right ventricle), and surgical treatment has been controversial, but most authorities now suggest that repair should be undertaken early, within 48h of the rupture.

Papillary muscle rupture

Papillary muscle rupture typically occurs in association with inferior MI, and presents dramatically with pulmonary oedema, hypotension and cardiogenic shock. A murmur of acute mitral regurgitation may be soft or inaudible, especially when cardiac output is low.

Echocardiography, either transthoracic or transesophageal, usually makes diagnosis. Haemodynamic monitoring with pulmonary artery catheterization may also be helpful. Management includes afterload reduction with nitroprusside and intra-aortic balloon pumping as temporizing measures. Inotropic or vasopressor therapy may also be needed to support cardiac output and blood pressure. Definitive therapy, however, is surgical valve repair or replacement, which should be undertaken as soon as possible since clinical deterioration can be sudden.

Right ventricular infarction

RV infarction occurs in up to 30% of patients with inferior infarction and is clinically significant in 10%. The combination of a clear CXR with jugular venous distention in a patient with an inferior wall MI should lead to the suspicion of a co-existing RV infarct. The diagnosis is substantiated by demonstration of ST-segment elevation in the right precordial leads (V_3R–V_5R) or by characteristic haemodynamic findings (elevated RA and RV end-diastolic pressures with normal to low wedge pressure and low cardiac output). Echocardiography can demonstrate depressed RV contractility.

RV preload should be maintained with fluid administration, but overdilation of the RV can compromise LV filling and cardiac output, and so inotropic therapy with dobutamine may be more effective in some patients. Maintenance of AV synchrony is also important to optimize RV filling. For patients with continued haemodynamic instability, intra-aortic balloon pumping may be useful to decrease RV wall stress and increase right coronary perfusion pressure. Reperfusion of the occluded coronary artery is also crucial. Patients with cardiogenic shock on the basis of RV infarction have a better prognosis than those with left-sided pump failure. This may be due in part to the fact that RV function tends to return to normal over time with supportive therapy, although such therapy may need to be prolonged.

Discharge regimen

Secondary prevention with therapeutic lifestyle modification, smoking cessation, blood pressure control (<130/80mm Hg) weight loss, exercise, control of diabetes (goal HgA1c <7%) should be provided to all patients at the time of discharge. Explanation of benefits and side effects of medications prescribed, as well as those to avoid (sildenafil, etc.) should be given. All patients should be discharged on ASA, β-blockers, ACE inhibitor or ARB, and statins unless contraindicated. Eplerenone may be given when indicated, and nitrates used as needed. The optimal duration of dual antiplatelet therapy is controversial, and depends on the type of reperfusion strategy (fibrinolytic or PCI) and the type of stent (bare metal or drug-eluting). For patients who undergo mechanical reperfusion, clopidogrel and ASA should be continued for at least 9–12 months. The greatest risk for very late stent thrombosis with drug-eluting stents is premature discontinuation of dual antiplatelet therapy.

Further reading

ACC guidelines STEMI `http://www.acc.org/qualityand-science/clinical/guidelines/stemi/Guideline1/index.pdf`

Antman EM, Anbe DT, Armstrong PW, *et al.* ACC/AHA guidelines for the management of patients with ST-elevation myocardial infarction—executive summary. A Report of the American College of Cardiology/American Heart Association Task Force on Practice Guidelines. *Circulation* 2004; 110: 588–636.

Boersma E, Mercado N, Poldermans D, *et al.* Acute myocardial infarction. *Lancet* 2003; 361: 847–58.

Chen ZM, Pan HC, Chen YP, *et al.* Early intravenous then oral metoprolol in 45,852 patients with acute myocardial infarction: Randomised placebo-controlled trial. *Lancet* 2005; 366: 1622–32.

Keeley EC, Boura JA, Grines CL. Primary angioplasty versus intravenous thrombolytic therapy for acute myocardial infarction: a quantitative review of 23 randomised trials. *Lancet* 2003; 361: 13–20.

National Registry of Myocardial Infarction `http://www.nrmi.org/index.html`

Van de Werf F, Ardissino D, Betriu A, *et al.* Management of acute myocardial infarction in patients presenting with ST-segment elevation. The task force on the management of acute myocardial infarction of the European Society of Cardiology. *Eur Heart J* 2003; 24: 28–66.

Acute heart failure: assessment

Definition

Acute heart failure (AHF) is defined as rapid onset or change in heart failure (HF) signs and symptoms resulting in the need for urgent therapy. AHF may occur with or without previous cardiac disease. The cardiac dysfunction can be related to systolic or diastolic dysfunction, to abnormalities in cardiac rhythm or to preload and afterload mismatch. This is a heterogeneous syndrome that has many different aetiologies and, as such, it is the result of diverse pathophysiological processes and encompasses a large spectrum of patients.

Most of our knowledge about AHF comes from studies made with in-hospital HF patients, but several recent publications challenged some of the traditional views by looking at admission data (Table 18.7.1)

Epidemiology and incidence

In the USA, each year, HF is the primary diagnosis of 1 million admissions within 3 million admissions with primary or secondary diagnosis of HF per year. It is a disease with a huge burden, with an in-hospital all-cause mortality of 10–16%, and a readmission rate of 20–25% at 90 days that goes up to 50% by 6 months; survival ranges from 80% at 2yrs for patients rendered free of congestion to <50% at 6 months for patients with refractory symptoms, and 75% of US HF annual expenditure is spent during the recurrent hospitalizations. Its incidence increases with age, and at >75yrs this incidence increases more steeply.

Table 18.7.1 Patient characteristics in major AHF registries

	ADHERE, *n* = 163 447	OPTIMIZE, *n* = 48 612	EHFS-II, *n* = 3580	EFICA, *n* = 599	Italian AHFS n = 2807
Mean age	75	73	70	73	73
Women %	52	52	39	41	39
New onset HF %	25	13	37	34	44
Preserved LVEF	50,4 %	49%	34% (<45%)	27% (<45%)	34

HF aetiologies

The Acute Decompensated Heart Failure National Registry (ADHERE) showed that the major reasons for HF hospitalizations in the USA are worsening chronic HF (70%), *de novo* AHF (25%) and advanced/end-stage HF (5%). In this series of the most common co-morbid conditions were hypertension (73%), CAD (57%) and diabetes (44%).

Almost 2/3 of AHF patients have a history of CAD, and >30% of these patients had prior myocardial ischaemia. Interestingly, several continental differences exist. More patients in the USA have hypertension (72% vs 53%), diabetes (44% vs 27%) and renal insufficiency (30% vs 17%), with fewer having AF (31% vs 43%) than in Europe.

Women admitted with AHF appear to have less CAD and more hypertension than men, but a similar rate of AF (30%), diabetes (40%) and anaemia (35%). 40% of men and 30% of women have an intraventricular conduction delay (QRS >120ms), and approximately 20% have decreased serum sodium (less than 136 mEq/L).

Table 18.7.2 Aetiologies of AHF

Decompensation of pre-existing chronic heart failure (CAD, myopathic, valvular)
Acute coronary syndromes
MI/UA with large extent of ischaemia and ischaemic dysfunction
Mechanical complication of AMI
Right ventricular infarction
Hypertensive crisis
Acute arrhythmia
Ventricular tachycardia, ventricular fibrillation
Atrial fibrillation or flutter
Other supraventricular tachycardia
Valvular regurgitation
Endocarditis
Rupture of chordae tendinae
Worsening of pre-existing valvular regurgitation
Severe aortic valve stenosis
Acute severe myocarditis
Cardiac tamponade
Aortic dissection
Post-partum cardiomyopathy
High output syndromes
Septicaemia
Thyroid storm
Severe anaemia
Shunt syndromes

History and examination

HF symptoms and signs are usually dominated by those related to congestion, due to elevated filling pressures. High left-sided filling pressures cause lung congestion noticeable as dyspnoea, orthopnoea or paroxistical nocturnal dyspnoea, lung rales, noticeable S3 or loud P2.

Elevated right-sided filling pressures cause anorexia, early satiety, abdominal fullness, discomfort when bending, high jugular venous pressure (JVP), oedema in pending regions or ascites, related to venous congestion in the liver, kidney, intestine, jugular veins or lower extremities.

Symptoms and signs attributable to low resting cardiac output are less common and usually include prostration or fatigue, low blood pressure, narrow pulse pressure, ACE inhibitor-related symptomatic hypotension, cold extremities, sleepiness, *pulsus alternans* or low urine output. Usually low resting cardiac output symptoms appear in an advanced stage of chronic HF.

ESC/ESICM classification

In 2005, the ESC and the ESICM proposed a new classification for AHF syndromes in the above-mentioned guidelines. In this classification, AHF is presented in 6 distinct clinical conditions:

1. **Acute decompensated HF *de novo* or decompensation of chronic HF:** signs and symptoms of AHF, which are mild and do not fulfil criteria for cardiogenic shock, pulmonary oedema or hypertensive HF.
2. **Hypertensive AHF:** signs and symptoms of HF accompanied by high blood pressure and relatively preserved LV function with signs and symptoms of congestion.

3 **Pulmonary oedema:** AHF accompanied by severe respiratory distress and usually SpO_2 <90% on room air prior to treatment.
4 **Cardiogenic shock:** cardiogenic shock defined as evidence of tissue hypoperfusion induced by HF after correction of preload. It is characterized by reduced blood pressure (SBP <90mm Hg or a drop of MAP >30mm Hg) and/or low urine output (<0.5ml/kg/h) with a pulse rate >60 bpm with or without evidence of organ congestion.
5 **High output failure** characterized by high heart rate with warm periphery, pulmonary congestion and sometimes with low BP, i.e. in septic shock.
6 **Right HF** characterized by low output syndrome with increased JVP, increased liver size and hypotension.

Clinical classification of 3580 patients hospitalized for AHF in 30 European countries according to these guidelines in the EHS-II divided AHF patients into **decompensated HF** (65%), **pulmonary oedema** (16%), **HF and hypertension** (11%), **cardiogenic shock** (4%) and **right HF** (3%). Coronary heart disease, hypertension and AF were the most common underlying conditions. In the Italian survey on AHF in 2807 patients, the clinical profiles according to the above-mentioned ESC guidelines were acute pulmonary oedema in 49.6% of patients, worsened NYHA functional class in 42.7% and cardiogenic shock in 7.7% of cases. More than half (56%) had worsening chronic HF, and an EF >40% was found in 34% of cases.

Classification based on SBP at admission

In the USA, in-hospital outcomes of 48 612 adult patients with HF showed that most patients with AHF present with specific sets of symptoms that can be classified into 3 main types of HF according to the patient's blood pressure at the time of presentation. This classification is mostly based on the recent evidence that a strong inverse relationship was noted between SBP and short- and long-term outcome: the higher the SBP at admission, the lower are short- and long-term morbidity and mortality. In addition, these subgroups have different clinical signs at admission and need different therapeutic targets:

Hypertensive AHF

Most patients admitted to hospital with AHF have a normal-to-high SBP. The elevated blood pressure may develop rapidly and is possibly related to increased sympathetic tone. It results in neurohormonal activation and increased LV afterload with impairment of cardiac function. Because symptoms may develop abruptly, these patients tend to be euvolaemic or mildly hypovolaemic, and present with pulmonary rather than systemic congestion (e.g. peripheral oedema). In these patients, with often preserved LV systolic function, pulmonary oedema is not caused by fluid accumulation but rather fluid redistribution that is directed into the lungs because of AHF. These patients are older, more likely to be women and have a higher incidence of hypertension, LV hypertrophy and diabetes than patients admitted with AHF and systolic dysfunction.

Normotensive AHF

The other common type of AHF is characterized by a normal SBP, usually with a history of progressive or chronic HF. In these patients, symptoms and signs develop gradually, over days or weeks, and pulmonary and systemic congestion (jugular venous distension, pulmonary rales and peripheral oedema) are usually present. They usually have a reduced EF. Despite high LV filling pressures they may present several degrees of pulmonary congestion (clinical and/or radiographic) but some may have minimal pulmonary congestion.

Hypotensive AHF

A small percentage of patients with AHF present with low SBP (2–8% of patients); typically presents with low cardiac output and signs of organ hypoperfusion, clinical pulmonary oedema (3% of patients) or cardiogenic shock (<1% of patients).

HF with preserved LVEF

In the major recent AHF registries, 30–50% of AHF patients showed preserved EF (Table 18.7.1). Hypertension-induced LV diastolic dysfunction often occurs in the ICU or emergency room. In the emergency room, Ghandi *et al.* compared the echocardiographic findings at admission and after 2–3 days of treatment in patients presenting for an acute pulmonary oedema in the context of severe arterial hypertension. The authors found no difference in LVEF between the acute episode and after 24 and 72h of adequate treatment. Furthermore, 50% of the patients admitted with an acute pulmonary oedema had preserved EF, and 89% of the patients who had a preserved EF after treatment also had no sign of systolic dysfunction during the acute episode. In addition, the authors suggested that acute diastolic failure might also be the major mechanism of decompensation in patients with baseline systolic dysfunction. Similar findings can be observed in the ICU. Of note, myocardial ischaemia is an important mechanism of LV diastolic dysfunction. Several factors including pain-induced sympathetic activation (tachycardia, hypertension), shivering, anaemia, hypovolaemia and hypoxia, may alter myocardial oxygen balance, leading to impaired ventricular relaxation and abnormal compliance.

Renal function and HF

Impaired renal function was shown to be a stronger predictor of mortality than impaired LVEF or NYHA class in advanced HF, and it is associated with increased plasma levels of natriuretic peptides. In these patients, impaired renal function is not related to LVEF.

Even mild or moderate decreases in renal function have been shown to correlate with significant morbidity and mortality in patients with asymptomatic and symptomatic congestive HF.

In Europe, nearly 1/3 of patients hospitalized for decompensated HF develop worsening renal function during hospitalization, excluding patients who have a major in-hospital complication likely to compromise renal function. Such patients have longer duration of admissions, but a similar mortality and re-hospitalization rate, to those without worsening renal function (if patients experiencing a major in-hospital complication are excluded). The risk of worsening renal function in these patients is associated with serum creatinine levels on admission, pulmonary oedema and a history of AF.

Diagnosis—immediate questions

Does this patient has HF?

The diagnosis of AHF is based on the symptoms and clinical findings, supported by appropriate investigations such as ECG, CXR, biomarkers and Doppler echocardiography.

Up to 75% of AHF patients will have at presentation a previous diagnosis of HF, and the available information may help the clinician. Dyspnoea is a common presenting symptom in patients with AHF syndromes.

Dyspnoea is the primary reason that patients present for medical care with AHF. In the ADHERE (n = 163 447) and OPTIMIZE-HF (n = 48 612) registries, 89 and 90% of patientsm respectively, initially presented with a complaint of dyspnoea.

Dyspnoea on exertion is the most sensitive symptom (negative likelihood ratio 0.45, 95% CI 0.35–0.67), whereas paroxysmal nocturnal dyspnoea is the most specific (positive likelihood ratio 2.6, 95% CI 1.5–4.5). Elevated JVP is the best indicator for identifying acute decompensated heart failure (positive likelihood ratio 5.1, 95% CI 3.2–7.9, negative likelihood ratio 0.66, 95% CI 0.57–0.77), although measurement of JVP by clinicians is notoriously inaccurate. A murmur may point to a new valvular disease or a complication of a previously known heart disease. An auscultated S3 gallop is not only diagnostic for AHF but predicts an increased risk of subsequent adverse events. Both ventricular gallops and jugular venous distension are limited by interobserver variation and low sensitivity.

In the emergency department, rapid measurement of brain natriuretic peptide (BNP) used in conjunction with other clinical information is useful in establishing or excluding the diagnosis of congestive HF in patients with acute dyspnoea, and improves the evaluation and treatment of patients with acute dyspnoea, thereby reducing the time to discharge and the total cost of treatment. In patients with acute shortness of breath, HF patients have higher mean levels of both BNP or NT-proBNP blood levels (see cardiac peptides below).

Although the pulmonary artery catheter may provide a good measure of filling pressures and an estimate of cardiac output in the patient in shock, therapy to reduce volume overload during hospitalization for heart failure led to marked improvement in signs and symptoms of elevated filling pressures with or without the PAC. Addition of the PAC to careful clinical assessment increased anticipated adverse events, but did not affect overall mortality and hospitalization.

What is the aetiology?

The HF aetiology is the next question to answer as it may imply specific management.

Are there any precipitating factors?

The presence of any precipitating factors should be sought as its correction may be of most importance to stabilize the patient, such as a hypertensive emergency, anaemia, dysrhythmia or infection (Table 18.7.3).

Table 18.7.3 AHF precipitating factors

Lack of compliance with medical treatment
Acute arrhythmia
Hypertensive crisis
Volume overload
Infection, particularly sepsis
Severe brain insult
Major surgery
Reduction in renal function
Asthma
New medications (excess β-blockade)
Alcohol abuse
Drug abuse
Phaeochromocytoma

Are there other conditions/co-morbidities that may contribute to the picture?

Patients with AHF also have significant cardiac and non-cardiac underlying conditions that may not be the main aetiology but may contribute to the pathogenesis of AHF, including CAD (ischaemia, hibernating myocardium and endothelial dysfunction), hypertension, AF and type II diabetes mellitus. Many patients have other complications of atherosclerosis, hypertension or diabetes, while other conditions share a common aetiology such as smoking-related chronic pulmonary disease or renal vascular disease. Some co-morbidities are complications of HF or the combination of HF, its underlying aetiology and advanced age, such as renal impairment, stroke, and atrial and ventricular arrhythmias. Patients with renal failure are less likely to be prescribed efficacious therapies, but have better outcomes if they receive these medications.

The importance of certain co-morbidities as independent predictors of poor outcome showed the importance of considering them as potential therapeutic targets, such as anaemia or obstructive sleep apnoea.

Troponin, worsening renal function, hyponatraemia, lung congestion persistence after initial treatment and low SBP have all been described as the main prognostic factors in AHF.

Hypertensive, normotensive or hypotensive?

Most patients with AHF present with either normal SBP or elevated blood pressure. Patients who present with elevated SBP usually have pulmonary congestion and a relatively preserved LVEF, and have symptoms that typically develop abruptly, with severe lung congestion and minimal weight gain often being seen in elderly women. Their response to therapy is usually rapid. Patients with normal SBP presenting with systemic congestion and reduced LVEF are usually younger, with a history of chronic HF, and have symptoms that develop gradually over days or weeks. Usually they present significant weight gain with oedema, liver and renal dysfunction, and hyponatraemia. Their lung congestion may not be so evident and, although they may improve with initial therapy, they will continue to have systemic congestion during the next days.

Systolic dysfunction or preserved EF?

The patient should be classified as soon as possible according to previously described criteria for systolic and/or preserved dysfunction, and by the characteristics of left or right HF.

Investigations

ECG

Besides signs of heart disease, the ECG may provide important aetiological information such as ACS or rhythm disturbances.

Chest X-ray

Although chest radiography is routine in the evaluation of patients with shortness of breath and a quick and inexpensive examination, ~1 of every 5 patients admitted from the emergency department with AHF have no signs of congestion on chest radiography, and patients lacking signs of congestion on emergency department chest radiography were more likely to have an emergency department non-HF diagnosis than patients with signs of congestion in the ADHERE registry.

Cardiac peptides

When the heart muscle cell is stretched, as in HF, the cardiac peptide, NT-proBNP, is released into the bloodstream.

Patients with HF have increased blood levels of NT-proBNP, and the worse the disease, the higher the NT-proBNP level.

Taken together with clinical information, BNP is a quantitative marker of HF that summarizes systolic and diastolic LV dysfunction, as well as valvular heart disease and RV dysfunction.

In all patients presenting with dyspnoea to emergency services, a history, physical examination, CXR and ECG should be undertaken, together with laboratory measurements that include BNP. The knowledge of a patient's baseline BNP level may further improve emergency department physician diagnostic accuracy.

BNP levels should be interpreted as a continuous variable. However, for reasons of simplicity, the use of cut-off values makes sense. When using cut-off values in patients with acute dyspnoea, one should apply two: one to 'rule out' (<100) and one to 'rule in' HF (>400). The grey zone area needs extra physician attention and ancillary testing. This grey zone (100–400pg/ml) represents 25% of dyspnoeic patients, 75% of whom will have HF as the ultimate diagnosis. This HF tends to be mild. The overall prognosis for dyspnoeic patients with BNP levels in the grey zone is good and may help risk-stratify patients for admission or discharge.

There seems to be a linear relationship between BMI and BNP. Patients who are obese or very obese should have their BNP multiplied by 2.0 to obtain a BNP level of similar severity to those of normal weight. BNP levels in the dyspnoeic patient do not have to be adjusted for age or gender. However, to optimize diagnostic accuracy, adjustments should be made for renal dysfunction and obesity.

One should not forget that both BNP and NT-proBNP blood levels are markers of heart muscle cell stretch, and there may be causes other than HF to justify their increased levels, either of cardiac origin as in ACS, hypertension, LV hypertrophy or valvular heart disease, or of non-cardiac origin, such as pulmonary embolism, pulmonary hypertension or sepsis.

Blood gas analysis, lytes, renal function, routine haematology

Pulse oximetry is a valuable option for immediate evaluation of oxygenation, but if the patient presents with signs of compromised peripheral perfusion or fatigue, blood gas analysis is useful in order to evaluate acid–base and lactate status, and to follow the response to treatment. Electrolyte abnormal values are often associated with rhythm disturbances, may be the result of abnormal renal function or drug administration and are often administrated to compensate the use of some drugs. Anaemia is a common precipitating cause, and AHF may just be the symptom translation of anaemia that may benefit from treatment.

Echocardiography

When it comes to HF, clinical examination alone may be an inaccurate diagnostic approach. Ultrasound examination of the heart, echocardiography, is widely accepted as an objective diagnostic tool in characterizing cardiac dysfunction. Besides ventricular function, evaluation echocardiography may provide early aetiological information, such as ischaemic regional motion abnormalities that could not yet be seen in the ECG, signs of muscular, valvular or pericardial disease. It should be done in every patient as soon as possible. Limited emergency echocardiography to evaluate wall motion and EF performed by emergency physicians has been shown to correlate well with definitive testing.

Other investigations

As appropriate, depending on the HF type and severity. Patients with ACS or serious mechanical cardiac disorders should proceed rapidly to angiography and catheterization for evaluation and therapeutic measures, including surgery or PCI.

Further reading

Adams KF, Jr, Fonarow GC, Emerman CL, *et al.* Characteristics and outcomes of patients hospitalized for heart failure in the United States: rationale, design, and preliminary observations from the first 100,000 cases in the Acute Decompensated Heart Failure National Registry (ADHERE). *Am Heart J* 2005; 149: 209–16.

Binanay C, Califf RM, Hasselblad V, *et al.* Evaluation study of congestive heart failure and pulmonary artery catheterization effectiveness: the ESCAPE trial. *JAMA* 2005; 294: 1625–33.

Cleland JG, Swedberg K, Follath F, *et al.* The EuroHeart Failure survey programme-- a survey on the quality of care among patients with heart failure in Europe. Part 1: patient characteristics and diagnosis. *Eur Heart J* 2003; 24: 442–63.

Dries DL, Exner DV, Domanski MJ, *et al.* The prognostic implications of renal insufficiency in asymptomatic and symptomatic patients with left ventricular systolic dysfunction. *J Am Coll Cardiol* 2000; 35: 681–9.

Gandhi SK, Powers JC, Nomeir AM, *et al.* The pathogenesis of acute pulmonary edema associated with hypertension. *N Engl J Med* 2001; 344: 17–22.

Gheorghiade M, Abraham WT, Albert NM, *et al.* Systolic blood pressure at admission, clinical characteristics, and outcomes in patients hospitalized with acute heart failure. *JAMA* 2006; 296: 2217–26.

Maisel AS, Krishnaswamy P, Nowak RM, *et al.* Rapid measurement of B-type natriuretic peptide in the emergency diagnosis of heart failure. *N Engl J Med* 2002; 347: 161–7.

Mueller C, Scholer A, Laule-Kilian K, *et al.* Use of B-type natriuretic peptide in the evaluation and management of acute dyspnea. *N Engl J Med* 2004; 350: 647–54.

Nieminen MS, Bohm M, Cowie MR, *et al.* Executive summary of the guidelines on the diagnosis and treatment of acute heart failure: the Task Force on Acute Heart Failure of the European Society of Cardiology. *Eur Heart J* 2005; 26: 384–416.

Nieminen MS, Brutsaert D, Dickstein K, *et al.* EuroHeart Failure Survey II (EHFS II): a survey on hospitalized acute heart failure patients: description of population. *Eur Heart J* 2006; 27: 2725–36.

Acute heart failure: management

Introduction

AHF is defined as gradual or rapid change in HF signs and symptoms, resulting in a need for urgent therapy. The vast majority of patients present with dyspnoea, due to increased LV filling pressures, with or without low cardiac output, with reduced or preserved EF.

Until recently, the clinical characteristics, management patterns and outcomes of patients admitted with AHF have been poorly defined, due to lack of specific data. AHF syndromes have traditionally been viewed as part of the chronic HF natural evolution, and lung congestion is often regarded as aconsequence of volume overload and/or low cardiac output, usually precipitated by dietary indiscretion and/or medication non-adherence, but several large AHF registries shed new light on the way we see and manage AHF.

Yet, admission SBP has been show to be an independent predictor of morbidity and mortality in patients with AHF with either reduced or relatively preserved systolic function. High SBP patients were more likely to have preserved systolic function, while patients with low SBP at admission had 3–4 times higher in-hospital and post-discharge mortality rates. Low SBP (<120mm Hg) at hospital admission identifies patients who have a poor prognosis despite medical therapy. This is a marker of advanced HF in a patent that usually has a history of cardiac disease, shows peripheral oedema, enlarged liver, decreased renal and liver function and hyponatraemia.

The problem: increased intracardiac diastolic pressure and oxygen disrupted balance

The heart pumping function maintains low intracardiac diastolic pressures allowing systemic and pulmonary venous return. Increased LV diastolic pressures lead to pulmonary congestion and poorer oxygenation. Increased RV diastolic pressures lead to peripheral oedema, liver, kidney and mesenteric vein increased pressures, with decreased function in these organs. Because they share a common septum, increased pressures in one side of the heart push the septum, increasing pressure and decreasing telediastolic volume in the other side, further compromising stroke volume and cardiac output. This is particularly important with hypoxia, consequent to lung congestion, which may markedly increase PVR, causing an increase in RV end-diastolic pressure that will further contribute to increased LV end-diastolic pressure and decreased LV diastolic volume. If there is deterioration in ventricular filling, as in HF with preserved EF, pressure is increased from the beginning of diastole. If the systolic function is compromised, the heart will try to maintain its output at the cost of increased diastolic ventricular volume, and the pressure goes up.

Increased intracardiac diastolic pressure increases wall tension, decreasing at the same time coronary blood flow when the oxygen consumption is greater. In the AHF patient with lung congestion, this becomes more noticeable due to poorer blood oxygenation, and, in each episode, the heart oxygen balance is further compromised by decreased myocardial perfusion due to increased diastolic pressures, increased heart rate or arrhythmia, with further impairment of cardiac contractility, enhancing the process of pulmonary congestion, thus contributing to ongoing irrevocable myocardial damage. In the later stage of chronic HF where low cardiac output is more prevalent, low BP adds a critical component, especially in patients with CAD, aggravating myocardial perfusion. In each episode, the bigger the oxygenation compromise, the bigger the hypotension, the greater myocardial damage will happen.

New arrhythmia during an exacerbation of HF identifies a high risk group with higher in-hospital and 60-day morbidity and mortality. Thus, each episode of AHF contributes more myocardial damage and worsens long-term prognosis.

AHF initial management

Goals for AHF patient management

- Immediate—improve symptoms
  - Restore oxygenation and improve organ perfusion
  - Avoid or limit cardiac, renal and other organ damage
- Intermediate—stabilize patient and optimize treatment
  - Initiate life-saving therapies
- Long-term—disease management
  - Prevent early readmission
  - Improve symptoms and survival

As in other medical emergencies, AHF needs a rapid, initial integrative approach where assessment and management are provided in the shortest time, in a parallel way, in order to stop an episode that continues damaging the heart after presentation, and, like thrombolysis or aspirin in patients with AMI, short-term intervention can lead to long-term benefit.

The immediate priority in AHF patients should be the stabilization of the respiratory failure to restore oxygenation and prevent further deterioration. The initial therapy for patients with AHF should improve symptoms and haemodynamics without causing myocardial injury that may adversely affect post-discharge morbidity and mortality. Several common therapies such as loop diuretics, morphine, inotropes or inodilators have long been used as first-line therapy without sound evidence from randomized studies on their benefit on morbidity or survival. However, all patients are not created equal, and in euvolaemic or hypovolaemic patients, loop diuretics may induce marked decreases in SV and cardiac output, hypotension or worsening renal function, while inodilators used in patients with preserved systolic function may increase mortality and hospital stay.

Several therapies in AHF management have an unacceptably high incidence of hypotension that may *per se* increase cardiac, renal and other organ damage. Their use should require frequent, or preferably, continuous BP monitoring and pre-emptive measures to avoid it.

If arrhythmia is likely to be the cause of pulmonary oedema or ACS, one should consider emergency cardioversion. Bradycardia should be addressed if it is the cause of symptomatic low cardiac output.

Patients with ACS or serious mechanical cardiac disorders should proceed rapidly to angiography and catheterization for therapeutic measures, including PCI or surgery.

NIV should be given early to every patient admitted with AHF, as it is the only tool with proven improvement in morbidity and mortality. If the respiratory acidosis is associated with mental status changes, endotracheal intubation and mechanical ventilation should be considered, as NIV needs patient cooperation. Signs of poor organ perfusion should be addressed immediately as in any acute circulatory failure.

Hypertensive AHF—congestive form with preserved SBP and likely preserved LVEF

Most patients admitted to hospital with AHF have a normal-to-high SBP. In the recently published Italian survey on AHF, up to 43% of patients had an SBP >140mm Hg. The elevated BP usually develops rapidly and is possibly related to increased sympathetic tone. It results in neurohormonal activation and increased LV afterload with impairment of cardiac function. Because symptoms develop abruptly, these patients tend to be euvolaemic or sometimes mildly hypovolaemic, due to their usual therapy, and present with pulmonary rather than systemic congestion, often with severe pulmonary oedema. Most patients are older, more likely to be women, to have a higher incidence of hypertension, LV hypertrophy, diabetes and to show AF in their first ECG than patients admitted with AHF and systolic dysfunction.

In a landmark paper, Gandhi *et al.* found that in patients with pulmonary oedema presenting to the emergency room with high blood pressure, the echocardiographic EF was almost within the normal range (EF = 0.5 ± 0.15).

In these patients, capable of maintaining high SBP, who present with pulmonary oedema, hypertensive crisis or exacerbated HF with high blood pressure, pulmonary oedema is not caused by fluid accumulation but rather by fluid redistribution that is directed into the lungs because of HF caused by a combination of progressive excessive vasoconstriction superimposed on reduced LV functional reserve.

Recent data suggest that this combination of events in which an inappropriate increase in SVR is met with insufficient systolic and diastolic myocardial functional reserve leads to an acute afterload mismatch. A vicious cycle is established by which impaired function is met with inappropriately high resistance, causing additional impairment in contractility. This increased SVR leads to increased LV diastolic pressures, which are transferred backwards to the pulmonary veins leading to pulmonary oedema.

Reduced systemic oxygen saturation leads to further impairment of cardiac contractility, enhancing the process of pulmonary oedema. The combination of increased pulmonary venous pressure, decreased oxygen saturation and sympathetic activity induces a marked increase in PVR, causing an increase in RV end-diastolic pressure that will further contribute to increased LV end-diastolic pressure and decreased LV diastolic volume.

Therefore, the immediate treatment of these AHF patients should favour the administration of strong, fast-acting IV vasodilators such as nitrates or nitroprusside instead of diuretics. This is not the usual practice. In the ADHERE registry, 88% of AHF patients received IV loop diuretics, with 64% receiving it as monotherapy.

The results of a prospective study comparing predominant IV isosorbide dinitrate with predominant frusemide in the treatment of patients presenting with pulmonary oedema showed that in all primary and secondary end-point measures, patients treated by high-dose frusemide faired significantly worse than patients treated with lower doses of frusemide and high-dose nitrates with fewer numbers of deaths, adverse events, need for mechanical ventilation or MI. The initial management of hypertensive AHF patients should include:

- NIV
- Immediate sublingual or inhaled nitrates
- Cautious diuretic use as they are euvolaemic or often mildly hypovolaemic due to their usual medication
- If BP persists >160/100 start IV vasodilator
- If BP persists <160/100 estimate severity of illness:
  - **Low risk**: good response to treatment, adequate urine output, SBP >90, SBP <210, troponin negative. Admit to intermediate care with close surveillance
  - **High risk**: poor response to treatment, inadequate urine output, SBP <90, SBP >210, troponin elevated, tachycardia, high respiratory rate, persistent hypoxia, increased Uurea or creatinine. Admit to ICU

According to their evolution patients may go from intermediate care to ICU or from ICU to intermediate care.

After initial stabilization, baseline therapy should be directed at reducing recurrent episodes of AHF, by prevention of repeated episodes of excessive vasoconstriction along with efforts to optimize cardiac function.

Normotensive AHF—systolic dysfunction

This other common type of AHF is characterized by a normal SBP, usually with a history of progressive or chronic HF and often with multiple AHF events. In these patients, symptoms and signs develop gradually, over days or weeks, and pulmonary and systemic congestion (jugular venous distension, hepatomegaly, pulmonary rales and peripheral oedema) are usually present. They usually have a weight above their normal dry weight and they often know that they have a reduced EF. Despite high LV filling pressures, they may present several degrees of pulmonary congestion (clinical and/or radiographic) but some may have minimal pulmonary congestion with signs of RV failure. These patients often present with hyponatremia, increased urea and creatinine, and sometimes discrete signs of liver dysfunction.

In these patients, volume overload is central to the pathophysiology of most episodes of acute decompensated HF. Loop diuretics should be the mainstay of their therapy because they produce significantly more natriuresis than other diuretics, particularly in the setting of decreased GFRs. IV loop diuretics may show a substantial difference, because increased mesenteric venous pressure may decrease the absorption of oral diuretic administration. The initial management of these patients should include:

- NIV
- IV loop diuretics
- Estimate severity of illness:
  - **High risk:** poor response to treatment, renal dysfunction, diuretic resistance, elevated SBP, troponin elevated, low urine output. Admit to ICU.
  - **Non-high risk**: good response to treatment, normal renal function, normal SBP, troponin negative, adequate urine output. Admit to intermediate care with close surveillance.
  - **Hypotensive AHF**: see below
- Start IV vasodilator
- If worsening or lack of improvement admit to ICU and consider additional monitoring and therapy.

These patients need time progressively to increase neurohumoral antagonism with some negative fluid balance for symptom improvement. Excessive negative fluid balance may induce hypotension with vasodilatation or β-blocker use.

Hypotensive AHF

Patients admitted to hospital with AHF and low BP represent a subgroup with high in-hospital and post-discharge mortality rates. These patients present with evidence of low cardiac output, decreased perfusion, cool extremities, altered mental status and hypotension. The reduction in cardiac function is not met by an adequate increase in PVR, leading to significant decrease in blood pressure and end-organ perfusion. The treatment of cardiogenic shock should be directed at improving cardiac performance (by optimizing filling pressure, intra-aortic balloon pump and immediate revascularization) and administration of peripheral vasoconstrictors.

Most of these patients require IV inotropic therapy. However, the use of current IV inotropes has been associated with risk for hypotension, atrial and ventricular arrhythmias and possibly increased post-discharge mortality, particularly in those with CAD.

The initial management of hypotensive AHF patients should include:

- NIV
- Consider fluid challenge
- Start IV inotrope/inodilator
- Admit to ICU
- Consider vasopressor for maintaining coronary perfusion
- Assess response to therapy:
  - If adequate response with improvement of peripheral perfusion, increasing urine output, decreasing acidosis or lactatem consider transfer to intermediate care with close surveillance
  - If pulmonary congestion, persistence of decreased perfusion, low urine output, persistent acidosis or lactatem start IV vasodilator. Consider more invasive monitoring. If severe hypervolaemia, consider diuretic or ultrafiltration

Further reading

Atherton JJ, Moore TD, Lele SS, *et al*. Diastolic ventricular interaction in chronic heart failure. *Lancet* 1997; 349: 1720–4.

Benza RL, Tallaj JA, Felker GM, *et al*. The impact of arrhythmias in acute heart failure. *J Card Fail* 2004; 10: 279–84.

Fonarow GC. The Acute Decompensated Heart Failure National Registry (ADHERE): opportunities to improve care of patients hospitalized with acute decompensated heart failure. *Rev Cardiovasc Med* 2003; 4 (Suppl. 7): S21–30.

Gandhi SK, Powers JC, Nomeir AM, *et al*. The pathogenesis of acute pulmonary edema associated with hypertension. *N Engl J Med* 2001; 344: 17–22.

Gheorghiade M, Abraham WT, Albert NM, *et al*. Systolic blood pressure at admission, clinical characteristics, and outcomes in patients hospitalized with acute heart failure. *JAMA* 2006; 296: 2217–26.

Gheorghiade M, Filippatos G. Reassessing treatment of acute heart failure syndromes: the ADHERE Registry. *Eur Heart J* 2005; 7 (Suppl B): B13–9.

Gheorghiade M, Zannad F, Sopko G, *et al*. Acute heart failure syndromes: current state and framework for future research. *Circulation* 2005; 112: 3958–68.

Nieminen MS, Bohm M, Cowie MR, *et al*. Executive summary of the guidelines on the diagnosis and treatment of acute heart failure: the Task Force on Acute Heart Failure of the European Society of Cardiology. *Eur Heart J* 2005; 26: 384–416.

Tavazzi L, Maggioni AP, Lucci D, *et al*. Nationwide survey on acute heart failure in cardiology ward services in Italy. *Eur Heart J* 2006; 27: 1207–15.

Zannad F, Mebazaa A, Juilliere Y, *et al*. Clinical profile, contemporary management and one-year mortality in patients with severe acute heart failure syndromes: The EFICA study. *Eur J Heart Fail* 2006; 8: 697–705.

Bacterial endocarditis

Introduction

The reported incidence of infective endocarditis (IE) in the Western world is 1.8–6.2 per 100 000, population with men more commonly affected than women and a rising incidence with age to >10 per 100 000 for people aged >50yrs. IE predominantly affects those individuals with structural cardiac lesions who develop a bacteraemia with organisms likely to cause endocarditis. Further risk factors include any conditions likely to result in bacteraemia (immunosuppression, diabetes, poor dental hygiene, chronic haemodialysis, chronic alcoholism). Endocarditis may be caused by bacterial organisms or fungi, or may be culture negative (5–10%). Culture-negative endocarditis may be due to concomitant antibiotic therapy, fungal organisms or slower growing organisms. Endocarditis may result from non-infective causes, e.g. SLE, or in malignant disease.

Pathogenesis

Endocarditis can affect native valves and prosthetic valves, and usually normal cardiac tissue is resistant to infection. Transient bacteraemia is very common, and the immune system plays an effective role in preventing endocarditis. Endothelial damage results in platelet and fibrin deposition forming a non-bacterial thrombotic lesion (vegetation). When a bacteraemia occurs from any potential source, e.g. intravascular catheter, post-dental work, wound infections, urinary and respiratory tract infections, these vegetations can be colonized.

Clinical features

The clinical features of bacterial endocarditis will depend on a number of factors including the nature of the underlying lesion and the virulence of the infecting organism. Acute bacterial endocarditis presents as a sudden illness characterized by high temperatures, rigors, exhaustion, weakness and collapse. Patients are frequently very unwell. Subacute endocarditis tends to present in a more insidious non-specific manner with symptoms of anorexia, weight loss, fever, myalgia, arthralgia or fatigue.

The clinical features of IE are due to:

- Bacteraemia/septicaemia—fever, rigors, chills, malaise, anorexia, confusion, arthralgia.
- Tissue destruction—valvular incompetence, root and myocardial abscess (20–40%), prosthetic valve dehiscence, heart block, cardiac failure.
- Embolic phenomena—occur in 50% cases of infective endocarditis resulting in: cerebrovascular accident (CVA), acute peripheral limb ischaemia, MI, TIAs, spleen and kidney infarction, PE and mycotic aneurysms (2–15%).
- Immunological phenomena—splinter haemorrhages (5–15%), Osler's nodes (5–10%) (tender nodes in pulp of fingertips), Janeway lesions (10–20%) (macules on palms or wrists), vasculitis rash, Roth spots (flame-shaped haemorrhages in the retina), arthralgia, nephritis, splenomegaly (30–50%).

Table 18.9.1 outlines commonly useful investigations. The diagnosis of IE is based on the combination of clinical, microbiological and echocardiographic findings. Definite IE is diagnosed on (1) pathological criteria where microorganisms are found by culture or histology in an embolized vegetation, an intracardiac abscess or (2) clinical criteria—these are described in the Duke classification (Table 18.9.2). Two major criteria, one major and three minor criteria, or five minor criteria confirm the diagnosis. Possible IE may be diagnosed where there are findings that fall short of the definite criteria but the diagnosis is not rejected. IE diagnosis is 'rejected' when there is a sound alternative diagnosis, or the manifestations have resolved with antimicrobial treatment for <4 days, or there is no pathological evidence of IE at surgery or autopsy.

Table 18.9.1 Investigations

Blood cultures (90% yield positive culture; 10% are sterile)
FBC, differential, ESR and CRP
CXR and ECG
Echo TTE (transthoracic) and/or TOE (transoesophageal)
Renal function (including urinalysis)
Infection-related antiphospholipid antibodies
Special cultures for *Coxiella*, *Bartonella* and mycoplasma if initial cultures are negative
Pre-operative MRSA screen

Common sites of infection

- Prosthetic valves
- Left-sided structures (>85%)
  - Aortic lesions (55–60%)
  - Mitral lesions (25–30%)
  - Mitral + aortic lesions (15%)
- Right-sided structures (10–15%)

Treatment

IE causes significant morbidity and mortality. Prevention is a priority, although early diagnosis and appropriate therapy are essential. Once the diagnosis is established, treatment should be commenced according to local guidance or directed by microbiological advice. Treatment should be initiated once blood cultures have been taken, and subsequently adjusted once the results are known. Early involvement of cardiologists, microbiologists and cardiac surgeons is advisable.

The majority of endocarditis is caused by streptococcal organisms (50–70%) with *S. viridans* accounting for half of these; staphylococcal organisms account for 25%, although in IV drug abusers this increases to ~60%, with associated increases in fungal and anaerobic organisms, and enterococci (10%).

Empirical treatment depends on the likely organism.

- Acute onset (often staphylococcal organisms)—flucloxacillin (8–12g IV daily in 4–6 divided doses) plus gentamicin (1mg/kg body weight IV 8 hourly, modified according to renal function).
- Gradual presentation (often α-haemolytic streptococcal organisms)—penicillin (7.2g IV daily in six divided doses) or ampicillin/amoxicillin (2g IV 6 hourly) plus gentamicin (1mg/kg body weight 8 hourly IV, modified according to renal function).
- Patients with penicillin allergy, intracardiac prosthesis or suspected MRSA—vancomycin (1g 12 hourly IV, modified according to renal function) plus rifampicin

Table 18.9.2 The Duke classification.

Major criteria	
Positive blood culture of organisms known to cause IE from 2 separate blood cultures.	
Persistently positive blood cultures	In 2 blood cultures drawn >12h apart
	In all of 3 or majority of 4 separate blood cultures with the first and last drawn over 1h apart
Evidence of endocardial involvement	
Positive echocardiographic findings	Mobile intracardiac mass on valve or supporting structures or in the path of a regurgitant jet, or on implanted material.
	Abscess
	New dehiscence of prosthetic valve or new valve regurgitation
Clinical evidence of new valvular regurgitation	
Positive serology	e.g. Q fever, *Bartonella* spp, *Chlamydia* Spp
Positive identification of a microorganism	Using molecular biology methods
Minor criteria	
Predisposition	Predisposing heart lesion or IV drug abuse
Fever	Temperature >38.0°C
Vascular phenomena	Arterial emboli, septic pulmonary infarcts, mycotic aneurysm, intracranial haemorrhage, conjunctival haemorrhage, Janeway lesions, new finger clubbing, splinter haemorrhages, splenomegaly
Immunological phenomena	Glomerulonephritis, Osler's nodes, Roth spots, +ve rheumatoid factor, raised ESR (>1.5× normal) raised CRP (>100mg/dl)
Microbiological evidence	Positive blood cultures but not meeting major criteria

(300–600mg 12 hourly by mouth) plus gentamicin (1mg/kg body weight 8 hourly IV, modified according to renal function).

Surgery is indicated in up to 25–30% of infections. These tend to be in those with life-threatening congestive HFor shock due to valvular heart disease, or those with prosthetic valve endocarditis. Early intervention may be associated with improved outcome.

Antibiotic therapy should be continued for 4–6 weeks. Response to treatment should be carefully monitored with repeated evaluation of clinical state and laboratory investigations.

Mortality

Overall mortality remains at ~20%. Prosthetic valve endocarditis carries an even higher mortality rate (26–70%). Right-sided endocarditis is usually related to IV drug abuse and carries a more favourable mortality risk at 4–5%. IE with staphylococcal organisms or with fungi have a high associated mortality (50%) when compared with enterococci (25%) or streptococci (15%).

Prophylaxis

People with predisposing factors for bacterial endocarditis include those with prosthetic heart valves, previous bacterial endocarditis, acquired valvular heart disease with stenosis or regurgitation, structural congitential heart disease (excluding fully repaired atrial and venticular septal defects and patent ductus arteriosous), and hypertrophic cardiomyopathy. At present antibiotic prophylaxis against infective endocarditis is *not* recommended for people undergoing dental procedures and other invasive clincial procedures involving the respiratory, genitourinary (including urological, gynaecological, obstetric procedures, and childbirth), and the upper and lower gastrointestinal tracts. Recommendations may change, and it is wise to consult a national formulary.

Episodes of infection in those at risk of infective endocarditis should be investigated and treated promptly to reduce the risk of endocarditis developing. If a person at risk of infective endocarditis is receiving antimicrobial therapy because they are undergoing a procedure at a site where there is a suspected infection, the person should receive an antibiotic that covers organisms that cause infective endocarditis.

Further reading

NICE clinical guideline 64. Prophylaxis against infective endocarditis: antimicrobial prophylaxis against infective endocarditis in adults and children undergoing interventional procedures. March 2008.

Chapter 19

Renal disorders

Chapter contents

Prevention of acute renal failure

Acute kidney injury (AKI) often complicates the course of critical illness and was previously considered as a marker rather than a cause of adverse outcomes, it is independently associated with an increase in both morbidity and mortality. The major causes of AKI in the ICU include hypoperfusion, sepsis and direct nephrotoxicity, with the common aetiology believed to be a change in intrarenal haemodynamics with resultant acute tubular dysfunction and oxidant stress. Treatment of established acute renal failure in the ICU entails the use of RRT by means of various modalities, although this therapy itself carries an inherent morbidity and risk. Therefore, preventing or minimizing renal injury should confer a benefit to patients. Consequently, several pharmacological interventions have been tried to treat AKI. These interventions can be separated into measures influencing renal perfusion and measures modulating intrarenal pathophysiology.

Optimizing renal perfusion

Volume expansion, inotropes, vasopressors

Improvement of renal function associated with hypovolaemia may be demonstrated by correcting volume status. The beneficial effect of prophylactic volume expansion has repeatedly been demonstrated for contrast-induced nephropathy (CIN), with normal saline showing some superiority over half-normal saline. Recent investigations indicate additional protection against CIN using isotonic bicarbonate solutions (i.e. 150mmol/l sodium bicarbonate) compared with normal saline.

In addition to the conventional inotropes dobutamine and dopexamine, the use of the new PDE inhibitor with myocardial calcium sensitizer activity, levosimendan, may improve renal function in patients with acute decompensated HF. Moreover, application of vasopressors in the setting of sepsis-associated AKI has shown some benefit, although studies investigating this aspect are small and mostly uncontrolled.

(Selective) renal vasodilators

Renal or low dose dopamine, though previously widely used, is now known to be ineffective in improving renal function though it may cause a diuresis initially, and in fact may worsen renal perfusion in patients with acute renal failure as determined by renal resistive indexes. Despite showing promising results in pilot studies of contrast nephropathy and sepsis-associated AKI, selective dopamine A_1 agonists such as fenoldopam have failed to provide significant nephroprotection in larger studies of either early acute tubular necrosis or CIN.

Prostaglandins (PGs) have been investigated mainly in the setting of contrast nephropathy. Both PGE and PGI (Iloprost) administered IV resulted in an attenuated rise of serum creatinine after application of contrast media. Major adverse events such as hypotension as well as flush and nausea at higher doses limit the extensive use of these substances.

Natriuretic peptides improve renal blood flow by causing afferent glomerular dilatation resulting in increased GFR and urinary sodium excretion. BNPs additionally inhibit aldosterone. Atrial natriuretic peptide (ANP) has been used in small human studies and shown to attenuate the rise in serum creatinine in ischaemic renal failure or in AKI after liver transplantation, but it has been ineffective in large RCTs of both non-oliguric and oliguric acute tubular necrosis. A recent study applying low-dose BNP (neseritide) conferred preservation of renal function in patients with chronic kidney disease stage 3 undergoing cardiopulmonary bypass surgery.

Currently the most promising preliminary reports exist for the adenosine antagonist theophylline for CIN as well as some forms of nephrotoxic AKI such as cisplatin-associated renal dysfunction. A randomized placebo-controlled trial in neonates with perinatal asphyxia showed a significant increase in creatinine clearance after a single dose of theophylline within the first hour of birth.

Modulation of renal physiology

Renal metabolism, tubular obstruction

Loop diuretics have been extensively investigated. They reduce oxygen consumption in the medulla in both animals and healthy volunteers. An RCT performed in established renal failure could not demonstrate improvement in outcome. Application of very high doses of frusemide, on the other hand, significantly increases the risk of serious adverse events such as hearing loss.

Oxygen radical damage

Several roles have been proposed for reactive oxygen species under both normal and pathological conditions, with the NAD(P)H oxidase system believed to be pivotal in their formation and instrumental in the development of certain pathophysiological conditions in the kidney. Under certain circumstances there may be a role for antioxidant supplementation with agents such as NAC, the antioxidant vitamin E (α-tocopherol), vitamin C (ascorbic acid) and selenium.

NAC has been investigated in multiple trials, especially in the setting of CIN. Despite several reports showing prevention of CIN when evaluating this substance, meta-analysis has been inconclusive. Furthermore, NAC was ineffective in other settings of AKI such as major cardiovascular surgery or sepsis.

Finally, studies of IV NAC in both human volunteers and patients receiving contrast media showed a decrease in serum creatinine which was not reflected by concomitant changes of cystatin C which is considered the more sensitive marker of early changes in GFR than serum creatinine.

Mannitol, an osmotic diuretic with oxygen radical-scavenging properties, has been investigated in randomized trials for the prevention of CIN but proved to be of no benefit compared with general measures such as volume expansion. Some authors favour mannitol for treatment of AKI following crush injuries, but there have been no RCTs to substantiate this use of mannitol.

Selenium is another antioxidant showing free radical scavenger properties. Selenium supplementation reduces oxidative stress, intranuclear factor-B translocation and cytokine formation, as well as tissue damage, and normalizes all known selenoenzymes including intracellular glutathione peroxidase and thioredoxin reductase. It was thought that selenium supplementation decreased the requirement for renal rescue therapy, but this finding has not been reproduced in a prospective RCT in septic shock.

Cocktails of antioxidants have been investigated in several small studies showing conflicting results. In one randomized trial in patients undergoing elective aortic aneurysm repair, use of an antioxidant cocktail resulted in an increased creatinine clearance on the second post-operative day, but the incidence of renal failure was very low.

Ascorbic acid given orally 2h pre-contrast in a single-centre trial appeared to protect against the development of CIN.

Renal regeneration and repair

Since the duration of AKI may be significantly influenced by the time renal (tubular epithelial) cells need for regeneration, several growth hormones including insulin-like growth factor (IGF-1), hepatocyte growth factor (HGF) and endothelial growth factor (EGF) have been investigated with limited success in animal experiments. However, investigations in established renal failure in humans did not demonstrate a significant improvement in renal recovery. Also a multi-centre PRCT in 72 patients with acute renal failure similarly failed to show an effect of IGF-1 on renal recovery.

Erythropoietin (EPO) not only stimulates erythroid progenitor cells but it is also a tissue-protective cytokine that mediates local antiapoptosis and differentiation-inducing effects in response to injury. Animal data do suggest a renoprotective effect of EPO in both ischaemic and toxic acute renal failure, and human studies are currently being undertaken.

Conclusion

Pharmacologicalo prevention and treatment of AKI have been shown to have very limited success, and on the basis of current evidence they can only have a weak recommendation. Adequate haemodynamic management by volume expansion and vasopressors/inotropes and some renal vasodilators such as theophylline are all reasonable interventions that may be employed in the prevention of AKI.

Further reading

Abassi ZA, Hoffman A, Better OS. Acute renal failure complicating muscle crush injury. *Semin Nephrol* 1998; 18: 558/

Angstwurm MW, Engelmann L, Zimmermann T, *et al.* Selenium in Intensive Care (SIC): results of a prospective randomized, placebo-controlled, multiple-center study in patients with severe systemic inflammatory response syndrome, sepsis, and septic shock. *Crit Care Med* 2007; 35: 118–26.

Bagshaw SM, Ghali WA. Theophylline for prevention of contrast-induced nephropathy: a systematic review and meta-analysis. *Arch Intern Med* 2005; 165: 1087–93/

Briguori C, Airoldi F, D'Andrea D, *et al.* Renal insufficiency following contrast media administration trial (REMEDIAL): a randomized comparison of 3 preventive strategies. *Circulation* 2007; 115: 1211–7.

Spargias K, Alexopoulos E, Kyrzopoulos S, *et al.* Ascorbic acid prevents contrast-mediated nephropathy in patients with renal dysfunction undergoing coronary angiography or intervention. *Circulation* 2004; 110: 2837–42.

Wijnen MH, Vader HL, Van Den Wall Bake AW, *et al.* Can renal dysfunction after infra-renal aortic aneurysm repair be modified by multi-antioxidant supplementation? *J Cardiovasc Surg* 2002; 43: 483–8.

Diagnosis of acute renal failure

Acute renal failure is characterized by an abrupt deterioration in renal function usually manifested as a drop in GFR and/or urine output.

More than 30 definitions of acute renal failure do exist, and most of them relate to absolute or relative changes in serum creatinine. However, acute renal failure should be rather regarded as the end-point of a continuum of deteriorating renal function called AKI. In 2004, the RIFLE criteria were established by the Acute Dialysis Quality Initiative (ADQI). On the basis of either increase of serum creatinine or reduction in urine output as a sensitive marker of renal dysfunction, acute renal injury is classified into risk, injury and failure, with two additional classes loss and ESKD (end-stage kidney disease) defined by the requirement for RRT for >4 weeks and >3 months, respectively (Table 19.2.1). RIFLE relies on prior knowledge of the baseline creatinine. The requirement for RRT has not been explicitly defined, although it was discussed in the original ADQI document. The major problem with RIFLE is lack of a defined time fame in which an increase in serum creatinine should occur to be classified as 'acute'. To overcome this problem, a modified RIFLE classification was proposed in 2007, where determination of at least 2 serum creatinine values within an observation period of 48h was suggested. An increase in serum creatinine of >0.3 mg/dl or of at least 150% was required for diagnosis of AKI (resulting in RIFLE risk or stage 1, respectively). Further classification was performed according to relative increase in serum creatinine (Table 19.2.1). Finally, the requirement for RRT was considered to be classified as RIFLE failure (or AKI stage 3). Although initially not designed as an outcome predictor, several studies validated RIFLE with respect to severity of AKI and impaired survival.

Table 19.2.1 Modified RIFLE according to AKI stage.

Stage	Creatinine criteria	Urine output criteria
AKI stage 1 (modified RIFLE risk)	Serum creatinine >0.3mg/dl (>26.4μmol/l) or increase to ≥150–200% (1.5- to 2-fold) from baseline	<0.5ml/kg/h for >6h
AKI stage 2 (modified RIFLE injury)	Increase serum creatinine to >200–300% (>2- to 3-fold) from baseline	<0.5ml/kg/h for >12 h
AKI stage 3 (modified RIFLE failure)*	Increase serum creatinine to >300% (>3- fold) from baseline (or serum creatinine ≥4.0mg/dl (≥354μmol/l with an acute rise of at least 0.5mg/dl (44μmol/l)	<0.3ml/kg/h x24 h or anuria x12h

*Individuals requiring RRT are considered to be classified as stage 3 (modified RIFLE failure).

Characterization of acute renal failure into pre-renal azotaemia, renal failure and post-renal obstruction is not explicitly discussed in current acute renal failure/AKI classification systems. It appears that in critically ill patients especially, the discrimination between pre-renal azotemia and so called acute tubular necrosis (ATN) appears to be neither represented by histological findings nor relevant in terms of pathophysiology. Nevertheless, exclusion of post-renal obstruction as a first step and discrimination between volume-responsive AKI and volume-unresponsive AKI is still of clinical relevance in daily practice and should be continued.

Parameters of glomerular function

Serum creatinine

Loss in GFR is reflected by an increase in serum creatinine.

Cystatin C

Cystatin C is a small (13kDa) molecule produced by nucleated cells and freely filtered by the glomerulus. Due to its small volume of distribution, small chages in GFR are reflected by an increase in cystatin C. Cystatin has been evaluated in patients, in whom reduced muscle mass results in a falsely low serum creatinine value, e.g. patients with liver cirrhosis.

Urine analyses

Urinary sediment

Urinary analysis is only of limited value for diagnosis of acute renal failure in critically ill patients. However, urinary sediment is still helpful in the differential diagnosis of renal impairmentn discriminating acute renal failure from other acute glomerular diseases (e.g. rapidly progressive glomerulonephtis, acute interstitial nephritis; see Table 19.2.2). 'Muddy brown casts' or tubular cells may be indicative of acute renal failure (so-called acute tubular necrosis); however, a benign sediment does not exclude ARF.

Leucocyturia, especially eosinophiluria is usually attributed to acute interstitial nephritis.

Table 19.2.2 Urinary analysis for AKI/acute renal failure.

	Pre-renal azotaemia	Acute renal failure (ATN)	Glomerular disease (e.g. GN)
Urinary sediment	Benign	'Muddy brown' casts	Nephritic (erythrocyte casts)
		Tubular epithelial cells	
Urinary osmolality	>500	<350	?
Urinary sodium	<10mmol/l	>20mmol/l	?/low
Urine/S-creatinine ratio	>40	<20	?
S-urea/ creatinine ratio	>40:1	20–30:1	<40:1
FE_{Na}	<1%	>2%	?
FE_{Urea}	<35%	≥35%	?

ATN = acute tubular necrosis; FE = fractional excretion; GN = glomerulonephritis

Urinary electrolytes

Reduced urinary sodium and urea excretion may be diagnostic of renal hypoperfusion. The calculation of fractional sodium excretion (FE_{Na}) or FE_{Urea} (see below) is recommended, with values <1% and <35%, respectively, being considered as indicative for renal hypoperfusion. Whereas FE_{Na} is increased despite hypoperfusion when using diuretics, FE_{Urea} is not influenced by medical natriuresis. Neither of these parameters, however, can be considered reliable in sepsis. Neither decreased FE_{Na} nor FE_{Urea} can be used to rule out acute renal failure reliably.

Fractional sodium/urea excretion

$$FE_{Na}\,(\%)^{*} = \frac{U_{Na}{}^{*}\,P_{Cr}}{P_{Na}{}^{*}\,U_{Cr}} {*}100$$

* For FEUrea, use urea values instead of sodium.

FE_{Na}: pre-renal if <1%

FE_{Urea}: pre-renal if <35%

Biomarkers

Several biomarkers have been investigated in terms of their usefulness to predict acute renal failure earlier than standard parameters. These are either enzyme activities of enzymes released by tubular cells or surface proteins only present in renal tubular cells:

The release of (large molecular) proteins from renal epithelial damage has been used for early diagnosis of renal tubular damage for decades. The ost widely applied enzyme was *N*-acetylglucosaminidase (NAG) also successfully investigated in critically ill patients. Determination, however, is costly and mostly not automated.

Neutrophil gelatinase-associated lipocalin (NGAL) is a 25kDa protein which is released in the kidney after ischaemia. In cardiac surgery in children and adults it can predict acute renal failure 24h earlier than creatinine .

KIM-1 is a surface protein expressed in proximal tubular cells in ischaemia. In humans it has been shown to be secreted in ischaemic renal failure. Both KIM-1 and NAG may be predictors for requirement for RRT.

NHE-3 (sodium/hydrogen exchanger Isoform 3), a membrane-bound protein is also found in the urine in ischaemic acute renal failure.

Finally IL-18 was found to predict mortality in patients with ARDS and acute renal failure.

Ultrasound

Renal ultrasound is helpful in excluding post-renal obstruction. Furthermore, it helps to discriminate acute damage from chronic damage kidneys. Acute renal failure typically is associated with bilaterally enlarged kidneys showing moderately enhanced parenchymal density. Chronically damaged kidneys are small, with clearly increased parenchymal density.

Acute renal failure is furtter characterized by increased resistive indices as determined by Doppler-flow measurements.

Further reading

Abosaif NY, Tolba YA, Heap M, *et al.* The outcome of acute renal failure in the intensive care unit according to RIFLE: model application, sensitivity, and predictability. *Am J Kidney Dis* 2005; 46: 1038–48.

Bellomo R, Ronco C, Kellum JA, *et al.* Acute renal failure—definition, outcome measures, animal models, fluid therapy and information technology needs: the Second International Consensus Conference of the Acute Dialysis Quality Initiative (ADQI) Group. *Crit Care* 2004; 8: R204–12.

Herget-Rosenthal S, Marggraf G, Husing J, *et al.* Early detection of acute renal failure by serum cystatin C. *Kidney Int* 2004; 66: 1115–22.

Kellum JA, Levin N, Bouman C, *et al.* Developing a consensus classification system for acute renal failure. *Curr Opin Crit Care* 2002; 8: 509–14.

Uchino S, Bellomo R, Goldsmith D, *et al.* An assessment of the RIFLE criteria for acute renal failure in hospitalized patients. *Crit Care Med* 2006; 34: 1913–7.

Parikh CR, Abraham E, Ancukiewicz M, *et al.* Urine IL-18 is an early diagnostic marker for acute kidney injury and predicts mortality in the intensive care unit. *J Am Soc Nephrol* 2005; 16: 3046–52.

Chapter 20

Gastrointestinal disorders

Chapter contents

Vomiting and gastric stasis/gastroparesis

Clinical features

Nausea usually precedes vomiting, and is generally associated with impaired gastric motility. Retching follows—the glottis remains closed and abdominal muscles and the diaphragm contract. Finally, the cardia relaxes and sustained contraction of the abdominal muscles produces vomiting. In surgical abdominal complaints, pain usually precedes vomiting, whereas the opposite is often the case with medical causes.

Causes

These are legion, but include:

- Any GI disorder, including intestinal obstruction (chronic vomiting without other abdominal symptoms is unlikely to be due to GI disease).
- Acute viral infections, e.g. influenza, Epstein–Barr virus, cytomegalovirus.
- Neurological disorders, e.g. raised ICP, meningitis, migraine, vestibular disturbances.
- Metabolic disorders, e.g. uraemia (although unlikely to be cause if blood urea <30mmol/l), hypercalcaemia, diabetic ketoacidosis.
- Drugs, e.g. opiates, cytotoxics, digoxin toxicity
- Pregnancy
- Psychogenic
- Post-surgery, especially gastric.
- Alcohol excess.

Evaluation

- History: important to differentiate vomiting from other, apparently similar entities, such as regurgitation, rumination, bulimia.
- Careful examination of patient (and drug chart).
- Fluid balance: signs of dehydration.
- Electrolyte/acid–base status: vomiting can cause hyponatraemia (excessive sodium losses in vomitus) *or* hypernatraemia (unreplaced losses of hypotonic GI fluids). Loss of H^+ and Cl^- produces hypochloraemic alkalosis. K^+ loss in the urine in exchange for H^+ exacerbates hypokalaemia. Treatment usually requires IV normal saline with potassium supplements to correct chloride and potassium deficits.

Investigations

- Routine bloods (including amylase, calcium)
- Arterial blood gases
- Pregnancy test
- Plain films: exclude intestinal obstruction.
- Oesophagogastroduodenoscopy: exclude peptic ulcer disease, malignancy.
- Barium series: exclude obstruction, superior mesenteric artery syndrome.
- Biliary ultrasound

Gastroparesis

Defined as a symptomatic, chronic disorder characterized by delayed gastric emptying and the absence of mechanical obstruction. Symptoms include early satiety, nausea, vomiting, bloating and upper abdominal discomfort. Gastric food retention can lead to bezoar formation. May be idiopathic (80% females), but risk factors for secondary gastroparesis include:

- type 1 diabetes
- abdominal surgery (vagotomy, fundoplication, bariatric surgery, heart/lung transplantation)
- hypothyroidism
- rheumatological disorders (e.g. scleroderma, SLE, amyloidosis)

Evaluation

- Gastric scintigraphy: gold standard for diagnosis. Performed after ingestion of a radiolabelled meal (usually ^{99m}Tc sulfur colloid cooked into test meal). Percentage radiolabel retention at 2–4h is compared with norms. Prokinetic agents, opiates and anticholinergics should be discontinued 48–72h prior to test, although serotonin receptor antagonists (e.g. ondansetron) can be continued. Despite widespread use, correlation with symptoms (both pre- and post-treatment) is poor.

Other means of evaluation are not widely available, but include:-

- Antroduodenal manometry: performed using nasogastroduodenal manometry probes in the fasting and postprandial periods. Typically there is a loss of antral contractility. Fasting migratory motor complexes are seen to originate from the small intestine, rather than from the stomach.
- Electrogastrography: cutaneous electrodes on the abdominal wall record gastric myoelectrical activity. Normal gastric slow wave frequency is ~3 counts/min. Deemed abnormal if dysrhythmias occur >30% of recording time, or solid meal ingestion fails to increase wave amplitude.
- Ultrasound: antral cross-sectional area used to assess gastric emptying. Non-invasive, but highly operator dependent.

Management

The management of gastroparesis is often disappointing and ineffective, but the following can be tried:

1. ***Dietary manipulation:*** frequent, small meals. Replace solids with soups (liquid emptying phase often preserved), low fat/fibre foods.
2. ***Optimize glycaemic control:*** hyperglycaemia alone can cause delayed gastric emptying in diabetic patients (although no long term studies to confirm symptom improvement with enhanced glycaemic control).
3. ***Antiemetics:***
   - Antidopaminergics, e.g. prochlorperazine. Act centrally on medulla oblongata (CTZ). Can be given in suppository/injectable form as well as orally.
   - Antihistamines, e.g. diphenhydramine. Act centrally on vestibular apparatus, and more often used for motion sickness.
   - Anticholinergics, e.g. hyoscine.
   - Serotonin (5-HT_3) receptor antagonists, e.g. ondansetron. Act centrally and on peripheral vagal afferents. Generally used as prophylaxis for chemotherapy/radiotherapy0induced vomiting, and post-operative symptoms. Role in gastroparesis less clear.

4 ***Prokinetics:***
- Metoclopramide: has prokinetic effects on proximal gut via 5-HT_4 agonist and weak 5-HT_3 antagonist action. Also central dopamine receptor antagonist, giving antiemetic effect. Loss of effectiveness with time and high incidence of CNS side effects (dystonias, drowsiness, Parkinsonism) limit use to the short term.
- Domperidone: peripheral D_2 receptor antagonist with similar prokinetic effects to metoclopramide, but less able to cross blood–brain barrier, therefore fewer CNS side effects. Improvements in gastric emptying may be transitory, with continued symptomatic relief being due to additional antiemetic properties.
- Erythromycin: macrolide antibiotic that acts via gastroduodenal motilin receptors, enhancing antral contractility. Most effective when given IV in severe refractory gastroparesis. GI side effects (nausea/vomiting/abdominal pain) can limit clinical effectiveness.
- Tegaserod: partial 5-HT_4 agonist. Enhances gastric emptying in healthy volunteers, but little evidence for effectiveness in gastroparesis.
- Cisapride: 5-HT_4 agonist with proven long-term effectiveness in increasing gastric emptying and improving symptoms. Withdrawn from market, however, due to action on cardiac potassium channels, leading to case reports of prolonged QT interval, cardiac arrhythmias and sudden death. Can still be prescribed on a named patient basis, provided there is no history of conduction defects or concurrent medications known to affect the QT interval.

For those patients with symptoms refractory to dietary manipulation, antiemetics and prokinetics, the following can be considered:

1 ***Enteral feeds/gastrostomy:*** placing a jejunostomy can be effective, both for nutrition and for the administration of medication, provided small bowel motility is preserved. A trial period of NJ feeding is sensible prior to jejunostomy placement. Gastrostomy tubes can assist in symptom control by allowing venting and draining of the stomach. Again the results of initial nasogastric decompression can help predict outcome.

2 ***Pyloric botulinum toxin:*** the increased pyloric tone seen in diabetic gastroparesis can be reduced (for a number of months) by pyloric botulinum toxin injection, but there are few studies as yet to support clinical effectiveness.

3 ***Gastric stimulation:*** electrodes are attached to the stomach at laparoscopy/laparotomy, and connected to a subcutaneous electrical stimulator. Gastric pacing uses stimulation at a rate slightly higher than the intrinsic slow wave frequency (~3 contractions/min) thus entraining gastric slow waves and accelerating gastric emptying. High frequency stimulation (12 contractions/min) has no effect on gastric emptying, but does appear to improve symptoms of nausea and vomiting. Currently the most effective combinations of stimulation parameters remain undefined. Promising symptomatic improvements have been reported, mainly in diabetic and idiopathic gastroparesis, but more experience is required.

Further reading

Lin Z, Forster J, Sarosiek I, McCallum RW. Treatment of gastroparesis with electrical stimulation. *Dig Dis Sci* 2003; 48: 837–48.

Parkman HP, Hasler WL, Fisher RS; American Gastroenterological Association. American Gastroenterological Association technical review on the diagnosis and treatment of gastroparesis. *Gastroenterology* 2004; 127: 1592–622.

Gastric erosions

Definition

Varies from mild erosions to ulcerations of the gastric mucosa.

Epidemiology

Found in patients with a critical illness, which can effect all ages and occur in acute and chronic disease states.

Incidence

The incidence quoted in the 1980s is below. The true incidence now is difficult to determine, but the perception is that it is very much less than it used to be.

1 Erosions ~40–50%
2 Ulcers ~5%
3 Macroscopic/clinically relevant bleeding <2%

Risk factors

1 Previous ulcer disease
2 Coagulopathy
3 Mechanical ventilation >48h
4 Previous factors (now questioned): head injury, multiple trauma, severe burns, sepsis/SIRS, hypotension, hypovolaemia, renal failure, hepatic failure

Prophylaxis

Gastric pH control, cytoprotective drugs, nutrition.

Reduced incidence is also probably due to:

1 Better ICU management
2 Better oxygen and fluid management
3 Early NG feeding
4 Improved analgesia
5 Treatment of coagulopathy

Pathology

The site is usually the fundus and body, rarely in the antrum, duodenum or oesophagus

1 Mucosal ulceration: superficial, eroding through to the muscularis mucosae only, little bleeding and heals rapidly.
2 Acute peptic ulceration: deep, through the muscular layer where the larger arteries reside, greater bleeding and slower to heal.

Factors which influence the risk of haemorrhage

1 Aspirin, NSAIDs, steroids
2 Alcohol
3 Anticoagulants and dextrans
4 Vitamin K deficiency and platelet defects
5 Vasoconstrictors

Local defence mechanisms include

1 The mucus barrier
2 Surfactants AND HCO_3 secreted by mucosa
3 H^+ reabsorbed by the mucosa is neutralized by blood-derived HCO_3

Shock states result in

1 Mucosal ischaemia
   - TNF causes thrombosis within the gastric mucosal vessels
   - Sympathetic redistribution of blood flow away from the splanchnic bed
2 H^+/pepsin/bile seep in and damage intracellular components
3 Mucosal necrosis leads to ulcer formation

Pepsin is still active unless pH >7

1 pH ~5–7: pepsin still dissolves clot
2 pH <5.4: pepsin prevents clot formation

NB: alkaline gastric contents are not necessary for prevention, and there is no evidence that hypersecretion of pepsin *per se* is responsible for erosions

Intracellular pH is probably more important than intragastric pH

Prostaglandins result in

1 Increased blood flow
2 Increased mucus production, and possibly mucus secretion
3 Decreased ulcer incidence and promotion of healing

Bile salt

Causes disruption of the mucosal barrier to occur, and prevention of duodenal reflux is associated with significant reduction in gastric ulceration.

Prevention

Acid/pepsin production reduced by	Mucosal resistance increased by
Enteral feeds	Enteral feeds
Prostaglandins	?Prostaglandins
Antacids	Sucralfate
H_2 blockers	

Treat stress factors

- Improve gut oxygen delivery
- Normovolaemia, adequate oxygenation and ventilation
- Maximize cardiac output and GI pressure

Nasogastric feeds as soon as possible

Especially high risk groups

- Head injury, major trauma, burns
- Prolonged IPPV
- Renal failure, hepatic failure
- Sepsis

Sucralfate or H_2 blocker where

- NG aspiration of blood/'coffee ground'
- Previous peptic ulcer disease

Omeprazole

- Clinical bleed on H_2 blockers
- Endoscopically proven ulceration not healing with H_2 blockers

Treatment: mild bleed

Maximize coagulation status/remove precipitants

1 Vitamin K
2 Stop heparin, NSAIDs other anticoagulants
3 Blood transfusion, FFP, platelets or other procoagulants

Antacids

Get pH >3.5 (ideally >7).

Sucralfate

H_2 blockers

1. Cimetidine, ranitidine and famotidine are competitive antagonists
2. Increase GI Gram-negative colonization and there is an associated increase of nosocomial pneumonia.

Omeprazole

1. Absorbed in the small intestine, short plasma half-life but effective for 24h
2. Binds irreversibly to fundic parietal cell H^+/K^+ ATPase. 20mg gives 65% inhibition at 4–6h and 25% inhibition at 24h
3. Results in hypergastrinaemia and potential enterochromafin hyperplasia

Prostaglandins

Aminocaproic acid

- 5g stat and 1g/h for 24h IV
- ~20–30% reduction in rebleeding
- ~40% reduction in mortality

Endoscopy for assessment

If major bleeding then proceed with

1. Resuscitation with airway and cardiovascular support. Will mainly require fluid resuscitation and reversal of precipitating factors.
2. Octreotide infusion; 100mcg stat, then 50mcg/h equally effective as sclerotherapy.
3. Pitressin infusion has questionable benefits in stress ulceration.
4. Endoscopic haemostasis: laser coagulation, electrocoagulation.
5. Surgery: partial or total gastrectomy in the setting of uncontrolled GI haemorrhage, but mortality is high in this group.

Nosocomial pneumonia

One of the potential adverse effects of increasing the gastric pH to prevent stress ulceration is that gastric bacterial growth may be encouraged. This has been associated with an increased rate of ventilation associated pneumonia.

Studies/evidence

Cook's metanalysis in 1994 recommended stress ulcer prophylaxis in critically ill patients who were mechanically ventilated or who had a coagulopathy. The evidence at the time supported the use of sucralfate over other agents, because of both a reduction in pneumonia and a possible reduction in mortality. Cook then went on in an RCT to compare ranitidine with sucralfate in 1200 critically ill patients. There was no difference in mortality (23%) or LOS. The ranitidine group had a clinically significant lower rate of GI haemorrhage, 1.7% vs 3.8% ($P = 0.02$). The VAP rates were 19.1% in the ranitidine group vs 16.2% in the sucralfate group ($P = 0.19$). A further metanalysis ($n = 7128$) concluded there was strong evidence of a reduction in clinically important GI bleeds with H_2 receptor antagonists. In addition, it suggested that sucralfate may be as effective in reducing bleeding as gastric pH-altering drugs, and is associated with lower rates of pneumonia and mortality. However, the data were insufficient to determine the net effect of sucralfate compared with no prophylaxis.

It may be best summarized that an observational study would give us the true incidence of gastric erosions, now that it is decreasing. Based on this, an RCT comparing no prophylaxis with ranitidine or sucralfate may give a definitive answer.

Cushing's ulcers occur in the oesophagus, stomach and duodenum, initially described by Cushing in association with coma of any cause. Now accepted as acute peptic ulceration in association with severe head injury and raised ICP. Results from increased vagally mediated gastric acid secretion and responds to H_2 blockade.

Curling's ulcer is a circumscribed (<2cm) duodenal ulcer in patients with >35% burns. Also results from gastric acid hypersecretion and responds to H_2 blockade.

Summary

Stress ulceration in the critically ill is managed by ensuring adequate resuscitation and early establishment of enteral feeding. If NG feeding is not established after 48h, 50mg IV ranitidine 8 hourly is recommended, but ensure there is increased surveillance for VAP.

Further reading

Cook D, Guyatt G, Marshall J, *et al.* A comparison of sucralfate and ranitidine for the prevention of upper gastrointestinal bleeding in patients requiring mechanical ventilation. Canadian Critical Care Trials Group. *N Engl J Med* 1998; 338: 791–7.

Cook DJ, Reeve BK, Guyatt GH, *et al.* Stress ulcer prophylaxis in critically ill patients. Resolving discordant meta-analyses. *JAMA* 1996; 275: 308–14.

Cook DJ, Reeve BK, Scholes LC. Histamine-2-receptor antagonists and antacids in the critically ill population: stress ulceration versus nosocomial pneumonia. *Infect Control Hosp Epidemiol* 1994; 15: 437–42.

Diarrhoea

This is the term used to describe an increased stool frequency with increased fluidity. Given that the differential diagnosis of diarrhoea is extremely broad, this chapter will concentrate on acute diarrhoea in the critical care setting.

Pathophysiology

The final cause of diarrhoea is imbalanced water/solute transport across the GI tract. The cause behind this imbalance can be divided into 4 pathophysiological mechanisms:

- Osmotic: failure of the gut to absorb osmotically active solutes results in retention of water within the gut lumen. In the critical care setting this may result from ingested compounds (e,g, Mg^{2+}-induced diarrhoea, certain laxatives), inefficient gut mucosa (e.g. bacterial overgrowth causing bile salt malabsorption) or inadequate gut length (short gut syndrome). It often involves a moderate volume of diarrhoea (500–1000ml/day) which improves with starvation.
- Secretory: increased secretion or reduced absorption of salts and water across the GI mucosa, the latter being more common. This can be caused for example by bacterial enterotoxins (*Vibrio cholerae*; enterotoxic *Escherichia coli*) and certain laxatives. It often involves a large volume of diarrhoea (>1000ml/day) which does not improve with starvation.
- Inflammatory: loss of mucosal integrity leading often to bloody diarrhoea if the colorectum is involved. All causes of colitis produce diarrhoea predominantly by this method.
- Dysmotility: impaired gut motility can occasionally cause diarrhoea, usually in the setting of ileus or, more commonly, the recovery from ileus, when copious retained water and electrolytes within the small bowel overwhelm the absorptive potential of the colon.

Clinical approach

History

Establish onset, duration, frequency, volume and consistency of stool. Additional characteristics such as colour, bloody, purulent or offensive are helpful. Dietary, drug and travel histories are vital. Past history of GI or immunosuppressive disease should be sought. Systemic symptoms such as fever, anorexia and weight loss may also be present

Examination

Evidence of dehydration, especially tachycardia and hypotension. Abdominal tenderness and especially localized peritonism are a concern and should raise suspicion regarding occult or impending perforation. Abdominal masses (e.g. Crohn's, intra-abdominal abscess) can be present. The abdomen may be distended and tympanitic, which is a concern in colitis. Inspection of the mouth and perineum may give clues to the aetiology of the diarrhoea (e.g. Crohn's), and rectal examination ensures the diarrhoea is not due to overflow from impaction, rectal tumours or pelvic abscesses.

Investigations in acute diarrhoea

Bloods

- *FBC*: raised WCC and differential may help to differentiate bacterial and viral infections
- *U&E*: evidence of renal failure; Na^+ and K^+ losses from the gut. Mg^{2+} and Zn^{2+} are also commonly depleted in prolonged diarrhoea.
- *LFTs*: may identify a protein-losing enteropathy
- *CRP*
- *Blood cultures*

Microbiology

- Stool culture and analysis for *C. difficile* toxin (CDT) in patients who have received antibiotics in the preceding few months. CDT remains positive in patients for some weeks even after successful treatment, and so assessment of recurrent infection is done on clinical grounds.
- *Rigid sigmoidoscopy* to exclude overt colitis, and biopsy to send for histology and culture. Occasionally pseudomembranes can be seen in *C. difficile* infection (pseudomembranous colitis)

Radiology

- *Abdominal X-ray (AXR)*: anyone with systemic features or abdominal tenderness. Repeat regularly if any suspicion of toxic megacolon
- *CXR*: anyone with localized peritonism
- *Flexible sigmoidoscopy* then colonoscopy if diarrhoea persists. Flexible sigmoidoscopy must be carried out with caution in anyone with evidence of acute colitis, and colonoscopy is contraindicated in these circumstances.

Common causes of diarrhoea in the critically ill

These can be summarized as infectious and non-infectious causes.

Infectious causes

Clostridium difficile is the most common infective cause in the critically ill, often due to antibiotic usage, especially cephalosporins and quinolones. In critically ill patients, *C. difficile* diarrhoea progresses to fulminant infective colitis in ~20% of cases. Risk factors include:

- Age >60–65
- Previous use of broad-spectrum antibiotics
- Underlying malignancy
- Renal or pulmonary disease
- Albumin <25mg/ml
- Previous antisecretory treatment proton pump inhibitors

Mortality is ~20% in fulminant pseudomembranous colitis.

Other significant infections include

- Campylobacter spp.
- Escherichia coli
- Salmonella enteritidis; Shigella spp.

Non-infectious causes

Drugs

A large number of drugs can cause diarrhoea, although antibiotics are the biggest cause in critically unwell patients. This is probably due to the reduction in GI bacterial load leading to an increased luminal carbohydrate concentration.

Supplementary feeding-related diarrhoea

The use of nasogastric/jejunal feeds is a well-recognized cause of diarrhoea. This may be due to high sodium content or concentrated feeds, leading to high osmolarity.

However, reducing the osmolarity of the feed seems to have little effect on the diarrhoea. A recent meta-analysis suggested enteral nutrition was no more likely to cause diarrhoea than parenteral nutrition.

Intestinal ischaemia

This can occur after particular operations (e.g. abdominal aortic aneurysm repair), but also as the result of splanchnic hypoperfusion in shocked patients on inotropes.

Overflow diarrhoea in pseudo-obstruction or impaction

Both faecal impaction and pseudo-obstruction can occur in critically ill patients. The former is often as a result of heavy opiate use coupled with immobility, and the latter as a result of systemic illness in any individual, but especially those immobile and neurologically impaired. This can be diagnosed by a combination of clinical examination which can mimic bowel obstruction and a cavernous rectum on per rectum examination. Copious gas and liquid are often released on per rectum examination, and a rigid sigmoidoscopy or contrast studies can be used to confirm the diagnosis.

Management

This depends upon the aetiology. The first step is resuscitation of a potentially dehydrated patient with electrolyte imbalance, especially hypokalaemia.

Infectious causes

Most GI infections are responsive to ciprofloxacin or metronidazole, and these can be used whilst waiting for sensitivities if infection is suspected. The treatment of *C. difficile* is with IV or oral metronidazole or oral vancomycin. IV vancomycin is not suitable. More recently oral and IV teicoplanin have been used. Recurrence rate is ~20%, but most will again respond to a 2nd course of antibiotics.

Non-infectious causes

Cessation of the offending drugs and slowing NG feeds is the treatment for diarrhoea caused by these agents. Occasionally a change in regimen is all that is required. Continuous pump-driven feeds as opposed to intermittent enteral feeding are beneficial in this respect. There seems to be no difference in rates of diarrhoea between gastric and jejunal feeding sites. Enriching enteral feeds with soluble fibre has also been shown to reduce the incidence and severity of diarrhoea in the critically ill. Pseudo-obstruction and faecal impaction can both be treated by limiting opioid drugs as much as possible and by a short course of stimulant oral and rectal laxatives. However, treatment of the underlying cause is essential to prevent recurrence. In intractable cases of pseudo-obstruction, 2mg neostigmine has been used with some success. Once infection and overflow have been excluded, an antimotility agent such as loperamide can be used, building up to 16mg daily.

Further reading

Bricker E, Garg R,Nelson R, *et al.* Antibiotic treatment for Clostridium difficile-associated diarrhea in adults. *Cochrane Database Syst Rev* 2005; (1): CD004610.

Gramlich L, Kichian K, Pinilla J, *et al.* Does enteral nutrition compared to parenteral nutrition result in better outcomes in critically ill adult patients? A systematic review of the literature. *Nutrition* 2004; 20: 843–8.

Montejo JC, Grau T, Acosta J, *et al.* Multicenter, prospective, randomized, single-blind study comparing the efficacy and gastrointestinal complications of early jejunal feeding with early gastric feeding in critically ill patients. *Crit Care Med* 2002; 30: 796–800.

Ponec RJ, Saunders MD, Kimmey MB. Neostigmine for the treatment of acute colonic pseudo-obstruction. *N Engl J Med* 1999; 341: 137–41.

Shang E, Geiger N, Sturm JW, *et al.* Pump-assisted versus gravity-controlled enteral nutrition in long-term percutaneous endoscopic gastrostomy patients: a prospective controlled trial. *JPEN J Parenter Enteral Nutr* 2003; 27: 216–9.

Sheth SG, LaMont JT. Gastrointestinal problems in the chronically critically ill patient. *Clin Chest Med* 2001; 22: 135–47.

Spapen H, Diltoer M, Van Malderen C, *et al.* Soluble fiber reduces the incidence of diarrhea in septic patients receiving total enteral nutrition: a prospective, double-blind, randomized, and controlled trial. *Clin Nutr* 2001; 20: 301–5.

Steevens EC, Lipscomb AF, Poole GV, *et al.* Comparison of continuous vs intermittent nasogastric enteral feeding in trauma patients: perceptions and practice. *Nutr Clin Pract* 2002; 17: 118–22.

Upper gastrointestinal haemorrhage (non-variceal)

Definition

Generally accepted to mean bleeding arising from anywhere between the proximal oesophagus and the ligament of Treitz (duodenojejunal flexure).

Clinical features

Upper GI bleeding typically presents with haematemesis and/or melaena. Fresh blood can appear unaltered per rectum (haemochezia) although this degree and rapidity of upper GI bleeding is usually accompanied by obvious haemodynamic compromise. The jet black, tarry appearance of melaena and its characteristically pungent smell is usually sufficient to distinguish it from the dark, often maroon colour and less offensive odour of more distal, colonic bleeding. The only sign in the critical care setting may be blood in nasogastric aspirates. Despite advances in endoscopic management, overall mortality remains at 8–10%.

Causes

- Peptic ulcer—duodenal or gastric (50–70%)
- Mallory Weiss tear
- Erosive gastritis/oesophagitis
- Dieulafoy lesions
- Stress-related mucosal damage
- Upper GI malignancy
- Vascular malformations (telangiectasia, gastric antral vascular ectasia (GAVE or watermelon stomach))
- Gastrointestinal stromal tumours (GISTs)

Risk factors

- *Helicobacter pylori*
- NSAIDs
- Aspirin
- Critical care.

Initial assessment

Severity is related to patient's age, co-morbidities, haemodynamic status, diagnosis and risk of rebleeding as assessed endoscopically. These can be quantified using the Rockall score (see Table 20.4.1). Early risk stratification into low and high risk groups is important for proper management, and allows prompt and safe discharge of patients in low risk groups.

Management

Management can be considered in a number of stages:-

Resuscitation

- Large bore IV access, urinary catheter.
- Bloods: FBC, U&Es (a raised urea:creatinine ratio indicates breakdown of blood in the GI tract, and hence an upper GI source), LFTs, cross-match, prothrombin time
- IV fluids (avoid normal saline if evidence of chronic liver disease)—otherwise no clear evidence for crystalloid vs colloid.
- Blood transfusion—f haemoglobin <10g/dl or signs of significant active haemorrhage.

Diagnosis

- Endoscopy—ideally within 24h in a mild/moderate bleed, and as soon as patient adequately resuscitated in severe bleeds. Ideally this should be in a fully equipped endoscopy suite with experienced staff, but severe bleeds in unstable patients require endoscopy in theatre with full monitoring/resuscitation equipment available and anaesthetic personnel present to ensure airway protection and provide general anaesthesia if required. There should be facilities to proceed directly to surgery if required. In young, fit patients with minor bleeds, endoscopy can be performed as an out-patient.
- Angiography/CT angiography—can be helpful if bleeding source not evident at endoscopy.

Immediate control of bleeding:

- Endoscopic injection with 1:10 000 adrenaline 4–16ml in quadrants around bleeding point. Usually reserved for ulcers with major stigmata of recent haemorrhage (see Table 20.4.1). Also for vascular lesions, Dieulafoy lesions. Fibrin glue/thrombin also effective but not widely available. Adherent clots should be dislodged by irrigation to allow appropriate treatment of underlying lesion. Consider repeat endoscopic therapy for rebleeding, or early planned repeat (12–24h) if suboptimal views/haemostatic results from initial procedure. Other endoscopic options include:
- Heat application—heater probes, multipolar caogulation (BICAP)—as effective as injection therapy, and some evidence of additional effectiveness if used in combination with adrenaline injection in active arterial bleeding.
- Mechanical clips—effective but need familiarity with use and can be tricky to deploy accurately, especially in duodenum.
- Surgery—for uncontrolled bleeding or significant rebleeds. Control of bleeding by simple under-running of vessel, although ligation of gastroduodenal/right gastroepiploic arteries may be required to achieve full control of duodenal ulcer bleed. Vagotomy unnecessary with advent of PPIs. Formal gastrectomy/ulcer excision are options for bleeding gastric ulcers, although simple under-running may be prudent in an unstable patient. May be required for bleeding gastric carcinoma/stromal tumour. Recurrent bleeding from the duodenal ulcer despite under-running may necessitate antrectomy, ideally with duodenal closure excluding the ulcer crater.
- Angiographic embolization (coils, foam)—generally reserved for complicated anatomy (e.g. post-surgical, pancreatic pseudoaneurysms), high anaesthetic risk patients, failed endoscopic/surgical treatment

Prevention of re-bleeding/future bleeding

Ulcers

- PPIs—given IV reduce risk of rebleeding and need for surgery, although no evidence for reduction in all-cause mortality. Profound gastric acid suppression (pH >6) best achieved with high dose IV PPI (e.g. IV omeprazole 80mg stat followed by 8mg/h infusion for 72h). This produces optimal conditions for clot stabilization, although overall evidence for superiority over other dosage regimes, e.g. once-daily IV PPI, is lacking.
- *Helicobacter pylori* eradication—90% of duodenal ulcers and 70% of gastric ulcers are *H. pylori* related. Eradication highly effective and further bleeding episodes rare.
- Discontinue NSAIDs, aspirin. If undesirable to stop NSAIDs, change to least damaging (e.g. ibuprofen) and continue PPI indefinitely.

Table 20.4.1 Severity scoring system for upper GI haemorrhage.

	Score			
Variable	**0**	**1**	**2**	**3**
Age (yrs)	**<60**	**60–79**	**≥80**	
Shock	No shock (SBP>100, pulse <100)	Tachycardia (systolic BP>100, pulse>100)	Hypotension (SBP <100, pulse >100)	
Co-morbidity	Nil major		Cardiac failure, ischaemic heart disease, any major co-morbidity	Renal failure, liver failure, disseminated malignancy
Diagnosis	Mallory Weiss tear, no lesion, no SRH	All other diagnoses	Malignancy of upper GI tract	
Major SRH	None or dark spot		Blood in upper GI tract, adherent clot, visible or spurting vessel	

Each variable is scored.

SRH = stigmata of recent haemorrhage.

Initial score 0-2 (low risk) 1% mortality, 3–5 (medium risk) 9% mortality, 6–7 (high risk) 17% mortality.

- Repeat endoscopy—unnecessary for *H. pylori*-related duodenal ulcers, but recommended for gastric ulcers to ensure healing and exclude malignancy (initially ~6/52 post-bleed), and for those continuing on NSAIDs.

Vascular malformations/Dieulafoy lesions:

- Usually respond to heater probe or argon plasma coagulation. May require multiple treatments, especially GAVE if extensive.

Malignancy

- External beam radiotherapy can be highly effective at controlling bleeding from gastric adenocarcinoma. Argon plasma coagulation/alcohol injection less effective.
- GISTs best treated by surgical excision but if metastatic or patient unfit consider GLIVEC.

Stress-related mucosal damage in critical care patients

- Mucosal ischaemia from splanchnic hypoperfusion exacerbated by positive pressure ventilation.
- Incidence of clinically significant bleeds probably <5%, but significantly increased mortality if occurs.
- Preventive measures include early enteral feeding and routine prophylaxis in high risk patients (>48h mechanical ventilation, coagulopathy, renal failure).
- H_2-receptor antagonists (e.g. ranitidine), sucralfate and PPIs (nasogastric, or more recently V) all effective in reducing clinically significant bleeds, with no firm evidence showing superiority of any one approach.

Further reading

Barkun A, Bardou M Marshall JK. Consensus recommendations for managing patients with nonvariceal upper gastrointestinal bleeding. *Ann Intern Med* 2003; 139: 843–57.

Lau JYW, Sung JJY, Lee KKC, *et al.* Effect of intravenous omeprazole on recurrent bleeding after endoscopic treatment of bleeding peptic ulcers. *N Engl J Med* 2000; 343: 310–6.

Leontiadis GI, Sharma VK, Howden CW. Proton pump inhibitor treatment for acute peptic ulcer bleeding. *Cochrane Database Syst Rev* 2006; (1): CD002094.

Stollman N, Metz DC. Pathophysiology and prophylaxis of stress ulcer in intensive care unit patients. *J Crit Care* 2005; 1: 35–45.

Bleeding varices

Gastro-oesophageal varices are present in ~50% of patients with cirrhosis. The incidence of bleeding from varices is between 5 and 15% per year. Despite advances in medical and endoscopic therapy, acute variceal bleeding is a medical emergency that carries an immediate mortality of 8% and a 20% chance of death after 6 weeks. Rarely, varices may develop secondary to portal or splenic vein thrombosis. The prognosis of patients with variceal bleeding secondary to non-cirrhotic portal hypertension is better than that of patients with cirrhosis once the acute episode is controlled. International guidelines for the management of patients with variceal bleeding have been published.

Assessment of the patient with variceal bleeding

Varices should be assumed to be the cause of upper GI bleeding in all patients with chronic liver disease until proven otherwise. The initial clinical assessment should focus upon haemodynamic state and resuscitation requirement. Patients with chronic liver disease have a high baseline cardiac output with reduced SVR, and are prone to hypotension. Encephalopathy may develop as a consequence of the bleed or a consequence of the decompensating illness.

Blood should be sent for FBC, clotting, renal and liver function. Cross-matched blood and clotting factors should be readily available (see below). Once the patient is stabilized, portal vein Doppler ultrasound to establish the direction of flow and to rule out thrombosis may be helpful.

General measures in management of variceal bleeding

Adequate IV access, with wide-bore peripheral cannulae, should be obtained as a priority. Standard practice is to inset two 14G cannulae on the antecubital fossae. CVP monitoring may be useful in guiding resuscitation, but absolute pressures may be falsely elevated in patients with ascites. The response of CVP (or mixed venous saturation) to a fluid load remains a useful measure.

Encephalopathy is common in cirrhotic patients and may be a consequence of the bleed or associated pathology. It is standard practice to give regular lactulose to prevent encephalopathy, although this recommendation is not evidence based. Endotracheal intubation may be necessary to ensure airway protection and is strongly recommended if prolonged therapeutic endoscopy or placement of a Sengstaken–Blakemore tube is planned.

Resuscitation

There is experimental evidence that vigorous resuscitation may provoke rebleeding and increase mortality. Published international guidelines therefore promote prompt but cautious blood volume resuscitation with the aim of maintaining haemodynamic stability, adequate renal and cerebral perfusion and a haemoglobin of ~8g/dl.

Correction of coagulopathy

Coagulopathy and thrombocytopaenia are common in patients with decompensated chronic liver disease. FFP should be infused if the prothrombin time is prolonged. Cryoprecipitate may be given if there is hypofibrinogenaemia. Recombinant activated factor VII did not improve outcome relative to standard therapy in a multi-centre placebo-controlled trial. A *post hoc* analysis of a subpopulation of patients with advanced liver disease and variceal bleeding did show reduced rebleeding and mortality. Platelet transfusion may be indicated if the platelet count is significant reduced.

Antibiotics

Bacterial infections may both precipitate and complicate variceal bleeding in patients with end-stage liver disease. Empiric antibiotic therapy reduces the risk of rebleeding and mortality from acute variceal haemorrhage. Broad-spectrum antibiotics with good Gram-negative cover such as a quinolone, third-generation cephalosporin or extended spectrum penicillin should be given routinely. The exact agent will depend upon local resistance patterns.

Balloon tamponade

In cases where endoscopic control of bleeding is not possible or when it will be some time before endoscopy will be possible, the use of balloon tamponade may be considered. Once passed, the gastric balloon of the Sengstaken–Blakemore tube should be inflated with water (± soluble contrast medium) and gentle traction applied by taping the tube to the side of the face. Effective control of bleeding will occur in 80–90% of cases. The risk of complications including oesophageal necrosis and perforation are high; therefore, definitive therapy must be performed within 24h. There is no evidence that the routine cooling of such tubes prior to use is helpful.

Medical reduction of portal pressure

Vasopressin is a potent splanchnic and peripheral vasoconstrictor that has been shown to reduce portal pressure. It has a short plasma half-life and must be given as a continuous infusion. It may be appropriate to give concurrent IV nitrates to ameliorate peripheral vasoconstriction. Terlipressin is a longer acting synthetic vasopressin analogue that can be given as a 4-hourly bolus. It is associated with fewer side effects than vasopressin. Somatostatin and analogues such as octreotide may also be given to reduce portal pressure in variceal bleeding.

Pharmacological therapy to reduce portal pressure is the first-line treatment in the management of variceal bleeding and should be initiated as soon as the diagnosis is suspected. Vasoactive drugs should continue for 2–5 days to reduce the risk of rebleeding.

Although propranolol is proven to reduce the risk of bleeding, β-blockade will reduce blood pressure and ameliorate the compensatory tachycardia induced by hypovolaemia. It is therefore contraindicated in the setting of an acute bleed but should be started once the initial episode is resolved.

Endoscopic therapy

Endoscopy is both diagnostic and therapeutic, and should be performed urgently once the patient has been transfused and stabilized. Guidelines recommend endoscopy is performed within 12h of admission to hospital.

A meta-analysis of 10 RCTs showed superior early control of bleeding from oesophageal varices with endoscopic band ligation relative to sclerotherapy. Variceal band ligation is the recommended form of endoscopic therapy, but sclerotherapy should be performed if band ligation is not technically feasible.

Bleeding from gastric varices is harder to control than bleeding from oesophageal varices. Injection of cyanoacrylate tissue glue is effective in achieving haemostasis and prevents rebleeds. Not all endoscopists are experienced in the use of tissue glue, and in this case consideration should be given to temporary balloon tamponade prior to transfer or definitive therapy.

Salvage therapy

Rebleeding from oesophageal varices, defined as further haematemesis or ongoing transfusion requirements >2h after endoscopic therapy, should be managed by repeat therapeutic endoscopy. If this is unsuccessful, consideration should be given to creation of a portal–systemic shunt. This may be performed radiologically (TIPS) or surgically. The aim is to reduce the portal venous pressure to <12mm Hg. Early TIPS and surgery have been shown to improve survival in high risk patients. The performance of both surgery and TIPS is dependent upon local expertise. All shunt procedures carry a risk of chronic encephalopathy.

TIPS is effective in control of gastric variceal bleeding in 90% of cases. The threshold for TIPS should be lower in bleeding from gastric than oesophageal varices.

Rectal varices

Bleeding from rectal varices is uncommon, and the evidence base of most treatments is limited. In addition to resuscitation and the correction of coagulopathy, empiric antibiotics and pharmacological therapy to reduce portal pressure should be given. Endoscopic therapy with band ligation or sclerotherapy can be attempted but may lead to recurrent bleeding from iatrogenic ulceration. Local tamponade with a urinary catheter inserted per rectum is effective but carries a significant risk of local necrosis if the balloon is left inflated. TIPS is effective in uncontrollable bleeding.

Further reading

Bosch J, Thabut D, Bendtsen F, *et al.* Recombinant factor VIIa for upper gastrointestinal bleeding in patients with cirrhosis: a randomized, double-blind trial. *Gastroenterology* 2004; 127: 1123-30.

de Franchis R. Evolving consensus in portal hypertension. Report of the Baveno IV consensus workshop on methodology of diagnosis and therapy in portal hypertension. *J Hepatol* 2005; 43: 167–76.

Garcia-Pagan JC, Bosch J. Endoscopic band ligation in the treatment of portal hypertension. *Nature Clin Pract* 2005; 2: 526–35.

Garcia-Tsao G, Sanyal AJ, Grace ND, *et al.* Prevention and management of gastroesophageal varices and variceal hemorrhage in cirrhosis. *Hepatology* 2007; 46: 922–38.

Vangeli M, Patch D, Terreni N, *et al.* Bleeding ectopic varices—treatment with transjugular intrahepatic porto-systemic shunt (TIPS) and embolisation. *J Hepatol* 2004; 41: 560–6.

Intestinal perforation

Patients suffering perforation of a GI viscus may present to the ICU under a variety of circumstances. Acute presentation is common when perforation is the primary diagnosis. However, perforation may also develop as a secondary phenomenon complicating critical illness.

GI perforation is associated with the development of sepsis. In addition, such a patient may undergo the further insult of surgical intervention to treat the underlying cause.

Whilst sepsis is a final common pathway following perforation, its presentation depends on the specific anatomical site. As such, there may be a variety of different signs, symptoms and investigative findings. The degree of sepsis also varies with the site of perforation, as the stomach and duodenal contents provide a fairly sterile, albeit highly caustic fluid, compared with the high bacterial load experienced in faecal peritonitis, a difference reflected in morbidity and mortality figures.

Causes

- Inflammation
  - Erosive, e.g. peptic ulcer, drug or chemical erosions
  - Autoimmune, e.g. Crohn's or vasculitides
  - Infective, e.g. diverticulitis, cholecystitis, *C. difficile* colitis
  - Ischaemia, e.g. Ischaemic colitis
  - Radiation, e.g. Radiotherapy
  - Unknown, e.g. Appendicitis
- Neoplastic, e.g. carcinoma of the colon
- Iatrogenic, e.g. endoscopy, anastomotic leak
- Trauma, e.g. blunt force or Boerhaave syndrome
- Mechanical, e.g. obstruction or pseudo-obstruction

Clinical approach

Presenting complaint

Primary presentations

As the majority of the GI tract is in the abdomen, symptoms of perforation are usually those of peritonitis. Pain is a common complaint, constant in nature and exacerbated by movement. Less commonly the oesophagus is perforated and a patient may complain only of pain in the chest or neck. Both groups of patients may suffer respiratory compromise either due to pain on movement of the diaphragm or due to pleural effusion, which is likely in oesophageal perforation.

Secondary presentations

Intestinal perforation may occur secondary to a period of critical illness. Pseudomembranous colitis presents with diarrhoea, either in immunocompromised patients or associated with antibiotics used to treat a previous source of sepsis. The colon becomes colonized with *C. difficile*, which causes diarrhoea by producing enterotoxins and cytotoxins.

The major risk factor for erosive gastritis is respiratory failure especially due to sepsis. It is suggested that erosive gastritis may occur as a result of compromised mucosal blood flow during critical illness, and raised end-expiratory pressures during ventilation decrease blood flow further. This prevents normal healing and also results in a decreased production of protective factors such as prostaglandins.

Drug history

A variety of drugs can lead to perforation. Commonly NSAIDs and steroids cause gastric or duodenal erosions, but this may also occur with other drugs such as methotrexate. Broad-spectrum antibiotics, chemotherapy or immunosuppressive medication can lead to pseudomembranous colitis which may perforate if megacolon develops.

Examination

- Signs of peritonitis
  - Rigid abdomen
  - Guarding
  - Percussion tenderness
- Distended abdomen
- Absent bowel sounds
- Shock secondary to sepsis
- Subcutaneous emphysema
- Loss of liver dullness to percussion

Peritonism may be absent in patients taking steroids or sedatives, or obese or frail elderly patients.

Investigations

Biochemical

Testing serum amylase is vital in the acute abdomen. This is a non-specific test, with values elevated in almost any acute abdominal pathology, but it is very rare for levels to be as high as 4 times the upper limit of normal as would be expected in pancreatitis. Pancreatitis must be excluded as it will initially contraindicate surgery.

Non-specific markers of inflammation such as CRP may be elevated, and electrolyte abnormalities or evidence of acute renal failure should be sought. A low albumin may be an indicator of both chronic and acute ill health.

Haematology

Other non-specific markers of inflammation and infection such as increased or decreased levels of either leucocytes or platelets may be present. Clotting abnormalities require correction, and preparations should be made to ensure that any required blood products are available, particularly if surgery becomes necessary.

Radiology

Plain X-ray is of some use in the initial work-up of patients. The classic feature of intraperitoneal perforation leads to free gas under the diaphragm on erect CXR in 80% of cases. In oesophageal perforations, a pneumomediastinum may be demonstrated. Gas will be seen in up to 60% of abdominal films, and normally only a supine film is available. Rigler's sign is the radiological effect of air on both sides of the bowel wall. Free gas also becomes visible against the contrasting density of the liver. Gas may highlight the inferior border of the liver or the ligamentum teres, or may be seen as bubbles between the liver and the anterior abdominal wall. If gas collects in the pouch of Rutherford Morrison, a triangular bubble may also be seen just medial and inferior to the 11th rib.

CT scanning has largely replaced contrast studies due to rapid advances in technology. However, water-soluble contrast studies remain useful in specific circumstances when free gas is expected to be present within a body cavity. This applies to situations when the peritoneum has been recently opened during surgery or during chest trauma, when a pneumothorax may co-exist with a ruptured oesophagus.

Treatment options

Conservative

Any septic collection must be adequately drained. If a cervical or thoracic perforation is particularly small, does not produce major sepsis and does not enter the pleural space it may be allowed to drain into the oesophagus whilst a NG tube drains the stomach. Intra-abdominal perforations can sometimes become walled off within an inflammatory mass. Examples of this include diverticular and appendix masses which are sometimes treated with IV antibiotics, enabling resolution of the inflammation prior to elective resection. Surgery may sometimes be avoided with the use of radiologically guided drains placed in intra-abdominal collections.

Operative

Oesophageal perforations in the cervical portion require drains placed at operation. If the perforation lies in the thoracic portion, a variety of treatment options are possible, including repair, diversion, diversion and exclusion or stenting. Common to these is the necessity to drain the pleural cavity using a large bore chest drain.

Intra-abdominal perforations will cause soiling of the peritoneum that must be washed out and drained. Decontamination of the abdominal cavity is followed by repair of the perforation, whose size and site will determine the nature of surgery performed. A small gastric or duodenal ulcer can be oversewn with an omental patch and this can be performed as an open or laparoscopic procedure. Small bowel perforation may be closed or a segment excised with primary anastomosis. Colonic perforation may be associated with major contamination, and segmental resection may be necessary. Traditionally, primary anastomosis is not performed because of the risk of anastomotic dehiscence. Instead the proximal colon is exteriorized as a colostomy (Hartman's procedure) and the rectal stump either exteriorized as a mucous fistula or simply oversewn. A Hartman's procedure can be reversed electively when the inflammatory process has completely settled, some 6–12 months later. A defunctioning ileostomy does not reduce the risk of a colonic perforation but mitigates against the effects should it occur. Subsequent reversal of an ileostomy is a relatively simple procedure which can be carried out a few weeks later and which rarely requires a full laparotomy.

In cases of severe contamination and inflammation, a laparostomy may be formed, whereby the laparotomy wound is left open and a 'Bogota' plastic bag or a vacuum dressing is sewn into the wound to maintain the moist, sterile environment in the abdomen. This allows the abdomen to be accessed for further washout and it provides an increased volume in the abdomen, thereby preventing abdominal compartment syndrome, which may occur when the abdomen is closed tightly over very inflamed and oedematous bowel. The laparaostomy can either be closed on return to theatre when the swelling has settled or can be closed over time with the assistance of a suction dressing.

Pseudomembranous colitis is normally successfully treated with conservative measures alone. However, should the patient develop a toxic megacolon, surgery may be considered to prevent or treat perforation or simply to remove the source of sepsis. There is no evidence for treating the colonic distension with colonoscopy, as might be done in psuedo-obstruction. Total colectomy and formation of ileostomy is the operation of choice, but mortality is high. Survival is improved with early surgery, but the morbidity and mortality associated with surgery make the decision to operate a matter of delicate timing.

Further reading

Chase CW, Barker DE, Russell WL, *et al.* Serum amylase and lipase in the evaluation of acute abdominal pain. *Am Surg* 1996; 62: 1028–33.

Koss K, Clark MA, Sanders DS, *et al.* The outcome of surgery in fulminant Clostridium difficile colitis. *Colorectal Dis* 2006; 8: 149–54.

Rubesin SE, Levine MS. Radiologic diagnosis of gastrointestinal perforation. *Radiol Clin North Am* 2003; 41: 1095–115,

Stollman N, Metz DC. Pathophysiology and prophylaxis of stress ulcer in intensive care unit patients. *J Crit Care* 2005; 20: 35–45.

Williams N, Everson NW. Radiological confirmation of intraperitoneal free gas. *Ann R Coll Surg Engl* 1997; 79: 8–12.

Intestinal obstruction

The generic term intestinal obstruction includes both small and large bowel obstruction. Untreated, obstruction may lead to perforation, discussed in Chapter 20.6. Large bowel is at risk of perforation if it becomes overdistended, whilst the small bowel will tend to perforate at an area of stricture or ischaemia created by the cause of the obstruction or venous congestion.

Obstructed bowel represents a single organ failure and leads to an array of metabolic sequelae that can necessitate a higher level of care. Patients may also require intensive monitoring following the operative management of the obstruction, which is often the only curative option.

Causes

Mechanical obstruction of the bowel will generally be caused by factors either within the bowel lumen, e.g. impacted foreign bodies, including faeces and gallstones; factors in the bowel wall, such as benign and malignant strictures; or factors outside the bowel wall, such as hernias, adhesions and congenital bands. Falling somewhere between these two final groups are problems such as volvulus and intussusception.

Ileus and pseudo-obstruction are conditions that are not distinguished as separate entities in continental Europe, and no biochemical distinction has been described. However, the terminology may be useful to describe the differing severity of a predictable dysmotility of the bowel, perhaps following surgery, and the progressive distension originally described by Ogilvie .

Clinical approach

History

Clinical presentation depends on the level of obstruction. More proximal ('higher') obstruction tends to lead to colicky abdominal pain and early onset of vomiting with relatively little abdominal distension. Small bowel obstruction presents in this manner. Vomitus is bilious if the obstruction lies distal to the sphincter of Oddi, and will appear increasingly faeculent at levels further down the ileum and colon. Unless there is a fistula between the small and large bowel the onset of faeculent vomiting will be a relatively late symptom. More distal ('lower') obstruction may present with insidious constipation, abdominal distension and relatively little pain or vomiting. Diarrhoea may be a sign of impending or subacute obstruction, whereas absolute constipation indicates established obstruction. In small bowel obstruction, constipation may be a late event. In general terms, vomiting tends to be the presenting feature in small bowel obstruction and constipation in large bowel obstruction.

In established intestinal obstruction, constant pain may simply reflect abdominal distension, but it may herald ischaemia indicative of impending perforation.

Past medical history

The two most common causes of small bowel obstruction in developed countries are abdominal hernias and post-surgical adhesions. Colorectal and gynaecological surgery are frequently associated with the development of post-surgical adhesions. Appendicectomy and pouch surgery are notorious for severe and extensive adhesions. A history of persistent change in bowel habit, weight loss and rectal bleeding could point to a colonic malignancy or inflammatory bowel disorder with associated stricturing.

Upper GI malignancy sometimes presents with obstruction and a history of dysphagia or early satiety. Non-bowel-related intra-abdominal malignancies may impinge on small bowel or colon, and are relevant in a comprehensive history.

Pseudo-obstruction can be initiated by various factors including electrolyte disturbance, hypothyroidism, sepsis or simply old age. Surgery itself, anaesthesia, analgesia and analgesic medication may all contribute to electrolyte disturbance. It is particularly common in the ICU setting because of the amalgamation of many of these factors.

Examination

- Evidence of dehydration
- Distended abdomen
- Irreducible hernias
- Non-specific tenderness
- Specific left iliac fossa tenderness (closed-loop obstruction)
- Palpable mass or lymphadenopathy, e.g. on per rectum examination
- Tympanic percussion
- Tinkling bowel sounds
- Absent bowel sounds

Investigations

Although a microcytic anaemia might suggest an underlying GI inflammatory or malignant process, routine blood tests are required to identify biochemical or haematological disturbances rather than to establish the diagnosis.

Radiology

Plain radiograph may reveal dilated loops of bowel and an absence of gas distal to the obstruction. Sometimes gas and fluid levels are visible. Small bowel loops are dilated if >3cm wide, and large bowel should be <6cm except at the caecum where 9cm is the acceptable limit. The specific point of colonic obstruction is often difficult to assess accurately on plain radiograph.

Occasionally, an obstructing hernia can be seen on plain films, and a soft tissue mass may be seen with intussusception. An important sign to note is the 'coffee bean sign' seen with closed-loop obstructions as these inevitably require urgent surgical decompression.

Contrast studies in small bowel obstruction may seem something of a paradox, but in adhesional obstruction water-soluble contrast passing through to the caecum within 4–8h of ingestion suggests that the patient has a subacute obstruction that is likely to resolve with conservative measures.

Treatment options

Conservative

The initial priorities are resuscitation and symptom control. Patients are likely to be suffering dehydration, and electrolyte disturbances should be corrected. An NG tube will decompress the stomach and limit vomiting, whilst a urinary catheter will help to assess fluid balance. Adhesional obstruction may settle with these simple measures. Combined surgical and medical gastroenterology care is essential in those patients with inflammatory bowel disease, where systemic steroids and broad-spectrum antibiotic therapy may be effective. There is a role for further immunosuppressive drugs in Crohn's disease, but this must be balanced with the risk of sepsis and so this a specialist decision.

Colonic volvulus can sometimes be reduced by rigid or flexible endoscope, with decompression tube placement if the bowel remains viable.

Pseudo-obstruction will normally resolve with correction of metabolic abnormalities, and neostigmine may promote a return of motility. 80% of severe cases will resolve with colonoscopy and decompression tube insertion, although some require a repeated procedure and there is a 3% risk of perforation each time.

Operative

Surgery is indicated if symptoms fail to settle with conservative measures, although the timing is still a matter of discussion in the literature. Water-soluble contrast studies in adhesional obstruction may indicate whether conservative measures are likely to be successful, but the timing of surgery remains an issue of debate, and requires experience. Specific time scales have been suggested, but none has been widely endorsed. The development of right iliac fossa tenderness in the presence of closed-loop distal colonic obstruction may indicate imminent caecal perforation and requires laparotomy.

Crohn's disease may produce strictures after the initial inflammatory event has settled, and these may require resection and anastomosis if the affected segment is too long to perform a stricturoplasty. Stricturoplasty involves making a longitudinal incision in the bowel wall across the stricture and then sewing the defect back together in a transverse plane. This is preferable for short strictures as it is a smaller operation and preserves bowel length.

High volvulus or malrotation may not resolve with conservative measures and usually require surgery. Delayed surgery for incarcerated hernias simply increases the likelihood of the bowel becoming compromised and resection required.

Obstructing tumours need either resection or a decompression operation, even if there is metastatic disease. Small bowel or right-sided colonic tumours can be excised with primary anastomosis, whereas left-sided colonic tumours are traditionally treated by Hartman's procedure. However, experienced surgeons may perform primary anastomoses, defunctioned by means of an ileostomy. Patients considered not to require resection may benefit from simple defunctioning, or from the positioning of a colonic stent.

Further reading

Abbas S, Bissett IP, Parry BR. Oral water soluble contrast for the management of adhesive small bowel obstruction. *Cochrane Database Syst Rev* 2005; (1): CD004651.

Ogilvie H. Large intestine colic due to sympathetic deprivation. *Br Med J* 1948; 2: 671–3.

Saunders MD, Cappell MS. Endoscopic management of acute colonic pseudo-obstruction. *Endoscopy* 2005; 37: 760–3.

Lower gastrointestinal bleeding

Acute lower GI tract haemorrhage is bleeding originating distal to the ileocaecal valve; however, brisk haemorrhage from the upper GI tract must also be considered.

If bleeding from the anal canal is excluded, then lower GI haemorrhage represents ~20% of all cases of GI haemorrhage. Bleeding due to haemorrhoids is a common occurrence, but only rarely will it cause major haemorrhage necessitating hospitalization.

In most patients, the bleeding is frequently relatively minor amounts, and can be investigated on an out-patient elective basis. This chapter will focus on the more infrequent profuse lower GI haemorrhage which requires urgent investigation and treatment.

Clinical approach

History

- Determine onset of the bleeding, along with its frequency and quantity. Patients and relatives find it difficult to ascertain the latter but using objective measures such as a spoon-full, eggcup-full, cup-full or bowl-full can help. Establish the colour and consistency of the blood; is it mixed in with the stool or just pure blood; are there any clots, etc.
- Ask about any associated symptoms such as a recent change in bowel habit, abdominal pain, weight loss or anorexia.
- Ascertain any previous episodes of GI haemorrhage, and any treatment given.
- Obtain a drug history focusing on any anticoagulant drugs including warfarin, clopidogrel and aspirin.

Examination: key points

The initial approach should be according to the ABCD system as for any critically ill patient, particularly looking for evidence of haemodynamic instability. Pale conjunctivae suggest clinical anaemia. Abdominal tenderness or masses may give clues as to the cause, and rectal examination confirms the presence and nature of blood and again may identify a cause.

Investigations

Bloods: the following should be taken routinely at the time of insertion of 2 large bore IV cannulae

- FBC: to establish haemoglobin and platelet concentration
- U&E: for evidence of renal failure. Note that an isolated elevated urea can indicate upper GI haemorrhage due to breakdown of haemoglobin in the GI tract.
- LFTs: derangement may give clues as to the presence of metastases.
- Clotting: abnormal clotting may be due to anticoagulant drugs, or may indicate the presence of disseminated intravascular coagulation (DIC).
- Group&save: vital to send this off early, and if the need for transfusion is obvious cross-match the necessary amount of blood and clotting products.

Proctoscopy: will confirm the presence of haemorrhoids, and may show evidence of recent bleeding.

Rigid sigmoidoscopy: to examine the rectum and distal sigmoid colon for evidence of mass lesions, colitis or diverticulae, and confirm the presence of blood.

Radiology: dependent on the causes being considered.

- AXR: may show mucosal oedema consistent with inflammatory bowel disease
- CXR: indicated in the presence of localized peritonism to examine for pneumoperitoneum.

Endoscopy: flexible sigmoidoscopy and colonoscopy are both excellent for imaging the colonic mucosa in a well prepared patient; however, visualization can be poor in the presence of profuse ongoing bleeding as clot and faeces will obscure the mucosa. Thus, in the acute setting they have a limited role, but can utilize diathermy or injection therapies to control the source of bleeding if it can be identified.

Arteriography: with bleeding rates of 1.0–1.5ml/min this technique can show extravasation of contrast into the lumen of the bowel and hence identify the source of bleeding. The superior mesenteric artery is selectively catheterized initially as it is usually found to be the source of the bleeding, but should this not be the case the inferior mesenteric artery can then be catheterized. Coil or sponge embolization can be used to arrest bleeding points; however, the risk of ischaemic colitis needs to be borne in mind.

Common causes to consider

The two most common causes are diverticular disease and angiodysplasia, with carcinoma of the colon and inflammatory bowel disease comprising a relatively small percentage of cases. Rarer causes to consider if the above are excluded include a bleeding Meckel's diverticulum, endometriosis and iatrogenic injury following endoscopic investigation of the colon.

Diverticular disease accounts for >50% of cases, with bleeding occurring from the rupture of nutrient vessels passing through the neck of the diverticulae. Vessel rupture is as a result of inflammation of/trauma to the colonic mucosa. The diverticulae are typically acquired herniations of the mucosa and submucosa through the muscularis, seen most commonly in the sigmoid colon (95–98%) although they can extend proximally and involve any part of the GI tract. These diverticulae are diagnosed in the non-acute setting via barium enema or endoscopic examination of the colon. The bleeding rarely needs treatment (<10%) and often stops spontaneously; however, long-term recurrence of the bleeding remains a substantial problem particularly in patients on anticoagulant drugs.

Angiodysplasia is responsible for 5–10% of cases, with bleeding due to overstretched, dilated fragile vessels running in the colonic mucosa. 80% of the vascular malformations occur on the right side of the colon, with the remaining 20% affecting the left-side and the sigmoid colon. Diagnosis requires angiography, as the endoscopic finding of a characteristic cherry-red spot is subtle and easy to miss in the profusely bleeding

Management

Resuscitation

First and foremost, the patient must be assessed and resuciated according to the ABCD approach.

- *Airway and breathing* are not normally a problem, but if there has been severe blood loss the patient can be tachypnoeic with low oxygen saturations due to severe anaemia.

- *Circulation* can be compromised with the patient tachycardic and hypotensive, depending on the volume of blood lost and the patient's ability to compensate for the loss. Two large bore IV cannulae must be sited, and blood taken simultaneously. In the presence of haemodynamic instability rapid infusion of crystalloid fluid should be commenced, whilst waiting for cross-matched blood to be made available. If the patient is severely unstable with ongoing haemorrhage, then O negative blood can be transfused, but this is rarely necessary. An arterial blood gas sample can give immediate information as to the degree of anaemia and acid–base status. A urinary catheter should be sited to monitor urine output in the unstable patient.
- *Disability* is not normally an issue unless the patient is severely hypotensive thus compromising their cerebral perfusion.
- *Exposure* and examination of the abdomen is necessary to elicit any abdominal tenderness or the presence of any masses. Rectal examination will confirm the presence of blood.

Once the patient is adequately resuscitated, then diagnostic tests can proceed as above.

80% of lower GI bleeds will settle spontaneously, and investigation as to the cause can be done electively. For the remainder that don't settle, immediate investigation and treatment is somewhat dependent on the services available locally. As mentioned previously, the role of colonoscopy in the presence of profuse active bleeding is contentious, and, if available, angiography and subsequent embolization is the preferred treatment option. If this is not available and the patient is unstable, then surgery is the only option. Without an identifiable source of bleeding, subtotal colectomy must be performed. If a source has been identified by endoscopy or angiography but not treated, then a targeted colonic resection can be performed aided by on-table washout. Surgery is preferable at an early stage, as mortality is increased with increasing transfusion requirement.

Further reading

Collins D, Worthley L. Acute GI bleeding: part I. *Crit Care Resusc* 2001; 3: 105–16.

Collins D, Worthley L. Acute GI bleeding: part II. *Crit Care Resusc* 2001; 3: 117–24.

Edelman D, Sugawa C. Lower GI bleeding: a review. *Surg Endosc* 2007; 21: 514–20.

Green B, Rockey D, Portwood G, *et al.* Urgent colonoscopy for evaluation and management of acute lower GI hemorrhage: a randomised controlled trial. *Am J Gastroenterol* 2005; 100: 2395–402.

Keeling W, Armstrong P, Stone PA, *et al.* Risk factors for recurrent hemorrhage after successful arterial embolization. *Am Surg* 2006; 72; 802–6.

Lim C, Shridhar I, Tan L, *et al.* Contrast CT in localization of acute lower GI bleeding. *Asian J Surg* 2006; 29: 92–4.

Strate L. Lower GI bleeding: epidemiology and diagnosis. *Gastroenterol Clin North Am* 2005; 34: 643–64.

Colitis

Colitis (and proctitis) describes inflammation of the colon (and rectum) of any aetiology. It usually presents with passing bloody stool with an associated increase in frequency. The consistency of stool often depends on the extent of the disease, with more extensive involvement often leading to an increased looseness of stool. Severe proctitis can, in fact, present with constipation, although the patient often passes blood and mucus independent of stool in these situations. Abdominal pain is more common in more extensive and severe disease and in ischaemic colitis. Systemic symptoms such as fever, anorexia and weight loss are more indicative of severe ulcerative colitis (UC) or Crohn's.

Abdominal examination is often unremarkable apart from mild tenderness. **Significant tympanitic distension or any evidence of peritonism are of great concern and need urgent attention.**

Differential diagnosis

See Figure 20.9.1.

- Ulcerative colitis
- Crohn's colitis
- Infective
  - Recent contact with infectious patient
  - *E. coli*, *Salmonella*, *Shigella*, *Campylobacter*, *Yersinia* are common causes
  - Recent antibiotic use; think *C. difficile* infection
- Diverticular colitis
  - Rectum looks normal in these patients
  - Bleeding diverticulae seen on endoscopy or diverticular disease noted on CT scan
- Radiation

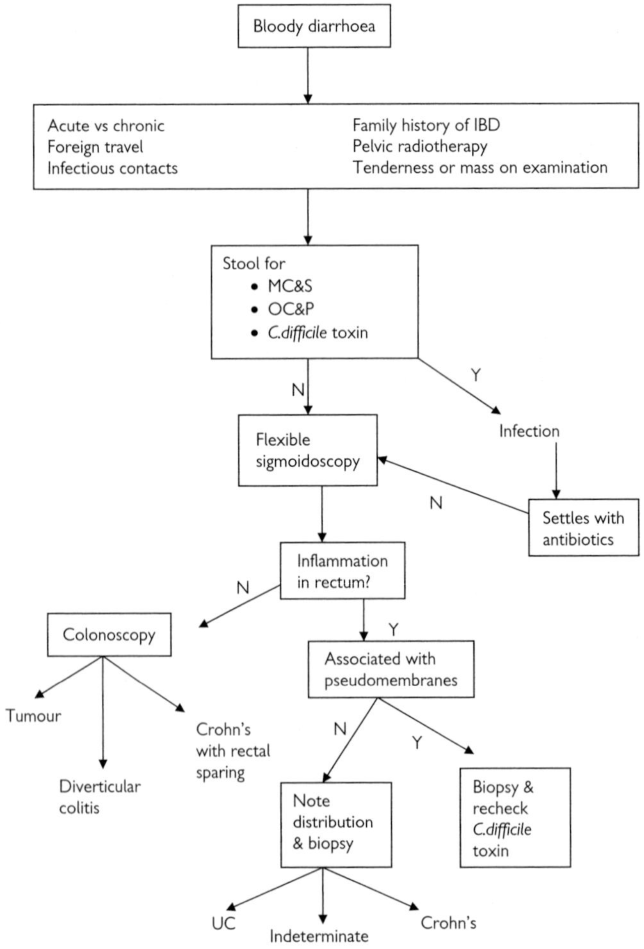

Fig. 20.9.1 Colitis flowchart.

- Ischaemic
  - Older person with known vascular disease or recent surgery for an abdominal aneurysm.
  - Often associated with significant abdominal pain
- Beçhet's enterocolitis
  - Associated past history of genital ulceration, arthropathy, uveitis

Investigation

Bloods

- Raised CRP, ESR, white cell count
- Low Hb, albumin
- Renal function in all patients presenting with severe acute colitis
- Autoantibodies if remaining doubts about diagnosis

Radiology

- AXR: vital in cases of severe acute colitis to exclude toxic dilatation of the colon. Oedema of the bowel wall can be seen as 'thumbprinting'.
- Erect CXR: f any suspicion of perforation

Other

- Cautious sigmoidoscopy and biopsy for histology
- Stool culture for: microscopy culture and sensitivity/ova and parasites/*C. difficile*

Management of severe acute colitis

Severe attacks are characterized by

- Stool frequency >6 times per day plus 1 of the following:
- Temperature >37.8°C
- Pulse >90bpm
- Hb < 10.5g/dl
- ESR >30mm/h

Management depends on the aetiology, but should include

- Frequent clinical evaluation including stool charts by gastroenterologists, surgeons & intensivists
- Daily blood (FBC, CRP, electrolytes, albumin) assessment
- Daily abdominal radiograph if any suspicion of colonic dilatation.
- IV electrolyte-rich fluid ± blood as required (beware hypokalaemia)
- Avoid antidiarrhoeal drugs (e.g. loperamide, codeine), opioids, anticholinergics and if possible NSAIDs, all of which increase the risk of perforation. Remember that significant pain may indicate perforation.
- Broad-spectrum antibiotics can be used in those showing signs of septic complications, except in bacterial causes where they should be targeted specifically to the infecting organism.

For acute severe UC also consider:

- High dose IV steroids (e.g. hydrocortisone 100mg qds) and topical steroids administered rectally (e.g. prednisolone enemas bd)
- IV cyclosporin if no significant improvement after 3 days, followed by oral cyclosporin when in remission (2mg/kg IV and 4–9mg/kg orally) or oral azathioprine (1.5–2.5mg/kg/day). This has been shown to reduce the colectomy rate in patients not responding to steroids, although there is a high relapse rate once the cyclosporin is stopped.
- Anticoagulation is essential in UC given the increased risk of DVT in these patients (e.g. SC tinazaparin 3500U once daily).
- After 3 days treatment, patients with stool frequency >8/day or a CRP >45 are unlikely to improve without a colectomy.
- Failure to improve within 5 days of treatment or deterioration within that period indicates that surgery is required—usually a subtotal colectomy with preservation of the rectum.

Complications of acute colitis

Toxic megacolon

Non-obstructive dilatation of colon >6cm in conjunction with pancolitis and systemic disturbance. Falling incidence. Patients are at greatest risk early after diagnosis—especially during the first attack. Often follows a prolonged attack of drug-resistant acute colitis. Precipitants are believed to include hypokalaemia, opioid analgesics, constipating drugs, anticholinergics and possibly superadded infections such as *C. difficile* and CMV. Examination reveals mild tympanitic distension, but any evidence of localized or generalized peritonism should be an indication for emergency surgery. Perforation has mortality of 40%. Criteria for diagnosis are:

- Diagnosis of colitis
- Radiographic evidence of colonic distension >6cm
- Fever >38°C
- Heart rate >120bpm
- Neutrophilia >10 x 10^9
- One of the following: anaemia, dehydration, electrolyte disturbance, hypotension, reduced GCS

Acute GI haemorrhage

Severe bleeds occurs in <5% of all colitis patients but accounts for ~10% of the emergency colectomies performed for UC. Risk of significant haemorrhage increases with the extent of the disease.

Further reading

Carter MJ, Lobo AJ, Travis SP, *et al.* Guidelines for the management of inflammatory bowel disease in adults. *Gut* 2004; 53 Suppl 5: V1–16.

Dunckley P, Jewell D. Management of acute severe colitis. *Best Pract Res Clin Gastroenterol* 2003; 17: 89–103.

Travis SP, Farrant JM, Ricketts C, *et al.* Predicting outcome in severe ulcerative colitis. *Gut* 1996; 38: 905–10.

Truelove SC, Witts LJ. Cortisone in ulcerative colitis; final report on a therapeutic trial. *Br Med J* 1955; 2: 1041–8.

Van Assche G, D'Haens G, Noman M, *et al.* Randomized, double-blind comparison of 4 mg/kg versus 2 mg/kg intravenous cyclosporine in severe ulcerative colitis. *Gastroenterology* 2003; 125: 1025–31.

Intra-abdominal sepsis

A septic focus present in the abdomen. Peritonitis (inflammation of the serosal membrane that lines the abdominal cavity and organs) may follow. It can be thought of as surgical or non-surgical.

Terminology

May be divided into primary, secondary and tertiary.

- Primary: spontaneous bacterial peritonitis—uncommon, almost exclusively found in patients with liver cirrhosis. Causative organism usually *E. coli*, *Enterococcus* or *Pneumococcus*. Treatment with β-lactam antibiotics.
- Secondary: related to pathological process in a visceral organ which can remain localized or focal, or become generalized, leading to peritonitis; may be further subdivided into operative and non-operative causes.
  - Operative: ruptured viscus—upper or lower bowel perforation, biliary obstruction, appendicitis, diverticulitis.
  - Non-operative: pancreatitis, enteritis, toxic megacolon.
- Tertiary: persistent or recurrent infection after initial treatment (usually laparotomy) has occurred, e.g. abscess and fistulae formation, pancreatic pseudocyst formation. These patients show ongoing sepsis with persistent organ failure and raised inflammatory markers. There may be frankly infected material from drains or they may have positive cultures.

Differential diagnosis

Includes causes of pain and raised inflammatory markers in the abdominal region, identifying problematic organ: bowel, tubo-ovarian, biliary tract and pancreas, renal tract. Importance placed on early identification of operative vs non-operative causes.

Symptoms and signs

- Onset: acute or insidious.
- Spectrum of disease: mild, limited (generally not seen on ICU) to severe systemic/septic shock.
- Sepsis—general malaise, pain, anorexia, nausea, fever
- Non-specific abdominal—pain, diarrhoea, hyperactive bowel sounds, peritonitis.

Investigations

- Blood tests: to aid diagnosis and establish severity of local and systemic illness include: FBC, U&E, glucose, LFT, Ca, amylase, CRP, clotting, lactate.
- ABG for PO_2, PCO_2, acid–base including base deficit.
- Microbiological specimens for culture.
- Radiology:
  1. Primary—ultrasound useful to aid paracentesis, ultrasound Doppler portal flow.
  2. Secondary—beware! In disease relating to bowel pathology CT and ultrasound give limited yield and increase time to laparotomy, which may be crucial.
  3. Tertiary—CT and contrast studies may be helpful in defining bowel leaks and collections which may be amenable to percutaneous drainage or require re-laparotomy.
- Surgery: laparotomy is frequently the investigation and treatment of choice.

Treatment

Principles of treatment are:

1. To correct the underlying cause—rapid surgery crucial if problem surgical.
2. Systemic antibiotics—to limit the infection as soon as possible.
3. Supportive therapy to limit/prevent complications from subsequent organ failure.

Important components are:

- Adequate and early resuscitation
- Broad-spectrum antibiotics—specific antibiotic once organism known.
- Surgery (laparotomy vs laparostomy, see abdominal compartment syndrome below).
- Supportive therapies, e.g. inotropes, respiratory support.
- Nutrition: enteral (consider NJ placement at laparotomy and feeding if NG feeding contraindicated); or parental nutrition.

Special considerations

Abdominal compartment syndrome may occur in the closed septic abdomen. An acute increase in intra-abdominal pressure results in organ dysfunction (especially renal, maybe hypotension or respiratory). The abdominal pressure can be measured via a urinary bladder pressure. If intravesical pressure is >25mm Hg laparostomy is indicated.

Further reading

Hutchins RR, Gunning MP, Lucas DN, *et al.* Relaparotomy for suspected intraperitoneal sepsis after abdominal surgery. *World J Surg* 2004; 28: 137–41.

Malbrain ML, Chiumello D, Pelosi P, *et al.* Prevalence of intra-abdominal hypertension in critically ill patients: a multicentre epidemiological study. *Intens Care Med* 2004; 30: 822–9.

Paugam-Burtz C, Dupont H, Marmuse JP, *et al.* Daily organ-system failure for diagnosis of persistent intra-abdominal sepsis after post-operative peritonitis. *Int. Care Med* 2002; 28: 594–8.

Rogers PN, Wright IH. Postoperative intra-abdominal sepsis. *Br J Surg* 1987; 74: 973–s5

Internet resources

Surviving Sepsis Campaign: `www.survivingsepsis.org`

Pancreatitis

Acute pancreatitis occurs with an incidence of ~100–200 per million of the population and represents a spectrum of disease ranging from a mild to a rapidly progressive illness with multi-organ dysfunction syndrome (MODS). Most patients (80–90%) settle with conservative management of IV fluids and analgesia. Gallstones or alcohol abuse are the most common causes of pancreatitis, and the eventual solution to preventing further attacks of pancreatitis may require cholecystectomy or an alcohol withdrawal programme. Those patients that do not settle with conservative management are a problem and may require the input of the critical care team.

Severe acute pancreatitis (SAP)

10–20% of patients admitted to hospital with pancreatitis will develop SAP. Of these, ~1/3 will develop infected necrosis of the pancreas which carries with it a mortality of up to 80%. In a study by Rau and colleagues in 2000, sterile necrosis was associated with a 33% incidence of multi-organ dysfunction (MOD) and a mortality of 6%, whereas infected necrosis was associated with an incidence of 81% MOD and 62% mortality.

A rise in *serum amylase* and clinical assessment are poor indicators of severity in the first 48h. *Ultrasound* has been used extensively to detect gallstones, but *contrast-enhanced CT* is now the investigation of choice and will detect early abscess formation and necrosis of the pancreas, confirm the diagnosis and reveal gallstones should they be present.

Endoscopic retrograde cholangiopancreatography (ERCP) is employed if available in the presence of jaundice.

The variation in management worldwide triggered the need for a multidisciplinary consensus conference in Washington in 2004 comprising 5 critical care societies:

- European Society of Intensive Care Medicine
- Society of Critical Care Mediciine
- American Thoracic Society
- European Respiratory Society
- Societe de Reanimation de Lange Francais

The aim was to try and simplify and rationalize the management of SAP. Evidence-based recommendations were developed by a jury of 10 people. There were 6 recommendations:

1. Admission to a critical care unit

These patients usually require early and aggressive *fluid resuscitation and adequate analgesia*. The use of epidural blockade has to be tempered by concern around the possiblity of the patients developing a coagulopathy. These patients are at risk of developing MODS and local complications of pancreatitis. They need close supervision and monitoring preferably in a critical care area. Lack of ICU beds may mean they are not admitted to an ICU until they require level 3 care and are often initially managed with the help of an *outreach* team.

Scoring systems used include the Ranson, Imrie and APACHE II.

Routine measurement of all or most of the parameters should be carried out in the first 48h, as well as regular clinical examination and evaluation of the patient with SAP. A Ranson score of >3/11 is associated with a mortality of 60%.

After adequate resuscitation, a CT scan of the abdomen (with IV contrast in the absence of contraindications) should be performed to confirm the diagnosis and, if possible, the CT should be repeated after a few days to identify local complications, such as necrosis which might not be visualized earlier.

2. Role of antibiotics

The routine use of prophylactic antibiotics in patients with necrotizing pancreatitis is not recommended.

Where an infected abscess has been demonstrated following fine needle aspiration (FNA) and in the presence of sepsis elsewhere, antibiotics should be prescribed according to local policies.

Selective decontamination of the digestive system has been proposed for patients with SAP; however, on the available evidence this technique is not routinely recommended. *Candida* infection of the pancreas is an independent risk factor for mortality; in a study by Hoerauf *et al.*, mortality was 12.5% when *Candida* was not grown, but 53.9% with *Candida* present in the pancreas.

3. Nutrition

There is no benefit in the routine use of TPN; early enteral feeding is increasingly used to maintain a high caloric intake. Early feeding via an NJ tube has been advocated as the method of choice and should probably be used, but the NG route should be attempted if this fails. It is reasonable to wait up to 7 days before TPN is started because of failure of the NJ and NG routes. Strict glycaemic control should be used, but the routine use of immune-enhanced feed is not recommended.

4. Indications for surgery

CT-guided FNA is recommended in order to determine whether necrotic pancreatic tissue has become infected. Only in the presence of infected pancreatic tissue and radiological evidence of gas should antibiotics and drainage/debridement be recommended. Drainage and debridement can be achieved percutaneously, laparoscopically or by laparotomy. Where appropriate, operative necrosectomy and/or drainage should be delayed at least 2–3 weeks to allow for demarcation of the necrotic pancreas. Delaying surgery is associated with increased survival; Mier *et al.* in 1997 demonstrated that mortality if surgery is performed in the first 72h is 56%, which reduces to 27% if surgery is delayed by at least 12 days.

5. Management of gallstone induced pancreatitis

Where pancreatitis is accompanied by jaundice, confirmed as obstructive by LFTs, then ERCP is often beneficial in removing a common bile duct stone. Care needs to be exercised to ensure that coagulation is restored to near normal prior to the procedure. If possible, ERCP should be performed within 3 days of admission. If ERCP cannot be accomplished because it is not technically feasible or available, alternative methods of biliary drainage must be considered.

6. Targeting inflammatory response

General measures used in the critically ill including tight blood glucose control, and lung protective ventilation strategies for patients with ALI, should be employed in patients with SAP. In the presence of severe sepsis, the patient with SAP can be managed according to Surviving Sepsis Campaign guidelines. This may necessitate consideration of the use of recombinant activated protein C (even though there is an as yet unproven concern that it may be responsible for causing retroperitoneal haemorrhage in patients with SAP).

Complications

Pancreatic abscess

Early scanning of patients who are failing to progress and appropriate treatment of necrosis should minimize the risk of an abscess forming. Abscess formation can occur some weeks after the initial attack, and rarely appears until the second week. Pain, persistent temperature, nausea, vomiting and a palpable mass could be indicators of either an abscess or a pseudocyst. A raised platelet count and a leucocytosis may be found on investigation. Imaging with CT is the gold standard, but an ultrasound in ICU may sometimes be necessary in a very ill patient. Treatment with percutaneous drainage is the ideal solution, but operation may be required where the collection is very extensive or not amenable to radiological intervention.

Pancreatic pseudocyst

Pseudocysts occur in 15–50% of patients after an attack of pancreatitis. There is usually no communication between the pancreatic duct and the psuedocyst. Intervention is only indicated if the cyst causes significant symptoms such as pain, vomiting, infection or inability to tolerate oral intake. Treatment is by endoscopic drainage or percutaneous aspiration and catheter drainage.

Outcome

Overall mortality from SAP is in the range of 7–10% but remains high in those in whom necrosis occurs; if necrosis is <30% of the pancreas, the mortality rate is 7%, whereas if the whole pancreas becomes necrotic mortality is of the order of 50%. SAP leads to death in ~25% of elderly patients.

Further reading

Hoerauf A, Hammer S, Muller-Myhsok B, *et al.* Intra-abdominal Candida infection during acute necrotizing pancreatitis has a high prevalence and is associated with increased mortality. *Crit Care Med* 1998; 26: 2010–5.

Mier J, Leon EL, Castillo A, *et al.* Early versus late necrosectomy in severe necrotizing pancreatitis. *Am J Surg* 1997; 173: 71–5.

Nathens Avery B, Curtis J, Randall MPH *et al.* Management of the critically ill patient with severe acute pancreatitis. *Crit Care Med* 2004; 32: 2524–36.

PACT module on Pancreatitis www.esicm.org

Ranson JH, Rifkind KM, Roses DF, *et al.* Prognostic signs and the role of operative management in acute pancreatitis. *Surg Gynaecol Obstet* 1974; 139: 69–81.

Surviving Sepsis Campaign www.survivingsepsis.org/

Acute acalculous cholecystitis

Definition

Acute acalculous cholecystitis (AAC) is inflammation of the gallbladder in the absence of gallstones.

Incidence

AAC accounts for 2–15% of all cases of cholecystitis undergoing cholecystectomy and up to 50–70% of cases in children.

In a mixed intensive care population, the incidence is 0.6–1%. In trauma patients, this may be up to 18%.

Risk factors

Men account for 80–90% of AAC seen after trauma or operation. Mean age in intensive care is 50–61yrs with a mean APACHE II score of 17.

Mortality is 50–85% without treatment, reduced by early diagnosis and intervention.

Organisms

Most commonly *E. coli* and *Klebsiella pneumoniae*. Other organisms implicated are *Enterococcus faecalis*, *Pseudomonas*, *Staphylococcus*, *Enterobacter*, anaerobes such as *Clostridium* or *Bacteroides*, or fungi. Anaerobes are particularly common in diabetics and patients >70yrs of age.

Pathogenesis

Opportunistic infections, e.g.

- Bacterial: Brucella, Coxiella, Leptospira, Mycobacterium tuberculosis, Salmonella, Mycoplasma, Vibrio cholerae
- Fungal: Candida spp.
- Parasitic: Leishmania, Plasmodium spp., Schistosoma spp.
- Viral: Epstein–Barr virus (EBV), CMV, varicella-zoster, Dengue virus

Gallbladder hypoperfusion and ischaemia

For example, shock due to trauma, multiple injuries, spinal injury, burns, recent operation particularly cardiopulmonary bypass, multi-system organ failure, congestive cardiac failure, haemodialysis

- Shock, use of vasopressors and low cardiac output result in splanchnic vasoconstriction leading to gallbladder ischaemia
- Mechanical ventilation with PEEP increases hepatic venous pressure decreasing portal perfusion
- Disturbed microcirculation may play a role due to intravascular coagulation and visceral atherosclerosis in vasculopaths and those with vasculitides, e.g. primary antiphospholipid syndrome, SLE, Sjogren's syndrome, Churg–Strauss, giant cell arteritis, polyarteritis nodosa, Henoch–Schonlein purpura
- Hepatic artery embolism in trauma or chemoembolization

Bile stasis leading to sepsis

- Opiate analgesics cause spasm of the sphincter of Oddi and induce increased biliary pressure
- Prolonged fasting or TPN (incidence up to 30%) inhibits gallbladder emptying, leading to bile stasis and toxic concentration of bile salts
- Obstruction, e.g. gallbladder polyp, multi-septate gallbladder, ampullary stenosis, tumour, *Echinococcus*, *Ascaria* spp.

Immunosuppression

For example, disseminated malignancy, chronic systemic disease, prolonged ICU stay, premature infants, HIV and AIDS often associated with *Cryptosporidium* or CMV, transplantation associated with Candida and CMV, bone marrow transplantation (incidence 4%),

Diagnosis

High index of suspicion and serial monitoring

The average stay of a patient with concurrent AAC in intensive care prior to diagnosis and subsequent cholecystectomy has been found to be as long as 19 days. Therefore, it is important to have a high index of suspicion and early radiographic evaluation. It has been suggested that trauma patients with a high Injury Severity Score >12 who are tachycardic and have required several units of packed red blood cells should be monitored by ultrasound for the development of AAC.

Symptoms and signs

- Fever or unexplained sepsis
- Right upper quadrant pain—only present in 25% of patients with AAC
- Recent jaundice
- Palpable right upper quadrant mass
- Ultrasound-induced Murphy's sign

Investigations

- Leucocytosis
- Elevated CRP
- Hyperamylasaemia
- Elevated aspartate aminotransferase (AST)

Ultrasound findings

- Thickened gallbladder wall >3.5mm
- Hydrops/pericholecystic fluid or subserosal oedema
- Sludge in gallbladder

These three have often been referred to as the diagnostic triad, although they are not pathognomonic for AAC and may be present in up to 50% of medical ICU admissions; therefore, correlation with clinical and laboratory parameters is required.

Special investigations

Cholescintigraphy involves IV administration of a 99mTechnetium-labelled analogue of iminodiacetic acid with hepatic uptake and subsequent concentration in bile. Failure to opacify the gallbladder is highly sensitive and specific for acute calculous cholecystitis due to cystic duct obstruction. In AAC, cholescintigraphy has a sensitivity of 79% and a specificity of 87%. False-negative results may occur because of cystic duct patency. False-positive results may occur because of fasting, liver disease or TPN, and may be as high as 30–40% in critically ill patients. Morphine-augmented cholescintigraphy may minimize false-positive results by increasing gallbladder filling by elevating the pressure in the common bile duct.

Morphine-augmented cholescintigraphy has the highest sensitivity for AAC of up to 90%, followed by CT with a sensitivity of 67% and ultrasound 27–30%. False positives occur when ascites or hypoalbuminaemia mimic a thickened gallbladder wall.

CT has the disadvantage of not being able to be performed at the bedside, but has the advantage of diagnosing other causes of intra-abdominal sepsis.

Laparoscopy in the ICU with local anaesthesia and IV sedation has also been used as a diagnostic tool.

Management

Optimization of haemodynamic status

Antibiotics according to cultures

Prophylaxis

Prophylactic measures include cholecystokinin or ceruletide. It is debateable whether these should be initiated in all ICY patients to promote gallbladder motility.

Laparoscopic cholecystectomy

This is essential for those with perforation/gangrene as these risk peritonitis.

It is safe and curative, even in the immunocompromised where the operative morbidity is 9.1%. Major complications are rare (4%) with a low morbidity of 12–13%, although this may rise to 14–30% in high risk patients.

CT- or ultrasound-guided percutaneous transhepatic cholecystostomy (PTC)

CT or ultrasound-guided PTC should be the management of choice in high-risk surgical candidates or elderly patients. PTC involves perforation of the gallbladder under ultrasound or CT guidance by a transhepatic approach to minimize the risk of bile peritonitis. A pigtail catheter is inserted into the gallbladder and irrigated with 5–10ml sterile saline daily to avoid occlusion. It is contraindicated in coagulopathy, ascites or colonic interposition.

In the elderly, PTC has been shown to result in prompt clinical improvement in 95% of patients, with morbidity and mortality each of 3%. Complications from PTC include haemorrhage, vagal reactions and hypotension from procedure-related bacteraemia, sepsis, bile peritonitis, pleural effusion, pneumothorax, respiratory distress, perforation of the intestinal loop, secondary infection or colonization of the gallbladder, and catheter dislodgement. During mean follow-up of 1.8yrs, no elderly patient with AAC developed a recurrent episode after catheter removal, and it has therefore been suggested that the drain may be removed 3 weeks after insertion without further intervention. It is important to perform cholecystocholangiography to ensure cystic duct patency prior to catheter removal.

ERCP

ERCP can be performed when surgery or PTC are contraindicated. This involves selective cannulation of the cystic duct and placement of a nasobiliary catheter within the gallbladder for drainage. Aspiration and lavage with 1% NAC dissolves luminal mucus and sludge. The complications are acute pancreatitis, cholangitis, intestinal perforation and haemorrhage.

Conservative management

In primary antiphospholipid syndrome the diagnosis is based on positive lupus anticoagulant or anticardiolipin antibodies. The treatment is LMWH and oral anticoagulants, not cholecystectomy.

AAC in SLE, Henoch–Schonlein purpura, Sjogren's syndrome and Churg–Strauss syndrome may be treated successfully with corticosteroid treatment alone, providing intestinal perforation has been excluded.

In children, serial ultrasound monitoring has been employed successfully in an attempt to avoid the need for cholecystectomy.

Complications

Clinical presentation is non-specific, resulting in a high incidence of gangrene (up to 63%), perforation (up to 15%), abscess (4%), ascending cholangitis, peritonitis, sepsis and death (up to 41%). Gallbladder perforation is particularly common in those with systemic diseases such as peripheral vascular disease, intrinsic heart disease or diabetes, and those who are chronically immunosuppressed. Cystic duct perforation has also been reported.

Further reading

Barie PS, Eachempati SR. Acute acalculous cholecystitis. *Curr Gastroenterol Rep* 2003; 5: 302–9.

Kalliafas S, Ziegler DW, Flancbaum L, *et al.* Acute acalculous cholecystitis: incidence, risk factors, diagnosis, and outcome. *Am Surg* 1998; 64: 471–5.

McChesney J, Northup P, Bickston S. Acute acalculous cholecystitis associated with systemic sepsis and visceral arterial hypoperfusion: a case series and review of pathophysiology. *Dig Dis Sci* 2003; 48: 1960–7.

Owen CC, Jain R. Acute acalculous cholecystitis. *Curr Treat Options Gastroenterol* 2005; 8: 99–104.

Vogt DP. Gallbladder disease: an update on diagnosis and treatment. *Cleveland Clin J Med* 2002; 69: 977–84.

Splanchnic ischaemia

Inadequate gut perfusion, due to imbalance of oxygen delivery compared with demand, leading to bowel damage and infarction if of sufficient duration. Splanchnic hypoperfusion is thought to have a significant impact on the outcome of many critically ill patients.

Pathophysiology

In shock, cardiac and CNS blood flow are maintained at the expense of the mesenteric circulation. Current hypotheses suggest that GI tract barrier function is impaired during periods of insufficient gut perfusion, leading to translocation of enteric bacterial endotoxin into the systemic circulation. A generalized inflammatory response is triggered, mediated by macrophage products, such as TNF-α, which is released as a result of endotoxin stimulation. Ultimately this can lead to multiple organ failure. Gut reperfusion may have similar deleterious effects as a result of oxidant-mediated damage.

Causes

- All forms of shock
- Burns
- Trauma; multiple injuries
- Compromised MI
- Haemodialysis with ultrafiltration.
- Abdominal compartment syndrome
- Occlusive mesenteric ischaemia due to a thromboembolic event. May be arterial, usually involving the superior mesenteric artery, venous or combined.
- Obstructive sleep apnoea
- Weaning from mechanical ventilation
- Protein malnutrition

Prevention

Prompt recognition/measurement of gut hypoperfusion and instigation of treatment.

Monitoring of intra-abdominal pressures (IAPs) every 1–2h in those at high risk of abdominal compartment syndrome and decompression prior to onset of end-organ failure can dramatically improve prognosis. Even mild elevations in IAP (>12mm Hg) worsen outcomes. Critical IAP values leading to higher incidences of complications are: ≥23mm Hg for delay in post-operative ventilatory weaning; ≥24mm Hg for renal dysfunction; and ≥25mm Hg for death. Non-surgical preventative measures may be used to reduce IAP prior to end-stage complications: sedation and pain control; gut emptying by NG tube placement, laxatives and enemas; neuromuscular blockade to relax the abdominal wall and improve organ perfusion; paracentesis in those with ascites or retroperitoneal collections; continuous haemofiltration in those with interstitial oedema. Continuous negative abdominal pressure devices have been designed, but require further research into their effects. Emergency surgery, i.e. formation of laparostomy, is required to prevent bowel ischaemia if IAP continues to rise and abdominal compartment syndrome develops. There are no established guidelines as to a cut-off pressure when surgery is necessary, and the pressure at which abdominal compartment syndrome occurs is dependent on host factors. The whole clinical picture should be taken into account, but early decompression may lead to improved outcomes. NB: fluid can re-accumulate beneath the dressings after formation of laparostomy, hence, continued IAP monitoring may be necessary.

Diagnosis

Rapid diagnosis and institution of treatment can significantly improve survival. Early clinical features include severe pain out of proportion to the physical findings. Peritonitis, fever, leucocytosis and lactic acidosis later develop.

Abdominal compartment syndrome may cause abdominal distension, shortness of breath, renal failure and syncope

Investigations

Gastric tonometry

Measures intraluminal pCO_2 as a measure of mucosal pCO_2 (and, hence, pH) in the GI tract via a catheter in the stomach. It monitors splanchnic hypoperfusion and can guide resuscitative measures according to gastric pH levels. Maintenance of gastric mucosal pH of ≥7.32 can reduce morbidity and mortality; however, there are difficulties in interpreting results, and some studies have shown no benefit of such monitoring. When initially introduced it was thought that this form of monitoring would be popular; however its use has been confined to a few centres.

Treatment

Clinical

- Deal with underlying cause
- Volume resuscitation: crystalloids or colloids; blood in cases of haemorrhagic shock. NB: those requiring >5l of fluid are at risk of abdominal compartment syndrome. Assessment of volume status is, therefore, vital. End-diastolic volumetric or echocardiographic indexes will give more accurate estimates than CVP and PAoP measurements in these patients.
- Vasoactive drugs. Abdominal perfusion pressure (APP = MAP – IAP) should be optimized. Inotropes may be necessary if APP <60mm Hg. Norepinephrine has no negative effects on gut perfusion. Avoid epinephrine and dopamine as they have been shown to reduce splanchnic perfusion.
- Early enteral nutrition, particularly containing immnunomodulating ingredients (e.g. glutamine and arginine), may improve clinical outcome in some clinical states.
- Surgery. Resection of ischaemic or gangrenous bowel; re-exploration at 24h may be advisable when demarcation of viable and non-viable bowel can be more obvious.

Experimental

- Small intestinal mucosal tissue oxygenation is improved after resuscitation with blood or gelatine infusions when compared with lactated Ringer's solution in pig models.
- Dobutamine and enoxamone (PDE inhibitor) and fenoldopam (dopamine D_1 receptor agonist) have been shown to maintain splanchnic blood flow during hypoperfusion in animal models.
- Dopexamine may be an option; no clinical study has shown a beneficial effect to date, and remains controversial.
- IL-1α. IV administration improves mesenteric blood flow in pig models.

Complications

- Bowel infarction
- Liver dysfunction. Hepatic arterial flow increases at times of reduced portal venous flow, thereby maintaining hepatic perfusion; however, this compensatory mechanism is limited, after which further decreases in splanchnic and/or systemic flow lead to liver failure.
- Sepsis
- Systemic inflammatory response leading to multi-organ failure

Outcome

Medical management may suffice in some cases; usually surgery is necessary and frequently life saving. However, survival is ~10–25% once the inflammatory response is fully developed.

Further reading

Ivatury RR, Diebel L, Porter JM, *et al.* Intra-abdominal hypertension and the abdominal compartment syndrome. *Surg Clin North Am* 1997; 77: 783–800.

Jakob SM, Clinical review: splanchnic ischaemia Crit Care 2002; 6: 306–12.

Kirton OC, Windsor J, Wedderburn R, *et al.* Failure of splanchnic resuscitation in the acutely injured trauma patient correlates with multiple organ system failure and length of stay in the ICU. *Chest* 1998; 113: 1064–9.

Lisbon A. Dopexamine, dobutamine and dopamine increase splanchnic blood flow: what is the evidence? *Chest* 2003; 123: 460S–3S

Malbrain MLNG, Chiumello D. Prevalence of intra-abdominal hypertension in critically ill patients: a multicentre epidemiological study. *Intensive Care Med* 2004; 30: 822–9.

Meier-Hellmann A, Reinhart K, Bredle DL, *et al.* Therapeutic options for the treatment of impaired gut function. *J Am Soc Neprhol* 2001; 12: S65–9.3S

Stechmiller JK, Treloar D, Allen N. Gut dysfunction in critically ill patients: a review of the literature. *Am J Crit Care* 1997; 6: 204–9.

Zakaria R, Garrison RN, Spain DA, *et al.* Intraperitoneal resuscitation improves intestinal blood flow following haemorrhagic shock. *Ann Surg* 2003; 237: 704–11.

Abdominal hypertension (IAH) and abdominal compartment syndrome

Our understanding of intra-abdominal hypertension (IAH) and the awareness of the potentially deleterious effects of abdominal compartment syndrome has increased markedly over the past decade

The anterior abdominal wall is compliant and distends to permit accommodation of a sudden increase in the intra-abdominal mass without a substantial increase in the IAP. However, as elasticity plateaus, further increase in the intra-abdominal contents will lead to a rise in the pressure.

The standard method for the measurement of IAP is directly by needle puncture into the abdominal cavity, e.g. at laparoscopy or during peritoneal dialysis. Indirect measurements can be obtained through a urinary bladder catheter or a balloon-tipped catheter inserted into the stomach.

Normal IAP is 5–7 mmHg in the critically ill patient. IAH is defined as a sustained or repeated pathological elevation of IAP >12mm Hg. IAH is graded as follows:

I	IAP 12–15mm Hg
II	IAP 16–20mm Hg
III	IAP 21–25mm Hg
IV	IAP >25mm Hg

The APP is calculated by the mean arterial pressure minus the intra-abdominal pressure; APP = MAP – IAP. The diagnosis of abdominal compartment syndrome is made when the peak IAP is >20mm Hg and/or the APP is <50mm HG during a minimum of two standardized measurements and there is associated single or multiple organ failure which was not previously present.

Aetiology of IAH/ abdominal compartment syndrome

The causes of raised IAP and IAH can be broken down to 4 main groups:

1 *Surgical.* Post-operative intra-abdominal or retroperitoneal haemorrhage, reduction of a large hernia, abdominal closure under excessive tension (e.g. oedematous or distended bowel), ileus secondary to leak or intra-abdominal leak/collection. prolonged pneumoperitoneum during laparoscopy.
2 *Medical.* Peritoneal dialysis, intra-abdominal infections, acute pancreatitis, ascites, pseudo-obstruction, generalized oedema from inflammatory process occurring outside abdomen.
3 *Post-traumatic.* Traumatic bleeding, visceral oedema from aggressive fluid resuscitation and external compression from body cast (e.g. MAST).
4 *Burns.* Third space loss from leaky capillaries and high volume fluid resuscitation.

Pathophysiology of organ dysfunction.

IAH adversely affects several organ systems.

1 *Respiratory*: lung compliance is reduced as is thoracic volume due to pressure on the diaphragm from below. The reduction in lung volume results in basal atelectasis. Parenchymal compression leads to infection. Pulmonary oedema follows and increased risk of ventilator-associated lung injury.
2 *Cardiovascular*: compression of the IVC and portal vein results in reduced venous return to the heart, a down and right shift of the Starling curve and commensurate fall in cardiac output. Decompression of the abdomen is shown to reverse the problem and improve cardiac function.
3 *Renal*: reduced cardiac output and tamponade of the kidneys combine to reduce renal perfusion. Tamponade is sufficient to reduce renal perfusion if the abdominal pressure exceeds 15mm Hg and results in anuria at IAP >30 mmHg.
4 *Alimentary system*: IAH reduces hepatic and splanchnic blood flow causing liver dysfunction and deterioration in gut function, mucosal acidosis and loss of gut barrier function
5 CNS: there is a correlation between IAP and ICP. Increased IAP lead to increased intrathoracic pressure, increased venous pressure and impedes venous return from the brain, causing a rise in the ICP.

Management

The reported mortality risk associated with abdominal compartment syndrome is 43%, and so it is important to be aware of, diagnose and treat the problem.

Appropriate treatment is based on 4 principles.

1 Serial monitoring of IAP
2 Optimization of organ function and systemic perfusion.
3 Medical therapy to reduce IAP can address the intra-abdominal contents by emptying the luminal contents of the intestine through gastric decompression and bowel purgation. Reduction of tissue oedema should be addressed. Intra-abdominal collections should be drained if possible. Abdominal wall tone can be reduced and, especially if there is pain or agitation, analgesia and sedation might be sufficient. The use of neuromuscular blockade to cause muscle relaxation may be required but is associated with increased ventilator-associated problems and ICU-related muscle wasting.
4 Surgical decompression should be considered for refractory IAH where the IAP is >20mm Hg or IAP is >15mm Hg and with evidence of organ dysfunction or ischaemia.

Surgical decompression of the abdomen leads to the problem of how to manage the open abdomen. Intra-abdominal viscera such as the small bowel can be inspected directly for viability or for perforation/leakage. However, an open abdomen exudes fluid and makes the nursing challenge more difficult, especially with regard to skin and wound care. Exposed bowel tends to desiccate and, combined with frequent dressing changes and contact with prosthetic materials, leads to serosal damage and the potential for bowel injury and fistula formation.

Fluid losses from the open abdomen are significant, and include the protein equivalent of 2g of nitrogen/day. This should be considered when thinking about fluid and electrolyte replacement. The reported fistula rate for patients with the open abdomen in the ICU is ~18%, and the incidence of anastomotic failure in this setting is ~10%. In the event of fistulation, then the management should involve an appropriate surgical team, fluid and electrolyte replacement, nutritional control, control of fistula effluent, relief of distal obstructions and possibly the use of octreotide.

The problems of management of the open abdomen have led to the use of several wound management systems. The Bogota bag, for example, can be sutured to the wound edges and has a tendency to rip and result in evisceration at a critical time. The currently preferred techniques are the Sandwich Pack Dressing and negative pressure suction therapy, as well as a dynamic closure system .

Once the acute problem is over, the abdomen may be closed up, but primary closure may not be feasible if there has been extensive tissue loss or retraction of the abdominal wall musculature. Reconstruction may involve the use of mesh prostheses, skin grafts and tissue expansion.

Further reading

Cheatham ML, Malbrain ML, Kirkpatrick A, *et al.* Results from the International Conference of Experts on Intra-abdominal Hypertension and Abdominal Compartment Syndrome II. Recommendations. *Intensive Care Med* 2007; 33: 951–62

De Laet I, Malbrain ML. Current insights, I Intra-abdominal hypertension and abdominal compartment syndrome. *Med Intensiva* 2007; 31: 88–99.

Malbrain ML, De Laet I, Cheatham M. Consensus conference definitions and recommendations on intra-abdominal hypertension (IAH) and the Abdominal compartment syndrome (ACS)—the long road to the final publications, how did we get there? *Acta Clin Belg Suppl* 2007; 1: 44–65.

Chapter 21

Hepatic disorders

Chapter contents

Jaundice

Jaundice (icterus) is the accumulation of bile pigments in serum and tissues including sclerae and skin. Jaundice is usually clinically detectable once serum bilirubin exceeds 50μmol/l. Hyperbilirubinaemia in the absence of primary hepatobiliary disease is common in the critically ill, occurring in 30% of patents spending >48h on the general ITU.

Causes of jaundice

The causes of jaundice are classically divided into pre-hepatic, hepatocellular and cholestatic causes, but overlap is common, especially in the critically ill.

Pre-hepatic jaundice

Pre-hepatic jaundice occurs when the liver's capacity to process bilirubin is exceeded. This is either related to excess breakdown of haem pigments in red cells or congenital abnormalities in the bilirubin conjugation pathway or bile salt export pump malfunction. Common causes of intravascular haemolysis include haemoglobinopathies, red cell membrane defects, microangiopathic haemolytic anaemia, drugs and sepsis. Because unconjugated bilirubin is not water soluble, it does not appear in the urine.

Gilbert's syndrome is a benign condition affecting 2–7% of the UK population and is characterized by mild unconjugated hyperbilirubinaemia in response to fasting or stress. Critical illness will almost inevitably precipitate hyperbilirubinaemia in patients with Gilbert's syndrome. Investigations including liver enzymes are normal. Other causes of congenital hyperbilirubinaemia including Dubin–Johnson, Rotor or Crigler–Najjar syndromes are rare. Mutations of the genes encoding the bile salt export pump underlying the familial intrahepatic cholestasis syndromes, which cause progressive cholestasis and liver damage, have recently been characterized.

Intrahepatic jaundice

Jaundice may be caused by hepatocellular dysfunction or intrahepatic cholestasis. Any cause of acute or chronic liver injury may cause jaundice. The most common causes in the UK are acute viral hepatitis (hepatitis A virus (HAV), CMV, EBV, rarely HBV or HCV) and drug reactions. Acute hepatitis with renal failure may complicate leptospirosis. Congestive hepatopathy occurs secondary to right heart failure or constrictive pericarditis. A salient cause of acute hepatocellular jaundice on the ITU is following an episode of hypotension, including that sustained secondary to hypovolaemia, or cardiac dysrhythmia. Jaundice may also occur both as a harbinger and as a marker of sepsis in the critically ill patient.

Idiosyncratic drug reactions may be predominantly hepatocellular (characterized by an elevated alanine aminotransferase (ALT)/aspartate aminotransferase (AST)) or cholestatic (rise in alkaline phosphatase). Drug-induced liver injury is unpredictable and may be difficult to diagnose since there can be considerable latency between drug intake and clinical presentation. Common hepatotoxic drugs are summarized in Table 21.1.1.

Table 21.1.1 Common causes of drug hepatotoxicity

Hepatocellular	Trazodone
Acarbose	Valproic acid
Allopurinol	**Mixed**
Amiodarone	Amitryptiline
Baclofen	Azathioprine
Disulfiram	Carbamazepine
Fluoxetine	Clindamycin
HAART	Enalapril
Halothane	Nitrofurantoin
Herbals including black cohosh, green tea extract, kava kava, germander	Phenobarbital
Isoniazid	Phenytoin
Ketoconazole	Sulfonamides
Lisinopril	Verapamil
Losartan	**Cholestatic**
Methotrexate	Amoxicillin-clavulanate
NSAIDs	Anabolic steroids
Omeprazole	Clopidogrel
Paroxetine	Erythromycin
Pyrazinamide	Irbesartan
Rifampicin	Oestrogens
Risperidone	Phenothiazines
Sertraline	Terbinafine
Statins	Tricyclics
Tetracyclines	

Extrahepatic jaundice

Extrahepatic jaundice occurs as a consequence of obstruction of the biliary tree distal to the biliary canaliculi. This may be secondary to:

- Gallstone disease:
  - Common bile duct stones
  - Cystic duct stones (Mirizzi's syndrome)
- Biliary strictures:
  - Cholangiocarcinoma
  - Benign biliary stricture
  - Primary sclerosing cholangitis
- Extrinsic compression:
  - Pancreatic carcinoma
  - Pancreatitis ± pseudocyst
  - Hilar lymphadenopathy

History and examination

Jaundice is a symptom, not a diagnosis. A cause for jaundice must always be sought. In hepatic and post-hepatic causes of jaundice, enterohepatic circulation of bile products is interrupted, hence stools will be pale whilst the urine is dark secondary to conjugated bilirubin. Pruritis is common. Right upper quadrant pain suggests either biliary obstruction or liver capsular stretching. Biliary obstruction may be complicated by cholangitis with fevers, rigors and features of sepsis. A history of biliary surgery or trauma may be apparent.

Risk factors for acute viral hepatitis should be sought. A full drug history including the use of over-the-counter, herbal or Chinese remedies, and recreational drug use is important.

Stigmata of chronic liver disease may be observed. Hepatomegaly is uncommon in chronic liver disease and suggests hepatic congestion, or infiltration. Splenomegaly suggests long-standing liver disease complicated by portal hypertension. A palpable gallbladder is suggestive of malignant biliary obstruction.

Investigations

Blood tests

LFTs confirm the diagnosis of jaundice and may differentiate between an obstructive and hepatocellular cause. Tests of liver synthetic function (albumin, prothrombin time) are important to stratify the severity of the liver injury. Deficiency of fat-soluble vitamins, including vitamin K, is common in cholestasis, so clotting may be deranged in the absence of significant synthetic dysfunction. In this instance, the prothrombin time corrects rapidly with (IV) vitamin K supplementation.

Viral studies (HAV IgM, HBVsAg, HCV Ab, CMV IgM, EBV IgM) should be tested in acute cases of jaundice. In early acute hepatitis C, antibody testing may be falsely negative. If clinical suspicion remains high, the diagnosis can be confirmed by testing for viral RNA.

Imaging

In the normal patient population, ultrasound is a sensitive method of diagnosing biliary obstruction, with a diagnostic accuracy of up to 79% for common bile duct stones. The technique is less accurate in the critically ill where biliary dyskinesia is common, but it is portable, non-invasive and does not require IV contrast, making it a suitable first-line investigation. CT imaging may diagnose the presence and level of biliary obstruction and is better at visualizing the pancreas than ultrasound. Magnetic resonance cholangiopancreatography (MRCP) is a highly T2-weighted MRI of the biliary tree that has impressive accuracy for the diagnosis of biliary tract stones. MRCP is of limited applicability to the critically ill.

Treatment

In pre-hepatic jaundice the underlying cause should be identified and treated appropriately. For intrahepatic causes of jaundice, care is supportive with treatment of the underlying condition.

Drug reactions

All drugs with the potential to cause jaundice or hepatotoxicity should be withdrawn. In practice on the ITU where critically ill patients are on multiple medications, this is rarely possible, but efforts should be made to stop as many drugs as possible or substitute for less hepatotoxic agents. In most cases of drug-induced hepatitis, the AST falls by 50% within 8 days of stopping the culprit drug, but liver injury may worsen or follow a protracted course. In cholestatic dug injury, it may take several months for LFTs to normalize. Rechallenge should not be performed. In cases of potential adverse effects secondary to antituberculous or antiretroviral drug regimens, expert advice should be sought.

Extrahepatic cholestasis

Sepsis is common in biliary obstruction, and broad-spectrum antibiotics with Gram-negative cover should be given. Coagulopathy corrects with parenteral vitamin K.

Decompression and drainage of the biliary tree is a priority in extrahepatic biliary obstruction. For patients who are stable, ERCP performed under sedation or general anaesthesia will allow dilatation and stenting of strictures and diagnostic cytology. ERCP is associated with a risk of pancreatitis, haemorrhage and cholangitis. In a recent audit of ERCP practice in England, >60% mortality was seen in patients of ASA class 5. Patients who are too unstable to tolerate ERCP should be referred for radiological percutaneous biliary drainage, with a view to definitive drainage and internalization once their clinical condition has improved.

Pruritis

Itching is common in obstructive jaundice. Troublesome symptoms may respond to oral antihistamines or cholestyramine (4g tds).

Further reading

Brienza N, Dalfino L, Cinnella G, *et al.* Jaundice in critical illness: promoting factors of a concealed reality. *Intensive Care Med* 2006; 32: 267–74.

Williams EJ, Taylor S, Fairclough P, *et al.* Are we meeting the standards set for endoscopy? Results of a large-scale prospective survey of endoscopic retrograde cholangiopancreatograph practice. *Gut* 2007; 56: 821–9.

Acute liver failure

Acute liver failure is a rare syndrome defined as the onset of liver dysfunction (manifest as jaundice, coagulopathy and encephalopathy) in a patient without known liver disease and an illness of <6 months duration. With the exception of a few rare causes, acute deterioration of chronic liver disease is not included in this definition. Although the incidence has declined following the introduction of blister packs and legislation limiting the amount that can be purchased, the most common cause of acute liver failure in the UK remains secondary to overdose of paracetamol (acetaminophen). In ~20% of cases no cause can be identified. The aetiology of acute liver failure is summarized in Table 21.2.1.

The presence of encephalopathy is required to diagnose liver failure, but this is an ominous, and frequently late, sign. Jaundice and synthetic dysfunction in a patient not known to suffer from liver disease should therefore be treated seriously. Acute liver failure is denoted hyperacute if the time from onset of jaundice to encephalopathy is <7 days, subacute if >4 weeks, and acute for intermediate durations.

Even with modern supportive care and emergency liver transplantation, mortality may exceed 50% even in specialist units. Patients' relatives should be counselled accordingly.

History and examination

The history and examination should be directed to finding the cause of the liver injury, identifying any co-morbidities that may influence the clinical course (including social factors that might contraindicate liver transplantation) and assessing the degree of damage to the liver and associated organ systems. A detailed drug history including use of over-the-counter and herbal medication should be taken. Any risk factors for exposure to waterborne or blood-borne hepatitis viruses including a travel history should be investigated. Other important questions include a family history of liver disease, organ-specific autoimmune syndromes, symptoms and risks for malignancy. Episodes of hypotension or collapse may be apparent.

There should be no signs of chronic liver disease on examination. The liver may be enlarged or collapsed. A careful examination for the presence or absence of encephalopathy should be undertaken. The pregnancy-related syndromes associated with acute liver failure occur in the third trimester.

Investigations

Recommended blood tests are summarized in Table 21.5.5. Liver imaging with ultrasound or CT will assess liver volume and exclude hepatic venous thrombosis. Slit lamp examination is useful to detect Kayser–Fleischer rings in acute Wilson disease. A CT brain scan may be considered to exclude other causes of deteriorating conscious level. A liver biopsy, usually via the transjugular route, may be helpful in the assessment of Wilson disease, autoimmune hepatitis or infiltrative hepatic malignancy, if the diagnosis is not clear from non-invasive testing.

Table 21.2.1 Common causes of acute liver failure

Drug toxicity (including paracetamol, amphetamine/ecstasy)
Acute viral hepatitis (hepatitis A, B, E)
Wilson disease
Autoimmune hepatitis
Acute fatty liver of pregnancy, HELLP syndrome
Acute hepatic ischaemia
Budd–Chiari syndrome
Malignant infiltration (lymphoma, breast and gastric cancers)
Toxins (*Amanita*)
Seronegative acute liver failure

Medical management

There is a risk of rapid deterioration in acute liver failure and therefore patients should be nursed in a high dependency environment and monitored closely for signs of decreasing conscious level. The advice of the local liver transplant centre should be sought with a view to an early transfer.

Patients with acute liver failure are nursed supine with 20° head-up tilt. GI bleeding is a recognized complication of acute liver failure, and prophylaxis against stress-induced gastric ulceration is routine. Mild hypothermia may prevent increased ICP in severe liver failure.

Nutrition/metabolic

Feeding, preferably enterally, should be instituted early. Hypo- and hyperglycaemia are common, and tight blood sugar control with IV glucose and insulin is important. Hypo-magnesaemia, hypophosphataemia and hypokalaemia are common and may require continuous supplementation. Lactic acidosis secondary to acute liver failure is an independent predictor of poor prognosis. Hyperlactaemia should be treated by ensuring adequate tissue perfusion. Severe lactic acidosis may be treated by high volume haemofiltration.

Sepsis

Sepsis, secondary to bacteria and fungi, is a common cause of clinical deterioration and death. Infections should be treated promptly and aggressively. Prophylactic broad-spectrum antibiotics with or without antifungals may reduce the risk of cerebral oedema.

Encephalopathy

Sedatives should be avoided if at all possible in the conscious patient due to the risk of accumulation. Sleep disturbance and disorientation may be signs of encephalopathy. Routine prophylaxis against seizures is not proven to be helpful. Propofol is the maintenance sedative of choice once mechanical ventilation is required.

Coagulopathy

There is a risk of bleeding secondary to coagulopathy and thrombocytopaenia. V vitamin K is usually given. Clotting factor support should be avoided in the absence of active bleeding unless the decision to list the patient for emergency liver transplantation has been made since this obscures one of the most important prognostic features. Venous and even arterial puncture or canulation is not an indication for clotting factor support.

Cardiovascular

Hypotension is common, and care must be taken to maintain renal and cerebral perfusion. Most patients are volume deficient at the time of presentation and require aggressive fluid resuscitation. Initial fluid replacement should be with colloid rather than crystalloid. There is no need for sodium restriction in acute liver failure. SVR is low, and hypotension resistant to volume replacement should be managed with vasopressor inotropes such as norepinephrine. Central venous access and monitoring is recommended in this situation. Pulmonary artery catheterization is not routine.

Adrenal insufficiency

Adrenal insufficiency is common in acute liver failure. IV hydrocortisone should be given to patients who do not have a satisfactory response to a short synacthen test.

Renal support

Acute renal failure is common and associated with poor prognosis. Acetaminophen has a direct nephrotoxic effect that peaks later than hepatotoxicity. Care should be taken to avoid dehydration, hypotension and potentially nephrotoxic agents. Continuous haemofiltration is associated with improved cardiovascular and intracranial parameters when compared with intermittent haemodialysis once renal failure is established.

Ventilation

Once grade III encephalopathy develops, endotracheal intubation should be performed. Ventilatory support should be provided according to standard protocols.

Specific therapies

If paracetamol overdose is suspected NAC should be instituted without delay. There may be some benefit from treatment even if 48h have elapsed since the time of ingestion. There is no evidence to suggest that the routine administration of NAC improves haemodynamic parameters, but it is common practice to start therapy with NAC in significant acute liver failure of any aetiology.

Specific therapies for causes of acute liver failure are infrequent and rarely subject to clinical trials. Lamivudine is given to patients with acute liver failure secondary to HBV infection, but there are no randomized trial data to support this. Aciclovir is given for acute liver failure secondary to acute herpes simplex hepatitis. Acute autoimmune hepatitis is an indication for steroids. There are case reports of improvement in acute liver failure secondary to lymphoma treated with chemotherapy. None of these therapies should delay listing for liver transplantation if poor prognostic criteria are met.

Liver transplantation

Liver transplantation is the only treatment proven to be of benefit in acute liver failure. Survival at 12 months after liver transplantation for acute liver failure is ~65%, significantly less than following transplantation for chronic liver disease. The majority of the excess risk is in the first month. There is a risk that patients with acute liver failure may deteriorate to a point that transplantation is not possible. Mortality rates whilst waiting for a suitable organ are up to 40%. Prognostic criteria for poor prognosis have been derived from historical cohorts of patients with acute liver failure and validated in large numbers of patients awaiting liver transplant. These criteria have high specificity for detecting those likely to die without liver transplantation, but are criticized for low sensitivity and low negative predictive value. Current UK criteria for super-urgent listing for liver transplantation in acute liver failure are summarized in Table 21.2.2.

Table 21.2.2 UK criteria for listing for super-urgent liver transplantation

Acetaminophen-induced acute liver failure, either:

1. Arterial pH <7.25 despite adequate fluid resuscitation or
2. Co-existing PT >100s or INR >6.5, creatinine >300mol/l or anuria, grade III–IV encephalopathy or
3. Serum lactate >3.5mmol/l on admission or >3.0mmol/l >24 h after overdose and after fluid resuscitation or
4. Two of 3 criteria from category 2 with clinical evidence of deterioration (e.g. increasing ICP, FiO_2 >0.5, increasing inotrope requirements) in the absence of clinical sepsis

Non-acetaminophen-induced acute liver failure:

1. Any grade of encephalopathy and any 3 of: unfavourable aetiology (idiosyncratic drug reaction, seronegative hepatitis), age >40yrs, jaundice to encephalopathy time <7 days, serum bilirubin >300 mol/l, PT >50s or INR >3.5
2. Hepatitis A or B, idiosyncratic drug reaction, seronegative hepatitis: PT >100s or INR >6.5 and any grade of encephalopathy
3. Acute presentation of Wilson disease or acute Budd–Chiari syndrome: coagulopathy and any degree of encephalopathy

The most common procedure in acute liver failure is whole organ cadaveric orthotopic liver transplantation. Auxiliary transplantation, in which a donor organ is implanted without recipient hepatectomy, has the advantage that immunosuppression can be withdrawn once liver function has recovered in the native organ. Living-related transplantation is limited because of the short window of opportunity to transplant.

Liver support systems

A number of systems utilizing hepatocytes or adsorption and dialysis techniques have been trialled in acute liver failure. Although minor improvements in encephalopathy score have been seen, no improvement in survival has been demonstrated.

Further reading

Hawton K, Simkin S, Deeks J, *et al.* UK legislation on analgesic packs: before and after study of long term effect on poisonings. *BMJ* 2004; 329: 1076.

Rahman T, Hodgson H. Clinical management of acute hepatic failure. *Intensive Care Med* 2001; 27: 467–76.

Bernal W, Donaldson N, Wyncoll D, *et al.* Blood lactate as an early predictor of outcome in paracetamol-induced acute liver failure: a cohort study. *Lancet* 2002;359: 558–63.

Liu JP, Gluud LL, Als-Nielsen B, *et al.* Artificial and bioartificial support systems for liver failure. *Cochrane Database Syst Rev* 2004; (1): CD003628.

Transplant UK. Guidelines for completing the super-urgent liver recipient registration form. 2005. https://www.uktransplant.org.uk/ukt/newsroom/bulletin/archive_bulletins/bulletin50/bulletin50-spring2004.pdf

Hepatic encephalopathy

Hepatic encephalopathy may occur in acute liver failure, acute on chronic liver failure or pose a long-term problem in cirrhosis. The aetiology of hepatic encephalopathy is poorly understood. Encephalopathy in acute and chronic liver disease has been considered to have separate causes, but this is now challenged. Clinical features are indistinguishable, but management is different. Hepatic encephalopathy is graded according to the West Haven criteria (Table 21.3.1). Once grade III encephalopathy is diagnosed, patients are at risk of airway compromise and should be electively intubated and mechanically ventilated.

Management of hepatic encephalopathy in acute liver failure

Acute liver failure is complicated by the development of intracranial hypertension. This arises as a consequence of cerebral oedema secondary to astrocyte accumulation of glutamine contingent upon hyperammonaemia, and cerebral vasodilatation with increased CBF. Cerebral oedema occurs in 35% of patients with grade III encephalopathy and acute liver failure, and in 65–75% of those in grade IV coma.

Patients with acute liver failure and encephalopathy should be discussed with the local liver transplant centre as a matter of urgency.

Monitoring

Clinical signs correlate poorly with ICP. Direct ICP monitoring provides useful clinical information and may lengthen survival, but has not been subject to randomized trials. Epidural catheters predispose to infection and a 1% chance of fatal haemorrhage, but are safer than subdural or intraparenchymal devices. Jugular bulb saturation <65% or <80% may predict an elevated ICP. Transcranial Doppler ultrasonography and other non-invasive methods of measuring cerebral blood flow are not reliable at monitoring ICP.

Treatment

ICP should be maintained <20–25mm Hg, and CPP (MAP – ICP) >50–60mm Hg. Airway suctioning and patient repositioning may cause surges in ICP and should be preceded by sedation bolus. Cooling to 32–33°C resulted in a mean reduction in ICP of 20mm Hg in 14 patients with acute liver failure and intracranial hypertension refractory to standard therapy. A multi-centre trial on the usefulness of moderate hypothermia in acute liver failure is underway. Lactulose, gut decontamination and enemata are not effective in treating encephalopathy secondary to acute liver failure.

Mannitol

IV mannitol (0.5–1g/kg bolus over 30min) reduces ICP by increasing serum osmolarity and improves survival in acute liver failure. Acute renal failure and oliguria reduce efficacy without haemofiltration to prevent fluid overload. Mannitol is contraindicated if plasma osmolarity >320mmol/l.

Table 21.3.1 West Haven staging of hepatic encephalopathy

I	Lack of awareness, euphoria or agitation, reduced attention span
II	Intermittent disorientation, drowsiness, inappropriate behaviour
III	Marked confusion, incoherent speech, reduced conscious level but rousable to voice
IV	Comatose with or without response to painful stimuli

Hypertonic saline

The administration of 30% hypertonic saline to raise serum sodium levels to 145–155mmol/l was associated with a reduced incidence of intracranial hypertension in a single small study.

Indomethacin

Indomethacin causes cerebral vasoconstriction and reduces ICP after head trauma, and may be useful in patients with acute liver failure. Side effects including nephrotoxicity limit its use in this setting.

Thiopentone

The barbiturate thiopentone causes cerebral vasoconstriction and may reduce ICP, but is associated with systemic hypotension and recurrence of intracranial hypertension on withdrawal.

Hyperventilation

Hyperventilation to reduce $PaCO_2$ is known to cause cerebral vasoconstriction and hence decreased CBF; however, this effect is transient. Prophylactic hyperventilation in acute liver failure does not reduce the incidence of intracranial hypertension or improve survival. Short periods of hyperventilation may be useful in controlling surges of ICP that do not respond to other therapies.

Corticosteroids

Although useful in treating some causes of intracranial hypertension, corticosteroids do not reduce ICP in acute liver failure. Corticosteroids may be indicated in a subgroup of patients with adrenal insufficiency secondary to acute liver failure.

Liver transplantation

Liver transplantation is the only therapy proven to improve survival significantly in acute liver failure complicated by hepatic encephalopathy. Liver support systems and isolated hepatocyte transplantation are not of proven survival benefit.

Management of hepatic encephalopathy in chronic liver failure

Chronic liver disease may be complicated by hepatic encephalopathy in a way that is clinically indistinguishable from that seen in acute liver failure. Although hyperammonaemia, abnormalities of GABAergic neurotransmission, elevated cytokine levels and even disturbances in CBF may be similar to those seen in acute liver failure, intracranial hypertension is not a feature of hepatic encephalopathy in chronic liver disease.

Hepatic encephalopathy may complicate any acute exacerbation of chronic liver disease, whether secondary to infection, GI bleeding, electrolyte disturbance, constipation or drug side effects. Chronic encephalopathy may develop in end-stage disease as a consequence of hepatoportal venous shunting, and is a complication of TIPS insertion.

Diagnosis

Hepatic encephalopathy is usually diagnosed clinically. Subtle encephalopathy may only be apparent on psychometric testing. Arterial ammonia levels lack both sensitivity and specificity. Slow waves (1.5–3Hz) on the EEG are a non-specific sign of metabolic encephalopathy. Visual provoked potentials may be prolonged in subclinical encephalopathy.

Patients with chronic liver disease who develop encephalopathy should be examined for evidence of constipation of GI bleeding. Bloods should be taken to exclude electrolyte abnormality, hypoglycaemia or signs of infection. A full septic screen including ascites cell count and culture is mandatory. Cerebral imaging (e.g. CT brain scan) may help to rule out focal intracerebral causes of altered sensorium.

Treatment

Management of encephalopathy is supportive, with attempts to correct the underlying cause of the acute deterioration. Infections should be treated aggressively.

Constipation

Non-absorbable disaccharides such as lactulose reduce colonic pH, alter gut flora in favour of *Lactobacillus* spp and sequester ammonia. A meta-analysis showed no significant effect on mortality or the development of encephalopathy with the use of lactulose over placebo.

In patients with encephalopathy, constipation should be prevented with regular purgatives (e.g. lactulose) to achieve 2 soft stools per day. Encephalopathy secondary to constipation may require enemata.

Gut decontamination

Neomycin does not reduce encephalopathy. Newer antibiotics such as rifaximin or vancomycin may be more effective, but predispose to bacterial overgrowth. A few small studies have suggested benefit from probiotics or synbiotics in patients with chronic low-grade encephalopathy.

Diet

Patients with chronic liver disease are usually malnourished and do not need to be protein restricted. There is no consensus on the role of branched chain amino acid supplements in the management of encephalopathy in chronic liver disease.

L-Ornithine L-aspartate (LOLA) converts L-ornithine to glutamate in muscle and utilizes ammonia to produce glutamine. LOLA reduces ammonia and may reduce encephalopathy; however, it is not licensed for use in the UK.

Benzoate

Benzoate is used in urea cycle disorders to reduce ammonia but has no effect on ammonia levels or degree of hepatic encephalopathy in liver disease.

Liver transplantation

Once encephalopathy has developed in a patient with chronic liver disease, referral for consideration of elective liver transplantation should be considered, once the acute illness has passed.

Further reading

Als-Nielsen B, Gluud LL, Gluud C. Non-absorbable disaccharides for hepatic encephalopathy: systematic review of randomised trials. *BMJ* 2004; 328: 1046.

Blei AT, Olafsson S, Webster S, *et al.* Complications of intracranial pressure monitoring in fulminant hepatic failure. *Lancet* 1993; 341: 157–8.

Jalan R, Damink SW, Deutz NE, *et al.* Moderate hypothermia for uncontrolled intracranial hypertension in acute liver failure. *Lancet* 1999; 354: 1164–8.

Kircheis G, Nilius R, Held C, *et al.* Therapeutic efficacy of L-ornithine-l-aspartate infusions in patients with cirrhosis and hepatic encephalopathy: results of a placebo-controlled, double-blind study. *Hepatology* 1997; 25: 1351–60.

Liu Q, Duan ZP, Ha DK, *et al.* Synbiotic modulation of gut flora: effect on minimal hepatic encephalopathy in patients with cirrhosis. *Hepatology* 2004; 39: 1441–9.

Murphy N, Auzinger G, Bernel W, *et al.* The effect of hypertonic sodium chloride on intracranial pressure in patients with acute liver failure. *Hepatology* 2004; 39: 464–70.

Polson J, Lee WM. AASLD position paper: the management of acute liver failure. *Hepatology* 2005; 41: 1179–97.

Tofteng F, Larsen FS. The effect of indomethacin on intracranial pressure, cerebral perfusion and extracellular lactate and glutamate concentrations in patients with fulminant hepatic failure. *J Cereb Blood Flow Metab* 2004; 24: 798–804.

Chronic liver failure

Cirrhosis is the end-stage of all chronic liver insults. Decompensation of cirrhosis leads to liver synthetic failure, hepatic encephalopathy and symptomatic portal hypertension. With modern standards of supportive care, the outcome of critically ill patients with chronic liver disease is significantly better than historical data, but long-term survival can often only be improved by liver transplantation.

Patients with chronic liver disease commonly present with an acute on chronic illness. Acute deterioration can be precipitated by bacterial or, less commonly, viral infection. Patients with hepatitis B may decompensate following acquisition of hepatitis D. Other causes of decompensation include GI bleeding, constipation, metabolic derangement, iatrogenic drug side effects, hepatocellular carcinoma and ongoing toxic liver insult including alcohol excess.

History and examination

Clinical history and examination should aim to determine both the underlying cause of liver disease (summarized in Table 21.4,1) and the reason for deterioration. A collateral history may be necessary if the patient is encephalopathic. A careful alcohol history including the remote past and recent binges is important. Alcohol dependence syndrome is not necessary to develop alcoholic liver disease. Risks for viral hepatitis (IV drug use, unsterilized tattooing equipment, receipt of blood products prior to the introduction of universal screening, occupational exposure, unsafe sexual practices, vertical transmission in patients from endemic areas) should be explored. A family history of autoimmune disease, diabetes or movement disorders may be helpful. A full drug history including over-the-counter and herbal remedies is necessary. Symptoms of encephalopathy, infection including spontaneous bacterial peritonitis, upper GI bleeding and constipation should be sought.

Examination may be salient for the features of chronic liver disease. Asterixis and other evidence of hepatic encephalopathy are important signs. Intravascular and extravascular fluid status including the presence of ascites and oedema should be carefully assessed.

Management of decompensated cirrhosis on the ITU

General features

The drug chart of all patients should be carefully reviewed for potentially toxic medication. Opiates and benzodiazepines accumulate and should be prescribed with care

Table 21.4.1 Causes of chronic liver disease in the UK

Alcohol excess
Hepatitis B and C infection
Autoimmune liver disease (autoimmune hepatitis, primary biliary cirrhosis, primary sclerosing cholangitis)
Non-alcoholic steatohepatitis
Hereditary haemochromatosis
Wilson's disease
α_1-Antitrypin deficiency
Budd–Chiari syndrome
Cystic fibrosis

and dose titrated to effect. Non-steroidal drugs should be avoided because of the risk of nephrotoxicity.

Constipation should be avoided, with regular lactulose (nasogastrically if necessary) titrated to achieve 2 soft stools per day. Regular enemata may be needed in acute encephalopathy.

Hyponatraemia is common despite total body sodium overload. Diuretic therapy should be curtailed, especially if there is evidence of renal failure. The management of severe hyponatraemia (serum sodium <120mmol/l) is difficult and controversial. In the presence of hypovolaemia, cautious plasma expansion with colloids may prevent deterioration of renal function.

Nutrition

Hypoglycaemia is common and responds to IV dextrose.

Patients with chronic liver disease are almost universally malnourished and are hypercatabolic as a consequence of acute illness. Early provision of nutrition, preferably via the enteral route, is a priority. Low sodium feeds are standard. It is normally neither necessary nor desirable to restrict protein intake. Oesopahageal varices are not a contraindication to the passage of a fine bore feeding NG tube, although this should be avoided in the days immediately following acute variceal bleeding.

Patients with alcoholic liver disease may present with Wernicke's encephalopathy (nystagmus, ophthalmoplegia, ataxia and confusion) secondary to thiamine deficiency. Acute, irreversible polyneuropathy may be precipitated by a carbohydrate load and is prevented with IV thiamine (usually as a multi-vitamin infusion).

Synthetic support

IV vitamin K will correct coagulopathy secondary to deficiency of vitamin K, which is common in chronic cholestasis. FFP and platelets may be necessary in acute haemorrhage. Cryoprecipitate and activated factor VII may be useful in severe blood loss and coagulopathy not responsive to standard measures.

There are no data to support the routine use of IV albumin in patients with chronic liver disease and hypoalbuminaemia.

Sepsis and spontaneous bacterial peritonitis

Sepsis is a common cause of decompensation in patients with chronic liver disease who are functionally immunosuppressed. Physicians should have a low threshold for empiric broad-spectrum antibiotics active against Gram-negatives and skin commensals ± antifungals. Antibiotics reduce rebleeding in variceal bleeding.

All patients with ascites and clinical deterioration should undergo diagnostic ascitic tap with samples sent for microscopy and inoculated in blood culture bottles. Bacterial peritonitis is diagnosed if the ascites neutrophil count is >250 cells/mm^3. Spontaneous bacterial peritonitis is usually monomicrobial. Coliforms, streptococci and enterococci are the most common organisms. Multiple organisms on culture are suggestive of intestinal perforation. There is no evidence to support total paracentesis in spontaneous bacterial peritonitis.

Adrenal dysfunction is common in cirrhotic patients with severe sepsis and may contribute to circulatory dysfunction.

IV hydrocortisone (100mg tds) improves haemodynamics, reduces vasopressor requirements and improves survival in cirrhotics with severe sepsis and a flat short synacthen test (see Chapter 27.9).

Bleeding

Upper GI bleeding is a common cause and consequence of decompensation in chronic liver disease because of coagulopathy, thrombocytopaenia, portal hypertension and critical illness-associated peptic ulceration. 50% is non-variceal. Early endoscopy, following haemodynamic stabilization, is diagnostic and potentially therapeutic. Propranolol should be given to all patients with varices as prophylaxis against bleeding if tolerated. The management of upper GI bleeding is discussed elsewhere (see Chapter 20.5). The management of non-variceal bleeding is as that of patients without liver disease.

Hepatic encephalopathy

Hepatic encephalopathy is discussed in the previous chapter.

Ascites

Ascites secondary to portal hypertension is suggested by a serum–ascites albumin gradient >11g/dl. Alternative diagnoses should be sought in high protein ascites, and treatment directed to the cause. Patients with chronic liver disease and ascites should be sodium restricted. Diuretic therapy with spironolactone (100mg/day increasing to maximum 400mg/day) ± frusemide (40mg/day to max 160mg/day) should be undertaken, with careful monitoring of electrolytes and renal function. Diuretics are stopped if serum sodium falls or creatinine rises. Patients who do not tolerate diuretics, or develop tense ascites (intra-abdominal pressure >20cm H_2O, signs of respiratory or ventilatory compromise, discomfort) may be treated with large volume paracentesis. Paracentesis <5l does not require albumin but should be followed by volume expansion with a synthetic colloid. Paracentesis >5l should receive 8g albumin per litre of ascites removed (e.g. 100ml 20% albumin per 3l ascites). The canula used to drain ascites should be removed after 6h.

Cardiovascular system

Patients with chronic liver disease have increased splanchnic blood flow and high cardiac output with low SVR, resulting in hyperaldosteronism and secondary sodium retention. Such patients are prone to hypotension, treatable initially with fluid challenges. There is debate about the ideal fluid resuscitation since sodium-containing fluids exacerbate ascites and peripheral oedema whilst dextrose worsens hyponatraemia. The opinion of the authors is that maintenance of renal and cerebral perfusion with colloids is the initial priority in resuscitation of the cirrhotic patient. Hypotension unresponsive to volume resuscitation is an indication for vasopressor inotropes such as norepinephrine.

Renal

Renal dysfunction is common in patients with chronic liver disease. Since hepatic protein turnover is reduced and muscle mass low, serum levels of urea and creatinine may remain within the normal ranges despite significant reductions in GFR. Renal failure may develop as a consequence of volume depletion, drug nephrotoxicity, sepsis, intrinsic renal disease or outflow obstruction. Renal failure in the absence of these factors, and persisting despite diuretic withdrawal, fluid challenge and treatment of sepsis, is termed hepatorenal syndrome (HRS). Type 1 HRS is characterized by a rapid decline in renal function frequently precipitated by severe sepsis or GI haemorrhage. It is historically associated with extremely poor prognosis. Type 2 HRS causes a milder and more slowly progressive decline in renal function, with severe ascites poorly responsive to diuretics. Survival of patients with type 2 HRS is less than that of non-azotaemic cirrhotics.

The administration of IV albumin (1g/kg then 20–40g/day) and terlipressin (0.5mg 4 hourly increasing to max 12mg daily) may reverse type 1 HRS in up to 58%. Long-term survival benefits are difficult to interpret because of a high rate of liver transplantation. Small studies suggest benefit of TIPS and extracorporeal albumin dialysis (MARS) in selected groups of patients. These therapies are not widely available. Type 2 HRS responds less well to albumin and vasopressors and is more prone to recurrence.

Alcoholic hepatitis

Acute alcoholic hepatitis occurs on the background of chronic alcohol excess. Liver biopsy invariably shows underlying hepatic fibrosis. Alcohol withdrawal should be avoided by reducing doses of chlordiazepoxide or benzodiazepines. Corticosteroids reduce mortality in patients with severe alcoholic hepatitis (discriminant function >32) in patients without acute bleeding or sepsis. Pentoxyfilline reduces the incidence of HRS and in-hospital mortality in alcoholic hepatitis.

Scoring systems for outcome

The mortality of cirrhotic patients with critical illness remains high, with in-hospital mortality rates of 44–74% in those requiring admission to ITU. Mortality is dependent not only on the severity of liver disease but also on the presence of cardiovascular or renal failure. Prognosis in the critically ill patient with chronic liver disease is more accurately predicted by ITU-specific scoring systems such as APACHE II or SOFA than the Child–Pugh score.

Liver transplantation

For patients with decompensated chronic liver disease and no reversible cause, liver transplantation is the only treatment proven to improve long-term survival. There is no provision for emergency liver transplantation for chronic liver failure in the UK. Patients should be discussed with the local transplant unit with a view to consideration of transplantation once the acute episode is passed. There is potential for significant improvement in liver function if patients with alcoholic liver disease achieve abstinence after recovery from their initial illness.

Further reading

Cowan M, Tilliard A, Cook M, *et al.* Morbidity and mortality associated with alcoholic liver disease following admission to St George's Hospital HDU/ICU. *Gut* 2006; 55 (Suppl 2): A46.

Fernandez J, Escorsell A, Zabalza M, *et al.* Adrenal insufficiency in patients with cirrhosis and septic shock: effect of treatment with hydrocortisone on survival. *Hepatology* 2006; 44: 1288–95.

McCullough AJ, O'Connor JF. Alcoholic liver disease: proposed recommendations for the American College of Gastroenterology. *Am J Gastroenterol* 1998; 93: 2022–36.

Moore KP, Aithal GP. Guidelines on the management of ascites in cirrhosis. *Gut* 2006;55 (Suppl 6): vi1–12.

Abnormal liver function tests

Enzymes

The liver contains a number of different enzymes that are released from damaged hepatocytes and can be detected in serum. The levels of such enzymes are frequently normal in patients with chronic liver disease, especially if there is little ongoing inflammation. Elevated liver enzymes may be considered hepatitic (i.e. a consequence of hepatocellular damage; raised AST and ALT), cholestatic (i.e. a consequence of biliary obstruction; raised alkaline phosphatase and γ-glutamyltransferase (γGT)) or mixed.

Aspartate aminotransferase/alanine aminotransferase

These are cytoplasmic hepatic enzymes that may be detected in excess in serum in liver disease with ongoing activity of any aetiology, but are most raised in hepatocellular injury. AST and, to a lesser extent, ALT are present in skeletal muscle and myocardium, thus myocardial necrosis and skeletal muscle damage should be excluded in cases of elevated aminotransferase levels (especially AST). AST may also be elevated in renal or intestinal infarction, pancreatitis or hypothyroidism. ALT is more specific for liver injury than AST. Causes of raised transaminases are summarized in Table 21.5.2.

The ratio AST/ALT may be used to differentiate the aetiology of liver disease. In acute viral hepatitis, the ratio is commonly <1, whereas in alcoholic liver disease the ratio is typically >2. An AST/ALT ratio >1 has been proposed as a marker of cirrhosis in chronic liver disease, but lacks sensitivity.

Alkaline phosphatase

Alkaline phosphatase is found in a number of tissues including liver, bone, intestine, kidney and placenta. Elevations in alkaline phosphatase occur in diseases affecting any of these organs and in normal pregnancy (Table 21.5.3). Although the tissue of origin can be determined by determining the predominant isoform of the enzyme, this is rarely necessary in clinical practice. In the liver, alkaline phosphatase is localized to the sinusoidal membrane, hence it is the primary enzyme raised in cholestatic liver disease, of intra- or extrahepatic aetiology. It is elevated to a lesser degree in hepatocellular injury.

γ-Glutamyltransferase (γGT)

γGT is located in the hepatocyte membrane and is a sensitive but non-specific marker of liver disease. It may be elevated in cholestatic, hepatocellular or infiltrative liver disorders. γGT may be elevated in patients with chronic alcohol abuse, and is sometimes used as a screening test for ongoing alcohol intake. This approach lacks sensitivity and is non-specific. Carbohydrate-deficient transferrin is not more accurate than γGT as a screening test for chronic alcohol abuse. γGT is also present in prostate tissue and may be elevated in prostate cancer.

Table 21.5.1 Normal values for liver function tests (values may differ slightly between laboratories)

Alanine aminotransferase	3–35 IU/l
Aspartate aminotransferase	3–35IU/l
Alkaline phosphatase	30–300IU/l
γ-Glutamyltransferase	10–50IU/l
Bilirubin	3–17μmol/l
Albumin	35–48g/dl
Prothrombin time	12–16s
Ammonia	15–45mcg/dl
Lactate	<1.5mmol/l

Table 21.5.2 Causes of elevated AST/ALT

Hepatocellular (ALT and AST)	Hepatitis (any cause) Drug-induced liver injury Impaired hepatic perfusion Biliary obstruction Hepatic congestion
Myocardial damage (AST>ALT)	Myocardial infarction Myocarditis
Skeletal muscle injury (AST>>ALT)	Trauma (including post-surgery) Rhabdomyolysis Myositis Muscular dystrophy
Renal necrosis (AST)	Renal infarct Trauma

Excretory liver function

Bilirubin is a byproduct of haem breakdown that is taken up by hepatocytes, conjugated and excreted into bile. Elevated bilirubin may occur as a result of haemolysis, hepatic disease or biliary obstruction.

Synthetic liver function

Albumin

Albumin, the most abundant serum protein, is synthesized exclusively in the liver, with a half-life of 15 days in health. Hypoalbuminaemia is a marker of poor synthetic liver function and is predictive of morbidity and mortality in chronic liver disease. Albumin is a negative acute phase marker, falling in acute illness as well as a consequence of renal or GI loss. Serum albumin below the normal level is almost universal in the critically ill, present in 98% of patients on admission to the general ITU.

Table 21.5.3 Causes of elevated alkaline phosphatase

Hepatobiliary	Extrahepatic biliary obstruction Intrahepatic cholestasis Primary biliary cirrhosis Hepatocellular damage
Bone	Healing fracture Metastatic tumour Paget's disease of bone Osteomalacia Physiological bone growth
Intestine	Intestinal infarction
Placenta	Normal pregnancy
Other	Sepsis Renal failure

Table 21.5.4 Causes of hyperlactataemia

Type A	Hypotension/cardiac arrest
	Regional infarction
	Septic shock
	Poisoning (e.g. ethylene glycol, methanol)
Type B	Liver failure
	Diabetes mellitus
	Renal failure
	Drugs, e.g. metformin
	Haematological malignancy
	Pancreatitis
	Thiamine deficiency
	Glucose-6-dehydrogenase deficiency
	Short bowel syndrome (D-lactate)

Clotting factors

Almost all the proteins that make up the coagulation cascade are produced by the liver. The PT is sensitive to low levels of factor VII, which, with a short half-life of 4–6h, is a sensitive test of liver synthetic function in the absence of vitamin K deficiency. Prolongation of the PT is predictive of mortality in both acute and chronic liver failure. Reduced factor V level is a poor prognostic marker in non-paracetamol acute liver failure.

Ammonia

Ammonia is produced throughout the body as the nitrogenous waste product of amino acid catabolism. The liver detoxifies ammonia to urea via the urea cycle prior to renal excretion. Ammonia levels rise as a consequence of hepatoportal shunting and may contribute to hepatic encephalopathy. Ammonia levels also rise in acute liver failure, Reye syndrome and rare inborn errors of metabolism.

Lactate

Lactic acid is produced by peripheral tissues, particularly skeletal muscle, brain and red cells as a byproduct of glucose metabolism, and metabolized by the liver and kidney. Blood lactate levels rise as a consequence of mitochondrial dysfunction secondary to tissue hypoxia or sepsis, or due to reduced hepatic perfusion or function. Lactic acidosis in the presence of tissue hypoxia is termed type A, whilst lactic acidosis secondary to reduced hepatic clearance is termed type B. Common causes of hyperlactataemia are summarized in Table 21.5.4. Hyperlactataemia is a poor prognostic sign in acute paracetamol-induced liver failure. Lactic acidosis is a common feature of critical illness in acute on chronic liver failure.

Dynamic tests of liver function

Dynamic LFTs assess the ability of the liver to metabolize or eliminate substrates over a short period of time. Dynamic liver function testing is superior to static tests (e.g. bilirubin, PT) in the assessment of liver function in critically ill patients with septic shock or following liver transplantation, but is not widely available.

Table 21.5.5 Suggested initial investigations for patients with acute liver injury

Urea and electrolytes
Glucose
Liver function tests (bilirubin, ALT/AST, alkaline phosphatase, γGT, albumin)
Creatine kinase
Full blood count
Prothrombin time/INR
Arterial blood gas
Arterial lactate
Paracetamol levels
Blood group
Toxicology screen
Viral hepatitis markers (anti-HAV IgM, HBsAg, anti-HBc IgM, anti-HEV IgM, anti-HCV Ab, anti-EBV IgM, anti-CMV IgM)
Autoimmune markers (immunoglobulin, antinuclear antibody, anti-smooth muscle antibody)
Caeruloplasmin
Pregnancy test

Indocyanine green clearance

Indocyanine green (ICG) is an infrared-absorbing, iodine-containing dye that is excreted unchanged in bile. Plasma levels can be measured non-invasively by transcutaneous infrared spectrophotometry. The rate of ICG clearance can be expressed as blood clearance or plasma disappearance rate. Normal values are >700ml/min/m^2 and >18%/min. ICG clearance is dependent upon liver perfusion, hepatocellular function and biliary excretion. Low ICG clearance predicts poor survival in cirrhotic patients listed for liver transplantation, dysfunction in the graft and worse outcome after liver resection. Reduced ICG clearance is an independent risk factor for mortality in critically ill patients without pre-existing liver disease with septic shock or acute respiratory distress.

Monoethylglycinxylidide (MEG-X) test

Lidocaine is metabolized to MEG-X via the cytochrome P450 system. MEG-X is assayed immediately before and 15min after an IV dose of lidocaine (1mg/kg). The MEG-X test therefore measures liver blood flow and hepatocellular function. Low rates of conversion of lidocaine to MEG-X are predictive of poor outcome in stable patients with cirrhosis, cirrhotic patients undergoing liver resection and critically ill patients with cirrhosis on the ITU. Measurement of MEG-X requires complex laboratory analysis, so it is not suitable as a bedside test. Accuracy is reduced by concurrent medication that induces or suppresses cytochrome P450.

Chapter 22

Neurological disorders

Chapter Contents

Agitation and confusion

Agitation and confusion are common features in critical illness. Agitation is a symptom or sign of numerous acute and chronic disease states that include pain, anxiety and delirium. Agitation is present in around half of ICU patients, with 15% experiencing severe agitation. Confusion may also be chronic or acute and arise from an overlapping set of pathological processes that includes hypoxia, hypotension, hypoglycaemia and dementia. It is possible to be agitated and not confused, and vice versa. Recognition and treatment of the underlying condition is of utmost importance, rather than treating the symptoms alone.

Acute confusional states are frequently the result of delirium. Delirium is defined as an acute change in mental status with a fluctuating course, characterized by inattention and disorganized thinking. It is acute cerebral insufficiency and should be considered as an organ failure (i.e. brain failure). Three subtypes of delirium exist.

1 Hyperactive (agitated, paranoid)
2 Hypoactive (inattentive, stuporous, withdrawn)
3 Mixed (fluctuates, hyperactive–hypoactive)

The incidence of delirium is reported to be between 15 and 80% in critical care patients. The pure hyperactive form only accounts for ~10% of delirium cases, with the mixed form accounting for a further 45% of cases. The hypoactive form can be missed completely or misdiagnosed as depression.

The presence of delirium and/or agitation increases the duration of mechanical ventilation and intensive care LOS. It is also associated with higher rates of adverse events, including a 3-fold increase in mortality.

The degree of sedative exposure, in particular to benzodiazepines, is predictive of delirium occurrence

Detection of delirium

Both the level and degree of clarity of a patient's consciousness require assessment. Consciousness level is judged using a subjective sedation–agitation scale, but a specific delirium screening tool must also be used to assess clarity. Agitation can commonly be the result of suboptimal analgesia, and thus pain must be thoroughly assessed. Sleep disturbances are associated with delirium, although it is unknown whether this is a cause or effect. Sleep disturbance may be an early marker for the development of delirium.

Sedation–agitation monitoring

The use of sedation–agitation scales to titrate doses of sedative drug infusions reduces the quantity of continuous sedatives delivered, the duration of mechanical ventilation and intensive care LOS. Numerous validated scoring systems are available, including the Richmond Agitation-Sedation Scale (RASS); Sedation Agitation Scale (SAS); and the Motor Activity Assessment Scale (MASS).

Sedation holds are beneficial in appropriate patients and reduce patient sedative exposure as well as LOS.

Delirium screening

Delirium screening tools have been developed for use in critical care patients, including the Confusion Assessment Method-Intensive Care Unit (CAM-ICU), Intensive Care Delirium Screening Checklist (ICDSC) and Delirium Detection Score (DDS). These do not all examine the same aspects of delirium, and this may explain the variability in delirium incidence when using different tools.

Analgesia evaluation

Often non-specific physiological parameters are utilized to guide analgesia, although behavioural aspects are more reliable. Systematic evaluation of pain and agitation using a behavioural pain score decreases the incidence of pain and agitation.

Sleep monitoring

Direct nurse assessment of nocturnal sleep time overestimates sleep quantity but provides a useful trend marker. Patient report allows sleep quality to be compared with the patient's own baseline, but a degree of caution is required as memory recall can be adversely affected by sedatives, delirium and sleep disturbance itself.

Prevention of delirium

Multi-factorial intervention programmes highlight the effectiveness of preventative strategies in elderly patients, although there is no specific evidence that these work in critically ill patients.

Non-pharmacological

Non-pharmacological measures essentially add up to good standards of basic nursing and medical care.

- Remove potential organic drivers, e.g. identify and treat hypoxia, infection, pain, etc.
- Provide support and orientation, e.g. named nurse, TV/radio, clock, calendar and daily schedule.
- Provide an unambiguous environment, e.g. allow clear day–night and activity–sleep cycles.
- Maintain competence, e.g. ensure patient has glasses, hearing aid, participates in range of motion exercises.

Pharmacological

Many drugs contribute to the incidence and severity of delirium. Drugs with antimuscarinic and/or dopaminergic activity are particularly deliriogenic. Changes in blood–brain barrier (BBB) permeability as a result of critical illness and changes in pharmacodynamics/pharmacokinetics due to multi-organ failure also increase the risk of developing delirium. Classes of drugs that are particularly culpable include:

- Antimuscarinic drugs—through overt or covert activity, e.g. hyoscine, amitriptyline, ranitidine, prednisolone.
- Dopaminergic drugs, e.g. levodopa.
- GABAminergic drugs, e.g. benzodiazepines.
- Drugs that suppress rapid eye movement (REM) sleep with the risk of REM rebound upon abrupt discontinuation, e.g. opioids, benzodiazepines, tricyclic antidepressants.

Treatment of delirium

When preventative measures fail and identified organic drivers have been or are in the process of being corrected, specific delirium treatment should be commenced and administered regularly.

Hyperactive/mixed delirium

Haloperidol

Haloperidol is currently the agent of choice, albeit on limited evidence. The initial dose is based on the patient's degree of agitation, age and hepatic function. Due to the fluctuating nature of the symptoms, it must be administered regularly during the period of delirium. The dose is reduced gradually as the patient stabilises.

Phenothiazines

Phenothiazines such as chlorpromazine are not recommended. Although probably of similar efficacy to haloperidol, they posses a less favourable side effect profile due to increased antimuscarinic and α-blocking activity.

Atypical antipsychotics

Evidence of efficacy in the critically ill is limited; however, olanzapine, risperidone and quetiapine probably have similar efficacy to haloperidol and offer an alternative where side effects occur, or in Parkinsonism. Olanzapine is the only atypical agent with an immediate release parenteral formulation suitable for acute control of symptoms.

Benzodiazepines

Benzodiazepines may predispose to, or aggravate delirium when used outside of the treatment of specific withdrawal deliria (e.g. alcohol). They should generally be avoided and restricted to irregular administration for control of dangerous psychomotor activity in severely disturbed patients. Short-acting agents such as midazolam can be used in these circumstances while awaiting the full effects of other interventions.

α_2 Agonists

There is growing interest in the use of agents such as clonidine and dexmedetomidine for treatment of delirium. Although some reports suggest that α_2 agonists may be useful in the treatment of hyperactive delirium, there are no supporting peer-reviewed publications.

Hypoactive delirium

Hypoactive delirium is more difficult to treat and is associated with a worse outcome.

Antipsychotics

Haloperidol or atypical antipsychotics in low doses may be of value.

Stimulants

Methylphenidate was reported to benefit cancer patients with hypoactive delirium in a small trial.

Night sedation

Benzodiazepines and other GABA agonists are not recommended in delirious patients.

Sedating antidepressants

Trazodone and mirtazapine have advantages over other sedating antidepressants such as amitriptyline, through reduced antimuscarinic activity and reduced adverse effects on sleep architecture.

Haloperidol

IV haloperidol may be useful in patients unable to utilize enteral routes.

Treatment of withdrawal syndromes

Withdrawal reactions should be considered and anticipated for medications introduced in the current admission as well as from the patient's usual chronic medication.

- Benzodiazepines. Adopt a withdrawal regimen over days to weeks in dependent patients.
- Opioids. Withdraw opioids slowly in dependent patients. Use adjunctive opioid-sparing analgesia when possible, e.g. paracetamol, gabapentin. Clonidine may reduce some withdrawal symptoms.
- Antidepressants. Restart medication as soon as possible, using the IV, buccal or rectal routes if necessary. Treat symptomatically if no alternative route.
- Alcohol. Replace thiamine. Benzodiazepines should be used in a tapering regimen. Adjunctive haloperidol may be needed for treatment of hallucinations.
- Nicotine. Consider nicotine replacement therapy (NRT) or clonidine. The safety of NRT in the critically ill has been questioned recently.
- Recreational drugs. Clonidine may be useful in the mixed picture of recreational drugs with or without adjunctive benzodiazepines.

Further reading

Brook AD, Ahrens TS, Schaiff RR, *et al.* Effect of a nursing-implemented sedation protocol on the duration of mechanical ventilation. *Crit Care Med* 1999; 27: 2609–15.

Brown TM. Drug-induced delirium. *Semin Clin Neuropsychiatry* 2000; 5: 113–24.

Carson SS, Kress JP, Rodgers JE, *et al.* A randomized trial of intermittent lorazepam versus propofol with daily interruption in mechanically ventilated patients. *Crit Care Med* 2006; 34: 1326–32.

Ely EW, Shintani A, truman B, *et al.* Delirium as a predictor of mortality in mechanically ventilated patients in the intensive care unit. *JAMA* 2004; 291: 1753–62.

Jaber S, Chanques G, Altairac C, *et al.* A prospective study of agitation in a medical-surgical ICU: Incidence, risk factors, and outcomes. *Chest* 2005; 128: 2749–57.

Lin SM, Liu CY, Wang CH, *et al.* The impact of delirium on the survival of mechanically ventilated patients. *Crit Care Med* 2004; 32: 2254–9.

Lundstrom M, Edlund A, Karlsson S, *et al.* A multifactorial intervention program reduces the duration of delirium, length of hospitalization, and mortality in delirious patients. *J Am Geriatr Soc* 2005; 53: 622–8.

Pandharipande P, Shintani A, *et al.* Lorazepam is an independent risk factor for transitioning to delirium in intensive care unit patients. *Anesthesiology* 2006; 104: 21–6.

Woods JC, Mion LC, *et al.* Severe agitation among ventilated medical intensive care unit patients: frequency, characteristics and outcomes. *Intensive Care Med* 2004; 30: 1066–72.

www.icudelirium.org

www.ics.ac.uk Standards: UKCPA Delirium document

Status epilepticus

Status epilepticus is defined as seizure lasting >30min, or as seizures that recur over 30min without the patient regaining consciousness between seizures. Any seizure type can evolve into status epilepticus, but this chapter focuses on tonic–clonic status epilepticus, which is a neurological emergency. Annual incidence is 18–28 cases per 100 000, and it occurs most frequently in children, patients with learning difficulties and patients with structural brain lesions (especially in the frontal lobes). It can develop in patients with established epilepsy (particularly in the context of drug withdrawal) or in *de novo* patients. Up to 5% of adults attending specialist epilepsy clinics experience one episode of status during the course of the epilepsy. Causes in *de novo* patients include trauma, cerebrovascular disease, tumours, encephalitis, alcohol and drug withdrawal, and toxic disturbances. Status accounts for up to 3.5% of admissions to neurological intensive care, and 0.13% of patients attending a university casualty department. Mortality is up to 20%, most often due to the underlying condition rather than the status itself. The longer the duration of the status, the greater the morbidity.

Treatment of status involves termination of the seizures, preventing recurrence once status controlled, management of the complications, and treatment of the underlying precipitant.

Complications of convulsive status epilepticus relate to either the cerebral and metabolic consequences of prolonged convulsions or the effects of treatment. They include tachyarrhythmias, pulmonary oedema, hyperthermia, rhabdomyolysis, aspiration pneumonia, myocardial ischaemia, pulmonary emboli, ARDS, cerebral hypoxia, electrolyte disturbance, metabolic acidosis and ultimately multi-organ failure. Drug treatments may cause respiratory depression, cardiac arrhythmias, hypotension and gastric paresis. Fluid resuscitation and inotropic support may be required. Therefore, rapid seizure control is mandatory.

Treatment of convulsive status epilepticus

General measures

- Secure the airway + oxygen ± intubate
- Set up 2 IV lines for administration of fluids and drugs Benzodiazepines should be given through a separate IV line
- Set up continuous ECG and BP monitoring
- Send blood for gases, FBC, electrolytes, glucose, calcium, LFTs, anticonvulsant blood levels
- Ensure that routine antiepileptic drug (AED) doses are maintained if already on medication
- IV glucose and/or thiamine if appropriate
- Treat complications
- Commence long-term anticonvulsant therapy
- Be vigilant that the patient is not in pseudostatus epilepticus

Immediate first-line medication (within 10min of presentation)

IV Lorazepam 0.07mg/kg body weight to a maximum of 4mg, which can be repeated. Ampoules (Ativan injection) contain 4mg in 1ml. Advantages: long duration of action, less likely to cause sudden hypotension or respiratory arrest because of lack of CNS accumulation after bolus dose. Disadvantages: rapid tolerance, therefore of no further benefit after 2 bolus doses. Should be used in preference to other benzodiazepines if available.

OR

IV Diazepam 10–20mg at a rate of 2–5mg/min (risk of apnoea with faster injection). Do not repeat more than twice, or to a total of >40mg because of risks of hypotension or respiratory depression.

Second-line medication (10–60min of presentation)

One of these should be instituted without delay if there is any suggestion that the status will not be halted by initial benzodiazepine. The choice depends on availability and whether the patient is already taking one of these medications on a regular basis.

IV fosphenytoin sodium (Pro-epanutin): fosphenytoin can be infused at 3 times the speed of phenytoin and is significantly better tolerated at infusion sites. It should be given in preference to phenytoin if available. As with phenytoin, it can cause hypotension and arrhythmias.

Dose: 15mg PE/kg at a rate of 100mg PE/min (PE = phenytoin equivalent units)

OR

IV phenytoin. Disadvantages: hypotension, arrhythmias, administration must be slow, effective blood levels not obtained until 20–30min after infusion commenced. Contraindications: AV block. Ampoules contain phenytoin 250mg in 5 ml, which should be diluted in normal saline to a concentration of no more than 10mg/ml. Check there is no precipitate. The infusion should be completed within 1h of mixing.

Dose: 15–18mg/kg at a rate not exceeding 50mg/min (<30mg in the elderly) because of the risk of fatal arrhythmia

AND/OR

If the status persists then give phenobarbitone.

IV phenobarbitone: may cause respiratory depression and hypotension. Contraindications: acute intermittent porphyria. Ampoules contain 200mg/ml. Must be diluted with water for injection to a concentration of not more than 20mg/ml.

Dose: 10mg/kg to a maximum of 1000mg at a rate of 100mg/min, followed by 1–4mg/kg/day

Some centres prefer to use a 3rd non-anaesthetic before induction of coma.

IV sodium valproate 25–45mg/kg bolus (up to 500mg/min), particularly if the patient is in non-convulsant status, where anaesthetic agents are preferably avoided.

Third-line treatment for refractory status (30–90min from presentation)

This should be instituted if the convulsion has continued for >60min. The patient should be intubated and ventilated (if not already undertaken). Ideally continuous EEG monitoring should be undertaken.

Thiopentone 100–250mg bolus, then 50mg bolus every 3min until burst suppression on EEG. Maintenance 3–5mg/kg/h.

OR

Propofol 2mg/kg bolus, then repeat bolus if necessary. Maintenance 5–10mg/kg/h.

Some units also use *midazolam infusions* before undertaking anaesthetic coma using the following regime: *0.2mg/kg bolus*, followed by a continuous infusion of 0.1–0.4mg/kg/h.

No systematic RCT of status epilepticus has yet been published to compare different anaesthetic agents directly in this circumstance. Therefore, the choice of agent depends on the preference of the intensive care physician.

Other drugs

Some patients remain highly resistant to treatment despite aggressive anaesthetic coma. There are some case reports of such patients finally responding to topiramate given enterally in doses of 300–1600mg, or enteral levetiracetam 500–3000mg/day (which is also now available in some countries in IV form).

Long-term anticonvulsant therapy must be given in conjunction with emergency treatment. The choice of drug depends on previous therapy, the epilepsy type and the clinical setting. Maintenance doses can be given orally via an NG tube and can be guided by serum level monitoring.

Specific cerebral monitoring

In prolonged status, and in comatose ventilated patients, motor activity may not be visible. Continuous EEG monitoring should be undertaken if possible, or at least daily EEG if available. This will monitor ongoing electrical seizure activity or burst suppression, which provides a target for the titration of anaesthetic therapy. Dosing is commonly set at a level that will produce burst suppression with interburst intervals of between 2 and 30s. Once the patient has been free of seizures for 12–24h and provided that there are adequate blood levels of concomitant AED medication, then the anaesthetic should be slowly tapered.

ICP monitoring is sometimes required in the presence of persisting, severe or progressive elevated ICP. The need for this is usually determined by the underlying cause rather than the status itself. IPPV, high dose corticosteroid therapy (dexamethasone 4mg every 6h) or mannitol infusion may be used if there is a danger of tentorial coning. Neurosurgical decompression or specific resective surgery is occasionally required.

Malignant status epilepticus

There are some patients who remain in status lasting weeks to months. Such patients are often young, female, and present *de novo* without any clear precipitant of focal underlying brain lesion. This condition is known as 'cryptogenic *de novo* refractory status epilepticus'. 'new-onset refractory status epilepticus' or 'malignant status epilepticus'. The presumed underlying cause is often thought to be a form of encephalitis, as the CSF in such patients often contains mononuclear cells.

Differential diagnosis: psychogenic status epilepticus

It must be remembered that not all that shakes is epilepsy. It has been estimated that up to 50% of patients admitted to ICUs with a diagnosis of status epilepticus actually have non-epileptic attack disorder, or 'pseudostatus'. The diagnosis should be suspected if a patient has had multiple presentations with suspected status, particularly if there is also a history of self-harming behaviour, deliberate overdose or frequent presentations with medically unexplained symptoms. Such patients are often younger, female, have lower CK levels and receive significantly higher doses of benzodiazepine, leading to respiratory failure. Clinical features of the non-epileptic episodes include pelvic thrusting, poorly controlled thrashing, back arching, eyes held tightly closed and head rolling. Serum prolactin levels are not always helpful, as prolactin levels normalize with prolonged true seizure activity. Ictal EEG and specialized knowledge of seizure semiology usually can differentiate the conditions, but these are often not available after hours in the emergency situation. These patients are at risk of iatrogenic complications from aggressive treatment for suspected true convulsive status.

Prognosis

The outcome after an episode of status epilepticus is poor, with mortality rates being as high as 10–20%. Predictors of mortality include old age, the underlying aetiology of the status, the lack of prior history of epilepsy, the requirement for barbiturate coma and the level of consciousness at presentation. There is also a risk of cognitive decline and late epilepsy.

Support groups

The National Society for Epilepsy: `www.nse.org.uk`

Epilepsy Foundation of America: `www.epilepsyfoundation.org`

Further reading

Holtkamp M. The anaesthetic and intensive care of status epilepticus. *Curr Opin Neurol.* 2007; 20: 188–93.

Holtkamp M, Othman J, Buchheim K, *et al.* Diagnosis of psychogenic nonepileptic status epilepticus in the emergency setting. *Neurology* 2006; 66: 1727–9.

Howard RS, Kullmann DM, Hirsch NP. Admission to neurological intensive care: who, when, and why? *J Neurol Neurosurg Psychiatry.* 2003; 74 Suppl 3: iii2–9.

Howell SJ, Owen L, Chadwick DW. Pseudostatus epilepticus. *Q J Med* 1989; 71): 507–19.

Rossetti AO, Logroscino G, Bromfield EB. A clinical score for the prognosis of status epilepticus in adults. *Neurology* 2006; 66: 1736–8.

Shorvon S. The management of status epilepticus. *J Neurol Neurosurg Psychiatry* 2001; 70 (Suppl II): ii22–7.

Shorvon S, Dreifuss F, Fish D, *et al.* The treatment of epilepsy. Oxford: Blackwell Science Ltd, 1996.

Walker MC. Status epilepticus on the intensive care unit. *J Neurol* 2003; 250: 401–6.

Walker M. Status epilepticus: an evidence based guide. *BMJ* 2005; 331): 673–7.

Meningitis

Definition
Meningitis is the term given to an inflammation of the meninges, the protective layers surrounding the brain and spinal cord.

The causes of this inflammation are multiple, and include infection, trauma, neoplastic, autoimmune and drug causes. The subsequent inflammatory response may cause damage to the adjacent structures and hence cause neurological damage and the potential for death, and as such requires prompt investigation and treatment.

In most cases, meningitis is due to an infective aetiology, which can be bacterial, viral or fungal. Viral meningitis is the most common form and usually follows a benign course. However, bacterial meningitis is a serious disease that is associated with significant morbidity and mortality, and remains so despite attempts to reduce its effect.

Epidemiology and incidence
The incidence of bacterial meningitis is 3/100 000 (rates of *Haemophilus* and meningococcal type C infections are being reduced by ongoing vaccination campaigns).

Causes
The most likely bacterial pathogens as considered by patient age.

Age group	Causes
Neonates	Group B streptococci, *Escherichia coli*, *Listeria monocytogenes*
Infants	*Neisseria meningitidis*, *Haemophilus influenzae*, *Streptococcus pneumoniae*
Children	*N. meningitidis*, *S. pneumoniae*
Adults	*S. pneumoniae*, *N. meningitidis*, mycobacteria, cryptococci

Symptoms and signs
Variable presentation usually accompanied by corryzal symptoms in the prodromal phase. This is often followed by rapid clinical deterioration.

The triad of symptoms neck stiffness, altered mental state and fever are classical; however, these are only found in ~40% cases.

The most common symptoms are headache, neck stiffness and photophobia. Others include fever, phonophobia, diminished consciousness and seizures. Young infants may also present with fontanelle signs indicative of the disease process.

Other signs include the presence of a petechial, rapidly spreading rash often affecting the trunk and lower extremities which is indicative of *N. meningitides* (meningococcal) meningitis.

Eponymous signs
- Kernig's sign: pain elicited on passive flexion of knees which represents nuchal sensitivity.
- Brudzinski's sign: neck flexion causing lower limb flexion, especially in paediatric cases.

Whilst commonly performed, many authors question the validity of these tests.

Investigations
Investigations should be commenced concurrently with empiric antibacterial treatment if a diagnosis of meningitis is suspected.

These investigations include:
- FBC including differential
- U&E
- Blood glucose
- LFTs
- CRP assay
- Clotting studies
- ABG with serum lactate
- Blood cultures if pyrexia present
- Throat swab
- EDTA blood sample for PCR
- Urine for pneumococcal antigen
- Blood/ skin scraping of rash for urgent Gram stain
- ECG
- Consider lunbar puncture (LP)
- Consider CT

Definitive diagnosis may require CSF identification of a pathogen via LP. If there are no clinical contraindications to LP, a CT scan may not be required. A normal CT scan does not exclude raised ICP.

However, LP is contraindicated in the presence of raised ICP, due to the potential to cause brain herniation. LP is also relatively contraindicated in meningococcal septicaemia.

Lumbar puncture findings

Acute bacterial meningitis	Low	High	High, often >300/mm³
Acute viral meningitis	Normal	Normal or high	Mononuclear, < 300/mm³
Tuberculous meningitis	Low	High	Pleocytosis, mixed <300/mm³
Fungal meningitis	Low	High	< 300/mm³
Malignant meningitis	Low	High	Usually mononuclear
Subarachnoid haemorrhage	Normal	Normal or high	Erythrocytes

Many new diagnostic clinical tests are currently being evaluated in an attempt to distinguish bacterial meningitis from other causes of the disease rapidly. The Bacterial Meningitis Score can distinguish bacterial from viral meningitis (the weighted predictive points include a positive Gram stain, CSF protein >80mg/dl, peripheral absolute neutrophil count (ANC) >10 000 cells/mm^3, seizure at or before presentation and CSF ANC >1000 cells/mm^3).

Other tests include WBC, CRP and many CSF inflammatory markers.. No definitive test is currently available.

Management
The initial management of bacterial meningitis is to provide systematic support until an appropriate antibiotic regime has been implemented. However, in the initial phase of illness, bacterial and viral meningitis share many common features. In most circumstances, a broad-spectrum

antibiotic regime to combat the suspected bacterial meningitis is commenced, based on epidemiological analysis of likely pathogens. (see above)

Treatment

Bacterial meningitis is a medical emergency and has a high mortality rate if untreated.

Following initial recognition, prompt senior intervention is required.

Antimicrobial

- Cephalosporins (2g Ceftriaxone or Cefotaxime) remain the first-line antimicrobial agents.
- Ampicillin 2g IV qds may be added in patients in whom *Listeria monocytogenes* is suspected (age <3 or >55yrs).
- Vancomycin ± may be required if pneumococcal penicillin resistance is considered likely.

This may be changed on microbiological advice, once a pathogen has been identified.

Adjunctive

Adjunctive treatment of bacterial meningitis with steroids have been proven to reduce its mortality and morbidity, including the rates of severe hearing loss and other neurological sequelae

Some advocate the use of anticonvulsants and empirical antiviral therapies.

Organ support

Organ support via appropriate respiratory and cardiovascular treatment is most likely to be performed in a critical care environment. This may include:

- Volume resuscitation ± isotropic or vasopressor support in the presence of a systemic inflammatory response syndrome or shock
- Consider intubation and ventilation in refractory hypoxia
- Consider tight glycaemia control, low dose corticosteroid therapy and APC
- Correct electrolyte disturbances
- If signs of raised ICP treat with appropriate medical management including ensuring control of PaCO2, 30° bed-head elevation, normothermia and the prevention of seizures.
- Assess and treat sequelae.

Prognosis

Prognostic indicators of disease severity relate to the aetiology (bacterial, viral, etc.) and the clinical findings, along with the development of complications.

Holub *et al.* have proven the efficacy of CSF cortical levels as having prognostic predictive value in bacterial meningitis.

Viral meningitis

Viral meningitis is usually a self-limiting condition which responds to supportive treatment, fluids, antipyretics and analgesia. In some cases, including the immunocompromised, antiviral agents may be considered.

Fungal meningitis

Rare in the immunocompetent. *Cryptococcus neoformans* is the most common pathogen causing AIDS-related fungal meningitis. Treatment involves a prolonged course of antifungals.

Post-neurosurgical meningitis:

The most common bacterial pathogens are staphylococci and Gram-negative bacilli, especially in the presence of prosthetic material. Cephalosporins remain efficacious treatment, dependent on local microbiological advice. If *P. aeruginosa* is isolated or suspected, Ceftazidime is preferred.

In those patients with resistant pathogens, vancomycin or chloramphenicol may be considered.

Paediatric meningitis

The management of meningococcal disease in paediatric patients requires early senior specialist paediatric and/or intensive care clinicians.

A complete overview of the initial management is described by Pollard *et al.*

Public health considerations

- Bacterial meningitis is a Notifiable Illness. Ensure that CCDC have been informed of likely/proven case to ensure prophylaxis can be considered for contacts.
- Isolation of the patient for the first 24h on admission is considered beneficial.
- Notify microbiological staff.

Further reading

Beckham J, Tyler K. Initial management of acute bacterial meningitis in adults: summary of IDSA guidelines. *Rev Neurol Dis* 2006; 3: 57–60.

Hasbun R, Abrahams J, Jekel J, *et al.* Computed tomography of the head before lumbar puncture in adults with suspected meningitis. *N Engl J Med* 2001; 345: 1727–33.

Pollard AJ, Britto J, Nadel S, *et al.* Emergency management of meningococcal disease in children. *Arch Dis Child* 1999; 80: 290–6.

Nigrovic L, Kuppermann N, Malley R. Development and validation of a multivariable predictive model to distinguish bacterial from aseptic meningitis in children in the post-haemophilus influenzae era. *Pediatrics* 2002; 110: 712–9.

Provan D, Krentz A. Oxford handbook of clinical and laboratory investigation. Oxford: Oxford University Press. 2005.

Thomas KE, Hasbun R, Jekel J, *et al.* The diagnostic accuracy of Kernig's sign, Brudzinski's sign, and nuchal rigidity in adults with suspected meningitis. *Clin Infect Dis* 2002; 35: 46–52.

van de Beek D, de Gans J, McIntyre P, *et al.* Corticosteroids for acute bacterial meningitis. *Cochrane Database Syst Rev* 2007; (1): CD004405.

Intracerebral haemorrhage

Intracerebral haemorrhage (ICH) is an acute spontaneous extravasation of blood into the brain parenchyma.

Epidemiology

- ICH accounts for 10–30% of all strokes but is one of the major causes of stroke-related death and disability.
- >85% of cases of ICH occur as a primary event following spontaneous haemorrhage arising from rupture of small arteries and arterioles.
- The majority of primary ICH is associated with hypertension (60–70% of cases) or amyloid angiopathy (15% of cases).
- Around half of primary ICH occurs in the basal ganglia, one-third in the cerebral hemispheres and one-sixth in the brainstem or cerebellum.
- Secondary ICH is haemorrhage arising as a result of trauma, rupture of an intracranial aneurysm, an AV malformation or a coagulopathy.

Incidence

- 12–15 cases per 100 000 of the population
- More common in males, the elderly and in those of Asian and African ethnicity
- Incidence of ICH is significantly increased in patients receiving antiplatelet or anticoagulation therapy.

Risk factors

Hypertension (especially untreated), cerebral amyloid angiopathy, high alcohol intake and cocaine use are risk factors for ICH. The risk of antiplatelet drugs in general is unclear, but high-dose aspirin is associated with increased risk of ICH in the elderly, particularly in the presence of untreated hypertension. Warfarin anticoagulation increases the risk 5- to 10-fold.

Pathophysiology

ICH was previously considered a single haemorrhagic event, but it is now known that it is a complex, dynamic process involving three distinct phases: (1) initial haemorrhage, (2) haematoma expansion and (3) perihaematoma oedema. Two factors are of prime importance in disease progression and outcome. Haematoma expansion (often >33% original volume) may occur for several hours after the onset of symptoms and is an important cause of early neurological deterioration and a powerful predictor of adverse outcome. Peri-haematoma brain oedema starts early (in most cases within 3h from ICH onset) and evolves over many days. It occurs as a result of inflammation, cytotoxicity and blood–brain barrier disruption caused by release of thrombin and other coagulation end-products.

Diagnosis

ICH is usually associated with rapid onset focal neurological deficit and signs of raised ICP such as vomiting and decreased level of consciousness. Severe ICH may result in immediate unconsciousness. More than 90% of patients present with acute hypertension (>150/100mm Hg). Dysautonomia, including hyperventilation, tachycardia, central fever and hyperglycaemia, is also common. The differentiation between ICH and other forms of stroke cannot be determined by clinical status alone and must be confirmed by cranial CT or MRI scan.

Investigations

Cranial CT scan

- Urgent CT will confirm the diagnosis of ICH
- The cause of the ICH may be suggested by the pattern of bleeding
- The volume of the haematoma can be estimated
- Confirmation of extravasation of contrast into the haematoma predicts haematoma expansion

MRI scan

- MRI is as sensitive as CT for acute detection of ICH
- Generally used as a follow-up study to identify AV malformation, amyloid angiopathy or associated neoplasm.

Cerebral angiography

- Angiography is useful for confirming vascular causes of ICH such as AV malformation, dural AV fistula, cortical vein thrombosis or vasculitis
- Angiography should always be considered in young patients with no obvious risk factors for ICH.

Management

ICH should be treated as a medical emergency since delays in treatment are associated with worse outcome—the concept of 'time is brain' has recently been described Acute treatment includes airway management and control of blood pressure and ICP. Airway management is a priority when conscious level is impaired in order to protect the airway and facilitate mechanical ventilation to minimize secondary brain injury from hypoxaemia and hypercarbia. Mortality after ICH is reduced in patients cared for in specialist neurointensive care units.

Cardiovascular control

- Hypertension is common in the first 6h after ICH even in previously normotensive patients.
- Treatment of excessive hypertension should balance the risks of hypertension-related haematoma expansion against excessive reduction in CPP and peri-haematoma ischaemia.
- Blood pressure targets should be individualized but, in general terms, blood pressure should not be treated unless >180/105mm Hg.
- In all cases SBP should be maintained >90mm Hg.

Control of intracranial pressure

Emergency measures to control ICP are required for comatose patients or those who develop clinical signs of brainstem herniation.

Medical management

- Standard methods of ICP control include 30° head-up tilt, mannitol or hypertonic saline.
- Although osmotic agents successfully reduce acute elevations in ICP, there is no evidence that they reduce mortality or disability after ICH.

Neurosurgery

- Neurosurgical intervention after ICH remains controversial
- The STICH (Surgical Trial in Intracerebral Haemorrhage) trial showed no outcome benefit of evacuation of a supratentorial haematoma within 72h of ICH. Although

STICH challenges the view that early neurosurgery is an effective treatment for ICH, it does not confirm that surgery is useless in all cases because patients who might have benefited from emergency surgery were excluded from the study. Certain subgroups, such as younger patients with lobar haemorrhages causing significant mass effect, might therefore derive some benefit from surgery. Furthermore, because the mean time to surgery was >24h, STICH does not exclude the possibility that ultra-early surgery might have a role in some patients.

- Patients with cerebellar haemorrhages >3cm in diameter benefit from emergency surgical evacuation because of the high risk of early deterioration.
- Placement of an external ventricular drain may be life-saving in the presence of hydrocephalus.

Haemostatic therapy

Recent evidence suggests that rapid correction of coagulopathy and enhancement of coagulation variables in the absence of coagulopathy can play a significant role in the acute treatment of ICH and is associated with improved outcome.

- The high incidence of early haematoma expansion, combined with the relationship between haematoma volume and outcome after ICH, represents a potential target for acute therapeutic intervention.
- Recombinant activated factor VII (rFVIIa) is a potent initiator of haemostasis approved for treatment of bleeding in patients with haemophilia resistant to factor VII replacement.
- In a preliminary study of 399 patients with ICH, rFVIIa administered within 4h of onset of symptoms reduced haematoma expansion by 50%, reduced mortality by 38% and improved functional outcome at 90 days. These benefits occurred despite a 5% increase in the frequency of thromboembolic adverse events.
- The recently concluded phase III FAST study (Factor VIIa for Acute Hemorrhagic Stroke Treatment) confirmed the efficacy of rFVIIa in controlling intracerebral bleeding and reducing haematoma volume but, in contrast to earlier studies, did not demonstrate a reduction in mortality or disability in survivors.
- There is some evidence from a *post hoc* analysis of the FAST data that rFVIIa might be effective in a subgroup of younger patients (<75yrs) when administered within 3h of onset of symptoms.

Reversal of anticoagulation

Warfarin anticoagulation massively increases the risk of ICH, doubles the mortality and increases the risk of progressive bleeding and clinical deterioration. Emergency reversal of oral anticoagulant therapy is recommended in warfarin-associated ICH despite the risks of thromboembolic complications.

- Vitamin K should be administered immediately
- Coagulation factors should be given simultaneously as it takes several hours for vitamin K to achieve maximal effect.
- FFP should be infused until normal coagulation indexes are restored. FFP volumes between 800 and 3500ml may be required
- Large infused volumes may precipitate circulatory overload, and prothrombin complex concentrates may be used in patients in whom a large volume of FFP is contraindicated.
- rFVIIa is a promising candidate for the acute reversal of anticoagulation therapy but its short half-life is a drawback. However, evidence is currently limited and a controlled trial is needed.
- The optimal time for resumption of anticoagulation therapy after ICH has not been resolved. The risks and benefits of withholding or restarting treatment should be assessed for each patient individually.

Other intensive care management

- In addition to ventilatory support, blood pressure control and ICP monitoring, general supportive measures should be provided.
- Fever control is crucial since hyperthermia is associated with increased mortality and worse outcome in survivors.
- Seizures occur in ~10% of patients after ICH, and EEG monitoring is recommended in those at particular risk (e.g. lobar haematoma). Seizures should be treated aggressively, but there is no evidence that prophylactic anticonvulsant therapy improves outcome.
- Tight glycaemic control is essential.
- ICH patients are at high risk for thromboembolic complications. Dynamic compression stockings and intermittent calf compression should be initiated on admission to the ICU. SC heparin prophylaxis is controversial, although there is some evidence that it is not associated with increased risk of intracranial bleeding.
- Calorific intake should be maintained via the enteral route whenever possible.

Outcome

- 30–55% 6-month mortality overall, rising to 67% in patients receiving oral anticoagulant therapy
- Predictors of mortality include large ICH volume, older age, coma, requirement for mechanical ventilation, intraventricular extension and posterior fossa haemorrhage.
- Fewer than 20% survivors regain functional independence by 6 months.

Further reading

Diringer M, Edwards D. Admission to a neurologic/neurosurgical intensive care unit is associated with reduced mortality after intracerebral hemorrhage. *Crit Care Med* 2001; 29: 635–40.

Marietta M, Pedrazzi P, Girardis M, *et al.* Intracerebral haemorrhage: an often neglected medical emergency. *Intern Emerg Med* 2007; 2: 38–45.

Mayer S. Recombinant activated factor VII for acute intracerebral hemorrhage. *Stroke* 2007; 38: 763–7.

Mayer S, Rincon F. Treatment of intracerebral haemorrhage. *Lancet Neurol* 2005; 4: 662–72.

Rincon F, Mayer, S. Novel therapies for intracerebral hemorrhage. *Curr Opin Crit Care* 2004; 10: 94–100.

Subarachnoid haemorrhage

Aneurysmal subarachoid haemorrhage (SAH) is a neurological emergency with a high rate of complications and death.

Epidemiology

- SAH accounts for only 3% of all strokes but is one of the major cause of stroke-related death
- 80% of SAH is caused by a ruptured intracranial aneurysm

Incidence

- 6–8 cases per 100 000 of the population
- Peak incidence in the sixth decade of life

Diagnosis

SAH should be suspected in patients with sudden onset headache (often described as the 'worst imaginable' or like a 'hammer blow'), nausea, vomiting, photophobia and neck stiffness. Headache may be the only presenting feature in up to 40% of cases and may completely resolve within minutes or hours (sentinel headaches). Sentinel headaches should be investigated urgently as they may proceed to a serious SAH within 2–3 weeks. The diagnosis of SAH is more certain if the headache is accompanied by focal neurological signs, including third or sixth cranial nerve palsies, motor deficits or obtunded conscious level. Catastrophic SAH presents as sudden loss of consciousness.

Diagnosis

SAH is initially misdiagnosed in up to 50% of cases. The differential diagnosis includes migraine, tension headache and ischaemic or haemorrhagic stroke.

Grading of SAH

Several grading scales have been developed to describe the severity of SAH and assess prognosis. That described by the World Federation of Neurosurgeons (WFNS) is widely used and based on the GCS and presence or absence of a motor deficit.

- Grade 1: GCS 15 and no motor deficit
- Grade 2: GCS 14–13 and no motor deficit
- Grade 3: GCS 14–13 with motor deficit
- Grade 4: GCS 12–7 with or without motor deficit
- Grade 5: GCS 6–3 with or without motor deficit

Investigations

Cranial CT scan

- Urgent CT scanning should be performed in any patient with suspected SAH
- Fine cut CT is essential since small blood loads can easily be missed
- Characteristic high density areas are seen in the basal cisterns and throughout the CSF spaces
- CT also demonstrates the presence of cerebral oedema, hydrocephalus and intraparenchymal blood

Lumbar puncture

- LP should be performed in any patient with suspected SAH in whom the CT scan is equivocal or negative
- Diagnostic features for SAH include high CSF opening pressure, elevated red cell count and xanthochromia after 12h.

Cerebral angiography

- Four-vessel angiography is the gold standard for aneurysm identification, characterization of vascular anatomy and diagnosis of cerebral vasospasm
- Conventional angiography is a time-consuming investigation that is not risk free
- CT or MR angiography are non-invasive alternatives

Management

Following SAH, cardiorespiratory status should be stabilized and patients transferred to a specialist neuroscience unit. Patients benefit from multi-disciplinary neurointensive care where management is targeted at optimizing cardiovascular variables, securing the ruptured aneurysm, detecting and treating intracranial complications, including the prevention and treatment of cerebral vasospasm, and managing systemic complications.

Cardiovascular control

- Prior to control of the aneurysm, systemic blood pressure should be carefully controlled in the 'high normal' range to maintain cerebral perfusion whilst minimizing the risk of re-bleeding.
- Hypotension should be treated initially with IV fluids followed by vasopressors.
- Hypertension should only be treated if SBP exceeds 160mm Hg in a previously normotensive patient.

Prevention of re-bleeding

- Re-bleeding occurs in 7% cases and is prevented by early protection of the ruptured aneurysm
- Endovascular intervention is now the treatment of choice for the majority of aneurysms.
- Endovascular treatment is associated with a relative risk reduction of 22.6% and absolute risk reduction of 6.9% in death or long-term dependency compared with surgical clipping.

Hydrocephalus

- Hydrocephalus occurs in ~25% patients within a few days after SAH.
- Temporary external ventricular drainage may be indicated to relieve the hydrocephalus
- A minority of patients require long-term CSF diversion via a ventricular shunt

Vasospasm

With the current emphasis on early protection of ruptured aneurysms, cerebral vasospasm and delayed ischaemic neurological deficit (DIND) is the most common cause of mortality and morbidity after SAH. Aggressive preventative and treatment strategies for vasospasm are key components of the ICU management of SAH.

Pathophysiology

- Vasospasm peaks at 4–10 days after the ictus and persists for several days.
- The exact cause remains obscure but is related to blood load in the basal cisterns.
- Constituents of oxyhaemoglobin are likely spasmogenic factors, and several mechanisms co-exist, including release of endothelin, generation of reactive oxygen species and inhibition of NO. Histotological changes, including

adventitial inflammation and intimal hyperplasia, also occur in the affected vessels.

Diagnosis

- Vasospasm is detected clinically in conscious patients by a reduction in conscious level with or without a focal neurological deficit.
- Cerebral angiography is the gold standard for diagnosis of cerebral vasospasm.
- CT angiography is less invasive and may be combined with CT perfusion scanning to allow assessment of associated perfusion abnormalities
- Transcranial Doppler ultrasonography is routinely used in the bedside assessment of vasospasm.

Prevention and treatment

- Triple-H therapy (hypervolaemia, hypertension and haemodilution) is widely used to prevent and treat cerebral vasospasm after SAH.
  - Crystalloids and colloids should be infused (>3000ml/24h) to achieve a daily positive fluid balance
  - Supranormal systemic blood pressure is maintained using vasopressors/inotropes
  - Haemodilution is the most controversial component of triple-H therapy and is not universally applied
  - Triple-H therapy is effective in reversing DIND in many patients but the efficacy of prophylactic treatment to prevent vasospasm is less clear
  - Triple-H therapy is not a risk-free intervention and should be discontinued as soon as the DIND resolves.
- Endovascular treatments, including balloon angioplasty and intra-arterial infusion of vasodilating agents, are useful in patients with symptomatic vasospasm resistant to triple-H therapy.

Cerebral protection

Many pharmacological agents have been tested in clinical studies of SAH. Some have become established into clinical practice whereas others show considerable promise.

- Nimodipine, a specific antagonist of the L-type voltage-gated calcium channel, improves outcome after SAH and is administered routinely (60mg PO 4 hourly).
- Magnesium is a promising treatment, and small studies demonstrate a reduction in the incidence of DIND and improved outcome.
- Statins may reduce the incidence of vasospasm after SAH.
- Tirilazad has little effect on overall outcome after SAH but may have benefit in patients with poor neurological grade.
- Potential treatments include selective endothelin A receptor antagonists and PDE inhibitors.
- Gene therapy that targets the transcription of harmful protein products such as endothelin is also likely to be developed.

Antithrombotic agents

Microvascular thrombosis may contribute to DIND and, despite concerns about bleeding, there has been interest in the use of antithrombotic agents after SAH.

- Cisternal infusions of recombinant tPA or urokinase are safe and effective interventions to reduce CSF blood load.
- Antiplatelet drugs reduce the risk of DIND with a trend towards improved outcome, but further studies are required to determine the haemorrhagic risk.
- There are conflicting data on the relative benefits and risks of LMWH after SAH.
- Antithrombotic agents are currently only indicated in highly selected patients.

Systemic complications

Systemic complications occur in up to 79% of patients after SAH. and are independently associated with higher mortality and worse functional outcome in survivors.

- ECG changes and 'stunned' myocardium syndrome are likely to be related to endogenous catecholamine release and activation of adrenoceptors.
- Pulmonary complications occur because of pulmonary expression of a systemic inflammatory response, neurogenic pulmonary oedema and as a complication of triple-H therapy.
- Hyponatraemia is common after SAH and related to haemodilution, cerebral salt wasting syndrome or the syndrome of inappropriate antidiuretic hormone secretion.
- Fever, anaemia and hyperglycaemia are associated with increased mortality and poor functional outcome in survivors, and should be corrected.

Outcome

- SAH has an overall mortality rate of 51%
- 12% of patients die before they receive medical attention
- 33% of survivors need lifelong care and a further 46% have residual cognitive deficits that affect functional status and quality of life
- Prognosis depends on three factors—the grade of SAH, the success of the procedure to secure the aneurysm and the occurrence of sequelae, particularly cerebral vasospasm,

Further reading

Diringer MN. To clip or to coil acutely ruptured intracranial aneurysms: update on the debate. *Curr Opin Crit Care* 2005; 11: 121–5.

Janjua N, Mayer SA. Cerebral vasospasm after subarachnoid hemorrhage. *Curr Opin Crit Care* 2003; 9: 113–9.

Sen J, Belli A, Albon H, *et al.* Triple-H therapy in the management of aneurysmal subarachnoid haemorrhage. *Lancet Neurol* 2003; 2: 614–21.

Smith M. Intensive care management of patients with subarachnoid haemorrhage. *Curr Opin Anesthesiol* 2007; 20: 400–7.

Suarez J, Tarr R, Selman W. Aneurysmal subarachnoid hemorrhage. *N Engl J Med* 2006; 354: 387–96.

Wartenberg KE, Mayer SA. Medical complications after subarachnoid hemorrhage: new strategies for prevention and management. *Curr Opin Crit Care* 2006; 12: 78–84.

Wilson S, Hirsch N, Appleby I. Management of subarachnoid haemorhage in a non-neurosurgical centre. *Anaesthesia* 2005; 60: 470–85.

Ischaemic stroke

Introduction

Stroke is the third most common cause of death worldwide and is a major cause of disability. 85% of all strokes are ischaemic and, of these, 35% are due to large artery thromboembolism, 24% are caused by cardiac embolism (e.g. due to AF, mural thrombus post-MI or complicating endocarditis), 18% are due to small vessel disease, 18% are due to uncertain causes and 5% are due to rare causes (e.g. vasculitis, arterial dissection). The diagnosis of ischaemic stroke requires a compatible history (an abrupt onset of a focal neurological deficit) and neurological examination (a neurological deficit localized to a vascular territory), with supportive evidence from neuroimaging (which also excludes differential diagnoses such as tumour and haemorrhage), and blood testing to exclude hyper/hypoglycaemia, sepsis and other metabolic derangements. Some types of ischaemic stroke carry a particularly high mortality and morbidity rate, e.g. middle cerebral artery (MCA) with cerebral oedema and basilar thrombosis.

There are now time-critical treatments available that improve outcome after stroke: aspirin and thrombolysis. Therefore, ischaemic stroke should be considered a medical emergency. These treatments have resulted in a more aggressive approach to management, necessitating more active involvement of intensive care.

Aims of management in acute ischaemic stroke

- Identify diagnosis of ischaemic stroke
- Pay particular attention to onset time and vascular territory, e.g. MCA, basilar, posterior cerebral, lacunar syndrome
- Exclude haemorrhage (with CT)
- Consider other diagnoses, e.g. tumour, migraine, seizure, cerebral venous sinus thrombosis, encephalitis
- Determine eligibility for thrombolysis
- Establish neurological status and blood pressure parameters
- Determine aetiology and mechanism of stroke, e.g. carotid stenosis, AF, arteritis
- Prevent and treat complications
- Initiate secondary stroke prevention when appropriate, e.g. antiplatelet agents, cholesterol-lowering agents, blood pressure-lowering agents, carotid endarterectomy

Suggested criteria for admission to ICU

The following criteria are suggested for ICU admission:

- Need for monitoring neurological deterioration
  - Thrombolytic therapy
  - Large hemispheric infarction
  - Cerebellar infarction
  - Basilar artery brainstem stroke
  - Fluctuating neurological deficits
  - Reduced conscious state
  - Control of seizures
  - Management of raised ICP
  - Maintenance of CPP
- Need for airway management
  - Maintain patient airway
  - Manage airway secretions/pneumonia
- Need for intensive cardiovascular monitoring
  - Uncontrolled hypertension
  - Myocardial ischaemia, congestive heart failure, arrhythmias
  - In-hospital strokes after medical and surgical procedures
- Need for general management
  - Temperature control
  - Glycaemic control
  - Fluid management
  - Treatment of complications, e.g. sepsis, pulmonary embolism
  - Intubation for diagnostic or therapeutic procedures, e.g. MRI

Acute treatment of ischaemic stroke

Antiplatelet agents

There is good evidence that use of aspirin (150–300mg/day) commenced within 48h of the stroke reduces the risk of recurrent stroke and death, as well as increasing functional outcome. Aspirin should therefore be routinely commenced as soon as possible unless there is a clear contraindication, such as proven ICH or definite aspirin sensitivity (e.g. wheeze or skin rash on aspirin exposure). Note, however, that protocols for the use of IV tPA call for avoiding all antithrombotic therapy, including heparin and aspirin, for the first 24h after thrombolysis.

Anticoagulation

There is no proven benefit from the routine use of anticoagulants in the treatment of acute ischaemic stroke. Despite this, heparin is commonly used in patients with cardioembolic stroke, large vessel stroke progression and basilar artery thrombosis. There is evidence, however, for anticoagulation for early secondary prevention in patients with cardiac embolism. In this circumstance, a delay of up to 2 weeks is recommended to reduce the risk of haemorrhagic transformation, particularly in large strokes, before commencing heparinization and then warfarinization. There may be occasions where heparin may be appropriate, e.g. patients at high risk of thromboembolic disease, patients in AF or patients with stroke due to cerebral venous thrombosis.

Thrombolysis

Reperfusion of ischaemic brain as soon as possible may lessen the volume of permanently damaged brain and lead to a better clinical outcome. Thrombolytic therapy potentially improves perfusion by lysing the occluding thrombus. Thrombolytic therapy has now been shown to reduce significantly the death rate and the number of patients left severely disabled after ischaemic stroke. There is, however, a net increase in deaths in the first 7–10 days from ICH. Three thrombolytic agents have been trialled: IV tPA (recombinant tissue plasminogen activator—alteplase), intra-arterial prourokinase, and ancrod (an IV defibrinogenating agent). tPA has been the most extensively investigated, and is associated with more benefit and fewer risks. It is now approved for use by NICE and US FDA.

Importantly, there is a very narrow time rame for administration. Treatment must be instituted within 3h of a clearly defined time of onset of the ischaemic stroke (or the risk of ICH outweighs the potential benefits of clot lysis). In the near future, however, new MRI techniques will be able to identify patients who might benefit from treatment beyond 3h. The patient must have a moderate to severe neurological deficit without significant improvement. Absolute contraindications include any blood on pre-treatment CT, established infarction on CT, severe hypertension, surgery or trauma within 14 days and known coagulopathy. The NICE recommendations for administration are tPA infusion in a 0.9mg/kg (max 90mg) continuous IV infusion over 60min, with 10% of total dose as a bolus at the start of the infusion (over 2–3min). These patients need careful monitoring for any neurological or cardiovascular decline, and should be managed in specialist units. Follow-up CT scan should be performed after 24h, and aspirin should be commenced if haemorrhage excluded.

Intra-arterial tPA

There are theoretical advantages to using intra-arterial tPA compared with systemic administration. Local tPA may be safer and more effective, as a higher concentration of tPA is attained directly at the thrombus site with potentially minor systemic side effects. However, intra-arterial thrombolysis is limited to specialized centres. There are only a few small randomized trials addressing this technique, but there is evidence for efficacy in acute basilar occlusion. Acute basilar occlusion accounts for up to 10% of large-vessel stroke, with the fatality rate being the highest for all ischaemic stroke subtypes, up to 90%, with rapid progression to coma and death in many patients. Although no large randomized studies have been performed, there is evidence from small series that patients who undergo successful recanalization of the basilar artery by intra-arterial thrombolysis have lower mortality of 39%. There have also been some case reports of recanalization by intra-arterial thrombolysis up to 18h after the onset of the basilar occlusion with improved outcome.

Decompressive surgery

There are certain circumstances where neurosurgical intervention may be considered. Decompressive surgery involves the removal of a large part of the skull to allow space for the expansion of swollen brain tissue, which thereby reduces ICP, prevents fatal brain herniation, increases perfusion pressure to the brain that is still salvageable, and preserves CBF.

Patients with large supratentorial infarcts may deteriorate due to massive cerebral oedema, usually developing between 2 and 5 days. Recent pooled data from three randomized trials has demonstrated that in patients with malignant MCA infarction, decompressive surgery undertaken within 48h of stroke onset reduces mortality and increases the number of patients with a favourable functional outcome, particularly if the non-dominant hemisphere is involved. The decision to perform decompressive surgery should, however, be made on an individual basis in every patient

Large cerebellar infarctions may be associated with oedema, which can cause compression of the 4th ventricle, obstructive hydrocephalus, herniation and death. Therefore, cerebellar infarction associated with a declining level of consciousness constitutes a potential neurosurgical emergency. Surgical decompression of the posterior fossa or shunting may be required. As the level of consciousness is the most powerful predictor for outcome, patients with large cerebellar infarction should be observed on a stroke unit or ICU.

Other interventions

The use of hyperventilation, steroids and mannitol to treat raised ICP and cerebral oedema in ischaemic stroke is widespread, although clinical trials do not demonstrate improved survival or improved functional outcome Several potential neuroprotective agents have been studied, including calcium channel blockers, antioxidants and NMDA antagonists. Although trials have been completed, they are still of unproven clinical value. Research is currently ongoing into the potential benefits of therapeutic hypothermia.

Other important stroke syndromes

Cerebral venous sinus thrombosis

Cerebral venous sinus thrombosis should be considered as a cause of stroke in young women on the oral contraceptive pill, during pregnancy and puerperium, in association with intracranial, ear or sinus infections, in patients with cancer and haematological disorders, and in patients with other types of hypercoaguable states, such as inflammatory bowel disease, phospholipid antibody syndrome or severe dehydration. Headache and seizures are common, and should alert to the possible diagnosis. Papilloedema with focal neurology is not uncommon. MRI with MR venography or CT with CT venography are the investigations of choice to confirm the diagnosis. Formal angiography may also be required, particularly in a patient with smaller vein occlusions. Many centres recommend anticoagulation with heparin and then warfarin, although supportive evidence from randomized trials is lacking. Causes of late deterioration include extension of the thrombosis, raised ICP, seizures, systemic complications (pneumonia, PEs, sepsis) and complications of the associated hypercoaguable state.

Support groups

The Stroke Association: `www.stroke.org.uk`

American Stroke Association: `www.strokeassociation.org`

Further reading

Chen, ZM, Sandercock P, Pan HC, *et al.* on behalf of the CAST and IST Collaborative Groups. Indications for early aspirin use in acute ischaemic stroke: a combined analysis of 40,000 randomised patients from the Chinese Acute Stroke Trial and the International Stroke Trial. *Stroke* 2000; 31: 1240–9.

Gubitz G, Counsell C, Sandercock P, *et al.* Antiplatelet agents for acute ischaemic stroke. In: The Cochrane Library. Oxford: Update Software, 2000a.

Gubitz G, Counsell C, Sandercock P, *et al.* Anticoagulants for acute ischaemic stroke. In: The Cochrane Library. Oxford: Update Software, 2000b.

Kollmar R, Schwab S. Ischaemic stroke: acute management, intensive care, and future perspectives. *Br J Anaesth* 2007; 99: 95–101

National Institute for Health and Clinical Excellence. Final appraisal determination: alteplase for the treatment of acute ischaemic stroke. Issue date April 2007, `www.nice.org.uk`

Singh V. Critical care assessment and management of acute ischaemic stroke. *J Vascul Intervent Radiol* 2004; 15: S21–7.

Smith WS. Intra-arterial thrombolytic therapy for acute basilar occlusion. *Stroke* 2007; 28: 701–3.

Vahedi K, Hofmeijer J, Juettler E, *et al.* Early decompressive surgery in malignant infarction of the middle cerebral artery: a pooled analysis of three randomised controlled trials. *Lancet Neurol* 2007; 6: 215–22.

Wardlaw JM, del Zoppo G, Yamaguchi T, *et al.* Thrombolysis for acute ischaemic stroke. *Cochrane Database Syst Rev* 2003; (3): CD000213.

Warlow CP, Dennis MS, van Gijn J, *et al.* Stroke: a practical guide to management, 2nd edn, Oxford: Blackwell Science, 2001.

Guillain–Barre syndrome

Guillan–Barre syndrome (GBS) is an acute peripheral neuropathy with at least four subtypes. Acute inflammatory demyelinating polyneuropathy (AIDP) is the most common subtype, characterized by ascending and symmetrical weakness, areflexia and sensory and autonomic disturbances. Acute motor axonal neuropathy (AMAN) describes a purely motor deficit, and when sensory fibres are also involved the subtype is designated acute motor sensory axonal neuropathy (AMSAN). The Miller–Fisher variant of GBS is characterized by ataxia, opthalmoplegia and areflexia with little limb weakness.

Epidemiology

- 1.5 times more common in males than females
- Subtypes have different geographical variations
- Most cases are sporadic

Incidence

- 1–4 cases per 100 000 of the population
- Increases with age

Causes

GBS has an immune basis. In AIDP, antibodies generated in response to an infectious agent cross-react with myelin proteins and result in the characteristic inflammatory demyelination. Often the causative agent is not identified, but *Campylobacter jejuni* (40%), *Mycoplasma pneumoniae* (5%), CMV (15%), EBV and HIV have all been implicated. Some vaccines (influenza, rabies) and major surgery have also been associated with the development of GBS. In 10% of cases the axon itself is damaged by antibodies to gangliosides on the axolemma (AMAN and AMSAN subtypes).

Diagnosis

Diagnostic criteria have been established and are based on clinical features, elevated CSF protein concentration and nerve conduction studies. In the acute phase, the symptoms can be mistaken for a psychological problem, and a high index of suspicion of GBS must be present in all patients presenting with acute weakness.

Differential diagnosis

The differential diagnosis of GBS is wide.

Acute polyneuropathy

- Acute intermittent porphyria
- Heavy metal poisoning
- Poliomyelitis
- Diphtheria
- Lyme disease

Disorders of the neuromuscular junction

- Myasthenia gravis
- Botulism
- Diphtheria
- Poisoning—organophosphates, lead, shellfish

Miscellaneous

- Critical illness polyneuropathy
- Transverse myelitis
- Brainstem lesions
- Carcinomatosis
- Muscle disorders—rhabdomyolysis, periodic paralysis

Clinical features

GBS is preceded by a 'flu-like illness or gastroenteritis in 66% of cases. A symmetrical weakness evolves over a few days, usually after the antecedent symptoms have settled. Sensory symptoms and pain may pre-date the onset of weakness. The weakness reaches a peak within 2–4 weeks and, following a plateau phase lasting 3–4 weeks, resolves over a variable period.

Symptoms and signs

GBS is characterized by a progressive, ascending symmetrical limb weakness that evolves over a few days and may be heralded by distal paraesthesia, pain and numbness. In severe cases, the weakness may progress to quadriplegia. Reflexes are diminished or absent. Involvement of respiratory muscles may result in hypoventilation and dyspnoea, and 30% patients require mechanical ventilation. Facial nerve weakness is a frequent finding, but bulbar weakness is less common, although serious. Autonomic involvement results in sinus tachycardia, cardiac arrhythmias, postural hypotension, severe sweating, ileus and urinary retention.

Investigations

Vital capacity (VC)

- 4 hourly VC routinely, with more frequent assessment if clinical deterioration
- Transfer to ITU when VC is <20ml/kg
- Intubation if VC is <15ml/kg

Cerebrospinal fluid analysis

- CSF protein elevated in 80% patients after 1 week
- WCC usually normal.

Neurophysiology

- Nerve conduction studies are abnormal in 85% of cases within 1 week of onset of symptoms
- Nerve conduction studies can differentiate between demyelination (decreased conduction velocity) and axonal damage (decreased amplitude)

Microbiology and immunology

- Antibodies for *C. jejuni,* CMV, EBV, HSV, HIV, *M. pneumoniae* and atypical pneumonia
- stool for *C. jejuni* and poliovirus
- Serology—hepatitis A, B, C and atypical pneumonia
- Antiganglioside autoantibodies to delineate GBS subtypes

Neuroimaging

- MRI brain and spinal cord
  - cord compression
  - brainstem lesions

Other investigations

- B12 and folate
- Thyroid function tests
- Urinary porphyrins
- Paraprotein bands
- Drug and toxin screen

Autonomic tests

Cardiac monitoring and others as indicated.

Management

The treatment of GBS consists of general supportive care and specific treatment. Many patients require ICU admission.

Indications for admission to ICU

- Respiratory failure
- Bulbar weakness
- Autonomic instability
- Management of complications

Intubation and mechanical ventilation

- ARF occurs because of hypoventilation, inadequate airway protection and poor cough.
- Intubation indicated when clinical evidence of fatigue, pulmonary aspiration or VC <15ml/kg.
- Early intubation is indicated when bulbar and respiratory muscle weaknesses co-exist.
- Care should be taken during intubation to avoid bradycardia and large swings in blood pressure related to autonomic instability. Succinylcholine is avoided because of the risk of fatal hyperkalaemia.
- NIV is of limited value, and is contraindicated in the presence of bulbar palsy.
- Early tracheostomy is recommended in those who respond poorly to treatment or who are difficult to wean.

Autonomic support

- Cardiac arrhythmias and labile blood pressure should be treated promptly with standard agents.
- Resistant bradyarrythmias may require cardiac pacing.
- GI ileus occurs frequently but urinary retention is less common.

General supportive care

- Pneumonia is a frequent complication and usual preventative measures are mandatory.
- Thromboembolic disease is a major risk, and LMWH, graded support stockings and physiotherapy minimize the risk of DVT.
- Pain is often severe and distressing. In addition to simple analgesics, opioids and agents to treat neuropathic pain (e.g. gabapentin) may be required.
- Enteral feeding is possible in many patients. If there is a severe ileus, the stomach should be drained via a gastric tube, and parenteral nutrition and gastric ulcer prophylaxis started.
- Neurophysiotherapy, using passive flexion exercises and splints, is vital to prevent tendon shortening during the period of paralysis. Frequent turning and careful limb positioning are also necessary to prevent pressure sores and nerve palsies.
- Effective means of communication should be established in patients who are paralysed. Activities to occupy patients are also beneficial.
- Cognitive disturbance and depression are common in those with severe disease, and psychiatric input may be necessary.

Immunotherapy

Two immunomodulatory therapies, plasma exchange and IV immunoglobulin (IVIG), are equally effective treatments for GBS but there is no advantage in combining the two. Relapses can occur, and most patients respond to a second course of either plasma exchange or IVIG.

- Plasma exchange with 3–5 treatments over 5–8 days reduces the need for respiratory support, improves muscle strength and shortens the recovery period. Benefit is greatest when started within 7 days of disease onset. Total plasma exchange for a treatment episode is ~400ml/kg. The risks include hypotension, coagulopathy and hypocalcaemia, as well as catheter-related thrombosis and sepsis. Patients with dysautonomia or severe cardiovascular disease may not tolerate plasma exchange.
- IVIG is a pooled blood product of purified IgG administered at a dose of 400mg/kg daily for 5 days. It is more expensive than plasma exchange but is usually the favoured treatment option because of its ease of administration and fewer side effects, particularly line-associated infection. There is a small risk of thrombosis during treatment with IVIG, so patients should be well hydrated prior to treatment.
- Corticosteroids are ineffective treatment for GBS and increase mortality.

Outcome

- 80% of patients with demyelinating GBS have a good outcome at 1yr.
- 5–15% overall mortality rate with up to 20% of survivors remaining disabled.
- ICU mortality is ~5%.
- Prognosis is worse in the elderly and in those with severe motor deficit or who require prolonged mechanical ventilation.

Patient support group

The Guillain–Barre syndrome support group www.gbs.org.uk

Further reading

Ashbury AK, Cornblath DR. Assessment of current diagnostic criteria for Guillain–Barre syndrome. *Arch Neurol* 1990; 27: S21–4.

Green D. Weakness in the ICU: Guillain–Barre syndrome, myasthenia gravis and critical illness polyneuropathy/myopathy. *Neurologist* 2005;11: 338–47.

Hughes RA, Cornblath DR. Guillain–Barre syndrome. *Lancet* 2005; 366: 1653–66.

Hughes RA, Raphael JC, Swan AV, *et al.* Intravenous immunoglobulin for Guillain–Barre syndrome. *Cochrane Database Syst Rev* 2001; (1): CD002063.

Hughes RA, van der Meche FG. Corticosteroids for treating Guillain-Barre syndrome. *Cochrane Database Syst Rev* 2002; (3): CD001446.

Hughes, RAC, Wijdicks E, Barohn RJ, *et al.* Supportive care for Guillain–Barre syndrome. *Arch Neurol* 2005; 62: 1194–8.

van der Meche FGA, Schmitz PIM, Dutch Guillain-Barre Study Group. A randomized trial comparing intravenous immune globulin and plasma exchange in Guillain–Barre syndrome. *N Engl J Med* 1992; 326: 1123–9.

Myasthenia gravis

Definition

Myasthenia gravis (MG) is an autoimmune disease affecting the postsynaptic membrane of the neuromuscular junction.

Epidemiology

Mainly affects young females and older males.

Incidence

0.25–2.0 per 100 000 population

Causes

85% of patients with MG have IgG antibodies against postsynaptic skeletal muscle acetylcholine receptors (AChR), often associated with an abnormality of the thymus gland. Receptor degradation, decrease in receptor half-life and complement-related damage to the postsynaptic membrane are characteristic of MG. Antibodies against muscle-specific receptor kinase (MuSK) are present in the majority of MG patients without anti-AChR antibodies (seronegative MG).

Diagnosis

The diagnosis of MG is relatively straightforward and based on recognition of a typical pattern of weakness, involving some combination of extraocular, bulbar, facial, neck and limb muscles. The diagnosis is confirmed by neurophysiological investigations and detection of anti-AChR antibodies.

Differential diagnosis

The differential diagnosis of MG is wide.

Motor neuropathies

- Guillain–Barre syndrome
- Motor neuron disease
- Diphtheria

Myopathies

- Muscular dystrophy
- Acquired myopathies (including electrolye disorders)
- Mitochondrial disorders

Disorders of the neuromuscular junction

- Lambert–Eaton myasthenia syndrome (LEMS)
- Botulism
- Organophosphate poisoning

Other

- Brainstem lesions
- Cervical myelopathy
- Multiple sclerosis
- Thyroid disease

Risk factors

There are many drugs and other factors that can induce or exacerbate MG.

Drugs

- Proven effects—penicillamine, corticosteroids
- Probable effects—aminoglycosides, β-blockers, procainamide, ciprofloxacin, phenytoin, lithium
- Possible effects—anticholinergics, ampicillin, erythromycin, muscle relaxants, verapamil, chloroquine

Other factors

- Infection
- Trauma and surgery
- Pregnancy

Clinical features

MG is characterized by fatigable weakness of skeletal muscle. Classically the weakness worsens after exercise and in the evening, and is improved by rest. Ptosis, diplopia and blurred vision are the presenting features in 60% of cases. Proximal limb weakness is more common than distal weakness. Bulbar muscle weakness may also be prominent, and respiratory muscle weakness occurs in 20–30% of cases. In 15% of patients the disease is confined to the eyes (ocular MG).

Symptoms and signs

Ptosis, often partial and unilateral, is common and most prominent on sustained upward gaze. Weakness usually progresses from ocular muscles in a craniocaudal direction, with upper limb weakness being more common than lower. There are no objective sensory signs, and deep tendon reflexes are normal or brisk. Weakness of intercostals muscles and the diaphragm leads to dyspnoea which improves on sitting up. Respiratory deterioration can occur rapidly and respiratory rate and vital capacity (VC) should be closely monitored. Hypercapnea is a sign of impending respiratory failure but hypoxaemia occurs late. Involvement of bulbar muscles is characterised by a slurred nasal voice, difficulty with chewing and swallowing and may result in aspiration pneumonia.

Investigations

Electrophysiological tests

- EMG
  - baseline compound muscle action potential (CMAP) usually normal
  - decrement >10% in first 4–5 CMAPs on low frequency (2–3Hz) repetitive stimulation
  - 80% sensitive for diagnosis of generalized MG
- Single fibre EMG
  - recording of response to stimulation of a single fibre
  - more sensitive (>90%) than standard EMG
  - technically difficult

Autoantibodies

- More specific for diagnosis than EMG
- Anti-AChR antibodies
  - diagnostic for MG
  - positive in 100% of thymoma-associated MG, in 70–90% of generalized MG and in 60% of ocular MG
  - titres not related to severity of disease
- Anti-MuSK antibodies
  - positive in 70% of patients with seronegative MG.

Edrophonium (Tensilon®) test

- For urgent diagnosis of severe MG only
- 2–10mg edrophonium (short acting anticholinesterase) IV
- Improvement in muscle strength within 45s (lasting 5min) confirms MG
- Low sensitivity and specificity

- Pre-treatment with atropine minimizes risk of bradycardia and hypotension
- May increase pulmonary secretions and worsen respiratory failure

Neuroimaging

- CT/MRI chest
  - thymoma in 20% of MG patients
  - thymic hyperplasia in 70% of MG patients
- MRI brain to exclude
  - brainstem lesions
  - mass lesions compressing cranial nerves

Muscle biopsy

- Quantify AchR density
- Electron microscopy of neuromuscular junction
- Exclude mitochondrial disease

Other investigations

- Thyroid function
- Antinuclear antibody
- Antistriated muscle antibodies
- Genetic testing for hereditary MG

Treatment of MG

- Enhancement of neuromuscular transmission—anticholinesterase drugs
- Immunosuppression—corticosteroids and/or azothiaprine
- Thymectomy—thymoma or thymic hyperplasia
- Plasma exchange or IVIG for exacerbations

Myasthenic crisis

Myasthenic crisis occurs when the weakness is severe enough to require endotracheal intubation for mechanical ventilation and airway protection. 8–27% patients with MG experience a crisis, often in the early years after diagnosis. It is more common in those with bulbar weakness or thymoma, and may rarely be the presenting feature of MG. Myasthenic crisis should be differentiated from cholinergic crisis (caused by excessive anticholinesterase treatment) which is characterized by hypersalivation, abdominal pains and diarrhoea, but is extremely rare with modern management strategies.

Precipitating factors for myasthenic crisis

- Respiratory tract infection (30–40%)
- Pulmonary aspiration (10%)
- Trauma, including recent surgery
- Drugs
- Unknown (30–40%)

Intensive care management

The ICU management of MG consists of general supportive care and specific treatment.

Indications for intubation

- Bulbar palsy
- Respiratory failure
- VC <15ml/kg, irrespective of arterial blood gases

Respiratory support

- A trial of BiPAP may prevent the need for intubation and mechanical ventilation in the absence of hypercapnea and bulbar palsy
- Patients with overt hypercapnea or who fail BiPAP require mechanical ventilation
- Respiratory support should be weaned as soon as possible after the patient is free from crisis triggers and VC >10ml/kg
- Tracheostomy is often not required as the duration of intubation rarely exceeds 2 weeks
- Physiotherapy and antibiotics for chest infection/pneumonia—avoid aminoglycosides and other drugs that exacerbate MG

General support

- Thromboembolic prophylaxis
- Gastric ulcer prophylaxis
- Adequate calorific intake via enteral feeding
- Neurophysiotherapy

Anticholinesterase medication

- Not usually required in patients who are mechanically ventilated
- If required, pyridostigmine IV at 1/30 the oral dose is effective within 20min and lasts for up to 4h
- Routine medication should be restarted at half usual doses when weaning criteria are reached

Immunotherapy

The most useful treatments for myasthenic crisis are plasma exchange and IVIG (see also Chapter 22.7).

- Plasma exchange is often used as first-line treatment as it results in rapid improvement and reduces time on ventilation. Five to eight daily exchanges are performed until pulmonary function reaches 80% of predicted.
- Plasma exchange may be used as preparation for thymectomy in patients with respiratory muscle involvement
- IVIG given over 2–5 days in a total dose of 2g/kg is as effective as plasma exchange in myasthenic crisis.
- Long-term immunosuppression with corticosteroids or azothiaprine is required since the improvement with plasma exchange or IVIG is usually transient
- Azathioprine takes several months to 1yr to have maximum effect.

Thymectomy

- In patients with thymoma and thymic hyperplasia
- Not usually performed during myasthenic crisis
- Pre-operative establishment of long-term immunosuppressive therapy reduces risk of post-operative mysathenic crisis
- More effective in younger patients
- Improvement of symptoms in 85% patients at 1yr

Outcome

- 20–30% 10yr mortality for untreated MG
- Modern treatment results in excellent prognosis, with mortality rates approaching zero
- Myasthenic crisis has 5% mortality

Further reading

Green D. Weakness in the ICU: Guillain–Barre syndrome, myasthenia gravis and critical illness polyneuropathy/myopathy. *Neurologist* 2005; 11: 338–47.

Hirsch NP. The neuromuscular junction in health and disease. *Br J Anaesth* 2007; 99: 132–8.

Lacomis D. Myasthenic crisis. *Neurocrit Care* 2005; 3: 189–94.

Saperstein DS, Barohn RJ. Management of myasthenia gravis. *Semin Neurol* 2004; 24: 41–8.

ICU neuromuscular disorders

Motor weakness in an ICU patient may be related to a pre-existing neuromuscular disorder, a new-onset or previously undiagnosed neuromuscular disorder or develop as a complication of critical illness. Two syndromes of ICU-acquired weakness are recognized—critical illness polyneuropathy (CIP) and critical illness myopathy (CIM). CIP is an acute axonal sensory-motor polyneuropathy and CIM an acute primary myopathy. CIP and CIM frequently co-exist and a single term, critical illness neuromyopathy (CINM), is now used to describe this association. CINM can delay weaning from mechanical ventilation and impair physical recovery after critical illness.

Epidemiology

CINM is often associated with sepsis, MOF, hyperglycaemia, immobility and the use of corticosteroids, neuromuscular blocking drugs, aminoglycosides, cathecholamines and parenteral nutrition. It is more common in females than males.

Incidence

CINM is often unrecognized but affects between 25 and 80% of intensive care patients. Reported incidence depends on the criteria used for diagnosis and timing of the examination. Electrophysiological tests identify more patients than clinical examination. In patients with ICU stays >28 days, electrophysiological evidence of CINM is present in >90% patients up to 5yrs after discharge.

Causes

The exact aetiology of CINM is unclear, but inflammatory mediators, microcirculatory damage, direct neurotoxicity and hyperglycaemia have been implicated. In CIP, vascular and cellular events result in nerve cell energy failure and, initially, pure functional failure. With persisting critical illness and continuing cellular failure, histological changes in the nerve cell ensue. CIM is an acute primary myopathy (i.e. not secondary to muscle denervation) with a spectrum extending from functional impairment of muscle with normal histology to muscle atrophy and necrosis. Histological examination often reveals signs of both primary (necrosis) and secondary (denervation related) mypoathy, indicating that CIM and CIP co-exist.

Risk factors

- Sepsis, systemic inflammatory response syndrome and MOF are risk factors for CINM, which is strongly associated with the duration of MOF.
- Chronic corticosteroid use is an independent risk factor for CINM.
- Neuromuscular blocking drugs have adverse effects on muscle strength by two mechanisms—prolonged neuromuscular blockade because of drug or metabolite accumulation in the setting of renal or hepatic failure and a direct causal relationship to the development of CINM because of prolonged pharmacological denervation.
- There is an established link between hyperglycaemia and CINM.
- Severe electrolyte abnormalities, including hypokalaemia, hyperkalaemia, hypophosphataemia and hypomagnesaemia, may damage muscle and lead to CIM.
- Bed rest and immobility due to sedation may potentiate ICU-acquired weakness.

Diagnosis

Diagnosis of CINM is based on evaluation of the clinical setting and predisposing factors, neurological examination and electrophysiological investigations. Clinical diagnosis is not straightforward. Accurate motor and sensory testing is difficult or impossible in critically ill patients because of sedation, delirium, poor cooperation or limited communication.

Clinicians often predict poor or fatal outcome in critically ill patients who are comatose and paralysed in the absence of evidence of irreversible brain or spinal cord damage. CINM is a potentially reversible condition and patients should therefore be carefully identified to avoid unreasonably pessimistic prognostication. Clinical examination is less sensitive than electrophysiological confirmation and leaves a substantial number of patients with CINM undiagnosed. However, electrophysiological investigations detect cases of CINM that are of little or no clinical relevance.

Differential diagnosis

ICU-acquired weakness must be distinguished from weakness resulting from new onset or previously undiagnosed neurological disorders such as GBS, MG and brainstem or spinal cord lesions. Other rarer confounding diagnoses include poliomyelitis and other mypoathies, porphyria, rhabdomyolysis and atypical presentation of amyotrophic lateral sclerosis.

Clinical features

CINM presents as difficulty with weaning from mechanical ventilation or unexplained weakness in conscious patients following a critical illness. CINM is characterized by a symmetrical motor deficit in all limbs, ranging from mild paresis to quadriplegia. The facial muscles are usually spared, and the first manifestation is often a weak or absent limb withdrawal with a normal facial grimace on painful simulation. Deep tendon reflexes are reduced or absent, but normal reflexes do not rule out the diagnosis. Associated sensory loss is present in 50% of patients, but its evaluation is often limited by the patient's conscious state. Phrenic nerve involvement and intercostal muscle weakness contribute to difficulty in weaning from mechanical ventilation.

Symptoms and signs

These are often unreliable and can be confused with other conditions. CINM is a clinical diagnosis of exclusion and often unrecognized. The following features are useful indicators of other causes of weakness in ICU patients.

CNS involvement

- Asymmetrical neurological signs
- Cranial nerve palsy
- Altered mental status

Spinal cord involvement

- Sensory level
- Loss of anal tone and sphincter reflex

Neuromuscular disease

- Extremity weakness and wasting
- Hypotonia and hyporeflexia
- Autonomic dysfunction

Investigations

Electrophysiological tests

Comprehensive electrophysiological studies, including motor and sensory nerves conduction studies and needle EMG in upper and lower limbs, are able to differentiate between CIP and CIM. However, electrophysiological tests do not predict duration of mechanical ventilation or length of ICU stay.

- Nerve conduction studies
    - CIP is characterized by decreased CMAP and sensory nerve action potential with normal conduction velocity
    - abnormalities may be detected as early as 48h after the onset of critical illness
    - prolongation of CMAP suggests an associated myopathy
- EMG
    - CIM is diagnosed by abnormal EMG during voluntary contraction in conscious and cooperative patients
- Direct muscle stimulation (DMS)
    - differentiates between CIP and CIM in uncooperative patients
    - stimulating and recording electrodes are placed in the muscle distal to the end-plate zone
    - in CIP there is a reduced or absent CMAP on motor nerve stimulation but a normal response with DMS
    - in CIM the CMAP is reduced or absent after both motor nerve stimulation and DMS
    - technically difficult
- Other electrophysiological tests
    - phrenic nerve conduction studies and diaphragmatic EMG may be indicated in patients who fail to wean from mechanical ventilation

Muscle biopsy

- Not used routinely because it is invasive and the results are not immediately available
- Myosin/actin ratio reduced in CIM
- Three types of histological changes are recognized—acute necrotizing, thick myosin filament loss and fibre atrophy
- Allows diagnosis of other causes of muscle pathology

Neuroimaging

- MRI of the spinal cord and brain to exclude cord compression and brainstem lesions

Other

- Serum CK—variably raised but may be normal

Prevention and treatment

There is no proven treatment for established CINM, and management focuses on prevention by avoidance of risk factors.

- Aggressive treatment of sepsis and MOF minimizes the risk of developing CINM, shortens its duration and reduces severity in established cases.
- The link between elevated blood glucose levels and CINM is well established. Tight glycaemic control with insulin infusion is associated with a 50% reduction in the evolution of CIP and mortality benefit in critically ill surgical patients. Tight glycaemic control in medical ICU patients results in a smaller reduction in the incidence of CIP but significant reductions in the duration of mechanical ventilation.
- Use of corticosteroids should be restricted to conditions in which they have been proven to have a significant impact on morbidity and mortality.
- Neuromuscular blocking drugs should also be used only for selected indications, such as difficult to ventilate patients and intractable intracranial hypertension, and only when all other means have failed. If the clinical condition permits, daily interruption of neuromuscular blocking drugs is recommended to reduce the risks associated with prolonged pharmacological denervation.
- Sedation protocols designed to minimize the use of sedatives and analgesics decrease the duration of mechanical ventilation and possibly the incidence and severity of CINM.
- Strategies to mobilize patients with passive stretching or active exercise seem reasonable given their relative safety.
- Electrolyte disorders, including phosphate and magnesium depletion, should be controlled throughout the entire critical care episode.
- Although not proven, adequate nutrition seems a necessity to prevent catabolism and muscle wasting.
- IVIG might reduce the development of CINM, but more studies are required before this treatment can be recommended.

Outcome

- CINM is an independent predictor of prolonged mechanical ventilation and increased ICU mortality and LOS.
- Complete functional recovery occurs in ~70% of patients.
- Muscle wasting and weakness are common in survivors of critical illness, and some remain severely disabled.
- Mild disabilities persist in patients with seemingly good recovery. These include reduced or absent reflexes, glove and stocking sensory loss, muscle atrophy, dysasthesia and foot drop.

Further reading

De Jonghe B, Sharshar T, Lefaucher JP, *et al.* Paresis acquired in the intensive care unit: a prospective multicenter study. *JAMA* 2002; 288: 2859–67.

Dhand UK. Clinical approach to the weak patient in the intensive care unit. *Respir Care* 2006; 51: 1024–40.

Fletcher SN, Kennedy DD, Ghosh IR, *et al.* Persistent neuromuscular and neurophysiologic abnormalities in long-term survivors of prolonged critical illness. *Crit Care Med* 2003; 31: 1012–6.

Latronico N, Peli E, Botteri M. Critical illness myopathy and neuropathy. *Curr Opin Crit Care* 2005; 11: 126–32.

Latronico N, Shehu I, Seghelini E. Neuromuscular sequelae of critical illness. *Curr Opin Crit Care* 2005; 11: 381–90.

Schweickert W, Hall J. ICU-acquired weakness. *Chest* 2007; 131: 1541–9.

Tetanus

Tetanus is a toxin-mediated disease caused by the bacterium *Clostridium tetani* resulting in:

- Skeletal muscle rigidity and spasm
- Autonomic nervous system instability

The disease is completely preventable by vaccination, and in recent years global vaccination initiatives in infants and young women have begun to have an impact on the disease incidence. Nevertheless, in the developing world, tetanus continues to be a common cause of mortality and morbidity of neonates, children and young adults.

In countries with well established vaccination programmes, the disease is rare and usually occurs in the elderly or certain 'high risk' groups such as IV drug users.

In either setting, mortality from severe disease is high and good outcome is dependent on high quality care.

Aetiology

C. tetani is an anaerobic Gram-positive bacterium which produces a highly potent toxin. Infection occurs after contamination of a wound with the bacterial spores. These are found throughout the environment, particularly in soil or human/animal faeces. Wounds can be very minor abrasions, and in ~25% of cases no wound is apparent by the time symptoms occur. Tetanus toxin prevents synaptic release of neurotransmitter from the presynaptic GABAergic inhibitory interneurons, resulting in uncontrolled motor neuron activity and thus the characteristic increased muscle tone and spasm. Similarly disinhibited autonomic (predominantly sympathetic) nervous system activity is seen, producing cardiovascular instability.

Presentation

The most common features from the history at presentation are:

- Lockjaw
- Muscle stiffness
- Back pain
- Difficulty swallowing
- There may or may not be any history of injury.

In neonates, the illness usually presents as difficulty in feeding.

Examination should look for

- Trismus: if not apparent this can be precipitated using the spatula test—where a patient with facial involvement will reflexly bite down on a spatula placed in the mouth)
- Risus sardonicus from facial muscle spasm (pathognomonic)
- Muscle spasms, or abdominal rigidity (continuous)
- Check airway and respiratory compromise as laryngeal spasm is common and rapidly fatal if untreated
- Source of infection
- Heart rate, blood pressure, temperature—also indicators of prognosis

There is no diagnostic test to confirm tetanus. In some cases *C. tetani* can be cultured from the wound, but in most the diagnosis is purely a clinical one principally based on the presence of muscle rigidity and spasms.

Special investigations should be ordered according to the clinical indications. In addition to routine blood tests, the following are helpful:

- ABG
- CXR (aspiration is common)

Natural history

Historically two periods have been used to characterize the progression of tetanus disease:

- Incubation period: the asymptomatic period from infection to the first symptom (typically 7–10 days). This cannot be calculated if no entry wound is found.
- Period of onset: the period from first symptom to first spasm (typically 24–72h).

Shorter periods are associated with more rapidly progressing and severe disease. More accurate prognosis can be calculated using specific prognostic scores.

Tetanus gradually increases in severity over 1 or 2 weeks, with spasms reaching maximum intensity during the second week, and maximal autonomic disturbance during the second and third weeks. These gradually improve, although muscle rigidity may persist for up to 6 weeks. A recurrence of spasms or worsening of severity may suggest a persistent source of *C. tetani* infection.

Differential diagnosis

- Strichnine poisoning
- Dystonic reactions to antidopaminergic drugs
- Surgical acute abdomen
- Oropharyngeal infection
- Hypocalcaemia or meningoencephalitis in neonates

Management

Airway management is paramount, but particular care must be taken to avoid provoking laryngeal spasm during laryngoscopy. If sufficient experience is available, primary tracheostomy is recommended.

Conventionally antitoxin is given SC, but recent studies and a meta-analysis have indicated that intrathecal administration of human immunoglobulin reduces disease progression and severity.

Standard first-line drugs are IV benzodiazepines (commonly diazepam or midazolam) and high doses are commonly required—often >100mg/24h. In severe disease, neuromuscular blocking agents are also necessary. Due to cardiovascular instability, chose an agent without significant cardiovascular effects.

Magnesium sulfate can be used as an adjunct. It is also useful as it improves cardiovascular instability. Target therapeutic range of serum levels 2–4mmol/l.

Cardiovascular instability is difficult to manage due to rapid fluctuations in peripheral resistance. Agents with short half-lives are necessary, but heavy sedation and adequate spasm control are also of benefit.

Any source of infection should be carefully cleaned and debrided. Deep or internal sources of infection are associated with worse prognosis.

A full primary immunization course of DT (<7yrs old) or dT (≥7yrs) is required in all patients.

Further reading:

Farrar JJ, Yen LM, Cook T, *et al.* Tetanus. *J Neurol Neurosurg Psychiatry* 2000; 69: 292–301.

Kabura L, Ilibagiza D, Menten J, *et al.* Intrathecal vs. intramuscular administration of human antitetanus immunoglobulin or equine tetanus antitoxin in the treatment of tetanus: a meta-analysis. *Trop Med Int Health* 2006; 11: 1075–81.

Thwaites CL. Tetanus. Curr Anaesth Crit Care 2005; 16: 50–7.

WHO. Tetanus vaccine. *Wkly Epidemiol Rec* 2006; 81: 198–208.

Botulism

Botulism is an acute, potentially life-threatening descending motor paralysis affecting primarily cranial, respiratory and autonomic nerves caused by exotoxin released from the bacterium *Clostridium botulinum*. It was first described in the early 19th century after an outbreak related to contaminated sausages, and was named after the Latin for sausage, botulus. Although a relatively rare cause of a proximal, neuroparalytic syndrome, it is important that clinicians recognize the different patterns of clinical presentation since timely use of specific antitoxin therapy significantly reduces mortality and morbidity.

Bacteriology

C. botulinum includes a number of genetically distinct Gram-positive, rod-shaped, anaerobic, spore-forming bacteria each of which produces antigenically specific neurotoxins. The organisms are found worldwide and can be isolated from soil, vegetables, fish and putrid foods. The spores are heat resistant and survive boiling water for several hours. The anaerobic, acidic conditions at ~30°C associated with canning, smoking and fermentation encourage germination of the spores, bacterial growth and toxin production.

Toxins

Of the eight toxins identified, three (A, B, E) are particularly associated with human disease. The toxins are denatured at temperatures >80°C. Botulinum toxin is the most potent bacterial toxin: 1g aerosolized is potentially capable of killing >1 million people.

Mechanism of action

The antigenically distinct toxins have a similar mechanism of action but vary in both species specificity and severity of clinical manifestations produced. Toxin is absorbed across mucous membranes, spreads via the bloodstream and binds to a specific receptor at cholinergic transmitter sites. Once bound, the toxin enters the cytoplasm and irreversibly blocks acetylcholine release from the presynaptic terminal, thereby blocking impulse transmission at neuromuscular junctions, autonomic ganglia and parasympathetic nerve terminals. Cranial nerves are preferentially affected as toxin binds more rapidly to sites with rapid cycles of depolarization and repolarization. Sensory nerves and adrenergic synapses are not affected, and the toxin does not cross into the CSF. Recovery takes up to 6 months and requires 'sprouting' of nerve terminals to form new motor endplates.

Clinical presentation

There are four clinical patterns of botulism determined by the route of exposure and site of toxin production:

- ***Foodborne***: eating food contaminated with toxin
- ***Infant***: spores colonize GI tract with *in vivo* toxin production—mainly in infants <6 months; rarely occurs in adults with a pre-existing GI disorder
- ***Wound***: infection of deep wounds or abscesses with *in vivo* toxin production, particularly heroin addicts
- ***Inhalation***: aerosolized toxin as could be used in a terrorist attack

Epidemiology

Traditionally infant botulism has been the most common clinical presentation reported. Adult outbreaks are sporadic, generally involving small numbers of people who have eaten toxin-contaminated food. Although the incidence of foodborne and infant botulism has been constant over the past 30yrs, wound botulism, particularly in California, has increased markedly mainly amongst drug abusers injecting black tar heroin by IM or SC injection ('skin-popping').

Foodborne botulism

Symptoms

Typically develop 12–48h after eating toxin-contaminated food. The severity and rate of progression reflects the toxin load, although individual susceptibility to the toxin varies considerably. Prodromal symptoms include nausea, vomiting, dry mouth and abdominal distension reflecting autonomic nerve dysfunction, after which cranial and respiratory nerve dysfunction manifest as diplopia, dysphonia, dysarthria and dysphagia, difficulty holding up the head and increasing respiratory distress. A symmetrical descending motor weakness follows initially affecting the trunk and proximal limb muscles. Smooth muscle paralysis may lead to constipation and urinary retention. Sensation is not affected.

Examination

Autonomic nerve involvement may be widespread resulting in:

- hypotension without compensatory tachycardia
- urinary retention
- abdominal distension with intestinal ileus
- dry mouth
- pupils 4–8mm with absent light and accommodation reflexes

Cranial nerve involvement results in ophthalmoplegia, particularly lateral rectus palsy, nystagmus, ptosis, dysarthria and difficulty in swallowing, protruding the tongue or shrugging the shoulders. Corneal and gag reflexes are preserved and facial muscles may be spared.

Phrenic nerve involvement and respiratory muscle weakness may occur early and develop rapidly. Limb involvement starts proximally and involves the arms first, producing a lower motor neuron flaccid paralysis.

Important normal findings are preserved cortical function, intact sensation and absence of fever.

Infant botulism

Occurs in infants under 6 months, but there can be considerable variability in the severity and presenting picture, presumably related to the extent of gut colonization and subsequent toxin production and the individual host response. Classically related to eating contaminated raw honey, it generally starts with constipation progressing over 3–10 days to produce a 'floppy infant' who feeds poorly with a weak cry and evidence of respiratory distress. Cranial nerve involvement with new squint, ptosis and head and facial weakness predicts a more severe course and warrants close monitoring of ability to protect the airway and progressing respiratory muscle weakness. Most infants recover quite rapidly without requiring intubation or respiratory support, but the more severe cases may run a relapsing course and full recovery may take many months.

Wound botulism

Caused by colonization of wounds following trauma or associated with drug abuse using SC injection ('skin-popping') particularly with black tar heroin. *In vivo* toxin production occurs after about 10 days. There are usually no prodromal GI symptoms and there may be fever and a leucocytosis.

Diagnosis

Most clinicians will rarely see a case, making diagnosis difficult particularly the first case in an outbreak, since autonomic and cranial nerve signs may be missed in what is apparently a GI problem. Also 'skin-popping' drug abusers with wound botulism may be admitted with an overdose and be intubated before careful neurological examination can be performed. Botulism should always be considered in patients with a relevant history who develop cranial nerve abnormalities and a symmetrical descending paralysis without sensory signs.

Differential diagnosis

Several other conditions have similar neurological features to adult foodborne and wound botulism. These are listed below with key distinguishing features:

- Miller–Fisher syndrome—a descending form of GBS. Limb weakness before respiratory failure; prominent ataxia; sensory changes; raised CSF protein
- Myasthenia Gravis. Lengthy history of fatiguable weakness, particularly in the evening; no autonomic features; normal pupillary responses.
- Lambert-Eaton Myasthenic Syndrome. Proximal leg weakness is an early sign; weakness improves with exercise; ptosis common but ophthalmoplegia and bulbar involvement are rare
- Tick paralysis. Complete ophthalmoplegia, check for presence of tick
- Brainstem CVA causing bulbar palsy
- Diphtheria. Presence of pharyngeal membrane; nasal discharge; fever and foetor; paralysis occurs late.
- Paralytic rabies. History of animal bite; fever; headache; local paraesthesiae; ascending asymmetrical paralysis starting in bitten limb
- Poisoning. Atropine excess; organophosphate; hypermagnesaemia; snake bites with neurotoxic venom (cobras, kraits, sea snake)

Investigations

1. Mouse bioassay for toxin in patient's serum, urine, gastric aspirate or in suspected food if available. Involves intraperitoneal injection of 0.5ml of sample with and without trivalent antitoxin into mice. Mice not given the antitoxin develop botulism and die in 2–3 days. Toxin can be measured directly by ELISA, but only available in specialist centres.
2. Neurophysiological studies show reduced amplitude muscle action potentials that enhance after tetanic stimulation, and normal nerve conduction velocities. Post-tetanic exhaustion does not occur, and this is only found in botulism and hypomagnesaemia.
3. Beware the use of the edrophonium (Tensilon) test to exclude MG as there are often false-positive results in patients with botulism
4. In wound botulism, samples should be sent for *C. botulinum* culture and the wound/abscess should be thoroughly debrided.
5. Serum samples are frequently negative in infant botulism, and diagnosis relies on positive stool culture.

Management

Patients with dyspnoea or clinical signs of respiratory distress (tachypnoea, use of accessory muscles) should be closely monitored with 6 hourly FVC, pulse oximetry and careful observation of bulbar function. Arterial blood gases should be performed. A 70kg adult with FVC falling below 1.2l will have a weak cough, difficulty clearing secretions, and progressive tachypnoea and respiratory distress. At this stage, the patient may require intubation and should be in a critical care area and kept nil by mouth so that urgent intubation can be safely performed as respiratory function may suddenly deteriorate. Respiratory failure is the main cause of death in botulism.

There is no evidence that antibiotics are beneficial in the early stages of foodborne botulism but may become appropriate later if nosocomial infection, particularly pneumonia, develops. Benzylpenicillin or metronidazole should be given to patients with wound botulism to cover other potential clostridial infections. Avoid aminoglycoside antibiotics which can potentiate the neuromuscular blockade.

Drugs that reverse neuromuscular blockade are ineffective, although guanidine, which increases acetylcholine release, may have a role, but it remains experimental.

Specific treatment

Specific trivalent (A, B, E) equine antitoxin should be given to all adults as soon as a clinical diagnosis is made. Therapy should not be delayed until the bioassay results are available since this takes several days and the antitoxin is ineffective once the circulating toxin has bound to the cholinergic receptor. Studies have shown reduced mortality and morbidity with the timely use of antitoxin. Anaphylaxis and serum sickness can occur, and an intradermal test dose is recommended although most serum reactions will not be predicted by this test. Infants <1yr old and patients with evidence of allergy to equine products should be given human derived antitoxin.

Key messages

- Consider botulism in patients presenting with symmetrical descending flaccid paralysis, cranial nerve palsies, autonomic dysfunction, and normal sensation.
- Obtain history of food exposure and drug abuse
- Give antitoxin as soon as diagnosis clinically suspected

Further reading

Arnon SS, Schechter R, Maslanka SE, *et al.* Human botulism immune globulin for the treatment of infant botulism. *N Engl J Med* 2006; 354: 462-71S.

Jin R, Rummel A, Biz T, *et al.* Botulinum toxin B recognizes its protein receptor with high affinity and specificity. *Nature* 2006; 444: 1092–20.

Schreiner MS, Field E, Ruddy R. Infant botulism: a review of 12 years' experience. *Pediatrics* 1991; 87: 159–65.

Werner SB, Passaro D, McGee J, *et al.* Wound botulism in California, 1951–1998: recent epidemic in heroin injectors. *Clin Infect Dis* 2000; 31: 1018–24.

Neurorehabilitation

Expert care in critical illness scenarios is producing more survivors. Investment in this care must be matched by investment in rehabilitation and vocational services to return people to optimal health states and full participation in society.

Morbidity and mortality is poor

The morbidity and mortality of individuals surviving >14 days ventilation was found in a study by Combes *et al.* to be poor, with only 197 survivors out of 347 achieving discharge from hospital. Of these, there were 99 long-term survivors who had impaired quality of life compared with a matched general population. There has been scant attention given to rehabilitation aspects and long-term functional outcome of people with critical illness polyneuropathy. In 2004, Van der Schaaf reported a small prospective study in which he found that most survivors of CIN had restrictions of functional abilities, reduced quality of life, autonomy and participation, and he recommended prolonged rehabilitation treatment to improve functional outcome, participation and social integration.

Rehabilitation improves outcome

Evidence of the benefits of a rehabilitation programme is growing. The most severely affected will not get back home without an intensive in-patient programme in a specialist facility. There are stringent efforts being made now to collect data to confirm the benefit of a range of rehabilitation interventions. Jones *et al.* reported the effectiveness of a 6 week self-help rehabilitation manual in an RCT, and Elliott *et al.* have set up an RCT of an 8 week individualized physical and psychological programme for survivors of critical illness.

Critical illness impairments

- Immobility: this causes muscle and tendon structure changes within 7 days, producing soft tissue shortening and contractures, reduces bone density, compromises skin integrity and predisposes to further complications including DVT, PE and respiratory infection
- Lung damage including pulmonary fibrosis due to prolonged ventilation, ARDS and PE, may reduce delivery of oxygen to re-covering nerve cells.
- Critical illness polyneuropathy and myopathy.
- Hypoxic, ischaemic or embolic damage to brain or spinal cord, causing the typical and easily recognized features of stroke, paraplegia, or tetraplegia, and the less obvious cognitive, memory and dysexecutive states, often a feature of watershed infarcts and severe hypotensive and hypoxic episodes. Vascular insults can also produce cauda equina syndrome, radiculopathies and peripheral nerve lesions.
- Multi-organ failure.
- Emotional and behavioural changes, sometimes linked to subtle cognitive changes, but can be part of a disabling post critical illness stress disorder.

Can you spot it early?

In the ICU some patients are unexpectedly difficult to wean off ventilation, and this is the early clue to look for neurological impairment and neuromuscular breathing difficulties. Latronica *et al.* reviewed the impact of CIN and CIP, and found it delayed weaning by 2–7 times and was associated with chronic long-term disability. 28% had severe disability with tetra- or paraplegia, and, although 68% recovered functional independence, many had persisting mixed sensorimotor symptoms and signs with footdrop muscle atrophy, peripheral sensory loss and painful hyperaesthesiae. Survivors of polytrauma or major complex surgery often have a critical illness picture superimposed on their primary pathology and are at increased risk of poor recovery. Additional problems of the patient soon to leave ICU that contribute to the overall picture of disability and dependence include the tracheostomy, catheters, drips and NG tubes or PEGs. Bowels may be incontinent, and sleep pattern is severely disrupted.

Rehabilitation starts in ICU

The human form soon resembles a banana shape if left paralysed, lying supine on a yielding pressure-relieving mattress with loss of lumbar lordosis, and development of hip, shoulder and ankle contractures. Pressure sores may be avoided, but at a structural cost with much soft tissue shortening.

1. Maintain passive range of movement at all joints
   This includes neck and back in addition to the usually targeted upper and lower limb joints.
2. How?
   Active hands-on therapy, supplemented by a postural regime including side and prone lying, and splinting to protect very vulnerable joints, e.g. ankles.
3. Maintain baroreceptor sensitivity
   This is not easy but a periodic head-up posture and tilt-tabling helps with this and neck and trunk mobilization.

Risks in severe acquired brain injury

These include early and severe generalized spasticity. Enthusiastic early treatment for this may prevent severe disabling contracture development. Multi-disciplinary management of severe spasticity includes the following:

- IM botulinum toxin injections
- Oral antispasticity medication
- Stretching physiotherapy
- Splinting regime
- Antispasticity postural regime

Access to neurorehabilitation expertise at this stage is vital.

A severe catabolic state with major weight loss, muscle wasting and mobilization of calcium from the skeleton is another particular complication of severe polytrauma with brain or spinal cord injury. Catabolism and immobility combined with muscle or joint trauma predispose osteoporosis, nephrolithiasis and heterotopic ossification (HO). Prevention of these complications may not always be possible. Up to 80% of individuals with brain injury causing impaired consciousness for at least 1 month will have HO compared with 10–20% with briefer loss of consciousness but requiring hospitalization and rehabilitation.

The treatments for catabolic state and early HO include providing calorific needs + 1000 kcal, following a physiotherapy regime, and use of antiinflammatory drugs.

Late HO requires ongoing physiotherapy supplemented rarely by orthopaedic interventions in the most severe cases.

Communication and emotional needs

Communication needs should be addressed as soon as the patient is conscious in ICU. Those with a tracheostomy will need aids provided early to facilitate asking questions and permitting communication with those around them. It also allows early assessment of cognitive and emotional status, which will influence outcome. If there is evidence of significant communication impairment, a speech and language therapist should be involved and will usefully spend time with both the patient and their relatives.

Leaving ICU

All patients with severe critical illness, a neuromyopathy, focal neurology of brain or spinal cord, obvious neurocognitive and psychological impairments should be considered for referral to a specialist neurorehabilitation facility as early as possible. It can be difficult to meet the needs of such patients on general medical wards where there may be little therapy and no equipment. Being discharged on to a general ward with a severe CIN, or a new paraplegia, can be distressing and depressing after the ICU experience. The patient is no longer the centre of attention, has to compete for staff time to receive basic care, feels abandoned, and may be highly dependent and frightened. Their relatives are often similarly worried and initially take on the ICU staff role by camping out on the ward. It is helpful if relatives can meet members of the rehabilitation team early rather than late, and visit the unit, which may not be in the same hospital.

How to do it

Moving into rehabilitation should give the patient the opportunity to work on impairments, reduce disability and develop a discharge plan. It is a simple problem-solving process, and depends on team work and clarity of thinking. The key qualities of successful rehabilitation team members are good communication skills, expertise and flexibility. Each patient has a personalized rehabilitation plan which includes:

1. Meeting ongoing surgical and medical needs
2. Assessing and observing cognition, communication skills and emotional state
3. Assessing physical impairments and functional deficits
4. Appraisal of the social situation, home environment and potential for later return to work

Knowledge of these permits the development of a rehabilitation programme and discharge plan which should include

1. Expected outcome—managing expectations
2. Identification of discharge destination
3. Expected date of discharge
4. Advice on work and driving
5. Referral on to community resources. This should be according to need but is often modified by availability.

Goal planning

This is the key to active, outcome-driven rehabilitation and can be used to bridge the gap between hospital and home, with the patient being an active driver of the process, and on discharge taking full responsibility to set goals to achieve continuing recovery after discharge. 'SMART' goals (Specific, Measurable, Appropriate, Relevant, Timely) are informed by experienced staff who have a reasonable knowledge of expected outcome, and by the patient and family, who have a better understanding of the contextual factors, the home and vocational environment.

Fatigue, pain and graded therapy

Initial attempts to work with the patient fresh out of ICU often stall, with problems with pain, low blood pressure, fatigue, balance disorders, compounded by loss of diurnal sleep–wake pattern and emotional reactions to the illness. There is a constant fine tuning initially as the therapist and patient begin to work out a programme that both can stick to. Certain pieces of equipment such as graded power-assisted pedals (e.g. MotoMed) are invaluable. Fatigue and pain remain the great limiters of recovery, and are associated with learned dependency, chronic fatigue states and secondary gain. That is why it is so important to have access to active rehabilitation early after the illness to prevent negative behavioural traits prevailing. Self-help programmes must include graded exercises, goal setting and regular review.

Cognitive problems affect outcome

Failure to motivate a self-directed recovery programme is often due to unrecognized cognitive problems, slowed information processing, short-term memory impairment and reduced new learning and executive skills. These problems reduce insight, intitiative, attention and concentration. Psychology input to the patient and the team can support new learning strategies recovery and adaptation.

The talking therapies

There are many. Cognitive behavioural treatment (CBT), Person-centred therapy (CPT), solution-focused brief therapy (SFBT), rewind theory and others all have their advocates. Counselling treatments encourage adjustment using a spectrum of methods that span reflective through to directive techniques. Most are based on frequent sessions, identifying negative patterns of behaviour and desired changes. Anxiety or depressive illness may also respond well to short-term pharmacological therapy.

Novel home-based therapies

In the future, traditional therapist-based services may be supplemented by virtual environments, teletherapy, portable robotic devices employing errorless learning systems and positive feedback. These methods are unlikely to be superior, but can enrich and vary the exercise environment and allow the patient greater control and application.

Further reading

Combes A, CostaMA, Troillet JL, *et al.* Morbidity, mortality and quality of life outcomes of patients requiring 14 days of mechanical ventilation. *Crit Care Med* 2003; 315: 1373–81.

Elliott D, McKinley S, Alison JA, *et al.* Study protocol: home based physical rehabilitation for surviviors of a critical illness. *Crit Care* 2006; 10: R90.

Jones C, Skirrow P, Griffiths RD, *et al.* Rehabilitation after critical illness: a randomised controlled trial. *Crit Care Med* 2003; 31: 2456–61.

Latronica N, Shehu I, Seghelini E. Neuromuscular sequela of critical illness polyneuropathy. *Curr Opin Crit Care* 2005; 11: 381–90.

Van der Schaaf M, Beelen A, de Vos R. Functional outcome in patients with critical illness polyneuropathy *Disabil Rehabil* 2004; 26: 1189–97.

Hyperthermias

Under normal circumstances, body temperature is closely controlled around a set point close to 37°C by balancing heat production and loss. Pyrexia can be a complicating factor in critical illness or a reason for admission to intensive care in its own right. The term hyperthermia is often used interchangeably with hyperpyrexia but can more accurately be defined:

Hyperpyrexia describes a situation in which the set point for temperature is raised, e.g. by infection.

Hyperthermia is an elevation of body temperature due to an inability of control systems to function. This results from an imbalance between factors making the body hot and those allowing it to cool.

Physiological effects of pyrexia

Cardiovascular

A high central temperature is associated with tachycardia, elevated cardiac output, low SVR and hypotension. This picture is seen when a patient in early sepsis is initially fluid resuscitated; failure to resuscitate adequately would result in the same patient being peripherally cold and clammy.

Metabolic

Tissue oxygen demand is increased in association with a rise in metabolic rate. Part of the effect on tissue oxygenation will be offset by a right shift in the oxyhaemoglobin dissociation curve, increasing availability of oxygen.

Immunological

Temperature-sensitive pathogens are compromised by a rise in body temperature, while leucocyte activity is enhanced, thus promoting response to infection.

Pyrexia complicating critical illness

The most likely cause of pyrexia in a critically ill patient is response to sepsis. Temperature is regulated in the hypothalamus. Cytokine release during sepsis results in activation of the arachidonic acid pathway and stimulation of heat production via PGE_2. Some of the effects of pyrexia may confer a survival benefit, but there comes a time when benefits are offset by disadvantages.

Management of pyrexia

Minimize heat gain

Unwanted heat gain should be minimized by considering environmental factors such as sunlight, poor room ventilation, excessive bed clothing and overly warm humidification circuits. Intensive care rooms should have controllable temperature settings. Some patient cooling techniques may be impeded by shivering. If a patient does not require muscle relaxation for other reasons chlorpromazine may limit shivering.

Treat obvious cause

Infection should be investigated and treated, e.g. by drainage of collections and use of broad-spectrum antibiotics, or targeted therapy if possible.

Drug therapy

There are several ways in which drugs can be used to lower body temperature:

- An elevated set point for temperature can be reset by antipyretic drugs such as paracetamol.
- Excessive heat production is a feature of some syndromes. Dantrolene is a drug that facilitates relaxation of muscle through its effect on intracellular calcium metabolism. This switches off heat production in conditions such as malignant hyperthermia.
- Cooling will be inhibited by drugs that adversely affect normal heat loss mechanisms such as anticholinergic agents which inhibit sweating.

Physical methods of cooling

Simple methods of cooling rely on enhancing normal heat loss. Evaporative losses can be encouraged using a fan and sponging the skin. Direct cooling of the skin can be achieved by using cold packs, but these may cause skin damage and will be ineffective if they cause vasoconstriction. Specially designed cooling blankets based on cold water or air circulation are safe and more effective. Irrigation of various body cavities with cold fluid has been described, most commonly the bladder and stomach.

Extracorporeal cooling

Special systems are available, but the majority of ICUs can rapidly deploy equipment they already have. Venovenous diafiltration in its various guises is a common form of RRT. Usually these systems are heated in an attempt to prevent heat loss. Some patients with marked pyrexia may benefit from connection to an extracorporeal circuit of this nature even when not in renal failure.

Purpose-built cooling systems

The desire actively to cool cardiac arrest patients has resulted in the availability of a number of specially designed cooling systems. One of these is based on the use of an intravascular catheter with a specially designed cuff through which cool water is circulated. Alternative designs include tents that surround the patient paying special attention to cooling of the neck region. A common characteristic of these systems is incorporation of sophisticated monitoring and control features.

Heat stroke

When the normal methods of heat loss are overwhelmed an individual will gradually become hot and dehydrated. Heat stroke is typically seen in patients with compromised heat control systems such as the very young and old or when healthy individuals exercise in hot and humid environments. Heat stroke is diagnosed in a hyperthermic patient with significant neurological impairment such as altered consciousness or convulsions. These patients may or may not be sweating.

MODs with rhabdomyolysis, disorders of clotting, renal and liver failure have all been described. In less severe cases, attention should be given to monitoring serum sodium and blood glucose, which can be high or low.

Treatment involves basic resuscitation, removing the patient from the source of heat and rapidly facilitating cooling. Speed of fluid resuscitation should be guided by clinical assessment, with invasive monitoring if necessary. Choice of fluid may be guided by electrolyte determination with special attention to the possibility of sodium depletion. Antipyretic agents are not indicated as abnormal body temperature control mechanisms are not a feature of heat stroke.

Hyperthermia syndromes

A number of serious hyperthermia syndromes that require admission to intensive care are remarkable not only for their similarities, such as high mortality if not treated aggressively, but also their differences.

Neurolept malignant syndrome

This is an idiosyncratic reaction to antipsychotic medication. A wide range of drugs have been implicated such as haloperidol, promethazine, risperidone and clozapine. A common feature of drugs precipitating the syndrome is their inhibitory effect on central dopaminergic receptors.

Typically the syndrome develops within the first week of commencing medication. It is seen most frequently in young adult males. The syndrome is characterized by muscle rigidity, delirium and agitation. Temperature elevation is seen, but may not be marked. Patients often have autonomic disturbance such as hypertension.

Rhabdomyolysis leading to renal failure is an important complication. Laboratory investigations often show a leucocytosis, high creatinine kinase and liver dysfunction.

Once the syndrome is recognized, any potential precipitating agent should be withdrawn and pyrexia and autonomic dysfunction should be managed symptomatically. Strategies should be implemented to minimize the effects of rhabdomyolysis and to protect renal function. Maintenance of an alkaline diuresis is probably more effective that other forms of therapy. Mannitol is advocated by some, but should only be used where dehydration is not a concern.

Drugs to target the pathological process have been used such as bromocritptine, which is a dopamine agonist, and dantrolene, which should block the metabolic production of heat; their role remains unclear.

Ecstasy toxicity

Hyperthermia is a well recognized complication of Ecstasy toxicity. The syndrome can be seen in some patients after taking a single tablet. Ecstasy is an amphetamine derivative, but tablets may be contaminated with other substances such as the hallucinogenic agent mescaline. Ecstasy is thought to have a stimulant effect through central release of dopamine. This is associated with sympathetic overactivity causing tachycardia, hypertension and hyperthermia. Hallucinogenic effects are related to an initial release then depletion of serotonin in the brain which causes euphoria, increased energy, altered time perception and other psychological changes which encourage an increase in sociability.

Frequently the drug is taken in environments such as 'all-night raves' where large numbers of individuals congregate and dance for many hours on end. The drug's tendency to cause hyperthermia is aggravated by the hot environment, exercise over a number of hours and inadequate fluid intake.

A severe toxic response to Ecstasy is associated with loss of consciousness, seizures and a marked elevation in body temperature similar to heat stroke. Similar complications occur, including rhabdomyolysis, renal failure and DIC. Hepatic damage can be seen in association with the initial insult or may develop some weeks later. This can progress to acute fulminate liver failure requiring transplantation. Management of ecstasy toxicity is similar to other hyperthermias, with concentration on cooling, adequate fluid resuscitation and prevention of renal failure. Dantrolene has been used in this condition.

Malignant hyperthermia (MH)

Although rare, MH is well known to anaesthetists as it is an important preventable cause of mortality under anaesthesia.

MH is caused by an abnormality of calcium metabolism in muscle, resulting in sustained contraction and development of a hypermetabolic state. It is inherited as an autosomal dominant with incomplete penetrance. Genetic mutations have been demonstrated in some patients, including several different mutations of the ryanodine receptor. MH occurs when the patient is exposed to a trigger agent such as a volatile anaesthetic or suxamethonium. It may present clinically with muscle rigidity expressing itself as master spasm causing difficult intubation or as evidence of a hypermetabolic state detected with routine anaesthetic monitoring. During anaesthesia, the first signs of MH include an unexpected rise in end-tidal carbon dioxide, tachycardia, hypoxia and cyanosis. This may be accompanied by ECG abnormalities and a temperature rise. Blood gas analysis shows worsening acidosis.

Clinically the patient rapidly deteriorates with marked hyperthermia and severe metabolic derangement due to muscle cell damage. If they survive long enough without treatment, renal failure, myoglobinurea and other signs of a severe hyperthermia develop.

The Association of Anaesthetists guidelines for treatment stress the need to halt the process by discontinuing trigger agents, administering dantrolene initially 2–3mg/kg and using active cooling. Dantrolne administered IV acts directly on the ryanodine receptor. Once the process is halted, the patient requires monitoring and symptomatic treatment including correction of acidosis with sodium bicarbonate, treatment of hyperkalaemia and alkaline diuresis. Following admission to intensive care, management needs to concentrate on monitoring for the possibility of compartment syndrome due to oedematous damaged muscle and recrudescence of MH.

Further reading

Association of Anaesthetists of Great Britain and Ireland. Management of a Malignant Hyperthermia Crisis. 2007. http://www.aagbi.org/publications/guidelines/docs/malignanthyp07amended.pdf

Chapter 23

Haematological disorders

Chapter contents

Bleeding disorders

Acquired bleeding disorders

Consumptive coagulopathy (DIC)

Inappropriate activation of the coagulation process. Usually presents as haemorrhage, but 5-10% may show microthrombi (e.g. digital ischaemia).
Clinical associations: sepsis, trauma, obstetric emergencies, malignancy, hepatic failure, toxic reactions (e.g. transfusion reactions, snake bites)

Diagnosis: Thrombocytopenia, prolonged prothrombin time (PT) and activated partial thromboplastin time (aPTT), hypofibrinogenaemia, elevated fibrin degradation products (FDPs) or D-dimers.

Management: Treat the underlying disorder.

In bleeding patients, platelet transfusion and replacement of coagulation factors with FFP and cryoprecipitate is indicated to maintain the platelet level >50 x 10^9/l, PT and APTT <1.5 times the normal control time and fibrinogen >1g/l.

The use of heparin is controversial. Low dose UFH (300–500U/h) has been used in patients with thrombotic manifestations (e.g. gangrene), but caution should be exercised as it can provoke haemorrhage.

Activated protein C (Drotrecogin alfa activated) has been shown to reduce mortality in certain cases of overwhelming sepsis.

Dilutional coagulopathy (massive blood transfusion)

Defined as the loss of one blood volume within a 24 h period. (Normal adult blood volume is ~7% of the ideal body mass, i.e. 5l.)

Coagulation factor deficiency is unlikely until 80% of the blood volume has been replaced.

Maintain the platelet count >50 x 10^9/l, PT and aPTT <1.5 times the normal control time and fibrinogen >1g/l.

Recombinant FVIIa (rVIIa) has been used in uncontrolled bleeding associated with trauma, although the results of RCTs have been disappointing. Doses have ranged from 50 to 200mcg/ kg.

Bleeding in the anticoagulated patient

Oral anticoagulants (e.g. warfarin)

Major bleeding on warfarin is ~3%/yr.

Treatment of overanticoagulation is with vitamin K (10mg IV).

If haemorrhage is present, then FFP (12–15ml/kg) or prothrombin complex concentrate (PCC) may be indicated. Haematological advice should be sought prior to the use of PCC due to thrombogenicity.

Parenteral anticoagulants (e.g. heparin, lepirudin, danaparoid)

UFH has a short half-life (30–60min) and can be reversed by protamine (1mg for each 100U heparin).

LMWH has a half-life of 3–8h. Protamine can only reverse 50–70% of the dose.

Lepirudin has a half-life of 30–60min. Danaparoid has a half-life of 24h. These drugs are principally used in cases of HIT. There are no reversal agents for Lepirudin and Danaparoid. However, haemofiltration has been used in cases of lepirudin overdose. rVIIa has been used to minimize bleeding complications of both drugs.

Antiplatelet therapy (e.g. aspirin, ticlopidine, clopidogrel, tirofiban, abciximab)

Tirofiban has a half-life of 10–15min and is renally excreted. The biological half-life of abciximab is 18h. Aspirin is an irreversible inhibitor, so is effective for the lifetime of the platelet (~7 days).

If haemorrhage occurs with any of these drugs, then treatment is with platelet transfusions.

Thrombocytopenia

Low automated platelet counts should be confirmed by blood film examination.

True thrombocytopenia is the result of decreased platelet production (e.g. bone marrow hypoplasia or marrow infiltration), platelet sequestration (hypersplenism) or increased platelet destruction (immune or non-immune). Immune causes include SLE and drugs such as quinine and heparin. Non-immune causes include microangiopathic haemolytic anaemias such as thrombotic thrombocytopenic purpura (TTP) and DIC. Septicaemia without DIC can cause thrombocytopenia. Drugs such as pipericillin may induce marrow aplasia and consequent thrombocytopenia.

Platelet transfusions are contraindicated in TTP and HIT. TTP is treated with plasma exchange. HIT requires cessation of heparin and therapy with an alternative anticoagulant.

Immune thrombocytopenia is treated with steroids (1mg/kg/day prednisolone), IVIG (1g/kg/day for 2 days) or IV anti-D (75mcg/kg) in Rh(D)-positive individuals with functioning spleens. In the face of major bleeding, steroids together with immunoglobulin or anti-D may be given and then platelets can be transfused.

Platelet refractoriness is commonly non-immune, due to sepsis, drugs or splenomegaly. If no clinical reason can be determined, then human leucocyte antigen (HLA) antibodies should be sought in conjunction with haematological advice. Provision of HLA-matched platelets may improve transfusion response.

Liver disease

All coagulation factors (except von Willebrand factor (vWF)) are synthesized in the liver. Reduced synthetic function of the liver results in prolongation of the screening tests of coagulation (particularly the PT). In cholestatic liver disease there is reduced absorption of lipid-soluble vitamins, so reduced levels of vitamin K-dependent coagulation factors. Failure of the normal enzymatic removal of sialic acid from fibrinogen results in dysfibrinogenaemia.

Treatment of bleeding in the context of liver disease will be determined by the results of coagulation tests (PT, aPTT, thrombin time (TT) and fibrinogen). Vitamin K should be given to aid synthesis of coagulation factors. FFP, cryoprecipitate and platelet transfusions may also be needed.

PT is used as an indicator for orthotopic liver transplantation. FFP will artificially correct a prolonged PT and so should be avoided in potential transplant candidates.

Renal disease

Platelet function is impaired in uraemia. Treatment of the anaemia associated with renal disease partially corrects the prolonged bleeding time. 1-Deamino-D-arginine vasopressin (DDAVP) has also been shown to reduce the bleeding time.

Alcohol

Excessive alcohol intake inhibits platelet aggregation and prolongs the bleeding time. Alcohol-induced cirrhosis results in a hypocoagulable state due to reduced synthesis of coagulation factors.

Vitamin K deficiency

Vitamin K is essential for the synthesis of fully functional coagulation factors II, VII, IX, X, protein C and protein S. Patients with a poor diet, malabsorption or those requiring TPN may become deficient. In addition, absorption may be reduced in cholestatic liver disease. Consequences can be prevented by the IV administration of vitamin K (10mg weekly).

Hypothermia and acidosis

Most of the coagulation factors are enzymes or cofactors in enzymatic reactions.

Their activity is greatest at physiological temperature and pH.

Pre-warmed fluids should be used in resuscitation of the trauma patient.

pH has been shown to be of greater importance than temperature in the likelihood of success with rVIIa.

Cardiopulmonary bypass and cardiac disease

The extracorporeal circuit is routinely heparinized with UFH to prevent thrombosis during cardiac bypass. Heparin is reversed at the end of the operation by infusion of protamine. However, excess use of protamine can result in a consumptive coagulopathy and haemorrhage. Following initial neutralization by protamine, heparin may be detected 2–6h later in the circulation due to the release of extravascular sequestered heparin.

Thrombocytopenia frequently occurs due to platelet damage in the extracorporeal circuit. This is usually self-limiting and corrects within 2–3h.

Aprotinin has been shown to reduce haemorrhage in high-risk cardiac patients but other risks may outweigh benefit.

Cardiac patients are often taking antiplatelet agents pre-operation, and so transfusion of platelets may be indicated irrespective of the absolute count.

Paraproteinaemia and amyloidosis

High levels of circulating immunoglobulins may impair platelet function. Immunoglobulins may have activity as inhibitors of coagulation factors (see below).

Paraproteinaemia may be associated with AL amyloidosis. This may infiltrate small blood vessels and result in haemorrhage.

Acute promyelocytic leukaemia

In this specific category of acute myeloid leukaemia, the leukaemic cells are believed to express high levels of tissue factor which predisposes to DIC. Coagulation screening tests are deranged. Aggressive transfusion of FFP, cryoprecipitate and platelets is often necessary.

Acquired von Willebrand syndrome

This has been described in association with myeloproliferative disorders (usually only when the platelet count is $>1000 \times 10^9$/l), paraproteinaemia and B-lymphoid malignancies. Control of the underlying disease stops the haemorrhagic phenotype.

Coagulation factor inhibitors

These are autoantibodies directed against a coagulation factor. They can appear *de novo* (acquired haemophilia) or result from exposure to factor concentrate in a congenital haemophiliac. They result in decreased activity of that factor and usually present with haemorrhage. In acquired haemophilia, they may be associated with autoimmune disease, malignancy, drugs or post-partum.

Treatment must include that of the underlying disorder (e.g. immunosuppression) and management of haemorrhage. Patients may be resistant to coagulation factor concentrates, and a bypassing agent (such as FEIBA or rVIIa) may be needed.

Congenital bleeding disorders

Haemophilia A and B

The severity of haemorrhage is inversely correlated with the coagulation factor level. Haemarthroses and muscle haematomas are the most common sites of bleeding. However, in the ITU setting, trauma and surgery are most likely to result in life-threatening haemorrhage if not managed appropriately. Treatment is with recombinant or plasma-derived factor VIII (FVIII) or IX, either by continuous infusion or by repeated bolus injections. Trough levels of the relevant factor should be measured to guide dosing.

Inhibitors may develop, and management is as for acquired haemophilia (see above).

von Willebrand disease

This is the most common inherited bleeding disorder, with a prevalence of 1%. vWF promotes the binding of platelets to damaged subendothelium and, as a carrier of FVIII, it helps to localize the haemostatic reaction to the site of injury.

von Willebrand disease usually results in mucosal bleeding. Life-threatening haemorrhage is unusual. Treatment is with DDAVP or intermediate purity FVIII concentrate.

Platelet disorders

These are characterized by mucosal bleeding and excessive haemorrhage following surgical challenge. They usually respond to DDAVP, but platelet transfusion may be needed. rVIIa has also been used.

Autosomal recessive coagulation disorders

Haemorrhage is usually less severe than in haemophilia A or B. Treatment is with the appropriate factor concentrate or FFP.

Hereditary haemorrhagic telangiectasia

This disorder results in the proliferation of abnormally fragile blood vessels. Bleeding occurs following minor trauma. It may be associated with cerebral and pulmonary AV malformations. Haemorrhagic episodes may be reduced by oral oestrogens.

Ehlers–Danlos syndrome

This and other connective tissue disorders may present with skin haemorrhage. Abnormal collagen results in recurrent stretching of the skin and subsequent bleeding. Treatment of haemorrhagic episodes is with platelet transfusion.

Further reading

British Committee for Standards in Haematology, Blood Transfusion Task Force. Guidelines for the use of platelet transfusions. *Br J Haematol* 2003; 22: 10–23.

Dempfle C-E. Coagulopathy of sepsis. *Thromb Haemost* 2004; 91: 213–24.

Hoffman M, Monroe DM, 3rd. A cell-based model of hemostasis. *Thromb Haemost* 2001; 85: 958–65.

Mittal S, Watson HG. A critical appraisal of the use of recombinant factor VIIa in acquired bleeding conditions. *Br J Haematol* 2006; 133: 355–63.

Stainsby D, MacLennan S, Thomas D, *et al.* Guidelines on the management of massive blood loss. *Br J Haematol* 2006; 135: 634–41.

Anaemia in critical care

Definition

Anaemia is defined as a haemoglobin concentration in the blood of <13.5g/dl in an adult male and <12g/dl in an adult female.

Anaemia is a frequent finding in the critically ill. 50% of patients are anaemic on admission to the ICU, and this figure rises to 95%. by the third day. These patients are extensively transfused, and ~50% will receive at least 5 units of packed red cells.

Pathogenesis

Anaemia in the critically ill is multi-factorial. Primary factors include blood loss from trauma, GI bleeding, continued blood loss after surgery and RRT. The anaemia is compounded by impaired red cell synthesis and intensive phlebotomy. The reason for reduced red cell production is unclear. Patients have anaemia of chronic disease, i.e a low serum iron and total iron binding capacity with a high serum ferritin. The fall in serum iron concentration is precipitated by a rise in hepcidin. Hepcidin inhibits cellular efflux of iron by binding to and inducing degredation of ferroportin, the sole iron exporter in transporting cells. Hepcidin synthesis is greatly increased during inflammation under the influence of the proinflammatory cytokine IL-6. Erythropoesis is further impaired by the reduced release of erythropoietin and by a blunted marrow response to its action. Previous studies suggest that decreased serum iron may be protective against infection and possibly mycobacteria.

Consequences of anaemia

End-organ function is dependent on the adequate delivery of oxygen to cells, due to appropriate cardiac output and arterial oxygen content. Arterial oxygen content is directly proportional to the concentration of haemoglobin. When haemoglobin concentration decreases, oxygen-carrying capacity is reduced. If the intravascular volume is preserved, increased cardiac output maintains adequate tissue oxygen delivery. In addition, there is a rightward shift of the haemoglobin–oxygen dissociation curve where oxygen is more preferentially released to the tissues. Oxygen delivery is redirected from non-vital organs such as the splanchnic bed. Studies in healthy adults show that these mechanisms can safely compensate until the haematocrit falls below 10% (this roughly equilibrates to a haemoglobin of 5g/dl). Below this level, oxygen deficit leads to significant organ impairment. Anaemia may impair recovery from illness. The critically ill are particularly susceptible to the deleterious effects of anaemia as the cardiac output is impaired in a substantial proportion of patients. These basic and logical assumptions have driven transfusion practice for many years.

Approach to the investigation of anaemia

The initial approach should focus on determining the severity of the anaemia and the rapidity with which it has developed. Classically anaemia is characterized as microcytic, normocytic and macrocytic. This is a useful framework on which to base further investigations. A blood film will rapidly provide evidence of haemolysis, iron deficiency, B12 or folate deficiency, underlying malignancy, a microangiopathic haemolytic anaemia or underlying haemoglobinopathy. These conditions may pre-date the condition prompting ICU admission and may significantly complicate individual patient care. The reticulocyte count provides an assessment of red cell production.

Microcytic anaemia	**Normocytic anaemia**	**Macrocytic anaemia**
Low MCV and MCH	*Normal MCV and MCH*	*High MCV*
Iron deficiency	Acute blood loss	B12 and folate deficiency
Anaemia of chronic disease	Anaemia of chronic disease	Drugs
Thalassaemia trait	Hypothyroidism	Haemolysis
	Hypopituitarism	Myelodysplastic syndrome
	Mixed B12 and iron deficiency	

MCH = mean corpuscular haemoglobin; MCV = mean corpuscular volume.

Classification of anaemia

Management of anaemia in critical care

Pre-existing causes of anaemia can be rapidly diagnosed and the appropriate treatment started. The anaemia of critical illness is managed with supportive transfusion therapy. The CRIT and the Anaemia in Blood Transfusion in Critical Care (ABC) studies show that red cell transfusion is independently associated with an increased mortality. This research builds on the earlier finding by Hérbert of a trend toward a decreased mortality in critically ill patients who were randomized to receive a restrictive vs a liberal transfusion strategy. These studies form the basis of the current National Blood Service (NBS) recommendation of withholding transfusion until the haemoglobin falls below 8.0g/dl. Specific exclusions apply to patients with active ischaemic heart disease or severe sepsis or those who are actively bleeding. To confuse matters further, the SOAP study showed no association between increased mortality and blood transfusion. The beneficial effect of leucodepletion has been suggested as the explanation for the conflicting results seen with the SOAP data and the previous studies. Leucodepletion reduces the risks of transmission of cell-associated viruses, prion transmission, transfusion-related febrile reactions and transfusion-related ALI. Therefore, by making transfusion safer, the threshold may rise. With the continued debate regarding the risk:benefit ratio of the transfusion threshold need to be more closely evaluated. A single measure of a target haemoglobin is easy to apply but probably too simplistic. The optimal haemoglobin concentration will vary for individuals, and some consideration of the serum lactate and mixed venous oxygen saturation may be used in the future to help further evaluate the need for transfusion.

Once a decision to transfuse has been made, there are no data to guide the number of red cell units that should be transfused. Single unit transfusions are of little clinical benefit and place increased logistical demands on local transfusion services, and are usually not recommended. There is no evidence to show that single unit transfusions reduce the overall number of transfusions an individual patient receives. However, single unit transfusions are easier to give in patients with brittle cardiorespiratory function. There is a reduced risk of smaller volumes tipping the patient into or exacerbating pulmonary oedema. The number of blood donors is continuing to fall, and should the blood supply become limited this assumption will be challenged.

Measures to minimize blood loss in the ICU

An effective measure to reduce blood loss includes where possible trying to restrict phlebotomy and minimize blood wastage. It has been estimated that blood gas (ABG) sampling and routine phlebotomy account for 40–80ml of blood loss daily. This equates to ~300–600ml of blood a week. A large part of this volume (up to 50%) can be accounted for with regular ABG testing. New in-line blood conservation pressure transducer systems for blood gas monitoring reduce blood wastage as there is no dead space loss. These systems reduce the need for transfusion and are theoretically safer for both staff and patients, with less risk of catheter-related infections and potential needle stick injuries. They may be applied to venous sampling in the future.

Post-operative strategies for optimizing the appropriate use of antifibrinolytics, FFP and platelets can reduce blood loss. Where possible, elective surgery should be delayed in anaemic patients. Surgery in these patients is associated with an increased mortality. Treating anaemia before surgery has been shown to reduce mortality.

Erythropoietin

Given the deleterious effects associated with red cell transfusion, there has been considerable interest in the role of erythropoietin in reducing the need for red cell transfusions. Despite resulting in a modest increase in haemoglobin, erythropoietin has not been shown to reduce the incidence of red cell transfusion in the critically ill. There is a role in those patients who decline red cell transfusion and those patients who have previously established renal failure.

Conclusion

Anaemia is very common in the critically ill. Recent research has shed new light on the aetiology of the anaemia in critical illness and its management. Transfusion remains very safe, but whenever possible measure should be taken to try to minimize excessive phlebotomy and critically evaluate the need for transfusion in individual patients.

Further reading

Corwin HL, Gettinger A, Pearl RG, *et al.* The CRIT Study: anaemia and blood transfusion in the critically ill—current clinical practice in the United States. *Crit Care Med* 2004; 32: 39–52.

Ganz T. Hepcidin and its role in regulating systemic iron metabolism. *Hematology* 2006; 29–35.

Hébert PC, Wells G, Blajchman MA, *et al.* A multicentre, randomised, controlled clinical trial of transfusion requirements in critical care. *N Engl J Med* 1999; 340: 409–17.

Hill SR, Carless PA, Henry DA, *et al.* Transfusion thresholds and other strategies for guiding allogeneic red blood cell transfusion. *Cochrane Database Syst Rev* 2002; (2): CD002042.

Vincent JL, Baron JF, Reinhart K, *et al.* Anaemia and blood transfusion in critically ill patients. *JAMA* 2002; 288: 1449–507.

Vincent JL, Piagnerelli M. Transfusion in the intiensive care unit. *Crit Care Med* 2006; 34: S96–101.

Sickle cell anaemia

Sickle cell disease (SCD) is the group of disorders associated with the abnormal sickle haemoglobin. Homozygous sickle cell anaemia (HbSS) is the most common form, whilst the double heterozygote conditions of HbSC, HbSβthalassaemia and HbS/Punjab also cause sickling disease. The sickle gene is estimated to be present in 8% of African-Americans. There are an estimated 15 000 patients in the UK. Whilst the life expectancy is improving, many patients are dying in their early forties. The leading cause of death is acute chest syndrome, which is also the most frequent cause precipitating ICU admission.

Pathogenesis

SCD is an autosomal recessive disorder where substitution of valine for glutamic acid in position 6 of the β-globin chain results in the abnormal haemoglobin. There is polymerization of HbS molecules within the red cell as a result of hypoxia. These polymers distort the erythrocyte, causing it to acquire the classical sickle shape with a marked reduction in flexibility. This leads to microvascular occlusion and hence a sickle cell crisis. SCD causes a chronic haemolytic anaemia. The sex distribution is equal. In the UK, universal neonatal screening is being implemented and so most British-born cases are identified early.

Clinical approach

The clinical manifestations of the disease vary amongst patients. Painful vaso-occlussion is the most common clinical feature. Visceral sequestration crises can affect any organ system, resulting in chest crises, splenic sequestration, and hepatic and girdle sequestration. Painful vaso-occlusive crises may cause infarcts in the bones, lungs and even the brain. The most serious manifestation is stroke, which can be either haemorrhagic or ischaemic. Stroke warrants an immediate exchange transfusion. SCD can also present with aplastic crisis due to an infection (classically parvovirus) causing transient red cell aplasia. Due to the shortened red cell survival in SCD, this may lead to a precipitous drop in the haemoglobin level. The heart may be involved, with chronic anaemia and microinfarcts leading to haemosiderin deposition within the myocardium, leading to ventriclular dilatation. Cholelithiasis may be asymptomatic or require acute surgical intervention. The kidneys lose concentrating capacity, which results in the loss of large volumes of fluid further exacerbating the dehydration. Proteinuria is common in older patients. Renal failure may ensue. The spleen undergoes repeated infarction, and over time becomes fibrotic and shrinks. Hence patients with SCD are regarded as asplenic. Pneumococcal infections are common. Attention must be paid to antibiotic prophylaxis and regular vaccination. Pulmonary hypertension has recently been reported as a common complication in SCD and is associated with a high mortality.

Examination

There are no specific exam findings. The patient is often icteric, the mucus membranes are pale and a systolic murmur is sometiems present. The spleen may be enlarged in younger patients. Evaluation must be undertaken for pulmonary hypertension as this may be present in as many as 60% of patients.

Investigations

If a diagnosis of SCD is in question, haemoglobin electrophoresis will rapidly confirm the diagnosis and delineate between HbSS, HbSC and HbSβthalassaemia. A reticulocyte count is useful to exclude aplastic crises. The HbA/HbS% should be measured. The urine should be examined for proteinuria. CXR is mandatory, and an echocardiogram should be considered.

Management 'general principles'

Morphine is the drug of choice for pain relief and can be given IV. In the ICU, patient-controlled analgesia (PCA) or intermitted SC injections are appropriate. PCA has been shown to provide superior pain relief, although there are concerns that patients may receive increased doses of morphine leading to respiratory depression and the potentially increased risk of a chest crisis. Pethidine should not be used because of its greater addictive potential and associated risk of seizures. Constipation should be pre-empted with the use of regular laxatives. When pain control is improved, the morphine should be weaned and converted to an equivalent oral dose. NSAIDs are effective at reducing deep bone pain when used in conjunction with strong opiates. IV fluids should be given to correct any dehydration, which will promote HbS polymerization.

All sickle cell patients should be regarded as asplenic and receive broad-spectrum antibiotics if an infection is suspected. Penicilllin prophylaxis daily should be continued throughout life. As a general principle, SCD patients should be immunized against hepatitis B and *Pneumococcus*, meningitis and *Haemophilus*.

Hydroxyurea (HU), now known as hydroxycarbamide (HC), increases the production of fetal haemoglobin (HbF). This reduces the rate of sickling. HC can produce reversible myelosupression and we routinely suspend its use in those patients who are admitted with severe illness. The HC is restarted immediately prior to discharge.

Transfusion in sickle cell anaemia

Although anaemia is a constant feature in SCD, the patients tolerate the anaemia well. The indications for an emergency transfusion include:

Top up transfusion: (aims to raise Hb by 2–3g/dl)

- Aplastic crisis
- Acute splenic sequestration

Exchange transfusion

- Acute stroke
- Acute chest syndrome
- Severe sepsis
- Hepatic sequestration
- Priapism (if surgical treatment has failed)
- Acute multi-organ failure

Despite profound anaemia, the amount of blood that can be given as a 'top up' is limited due to concerns over possible hyperviscosity. HbS-containing cells are hyperviscous and have poor flow characteristics which are exacerbated by the transfusion of HbA-containing red cells. Practically, the post-transfusion haemoglobin should not exceed 10g/dl. Exchange blood transfusion produces rapid and sometimes dramatic improvements in biological and oxygenation parameters. By removing red cells, the concerns over hyperviscosity are circumvented. The proportion of HbA/HbS red cells should be measured pre- and post-exchange. The major disadvantage of exchange transfusion is the increased donor exposure, with a greater risk of infection and alloimunization. To try to prevent immunization, patients with SCD should be transfused ABO-compatible blood with matching of their Rh C, D, E and Kell antigens. This approach reduces the probability of alloantibody formation. The exchange can either be performed manually or with an apheresis machine. In the critically ill, an automated exchange is preferable as it is relatively quick, taking ~2h, and provides more control, achieving a target final Hb, %HbS and fluid balance. There is less fluctuation in the circulating volume and it is probably safer in patients with haemodynamic compromise. However, there is no evidence directly comparing an automated exchange with a manual exchange. The major advantage of a manual exchange is that less training is required without the need to use an apheresis machine. For both techniques, a 1.5 red cell volume exchange is regarded as the best volume to achieve a maximum reduction in HbS red cells. The patient's red cell volume is equal to the pre-transfusion haematocrit multiplied by the estimated blood volume (70ml/kg for an adult

The acute chest syndrome

This is a common complication and the most frequent crisis requiring ICU support. It may be precipitated by infection, hypoventilation and atelectasis, pulmonary oedema or bonchospasm. Acute chest syndrome may present post-operatively, and is the most common cause of post-operative death in SCD. Careful perioperative management is required. Acute chest syndrome is diagnosed when a new pulmonary infiltrate is detected on a CXR involving at least one complete lung segment with the addition of either chest pain, fever >38.5°C, tachypnoea or hypoxaemia with a pO_2 <9mm Hg. Life-threatening respiratory compromise can occur. The acute treatment of acute chext syndrome is supportive. In addition to the general measures mentioned above, patients with acute chest syndrome should receive treatment with inhaled bronchodilators. NIV has been a significant step forward in the management of acute chest syndrome, reducing the requirement for mechanical ventilation, and should be started early if possible in the management of an acute chest crisis. The primary treatment remains prompt exchange transfusion. There is no evidence for the routine use of anticoagulation.

Pulmonary hypertension

This is defined as a raised pulmonary artery pressure of >25mm Hg on catheterization. This roughly equates to a tricuspid regurgitant jet velocity of 2.5m/s on echocardiography. Haemolysis results in the release of free haemoglobin which scavenges NO and catalyses the formation of reactive oxygen species. Asplenia increases the circulation of platelet-derived mediators which promote pulmonary microthrombosis and adhesion of red cells to the pulmonary vasculature. Repeated episodes of regional pulmonary hypoxia produce progressive tissue damage and alteration of the pulmonary vasculature, ultimately leading to pulmonary hypertension. Pulmonary hypertension is a frequent finding at autopsy, and may be present in as many as 60% of patients with SCD. Symptoms tend to be absent until irreversible damage has occurred and the patient complains of shortness of breath. Patients with SCD and pulmonary hypertension have been successfully treated with infusions of prostacyclin or sildenafil. Echocardiography should be considered on all patients with SCD admitted to the ICU to exclude the presence of occult pulmonary hypertension.

Surgery

There is a high risk of post-operative complications and an ~1% mortality among SCD patients undergoing elective surgery. In these patients, an elective exchange transfusion may be undertaken in an attempt to try to reduce this mortality. However, in patients with a low haemoglobin, top up transfusion has been shown to be as good as a red cell exchange. Extrapolating this to critically ill patients, it would appear reasonable to consider an exchange transfusion in any critically ill SCD patient prior to a surgical procedure. Post-operatively, scrupulous care must be taken to monitor oxygenation and hydration in an attempt to prevent a crisis. A series of patients undergoing elective cholecystectomy with SCD received CPAP for the first 24h post-operatively. Only one patient developed a chest crisis. The remaining patient responded well to a prolonged course of CPAP. Incentive spirometry has also been shown to reduce the incidence of chest crises. Dehydration increases the relative concentration of the abnormal HbS within the red cell, increasing the chances of polymerization.

SCD patients have a prothrombotic profile and thus should receive thromboprophylaxis when acutely ill and perisurgery.

Conclusion

Patients with SCD present specific challenges when critically ill. However, with the development of improved transfusion strategies and the use of NIV, the prognosis is continuing to improve in this challenging patient group. Successful care is reliant on close communication between the critical care and haematology teams.

Further reading

Howard J, Gabriel I. Pulmonary complications of sickle cell disease. *Airways J* 2005; 3: 001.

Hoffbrands AV, Pettit JE, Moss PAH. Essential haematology. Oxford: Blackwell Science.

Mak V, Davies SC. The pulmonary physician in critical care * Illustrative case 6: acute chest syndrome of sickle cell anaemia. *Thorax* 2003; 58: 726–8.

Platt OS, Brambilla DJ. Mortality in sickle cell disease. Life expectancy and risk factors for early death. *N Engl J Med* 1994; 330: 1639–44.

Vichinsky EP, Haberkern CM, Neumayr L, *et al.* A comparison of conservative and aggressive transfusion regimens in the perioperative management of sickle cell disease. The Preoperative Transfusion in Sickle Cell Disease Study Group. *N Engl J Med* 1995; 333: 206–13.

Haemolysis

The normal red cell survives for 120 days in the circulation. If the bone marrow is healthy, then red cell survival can be reduced by as much as 8-fold without developing significant anaemia. However, if red cell survival is <15 days, anaemia is inevitable.

Premature destruction occurs due to abnormal red cell structure, excess physical trauma to the cells or because the cells have become abnormally rigid, or via immune mechanisms—complement can punch large holes in the membrane, or IgG-coated cells are removed by the reticuloendothelial system. Constant haemolysis results in splenomegaly.

General approach to haemolysis

1. Is there increased red cell production?
   - Blood film—polychromasia, macrocytosis
   - Raised reticuloyte count
2. Is there increased red cell destruction?
   - Elevated bilirubin level
   - Elevated LDH
   - Elevated faecal and urinary urobilinogen
   - Reduced haptoglobins
3. Is the haemolysis intravascular?
   - Elevated plasma haemoglobin
   - Methaemoglobin present
   - Haemoglobinuria
   - Urinary haemosiderin if a chronic condition
4. Why are the cells being destroyed?
   - Genetically determined
     - Morphology looking for sickle cells, spherocytes, etc.
     - Haemoglobinopathy analysis
     - Enzyme deficiency, glucose-6-phosphate dehydrogenase (G-6-PD) being most common in UK
   - Acquired
     - Immune—do a Coombs test, if clinical suspicion high, repeat if negative.
     - Non-immune—trauma, valve prosthetic leak, liver disease, parasitic disorder, bacterial infection, physical agents, Hypersplenism, microangiopathic haemolytic anaemia.

Haemolytic conditions particularly relevant to critical care

Glucose-6-phosphate dehydrogenase deficiency

This X-linked deficiency makes red cells vulnerable to oxidative damage. It is widely distributed and has a high prevalence in Africa, Southern Europe, the Middle East, Asia and Oceana. Most individuals are asymptomatic but risk haemolytic anaemia with

1. Drugs (antimalarials, sulfonamides, aspirin, ciprofloxacin, etc.)
2. Infections
3. Fava beans

The anaemia is largely due to intravascular haemolysis; the blood film shows the features of acute haemolysis along with 'bite cells' (bits of cell bitten away) and Heinz bodies (denatured haemoglobin).

The diagnosis is made by demonstrating decreased levels of G-6-PD.

Immune haemolysis

Alloimmune haemolysis

IgM antibodies fix complement and cause intravascular haemolysis, as seen with blood transfusion of an ABO mismatch. Pre-formed anti-A or anti-B will bind to transfused red cells causing instantaneous intravascular haemolysis, with shock and renal failure. Over 20% of patients with ABO incompatibility die.

IgG antibodies bind to red cells, and red cell destruction occurs in the spleen (extravascular), e.g. if a patient develops anti-D or anti-Kell antibodies. Due to the time taken to develop these antibodies, this occurs 7–10 days after transfusion.

Autoimmune haemolysis

These may be 'warm' due to the presence of antibodies active at 37°C or cold when the antibodies are active at 40°C. Both are uncommon and should be referred to a haematologist.

Non-immune

Damage to red cells due to oxidative stress is common in patients in critical care, brought about by drugs, physical damage such as burns, and infection.

Fragmentation of red cells by mechanical trauma occurs either with

- Cardiac haemolysis', when foreign material is in contact with the blood such as haemofiltration, the intra-arotic balloon pump and the ventricular assist device, or when there is a para valvular leak.
- Microangiopathic haemolytic anaemia. When blood vessels are partially blocked by fibrin strands of platelets, arteritis, fibriniod necrosis or malignant cells. (see Table 23.4.1)

Table 23.4.1 Microangiopathic haemolytic anaemia

Disease	Underlying Pathology
Malignant hypertension	Fibrinoid necrosis
Haemolytic–uraemic syndrome	Renal microthrombi
Thrombotic thrombocytopenia purpura	Platelet aggregates
Disseminated intravascular coagulation	Microthrombi
The vasculitides (polyarteteritis, Wegeners, SLE)	
Meningoccocal sepsis	Microthrombi/DIC
Homograft rejection	Microthrombi
Pre-eclampsia	Fibrinoid necrosis ± DIC

Haemolytic–uraemic syndrome (HUS) is a triad of thrombocytopenia, haemolysis and renal failure. There may be associated multi-organ disease including enterocolitis, neurological complications, liver, pancreatic and cardiac dysfunction. The epidemic form (D+) is associated with a prodromal illness, bloody diarrhoea and verotoxin enterococcal (verocytotoxin-producing *Escherichia coli* (VTEC)) infection. Rare sporadic or atypical cases have no prodrome and may be associated with HIV, CMV or bacterial infection. Secondary cases of HUS include post-solid organ or bone marrow transplantation, drug exposure (pentostatin, cyclosporin, mitomycin C, heroin and quinine), malignancy, pregnancy and familial complement factor H deficiency or other complement defects.

Early stool culture is essential for the diagnosis of VTEC-associated HUS. Other investigations are as for TTP. Management involves meticulous fluid and electrolyte balance, and blood pressure control, with renal dialysis as required. Antimotility drugs and antibiotic treatment adversely affect the outcome and should be avoided. At present there is no conclusive evidence that either FFP or plasma exchange improves outcome. Adjuvant treatment with antiplatelet agents, anticoagulation, antifibrinolytics or IVIG is not recommended.

TTP

Thrombotic thrombocytopenic purpura (TTP) is a clinical diagnosis characterised by thrombocytopenia, microangiopathic haemolytic anaemia, fluctuating neurological signs, renal impairment and fever.

Excessive platelet aggregation results in platelet microvascular thrombi, which particularly affect the cerebral circulation. This is mediated by ultra-large von Willebrand factor (vWF) multimers due to a deficiency of vWF cleaving protease (vWF-CP), also known as ADAMTS13. Deficiency of vWF-CP activity may be;

- genetic—absence of the enzyme
- acquired—presence of an autoantibody to vWF-CP.

Coagulation profiles are usually normal. Secondary DIC due to prolonged tissue ischemia is an ominous prognostic indicator.

Specialised units CAN measure levels of vWF-CP and its inhibitor to confirm the diagnosis of TTP, but results are not available quickly. IF TTP is suspected they must be treated immediately and the diagnosis must be confirmed or refuted retrospectively. Delay in treatment may result in sudden death due to thrombotic occlusion of the coronary arteries.

A panel of investigations required in a suspected case of TTP includes:

- FBC and film
- Reticulocyte count
- Clotting screen including fibrinogen and D-dimers
- Urea and electrolytes
- Liver function tests
- Lactate dehydrogenase
- Urinalysis
- Direct antiglobulin test
- HIV and hepatitis serology

Single volume daily plasma exchange should be commenced immediately. Theoretically plasma exchanges using cryosupernatant or solvent–detergent prepared FFP (both deficient in high MW von Willebrand factor multimeric forms hence less likely to stimulate further thrombosis) may be more efficacious than using standard fresh frozen although there is no clinical data to support this currently. Daily plasma exchange should continue for a minimum of 2 days after complete remission.

Adjuvant pulsed methylprednisolone 1g IV daily for 3 days can be considered. Low dose aspirin (75mg daily) should be commenced on platelet recovery (platelet counts > 50 x 109/l). Red cell transfusion according to clinical need. Folate supplementation is required.

Platelet transfusions are contraindicated unless there is life-threatening haemorrhage. In refractory disease intensification of plasma exchange should be considered. The use of Ritoximab is emerging as a major advance in the management of acquired TTP.

References

Allford SL, Hunt BJ, Rose P, Machin SJ; Haemostasis and Thrombosis Task Force, British Committee for Standards in Haematology. Guidelines on the diagnosis and management of the thrombotic microangiopathic haemolytic anaemias. *Br J Haematol.* 2003 Feb;120(4):556–73.

Hoffman PC. Immune hemolytic anemia–selected topics. *Hematology Am Soc Hematol Educ Program.* 2006:13–8.

Disseminated intravascular coagulation

DIC is not a disease or a symptom but a syndrome which is always secondary to an underlying disorder. It is characterized by a systemic activation of the blood coagulation system, which results in the generation and deposition of fibrin, leading to microvascular thrombosis in various organs and contributing to the development of MOF. Consumption and subsequent exhaustion of platelets and coagulation proteins may result in severe bleeding complications. In the UK, bacterial sepsis, trauma and obstetric calamities are the common causes of DIC. Worldwide, snake bites are the major cause.

Pathogenesis of DIC

Tissue factor, dysfunctional physiological anticoagulant pathways and impaired fibrinolysis all contribute to widespread fibrin deposition. In sepsis, the generation of TNF and IL-1 lead to expression of tissue factor on monocytes and endothelial cell activation. In meningococcal sepsis, it has been shown that the level of tissue factor present on monocytes is predictive of outcome. PAI-1 gene polymorphisms which produce poor fibrinolysis are associated with increased mortality.

DIC is a clinicopathological diagnosis. It cannot be made in the haemostasis laboratory as several other conditions such as liver disease will produce the same haemostatic picture—prolongation of aPTT and INR, and low fibrinogen and platelet count (all due to consumption), and elevated D-dimers. In liver disease, this same picture reflects lack of production of haemostatic factors, as in patients with massive blood loss, where the mechanism is loss of haemostatic factors. Hyperfibrinolysis can also tend to produce a similar picture, although the fall in platelet count tends to be less severe.

A scoring system that uses simple laboratory assays is a strong independent predictor of outcome in intensive care patients (see Taylor *et al.*). The keystone of management is the specific and forceful treatment of the underlying disorder. Once the triad of DIC, hypoxia and acidosis has developed, the prognosis is poor, and so aggressive management is required to prevent this stage. Plasma and platelet substitution therapy, anticoagulation and the restoration of anticoagulant pathways are also beneficial in experimental and clinical studies.

Management of DIC is to replace the missing haemostatic factors:

- If aPTT and/or INR >1.5 of normal give FFP 15ml/kg
- If fibrinogen <1.5 g/dl give cryoprecipitate
- If platelets <50 x 10^9/l give a pool of platelets

Constant repeated monitoring of haemostasis with coagulation screen and FBC is indicated. Antifibrinolytics are contraindicated as the lysis of thrombus is essential for resolution of DIC.

In profoundly prothrombotic DICs such as meningococcal sepsis, there is a theoretical argument to give an anticoagulant to switch off the prothrombotic effect of tissue factor on the monocytes. Options include giving supplementary antithrombin, APC and IV heparin. A haematologist should be consulted for advice as there are no clinical trials in this area.

Further reading

Bernard GR, Vincent JL, Laterre PF *et al.* Efficacy and safety of recombinant human activated protein C for severe sepsis. *N Engl J Med* 2001; 344: 699–709.

Hermans PW, Hazelzet JA. Plasminogen activator inhibitor type 1 gene polymorphism and sepsis. *Clin Infect Dis* 2005; Suppl 7: S453–8.

Levi M. Current understanding of disseminated intravascular coagulation. *Br J Haematol* 2004; 124: 567–76.

Osterud B, Bjorklid E. The tissue factor pathway in DIC. *Semin Thromb Haemost* 2001; 27: 605–17.

Taylor FBJ, Toh CH, Hoots K, *et al.* Towards a definition, clinical and laboratory criteria and a scoring system for disseminated intravascular coagulation. *Thromb Haemost* 2000; 86: 1327–1330.

Neutropenic sepsis

A fever of >38°C in a neutropenic patient is a medical emergency. Immediate assessment with prompt initiation of broad-spectrum antibiotic therapy is essential. Neutropenic sepsis remains the most common life-threatening complication of treatment with chemotherapy, and the most frequent reason for patients receiving chemotherapy to require ICU admission. Although improving, critically ill patients with neutropenic sepsis continue to have poorer outcomes when compared with matched patients without malignancy. Access to ICU care may be restricted because of the perceived increased mortality and poor outcomes. A multi-disciplinary approach is required to optimize management.

Definition

A diagnosis of neutropenic sepsis is made when a patient has a neutrophil count <1.0 x 10^9/l, and either a single oral temperature >38.5°C, or 38°C sustained for ≥1h. For practical purposes, unexplained hypotension without fever, or new onset confusion should also require urgent evaluation and treatment.

Pathogenesis

Chemotherapy has a direct toxic effect on the bone marrow, causing pancytopenia. Many haematological malignancies infiltrate the bone marrow compromising haematopoiesis. Both chemotherapy and malignancy cause disordered T-cell and B-cell function, further contributing to immune dysfunction.

Clinical approach

History

- The type of malignancy, disease state (active/remission), recent chemotherapy, presence of graft vs host disease (GvHD) must be documented. These factors have all been shown independently to affect outcome and may lead to significant alterations in care.
- Patients from Eastern Europe, the Middle East, Far East or the Indian subcontinent should be considered at risk of TB especially if they have not received TB prophylaxis with chemotherapy

Examination

- Identify the site of infection to guide evaluation and treatment. Neutropenic patients deteriorate rapidly and are susceptible to unusual infections presenting in an atypical fashion.
- Look for signs of infection around tunnelled venous catheters, the mouth for mucositis and dental abscesses, the perianal area for infection. Rectal examinations risk introducing further infection and are not recommended.
- Hypotension without fever or general malaise can still be due to severe sepsis.

Investigations

- Blood cultures should be taken from all the lumens of a tunnelled venous line, and in addition peripheral cultures taken; sputum and urine culture, and CXR are all essential.
- A high resolution CT (HRCT) of the chest and sinuses (HRCT remains the most sensitive and specific way of diagnosing fungal chest infections in neutropenic patients.)
- Ultrasound of the abdomen looking for hepatosplenic candidiasis

Initial treatment

It is imperative that broad-spectrum antibiotics are started promptly. The UK national service framework requires that all such patients should receive antibiotics in <1h following admission. In practice, most units would aim to have initiated treatment within 20min. Obtain the appropriate cultures prior to the initiation of antibiotic therapy, but antibiotic therapy must not be overly delayed.

Microbiological approach

Infection control measures

These patients are at extremely high risk of contracting other infections. Scrupulous attention must be paid to hygiene and, if possible, they are best managed in side rooms preferably where high efficiency particulate air (HEPA) filter units are installed.

Bacterial infection

Look for previous micriobiological history and any prior colonization with MDR organisms. This may lead to alteration of the empiric treatment protocol. Gettting the antibiotic choice right first time improves outcome—choosing the wrong antibiotics in this patient group may be rapidly fatal.

Prior to the 1980s, Gram-negative bacilli were the predominant organisms causing infection in neutropenic patients. Now Gram-positive infections account for up to 60–70% of identified bacteraemias.

Empiric treatment is with an antipseudomonal penicillin and an aminoglycoside. Single daily dosing of aminoglycosides is favoured since it is more efficacious and associated with less ototoxicity and nephrotoxicity. Some authors argue that the addition of aminoglycoside therapy only increases the incidence of side effects, but the addition of an aminoglycoside to ceftazadine monotherapy gives better Gram-negative cover. Carbapenems have very broad-spectrum activity and can be used as first-line monotherapy but are generally held as second line. There are no RCTs of one antibiotic regimen compared with another, and the precise regimen used should be decided locally. Vancomycin is frequently used as second-line agent; however, if the risk for MRSA is high, it should be initiated as first line.

A response to first-line antibiotics should occur within 48h. If not, they should be changed to second-line antibiotics. If pyrexia persists after 96h, consideration must be given to antifungal therapy. There are no firm rules as to the duration of antibiotic therapy; however, many centres continue antibiotics until the neutrophil count has recovered to >0.5–1.0 x 10^9/l. Prolonged courses of broad-spectrum antibiotic increase the chances of developing multi-resistant organisms. If a specific organism with known sensitivities is cultured, it is appropriate to narrow the antibiotic spectrum to minimize the chances of producing multi-resistant organisms. This approach is controversial as neutropenic patients may be infected with more than one organism; infection with two organisms is reported in up to 19% of patients. No attempt should be made to de-escalate therapy if the patient has mucositis; the risk of multiple infections is too high.

Fungal infection

This remains a considerable diagnostic and therapeutic challenge in neutropenic patients and a major cause of morbidity and mortality. Autopsy studies suggest that invasive fungal infections are found in up to 40% of haematology patients. The most common fungal infections are *Candida* and *Aspergillosis*.

Invasive candidiasis in the neutropenic patient is usually associated with well defined risk factors including, a prolonged duration of neutropenia, mucositis, corticosteroids, prolonged use of broad-spectrum antibiotics and the presence of a central venous line. The overall mortality for *Candida* infections approaches 60%. Treatment involves removal/replacement of any in-dwelling lines (including tunnelled lines) and treatment with either a lipid formulation of amphotericin B or either voriconazole or caspofungin. The data regarding caspofungin are encouraging, and it may well become the first line. Treatment should continue for a minimum of 14 days, and should only be stopped if the neutrophil count has recovered.

Invasive aspergillosis is probably the most serious infection in neutropenic patients, occasionally proving exceptionally difficult to treat. In bone marrow transplant recipients, the mortality is reported to be >80%. The use of high dose steroid or other immunosuppression and GvHD are well defined risk factors. Recovery of bone marrow function is critical for survival, and ultimately antifungal agents are temporary holding measures awaiting immune regeneration; granulocyte colony-stimulating factor (G-CSF) should be used. The traditional treatment has been high dose liposomal amphotericin B. Voriconazole was found to have an increased response rate with a lower mortality rate and a reduced incidence of adverse reactions, and some centres recommend voriconazole as first-line treatment. Liposomal amphotericin has a broader spectrum of action. Caspofungin has been used as salvage therapy or when patients are intolerant of the other medications. Antifungal therapy should continue until all signs and symptoms of the infection have resolved for at least 2 weeks and the neutrophil count has recovered.

Given the high mortality rate of invasive fungal infection there has been considerable interest in the use of combination therapy, with potential synergy between antifungal agents to enhance fungal killing. The cost of such therapy is extremely high and has not been studied in an RCT.

Viral infections

Viral infections are also an important cause of morbidity and mortality in neutropenic patients. The difference in the incidence and outcome of viral infections varies widely between patient groups. The most vulnerable group of patients are those who have received bone marrow transplants and require ongoing immunosuppression. CMV, HSV, varicella-zoster virus, respiratory syncytial virus and influenza viruses are the more frequent pathogens. CMV infection is a frequent complication following a bone marrow transplant—reactivation of latent infections in patients who were seropositive prior to their transplant. Pre-emptive therapy based on PCR screening is conducted by bone marrow transplant units. Indications for treatment include a high CMV or rising CMV titres; treatment is with either foscarnet or ganciclovir. Waiting for the emergence of symptoms is frequently fatal. Treatment should continue until two consecutive negative CMV blood PCR results are obtained.

Blood product support

Patients with haematological malignancies require extensive blood product support. Each patient receiving chemotherapy who has special transfusion requirements should have a record of their transfusion status stored with their local blood bank.

Thrombocytopenia

Thrombocytopenia presents many practical difficulties in a critical care environment. For a 'severe sepsis patient' the platelet count should be maintained above 20×10^9/l. Below this level there is a progressive and substantially increased risk of spontaneous bleeding. Many patients will require daily platelet support and some become refractory to platelet transfusion. Pethidine 50mg SC is an excellent antipyretic agent which can be used to cover mild febrile reactions; with platelets, however, there is a risk of seizures related to the accumulation of its metabolites. In ICU, chlorpheniramine is probably the safest agent to cover platelet reactions. Frequently platelet transfusions are co-administered with hydrocortisone; this should not be used routinely in the ICU, since patients are already profoundly immunosuppressed and additional doses of steroid further impair immunity as well as exacerbating problems with glycaemia and adrenal suppression.

Invasive procedures

It is not always practical to aim for a platelet count of 100, and a count of 50 should be acceptable for most procedures (CVP line placement, Hickman line removal, paracentesis, NG tube insertion, bronchoscopy). A platelet count >100 is required for major surgery.

Irradiated blood products are needed for all bone marrow transplant recipients, patients with Hodgkin's disease and those who have received purine analogues or alemtuzumab. There have been no reported cases of transfusion-associated GvHD since the initiation of leucodepletion, but care must be taken as transfusion-associated GvHD is regarded as universally fatal. FFP and cryoprecipitate are not cellular products and therefore do not need to be irradiated.

CMV-negative blood products should be requested for all potential candidates or recipients of a bone marrow transplant who are CMV negative prior to transplant. There is no need for CMV-negative products if the patient was seropositive prior to their transplant.

Granulocyte-colony stimulating factor

G-CSF is given once daily as an SC injection, stimulating the production of WBCs. It accelerates recovery from neutropenia after chemotherapy, reducing the frequency of infections and the duration of neutropenia. There is no evidence to suggest a substantial benefit in the critically ill. One study showed no difference in the depth or duration of neutropenia, or survival with the use of G-CSF. As there is no evidence to suggest that G-CSF causes additional harm and there is a potential theoretical benefit, most haematologists support its use.

Dosage

Theoretically (no evidence and costly) there is potentiallly reduced adsorption of G-CSF in patients receiving vasopressors so in patients receiving either adrenaline or norepinephrine the dose of G-CSF should be doubled. G-CSF can be stopped when the neutrophil count is $>1.0 \times 10^9$/l for two consecutive days. G-CSF should be restarted if the count drops below this level.

Nutritional support

Enteral nutrition should be considered early. Patients with malignant disease and who have received chemotherapy are frequently malnourished and have lost a significant proportion of their body weight. Inadequate nutritional support contributes significantly to mortality. Mucositis makes oral feeding extremely difficult, and it is virtually impossible to maintain a satisfactory calorific intake.

Organ-supportive therapy

Mechanical ventilation and intubation has been shown to impact negatively on the survival of critically ill haematology patients. The reported mortality of ventilated neutropenic patient's ranges from 85 to 94%. The major cause of death in ventilated patients is septic shock and MOF rather than hypoxaemia. These poor outcomes must be tempered by the fact that several studies have now shown improved overall survival in patients requiring ventilatory support. The cause of this improved survival is attributable to the increased use of NIV and the use of lung protective ventilatory strategies. Each patient needs to be evaluated on a case-by-case basis, with close liaison between the attending intensivist and haematologist to ensure patients with limited chances of survival are not inappropriately treated.

Renal replacement therapy is also associated with an increased mortality rate of 67% when used in neutropenic patients. In patients requiring combined RRT and mechanical ventilation, the mortality is extremely high. The data on this patient group are limited, but one study reports a 5% survival

Tunnelled venous lines

Reliable venous access is essential, and the majority of patients have tunnelled venous lines. These devices are associated with a significant potential for iatrogenic bacteraemia and candidaemia. The two main causes of line infection are inadequate insertion technique resulting in early infection and poor handling/manipulation of the line. Colonization can also develop from haematogenous spread from an established infection. Suspicion of line sepsis must always be high in neutropenic patients. If in doubt of the source, the line should be removed and a fresh catheter placed at a new site. If the tunnel of a long-term catheter appears infected the device should be removed. Multiple studies have reported the use of antibiotics to treat infected long-term catheters. These studies generally exclude neutropenic patients and report success rates of 60–90%. As a general rule, the tunnelled line of any neutropenic patient should be removed if they are admitted to ICU with severe sepsis. This should be mandatory if there is bacteraemia, or evidence of MRSA or fungal (*in particular candida*) colonization of the line.

Conclusion

There will continue to be an increasing demand for critical care resources for these patients. Currently neutropenic patients with severe sepsis have poor outcomes, but there is much scope for further improvement in the treatment of this challenging patient group.

Further reading

Azoulay E, Alberti C, Bornstain C, *et al.* Improved survival in cancer patients requiring mechanical ventilatory support: impact of non-invasive ventilatiory support. *Crit Care Med* 2001; 29: 519–25.

Benoit D, Depuydt P, Peleman RA, *et al.* Documented and clinically suspected bacterial infection precipitating intensive care admission in patients with haematological malignancies: impact on outcome. *Intensive Care Med* 2005; 31: 934–42.

Bow E. Of yeasts and hyphae: a hematologist's approach to antifungal therapy. *Hematology* 2006; 361–7.

Brunet F, Lanore J, Dhainaut JF, *et al.* Is intensive care justified for patients with haematological malignancies? *Intensive Care Med* 1990; 16: 291–7.

Donovitz G, Makii D, Crnich CJ, *et al.* Infections in the neutropenic patient—new view of an old problem. *Hematology* 2001; 113–39.

Hilbert G, Gruson D, Vargas F, *et al.* Noninvasive ventilation in immunosupressed patients with pulmonary infiltrates, fever and acute respiratory failure. *N Engl J Med* 2001; 344: 481–7.

Pene F, Aubron C, Azoulay E, *et al.* Outcome of critically ill allogeneic stem-cell transplant recipients: a reappraisal of indications for organ failure supports. *J Clin Oncol* 2006; 24: 643–9.

Rebulla P, Finazzi G, Marangoni F, *et al.* The threshold for prophylactic platelet transfusions in adults with acute myeloid leukaemia. *N Engl J Med* 1997; 337: 1870–5.

Wade J. Viral infections in patients with hematological malignancies. *Hematology* 2006: 368–74.

Haematological malignancies in the ICU

Patients with haematological malignancies may present to ICU due to disease-related complications or treatment issues. Over the last few decades therapeutic interventions for leukaemias and lymphomas have evolved and pose new challenges to clinicians.

Though the management of patients with haematological malignancies with acute complications is similar to any critically ill patient, it is important to discuss the following key issues before intensive care admission.

- The type of the malignancy including staging.
- Severity of the illness and immediate management.
- Is the symptom related to malignancy or a side effect of treatment?
- Further treatment options for the disease and prognosis.
- Communication with the patient and family regarding their wishes.

Complications of haematological malignancies

Neutropenia and infection

Neutropenia is one of the most common complications due to underlying disease or cytotoxic treatment. These patients are susceptible to infections with Gram-negative bacteria, staphylococci and fungi. As a consequence, patients may present with septicaemic shock and MOF.

Metabolic complications

Hyperuricaemia, hyperkalaemia, hyperphosphataemia and hypocalcaemia are consequences of tumour lysis syndrome (TLS), which is due to the release of intracellular purines, phosphates and potassium from rapidly proliferating tumour cells. TLS is commonly observed in solid tumours. This may occur spontaneously or with the initiation of chemotherapy. Other metabolic complications include hypercalcaemia and hyponatraemia.

Haemorrhagic complications

Thrombocytopenia and abnormal coagulation, including DIC secondary to disease process or treatment, may lead to severe bleeding, e.g. acute GI and cerebrovascular haemorrhages. Thrombocytopenia is a common complication with platelet count <10 000/mm^3. Haemorrhagic complications may occur due to platelet dysfunction rather than actual platelet count.

Leucostasis

A serious complication with a leucocyte count >100 000/μl. The high count may lead to capillary stasis and tissue hypoxia.

Chemotherapy-induced toxicity

Chemotherapy for leukaemias and lymphomas can be toxic and lethal, with myelosuppression, metabolic complications, immunosuppression and cardiac dysrhythmias. All chemotherapy drugs have distinct side effect profiles.

Haemopoietic cell transplantation (HCT) and GvHD

An increasing number of haematological malignancies receive HCT. Failure of allogenic HCT may result in graft rejection or GvHD, with serious consequences. GvHD results from donor-derived T cells that react with recipient tissue antigens. The clinical presentation of acute GvHD involves skin rashes, liver dysfunction and various GI symptoms. Patients are also susceptible to respiratory infections and sepsis.

Mechanical complications

SVC syndrome, as a result of impaired venous return through the SVC to the right atrium, is seen in lymphomas. Pericardial effusion and cardiac tamponade may spontaneously develop in patients with leukaemia and lymphoma. Epidural cord compression with neurological affects is a rare but serious complication seen in patients with lymphoma and myeloma.

Principles of management

- Profound neutropenia necessitates prophylaxis with antibacterial, antifungal and antiviral agents. Adjunctive measures include early intervention with G-CSF to hasten haemopoietic cell recovery. If vascular catheter-related infection is suspected the catheter should be removed. Septicaemic shock and MOF should be treated aggressively with sepsis treatment strategies. Individual units may follow their own antibiotic guidelines.
- Respiratory failure requiring tracheal intubation and mechanical ventilation have very poor outcome. Recent studies have shown that early intervention with NIV reduces the need for intubation with better ITU outcome.
- Management of TLS includes allopurinol, to inhibit xanthine oxidase and uric acid crystal formation, aggressive IV fluid hydration and alkalization of urine. Patients with metabolic derangements need monitoring and optimization of electrolyte imbalance. Patients with acute renal failure will benefit from early haemofiltration.
- Regular transfusion of blood and clotting products are indicated in patients with haemorrhagic complications. The management of patients with thrombocytopenia depends on the severity of the underlying defect, the extent of bleeding, the type of invasive procedures, and the risks associated with treatment. Platelet transfusion should be limited to severe thrombocytopenia with complication in order to avoid platelet refractoriness.
- Leucopheresis is indicated in severe leucostasis to decrease the tumour cell burden without inducing lysis.
- Chemotherapy may have to be instituted during acute critical illness to control the active disease.
- High dose methylprednisolone is the primary therapy of acute GvHD. The initial course is 2mg/kg/day for 14 days and, if the symptoms are controlled, steroid weaning should be considered. Chronic GvHD patients need long-term steroid therapy with or without immunosuppressants.
- The management of mechanical complications depends on the aetiology, the severity of symptoms and the disease prognosis. Chemotherapy is the treatment of choice for SVC syndrome. Cardiology intervention with pericardiocentesis may be indicated in acute cardiac tamponade. Therapeutic options for epidural cord compression include corticosteroids, surgery and radiation.
- Regular consultation with haematology and oncology teams to discuss appropriateness of the treatments and also prognosis..

Outcome and prognosis

Despite the recent advances in ITU management, mortality and morbidity in this group of patients are relatively high. The factors associated with poor outcome include respiratory failure requiring mechanical ventilation, MOF needing vasopressors and haemofiltration, established GvHD, persistent neutropenia and high APACHE II score. Overall mortality and outcome are likely to depend on the severity of the organ dysfunction rather than the type of the disease.

Further reading

Sekeres MA, Stone RM. Acute leukemias In: Irwin RS, Rippe JM, eds. Intensive care medicine, 5th edn. Philadelphia, PA: Lippincott Williams & Wilkins, 2003: 1295–302.

Montgomery BR, Thompson JA. Oncologic emergencies In: Irwin RS, Rippe JM, eds. Intensive care medicine, 5th edn. Philadelphia, PA: Lippincott Williams & Wilkins, 2003: 1302–13.

Negrin RS, Blume KG Allogenic and autologous hematopoietic cell transplantation. In: Beutler E, Lichtman MA, Coller BS, Kipps TJ, ed.s Williams hematology, 6th edn. New York: McGraw-Hill, 2001: 209–47.

Pawson H, Jayaweera A, Wigmore T. Intensive care management of patients following haematopoietic stem cell transplantation. *Current Anaesthesia and Critical Care* 2008; 19(2): 80–90.

Coagulation monitoring

Coagulation screen

Prothrombin Time (PT) is prolonged in deficiencies of factors II, V, X, VII.

Activated Partial Thromboplastin Time (APTT) is prolonged in deficiencies of factors II, V, X, VIII, IX, XI, XII. It is also prolonged in the presence of heparin and in patients with a lupus anticoagulant.

Thrombin Time (TT) is prolonged in hypo- and dysfibrinogenaemia, in the presence of heparin, and in the presence of fibrin degradation products. Heparin contamination can be confirmed if the prolonged thrombin time is corrected by the addition of reptilase.

The Bleeding Time has been largely superseded by the PFA-100®. This test indicates global platelet function in a high-shear environment. Interpretation of prolonged times must be made in the light of the clinical situation and other coagulation tests. The test should only be requested following liason with a haematologist.

Normal screening tests may not mean that patient has normal haemostasis in vivo (e.g. mild haemophilia A). Conversely, abnormal tests may not mean that there is a risk of clinical haemorrhage (e.g. lupus anticoagulant).

Specific factor assays (e.g. monitoring haemophilia A)

For major operations, factor levels should be maintained at 50-100% for 7-10 days. This can be achieved by an initial bolus to bring the level to 100% and then either continuous infusion or twice daily dosing (once daily for haemophilia B) with the appropriate factor concentrate. Factor assays should be performed to guide dosage.

Anaemia

Erythrocytes facilitate the interaction of platelets with the vessel wall, so increasing the haematocrit can correct an increased bleeding tendency.

Thrombocytopenia

Increased bleeding is unlikely to occur until the platelet count falls to 50 x 10^9/l, unless there is concurrent anti-platelet therapy. There is an increased risk of spontaneous life-threatening bleeding at counts below 10 x 109/ L. In the presence of sepsis, the transfusion threshold should be raised to 20 x 10^9/l.

Laboratory control of oral anticoagulants

Warfarin anticoagulation is monitored using the INR (international normalised ratio). For the majority of indications an INR of 2.0–3.0 is effective.

It is usually sufficient to stop warfarin three days prior to invasive surgery and restart the usual maintenance dose on the evening of the surgery. The three day period usually needs to be covered by heparin anticoagulation.

Laboratory control of parenteral anticoagulants (heparin, danaparoid, lepirudin, bivalirudin)

Anti-Xa

This is used primarily to monitor LMWH (low molecular weight heparin) as LMWH does not affect the APTT. It is the test of choice for monitoring UFH (unfractionated heparin) if a lupus anticoagulant is present or if the APTT appears to be resistant to heparinisation. Testing should be performed three hours after the injection.

Anticoagulant	Test for monitoring	Therapeutic window
UFH	APTT	2–3 times normal control
LMWH	Anti-Xa	Prophylactic: 0.2–0.4 IU/ml Therapeutic: 0.4–1.0 IU/ml
Danaparoid	Anti-Xa	0.5–0.8 IU/ml
Lepirudin	APTT	1.5–3 times normal control
Bivalirudin	ACT	> 350 seconds

Near patient testing devices are available.

Difficulties with heparin management

Acute phase response

Fibrinogen, von Willebrand factor and FVIII are acute phase proteins. They will be raised in inflammatory conditions. This can result in a resistance of the APTT to prolongation by therapeutic dose unfractionated heparin. In this case, monitoring of anticoagulation by anti-Xa levels is appropriate.

Antithrombin deficiency

In antithrombin deficiency states (e.g. severe sepsis), true heparin resistance may occur and adequate anticoagulation may require replacement with antithrombin concentrate or fresh frozen plasma in addition to heparin. Note that some anti-Xa assays are sensitive to the amount of antithrombin in patient plasma. Haematological advice will be necessary.

Near-patient testing

ACT

Whole blood clotting time is used for monitoring high doses of heparin (e.g. when on cardiopulmonary bypass). It is likely to be inaccurate if the patient has an inhibitor (e.g. lupus anticoagulant). ACT needs to be interpretated with caution in the presence of aprotinin and in critically ill patients

PT and APTT devices

These are designed to test patients on anticoagulants (e.g. Coaguchek®).

Thromboelastography

This is seen as a global test of coagulation as it uses whole blood rather than plasma. The thromboelastogram® works on the principle that the physical properties of a blood clot indicate whether under, over, or normal activity of the haemostatic system is present. Clot formation is recorded graphically. Parameters of the trace indicate activity of platelets, coagulation factors, and fibrinolysis and so can aid appropriate product transfusion. It is used primarily in liver and cardiac surgery.

The time to commencement of fibrin formation is measured as the r-time. An increased r-time has been used as an indication for FFP infusion. A decrease in the maximal clot strength (MA) is used to guide platelet transfusion. A reduction in the α-angle suggests the need for cryoprecipitate. The additional use of heparinase in the system may guide protamine dosage.

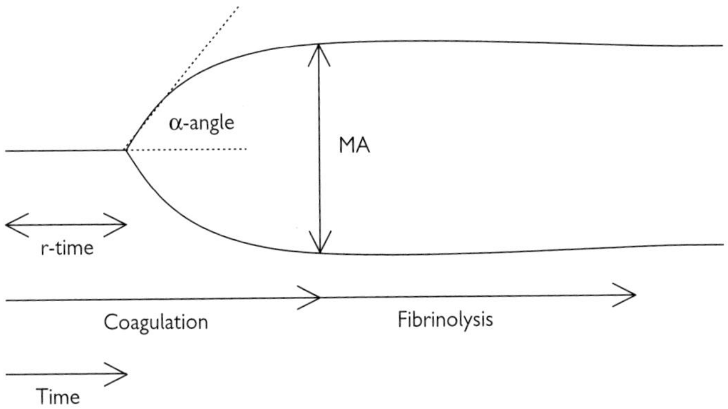

Fig. 23.8.1 Thromboelastogram® trace. The r-time (normal range 4–8minutes), α-angle (normal range 47–74°), and MA (maximal amplitude, normal range 55–73mm) are shown.

References

Anderson JA, Saenko EL. Heparin resistance. *Br J Anaesth* 2002; 88(4):467-9.

Baglin T, Barrowcliffe TW, Cohen A, Greaves M. Guidelines on the use and monitoring of heparin. *Br J Haematol* 2006;133(1): 19-34.

Chee Y, Crawford, JC, Watson HG, Greaves M. Guideline on the assessment of bleeding risk prior to surgery or invasive procedures. BCSH; 2007. www.bcshguidelines.com/pdf/Coagscreen200107.pdf

Hayward CP, Harrison P, Cattaneo M, Ortel TL, Rao AK. Platelet function analyzer (PFA)-100 closure time in the evaluation of platelet disorders and platelet function. *J Thromb Haemost* 2006;4(2): 312-9.

Rochon AG, Shore-Lesserson L. Coagulation monitoring. *Anesthesiol Clin* 2006;24(4):839-56.

Luddington RJ. Thrombelastography/ thromboelastometry. *Clin Lab Haem* 2005;27:81-90.

Chapter 24

Metabolic disorders

Chapter contents

Electrolyte disorders

The physiology, aetiology, clinical features and management of potassium, magnesium, calcium and phosphate disorders in the critically ill.

Potassium

98% of total body potassium (K^+) is intracellular, with only 2% located in the extracellular fluid. The potassium ratio between intracellular and extracellular fluid is the major determinant of resting membrane potential. Potassium concentration in plasma is maintained within tight limits, between 3.5 and 5.0mmol/l.

Potassium is mostly absorbed by diffusion from the GI tract. It is excreted by the kidney. A smaller amount (10%) is excreted through the GI tract. Control of extracellular potassium is achieved by:

- Insulin—drives K^+ into cells via Na/K ATPase
- β_2-Adrenoceptor agonists—drive K^+ into cells
- Acid–base status—exchange of H^+ for K^+
- Osmolality—increase causes K^+ to be dragged extracellularly
- Mineralocorticoids – drive K^+ into cells

Hypokalaemia

Hypokalaemia is defined as a serum potassium concentration <3.5mmol/l, and is severe if <2.5mmol/l.

Causes

- Inadequate K^+ intake: if <1g/day
- Intracellular shift of K^+: metabolic alkalosis, β_2 agonists, insulin, theophyllines
- Increased K^+ loss: drugs (loop/thiazide diuretics, corticosteroids, aminoglycosides, amphotericin B), hypomagnesaemia, RRT, GI losses (diarrhoea, fistulae, NG suctioning), hyperaldosteronism.

Clinical features

Mild hypokalaemia is often asymptomatic. Hypokalaemia <2.5mmol/l patients can develop generalized weakness, nausea, vomiting and constipation. Some patients can develop an ascending paralysis. Rhabdomyolysis can also occur. Cardiac arrhythmias are the most worrying effect of hypokalaemia, and are more common in patients with underlying heart disease and those on digoxin. ECG changes seen in hypokalaemia can vary, with U waves, ST depression, T wave flattening or inversion all seen.

Management

Potassium replacement is the mainstay of treatment. As a guide, a 0.3mmol/l fall in serum potassium corresponds to a 100mmol total body deficit. This is unreliable when hypokalaemia has been caused by intracellular shift of K^+.

Potassium chloride can be administered orally or through a nasoenteric tube in divided doses up to 100mmol/day. Potassium phosphate and potassium bicarbonate are alternatives in the presence of hypophosphataemia and acidaemia, respectively. Oral potassium supplementation has an unpleasant taste, and may cause GI erosion.

IV potassium supplementation will rapidly correct hypokalaemia. When administering potassium through a peripheral vein, the concentration should not exceed 80mmol/l, as it may cause pain and thrombophlebitis. Adminstration through a central venous line allows higher concentrations to be used. The rate of infusion of potassium **should not exceed 20mmol/h,** although rates as high as 60mmol/h have been used in emergency situations. Rapid infusion is dangerous as it can lead to VF.

In patients with renal impairment, the dose should be halved, and serum levels checked to assess response to therapy. Potassium should not be diluted in dextrose as it can increase intracellular potassium shift by stimulating insulin release.

Potassium-sparing diuretics can be used in the prevention of hypokalaemia, but are of limited use in the acute setting.

If hypomagnesaemia co-exists with hypokalaemia, it should be corrected as it can cause refractory hypokalaemia.

Hyperkalaemia

Hyperkalaemia is defined as a serum potassium level >5.0mmol/l, and may be life threatening if >6.5mmol/l.

Causes

- Increased K^+ intake: iatrogenic
- Extracellular shift: acidaemia, hyperosmolality, β_2-adrenoceptor antagonists, insulin deficiency, succinylcholine, digoxin overdose, rhabdomyolysis.
- Decreased renal excretion
  - renal failure
  - mineralocorticoid deficiency (Addisons disease, isolated aldosterone deficiency, renin deficiency, drugs, e.g ARBs, ACE inhibitors, NSAIDs)
  - mineralocorticoid resistance (spironolactone, trimethoprim, tubulointerstitial disease)
- Pseudohyperkalaemia: release of intracellular K^+ during phlebotomy or storage of blood, haemolysis, thrombocytosis, leucocytosis.

Clinical features

Hyperkalaemia is often asymptomatic at levels <6.5mmol/l, and may first be detected on routine blood sampling. The symptoms are related to muscle and cardiac disturbances. Generalized weakness, muscle twitching, cramping and ascending paralysis can occur. Arrhythmias occur, which can include bradycardias, VF and asystole. ECG changes include peaked T waves, PR interval prolongation, QRS complex widening, QT interval shortening, leading eventually to the sine wave which precedes VF.

Management

The management of hyperkalaemia is dependent on the presence of symptoms and on the presence of ECG changes.

In asymptomatic patients with no ECG changes, the initial management is to stop exogenous sources of potassium and all drug therapies which may increase potassium. Serum potassium should be rechecked.

In a symptomatic patient, or those with ECG changes, therapies can act in several ways.

- Membrane stabilization
- Increase intracellular shift of K^+
- Increase K^+elimination
- GI binding of K^+

Potassium levels should be monitored at least every 6h in patients with hyperkalaemia.

Treatment	Dose	Mechanism of action
Calcium gluconate	10% 10ml over 5–10min	Membrane stabilization
Insulin	10U in 50ml 50% dextrose	Intracellular shift
Sodium bicarbonate	50–100mmol	Intracellular shift
Salbutamol	5mg nebulized	Intracellular shift
Furosemide	20–250mg IV	Increased elimination
Haemodialysis		Increased elimination
Sodium polystyrene sulfonate	30g oral or rectal, then 15mg 3x day	GI binding

Magnesium

The majority (99%) of magnesium is found intracellularly in bone, muscle and soft tissue. Normal serum levels are 0.7–1.05mmol/l. It acts as a physiological antagonist to calcium and is a cofactor in all ATP reactions and numerous other enzyme reactions.

Absorption of magnesium is through the small intestine. It is reabsorbed by the kidney, so that only 1% of filtered magnesium is excreted in the urine. Parathyroid hormone increases GI absorption and reduces renal excretion, whereas renal excretion is increased by aldosterone.

Magnesium is used therapeutically in acute severe asthma, torsades de pointes, digoxin toxicity, atrial and ventricular arrhythmias, pre-eclampsia and eclampsia. Its use following AMI is debatable.

Hypomagnesaemia

Hypomagnesaemia is defined as a serum Mg^{2+} <0.7mmol/l, although serum levels do not correlate well with intracellular levels. It may occur in up to 65% of critically ill patients, and has been associated with an increased mortality.

Causes

- Inadequate intake: malnutrition, alcoholism
- Excess GI losses: NG tube, small intestine disease, malabsorption, diarrhoea
- Renal loss: aminoglycosides, amphotericin, dopamine, diuretics
- Chelation: citrate in blood transfusion
- Redistribution: refeeding syndrome, catecholamines.

Clinical features

Cardiovascular features of hypomagnesaemia include hypertension, angina and arrhythmias (typically torsades de pointes). The neuromuscular signs are of stridor, dysphagia, myoclonus and tetanus. Seizures and coma can also be seen. Hypomagnesaemia is associated with hypokalaemia, and hypocalcaemia

Management

Oral or IV supplementation; oral magnesium is poorly tolerated—GI upset. IV doses of 8–64mmol can be used, at a maximum infusion rate of 8mmol/h in asymptomatic patients. In severe symptomatic hypomagnesaemia, 8mmol can be given over 5min. Smaller doses may be necessary in renal failure.

Hypermagnesaemia

Hypermagnesaemia is a plasma concentration >1.05mmol/l. It is usually iatrogenic.

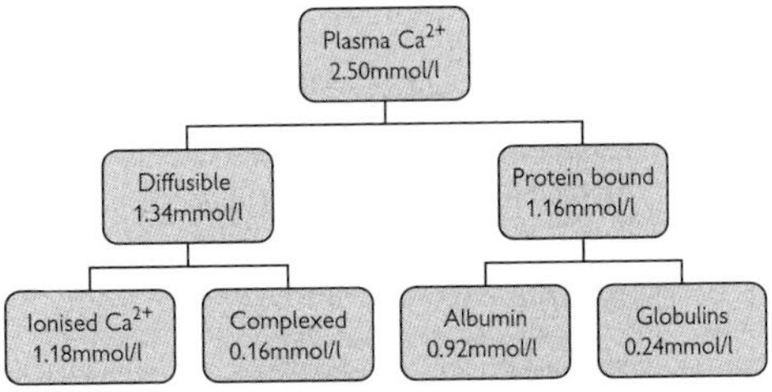

Causes

- Iatrogenic
- End-stage renal disease.

Clinical features

Usually well tolerated, but it can cause nausea and vomiting. Deep tendon reflexes are lost, and at higher levels respiratory paralysis can occur. Cardiovascular symptoms are of hypotension, bradycardia and increased PR interval and/or QRS duration on the ECG.

Management

Stop magnesium administration. If necessary, systemic effects can be antagonized in severe cases by IV calcium (e.g. calcium chloride 0.5–1mg over 5–10min). Its excretion can be increased by fluid administration, loop diuretics or haemodialysis.

Calcium

Calcium is integral to excitation–contraction coupling in myocardial, smooth and skeletal muscle. It is also essential in bone metabolism, cardiac automaticity, coagulation, hormone secretion and nerve conduction.

99% of the body's calcium is skeletal, <1% is in the plasma. Total plasma calcium level is 2.5mmol/l, and 40–50% is bound to plasma proteins. Calcium binding to plasma proteins is reduced by metabolic acidosis.

Calcium is absorbed from the GI tract in a process regulated by 1,25-dihydroxycholecalciferol. Parathyroid hormone and 1,25-dihydroxycholecalciferol promote Ca^{2+} release from bone stores. It is excreted in the kidneys, where it is filtered then 99% reabsorbed.

Hypocalcaemia

Falsely low plasma calcium levels can occur in the presence of hypoalbuminaemia, therefore ionized Ca^{2+} or corrected serum Ca^{2+}should be used. Hypocalcaemia is defined as a serum calcium <2.0mmol/l or an ionized Ca^{2+} <1.1mmol/l.

$$\text{Corrected } Ca^{2+}(\text{mmol/l}) = \text{measured} \times [40 - \text{albumin(g/l)}] \times 0.02$$

Causes

- Septic shock
- Renal insufficiency
- Hypomagnesaemia, hyperphosphataemia
- Malignancy
- Pancreatitis
- Rhabdomyolysis
- Hypoparathyroidism
- Pseudohypoparathyroidism
- Post-parathyroidectomy
- Vitamin D deficiency

Clinical features

Neuromuscular features predominate, with paraesthesia, muscle cramps, tetany, laryngospasm and seizures. Cardiovascular features include hypotension, bradycardia and prolongation of the QT interval.

Management

Chronic hypocalcaemia is treated with oral calcium supplementation. In severe hypocalcaemia or symptomatic patients, rapid correction is indicated. This is achieved using IV calcium gluconate 10% 10ml (94mg Ca^{2+}) or calcium chloride 10% 10ml (272mg Ca^{2+}) over 10min. It should be remembered that calcium salts are irritant to veins, so should ideally be given through central venous access. Calcium salts can precipitate if infused with sodium bicarbonate. Calcium administration to patients on digoxin may cause toxicity, so extra monitoring is needed.

Other considerations are to check and correct hypomagnesaemia, and to correct hypocalcaemia prior to correcting acidosis. Hyperphosphataemia may occur with hypocalcaemia, and administration of calcium can lead to precipitation of calcium phosphate in tissues. Therefore, if hyperphosphataemia is present, a phosphate binder should be given.

Hypercalcaemia

Hypercalcaemia is defined as a total serum calcium concentration >2.55mmol/l.

Causes

- Primary hyperparathyroidism
- Malignancy
- Drugs: thiazide diuretics, lithium, vitamin D toxicity, theophylline
- Hyperthyroidism
- Immobilization
- Rhabdomyolysis
- Granulomatous disease: tuberculosis, sarcoidosis
- Familial hypercalcaemia
- Phaeochromocytoma.

Clinical features

The symptoms of hypercalcaemia usually correlate with the speed and severity of calcium rise. Mild hypercalaemia is usually asymptomatic. At higher Ca^{2+} levels neurological symptoms occur: depression, weakness, lethargy, even coma. GI effects of nausea, vomiting and anorexia can be seen. The cardiovascular effects are hypertension and arrhythmias. Nephrogenic diabetes insipidus may cause hypovolaemia. Nephrolithiasis, metastatic calcification and renal failure may be seen with chronic hypercalcaemia.

Management

Mild-moderate hypercalcaemia (Ca^{2+} 2.58–3.23mmol/l)

- Hydration
- Mobilization
- Stop medications which may cause hypercalcaemia
- Surgery if due to primary hyperparathyroidism.

Severe hypercalcaemia (Ca^{2+} >3.24mmol/l)

- Volume repletion: IV 0.9% sodium chloride 200–300ml/h
- Enhance renal excretion:
  - furosemide 40–100mg 1–4 hourly
  - haemodialysis
- Reduce bone resorption: bisphosphonates will reduce Ca^{2+} levels over days
  - Etidronate 7.5mg/kg/day over 4h for 3–7 days
  - Pamidronate 60–90mg over 4h
- Treat underlying disease: parathyroidectomy in hyperparathyroidism
- Other treatments: glucocorticoids, plicamycin, calcitonin and gallium nitrate have been used.

Phosphorus

Phosphorus is found predominantly (85–90%) in the skeleton. It is a vital constituent of ATP, cAMP and 2,3-diphosphoglycerate. In serum, phosphorus is mostly present as phosphate, and normal levels are 0.8–1.4mmol/l. GI absorption of phosphorus is increased by 1,25-dihydroxycholecalciferol. Phosphorus is filtered through glomeruli, and 85–90% reabsorbed in the proximal tubule. This process is inhibited by parathyroid hormone.

Hypophosphataemia

Hypophosphataemia is defined as a serum phosphate <0.75mmol/l, severe if <0.4mmol/l. It is worse in the presence of hypomagnesaemia.

Causes

Redistribution

- Refeeding following malnutrition
- Respiratory alkalosis
- Sepsis
- Drugs: insulin, epinephrine, glucose

Reduced GI absorption

- Malabsorption
- Vitamin D deficiency
- Diarrhoea

Urinary excretion

- Hyperparathyroidism
- Renal tubular disorders
- Renal transplantation
- Metabolic or respiratory acidosis

Clinical features

Hypophosphataemia can cause a wide range of symptoms. Cardiac contractility is reduced and cardiomyopathy can occur. Respiratory function is impaired through a reduction in diaphragmatic contractility. Haemolysis and thrombocytopaenia also occur. CNS effects range from paraesthesia to seizures and coma. There may be paralysis and weakness of skeletal muscle. Tissue hypoxaemia is mediated by reduced 2,3-DPG causing increased haemoglobin affinity for oxygen.

Management

Serum phosphate concentrations should be kept within normal limits. Oral phosphate supplementation can be achieved with sodium or potassium phosphate. They may cause diarrhoea and may not be absorbed. IV phosphate supplementation can be used in symptomatic patients and those with severe hypophosphataemia. Potassium or sodium phosphate can be used, diluted in 0.9% sodium chloride and infused over 6h to reduce the incidence of thrombophlebitis and severe hypocalcaemia. Patients with renal failure should receive 50% of the usual dose, although those on continuous RRT may have higher phosphate requirements.

Hyperphosphataemia

Serum phosphate levels >1.45mmol/l define hyperphosphataemia.

Causes

Factitious

- Haemolysis

Increased intake

- Iatrogenic: excess phosphate administration

Increased release from cells

- Respiratory or metabolic acidosis
- Rhabdomyolysis
- Tumour lysis syndrome
- Bowel infarction

Reduced excretion

- Renal insufficiency
- Hypoparathyroidism

Clinical features

A rapid increase in serum phosphate levels causes hypocalcaemia and tetany. A serum calcium x serum phosphorus >4.6mmol^2/l^2 is associated with increased risk of tissue deposition of calcium phosphate.

Management

The optimum management of hyperphosphataemia is to treat the underlying cause. Oral phosphate binders can reduce GI absorption.

Further reading

Bushinsky DA, Monk R Electrolyte quintet: calcium. *Lancet* 1998; 352: 306–11.

Halperin ML, Kamel KS. Electrolyte quintet: potassium. *Lancet* 1998; 352: 135–40.

Kraft MD, Btaiche IF, Sacks G, *et al*. Treatment of electrolyte disorders in adult patients in the intensive care unit. *Am J Health Syst Pharm* 2005; 62: 1663–82.

Rastergar A, Soleimani M. Hypokalaemia and hyperkalaemia. *Postgrad Med J* 2001; 77: 759–64.

Weisinger JR, Bellorin-Font E. Electrolyte quintet: magnesium and phosphorus, *Lancet* 1998; 352: 391–6.

Hyponatraemia

Hyponatraemia is defined as a serum sodium <135mmol/l. Since most critically ill patients in the ICU have an impaired capacity of renal water excretion, hyponatraemia is almost always caused by an excess of total body water. Hyponatraemia due to an excess of total body water will not normalize with supplementation of saline. Hyponatraemia needs to be corrected quickly in the presence of neurological symptoms (convulsions or coma), which is often the case when hyponatraemia has developed rapidly. Correct rapidly if onset rapid, correct slowly if onset slow. If correction of hyponatraemia is too rapid or too much it may precipitate the development of central pontine demyelination with permanent neurological damage.

Clinical features

Clinical features are secondary to intracellular cerebral oedema and increased ICP, are variable in presentation and depend strongly on the speed of serum sodium decrease. In sedated, mechanically ventilated intensive care patients, clinical features may be undetectable on clinical examination.

- Serum sodium <120mmol/l (acutely): headache, agitation, nausea, vomiting, and lethargy
- Serum sodium <120mmol/l (chronic): clinical features may be totally absent
- Serum sodium <110mmol/l: convulsions, coma

Differential diagnosis

1. Decreased circulating volume (GI or renal loss, burn wounds, heart failure, liver cirrhosis)
2. Syndrome of inappropriate ADH secretion (SIADH) (post-operative, pulmonary diseases, neuropsychiatric, intoxication, malignancy)
3. Adrenal insufficiency
4. Diuretic use (mainly thiazide)
5. Cerebral salt wasting (mainly in the case of SAH)
6. Renal failure
7. Excessive water intake
8. Salt-losing nephritis
9. Transurethral resection of prostate (TURP) syndrome
10. Hypothyroidism

Laboratory analysis

Plasma osmolality, urine osmolality and urine sodium.

When indicated: potassium, creatinine, urea, glucose, urine-acid, TSH, FT4.

Diagnosis

Plasma osmolality is always decreased (<280mOsm/kg) and therefore urine osmolality should be low. A very low urine osmolality is invariably present in hyponatraemia due to excessive water intake and TURP syndrome. Any urine osmolality >100mOsm/kg is abnormal in this situation. In combination with a low urine sodium (<25mmol/l) it is indicative of decreased circulating volume. A normal or increased urine sodium (>40mmol/l) suggests SIADH, adrenal insufficiency, diuretic use, renal failure, cerebral salt wasting, salt-losing nephritis or hypothyroidism.

Therapy

The pace of correction is determined by the presence of clinical manifestations and their severity. Treat a specific cause. Supportive therapy should be provided if necessary. Patients with symptomatic hyponatraemia due to decreased circulating volume, adrenal insufficiency or diuretic use require saline infusion.

Urine osmolality (mOsm/kg)	Urine sodium (mmol/l)	Cause
<100	<25	Excessive water intake, TURP syndrome
>100	<25	Decreased circulating volume
>100	>40	SIADH, adrenal insufficiency, diuretic use, renal failure, cerebral salt wasting, salt-losing nephritis, hypothyroidism

Infusate	Infusate Na^+ (mmol/l)
5% sodium chloride in water	855
3% sodium chloride in water	513
0.9% sodium chloride in water	154

In the case of SIADH, congestive heart failure and excessive water intake, the patient requires water restriction and close observation. Severe symptoms call for infusion of hypertonic saline, if necessary in combination with furosemide. Isotonic saline is not helpful in this condition.

In general, a serum sodium >120mmol/l is asymptomatic, rapid correction is unnecessary and should not exceed 0.5mmol/l/h. In case of symptomatic hyponatraemia with serious neurological manifestations, rapid correction at a rate of 1–2mmol/l/h is indicated until cessation of life-threatening manifestations or the achievement of a serum sodium concentration of 120mmol/l, and no faster than 0.5mmol/l/h once this value is achieved. The targeted rate of correction should not exceed 10mmol/l on any day of treatment.

The rate of infusion of saline solutions can be derived by applying the formula:

$$\text{Change in serum Na}^+ = \frac{\text{infusate Na}^+ - \text{serum Na}^+}{\text{total body water} + 1}$$

which estimates the effect of 1l of infusate on serum sodium. Dividing the change in serum sodium targeted for a given treatment period by the result of the formula determines the volume of infusate required and the rate of infusion. The sodium concentrations of commonly used infusates are presented above. The estimated total body water (in litres) is calculated as a fraction of body weight, 0.6 and 0.5 in non-elderly men and women, respectively; and 0.5 and 0.45 in elderly (age >65ys) men and women, respectively.

Further reading

Adrogué HJ, Madias NE. Hyponatremia. *N Engl J Med* 2000; 342: 1581–9.

Rose BD. Clinical physiology of acid–base and electrolyte disorders. 4th edn. New York: McGraw-Hill, 1994.

Hypernatraemia

Hypernatraemia is defined as a serum sodium >145mmol/l. It is always associated with hypertonic hyperosmolality, which causes cellular dehydration. Hypernatraemia is caused by net water loss or excessive sodium gain. The latter usually develops as a iatrogenic condition due to administration of sodium bicarbonate or chloride. Normally the thirst response corrects water depletion, but critically ill patients in the ICU are often sedated and intubated and therefore unable to obtain water. Although infrequent in a general hospital population, hypernatraemia occurs frequently in the ICU mainly due to pure water deficit.

Clinical features

Hypernatraemia usually produces symptoms if the serum sodium exceeds 155–160mmol/l and mainly when the increase in the serum sodium concentration is large or occurs rapidly. Clinical features include pyrexia, restlessness, irritability, drowsiness, lethargy, confusion and coma. Convulsions are uncommon, except in cases of inadvertent sodium loading or aggressive rehydration. Brain shrinkage induced by hypernatraemia can cause vascular rupture, with cerebral bleeding or SAH. The diminished extracellular fluid may reduce cardiac output, thereby reducing renal perfusion, leading to pre-renal failure.

Differential diagnosis

1 Net water loss
  a Pure water
    - insensible losses (respiratory or dermal)
    - hypodipsia
    - neurogenic diabetes insipidus (post-traumatic, caused by tumours, cysts or TB, idiopathic, caused by aneurysms, meningitis, encephalitis or GBS)
    - nephrogenic diabetes insipidus (congenital, hypercalcaemia, hypokalaemia, drugs mainly lithium, foscarnet, amphotericin B, renal diseases such as pyelonephritis, medullary sponge kidney or polycystic kidney)
  b Hypotonic fluid
    - renal causes (loop diuretics, osmotic diuresis driven by urea, mannitol or glucose, post-obstructive diuresis, polyuric phase of acute tubular necrosis, intrinsic renal disease)
    - GI causes (diarrhoea, vomiting, lactulose use, enterocutaneous fistulas, NG drainage)
    - cutaneous causes (excessive sweating, burns)

2 Hypertonic sodium gain
  a Hypertonic sodium chloride infusion
  b Hypertonic sodium bicarbonate infusion
  c Hypertonic feeding preparation or ingestion
  d Primary hyperaldosteronism
  e Cushing's syndrome

Laboratory analysis

Urine osmolality.

When indicated: plasma osmolality, urine sodium, potassium, urea, glucose, creatinine, bicarbonate, and blood gas analysis.

Diagnosis

The patient history and medication/infusions will often give clues to the probable cause of hypernatraemia. Physical examination for signs of dehydration (mucous membranes, skin turgor), blood pressure, CVP if available, orthostatic changes and heart rate will give an indication of the extracellular fluid volume of the patient. Together with urine osmolality, sufficient information for a diagnosis is available in most cases. Urine osmolality should be maximal (i.e. 800–1000mOsm/kg) when hypernatraemia is present due to pure water deficit or sodium gain. In the case of large urine volume and urine osmolality <300mOsm/kg, diabetes insipidus is diagnosed.

Urine osmolality (mOsm/kg)	Cause
<300	Diabetes insipidus
>300 to <800	Osmotic loss
>800	Pure water deficit or sodium gain

Therapy

Therapy must focus on the underlying cause and on correcting the hypertonicity. Supportive therapy should be provided if necessary. Treat a specific cause. Isotonic saline is unsuitable for correcting hypernatraemia—the sole indication is hypotension, in which case normotension is achieved by supplementation of 0.9% sodium chloride IV. Thereafter only hypotonic fluids should be administered. For pure water depletion, the treatment is administration of water, orally if possible. If IV fluid is required, 5% dextrose or hypotonic saline solutions are administered guided by urine output and plasma sodium. Since rapid rehydration may give rise to cerebral oedema, the fall in serum sodium should be no greater than 2mmol/l/h, with a maximum correction of 10 mmol/l/day. Initially check serum sodium concentration every 2–4h until <150mmol/l.

In the case of diabetes insipidus, desmopressin may be necessary while awaiting the effect of treatment of the underlying cause.

After selecting the appropriate infusate, the rate of infusion can be derived by applying the formula:

$$\text{change in serum Na}^+ = \frac{\text{infusate Na}^+ - \text{serum Na}^+}{\text{total body water} + 1}$$

which estimates the change in the serum sodium concentration caused by the retention of 1l of any infusate. Dividing the change in serum sodium concentration targeted for a given treatment period by the result of the formula determines the volume of infusate required and the rate of infusion. The sodium concentrations of commonly used infusates are presented below. The estimated total body water (in litres) is calculated as a fraction of body weight, 0.6 and 0.5 in non-elderly men and women, respectively; and 0.5 and 0.45 in elderly (age >65yrs) men and women, respectively.

Infusate	Infusate Na^+ (mmol/l)
5% dextrose in water	0
0.2% sodium chloride in 5% dextrose in water	34
0.45% sodium chloride in water	77
Ringer's lactate solution	130
0.9% sodium chloride in water	154

Further reading

Adrogué HJ, Madia NE. Hypernatremia. *N Engl J Med* 2000; 342: 1493–99.

Rose BD. Clinical physiology of acid–base and electrolyte disorders. 4th edn. New York: McGraw-Hill, 1994.

Categorizing metabolic acidoses

The human body produces acid quite readily, and employs a number of mechanisms designed to maintain normal arterial pH between 7.35 and 7.45 (e.g. respiratory compensation for volatile acid (CO_2) production, renal excretion to compensate for fixed acid production). Any pathology which compromises these compensatory mechanisms will produce an acidosis. Disorders of CO_2 are characterized as respiratory acidoses/alkaloses, while disorders of all other factors are characterized as metabolic acidoses/alkaloses, which includes disorders of weak and strong acids and bases.

Metabolic acidoses occur when the serum pH falls below 7.35, and typically are categorized as either pure vs mixed (dependent on whether there is one or multiple processes producing acidaemia), or anion gap (AG) vs non-AG acidoses (dependent on the presence or absence of unmeasured anions in the blood). AG acidoses produce changes in the AG, where AG = $\{[Na^+] + [K^+] - [Cl^-] - [HCO_3^-]\}$. Typically, the AG = 8–12mEq/l, and represents the relative 'gap' between unmeasured cations (generally magnesium, and calcium) and unmeasured anions (generally plasma proteins, phosphate, sulfate, lactate and organic anions). An abnormal AG indicates the presence of unmeasured, pathophysiological anions such as lactate, ketones, sulfate, etc. A high AG can indicate a metabolic acidosis due to an accumulation of organic acids or toxins (e.g. salicylate) The AG is insensitive, and can vary in critically ill patients based on changes in albumin concentration or unmeasured cations, the addition of abnormal cations (e.g. lithium, immunoglobulins), hyperviscosity and hyperlipidaemia. Additionally, the 'normal' AG range may vary from patient to patient. A corrected anion gap (AGc) is more sensitive for estimating unknown anions and is given by the equation:

$$AGc = \{[Na^+] + [K^+] - [Cl^-] - [HCO_3^-]\} - \{2[\text{albumin (g/dl)}] + 0.5[PO_4^{2-}\text{(mg/dl)}] + [\text{lactate}]\}$$

Or for international units:

$$AGc = \{[Na+] + [K^+] - [Cl^-] - [HCO_3^-]\} - \{0.2[\text{albumin (g/l)}] + 1.5[PO_4^{2-}\text{(mmol/dl)}] + [\text{lactate}]\}$$

AG acidoses refer to acidemias that increase the AG, and include acidoses induced by:

- Methanol
- Uraemia
- Diabetic ketoacidosis
- Paraldehyde, phenformin
- Isopropyl alcohol, isoniazid
- Lactic acidosis (patients should also be evaluated for shock)
- Ethylene glycol, ethyl alcohol
- Salicylates
- Hyperalbuminaemia, administered anions

Non-AG/normal AG acidoses are essentially abnormalities in chloride regulation (hyperchloraemic acidoses), and include acidoses due to:

- Diarrhoea
- Renal tubular acidosis (proximal or distal)
- Carbonic anhydrase inhibitors
  - Acetazolamide
  - Mefenamic acid
- Ureteral diversion,
  - Ureterosigmoidostomy,
  - Ileal bladder or ureter
- Post-hypercapnia
- Renal failure
- Acidifying agents
  - Ammonium chloride
  - Calcium chloride
  - Arginine
- Sulfur toxicity
- For explanations of the mechanism of these acidoses, see Chapter 24.5. In addition to the AG, standard base excess (SBE) is commonly employed to quantify the metabolic component of a given acid-base disorder.

Standard base excess

The SBE is calculated by SBE = HCO_3 – 24.4) + (8.0Alb + 0.30Phos) x (pH 7.4); the typical reference range is –2.0 to +2.0mEq/l, with SBE less than –2.0mEq/l indicating metabolic acidosis and SBE >2.0mEq/l indicating metabolic alkalosis. The offset of the calculated SBE from zero indicates approximately how much compensation is needed to restore homeostasis. Recent research and clarification have shown that the change in SBE equals the change in strong ion difference (SID).

Strong ion difference (SID) and strong ion gap (SIG)

The SID can be calculated by the difference between the sum of strong cations and sum of strong anion concentrations—the apparent SID (SIDa). The effective SID can be calculated by the difference between the sum of the concentrations of weak acids $[A^-]$ and the bicarbonate concentration $[HCO_3^-]$ (SIDe). The strong ion gap (SIG) is a quantitative methodology for determining unmeasured ions based on the difference between SIDa – SIDe = SIG.

Normally, SIDa = SIDe and SIG=0; if SIDa ≠ SIDe, unmeasured ions must be present (anions if SIDa > SIDe, cations if SIDe > SIDa). The SIG does not change in relation to pH alterations or albumin concentration. The AGc approximates SIG.

Epidemiology

Because metabolic acidoses typically occur as the result of other pathophysiology, the incidence and prevalence of the disorders are difficult to characterize. However, metabolic acidosis is quite common in the critically ill and injured.

Causes

Acid–base disturbances are caused by pCO_2, the total weak acid (A_{tot}) and/or the SID present.

According to physical chemical principles:

- In plasma only three independent variables determine hydrogen ion concentration (pH):
  1. strong ion difference (SID)
  2. partial pressure of carbon dioxide (pCO_2)
  3. total weak acid concentration (A_{tot})
- All buffering mechanisms, such as respiratory compensatory mechanisms, blood buffers and ion excretion through the kidneys regulate pH only by modulating the above three independent variables.

- The kidneys primarily modulate the SID by regulating the excretion of chloride (Cl^-) ions. Each Cl^--ion that is filtered but not reabsorbed increases the SID, which subsequently increases the pH.
- Renal ammoniagenesis occurs to allow the co-excretion of Cl^- without Na^+ or K^+ excretion. This is achieved by supplying a weak cation (NH_4^+) to excrete with Cl^-, thereby decreasing the SID.

Risk factors

- Fluid loading with saline (greater Cl^- increase relative to sodium produces hyperchloraemic acidosis)
- Bicarbonate loss (diarrhoea)

Clinical features

Pure metabolic acidoses are diagnosed by the presence of acidaemia (arterial pH <7.35), hypobicarbonataemia (HCO_3^- <22mmol/l), hypocarbia (PCO_2 <40mm Hg) and a reduced SBE (less than –3mEq/l). Mixed metabolic acidoses or a mixed acidosis/alkalosis may produce the appearance of balanced acid–base status. Electrolyte levels can offer clues to acid–base status, but require confirmation by ABG measurements.

Treatment/management

Metabolic acidoses frequently occur as sequelae of other pathologies; the best means of treatment for metabolic acidosis is to treat the underlying cause. General guidelines:

- Many metabolic acidoses are acute, self-limiting and do not require specific therapies (e.g. lactic acidosis due to exercise or seizures will resolve with rest). Acute metabolic acidoses can also resolve via respiratory compensation (reduction of pCO_2). Treatment of acute acidosis with $NaHCO_3$ is not recommended, is of dubious benefit and may be harmful in some patients.
- Acidoses due to toxin ingestion require separate interventions (e.g. methanol ingestion requires therapeutic intervention for both the methanol and the subsequent acidosis).
- Chronic acidoses (e.g. those due to renal injuries or chronic mineralocorticoid disorders) require therapy to restore the SID (e.g. oral $NaHCO_3$).
- Distal renal tubular acidosis is associated more frequently with severe acidosis and hypokalaemia than is proximal renal tubular acidosis. Non-HCO_3 buffers *may* be effective in severe metabolic acidosis.
- In severe metabolic acidosis, continuous RRT may be needed. Additionally, limited data suggest that non-bicarbonate buffers may be effective.
- In acidosis complicated by hypokalaemia, K^+ must be corrected *before* the pH is corrected (serum [K^+] will fall precipitously if pH is corrected first).

Complications

Potential clinical sequelae of metabolic acidoses include:

Cardiovascular changes

- Decreased inotropy
- Conduction defects
- Arterial vasodilation
- Venous vasoconstriction

Electrolyte imbalances

- Hyperkalaemia
- Hypercalcaemia
- Hyperuricaemia

Gastrointestinal effects

- Emesis

Immunological changes

- Changes in inflammatory mediators

Metabolic changes

- Protein wasting
- Bone demineralization
- Catecholamine, parathryroid hormone and aldosterone stimulation
- Insulin resistance

Neuromuscular changes

- Respiratory depression
- Decreased awareness

Decreased oxygenation

- Decreased oxy-Hb binding
- Decreased 2,3-DPG (late)

Further reading

Androgue H, Madias N. Management of life-threatening acid–base disorders. First of two parts. *N Engl J Med* 1998; 338: 26–34.

Androgue H, Madias N. Management of life-threatening acid-base disorders. Second of two parts. *N Engl J Med* 1998; 338: 107–11.

Kellum J. Closing the gap on unmeasured anions. *Critical Care*. 2003; 7: 219–20.

Kellum J. Determinants of blood pH in health and disease. *Critical Care*. 2000; 4: 6–14.

Kellum J, Song M, Li J. Science review: extracellular acidosis and the immune response: clinical and physiological implications. *Crit Care* 2004; 8: 331–6.

Schlichtig R, Grogono AW, Severinghaus JW. Human $PaCO_2$ and standard base excess compensation for acid-base imbalance. *Crit Care Med* 1998; 26: 1173–9.

Wooten EW. Science review: quantitative acid–base physiology using the Stewart model. *Crit Care* 2004; 8: 448–52.

Metabolic acidosis aetiology

Pure metabolic acidosis is characterized by

- Acidaemia (arterial pH <7.35)
- Hypobicarbonatqemia (HCO_3^- <22 mmol/l)
- Hypocarbia (PCO_2 <40mm Hg) and a
- Decreased SBE (less than −3mEq/l)

Metabolic acidoses are categorized according to the presence or absence of unmeasured anions—which are routinely detected by examining the plasma electrolytes and calculating the AG.

Metabolic acidosis with an increased AG

Lactic acidosis

During critical illness, lactate is the most important cause of metabolic acidosis and correlates with outcome in patients with haemorrhagic and septic shock. The assumption that hypoperfusion is the most likely cause has been seriously challenged, especially in well resuscitated patients. The aetiology of hyperlactataemia during critical illness is complex, multi-factorial and arises due to several mechanisms (Table 24.5.1). Lactate is released from the mesentry during gut ischaemia and from the lungs during ALI. Hyperlactataemia in sepsis usually occurs as a consequence of increased aerobic metabolism rather than tissue hypoxia. Lactate production alters cytosolic, and hence mitochondrial redox state such that the increased NADH/NAD supports oxidative phosphorylation as the dominant source of ATP production. Catecholamines, especially epinephrine, result in lactic acidosis presumably by stimulating cellular metabolism (e.g. increased hepatic glycolysis and muscle Na^+,K^+ ATPase) and is a common source of lactic acidosis in the ICU.

Table 24.5.1 Mechanisms of hyperlactataemia during critical illness.

Tissue hypoxia
Hypodynamic shock
Organ ischaemia
Hypermetabolism
Increased aerobic glycolysis
Increased protein catabolism
Hematologic malignanciesal
Decreased clearance of lactate
Liver failure
Shock
Inhibition of pyruvate dehydrogenase
Thiamine deficiency
Endotoxin

Treatment

- Treatment of underlying cause is the most important measure to correct lactic acidosis; however, this may not always be possible.
- Therapy aimed at increasing oxygen delivery may not always be effective.
- Although treatment with sodium bicarbonate and dichloroacetate (the enzyme that stimulates pyruvate dehydrogenase (PDH)) improves pH, they do not improve outcome; nevertheless, Na-bicarbonate is used particularly when lactic acidosis is severe or refractory.

Ketoacidosis

Ketones are formed by β-oxidation of fatty acids, a process inhibited by insulin. In insulin-deficient states (e.g. diabetes), ketogenesis is accelerated due to high glucose-induced osmotic diuresis which may lead to volume contraction. This state is associated with elevated cortisol and catecholamine secretion, which further stimulates free fatty acid production. In addition, increased glucagon, relative to insulin, leads to decreased malonyl co-enzyme A and increased carnitine palmityl acyltransferase, the combination of which increases ketogenesis. Ketone bodies include acetone, acetoacetate and β-hydroxybutyrate. Both acetoacetate and β-hydroxybutyrate are strong anions that decrease the SID and increase the H^+ concentration. Ketoacidosis may result from diabetes (DKA) or alcohol (AKA).

Diagnosis

- Diagnosis is established by measuring serum ketones.
- Nitroprusside reaction only measures acetone and acetate, but not β-hydroxybutyrate.
- Measured ketosis is dependent on the ratio of acetoacetate to β-hydroxybutyrate.
- Ketones may even appear to increase as β-hydroxybutyrate is converted to acetoacetate during treatment.

Treatment

- The treatment of DKA includes insulin and large amounts of isotonic IV fluids
- Potassium replacement is often required
- Fluid resuscitation reverses the hormonal stimuli for ketone body formation and insulin allows for the metabolism of ketones and glucose
- Sodium bicarbonate is rarely necessary and should probably be avoided except in extreme cases
- Response to therapy is observed by monitoring pH and AG more than by the assay of serum ketones
- The treatment of alcoholic ketoacidosis consists of fluids and glucose instead of insulin. Thiamine must also be given to avoid precipitating Wernicke's encephalopathy

Renal failure

Renal failure allows the build up of sulfates and other acids, thereby increasing the AG. Uncomplicated renal failure rarely produces severe acidosis except when it is accompanied by high rates of acid generation such as from hypermetabolism. In all cases, the SID is decreased and is expected to remain so unless some therapy is provided. Haemodialysis will permit the removal of sulfate and other ions and allow normal Na^+ and Cl^- balance to be restored, thus returning the SID to normal. However, patients not yet requiring dialysis and those who are between treatments often require some other therapy to increase the SID. Sodium bicarbonate is used as long as the plasma Na^+ concentration is not already elevated. Other options include Ca^{2+} which usually requires replacement. Ca^{2+} replacement cannot increase the SID much given the rather narrow range of free Ca^{2+}.

Poisons

Metabolic acidosis with an increased AG is a major feature of various types of drug and substance intoxications. It is important to recognize these disorders so that specific therapy can be provided rather than to treat the acid–base disorder that they produce. The use of the osmolar gap can often detect toxins with high osmolality (e.g. methanol).

Unknown causes

Recently, some unknown causes of an increased AG have been reported in non-ketotic hyperosmolar state of diabetes, sepsis, liver disease and in experimental animals given endotoxin. Also unknown cations appear in the blood of some critically ill patients; the significance of these is unknown, but increased mortality has been reported in some studies.

Non-anion gap (hyperchloraemic) acidoses

Hyperchloraemic acidosis occurs as a result of either an increase in Cl^- relative to strong cations, especially Na^+, or the loss of cations with retention of Cl^-. When acidosis occurs, the normal response by the kidney is to increase Cl^- excretion. Failure to do so identifies the kidney as the source of acidosis. Extrarenal hyperchloraemic acidoses occur as a result of exogenous Cl^- loads (iatrogenic acidosis—aline) or because cations are lost from the lower GI tract without proportional loss of Cl^-.

Renal tubular acidosis

Examination of the urine and plasma electrolytes and pH, and calculation of the urine SIDa allows one to diagnose most cases of renal tubular acidosis correctly. However, caution must be exercised when the plasma pH is >7.35 because this may turn off urine Cl^- excretion. In such circumstances, it may be necessary to infuse sodium sulfate or furosemide. These agents stimulate Cl^- and K^+ excretion, and may be used to unmask the defect and to probe K^+ secretory capacity. The defect in all types of renal tubular acidosis is the inability to excrete Cl^- in proportion to Na^+, although the reasons vary by type. Treatment is largely dependent on whether the kidney will respond to mineralocorticoid replacement or whether there is loss of Na^+ that can be replaced as sodium bicarbonate.

Gastrointestinal acidosis

Diarrhoea significant enough to produce a hyperchloraemic metabolic acidosis is usually difficult to miss. Fluid secreted into the gut lumen contains higher amounts of Na^+ than Cl^-, similar to the differences in plasma. Extremely large losses of these fluids, particularly if volume is replaced with fluids containing equal amounts of Na^+ and Cl^-, will result in a decrease in the plasma Na^+ concentration relative to the Cl^- concentration and a decrease in the SID. Such a scenario can be avoided if solutions such as lactated Ringer's are used instead of water or saline. Ringer's solution has a more physiological SID and therefore does not produce acidosis except in rare circumstances.

Iatrogenic acidosis

Two of the most common causes of a hyperchloraemic metabolic acidosis are iatrogenic, and both are due to administration of chloride. Modern parenteral nutrition formulas contain weak anions such as acetate in addition to Cl^- and the balance of each anion can be adjusted depending on the acid–base status of the patient. If sufficient amounts of weak anions are not provided, the plasma Cl^- concentration will increase, decreasing the SID and resulting in acidosis. A similar condition may arise when saline is used for fluid resuscitation, resulting in a so-called 'dilutional acidosis'. The clinical implication for management of patients in the ICU is that when large volumes of fluid are used for resuscitation they should be more physiological than saline. One alternative is lactated Ringer's solution. This fluid contains a more physiological difference between Na^+ and Cl^- concentrations and thus the SID is closer to normal (~28mEq/l compared with saline which has a SID of 0mEq/l).

Unexplained hyperchloraemic acidosis

Critically ill patients sometimes manifest hyperchloraemic metabolic acidosis for unclear reasons. Often these patients have other co-existing types of metabolic acidosis, making the precise diagnosis difficult. For example, some patients with lactic acidosis have more acidosis than can be explained by the increase in lactate concentration, and patients with sepsis and acidosis frequently have normal lactate levels. Often, unexplained anions are the cause, but also quite often there is a hyperchloraemic acidosis. Experimental evidence in endotoxemic animals suggests that as much as a third of the acidosis is still unexplained. A potential explanation for this finding is the partial loss of Donnan equilibrium between plasma and interstitial fluid. The severe, accompanying, capillary leak results in loss of albumin from the vascular space, necessitating the movement of another ion to maintain charge balance between the two compartments. If Cl^- moves into the plasma space to restore charge balance, a strong anion would be replacing a weak anion and a hyperchloraemic metabolic acidosis would result.

Further reading

Alberti KGMM. Diabetic emergencies. *BMJ* 1989; 45: 242–63.

Cooper DJ, Walley KR, Wiggs BR, *et al.* Bicarbonate does not improve hemodynamics in critically ill patients who have lactic acidosis: a prospective, controlled clinical study. *Ann Intern Med* 1990; 112: 492–8.

Gore DC, Jahoor F, Hibbert JM, *et al.* Lactic acidosis during sepsis is related to increased pyruvate production, not deficits in tissue oxygen availability. *Ann Surg* 1996; 224: 97–102.

Kellum JA. Determinants of blood pH in health and disease. *Crit Care* 2000; 4: 6–14.

Kellum JA, Kramer DJ, Lee KH, *et al.* Release of lactate by the lung in acute lung injury. *Chest* 1997;111: 1301–5.

Stewart PA. Modern quantitative acid–base chemistry. *Can J Physiol Pharmacol* 1983; 61: 1444–61.

Weil MH, Afifi AA. Experimental and clinical studies on lacate and pyruvate as indicators of the severity of acute circulatory failure (shock). *Circulation* 1970; 41: 989–1001.

Metabolic alkalosis

The normal range of blood pH is between 7.35 and 7.45, with >7.45 indicating alkalaemia. When alkalaemia is a result of loss of volatile acids such as CO_2 it is classified as a respiratory alkalosis, while alkalaemia arising from non-CO_2 causes (e.g. strong ion imbalances) is classified as metabolic alkalosis. Metabolic alkaloses follow the same physical–chemical principles as metabolic acidoses (see Chapter 24,4).

In broad terms, metabolic alkalosis can result as a consequence of an inappropriately large strong ion difference (SID). SID may be increased by the loss of anions in excess of cations (e.g. vomiting, diuretics) or, rarely, by administration of strong cations in excess of strong anions (e.g. Na^+ together with a metabolizable anion such as citrate, bicarbonate, lactate or acetate).

Metabolic alkaloses can be divided into two broad categories: chloride-responsive and chloride-resistant. The urine Cl^- concentration can be used to help narrow the differential diagnosis. In chloride-responsive metabolic alkalosis, Cl^- losses in excess of Na^+ increase the SID. Chloride-resistant alkalosis results in a urine Cl^- concentration >20mmol/l and is usually caused by mineralocorticoid excess or active diuretic use.

Epidemiology

Metabolic alkaloses frequently occur as sequelae to other acute and chronic conditions; the incidence and prevalence will vary dependent upon the underlying aetiology of the metabolic disorder. Acute metabolic alkaloses are more frequent than chronic alkaloses.

Causes

There are four mechanisms that result in increases in SID and consequent metabolic alkalosis:

1 *Severe depletion in free water induces a parallel increase in Na^+ and Cl^-.* The relative plasma concentration of Na^+ becomes greater than that of Cl^-, increasing the SID.

2 *Any disorder that leads to Cl^- loss from the GI tract or urine in excess of Na^+.* Common causes include:
- Diuretic use (or abuse)
- Vomiting or gastric drainage
- Chloride-wasting diarrhoea (villous adenoma)
- Chronic respiratory failure and elevated pCO_2 (post-hypercapnic metabolic alkalosis caused by compensatory renal Cl^- loss).
- All forms of mineralocorticoid excess can produce renal Cl^- wasting and chronic metabolic alkalosis: primary hyperaldosteronism (Conn's syndrome), secondary hyperaldosteronism, Cushing's syndrome, Liddle's syndrome, Bartter's syndrome, exogenous corticoids and excessive liquorice intake.

3 *Na^+ administration in excess of Cl^-.* Administration of non-chloride sodium salts can occur via:
- Massive blood transfusions (sodium citrate)
- Parenteral nutrition (sodium acetate)
- Plasma volume expanders (acetate or citrate)
- Ringer's solution (sodium lactate)
- Overzealous use of sodium bicarbonate

4 *A severe deficiency of intracellular cations such as magnesium or potassium.* This deficiency primarily decreases intracellular Cl^- and secondarily reduces total body Cl^-; this results in an increased net SID.

Clinical features

Metabolic alkalosis usually manifests by:
- Alkalaemia (arterial pH >7.45)
- Hyperbicarbonataemia (HCO_3^- >26mmol/l)
- Hypercarbia (PCO_2 >40mm Hg) and an increased SBE (>3mEq/l).
- Urine chloride:
  - Cl-responsive: urine chloride <10mmol/l
  - Cl-resistant: urine chloride >20mmol/l

Assessment of metabolic alkalosis should include examination of the extracellular fluid volume, including, recumbent/upright blood pressure, skin turgor, capillary refill, and CVP measurement to assess volume status.

Symptoms and signs

Metabolic alkalosis causes changes in central and peripheral nervous system function (e.g. confusion, obtundation, seizures, paraesthesias, etc.) muscular cramping and/or tetany, arrhythmias and hypoxemia. A family history may reveal an underlying cause associated with a mineralocorticoid excess (e.g. Cushing's or Liddle's syndrome). In these instances, acute metabolic alkalosis is generally ruled out and the attention should turn to chronic alkalosis.

Management

Serum electrolytes, ABG values and urine chloride should be reviewed. There may be a concomitant respiratory component involved, and the expected arterial pCO_2 value associated with metabolic alkalosis should be calculated by using the HCO_3^- concentration or the SBE.

$$pCO_2 = (0.7 \times HCO_3^-) + 21 \text{ or,}$$

$$pCO_2 = 40 + (0.6 \times SBE)$$

A measured pCO_2 value >2mm Hg more than the derived expected value indicates respiratory acidosis while a pCO_2 value <2mm Hg indicates respiratory alkalosis.

Treatment

Treat the underlying aetiology. The recognition of the disorder and the subsequent differential diagnosis (chloride-responsive or chloride-resistant) are essential first steps. Based on the aetiology, attention should be given to the reversal of Cl^- depletion, volume restoration and preventing additional losses.

Chloride-responsive alkalosis:

- **Diuretic-induced metabolic alkalosis is the most common acute metabolic alkalosis.** Saline should be administered in this instance. A 0.45% saline solution is effective at reversing the free water deficit and relative chloride depletion (this solution will actually reduce the [Cl^-] but, since it reduces [Na^+] more, SID will fall. Several litres may be required throughout the first days of treatment. If hypokalaemia is present with volume depletion, 20–40mEq/l of KCl can be added to 0.45% saline or given separately. Additionally, diuretics should be discontinued.
- In patients with underlying renal failure or risk for volume overload, 0.1M HCl (100mmol Cl^-/l) can be administered with caution via a central venous line to treat the Cl^- depletion. A repeat evaluation of the metabolic alkalosis is recommended after each litre is infused.

Table 24.6.1 Common causes of metabolic alkalosis

Chloride responsive:
Gastric losses (e.g. vomiting, mechanical drainage, bulimia)
Post-chloruretic diuretic use (e.g. bumetanide, chlorothiazide, metolazone, etc.)
Diarrhoeal states (e.g. villous adenoma, congenital chloridorrhoea)
Post-hypercapneic state
Gastrocystoplasty
Cystic fibrosis
Post-organic acidosis
Milk-alkali syndrome
Select antibiotics (e.g. carbenicillin, gentamicin, penicillin, ticarcillin)
Sodium bicarbonate loading
Excess cation administration:
Sodium salt administration (acetate, citrate)
Blood transfusions
Plasma volume expanders
Sodium lactate
Parenteral nutrition
Chloride resistant:
Mineralcorticoid excess
Excessive licorice consumption (glycyrrhizic acid and carbenoxolone)
Bartter syndrome
Cushing syndrome
Liddle syndrome
Gitelman syndrome
Hyperaldosteronism (primary and secondary)
Antineoplastic drugs (e.g. cisplatin)
Miscellaneous (unknown aetiologies or able to result in resistant and responsive alkalosis):
Prolonged diuretic usage
Prolonged laxative usage
Ion imbalances:
Hypoalbuminaemia
Hypophosphataemia
Hypokalaemia
Hypomagnesaemia

- Metabolic alkalosis in the presence of volume overload (e.g. in the presence of congestive heart failure) is best treated with potassium chloride solutions. If diuresis is necessary, K^+-sparing diuretics (e.g. spironolactone), which also spare Cl^- concentrations, can be used in therapy. Alternatively, in persons with adequate renal function, a carbonic anhydrase inhibitor such as acetazolamide can be administered at a rate of 250–500mg bid. Acetazolamide is associated with Na^+ excretion in excess of Cl^- excretion, thus a net increase in SID. Acetazolamide also increases K^+ secretion, making it useful if K^+ is elevated. Complications of acetazolamide use are hypokalaemia and metabolic acidosis.
- In patients actively losing gastric fluid, H_2-blockers and/or PPIs are useful in treatment as they reduce gastric Cl^- loss.
- If severe, additional interventions such as RRT may be required. Renal failure and acetazolamide-resistant volume overload are common indications for dialysis. Peritoneal dialysis should use normal saline with electrolyte concentrations as indicated. Haemodialysis should incorporate low HCO_3^- concentrations for the dialysate.

Chloride-resistant alkalosis:
Cases of chloride-resistant metabolic alkalosis are most commonly seen in the chronic state, but can occur acutely (e.g. glycyrrhizic acid). Aetiologies involving hypokalaemia and hypomagnesaemia warrant the appropriate electrolyte repletion. Glycyrrhizic acid-induced alkalosis is usually self-correcting upon the discontinuation of ingestion. K^+-sparing diuretics may also be given if there is no improvement.

Hypoalbuminemic alkalosis
In theory, a reduction in weak acids (typically albumin) will induce metabolic alkalosis. However, hypoalbuminaemia results in a decreased SID (principally through renal Cl^- excretion. Thus, a 'normal'" SID in the face of hypoalbuminaemia is in fact abnormally high. Acute hypoalbuminaemia would result in acute alkalosis until renal compensation can occur but, in practice, acute hypoalbuminaemia is almost always due to crystalloid resuscitation and the resulting pH is a function of both the dilution of albumin and changes in SID (see Chapter 24.5).

Complications

Alkalosis may be less well tolerated than acidosis since relatively mild increases in arterial pH may cause adverse clinical effects, especially if the alkalaemia developed rapidly (e.g. seizures and respiratory depression may occur when arterial pH is brought to 7.60).

- Alkalosis affects tissue oxygenation by decreasing the tendency of haemoglobin to release oxygen in tissue capillaries. Concomitant with these shifts, intracellular alkalosis can increase oxygen demand by stimulating glycolysis. Increased oxygen demand coupled with decreased oxygen delivery exacerbates tissue hypoxia.
- Alkaloses can produce ion deficiencies and excess (e.g. hypokalaemia, hypophosphataemia, hypercarbia, hyperbicarbonataemia, etc.), which increase the risk of morbidity and mortality. These abnormalities can alter neuromuscular excitability and coronary blood flow, produce seizures, impair enzymatic function, alter cardiac inotropy, increase the accumulation of organic acids and exacerbate drug toxicity (e.g. digoxin).
- Compensatory hypoventilation resulting in increased pCO_2 can result in CNS depression and pulmonary hypertension. The consequences of decreased levels of oxygen delivery throughout the system can, in cases of severe alkalosis, be quite serious (pH >7.60).
- The cardiovascular response to metabolic alkalosis is primarily vasoconstriction and a subsequent decrease in coronary blood flow. Transient increased cardiac inotropy may result. In some instances, cardiac arrhythmias may be detectable.
- Neurologically, metabolic alkalosis may induce delirium, apathy, neuromuscular excitability or, in more severe instances, seizures.

Further reading

Kaplan LJ, Frangos S. Clinical review: acid–base abnormalities in the intensive care unit. *Crit Care* 2005; 9: 198–203.

Kellum JA. Clinical review: reunification of acid–base physiology. *Crit Care* 2005; 9: 500–7.

Kellum JA. Diagnosis and treatment of acid–base disorders. Textbook of critical care medicine. Philadelphia: Elsevier, 2005.

Morgan TJ. Clinical review: the meaning of acid–base abnormalities in the intensive care unit—effects of fluid administration. *Crit Care* 2005; 9: 204–11.

Neligan PJ, Deutschmann CS. Acid–base balance in critical care medicine. *Contemp Crit Care* 2004; 216: 1–9.

Stewart P. Modern quantitative acid–base chemistry. *Can J Physiol Pharmacol* 1983; 61: 1444–61.

Glycaemic control in the critically ill

Hyperglycaemia is common in acute illnesses, irrespective of diabetic status. Moderate hyperglycaemia has been considered beneficial, ensuring adequate glucose as an energy source for organs that do not require insulin for glucose uptake—the brain and the immune system. However, even a moderate hyperglycaemia is related to adverse outcome as has been shown in a study on tight glycaemic control in the critically ill.

Clinical studies

In a surgical ICU, tight glycaemic control had beneficial effects on both mortality and morbidity. Comparison was made between conventional insulin use with a mean blood glucose of 8.3–9.9mmol/l and intensive insulin therapy, with blood glucose levels between 4.4 and 6.1mmol/l (mean blood glucose levels of 5.0–5.5mmol/l).

In 2006, the effects of tight glycaemic control in the medical ICU showed that tight glycaemic control significantly reduced morbidity, (mortality reduction did not reach statistical significance). In long-stay patients, maintaining normoglycaemia significantly reduced mortality and morbidity.

Effects of tight glycaemic control in the critically ill were:

- decreased mortality
- decreased length of ICU stay
- prevention of acute kidney failure, anaemia and hyperbilirubinaemia
- decreased need for prolonged mechanical ventilation and dialysis
- reduced incidence of critical illness polyneuropathy and/or myopathy
- reduced incidence of hyperinflammation and development of bloodstream infections
- improved long-term rehabilitation in patients with isolated brain injury
- improved long-term outcome of high risk cardiac surgery patients
- reduced costs

Tight glucose management was evaluated in a heterogeneous ICU population. Mean blood glucose was 7.3mmol/l in the protocol period, compared with 8.4mmol/l in the baseline period. There was a significant decrease in hospital mortality, length of ICU stay, development of new renal failure and red blood cell transfusions, as well as a reduction in medical costs.

In a predominantly surgical patient population, glucose levels maintained between 4.4 and 6.7mmol/l (mean 6.9mmol/l) resulted in a decreased incidence of nosocomial infections.

Mechanisms of actions of tight glycaemic control

- Prevents immune dysfunction
- Prevents sustained systemic hyperinflammation
- Improves dyslipidaemia
- Ameliorates muscle insulin sensitivity
- Protects the endothelium and mitochondrial ultrastructure and function.

Potential risks

Multi-variate logistic regression analysis of the surgical study indicated that blood glucose control rather than the insulin dose administered statistically explains most of the beneficial effects of tight glycaemic control. The risk of death was linearly correlated with the degree of hyperglycaemia. A reduction of blood glucose levels to <6.1mmol/l appeared to be crucial to gain most benefit on mortality and for the prevention of events that cause morbidity.

Controversy

The prospective VISEP trial—the insulin arm of the study—was stopped prematurely because the rate of hypoglycaemia in the intensive treatment group was considered unacceptably high (12.1%). The GLUCONTROL study to assess whether tight glycaemic control (4.4–6.1mmol/l) improves survival in a mixed population of critically ill patients was stopped early because of inadequate blood glucose control and risk of hypoglycaemia.

Both trials were underpowered for this effect.

Two large, randomized trails on the infusion of glucose together with insulin and potassium in patients with diabetes and MI (DIGAMI-2) and patients with AMI (CREATE-ECLA) failed to show clinical benefits of this treatment. In neither study was normoglycaemia achieved.

Conclusions: (1) strict glucose control is necessary to demonstrate benefits and (2) adequate power calculations are crucial to produce meaningful studies.

An ongoing study is the multi-centre trial 'Normoglycemia in Intensive Care Evaluation and Survival Using Glucose Algorithm Regulation' (NICE-SUGAR).

Hypoglycemia

Tight glucose control with insulin carries the risk of hypoglycaemia. Severe or prolonged hypoglycaemia can cause convulsions, coma and irreversible brain damage, as well as cardiac arrhythmias. In the surgical population the risk of hypoglycaemia (glucose ≤2.2mmol/l) increased from 0.8 to 5.1% with intensive insulin therapy and from 3.1 to 18.7% in the medical ICU population. Patients with sepsis appeared to be susceptible to the development of hypoglycaemia. These brief episodes of hypoglycaemia were not associated with obvious clinical problems: hypoglycaemia did not cause early deaths, and only minor immediate and transient morbidity was seen in a minority of patients, and no late neurological sequellae occurred among hospital survivors. The risk of hypoglycaemia did coincide with a higher risk of death in both conventional and intensive insulin groups. In a recent study, no causal link was found between hypoglycaemia in the ICU and death. These observations suggest that hypoglycaemia in ICU patients who receive intensive insulin therapy may merely identify patients at high risk of dying rather then representing a risk on its own.

Conclusion

Maintaining normoglycaemia with intensive insulin therapy improves survival and reduces morbidity in surgical and medical ICU patients. Current evidence is in favour of controlling blood glucose levels below 6.1mmol/l in the ICU, despite a higher incidence of hypoglycaemia.

Further reading

CREATE-ECLA Trial Group Investigators. Effect of glucose–insulin–potassium infusion on mortality in patients with acute ST-segment elevation myocardial infarction: the CREATE-ECLA randomized controlled trial. *JAMA* 2005; 293: 437–46.

Glucontrol study: comparing the effects of two glucose control regimens by insulin in intensive care unit patients. Available from http://www.clinicaltrials.gov/ct/show/NCT00107601.

Hermans G, Wilmer A, Meersseman W, *et al.* Impact of intensive insulin therapy on neuromuscular complications and ventilator dependency in the medical intensive care unit. *Am J Respir Crit Care Med* 2007; 175: 480–9.

NICE-SUGAR study: normoglycemia in intensive care evaluation and survival using glucose algorithm regulation. Available from http://www.clinicaltrials.gov/ct/show/NCT00220987.

Van den Berghe G, Wouters P, Weekers F, *et al.* Intensive insulin therapy in critically ill patients. *N Engl J Med* 2001; 345: 1359–67.

Van den Berghe G, Wilmer A, Hermans G, *et al.* Intensive insulin therapy in the medical ICU. *N Engl J Med* 2006; 354: 449–61.

Van den Berghe G, Wilmer A, Milants I, *et al.* Intensive insulin therapy in mixed medical/surgical ICU: benefit versus harm. *Diabetes* 2006; 55: 3151–9.

Diabetic ketoacidosis

Diabetic ketoacidosis (DKA) is a medical emergency that is characterized by hyperglycaemia, ketosis and acidosis

This disorder primarily occurs in people with type 1 diabetes but also occurs in patients with type 2 diabetes.

Pathogenesis

Ketoacidosis is a state of uncontrolled catabolism associated with insulin deficiency. The absence of insulin causes an increase in hepatic glucose production, leading to hyperglycaemia. It also accelerates hepatic fatty acid breakdown producing excess ketone bodies, which leads to ketoacidosis. Concurrent osmotic diuresis and vomiting enhance fluid and electrolyte depletion. Subsequent renal hypoperfusion results in impaired excretion of ketones and hydrogen ions, and the cycle self-perpetuates.

Causes

- Previously undiagnosed diabetes
- Stress of a concurrent illness
  - Most commonly UTI or pneumonia
- Interruption of insulin therapy
  - 25% of hospital admissions due to DKA are because the patient omitted their insulin
- Drugs
  - Corticosteroids
  - Thiazide diuretics
- Alcohol or substance abuse

Clinical presentation

The symptoms and signs of DKA are related to hyperosmolality, volume depletion and metabolic acidosis.

History

- Typically a 2–3 day history of gradual deterioration, perhaps precipitated by infection

Symptoms

- Polyuria and polydipsia
- Weight loss
- Vomitting
- Abdominal pain
  - Can mimic peritonitis
- Those of a concurrent infection/precipitating cause.

Signs

- Volume depletion and shock
  - Hypotension, tachycardia, cool peripheries, low JVP, dry mucous membranes, increased skin turgor
- Acidosis
  - Kussmaul respiration, 'fruity odour' (specific to ketoacidosis)
- Neurological
  - Lethargy, visual disturbance, altered level of consciousness, seizures, coma

Investigations

- Blood
  - FBC
  - U&E, glucose, LFT, CRP, amylase, osmolality
  - Culture
  - ABG (including lactate)
- Urine
  - Dipstick for ketones
  - Microscopy and culture
- CXR
- ECG

Immediate management

Dehydration is more life threatening than the hyperglycaemia, so its correction takes precedence.

Fluid

The average fluid loss is 3–6l in DKA. The optimal rate at which fluid should be replaced is dependent upon the clinical state of the patient.

- 0.9% Saline should be used initially.
- Fluids should be infused quickly when patients are in shock.
- An average regime may be:
  - 1l in 30min
  - 1l in 1h
  - 1l in 2h
  - 1l in 4h
  - 1l in 6h
  - KCl should be added to each bag of fluid whilst monitoring the serum potassium level (see the electrolyte section)
- Patients who do not have an extreme volume deficit may be effectively re-hydrated at a rate of 500ml/h for the first 4h followed by 250ml/h for the next 4h.
- More rapid resuscitation may not be necessary and can delay correction of the acidosis.
- Switch to dextrose saline when the blood glucose falls below 12mmol/l.

NB: the fluid regimes set out above are a guideline for patients with DKA. Excessive fluid can precipitate cerebral oedema, and inadequate fluid can lead to renal failure. Fluid management needs to be tailored to each individual patient and monitored carefully throughout treatment

Electrolytes

Potassium

Renal and GI losses contribute to a marked potassium depletion. Despite this, the plasma potassium concentration is usually normal or, elevated at presentation (1/3 cases). This is due to initial hyperosmolality and insulin deficiency, which results in potassium movement out of the cells.

- There is a danger of hypokalaemia as glucose enters cells with insulin treatment
- Aim for a plasma K^+ of 4–5mmol/l
- If K^+ 3–4 mmol/l, aim to replace 40mmol KCl/h
- If K^+ 4–5.5 mmol/l, aim to replace 20mmol KCl/h
- Measure plasma K^+ every 2h
- Withhold K^+ if oliguric (rare) or if initial K^+ is >5.5mmol/l (the K^+ will fall quickly as glucose re-enters cells)

Sodium

Reversing hyperglycaemia with insulin will lower the plasma osmolality, cause water to move from the extracellular fluid into cells, and raise the plasma sodium concentration. Thus, a patient with a normal initial plasma sodium concentration may become hypernatraemic during therapy with insulin and 0.9% saline.

- 0.45% Saline is not, however, routinely used in the management of DKA

Phosphate

The plasma phosphate concentration may initially be normal or elevated, but phosphate depletion is rapidly unmasked following insulin therapy, frequently leading to hypophosphataemia.

- Most patients remain asymptomatic and phosphate administration is not indicated.

Insulin

Insulin lowers the plasma glucose concentration (primarily by reducing hepatic glucose production rather than enhancing peripheral utilization), decreases ketone production (by reducing both lipolysis and glucagon secretion) and may augment ketone utilization.

IV bolus

- 6–10U stat

Continuous IV infusion

- 50U of soluble insulin made up to 50ml with 0.9% saline to run through an infusion pump.
- Start infusion at 6U (6ml) per hour (10U (10ml) per hour if infection is present).
- Aim to lower the plasma glucose by ~3.5–7mmol/l/h.
- When the blood glucose is <12 mmol/l, switch to either an insulin sliding scale protocol or the patients standard insulin regime.
- A minimum infusion of 2U per hour should be continued until the ketoacidosis is corrected. This may require co-administration of 5% dextrose.

Both IM and SC insulin therapy are as effective as IV therapy, if the patient is not in shock. However, their use is not recommended by most Diabetologists. There is concern that the combination of volume depletion and secondary sympathetic activation decreases subcutaneous blood flow, resulting in reduced insulin absorption. As normal blood flow returns, absorption improves and initial persistent hyperglycaemia can turn into delayed hypoglycaemia.

Acid–base balance

Trials do not demonstrate any clinical benefit from the routine administration of sodium bicarbonate.

- Bicarbonate is not indicated when treating DKA
- Bicarbonate can raise pCO_2 (by decreasing acidaemic respiratory drive), thus reducing cerebral pH
- Bicarbonate slows the rate of recovery of ketosis
- Bicarbonate can lead to a post-treatment metabolic alkalosis.

Additional measures

- Pass an NG tube—to prevent gastric dilation and aspiration (essential in patients with reduced level of consciousness)
- Add broad-spectrum antibiotics if infection is suspected
- Insert a bladder catheter if no urine has passed after 2h
- Place a central venous line if the patient is in shock or elderly to assist the fluid management.

Ongoing management

- For the first 8h (at least):
    - Monitor glucose hourly
    - Monitior electrolytes 2 hourly
- Adjust K^+ replacement according to results
- Alter insulin infusion and fluid type when targets are reached (see immediate management section)
- Seek the underlying cause

Complications and pitfalls in DKA

- Patients may present with combined DKA and HONK (hyperosmolar non-ketotic)
- Initial potassium concentrations may be high but decrease rapidly after the initiation of treatment
- DKA may complicate type 2 diabetes mellitus as well as type 1 diabetes.
- Ketoacidosis is seen in a number of inborn errors of metabolism (often presenting in infancy) and in alcoholic and fasting ketoacidosis. It is unusual for the blood glucose to be raised in these conditions.

Prognosis

The mortality rate in patients with DKA is <5% in experienced centres.

NICE guidelines

`http://guidance.nice.org.uk/topic/endocrine`

Further reading

Adrogue HJ, Barrero J, Eknoyan G. Salutary effects of modest fluid replacement in the treatment of adults with diabetic ketoacidosis. Use in patients without extreme volume deficit. *JAMA* 1989; 262: 2108–13.

Fisher JN, Kitabchi AE. A randomized study of phosphate therapy in the treatment of diabetic ketoacidosis. *J Clin Endocrinol Metab* 1983; 57: 177–80.

Fisher JN, Shahshahani MN, Kitabchi AE. Diabetic ketoacidosis: low-dose insulin therapy by various routes. *N Engl J Med* 1977; 297: 238–41.

Kumar P, Clark M. Clinical medicine. Bailliere Tindall, 1994

Page, MM, Alberti, KG, Greenwood, R, *et al.* Treatment of diabetic coma with continuous low-dose insulin infusion. *BMJ* 1974; 2: 687.

Viallon A, Zeni F, Lafond P, *et al.* Does bicarbonate therapy improve the management of severe diabetic ketoacidosis? *Crit Care Med* 1999; 27: 2690–3.

Hyperosmolar diabetic emergencies

Hyperosmolar non-ketotic state (HNS) is a medical emergency, usually but not exclusively, in older patients with type 2 diabetes. They present with marked dehydration, a raised blood glucose (>50mmol/l) and often coma

Remember patients with type 2 diabetes can also present with DKA, and DKA and HNS can co-exist.

Pathogenesis

Non-ketotic coma occurs in patients with relative insulin deficiency and is usually precipitated by an acute illness (e.g. infection), MI or stroke. Increased secretion of counter-regulatory hormones (glucagon, catecholamines and cortisol) exacerbates insulin resistance and glucose production is unrestrained. The resulting rise in serum osmolarity (often >350mOsm/kg (normal 285–295mOsmol/kg)) causes an osmotic diuresis, volume depletion and haemoconcentration, further increasing blood glucose concentrations. Importantly endogenous insulin levels are sufficient to inhibit hepatic lipolysis and ketogenesis, hence the absence of ketoacidosis. This gradual nature of the development, over 7–10 days, causes profound dehydration throughout all volume compartments.

Causes

- Previously undiagnosed diabetes
- Stress of a concurrent illness
  - Most commonly UTI or pneumonia, MI, CVA
- Consumption of glucose-rich fluids (e.g. Lucozade)
- Drugs
  - Corticosteroids
  - Thiazide diuretics

Clinical presentation

The symptoms and signs of HNS are related to the degree of hyperosmolality and volume depletion. As the plasma osmolality rises to >330mOsmol/kg, neurological symptoms become more prominant

History

- 7–10 day history of gradual deterioration.

Symptoms

- Polyuria and polydipsia
- Lethargy
- Confusion
- Vomiting
- Those of a concurrent infection/precipitating cause.

Signs

- Neurological
  - Lethargy, altered level of consciousness, CVA, coma
- Volume depletion and shock
  - Hypotension, tachycardia, cool peripheries, low JVP, dry mucous membranes, increased skin turgor
- Vascular—MI, limb ischaemia (as a consequence of hyperosmolar state)

Investigations

- Blood
  - FBC
  - U&E, glucose, LFTs, CRP, amylase, osmolality
  - Cultures
  - ABG (including lactate)
- Urine
  - Dipstick (check for ketones which may be there in small quantities if patient has been fasting)
  - Microscopy and culture
- CXR
- Electrocardiogram

Immediate management

NB: although the management of HNS appears similar to that of DKA, there are important differences.

Patients must be managed in a HDU or ICU as they often present in a precarious state with a high potential to deteriorate.

Dehydration is more life threatening than the hyperglycaemia, but it needs to be corrected more slowly than in DKA.

Fluid

The average fluid loss is up to 8–10l in HNS. This is largely due to hyperglycaemic-induced osmotic diuresis. Due to the nature of patients with HNS, consideration must be made of co-morbidities such as cardiac failure when prescribing the fluid replacement regime.

- 0.9% Saline should be used initially.
- As a guide, a maximum starting rate of 15–20ml/kg/h (~1–1.5l in the average adult) may be appropriate, but is likely to need to be reduced after the first few hours.
- Potassium should be added to the fluid, but there may be exceptions (see electrolyte section).
- Subsequent choice for fluid replacement depends on the state of hydration, serum electrolyte levels and urinary output.
- Switch to 5% dextrose when the blood glucose falls below 12mmol/l.
- You should aim to clear the fluid deficit over the first 48h.

NB: the fluid regimes set out above are a guideline for patients with HNS. Excessive fluid can precipitate cerebral oedema, and inadequate fluid can result in renal failure. In patients with renal or cardiac compromise, monitoring of serum osmolality and frequent assessment of cardiac, renal and mental status must be performed during fluid resuscitation to avoid iatrogenic fluid overload.

Electrolytes

Potassium

Renal and GI losses contribute to a marked potassium depletion. Despite this, the plasma potassium concentration is usually normal or elevated at presentation (1/3 cases). This is due to initial hyperosmolality and insulin deficiency, which results in potassium movement out of the cells.

- There is a danger of hypokalaemia as glucose enters cells with insulin treatment
- Aim for a plasma K^+ of 4–5mmol/l
- If K^+ 3–4 mmol/l aim to replace 40mmol KCl per hour
- If K^+ 4–5.5mmol/l aim to replace 20mmol KCl per hour
- Measure plasma K^+ every 2h
- Withhold K^+ if oliguric or if initial K^+ is >5.5mmol/l (the K^+ will fall quickly as glucose re-enters cells)

Sodium

Reversing hyperglycaemia with insulin will lower the plasma osmolality, cause water to move from the extracellular fluid into cells, and raise the plasma sodium concentration. Thus, a patient with low or normal initial plasma sodium concentration may become hypernatraemic during therapy with insulin and 0.9% saline.

- 0.45% Saline is contraindicated. A rapid decrease in sodium concentration may precipitate severe cerebral oedema.

Insulin

It is often reported that patients with HNS may be particularly sensitive to insulin and require lower doses than patients with DKA, though studies have not proven this. The rapid decrease in blood glucose that may be seen in HNS is more likely to be related to correction of the severe hypovolaemia with fluid repletion. However, in order to prevent rapid changes in plasma osmolality, a more cautious approach to insulin administration in the first 2h is recommended, and stat dose at treatment induction should not be given.

Continuous IV infusion

- 50U of soluble insulin made up to 50ml with 0.9% saline to run through an infusion pump.
- Start infusion at 3U (3ml) per hour.
- Do not give initial bolus dose
- If, after 2h, the blood glucose is not falling fast enough, increase the infusion to 6U (6 ml) per hour.
- Aim to lower the plasma glucose by 3.5–7mmol/l/h.
- When the blood glucose is <12mmol/l, switch to either an insulin sliding scale protocol or the patients standard hypoglycaemic regimen.

Additional measures

- NG tube—to prevent gastric dilation and aspiration (essential in patients with reduced level of consciousness)
- Broad-spectrum antibiotics if infection is suspected
- Insert a bladder catheter
- Place a central venous line if the patient is in shock or elderly to assist the fluid management.

Anticoagulation

HNS results in a hypercoagulable state, increasing the risk of thromboembolism

- UFH or LMWH should be used formally to anticoagulate patients with HNS.

Ongoing management

- For the first 8h at least:
  - Monitor glucose hourly
  - Monitior electrolytes 2 hourly
- Adjust K^+ replacement according to results
- Alter insulin infusion and fluid type when targets are reached (see Immediate management section)
- Seek the underlying cause

Pitfalls of HNS

- Cerebral oedema is a complication of therapy that typically occurs within 24h after treatment has been initiated. Headache is the first clinical sign, but marked neurological dysfunction can develop. The condition is precipitated by rapid changes in serum osmolality and carries a high mortality and morbidity,
- Patients often have a concurrent lactic acidosis,

Prognosis

The mortality of patients with HNS is 30–35% and increases with age, medical co-morbidity, severity of metabolic derangement and degree of impairment of consciousness .

Unlike DKA, HNS is not an absolute indication for subsequent insulin therapy, and survivors may do well on oral agents with good diet control.

Further reading

Adrogue HJ, Barrero J, Eknoyan G. Salutary effects of modest fluid replacement in the treatment of adults with diabetic ketoacidosis. Use in patients without extreme volume deficit. *JAMA* 1989; 20; 262: 2108–13.

Kitabchi AE, Umpierrez GE, Murphy MB. Hyperglycemic crises in patients with diabetes mellitus. *Diabetes Care* 2003; 26 Suppl 1: S109.

Kumar P, Clark M. Clinical medicine. Bailliere Tindall 1994

Malone ML, Gennis V, Goodwin JS. Characteristics of diabetic ketoacidosis in older versus younger adults. *J Am Geriatr Soc* 1992; 40: 1100–4.

Newton CA, Raskin P. Diabetic ketoacidosis in type 1 and type 2 diabetes mellitus: clinical and biochemical differences. *Arch Intern Med* 2004;164: 1925–31.

Page MM, Alberti KG, Greenwood R, *et al.* Treatment of diabetic coma with continuous low-dose insulin infusion. *BMJ* 1974; 2: 687.

Rosenthal NR, Barrett EJ. An assessment of insulin action in hyperosmolar hyperglycemic nonketotic diabetic patients. *Clin Endocrinol Metab* 1985; 60: 607–10.

Thyroid emergencies: thyroid crisis/thyrotoxic storm

A rare life-threatening disorder associated with hyperthyroidism. Mortality may be as high as 30% with treatment. Characteristic features include: *hyperpyrexia, severe tachycardia, extreme restlessness* and *dehydration*.

Pathogenesis

Most commonly occurs in patients with undiagnosed or poorly controlled hyperthyroidism (usually Graves' disease) in association with a recognized precipitant. The exact pathogenesis is unknown but serum free thyroxine (T_4) or triiodothyronine (T_3) concentrations are increased.

Causes

- Graves' disease
- Toxic multi-nodular goitre
- Thyroid adenoma
- Trauma
- Excessive exogenous thyroid hormones

A thyrotoxic storm is usually precipitated by a trigger such as a severe infection, surgery, DKA, pulmonary thromboembolism or parturition. Less common precipitants include, radioiodine therapy (Jod Basedow phenomenon), radiocontrast dyes, salicylates, haloperidol and amiodarone administration.

Clinical presentation

Four major features

- Fever >38.5°C
- Sinus or supraventricular tachycardia
- Agitation, restlessness, emotional lability, confusion, psychosis, seizures and coma
- Diarrhoea, vomiting, abdominal pain, jaundice.

Occasionally patients present with profound exhaustion, tachycardia, hyporeflexia, severe myopathy, marked weight loss and hypotension. This rare variant is termed apathetic hyperthyroidism.

Symptoms and signs

The diagnosis of thyroid crisis is clinical. Treatment must start before biochemical confirmation of the condition is obtained, and mortality is high (10–30%)

- Goitre (thyroid gland findings can vary)
- Fever >38.5°C. Skin maybe moist and warm
- Cardiovascular: sinus tachycardia, AF, ventricular arrhythmias, systolic hypertension with a widened pulse pressure. Cardiomegaly and LV hypertrophy may be present
- Neurological: symptoms range from tremor and increasing restlessness to delirium, seizures, coma and death. Profound muscle weakness and rhabdomyolysis may occur
- GI: nausea and vomiting are common. Severe abdominal pain may indicate underlying GI precipitant. Jaundice is occasionally present.

Investigations

- FBC
  - leucocytosis
- Electrolytes
  - hypokalaemia, hypomagnesaemia, hypercalcaemia
- Glucose
  - hyperglycaemia
- LFTs
  - elevated transaminases, alkaline phosphatase and bilirubin
- Thyroid function tests
  - suppressed thyroid-stimulating hormone (TSH)
  - elevated T_4 and T_3 (concentrations do not correlate well with severity of condition)
- Blood cultures
- ABG
  - respiratory and metabolic acidosis
- Urine for microscopy and culture
- CXR
  - pulmonary oedema, cardiomegaly
- ECG
  - arrhythmias, LV hypertrophy

Immediate management

This is a medical emergency. Patients require immediate and aggressive supportive management in a critical care setting and early alleviation of the thyrotoxicosis.

Supportive therapy

- Oxygen: high flow humidified oxygen via mask and reservoir bag. Oxygen requirements will be markedly increased and the majority of patients will require intubation and ventilatory support to manage the severe respiratory and metabolic acidosis.
- Fluids: crystalloid resuscitation to replace losses associated with fever and underlying precipitants
- Potassium and magnesium frequently require replacement.
- Glucocorticosteroids. Thyrotoxicosis is associated with an increased requirement for and relative deficiency of corticosteroids. In addition, corticosteroids decrease the peripheral conversion of T_4 to T_3. Doses: hydrocortisone, IV 100mg every 6h or dexamethasone 2mg every 6h
- Active cooling. Temperatures can exceed 41°C, Cooling blankets and cold fluids are required.

Antithyroid drugs

Management of the thyrotoxicosis should be initiated with the resuscitation. A number of drug options are available. None is ideal in isolation.

- β-Adrenoceptor antagonist are critical in the management of thyroid storm. Non-selective agents antagonize the peripheral effect of thyroid hormones, decrease conversion of T_4 to T_3, albeit slowly, and reduce catecholamine hypersensitivity, β_1-selective agents are less effective peripherally. Higher doses than normal may be required because of increased clearance.
  - Propranolol: IV dose 0.5mg increments up to 10mg, PO dose 60–80mg 4 hourly.
  - Metoprolol: 2–5mg increments, up to 20mg IV or 100–200mg PO every 6h
  - Esmolol: bolus of 250–500mcg/kg followed by 50–200mcg/kg/min infusion
- Carbimazole: blocks the synthesis of thyroid hormone, 60–120mg orally, via NG tube or per rectum. Takes ~1h to start working. Can cause neutropenia at 1 month.
- Propylthiouracil: blocks the synthesis of thyroxine and the conversion of T_4 to T_3. 200mg every 4h orally, via NG tube or per rectum.

- Potassium iodide: blocks the synthesis and release of the thyroid hormones. Lugol's solution contains 130mg/ml. Dose 0.3ml diluted to 50ml every 8h via NG or per rectum.
  - Iodine-containing compounds should only be given at least 1h after the administration of a thionamide. Prior administration of iodine-containing compounds may exacerbate thyrotoxicosis. Thionamides; propylthiouracil, methimazole inhibit iodine uptake and utilisation.
- Lithium carbonate is a similar alternative for patients allergic to iodine. Lithium blood concentrations should be monitored.

Additional measures

- NG tube for the administration of oral medications
- Broad-spectrum antibiotics if infection is suspected.
- Invasive monitoring, central venous line, arterial blood pressure and cardiac output monitoring to guide fluid and management with inotropes and vasopressors.
- Digoxin. May be useful for rate control of atrial fibrillation in addition to β-blockade.
- Amiodarone. May be useful for the control of atrial fibrillation but should not be used prior to starting a thionamide because of potential aggravation of the thyroid crisis.
- Vitamin B complex. Vitamin B1 (thiamine) requirements are increased in thyrotoxicosis, and deficiency may be associated with peripheral neuropathies and Werncke's encephalopathy. Vitamin B12 (cobalamin) defiency may be associated with thyrotoxicosis.
- Dantrolene. Has been used to control the hyperpyrexia syndrome.
- Reserpine and guanethidine may be useful in thyroid crises resistant to propranolol.
- Plasmapheresis has been used successfully to remove excess thyroid hormones in resistant thyrotoxicosis.

Avoid

Drugs known to increase free T_3 and T_4 concentrations, notably: NSAIDs, heparin, furosemide, phenytoin, carbemazepine, benzodiazepines.

Pitfalls of thyrotoxic crisis

- Mortality is increased with failure to recognize the syndrome early. Differential diagnosis includes malignant hyperpyrexia syndromes (including illicit drug reactions) and severe sepsis. Supportive measures are common to all diagnoses.
- Avoid administering iodine-containing medications prior to initial doses of a thionamide.
- Avoid administration of medications with the potential to exacerbate the thyrotoxicosis (listed above).
- Patients may not have displayed all the signs of thyrotoxicosis prior to the thyroid storm being triggered.

Prognosis

Thyrotoxic crisis is rare, and delay in its recognition exacerbates the mortality. Once the crisis is under control, the patient's outcome depends on co-morbidities associated with the storm and definitive treatment of the underlying thyroid disease.

Further reading

Duggal J, Singh S, Kuchinic P, *et al.* Utility of esmolol in thyroid crisis. *Can J Clin Pharmacol* 2006; 13: 292–5.

Geffner DL, Hershman JM. Beta-adrenergic blockade for the treatment of hyperthyroidism *Am J Med* 1992; 93: 61–8.

Nayak B, Burman K. Thyrotoxicosis and thyroid storm. *Endocrinol Metab Clin North Am* 2006; 35: 663–86.

Parmar MS, Thyrotoxic atrial fibrillation. *Med Gen Med* 2005; 7: 74.

Tajiri J, Katsuya H, Kiyokawa T, *et al.* Successful treatment of thyrotoxic crisis with plasma exchange. *Crit Care Med* 1984; 12: 536–7.

Tietgens ST, Leinung MC. Thyroid storm. *Med Clin North Am* 1995; 79: 169–84.

Tsatsoulis A, Johnson EO, Kalogera CH, *et al.* The effect of thyrotoxicosis on adrenocartical reserve. *Eur J Endocrinol* 2000; 142: 231–5.

Thyroid emergencies: myxoedema coma

Myxoedema coma is the extreme decompensated form of hypothyroidism associated with one or more organ system dysfunction. This may include but does not demand deterioration in mental status. Many patients have neither non-pitting oedema nor coma. It is rare, but can have a very high mortality rate of 50–60% if recognized late. It presents at any age and in either sex, but is most common in winter in elderly women.

Pathogenesis

Although a number of patients will have a history of thyroid disease, radioiodine therapy or surgical thyroidectomy causing primary thyroid failure, many will have idiopathic primary hypothyroidism. Serum T_3 and T_4 are suppressed and TSH increased. The magnitude of changes does not correlate well with clinical presentation and can be very difficult to interpret in critical illness. More rarely (5%) patients will have hypothalamic or pituitary disease causing secondary thyroid failure

Precipitating factors

- Previously undiagnosed hypothyroidism
- Extreme cold weather
- Sepsis (pneumonia, UTIs)
- Trauma
- Cardiac or cerebrovascular events
- Drugs with antithyroid actions (e.g. amiodarone)
- CNS depressant drugs (including anaesthesia).
- Iatrogenic (i.e. failure to reinstate thyroid hormone replacement during hospitalization)

The diagnosis of hypothyroidism in critically ill patients is fraught with difficulty. Severe sepsis and a number of drugs (e.g. phenytoin, dopamine, corticosteroids and furosemide) interfere with thyroid hormone concentrations and assays

Clinical presentation

The clinical presentation of myxoedema coma is often non-specific, making the diagnosis difficult, and a high index of suspicion is required.

Three major features:

- Altered mental state: may range from apathy, neglect, decreased intellectual function to confusion, delirium or coma
- Hypothermia
- Clinical features of hypothyroidism.

History

There may be a history of prior thyroid disease, long-term thyroxine replacement therapy, previous thyroid surgery or radioiodine therapy.

Symptoms

- Hypothermia <35.5°C (may be profound, <30°C)
- Lethargy
- Cognitive dysfunction
- Confusion/depression/psychosis
- Those of a concurrent infection/precipitating cause.
- Anorexia/nausea
- Abdominal pain
- Urinary retention

Signs

- Neurological: Llethargy, altered level of consciousness, focal neurology, seizures, coma
- Cardiovascular: bradycardia, hypotension, cool peripheries, shock
- Respiratory: decreased respiratory rate, macroglossia, nasopharyngeal and laryngeal oedema
- GI: distended abdomen, absent bowel sounds, paralytic ileus, megacolon, dysphagia, aspiration
- Renal: urinary retention (bladder atony), oliguria
- Infection: signs of infection may be absent or masked because of hypothyroidism, but infection should always be suspected

Investigations

- Thyroid tunction tests. All patients with myxoedema coma have low free T_4 and T_3 blood concentrations
  - Primary hypothyroidism: low T_4 and T_3, high TSH
  - Secondary (pituitary dysfunction): low T_4 and T_3, low/low-normal TSH
  - Sick euthyroid: low or normal TSH, very low free T_3, low or normal free T_4, increased inactive rT_3
- Hypoglycaemia
- FBC: normocytic anaemia and leucopenia
- Clinical chemistry: hyponatraemia, hypophosphataemia, increased LDH and CK, hypercholesterolaemia
- Blood cultures
- ABG: hypoxaemia, hypercapnia and lactic acidosis.
- Urine microscopy and culture
- Urine sodium and osmolality: Na^+ is normal or increased, urine osmolality is increased relative to plasma osmolality

CXE: cardiomegaly and pleural effusions

ECG: slow rate, low voltage, prolonged QT and T wave inversion/flattening, conduction blockade.

Immediate management

NB: this is a medical emergency requiring admission to intensive care for complex multi-organ support.

Ventilatory support

- Oxygen
- Intubation and ventilation. Indications include: hypoventilation, hypoxia, respiratory and metabolic acidosis, airway obstruction (macroglossia and laryngeal oedema), reduced consciousness and precipitating respiratory infections.

NB: some patients may require ventilatory support for a prolonged period (several weeks)

Cardiovascular resuscitation

Hypotension and low cardiac output states are common.

- Intravascular volume is decreased by 10–20% despite an overall increase in total body fluid and sodium.
- Fluid resuscitation should be guided by central venous and cardiac output monitoring. The floatation of a pulmonary artery catheter may be warranted in cases complicated by cardiac disease
- Fluids should be warmed.
- Vasopressors and inotropes are required to maintain perfusion pressures and cardiac output. Resistance to β-adrenergic agents is common.

- Adrenal function is impaired. Give hydrocortisone 100mg IV early, at the initiation of therapy, followed by 50–100mg every 8h or 10mg/h hour continuous IV infusion.

NB: cardiovascular resuscitation can be complex because of the severity of both the metabolic derangement and concomitant cardiac disease. Give corticosteroids.

Warming

Hypothermia is common and may be profound. A low temperature thermometer is required for accurate recordings. Patients require warm fluids, warm inspired gases and external warming, e.g. warming blanket to achieve a temperature >34°C. Normothermia may not be achieved until thyroid hormones are restored.

NB: active warming will cause peripheral vascular dilatation and hypotension requiring increased fluid and vasopressor administration.

Electrolytes

Sodium (Na^+)

Hyponatraemia is common, caused by a failure to excrete excess water and may be severe (<120mmol/l). Correction should not exceed 12mmol/L/24h.

- 0.9% Saline is adequate replacement; hypertonic saline is not indicated.
- Once fluid resuscitation is complete, water restriction is usually sufficient to correct Na^+

Glucose

Hypoglycaemia can be severe, and requires early recognition and treatment.

- 25g IV glucose followed by an infusion (20–50% glucose) via central venous access, titrated to maintain normoglycaemia.

Thyroid hormones

Patients undoubtedly require thyroid hormone replacement to recover, but the optimum regimen remains controversial. Replacement is best achieved gradually; rapid replacement has been associated with sudden death from cardiac complications. In uncomplicated hypothyroidism, the agent of choice is oral T_4. In critically ill patients, oral T_4 may be inadequately absorbed and the peripheral conversion of T_4 to T_3 is markedly decreased. IV T_4 is not available in the UK. T_3 provides a more rapid correction of thyroid hormone function. Gradual replacement is recommended, and the following is a suggested regimen.

- T_3: initial IV dose 10–20mcg followed by 10mcg every 8–12h or a continuous IV infusion 20mcg/day, until the patient is established on an oral T_4 regimen.
- T_4: initial oral dose 250mcg, followed by 100mcg 24h later and 50mcg daily thereafter
- Adjust dosages according to clinical and laboratory findings.

NB: higher doses of hormones cannot be justified by the current literature. Although more rapid correction may be tolerated by young patients, the risk of adverse cardiovascular events is significant in the elderly, and mortality is increased.

Additional measures

- NG tube—to prevent gastric dilation and aspiration (essential in patients with reduced level of consciousness)
- Broad-spectrum antibiotics if infection is suspected
- Insert a bladder catheter

Pitfalls of myxoedema

- Adrenal insufficiency is a frequent association
- Hypoglycaemia must not be missed
- Warming may precipitate hypotension
- High dose thyroid hormone replacement may be complicated by serious cardiac events
- Patients do not absorb oral medications

Prognosis

Myxoedema coma is the rare extreme of a common condition. Diagnosis is often difficult, and a high index of suspicion is required. However, with best care, mortality can be decreased from 60%–25%.

Further reading

De Groot LJ, Dangerous dogmas in medicine: the nonthyroidal illness syndrome. *J Clin Endocrinol Metab* 1999; 84: 151–64.

Jordan RM, Myxedema coma. Pathophysiology, therapy, and factors affecting prognosis. *Med Clin North Am* 1995; 79: 185–94.

Kwaku MP, Burman KD, Myxedema coma, *J Intensive Care Med* 2007; 22: 224–32.

Peeters RP, Wouters PJ, Kaptein E, *et al.* Reduced activation and increased inactivation of thyroid hormone in tissues of critically ill patients. *J Clin Endocrinol Metab* 2003; 88: 3202–11.

Rodríguez I, Fluiters E, Pérez-Méndez LF, *et al.* Factors associated with mortality of patients with myxoedema coma: propective study in 11 cases treated in a single institution. *J Endocrinol* 2004; 180: 347-350.

Wartofsy L. Myxedema coma. *Endocrinol Metab Clin North Am* 2006; 35; 687–98.

Hypoadrenal crisis

Hypoadrenal crisis is a life-threatening condition that is difficult to diagnose, but easy to treat. The critically ill population are at higher risk, and therefore a high index of suspicion is appropriate.

Causes

A crisis can be precipitated *de novo* by acute failure of the hypothalamus, pituitary or adrenal glands, or as a result of smaller change in function of any part of the hypothalamo-pituitary–adrenal (HPA) axis on a background of chronic insufficiency. The causes are divided up on the basis of the organ they affect into: primary (adrenal), secondary (pituitary) and tertiary (hypothalamus).

Primary (Addison's disease)

Autoimmune adrenalitis

70–90% of cases are caused by autoimmune conditions. Polyglandular autoimmune syndrome I and II each include autoimmune adrenalitis (predominantly female). Autoimmune adrenalitis as an isolated autoimmune adrenal insufficiency is more common in males.

Infectious causes

As described by Thomas Addison, most cases were caused by TB with bilateral adrenal infiltration and destruction. Now this accounts for 7–20%. Active TB seeds to the adrenals via haematogenous spread. Disseminated fungal disease from histoplasmosis or paracoccidioidomycosis is a significant cause of adrenal failure in high risk areas. Patients who have developed AIDS are at risk of developing necrotizing adrenalitits secondary to CMV infection and infiltration by *Mycobacterium avium-intracellulare*, cryptococci or Kaposi's sarcoma.

Metastatic cancer

Metastatic inflitration of the adrenal glands is common, and 40–60% of patients with disseminated lung or breast cancer have adrenal deposits. Clinical manifestations are rare as most of the adrenal cortex must be destroyed before symptoms occur.

Adrenal haemorrhage/infarction

Risk factors:

- Stress states, especially sepsis. Haemorrhage is classically associated with meningococcal septicaemia (Waterhouse–Friderichsen syndrome). Similar findings from *Streptococcus pneumoniae*, *Neisseria gonorrhoeae*, *Escherichia coli*, *Haemophilus influenzae* and *Staphylococcus aureus* have also been reported.
- Anticoagulation use, especially heparin. Thrombocytopaenic patients in their middle/old age are at high risk
- Hypercoaguable states, especially antiphospholipid syndrome.

Drugs

There are a small number of drugs which inhibit cortisol production. These include aminoglutethimide, etomidate, ketoconazole, metyrapone and suramin. These agents are relatively safe in patients with normal HPA axis function.

Infiltrations

Both granulomatous and amyloid infiltrations can affect the adrenal.

Others

Irradiation of the adrenals. Iron deposits of haemochromatosis.

Secondary/tertiary

Acute failure of the pituitary or hypothalamus is rare. Causes include: neoplasms, haemorrhage, infarction, radiation damage and granulomatous infiltration.

Prolonged administration of glucocorticoids leads to HPA axis suppression. These patients are therefore at risk of developing a crisis if there is inadequate replacement and/or other causes of hypoadrenalism. Typically suppression occurs in regimes of >7.5mg prednisolone (or equivalent) daily for >2 weeks.

Clinical approach

Hypoadrenal crisis usually presents with shock. The shock is usually high output and dependent on vasopressors. It is often initially misdiagnosed as septic shock.

The clinical approach should be tailored to identify likely causes and to gather clues of preceding adrenal insufficiency as these will guide treatment after the initial crisis has been dealt with.

History—key points

Potential causes

- Severe stress: sepsis, burns, trauma, surgery
- Other autoimmune conditions, such as hypothyroidism or gonadal failure
- Foreign travel/potential contact with infectious diseases
- Steroid use: length of treatment/cessation/reduction
- Anticoagulation
- Drugs which interfere with steroid metabolism or synthesis (ketoconazole, etomidate, metayapone, phenytoin and suramin)
- Inherited clotting disorders
- Previous history of cancer
- Pregnancy
- Sudden onset flank or epigastric pain (suggestive of adrenal haemmorhage)

Symptoms of preceding adrenal insufficiency should be identified; these are very vague and include:

- Weakness/tiredness
- Anorexia
- GI symptoms: nausea, vomiting, constipation, abdominal pain, diarrhoea
- Salt craving
- Postural dizziness

Examination

The patient will have signs of high output shock. These obviously depend on the clinical situation and the treatments already underway.

In primary hypoadrenalism there will be hyperpigmentation of the skin that has been exposed to light, friction or pressure as a result of increased concentrations of adrenocorticotrophic hormone (ACTH).

Investigations

Haematology and biochemistry

There is usually a slight neutropenia with relative eosinophilia.

Hyponatraemia and hyperkalaemia are often found. Pure Addison's disease usually has a normal CRP and procalcitonin.

Hypoglycaemia is often a feature, especially if the defect is primary and so there is a high serum concentration of ACTH.

Endocrine

Measure initial cortisol and ACTH levels.

Primary adrenal failure—inappropriately low serum cortisol and very high serum concentrations of ACTH. In secondary or tertiary failure both levels would be inappropriately low. Assays for ACTH can be unreliable and results are slow to arrive, and therefore it is necessary to perform a stimulation test.

The short ACTH stimulation test can be run alongside emergency treatment for hypoadrenal crisis as it is not affected by dexamethasone. It provides a quick easy test for identifying most cases of adrenal insufficiency. A 250mcg IV bolus of ACTH (Synachthen) should be given and blood taken for cortisol at 30 and 60min. Cortisol concentration peaks of <18mcg/dl at 30 or 60min indicate that there is adrenal insufficiency.

This test has been shown in a large meta-analysis to have a 95% specificity and 97.5% sensitivity for primary hypoadrenalism. However, the sensitivity for secondary adrenal insufficiency was only 57%. Therefore, a positive result establishes the diagnosis of hypoadrenalism and a negative result can rule out primary hypoadrenalism, but not secondary or tertiary. Further tests such as the insulin-induced hypoglycaemia or the metyrapone test will be required to exclude secondary or tertiary hypoadrenal insufficiency.

ECG

There may be changes of hyperkalaemia

Radiology

Plain chest film may show a small heart. Further cross-sectional imaging can be undertaken in order to help reveal the cause of the event. Adrenal calcification can often be seen in tuberculous and fungal infiltration, and enlarged adrenals are seen in adrenal haemorrhage.

Management

Treatment should be instigated in cases where clinical suspicion of a crisis is high, and should not be delayed in order to make a diagnosis.

The aims of immediate treatment are to correct:

- Hypotension
- Electrolyte imbalance
- Cortisol deficiency

Initial treatment

1. Large bore IV access should be obtained and bloods taken for electrolytes, glucose, cortisol and ACTH.
2. 0.9% Saline should be infused quickly; 2 or 3l may be required. The patient must be monitored for signs of overload, preferably with CVP monitoring. Blood glucose should be monitored and corrected with dextrose run alongside the saline as necessary.
3. IV glucocorticoid must be given. The usual choice is 10mg of dexamethasone as it does not interfere with the cortisol measurements. Hydrocortisone can be substituted for dexamethasone after the first dose using the following regime:
    - Day 1 hydrocortisone 100mg 6–8 hourly
    - Day 2 hydrocortisone 100mg – 8 hourly
    - Day 3 hydrocortisone 100mg – 12 hourly
    - Day 4 maintenance regime.
4. ACTH (Synacthen) should be given at the same time for the short ACTH stimulation test, as detailed under investigations.
5. Further supportive measures and monitoring should be introduced as required.

There is no need to give mineralocorticoids acutely as the saline infused replaces the sodium and mineralocorticoids take several days to act.

Subsequent treatment

IV saline should be continued for ~24–48h at a slower rate. Once the saline infusion has finished, it is necessary to start mineralocorticoid replacement with fludrocortisone 0.1mg daily.

The cause of the adrenal crisis should be found and treated if possible. This may involve more extensive hormonal investigations.

Further reading

Addison T. On the constitutional and local effects of disease of the supra-renal capsules. London: Highley, 1855.

Dorin R, Qualls C, Crapo L. Diagnosis of adrenal insufficiency. *Ann Intern Med* 2003; 139: 194–204.

Falorni A,, Laureti S, De Bellis A, et al. Italian Addison network study: update of diagnostic criteria for the classification of primary adrenal insufficiency. *J Clin Endocinol Metab* 2003; 89: 1598–604.

Vedig A. Adrenocortical Insufficiency. In: Oh's intensive care manual. London: Butterworth Heinemann, 2004: 575–82.

Chapter 25

Poisoning

Chapter contents

Management of acute poisoning

Acute poisoning remains one of the most common medical emergencies, 5–10% of hospital medical admissions. In the majority of cases, the drug ingestion is intentional, but the in-hospital mortality remains low (<0.5%). There are specific antidotes available for a small number of poisons and drugs; in most intoxications, basic supportive care is the main requirement and recovery follows. Internet-based information services such as Toxbase are useful: http://www.spib.axl.co.uk.

General principles

The general principles of the management of poisoned patients are diagnosis, clinical examination and resuscitation, investigations, drug manipulation, specific measures and continued supportive care. In the more acute situations, these actions often have to be carried out simultaneously.

Airway and ventilation

In unconscious patients, tracheal intubation and airway protection is almost always necessary—a test is when a patient tolerates insertion of an oropharyngeal airway then intubate. Inadequate spontaneous ventilation, determined clinically or by blood gas analysis, obviously requires ventilatory support. Venous access should be established, and basic observations, including blood pressure, pulse rate, peripheral perfusion and urine output should be recorded.

Clinical examination

Full examination and look particularly for needle marks or evidence of previous self-harm. When no history is available, the diagnosis depends upon excluding other common causes of coma (such as ICH, intracranial infection or diabetic comas). Specific attention should be paid to the temperature, pupil size, respiratory and heart rate, as these may help to narrow the list of potential toxins.

Investigations

Initial investigations include:

- Urinalysis—with a sample kept for later analysis if required (rapid reaction dipsticks are available to screen for common drugs of abuse/recreational drugs; however, their reliability questionable).
- Basic biochemistry—significant renal insufficiency may alter drug elimination.
- ABG analysis—metabolic and/or respiratory acidosis are most common. Metabolic alkaloses are unusual.
- Anion gap = $([Na^+] + [K^+]) - ([Cl^-] + [HCO_3^-])$—it is normally 10–14. Ethanol, methanol, ethylene glycol, metformin, cyanide, isoniazid or salicylates are the most frequent causes of a high anion gap metabolic acidosis.
- Osmolal gap—the difference between the laboratory measured osmolality (Om) and the calculated osmolality (Oc). $Oc = 2(Na_+ + K_+) + Urea + Glucose$. The osmolal gap is normally <10. Causes of a raised osmolal gap are ethanol, methanol and ethylene glycol.
- CXR—inhalation of gastric contents is not uncommon.
- Drug levels—are rarely helpful except in paracetamol, salicylates, iron, digoxin and lithium poisonings.

Gut decontamination

Emesis

Ipecacuanha-induced emesis is no longer recommended since it is often ineffective at removing significant quantities of poison from the stomach, and it limits the use of activated charcoal (AC).

Gastric lavage

Unless performed within 1h of drug ingestion, it is no longer recommended. The amount of poison removed is insignificant, and lavage may only propel unabsorbed poison into the small intestine. Prior intubation is essential when laryngeal competence is absent or doubtful, especially because, in the majority of overdoses, pulmonary aspiration is more lethal than the ingested drug. Gastric lavage is contraindicated in ingestions of corrosives, caustics and acids; oesophageal or gastric perforation may occur.

Activated charcoal

AC remains the first-line treatment for most acute poisonings. Owing to its large surface area and porous structure, it is highly effective at adsorbing many toxins, with few exceptions. Exceptions include elemental metals, pesticides, strong acids and alkalis, and cyanide. It should be given swiftly to all patients who present within 1h of ingestion, although it is also acceptable to administer it after 1h if it follows an overdose of a substance that slows gastric emptying (e.g. opioids, tricyclic antidepressants (TCAs)). AC is given in 50g doses for adults and 1g/kg for children. It commonly causes vomiting; therefore, consider giving an antiemetic prior to administration. Repeated doses (4 hourly intervals) of AC can increase the elimination of some drugs, interrupting their enteroenteric and enterohepatic circulation. These include:

- carbamazepine
- theophylline
- digoxin
- quinine
- phenobarbitone
- dapsone
- some sustained-release preparations.

Whole bowel irrigation

Whole bowel irrigation involves administration of non-absorbable polyethylene glycol solution to cause a liquid stool and reduce drug absorption by physically forcing contents rapidly through the GI tract. It may have a role in treating large ingestions of drugs that are not absorbed by AC, such as large ingestions of iron or lithium, drug-filled packets/condoms ('body packers'), and ingestions of sustained-release or enteric-coated drugs.

Enhancing drug elimination

In the overwhelming majority of patients who present after an overdose, gut decontamination techniques and supportive care are all that is required. In a limited number of acute poisonings it may be necessary to consider methods to enhance elimination.

Urinary alkalinization

Urinary alkalinization may be useful for serious poisonings with:

- Salicylates
- Phenobarbitone (with repeated dose AC)
- Chlorpropamide
- Methotrexate

IV sodium bicarbonate (>1.26%) is infused to maintain a neutral balance and attempt to achieve a urine pH of ~7.5. The term urine alkalinization emphasizes that urine pH manipulation is the prime objective of treatment. It should be considered the treatment of choice for moderate to severe salicylate poisoning. Care must be taken to ensure the potassium does not fall rapidly.

Extracorporeal techniques

Extracorporeal techniques should be considered when there are clinical features of severe toxicity and failure to respond to full supportive care, coupled with poisoning by a drug that can potentially be cleared. Impairment of the normal route of elimination of the compound may also influence the decision. Haemoperfusion is rarely performed in most ICUs, and intermittent haemodialysis is often confined to renal units. Consequently, the use of continuous haemofiltration with or without dialysis, using filtration rates of >50–100ml/kg/h, is likely to be as equally effective.

Specific therapy of some common or difficult poisonings

Amphetamines (including 'Ecstasy' MDMA)

Clinical features

Symptoms of mild overdose include sweating, dry mouth and anxiety. Although the majority of Ecstasy patients are dehydrated, a proportion have hyponatraemia from drinking excess water. More severe features include hypertonia, hyper-reflexia, hallucinations and hypertension. Supraventricular dysrhythmias may follow, with coma, convulsions and the risk of haemorrhagic stroke. A hyperthermic syndrome may develop, leading to rhabdomyolysis, acute renal failure, DIC and MOF.

Treatment

AC should be considered up to 1h post-ingestion. Benzodiazepines are useful for agitated or psychotic patients and have a central effect in reducing tachycardia, hypertension and hyperpyrexia. If benzodiazepines fail to control hypertension, α-blockers, labetalol or direct vasodilators should be started. Hypertonic saline should be considered in severe hyponatraemia. Hyperthermia should be treated with cold fluids, physical cooling measures and, in the presence of convulsions, sedation, paralysis and ventilation. Dantrolene has been used in the treatment of Ecstasy-related hyperpyrexia, but it is better to direct treatment at the central mechanisms of thermoregulation.

Cocaine

Clinical features

Features of severe intoxication include hyper-reflexia, drowsiness and convulsions. Severe hypertension may cause ICH, and coronary artery spasm may result in MI or ventricular arrhythmias; fatalities generally occur early. Hyperthermia associated with rhabdomyolysis, renal failure and DIC may also occur.

Treatment

The toxic dose is variable and depends upon tolerance, presence of other drugs and route of administration, but ingestion of >1g can be fatal. Blood pressure and ECG monitoring should be instituted early and AC administered within 1h of ingestion. Benzodiazepines are used for agitated or psychotic patients and have a central effect in reducing tachycardia, hypertension and hyperpyrexia. If benzodiazepines fail to control hypertension, β-blockers, labetalol or vasodilators such as nitrates should be started. β-blockers are controversial and should be used with caution because of the risk of unopposed α stimulation. Hyperthermia should be treated in the standard manner (see Amphetamines above).

Household chemicals: bleach

Clinical features

Bleach usually contains 5–10% sodium hypochlorite and causes moderate irritation of the mucous membranes and oesophagus. Small accidental ingestions rarely cause more than nausea and vomiting; however, adults who deliberately ingest large quantities can develop oesophageal ulceration, haematemesis or perforation.

Treatment

Severe poisoning in adults requires IV fluids and endoscopy to reveal the extent of the injury.

Carbon monoxide

Clinical features

Neurological signs vary from mild confusion through to seizures and coma. A history of loss of consciousness may be the only indicator of significant poisoning. ST segment changes may be present on the ECG. In the absence of respiratory depression or aspiration, PaO_2 will be normal. It is essential that SaO_2 is measured directly by a co-oximeter, and not calculated. Cherry-pink skin is infrequently seen; cyanosis is far more common. Coma and/or carboxy-Hb levels >40% always indicate serious poisoning (smokers may have up to 10% carboxy-Hb without deleterious effects); however, delayed deterioration can occur in their absence.

Treatment

High flow oxygen (up to 100%) should be administered and continued until the carboxy-Hb level is <5%—this can take up to 24h. Hyperbaric oxygen (HBO), although often used, remains controversial. Trials of HBO vs normobaric oxygen have not shown statistical benefit in reducing neurological sequelae at 1 month. Considering the frequent logistical difficulties in transferring unconscious patients to an HBO centre, it cannot be recommended currently.

Methanol and ethylene glycol

Clinical features

Methanol and ethylene glycol are relatively non-toxic, but their ingestion is a medical emergency because of their metabolism (following a latent period of 12–18h) to formic and glycolic acid, respectively. These metabolites account for the metabolic acidosis, ocular toxicity, renal failure, coma, convulsions and mortality that are occasionally seen. Mild features include dizziness, drowsiness and abdominal pain. The osmolal and the anion gap are increased.

Treatment

AC does not adsorb either toxin. The metabolic acidosis should be treated with sodium bicarbonate and the serum electrolytes measured. Ethanol prevents formation of the toxic metabolites and historically has been the most common treatment. Yet, ethanol dosing is complex, requires repeated monitoring and has adverse effects. The recent introduction of fomepizole (4-methypyrazole), although expensive, has significantly simplified the treatment of ethylene glycol and methanol poisoning, and is now strongly recommended as first-line therapy. It has been shown to be safe and effective, with minimal adverse effects, and potentially prevents the need for haemodialysis in patients presenting with visual disturbances or severe acidosis. If the ethylene glycol blood concentration is >20mg/dl or if there is a good history of ethylene glycol/methanol ingestion with an osmolal gap >10, then patients should receive it. Folinic acid should also be given since it enhances the metabolism of formic acid.

Organophosphorus poisoning

Clinical features

Organophosphorus compounds have numerous complex actions; however, their major effect is inhibition of cholinesterase enzymes (especially acetylcholinesterase). This leads to accumulation of acetylcholine at both nicotinic and muscarinic receptors, and in the CNS. The onset, severity and duration of clinical features are dependent on the route of exposure and the agent involved. Early muscarinic clinical features include vomiting, abdominal pain, diarrhoea, miosis, diaphoresis, sweating, bronchoconstriction and hypersalivation. Respiratory muscle weakness, drowsiness and coma occur later, but are the major cause of death in the severely poisoned. In general, clinical features are more helpful than red cell cholinesterase measurements in determining toxicity, but measurements do confirm the diagnosis.

Treatment

If the compound has been ingested, gastric lavage can be attempted within 1h, followed by AC. Convulsions should be controlled by benzodiazepines, and atropine (sometimes in very large doses—up to 30mg in 24h) reduces many of the unpleasant symptoms. Cholinesterase reactivators such as pralidoxime are also helpful in symptomatic patients if given early, and duration of therapy is determined by clinical response.

Paracetamol

Clinical features

Nausea and vomiting may be the only features present in the first 24h. In normal adults, doses >10g may exceed the ability of hepatic glutathione to conjugate the toxic metabolite. Plasma concentrations >200mg/l at 4h or ≥50mg/l at 12h are usually associated with hepatic damage. Although severe hepatic injury has a 10% mortality, the majority of patients recover within 1–2 weeks.

Treatment

Measure drug levels, noting the time from ingestion, and administer AC as soon as possible even if >4h after overdose. NAC should be given in all patients with significant levels (see www.patient.co.uk/showdoc/40001390/). Treatment should begin at lower levels for those considered to be high risk (such as those who regularly consume alcohol, or patients taking enzyme-inducing drugs such as phenytoin, carbamazepine, phenobarbitone or rifampicin, or patients with conditions causing glutathione depletion, such as HIV, eating disorders, malnutrition or cystic fibrosis. Although an ingestion–treatment interval of <10h gives the best results, NAC can be given >24h from ingestion with clinical benefit. Expert opinion should be sought early on from a regional centre if liver failure is progressive since liver transplantation may become necessary.

Salicylates (aspirin)

Clinical features

Moderate toxicity occurs with serum concentrations 500–750mg/l (3600–5500μmol/l), and severe toxicity with concentrations >750mg/l. Serum concentrations alone do not determine prognosis. The elimination half-life increases significantly with increasing concentrations. Small reductions in pH produce large increases in non-ionized salicylate, which then penetrates tissues. Tinnitus, deafness, diaphoresis, pyrexia, hypoglycaemia, haematemesis, hyperventilation and hypokalaemia may all occur. Coma, hyperpyrexia, pulmonary oedema and acidaemia are reported as more common in fatal cases, which present late.

Treatment

Multiple dose AC may be effective, but is not established. Vitamin K and glucose are used to correct hypoprothrombinaemia and hypoglycaemia. Urinary alkalinization decreases the amount of non-ionized drug available to enter tissues, but is hazardous and should only be used for the most severe ingestions. Extracorporeal techniques are very effective in removing salicylates and correcting acid–base disturbance, and should be considered for severe cases.

Sedatives: benzodiazepines

Clinical features

Overdose is common, but clinical features are not usually severe unless complicated by other CNS depressant drugs (such as alcohol), pre-existing disease or the extremes of age. Toxicity commonly produces drowsiness, dysarthria, ataxia and nystagmus; however, agitation and confusion can occur.

Treatment

AC can be given if patients present within 1h of ingestion, yet supportive treatment is usually all that is required. Flumazenil is a specific antagonist, but its brief duration of action limits its use to diagnostic purposes. Moreover, flumazenil may cause other symptoms in patients who have ingested a cocktail of drugs (e.g. precipitation of fits in patients co-ingesting TCAs), consequently administration risks increasing morbidity and mortality.

Sedatives: opioids

Clinical features

Overdose is characterized by pinpoint pupils, drowsiness, shallow breathing and ultimately respiratory failure.

Treatment

AC may be effective for oral ingestions, otherwise treatment is supportive. Naloxone 0.1–0.4mg IV can be given by bolus and if there is an inadequate response, repeat doses may be required. Intubation and mechanical ventilation are required if respiratory failure is not rapidly reversed by naloxone.

Tricyclic antidepressants

Clinical features

TCAs are the leading cause of death from overdose in patients arriving at hospital alive, and account for ~50% of all overdose-related adult ICU admissions. Features include anticholinergic effects such as warm dry skin, tachycardia, blurred vision, dilated pupils and urinary retention. Severe features include respiratory depression, reduced conscious level and cardiac arrhythmias, fits and hypotension. Arrhythmias may be predicted by a QRS duration >100ms on the ECG; a QRS duration of >160ms increases risk of seizures. All forms of rhythm and conduction disturbance have been described, and are not necessarily predicted by the ECG. Toxicity is worsened by acidaemia, hypotension and hyperthermia.

Treatment

Continuous cardiac monitoring is essential, and multiple dose AC should be considered. Increasing arterial pH to ≥7.45 significantly reduces the available free drug, and this may avoid TCA toxicity. Mild hyperventilation and 8.4% sodium bicarbonate in 50mmol aliquots achieves this strategy, and may improve outcome. Bicarbonate should probably be given in all cases of QRS prolongation (even in the absence of metabolic acidosis), malignant arrhythmias, hypotension or metabolic acidosis. If arrhythmias occur, avoid Class 1a agents; lidocaine may be best. Benzodiazepines are the drug of choice for sedation, treatment of seizures and prevention of the emergence of delirium.

Further reading

American Academy of Clinical Toxicology; European Association of Poison Control Centres and Clinical Toxicologists. Position statement: gastric lavage. *Clin Toxicol* 1997; 35: 711–9.

American Academy of Clinical Toxicology; European Association of Poison Control Centres and Clinical Toxicologists. Position statement: whole bowel irrigation. *Clin Toxicol* 1997; 35: 753–62.

American Academy of Clinical Toxicology; European Association of Poison Control Centres and Clinical Toxicologists. Position statement and practice guidelines on the use of multi-dose activated charcoal in the treatment of acute poisoning. *Clin Toxicol* 1999; 37: 731–51.

American Academy of Clinical Toxicology and European Association of Poisons Centres and Clinical Toxicologists. Position paper: ipecac syrup. *J Toxicol Clin Toxicol* 2004; 42: 133–43.

Barceloux DG, Bond GR, Krenzelok EP, *et al.* American Academy of Clinical Toxicology practice guidelines on the methanol poisoning. *J Toxicol Clin Toxicol* 2002; 40: 415–46.

Buckley NA, Isbister GK, Stokes B, *et al.* Hyperbaric oxygen for carbon monoxide poisoning: a systematic review and critical analysis of the evidence. *Toxicol Rev* 2005; 24: 75–92.

Chyka PA, Seger D, Krenzelok EP, *et al.* American Academy of Clinical Toxicology; European Association of Poisons Centres and Clinical Toxicologists. Position paper: single-dose activated charcoal. *Clin Toxicol* 2005; 43: 61–87.

Hall AP, Henry JA. Acute toxic effects of 'Ecstasy' (MDMA) and related compounds: overview of pathophysiology and clinical management. *Br J Anaesth* 2006; 96: 678–85.

Proudfoot AT, Krenzelok EP, Vale JA. Position paper on urine alkalinisation. *J Toxicol Clin Toxicol* 2004; 42: 1–26.

Seger DL. Flumazenil—treatment or toxin. *J Toxicol Clin Toxicol* 2004; 42: 209–16.

Chapter 26

Shock

Chapter contents

Shock: definition and diagnosis

Shock, or acute circulatory failure, defines a state in which the delivery of oxygen and nutrients to the tissue is insufficient to meet basal metabolic needs, leading to tissue hypoxia, and, if persistent, to MOF and death. Shock results from tissue hypoperfusion and microcirculatory dysfunction, and should thus not be restricted to hypotension. Although frequent, hypotension is not mandatory for the diagnosis of shock. In the absence of hypotension, increased lactate levels may indicate tissue hypoperfusion and can be used to diagnose shock (at least at its initiation).

Clinical findings

Hypotension

Hypotension is defined by an SBP <90mm Hg or a MAP <65mm Hg, or requirement for vasopressor agents to maintain blood pressure above these levels.

Signs of perfusion alteration to the organs

Alteration in mental state: confusion, agitation, sometimes coma.

Oliguria: urine output <0.5ml/kg/h. Requires at least 1h to be diagnosed, and sometimes longer when the bladder is not catheterized.

Skin vasoconstriction (clammy skin): may be absent in distributive shock states.

Biological signs

Metabolic acidosis is due to excess of hydrogen ions due to ATP hydrolysis occurring during anaerobic metabolism.

Hyperlactataemia also occurs in response to hypoxia. In the absence of oxygen, pyruvate cannot enter the Krebs cycle and lactate is produced in large amounts. Normal values are close to 1mEq/l; values >2.0 suggest tissue hypoxia, values >4.0 are associated with a mortality rate >50%. Of note hyperlactataemia may also occur in the presence of oxygen (increased aerobic glycolysis in response to inflammatory processes) or may reflect past rather than ongoing tissue hypoxia when liver lactate clearance is decreased. In the early phases of shock, hyperlactataemia is highly suggestive of tissue hypoxia; at later stages, hyperlactataemia should be interpreted more cautiously.

Signs of organ dysfunction: decreased PaO_2, increased creatinine levels, hyperbilirubinaemia.

Increased tissue to arterial PCO_2 gradient. Tissue PCO_2 can be estimated in the stomach and in the sublingual area. An increased gradient (>10mm Hg) suggests tissue hypoperfusion. A gradient >20mm Hg may be associated with tissue hypoxia.

Classification of shock

Weil and Subin have classified shock into four categories: hypovolaemic, cardiogenic, obstructive and distributive. In this categorization of shock, the circulation is divided into its four essential components (Fig. 26.1.1):

- the vascular reservoir (hypovolaemic shock)
- the pump (cardiogenic shock)
- the conduits (obstructive shock)
- distribution of blood flow among and within the organs (distributive shock).

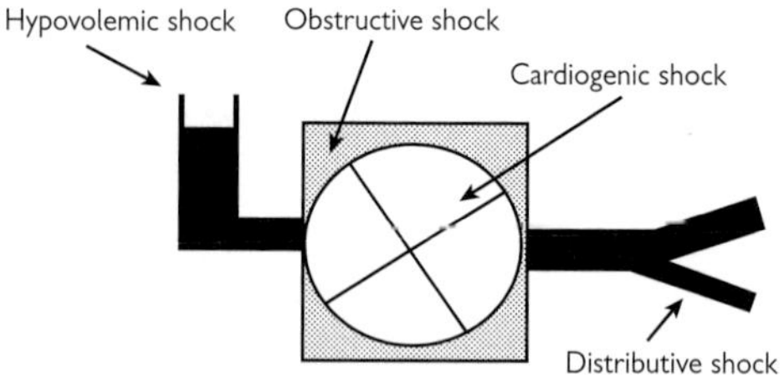

Fig. 26.1.1 The four categories of shock.

Identifying the type of shock is thus important as it helps to indicate what should be the target of the primary intervention. There may be some overlap between these presentations, as a patient with distributive shock may also present hypovolaemia and myocardial depression. These four presentations of shock cover multiple causes. Distributive shock includes septic shock, anaphylactic shock, pancreatitis and ischaemia–reperfusion injury. All these causes of distributive shock are characterized by a marked activation of inflammatory processes leading to the release of vasoactive substances.

How to diagnose the type of shock

Differentiation between the four categories of shock can be made using several haemodynamic monitoring tools, including a pulmonary artery catheter, cardiac echocardiography and pulse contour analysis. Whatever the technique used, classification of shock relies on the determination of cardiac output and evaluation of intravascular pressures or volumes (Fig. 26.1.2).

Measurement of cardiac output is essential to discriminate between the different types of shock: cardiac output and oxygen delivery are decreased (hypodynamic shock) in hypovolaemic, cardiogenic and obstructive shock, while it may be preserved and even increased in distributive shock (hyperdynamic shock).

To identify further the different components of hypodynamic shock, the determination of intravascular pressures (CVP) is essential: it is decreased in hypovolaemia, but increased in cardiogenic and obstructive shock. Of note, hypovolaemia can complicate any type of shock.

Echocardiography is mandatory to differentiate obstructive from cardiogenic shock (even though some indexes can be inferred from the pulmonary artery catheter or measurements of intravascular volumes with transpulmonary thermodilution) and to determine the exact cause of cardiogenic shock (contractility, valve disease).

The four types of shock

Hypovolaemic shock

Hypovolaemic shock is characterized by a profound reduction in blood volume. It is the most common source of shock, and can be due either to bleeding (trauma, digestive haemorrhage or other causes of blood losses) or to decreased plasma volume (dehydration most commonly due to diarrhoea or vomiting). Children are very sensitive to dehydration.

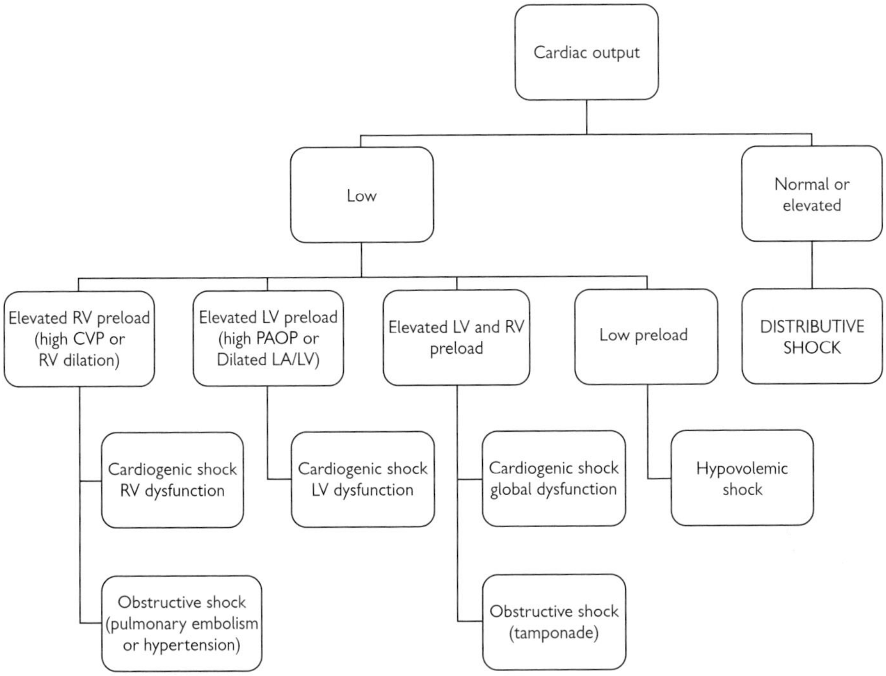

Fig. 26.1.2 The diagnostic tree.

The typical clinical presentation is a patient with hypotension, skin vasoconstriction and collapsed jugular veins.

The key haemodynamic findings are a decreased cardiac output, high systemic vascular resistances and low filling pressures. Haemoglobin can initially be maintained in haemorrhage.

Cardiogenic shock

Cardiogenic shock is due to a failure of the cardiac pump, related either to impaired contractile function or to valvular dysfunction. In addition, it can be global, affecting both right and left sides, or predominantly left or right sided. It is important to make a precise diagnosis of the cause of cardiogenic shock, as therapy may differ accordingly.

The typical clinical presentation is a patient with hypotension, skin vasoconstriction and dilated jugular veins.

Diagnosis: the haemodynamic definition of cardiogenic shock is based on the finding of a decreased and inadequate cardiac index (CI lower than $2.2 l/min/m^2$ and low SvO_2) in the presence of adequate preload and accompanied by signs of hypoperfusion (decreased blood pressure or elevated lactate levels). In this definition, it is important to evaluate cardiac output, and especially to determine that it is inadequate for metabolic needs (signs of inadequate tissue perfusion): indeed patients with chronic heart failure may present signs of decreased systolic function and dilated ventricules, but cardiac output can be preserved.

Evaluation of ventricular preload (pressure or echo measurements) is essential to rule out hypovolaemic shock, but also to differentiate right from left side dysfunction (Fig. 26.1.2). Intravascular pressures can either be invasively measured (central venous and pulmonary artery catheters) or estimated by echocardiography. Intravascular volumes can be estimated by echocardiography and transpulmonary thermodilution. Of note, the latter cannot differentiate left and right ventricular volumes.

Obstructive shock

Obstructive shock is due to obstruction of the cardiovascular system. The most common causes are PE and cardiac tamponade.

The typical clinical presentation is a patient with hypotension, skin vasoconstriction and dilated jugular veins. Pulsus paradoxus is frequent.

The typical haemodynamic presentation is a low cardiac output, high SVR, high filling pressures (right in PE, left in aortic dissection, bilateral in tamponade) and pulmonary hypertension in PE.

Echocardiography is extremely helpful to diagnose obstructive shock and its cause.

Distributive shock

Distributive shock is a complex syndrome characterized by profound cardiovascular derangements, associating a decreased vascular tone, myocardial depression, blood flow redistribution between organs and microcirculatory alterations. In addition, hypovolaemia is frequent in its early stages (fluid losses and venous blood pooling in the splanchnic area).

The typical clinical presentation is a patient with hypotension, skin vasodilation, and acrocyanosis or mottled skin.

The typical haemodynamic picture is a patient with normal to high cardiac output, low blood pressure and low indices of preload who fails to correct his haemodynamic profile after rapid volume infusion.

Further reading

Antonelli M, Levy M, Andrews PJ, *et al.* Hemodynamic monitoring in shock and implications for management: International Consensus Conference, Paris, France, 27–28 April 2006 *Intensive Care Med* 2007; 33: 575–90.

De Backer D Lactic acidosis *Intensive Care Med* 2003; 29: 699–702.

Weil MH, Shubin H. Proposed reclassification of shock states with special reference to distributive defects *Adv Exp Med Biol* 1971; 23: 13–23.

Hypovolaemic shock

Hypovolaemic shock is the most common source of shock; it often can easily be reversed, if detected early and provided its cause can be corrected.

Pathophysiology of hypovolaemic shock:

Hypovolaemic shock is due to a profound reduction in blood volume. Hypovolaemia is associated with an initial decrease in ventricular preload, but the almost immediate increase in endogenous catecholamines limits the decrease in stroke volume (by increasing contractility), while cardiac output is maintained by the compensatory increase in heart rate. The profound vasoconstriction also helps to redistribute blood volume from the peripheral to the central compartment, helping to maintain cardiac output and blood pressure. This venous constriction limits the decrease in preload by decreasing the amount of blood stored in large venous capacitance beds (mostly splanchnic veins, but also arm and leg veins). It also affects blood flow distribution, so that the limited amount of blood is redirected to the most vital organs. Blood flow to splanchnic organs, kidneys and the skin is markedly decreased, while brain and heart circulations are somewhat preserved. If hypovolaemia persists, these compensatory mechanisms are not sufficient and cardiac output and blood pressure decrease.

These compensatory mechanisms are clearly vital and beneficial in the short term, but unless the hypovolaemia is corrected they will begin to cause deleterious effects. The decrease in kidney perfusion may lead to renal damage and eventually acute tubular necrosis. Myocardial oxygen balance is threatened by the combination of tachycardia, increased contractility, and increased catecholamine levels in the context of decreased coronary perfusion (due to hypotension). This may lead to myocardial ischaemia and even to MI in patients with coronary lesions. The decrease in splanchnic perfusion may alter the gut defences and integrity, with the possibility of promoting translocation of bacteria and bacterial toxins, especially during the reperfusion phase.

Causes of hypovolaemic shock

There are many causes, ranging from bleeding (trauma, digestive haemorrhage or other causes of blood losses), to decreased plasma volume (dehydration, most commonly due to diarrhoea or vomiting) or tissue damage and fluid loss such as burns. Children are particularly sensitive to dehydration.

Clinical features

Presentation; tachycardia, skin vasoconstriction and acrocyanosis. Hypotension often occurs, but blood pressure can initially be preserved even with large fluid losses, especially in the young. Signs of tissue hypoperfusion are frequent (alteration in mental state, oliguria). Signs of dehydration or anaemia may be encountered, but these may sometimes be missing.

Key haemodynamic findings

Hypovolaemic shock is characterized by a decreased cardiac output, high SVR and low filling pressures. In patients on mechanical ventilation, large respiratory variations in pulse pressure and stroke volume can be observed. Venous O_2 saturation (mixed venous and central venous) is typically decreased. Lactic acidosis is frequent.

Haemoglobin levels can initially be maintained in haemorrhage and decrease only after initiation of fluid resuscitation or when shock is prolonged (volume mobilization from the extravascular compartment).

Therapy

Treatment includes control of the source of bleeding and fluid replacement (including red blood cell transfusions and coagulation factors). Vasopressor agents may be transiently required. Inotropic agents are usually not required, as contractility is preserved (with the exception of patients with underlying cardiac disease or heart trauma). It is recommended that therapy of haemorrhagic shock should not aim at full restoration of blood volume and blood pressure while the haemorrhage is not controlled. In bleeding patients, a systolic pressure of 90mm Hg is sufficient to preserve tissue perfusion while limiting the risk of bleeding. In bleeding patients with brain trauma, a systolic pressure of 120mm Hg should be attained to protect cerebral perfusion. Once bleeding has been stopped, resuscitation should aim at full restoration of tissue perfusion.

Vasopressor agents

Vasopressor agents should be used with caution. By improving blood pressure, these agents help to restore organ perfusion, including brain and coronary artery perfusion. The mechanism of action may mean that there is an additional increase in SVR, which may further compromise blood flow in some vascular beds (especially the skin, splanchnic region and kidneys). These agents should thus always be used at the lowest dose compatible with adequate organ perfusion, essentially buying time for correction of blood volume. Vasopressor agents should be weaned once blood volume has been restored, where possible. If vasopressor agents are still required after correction of hypovolaemia, one should think of an alternative cause of the hypotension (usually distributive shock, either from ischaemia–reperfusion or due to sepsis).

Adrenergic agents are still the most commonly used vasopressor agents. Dopamine, noradrenaline and adrenaline have variable effects on α and β receptors. Adrenaline and noradrenaline are the most potent agents. Noradrenaline has a strong and dose-dependent α effect accompanied by a weak β effect. Adrenaline has similar strong dose-dependent α and β effects. Dopamine has moderate α and β effects and a weak dopaminergic effect. The role of the dopaminergic effect can be questioned as there is no proof of a beneficial effect on splanchnic and renal perfusion, but there are data suggesting that the dopaminergic effect may be responsible for the endocrine effects of the drug. Noradrenaline and adrenaline are both very potent pressor agents; however, the inotropic, chronotropic and metabolic effects of adrenaline are stronger than those of noradrenaline. As patients with hypovolaemic shock are often tachycardic, noradrenaline should be preferred to adrenaline, although the impact on outcome of these differences have not been evaluated.

Non-adrenergic vasopressor agents, and especially vasopressin, may also have a place in the therapy of hemorrhagic shock. Experimental studies and case reports suggest that vasopressin may be more potent than adrenaline in restoring blood pressure in haemorrhagic shock due to liver laceration. This agent has the advantage of restoring blood pressure but decreasing portal blood flow and portal pressure, limiting the rate of bleeding. In other types of shock, this decrease in splanchnic blood flow is probably detrimental and this agent should be used cautiously. There are no adequate studies of the impact of vasopressin on outcome.

Caution is urged when applying sedation or analgesia to patients with hypovolaemic shock. These agents blunt the release of endogenous catecholamines, and induce vasodilation and myocardial depression. Ketamine, in contrast to other morphinic agents, is not associated with these unfavourable haemodynamic effects and is thus often considered as the analgesic agent of choice.

Positive pressure ventilation reduces ventricular preload, thereby exacerbating the haemodynamic alterations. Initially tidal volume and PEEP should be limited, and these should be progressively increased with caution.

The reperfusion phase

Reperfusion injury is common after recovery from severe hypovolaemic/haemorrhagic shock. Ischaemia–reperfusion injury is characterized by an activation of inflammation and coagulation, and release of reactive oxygen species. Although related to the severity of tissue hypoperfusion during the ischaemic phase, most of the histological lesions occur during the reperfusion phase. Reperfusion syndrome is characterized by a distributive shock, associated with severe microvascular and cellular alterations. Despite intense research, no specific therapy can actually be proposed. Supportive therapy is similar to the supportive therapy for distributive shock.

Further reading

Antonelli M, Levy M, Andrews PJ, *et al.* Hemodynamic monitoring in shock and implications for management: International Consensus Conference, Paris, France, 27–28 Apil 2006 *Intensive Care Med* 2007; 33: 575–90.

Bickell W, Wall M, Pepe PE, *et al.* Immediate versus delayed fluid resuscitation for hypotensive patients with penetrating torso injuries. *N Engl J Med* 1994; 331: 1105–9.

Meybohm P, Cavus E, Bein B, et al. Small volume resuscitation: a randomized controlled trial with either norepinephrine or vasopressin during severe hemorrhage. *J Trauma* 2007; 62: 640–6.

Cardiogenic shock

Definition, incidence, causes

Cardiogenic shock is defined as a state of inadequate tissue perfusion due to cardiac failure. Most commonly caused by pump failure in patients with AMI or mechanical complications of AMI (acute MR, ventricular septal defect, cardiac tamponade due to LV rupture, or pericardial effusion), or myocarditis, myocardial contusion, septic myocardial depression, LV outflow obstruction, stress-induced cardiomyopathy, intoxication with cardiodepressant substances (β-blockers, calcium channel antagonists, etc.). It occurs in 6–9% of patients with AMI. Shock is present on hospital admission in <1% of patients with AMI. In others, shock usually develops during the first days of hospitalization, most commonly in older women with previous CAD, concomitant peripheral arterial diseases and cerebrovascular disease, diabetes and hypotension, tachycardia and Killip class III or IV on admission .

Symptoms and signs

Often associated with anterior MI. Beside typical retrosternal pain, patients have symptoms and signs of severe tissue/organ hypoperfusion (cyanosis, cold and clammy skin, slow capillary refilling, mental changes, obtundation, oliguria) and pulmonary congestion (dyspnoea, tachypnoea, orthopnoea). Signs of tissue hypoperfusion are present in 92%, signs of pulmonary congestion in 70% and both in 68% of patients. Haemodynamic characteristics include tachycardia, hypotension, low cardiac output, elevated cardiac filling pressures, increased SVR and low mixed venous oxygen saturation (SvO_2). Hypotension, which is defined as an SBP <90mm Hg or decrease of MAP of >30mm Hg from the patient's normal level, is common in cardiogenic shock. It is the result of decreased stroke volume, which cannot be compensated by arterial vasoconstriction. The combination of low cardiac output and systemic vasoconstriction results in severe tissue hypoperfusion and decreased coronary artery blood flow, which further worsen the cardiac performance. In some patients with cardiogenic shock, systemic arterial vasodilatation is present, most probably because of the systemic inflammatory response with cytokine release and elevated NO level, which provokes further systemic and coronary hypoperfusion and directly decreases myocardial contractility.

Predominant RV failure complicates inferior MI with extension to the RV. It is characterized by hypotension and elevated RV filling pressure without pulmonary congestion. It is easily detected and confirmed by echocardiography, which shows an enlarged and hypokinetic RV.

Acute MR can be the consequence of ischaemic papillary muscle dysfunction or rupture of papillary muscle or chordae tendineae. Characterized by sudden and refractory pulmonary oedema, shock and new apical systolic murmur, it is associated with poor prognosis. A new systolic murmur, together with acute left to right shunt, is characteristic for ventricular septum rupture. Both complications of AMI are usually recognized and confirmed by TTE or TOE.

Cardiogenic shock is seen in stress-induced cardiomyopathy (tako-tsubo syndrome or transient apical ballooning), which occurs most commonly in post-menopausal women with normal coronary arteries after severe physical or emotional stress. Because of transient LV dysfunction and rapid recovery, prognosis is excellent.

The differential diagnosis of cardiogenic shock includes AMI or ischaemia associated with severe aortic stenosis. Haemorrhage during thrombolytic treatment can result in haemorrhagic shock, and septic shock can develop in patients with multiple intravascular lines. Recognition is important as these diagnoses need a different management approach

Diagnosis

The diagnosis and aetiology should be confirmed as soon as possible. Routine investigations include ECG, CXR and laboratory tests, which should include blood gas analysis, lactate and troponin measurement. Early TTE is mandatory for aetiological diagnosis and initial haemodynamic assessment in every patients with suspected cardiogenic shock. It enables rapid and reliable assessment of morphology, global and regional systolic function of the left and right ventricle, LV diastolic function, valvular morphology and function, and recognition of cardiac tamponade, PE and dissection of the proximal aorta. It is especially helpful for early diagnosis of mechanical complications of AMI. In the case of inadequate visualization or non-conclusive findings, TOE can be performed. Low LVEF and severity of MR on echo examination are important predictors for poor outcome.

Invasive haemodynamic measurements using an intra-arterial catheter and Swan Ganz pulmonary catheter allow haemodynamic diagnosis and continuous monitoring of haemodynamic variables (arterial pressure, CVP, PAP, PAOP, SvO_2, cardiac output, RV end-diastolic volume and EF), evaluation of the therapeutic effects and precise titration of the drugs. Invasive arterial pressure monitoring is mandatory in patients treated with vasopressors or vasodilators and patients with severe hypotension. The routine and early use of echocardiography significantly decreases the use of a pulmonary artery catheter; it is still useful and necessary in patients with unstable haemodynamics, those who do not respond to the treatment and those with progressive pulmonary congestion or hypotension.

In some centres, acute coronary angiography can be performed in cardiogenic shock due to AMI, allowing confirmation of the diagnosis and immediate interventional treatment.

Treatment

Cardiogenic shock necessitates ICU admission and intensive care monitoring and treatment: optimal oxygenation, correction of electrolyte and acid–base disturbances, tight glucose control, stress ulcus prophylaxis, early oral feeding, upright position in ventilated patients and sedation with analgesia. After obtaining the aetiological and haemodynamic diagnosis, patient should be haemodynamically stabilized by using fluid challenge in those without pulmonary oedema and vasopressors in those with hypotension unresponsive to fluids.

Preload should be assessed repetitively and optimized by giving boluses of crystalloid or colloid infusion. The changes of haemodynamic variables (heart rate, arterial pressure, CVP, PAOP, cardiac output, ScO_2) and oxygenation (SaO_2) should be monitored closely to prevent pulmonary oedema and hypoxaemia, and to evaluate the response to the treatment. Inadequate cardiac filling can be also provoked by intensive diuretic and vasodilator treatment and should be considered, recognized and corrected in every phase of acute heart failure and cardiogenic shock. Preload assessment is most accurately performed by measuring LV volume/area by echocardiography. Nevertheless, filling pressures (CVP and/or PAOP) are commonly used, despite the fact that they are poor measures of preload. The trends and responses to the treatment are much more important that the static measurements.

Vasoactive and inotropic drugs remain the mainstay of first-line treatment despite the fact that they are of very limited success. Commonly used vasopressor and inotropic drugs are listed in Table 26.3.1. In general, vasopressors increase afterload. Dobutamine tends to dilate but increases myocardial oxygen consumption. Both can negatively affect cardiac performance, especially in patients with ACS. Selection depends on degree of hypotension, impairment of contractility and presence or absence of pulmonary congestion. The absolute prerequisite for vasopressor and inotropic treatment is adequate cardiac preload. In hypotensive patients, dopamine is still often used as a first agent, but its effect is limited by increase of heart rate and elevation of pulmonary pressure. In patients with profound hypotension, norepinephrine is the most efficient vasopressor used. Dobutamine, which is the first-line inotropic agent, can be combined with nitroglycerin or sodium nitroprusside in patients with pulmonary congestion. Levosimendan, a new potent inotropic and vasodilator drug, which does not increase myocardial oxygen consumption, has been successfully used in cardiogenic shock. Frequent titration of various drugs to modify haemodynamic variables may be necessary, and cardiac output and its adequacy should be measured. Since the main indication for inotropic support is inadequate cardiac output, the measurement of adequacy is of utmost importance. The best way to monitor the adequacy is continuous measurement of SvO_2, which reflects the oxygen extraction rate. Monitoring the trend of cardiac output is helpful for evaluation of the treatment effect.

Mechanical support with an intra-aortic balloon pump (IABP) should be used in intractable shock. In profound shock or severe left heart failure, an IABP should be inserted even before using the drugs for haemodynamic stabilization. An IABP can rapidly stabilize the cardiogenic shock by improving coronary and systemic blood flow and reducing systolic afterload. However, without previous revascularization in patients with AMI (PCI, CABG or thrombolysis), the effect of an IABP is only temporary. Beside IABPs, other mechanical devices (LV assist device, percutaneous cardiopulmonary bypass with extracorporeal oxygenation, left atrial to femoral arterial ventricular assist device and impeller pump inside the catheter) can be successfully used in specialized centres.

Mechanical ventilation when necessary should be started early to reduce increased work of breathing and allow ventilation with high FiO_2 and PEEP. Positive inspiratory pressure often has favourable haemodynamic effects in patients with heart failure by decreasing venous return, and enhances LV ejection by decreasing LV afterload and hence reducing congestion. Weaning from a ventilator can be difficult in patients with LV failure and should be planned carefully. Close monitoring is mandatory.

In patients with AMI, antiaggregation with aspirin and clopidogrel is usually started together with heparin which prevents DVT and can maintain coronary artery patency.

Early thrombolytic therapy improves the outcome and reduces the incidence of cardiogenic shock in patients with STEMI and should be started as soon as possible. Alteplase, tenecteplase and reteplase are preferred, since they are more effective than streptokinase which is considerably less expensive. The contraindications for thrombolytic therapy should be checked before the treatment, and patients must be regularly examined for possible bleeding. However, thrombolysis alone is not effective in patients with cardiogenic shock unless it is used together with an IABP. If unsuccessful, thrombolysis and persistent shock patients should be referred for rescue PCI or CABG.

PCI significantly reduces early and late mortality from cardiogenic shock and is preferred to thrombolysis in patients with AMI complicated by cardiogenic shock. PCI should be performed as soon as possible in patients with cardiogenic shock, and an IABP can be inserted before or immediately after PCI. However, the outcome in patients treated by IABP is not significantly better and is related to the skill and frequency of using the device.

Experimentally, l-NMMA (tilarginine acetate), an inhibitor of nitric NOS was used to reverse the severe cardiogenic shock with vasodilation due to excessive cytokine and NO production. The results were promising in the small number of patients, but unfortunately they have not been confirmed in a new larger trial.

Prognosis

Mortality rate for cardiogenic shock was 80–90% in the 1970s and 1980s, but shows a continuous decrease with the use of aggressive reperfusion strategies and of the IABP. The mortality is now 55–65%, with the exception of unchanged high mortality in patients with ventricular

Table 26.3.1 Vasopressor and inotropic drugs

Drug	Dose	Heart rate	Contractility	Vasoconstriction	Vasodilation
Dopexamine	1–4μg/kg/min	++	+	0	+
Dopamine	1–5μg/kg/min	++	++/+++	++/+++	0
Norepinephrine	0.1–0.5μg/kg/min	+	++	++++	0
Epinephrine	0.1–0.5μg/kg/min	++++	++++	++++	++ at low dose only
Dobutamine	2–20μg/kg/min	++	++++	0	++
Milrinone	Bolus 50μg/kg over 10 minutes 0.375–0.75mcg/kg/min	+	+++	0	++
Levosimendan	Bolus 6–12mcg/kg 0.05–0.2μg/kg/min	+	++++	0	+++

septum rupture. Mortality is similar in patients with STEMI and NSTEMI. Predictors of mortality are increasing age, prior MI, severe clinical manifestation on admission, oliguria, low EF, and MR by echocardiography, three-vessel or left main coronary artery disease and unsuccessful revascularization.

Further reading

Antman EM, Anbe DT, Armstrong PW, *et al.* ACC/AHA guidelines for the management of patients with ST-elevation myocardial infarction. *J Am Coll Cardiol* 2004; 44: 671–719.

Babaev, A, Frederick, PD, Pasta, DJ, et al Trends in management and outcomes of patients with acute myocardial infarction complicated by cardiogenic shock. *JAMA* 2005; 294: 448–54.

Barron HV, Every NR, Parsons LS, *et al.* The use of intra-aortic balloon counterpulsation in patients with cardiogenic shock complicating acute myocardial infarction *Am Heart J* 2001; 141: 933–9.

Berger PB, Holmes DR, Stebbins AL, *et al.* Impact of an aggressive invasive catheterization and revascularization strategy on mortality in patients with cardiogenic shock in the Global Utilization of Streptokinase and Tissue Plasminogen Activator for Occluded Coronary Arteries (GUSTO-I) trial. *Circulation* 1997; 96: 122–7.

Cotter G, Kaluski E, Milo O, *et al.* LINCS: l-NAME (a NO synthase inhibitor) in the treatment of refractory cardiogenic shock: a prospective randomized study. *Eur Heart J* 2003; 24: 1287–95.

French JK, Feldman HA, Assmann SF, *et al.* Influence of thrombolytic therapy, with or without intra-aortic balloon counterpulsation, on 12-month survival in the SHOCK trial. *Am Heart J* 2003; 146: 804–10.

Hochman JS Cardiogenic shock complicating acute myocardial infarction: expanding the paradigm. *Circulation* 2003; 107: 2998–3002.

Picard MH, Davidoff R, Sleeper LA, *et al.*. Echocardiographic predictors of survival and response to early revascularization in cardiogenic shock. *Circulation* 2003; 107: 279–84.

The TRIUMPH Investigators. Effect of tilarginine acetate in patients with acute myocardial infarction and cardiogenic shock: The TRIUMPH randomized controlled trial. *JAMA* 2007; 297: 1657–66.

Anaphylactic shock

Anaphylactic shock is a life-threatening multi-system disorder, caused typically by an IgE-mediated type 1 hypersensitivity reaction.

The incidence of anaphylactic reactions is difficult to quantify (no consensus on definition); however, a recent symposium suggested that any 'allergic reaction that is rapid in onset and may cause death' is, by definition, anaphylactic.

It is estimated that 1 in 3000 in-patients (in the USA) suffer an anaphylactic reaction—1% of all anaphylactic reactions are fatal, so prompt recognition and treatment of the condition is essential.

Critical care clinicians are likely to encounter patients suffering anaphylaxis from drugs administered in the critical care setting or in patients referred to ITU following a reaction.

Pathophysiology

Allergy to a substance occurs via a number of steps.

1. On first exposure to an allergen, IgE antibodies specific to that allergen are produced by B cells.
2. These antibodies bind to mast cells and basophils and cause them to be 'sensitized'.
3. Further exposure to the allergen causes cross-linking of bound IgE, resulting in degranulation.

Mast cell degranulation leads to the release of a number of vasoactive mediators including histamine, prostaglandins, tryptase, platelet-activating factor and leukotrienes. The combined effect of these mediators is to produce vasodilatation, increased vascular permeability, oedema and, in cases of anaphylaxis, smooth muscle spasm in the respiratory and GI tracts. Chemotactic mediators are also released, attracting eosinophils to the site of inflammation.

Anaphylactoid-type reactions cause mast cell degranulation with release of mediators, as above, but do not involve IgE cross-linkage and so do not require prior exposure to the causative agent. Clinical features and management are identical to those of anaphylactic reactions.

Clinical approach

History

- In any patient presenting with unexplained collapse, it is essential to obtain an allergy history as soon as possible and to consider anaphylaxis in the differential diagnosis.
- Ascertain history of previous allergic reactions prior to exposing patients to any potential allergens.
- Of particular importance in the critical care setting is allergy to antibiotics.
- Allergy to kiwi fruit is of importance as cross-sensitivity to latex is well documented.
- Allergy to eggs or soya should prompt caution in the use of propofol as it contains soya bean oil and egg phosphatide.
- It must be remembered that although prior exposure to an allergen is usually necessary, cross-sensitivity may occur, e.g with penicillins and cephalosporins, and in the case of anaphylactoid reactions no prior exposure is required.

Symptoms and signs

Anaphylaxis is difficult to recognize in the unstable critically ill patient. The presenting features may be attributed to the critical illness. The intubated patient provides a diagnostic challenge as early features of anaphylaxis are likely to go unnoticed. Thus a high level of clinical suspicion must be maintained. It must be remembered that anaphylactic reactions, although typically rapid in onset, may occasionally develop over a number of hours.

Cutaneous

- Flushing
- Angioedema
- Urticaria

Respiratory

- Cough
- Hoarseness
- Stridor
- Bronchospasm
- If ventilated a sudden rise in airway pressures may be noted

Cardiovascular

- Palpitations
- Tachycardia
- Arrhythmias
- Hypotension
- Collapse

Differential diagnosis

Other conditions which should be considered when faced with the above symptoms and signs include:

- Acute asthma attack/bronchospasm
- Tension pneumothorax
- Myocardial infarction
- Airway obstruction
- Acute hypovolaemia

Table 26.4.1 Typical precipitants of anaphylaxis on ICU

Antibiotics—most commonly penicillins; cross-sensitivity of 10% with cephalosporins must be remembered
Plasma expanders—gelatins, starches, etc.
Muscle relaxants—suxamethonium and atracurium most commonly
Latex
Blood products—rare

Immediate management

- Stop administering any potential trigger agents; in a critical care setting classical triggers would include antibiotics (vancomycin is a well known trigger of anaphylactoid reactions), muscle relaxants (particularly suxamethonium), gelatins, latex and radiocontrast materials.
- ABC approach to assessment and resuscitation.
- 100% oxygen and obtain a definitive airway, i.e intubation, if necessary.
- Lie the patient flat and elevate the legs.
- Administer epinephrine in increments of 50mcg IV until blood pressure and/or bronchospasm improves, if IV

access has been lost, a bolus of 500mcg may be administered IM repeated after 10min as necessary.

- IV fluids should be administered to assist in blood pressure control.
- If the patient is known to be taking TCAs or MAOIs, it is advised that the dose of epinephrine used should be halved.
- If hypotension is refractory to epinephrine, vasopressin may be considered as an alternative agent.

Subsequent management

- An antihistamine should be given, usually chlorpheniramine 10–20mg IV.
- Hydrocortisone in a dose of 100–300mg IV should be given.
- A catecholamine infusion (epinephrine or norepinephrine) may be required, as cardiovascular instability may persist for hours.
- Nebulized salbutamol may be required to aid bronchodilatation; if persistent, IV salbutamol may be considered.
- Prior to extubation the cuff of the ETT should be deflated and an air leak appreciated to ensure adequate resolution of any airway oedema.

Investigations/follow-up

No investigations are helpful during the acute event and so should be deferred until the patient is stabilized.

Serum for a mast cell tryptase level should be taken ~1h post-reaction to obtain peak levels and 5h post-reaction to ensure the level is falling. Levels will be high in both true anaphylactic and anaphylactoid reactions. Serum tryptase has a half-life of 2.5h and a basal level of 0.8–1.5ng/ml; levels >20ng/ml may be seen in true anaphylaxis. It may also be useful to send blood for complement and IgE levels at this time.

Referral should be made to either a dermatologist or an immunologist with a detailed record of events including all drugs being administered, so that skin prick testing can be arranged to determine the cause of the reaction.

The reaction should be reported to the Committee on Safety of Medicines (CSM).

Patient advice

The patient should be given advice regarding what substances are potential triggers to avoid furthers attacks.

The importance of informing any medical staff who subsequently care for the patient about the nature of, and triggers for, their reaction must be stressed.

In some circumstances, depending on the trigger, it may be appropriate to prescribe a preloaded syringe of epinephrine for the patient to self-administer in case of further attacks; this decision would ideally be made by the immunologist following up the patient.

Further reading

Ewan PW. ABC of allergies: anaphylaxis. *BMJ* 2007; 316: 1442–5.

Neugut AI, Ghatak AT, Miller RL. Anaphylaxis in the United States: an investigation into its epidemiology. *Arch Intern Med* 2001; 161: 15–21.

Project team of the Resuscitation Council (UK). The emergency medical treatment of anaphylactic reactions for first medical responders and for community nurses. 2005. www.resus.org.uk

Sampson HA, Munoz-Furlong A, Campbell RL, *et al.* Second symposium on the definition and management of anaphylaxis: summary report—Second National Institute of Allergy and Infectious Disease/Food Allergy and Anaphylaxis Network symposium. *J Allergy Clin Immunol* 2006; 117: 391–7.

Stephenson TJ. Immunology and immunopathology. In: Underwood JCE, ed. General and systematic pathology, Edinburgh: Churchill Livingstone, 1996: 192–5.

Septic shock: pathogenesis

Septic shock is defined as sepsis-induced refractory hypotension despite adequate fluid resuscitation, along with the presence of hypoperfusion abnormalities or organ dysfunction. The hypotension is mainly due to a drop in SVR secondary to vasodilation. There is, however, often concurrent myocardial depression. It is the most severe end of a spectrum of syndromes caused by entry into the bloodstream of microbiological pathogens.

Toxins released by these pathogens invoke an inflammatory response by the host. This response must be a finely controlled balance of inflammation, coagulation and fibrinolysis. Loss of this balance may lead to septic shock.

Pathogens

Bacteria account for 90% of cases of sepsis in which pathogens are identified, fungi (mainly *Candida*) make up a further 5% (probably increasing, up to 20% in the USA) and mixed bacterial/fungal/viral infections make up the final 5%. In 30–40% of cases no pathogen is identified.

Gram-negative infection has been traditionally associated with development of septic shock. However, the proportion of cases caused by Gram-positive organisms has recently escalated. This is likely to be related to the increased instrumentation of patients.

Initiation of the disease process

Gram-negative sepsis

Endotoxin (lipopolysaccharide (LPS)) is the most investigated component in triggering Gram-negative sepsis. It is found in the cell wall of the bacteria and, following infection, binds to serum proteins. It then interacts with CD14 receptors found on the surfaces of various cells, including leucocytes and endothelia cells.

Gram-positive sepsis

A variety of toxins are harboured by different Gram-positive bacteria. These comprise cell wall components (such as lipoteichoic acid and peptidoglycan) and extracellular products (such as pore-forming enzymes and superantigens). Lipoteichoic acid interacts with CD14 receptors in a similar way to LPS, but the other products have a diverse range of toxic mechanisms.

One final pathway common to both Gram-positive and Gram-negative sepsis is via cell surface Toll-like receptors. These receptors activate nuclear transcription factors (such as NF-κB) which stimulate the nucleus to release cytokines and other inflammatory mediators. Whilst the cytokine profile of the two major forms of sepsis may differ slightly, the overall response, disease progression and mortality are similar.

Host response

Inflammation

Stimulation of macrophages initiates an inflammatory response to infection with the aim of destroying damaged tissue and promoting wound healing. This is followed by release of anti-inflammatory mediators to dampen the inflammatory response and maintain homeostasis. In sepsis, this balance is lost. Initially excessive inflammation leads to a procoagulant state, widespread endothelial dysfunction, MOD and shock. This is followed by excessive anti-inflammatory activity leading to immunosuppression and increased susceptibility to secondary infection.

Proinflammatory

Figure 26.5.1 shows a simplified overview of the inflammatory response. In reality, many complex physiological respsonses occur simultaneously. Macrophages release many inflammatory cytokines and mediators, e.g. IL-6, IL-1, TNF and NO. These in turn stimulate selectins which attract neutrophils to the site of inflammation and aid with their degranulation and adhesion to the endothelium. The cytokines also activate platelets and T lymphocytes which release further cytokines, eg. IL-2 and interferon-γ. The resulting endothelial damage results in release of tissue factor, which is a key link between the immune and coagulant systems and results in a procoagulant state.

Anti-inflammatory

Macrophages subsequently release anti-inflammatory mediators such as IL-10 and IL-13, which counteract the actions of IL-6, IL-1 and TNF. This response is often insufficient in the early stages of sepsis and excessive later in the disease.

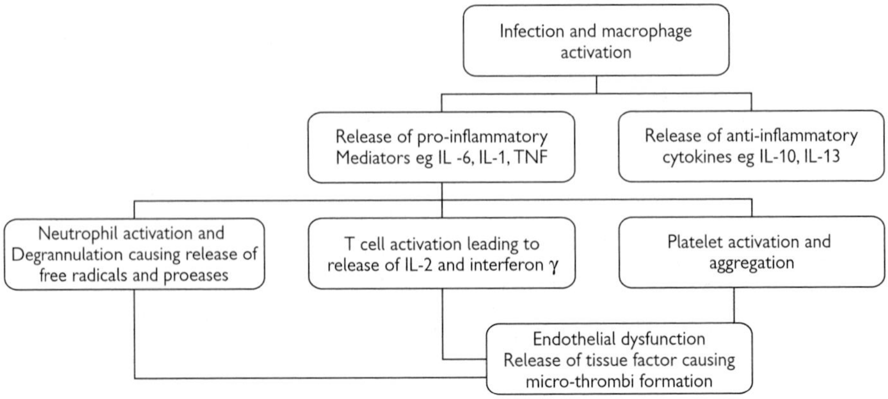

Fig. 26.5.1 Simplified view of the inflammatory response.

Vascular endothelium

The endothelium is a dynamic participant in cellular and organ function. During inflammation, activation or damage of endothelial cells results in increased capillary leak, allowing ingress of fluid migration of leucocytes to the point of injury. Endothelial damage also leads to release of tissue factor which stimulates coagulation and inhibits fibrinolysis. This response is usually then downregulated by anti-inflammatory and anticoagulant mediators expressed by the endothelium. However, in sepsis, excessive damage to the endothelium results in loss of this regulatory function, resulting in inappropriate cytokine release, thrombus formation, regional areas of vasodilation and vasoconstriction, shock and generalized tissue damage.

Coagulation

Sepsis induces a procoagulant state by several mechanisms. The interaction of neutrophils with platelets causes microthrombi formation. Damaged endothelium releases tissue factor which stimulates the coagulation cascade and deposition of fibrin. Endogenous anticoagulant factors such as protein C, antithrombin and heparin sulfate are depleted, and activation of plasminogen activator inhibitor-1 downregulates the production of plasmin and thus reduces fibrinolysis. This results in the laying down of thrombi in the microvasculature. It also, paradoxically, induces an increased tendency to bleeding due to consumption of procoagulant factors and platelets. The most severe form of coagulaopathy is the syndrome of DIC. The clinical significance of microthrombi is uncertain; however, thrombin is a highly potent proinflammatory mediator.

Nitic oxide

NO is produced by various cells primarily by NOS. Three types of NOS have been identified, endothelial constitutive NOS (ecNOS) neuronal NOS (nNOS) and inducible NOS (iNOS). ecNOS and nNOS are produced by healthy cells and play a part in normal regulation of blood flow and cell signalling. However, in the presence of inflammation, they are downregulated while iNOS production is upregulated. iNOS produces excessive NO for a prolonged period. The overproduction of NO causes mitochondrial inhibition and extensive systemic vasodilation which can be refractory to vasopressors. This, may lead to sustained hypotension, the defining feature of septic shock.

Mitochondria

In sepsis, organs can fail despite adequate tissue oxygen tensions. This implies a problem with oxygen utilization. 90% of oxygen utilization within most cells is mitochondrial respiration and generation of ATP. Inflammatory mediators including NO and other reactive species can impair mitochondrial function. The subsequent decrease in energy supply may lead to a fall in cellular metabolism manifest as organ dysfunction.

Endocrine

Septic shock is often associated with alterations in hormone expression. Thyroid and adrenal function are often depressed, and insulin resistance is common. Oestrogen levels are often high, and testosterone and leptin levels low. The presence of these endocrine abnormalities in septic shock is associated with a poor outcome, but causation remains unclear. While some studies have suggested correction of relative adrenal insufficiency and hyperglycaemia may improve outcome, this remains controversial

Mechanisms of shock

Hypotension in septic shock is cause by a combination of changes to the peripheral circulation and myocardial function. The peripheral circulation alters in three ways. Prostaglandins and NO cause peripheral vasodilation, cytokines increase capillary leak which results in intravascular hypovolaemia, and vascular smooth muscle becomes hyporeactive to sympathetic stimulation. The vascular hyporeactivity is a consequence of a combination of down regulation of α adrenergic receptors, excessive activation of potassium channels, disruption of intracellular calcium homeostasis and relative vasopressin deficiency. Although cardiac output is often increased in septic shock, there is good evidence of myocardial depression. This is caused by a combination of cytokines, NO and other myocardial depressant factors.

Necrotizing fasciitis

Necrotizing fasciitis is a bacterial infection of soft tissue that spreads insidiously along fascial planes. It may be divided according to the causative organism into type 1 or polymicrobial, type 2 caused by Group A β haemolytic *Streptococcus* and type 3 gas gangrene caused by clostridia. Types 1 and 3 commonly follow trauma or surgery whereas type 2 can occur *de novo*.

Pathophysiology

The spread through the fascial planes is facilitated by bacterial enzymes and toxins. Deep-seated infection causes vascular occlusion and tissue necrosis. Destruction of superficial nerves causes a characteristic anaesthesia. Group A β haemolytic *Streptococcus* release directly toxic streptococcal pyrogenic exotoxins which, combined with streptococcal superantigens, cause massive release of cytokines and septic shock. The pathogenicity is further enhanced by the expression of surface proteins M1 and M3 which facilitate adherence to tissues and inhibit phagocytosis by neutrophils. This combination gives the condition a mortality of 20–70%.

Further reading

Bone RC, Balk RA, Cerra FB, *et al.* Definitions of sepsis and organ failure and guidelines for the use of innovative therapies. The ACCP/SCCM consensus conference committee. American College of Chest Physicians/Society of Critical Care Medicine. *Chest* 1992; 101: 1644–55.

Brun-Buisson C, Doyon F, Carlet J, *et al.* Incidence, risk factors and outcomes of severe sepsis and septic shock in adults. *JAMA* 1995; 274: 968–74.

Kidokoro A, Iba T, Fukunaga M, *et al.* Alterations in coagulation and fibrinolysis during sepsis. *Shock* 1996; 5: 223–8.

McGill SN, Ahmed NA, Christou NV. Endothelial cells: role in infection and inflammation. *World J Surg* 1998; 22: 171–8.

Opal SM, Cohen J. Clinical Gram-positive sepsis: does it fundamentally differ from Gram-negative bacterial sepsis? *Crit Care Med* 1999; 27: 1608–16.

Sriskandan S, Cohen J. Gram-positive sepsis. Mechanisms and differences from Gram-negative sepsis. *Infect Dis Clin North Am* 1999; 13: 397–412.

Stewart TE, Zhang H. Nitric oxide in sepsis. *Respir Care* 1999; 44: 308–13.

Chapter 27

Infection and inflammation

Chapter contents

Pathophysiology of sepsis and multi-organ failure

Infectious agents entering the body lead to local inflammation, pus and abscess formation, and affect the whole body through systemic inflammation. Systemic inflammation is recognized by the presence of fever, abnormal WCC, and increased heart and respiratory rate, and is known as systemic inflammatory response syndrome (SIRS). If SIRS is due to infection (as distinct from other causes such as pancreatitis, burns or major trauma) it is defined as sepsis.

The body, or host, reacts to infection by two mechanisms, the innate and adaptive immune systems. The innate immune system comprises mast cells, phagocytes (macrophages, neutrophils and dendritic cells), basophils, eosinophils and natural killer cells, and defends the body by non-specifically reacting to foreign materials that enter the body. It also activates the adaptive immune system via T and B lymphocytes. The adaptive immune response is more specific, recognizes specific pathogens and generates immunity to them by antibodies. These two immune responses effectively combat minor infections. When this process becomes exaggerated sepsis results. In sepsis, three processes are involved,

1. Recognition of microbial material as foreign to the body.
2. Immediate release of histamine, bradykinin, serotonin and leukotrienes, causing vasodilatation of the local microcirculation and attracting neutrophils to form pus.
3. Leucocytes and other cells lyse, destroy and mop up foreign material and microbes, neutralizing the infectious challenge.

If local processes are overwhelmed, the invading organism is particularly virulent or treatment is inadequate, progression to systemic inflammation and sepsis occurs.

Sepsis can affect any major organ and potentially results in organ failure. Septic shock occurs when the effects of abnormal microcirculatory flow become apparent and perfusion of organs is affected. This is characterized by excessive vasodilatation, vascular hyporeactivity (decreased responsiveness to catecholamines) and variable degrees of myocardial depression, leading to hypotension that is unresponsive to fluid resuscitation. These changes result from excess NO, excessive activation of potassium channels and inappropriately low circulating levels of vasopressin.

Recognition of pathogenic materials in the body and regulation of genetic transcription

Pathogens have patterns of exogenous molecules on their surface, pathogen-associated molecular patterns (PAMPs). These include endotoxin (LPS), lipoproteins, outer membrane proteins, flagellin, fimbriae, peptidoglycan, peptidoglycan-associated lipoprotein and lipoteichoic acid. Other molecules become PAMPs when bacterial lysis occurs and heat shock proteins and fragments of DNA are released. PAMPs are recognized by Toll-like receptors (TLRs) and cytoplasmic 'pattern recognition receptors' (PRRs). TLRs are the key molecules embedded in cell membranes, which alert the immune system to the presence of microbes and trigger a host response. Thirteen TLRs have been identified and are the bridge between the innate and adaptive immune systems. Interaction between TLR and IL-1 receptors, so-called Roll-IL-1 receptors (TIRs), activate the transcription nuclear factor-κB (NF-κB), a protein complex found in all cell types. NF-κB is involved in the cellular responses to any damage from shear stress, cytokines, free radicals, ultraviolet irradiation, and bacterial or viral antigens. It upregulates expression of genes encoding proinflammatory mediators such as the cytokines and interleukins (IL-1 and IL-6) and also enzymes such as iNOS and cyclo-oxygenase-2 (COX-2). NF-κB regulates the immune response.

Pathogens also stimulate the arachidonic acid cascade, within endothelial cells generating further proinflammatory prostaglandins, thromboxanes and leukotrienes. Activated neutrophils also produce and release large quantities of proteases, hydrogen peroxide and reactive oxygen species.

Thus a 'storm' of pathological substances causes the characteristic effects of sepsis,

- Increased vascular permeability allowing the passage of fluid, plasma proteins and activated neutrophils into the extravascular space.
- Microcoagulopathy.
- Alterations in microvascular tone.
- Possible alteration in the epithelial tight junctions in the lung, liver and gut, thereby promoting translocation of bacteria into the circulation adding still further to the septic process and organ failure

The gross effect of these changes is hypovolaemia with interstitial oedema, blood flow redistribution and tissue hypoxia. Although antibiotics and/or surgical intervention 'cure' sepsis, adequate fluid loading to compensate for tissue 'leak', inotropic support to maintain cardiac output and good oxygenation are essential supportive treatments for advanced sepsis.

TLRs and NF-κB also show that there are significant genetic influences on a patient's response to infection and are important future areas of study.

Cytokine production

Cytokines are implicated in SIRS, inflammatory and immunological diseases and may be pro- or anti-inflammatory. They are small water-soluble proteins and glycoproteins which are produced very quickly by leucocytes, mast cells, epithelial cells and endothelial cells. Some enhance the microbiocidal effects of phagocytosing cells, recruit leucocytes to the site of infection, enhance haematopoesis, produce fever and induce most of the physiological changes associated with sepsis and septic shock.

Predominantly proinflammatory cytokines include IL-1, IL-12, IL-18, TNF-α, interferon-γ and granulocyte–macrophage colony-stimulating factor (GM-CSF). Proinflammatory cytokines contribute to the anti-infectious process but their excess production leads to tissue damage.

Anti-inflammatory cytokines are IL-4, IL-10, IL-13, interferon-α and transforming growth factor-β (TGF-β). Anti-inflammatory cytokines are useful in damping inflammation, but their excessive production may cause immunodepression.

Attempts at therapeutic cytokine administration have failed to modify sepsis, probably because the septic pathway is too complex to be influenced by the absence or presence of any one cytokine.

Immune cells (leucocytes)

Infection stimulates bone marrow production of leucocytes that are released into the blood as newly differentiated or immature cells. Chemotactic agents and adhesion molecules facilitate migration of activated leucocytes from the bloodstream to inflammatory tissues. These phagocytose and destroy infectious agents, while monocytes, tissue macrophages and other myeloid-derived cells release cytokines.

Leucocytes also release proteases, e.g. elastase, that play a pivotal part in combating infections. Increased concentrations of elastase found in plasma and bronchoalveolar lavage fluid might contribute to shock and organ dysfunction.

The terms anergy, immunodepression or immunoparalysis are also commonly used to describe the immune status of septic patients. *Ex vivo* studies suggest that the responsiveness of leucocytes to infection can be blunted by exposure to LPS and IL-10. Negative regulators of TLR-dependent signalling pathways probably exist but are not yet identified. Overwhelming sepsis does depress immune function.

Endothelium

Constitutive nitric oxide synthase (cNOS) is an enzyme secreted from within the endothelium to produce the potent vasodilator NO. NO acts to dilate pre-capillary sphincters at the entry to the microvascular capillaries regulating blood flow to tissues. In sepsis, this process is disrupted by NF-κB, stimulating production of an additional enzyme called iNOS which produces excess NO and thus excessive vasodilatation. The normal microvascular flow is disrupted and there is indiscriminate alteration of perfusion and increased vascular permeability. This contributes to the poor perfusion associated with septic shock, and tissue blood flow can be abnormal despite the appearance of a high cardiac output. Unfortunately, attempts to modulate cNOS have proved unsuccessful in improving clinical outcome from septic shock. Drugs which modify iNOS are not available.

Coagulation and sepsis

Coagulation and sepsis are interlinked. TNF-α, IL-1 and IL-6 are all capable of activating coagulation and inhibiting fibrinolysis. The procoagulant thrombin is capable of stimulating multiple inflammatory pathways. These interactions promote diffuse endovascular injury, MOD and death. The importance of APC in coagulation and sepsis is now known. Reduced levels of protein C are found in the majority of patients with sepsis. APC is an endogenous protein and is converted from its inactive precursor, protein C, by thrombin coupled to thrombomodulin. This conversion may be impaired during sepsis as a result of the downregulation of thrombomodulin by inflammatory cytokines, excess thrombin and a worse outcome from septic shock. APC promotes fibrinolysis, inhibits thrombosis and decreases inflammation. When supplemental APC is infused into patients with advanced sepsis, mortality is reduced.

Neuroendocrine function

Damage caused to tissues during sepsis is not purely due to ischaemic or haemorrhagic processes. Some tissues isolated from recovered patients are remarkably normal. More subtle changes induced by TNF, IL-1α, NO and reactive oxygen species inhibit the mitochondrial respiratory chain, reducing energy production through aerobic respiration. This is aggravated by malfunction of the sympathetic nervous system. This again emphasizes how complex the septic process is, and the interplay between the sympathetic nervous system, sympathomimetic drugs and organ metabolism in sepsis is incompletely understood.

Apoptosis

When an epithelial cell becomes infected its membranes may display a transmembrane ligand known as a Fas ligand. Fas ligands bind cytokines and kill the affected cell; thus this is a kind of 'suicide' mechanism for cells that become infected. This is a form of programmed cell death or apoptosis. This differs from necrosis, cell death resulting from injury. Fas bacteria-mediated epithelial cell apoptosis contributes to immune defences via activation of the Fas/Fas ligand system and thus can help the septic process by 'sacrificing' infected cells by use of cytotoxic T cells. The role of apoptosis in septic shock is unclear, but it may exacerbate or promote the cellular damage associated with sepsis.

Conclusion

Sepsis is a complex and multi-factorial disease. Normal immune and neuroendocrine systems that defend the body against infection can be overstimulated, and systemic inflammation occurs to the point that it affects the whole body and becomes detrimental. A cascade of disrupted microcirculatory blood flow, excess activation of coagulation and adversely affected organ function results. Understanding the complexity and controlling sepsis is one of the great medical challenges of our time.

Further reading

Bernard GR, Vincent JL, Laterre PF, *et al.* Efficacy and safety of recombinant human activated protein C for severe sepsis. *N Engl J Med* 2001; 344: 699–709.

Bone RC, Fisher CJ, Clemmer TP, *et al.* Sepsis syndrome: a valid clinical entity. Methylprednisoline Severe Sepsis Study Group. *Crit Care Med* 1989; 17: 389-93.

Boveris A, Alvarez S, Bustamante J, *et al.* Measurement of superoxide radical and hydrogen peroxide production in isolated cells and subcellular organelles. *Methods Enzymol* 2002; 349: 280–7.

Buckley JF, Singer M, Clapp LH. Role of KATP channels in sepsis. *Cardiovasc Res* 2006; 72: 220–30.

Kaisho T, Akira S. Toll-like receptors as adjuvant receptors. *Biochim Biophys Acta* 2002; 1589: 1–13.

Landry DW, Oliver JA. The pathogenesis of vasodilatory shock. *N Engl J Med* 2001; 345: 588–95.

Lopez A, Lorente JA, Steingrub J, *et al.* Multiple-center, randomized, placebo-controlled, double-blind study of the nitric oxide synthase inhibitor 546C88: effect on survival in patients with septic shock. *Crit Care Med* 2004; 32: 21–30.

Singer M, De Santis, V, Vitale D, *et al.* Multiorgan failure is an adaptive, endocrine-mediated, metabolic response to overwhelming systemic inflammation. *Lancet* 2004; 364: 545–8.

Thiemermann C. Nitric oxide and septic shock. *Gen Pharmacol* 1997; 29: 159–66.

Tsiotou AG, Sakorafas GH, Anagnostopoulos G, *et al.* Septic shock; current pathogenetic concepts from a clinical perspective. *Med Sci Monit* 2005; 11: RA76–8.

Vervloet MG, Thijs LG, Hack CE. Derangements of coagulation and fibrinolysis in critically ill patients with sepsis and septic shock. *Semin Thromb Hemostasis* 1998; 24: 33–44.

Yan SB, Helterbrand JD, Hartman DL, *et al.* Low levels of protein C are associated with poor outcome in severe sepsis. *Chest* 2001: 120: 915–22.

Infection control—general principles

The majority of patients admitted to critical care units will receive treatment for infection at some time. Around a third will develop a nosocomial infection; rates of health-care-associated infection are 3–5 times higher than for general ward patients. A variety of factors in ICU lead to increased risks of infection with and transmission of multi-resistant organisms. These include

1 critically ill (often imunosuppressed) patients
2 frequent use of in-dwelling devices
3 prescription of broad spectrum antimicrobials, often in combination
4 intensive nursing/medical contact that can lead to cross-transmission of organisms.

Hospital ICU infection control guidelines, although based on national and international guidelines, should reflect local conditions. The 'Winning Ways' report (UK) summarizes recommendations for reducing nosocomial infections.

Prevention of infection related to devices

Intravascular catheters

Approximately 39 per 1000 patients in English ICUs develop device-related bacteraemia, with the vast majority of these being due to CVCs. Catheter-related bloodstream infections (CR-BSIs) are most commonly caused by skin organisms that colonize the exit site and catheter hub. These may contaminate the catheter during insertion or be transferred from the hands of staff during care interventions. Coagulase-negative staphylococci such as *Staphylococcus epidermidis* are most commonly implicated, followed by *S. aureus*, *Candida* species and enterococci.

A range of techniques is associated with reduced rates of CR-BSI.

- During insertion the use of maximal sterile barriers including a sterile gown, sterile gloves and a large sterile drape reduces CR-BSIs. The skin should be cleansed with alcoholic chlorhexidine gluconate solution or with povodine-iodine if patients are sensitive to chlorhexidine.
- Single lumen catheters should be used unless multiple ports are essential for patient management, and a dedicated lumen should be kept exclusively for parenteral nutrition.
- A tunnelled line or implantable device should be used if vascular access is required for >3–4 weeks.
- Antimicrobial- or silver-impregnated lines are available and may be appropriate in patients requiring short-term central venous access and who are at high risk of CR-BSI, in situations where rates of CR-BSI remain high despite strategies to reduce them.
- Insertion of the line into a subclavian site appears to be associated with lower rates of infection than femoral or internal jugular sites, and should be used unless medically contraindicated.
- Central lines should not be replaced routinely but on evidence of infection. If a patient has a CR-BSI, then guide wire-assisted exchange should not be used for line replacement.

Ventilator-associated pneumonia

Nosocomial pneumonia has mortality rates of 20–50%. VAP rates can be reduced by methods to prevent aspiration, such as elevation of the patient's head to a 30–45° angle and avoiding gastric distension. NIV should be used when appropriate to avoid endotracheal intubation. The use of selective digestive decontamination remains controversial (see Chapter 27.7).

Diagnosis of VAP is difficult, but invasive diagnostic methods using quantitative culture of a bronchoscopic protected specimen brush or bronchoalveolar lavage samples can improve specificity of the diagnosis. These techniques have been associated with decreased antibiotic use without any increase in mortality.

Urinary catheters

Catheter-associated UTI is the most common nosocomial infection in hospitals, with cumulative rates increasing with length of time the catheter is *in situ*. The use of silver alloy catheters in hospitalized patients requiring short-term catheterization appears to reduce rates of catheter-associated UTI. Most importantly, local guidelines should be followed for care of urinary catheters, with early removal of the catheter if possible.

Prudent antimicrobial use

Empiric therapy, started after cultures are taken, is usually guided by local antibiotic policy. Proper collection of specimens and careful interpretation of culture results helps to differentiate between organisms that are contaminating specimens or colonizing the patient and organisms that are causing infection. Therapy should be adjusted to the narrowest spectrum effective antimicrobial based on culture results, and antibiotics should be stopped as soon as there is cure or if no evidence of infection is found.

Involvement of infectious disease or microbiology clinicians improves patient outcomes and decreases treatment costs in serious infections.

Local antibiotic policy

In ICU, the aim is to use the safest, most effective (and most economical) antimicrobials whilst reducing the risk of selection of bacterial resistance. Local antibiotic policies should be developed in collaboration by clinicians, microbiologists and pharmacists, and be regularly reviewed. They are based on the nature of the local patient population and must reflect the types and susceptibility patterns of pathogens circulating within the ICU, the hospital and the local community.

The implementation of antibiotic guidelines has been associated with stable antibiotic susceptibility patterns for Gram-negative and Gram-positive organisms. The use of narrow-spectrum antibiotics appears to be associated with lower resistance rates and fewer episodes of antibiotic-associated diarrhoea due to *Clostridium difficile*. Restricted use of specific antibiotics or antibiotic classes in association with other infection control measures have been used to halt outbreaks of antibiotic-resistant bacteria. Studies can be found to support and refute the benefits of antibiotic cycling, and it may be that antibiotic heterogeneity, achieved by 'mixing' antibiotics is more effective.

Prevention of transmission of infection

Hospital environmental hygiene

The most important source of transmitted infection is the hands of health workers, but almost every item of equipment in the ICU has been shown to be a source of nosocomial infection. The environment must be kept clean, and surfaces damp-dusted at least daily. Routine use of disinfectants is not necessary, but disinfection of isolation rooms or areas where patients with multi-resistant organisms have been nursed should be carried out as per local infection control recommendations.

Hand hygiene

Despite the hands being the most common vector for spread of infection, compliance rates of ICU hand washing procedures average 30–40%. Rates can be improved with the use of hand disinfection with alcohol-based antiseptic hand rubs which are highly effective and quicker to use. Hands that are visibly soiled should be washed in soap and water. Hand washing is more effective against certain diarrhoeal pathogens such as Norovirus and the spores of *C. difficile*. Hygienic hand wash refers to washing hands with an antiseptic agent added to the detergent, and should be used when prolonged reduction in microbial flora on the hands is required, such as before invasive procedures. Improvement in infection rates has been shown in response to improved hand hygiene compliance in descriptive studies and clinical trials.

Personal protective equipment

Appropriate use of aprons, gowns, gloves, protective eyewear and face masks protects staff and prevents transmission of microorganisms to patients. In the ICU, disposable gowns/aprons and gloves should be used for each patient care episode. Gloves must be discarded and hands decontaminated after each care activity for a patient. Particulate filter masks are worn when caring for patients with respiratory infections transmitted by airborne particles, such as *Mycobacterium tuberculosis* or epidemic influenza. Face masks and eye protection protect mucous membranes from splashes. Face masks have not been shown to protect patients from healthcare-associated infection during routine ward procedures. There are concerns, however, about the 'cloud' healthcare provider phenomenon whereby viral upper respiratory tract infection promotes transmission of pathogens such as MRSA which colonize the oropharynx. Some of this transmission may be prevented by face masks, although healthcare workers may provide better protection to their patients by staying away from work when unwell themselves.

Contact precautions/isolation

Two types of isolation (or barrier nursing) are used in the ICU setting: 'protective' or 'source'. Immunocompromised patients need protective isolation from pathogens circulating in ICU. Patients with communicable diseases or carrying multi-resistant bacteria are cared for in source isolation to protect other patients and staff from acquiring these pathogens. If isolation facilities are not available, other options of providing contact precaution may be used, such as cohorting. Although not an exhaustive list, some of the organisms that should prompt isolation include MRSA, *C. difficile*, vancomycin-resistant *Enterococcus* (VRE) and multi-resistant Gram-negative bacteria such as multi-resistant *Acinetobacter baumanii*.

Patients may be colonized with multi-resistant organisms but not manifest active infection, and so may not be recognized. Screening for these organisms on admission to ICU is important to provide appropriate isolation or cohorting of colonized patients. Up to 86% of VRE or MRSA-colonized patients will not be recognized except by active surveillance. New very rapid (hours) techniques are becoming available for screening.

Consult infection control team

The infection control team

- policy production
- education of staff
- practical advice
- audit in close collaboration with ICU staff.

Surveillance is an essential part of prevention and control. It helps to detect and define sources of cross-infection more rapidly and to evaluate control methods, and provides information for resource allocation in infection control. There are various ways this may be achieved, but surveillance is best conducted prospectively by staff trained in infection control.

Staffing

The strict application of barrier nursing techniques in ICU may break down during periods of understaffing or overcrowding, and this has been associated with outbreaks of nosocomial infection.

Occupational health

Staff should be up to date with vaccinations for hepatitis B, TB, influenza and varicella-zoster. Measles status is increasingly important.

Further reading

Emmerson AM, Enstone JE, Griffin M, *et al.* The Second National Prevalence Survey of infection in hospitals—overview of the results. *J Hosp Infect* 199; 32: 175–90.

Fagon JY, Chastre J, Wolff M, *et al.* Invasive and noninvasive strategies for management of suspected ventilator-associated pneumonia. A randomized trial. *Ann Intern Med* 2000; 132: 621–30.

Kollef MH. Is antibiotic cycling the answer to preventing the emergence of bacterial resistance in the Intensive Care Unit? *Clin Infect Dis* 2006; 43 Suppl 2: S82–8.

Molstad S, Cars O. Major change in the use of antibiotics following a national programme: Swedish Strategic Programme for the Rational Use of Antimicrobial Agents and Surveillance of Resistance (STRAMA). *Scand J Infect Dis* 1999; 31: 191–5.

Pearson ML. Hospital Infection Control Practices Advisory Committee. Guideline for the prevention of intravascular-device-related infections. *Infect Control Hosp Epidemiol* 1996; 17: 438–73.

Pittet D. Improving adherence to hand hygiene practice: a multidisciplinary approach. *Emerg Infect Dis* 2001; 7: 234–40.

Pratt RJ, Pellowe CM, Wilson JA, *et al.* epic2: national evidence-based guidelines for preventing healthcare-associated infections in NHS hospitals in England. *J Hosp Infect* 2007; 65 Suppl 1: S1–64.

Salgado CD, O'Grady N, Farr BM. Prevention and control of antimicrobial-resistant infections in intensive care patients. *Crit Care Med* 2005; 33: 2373–82.

Sherertz RJ, Bassetti S, Bassetti-Wyss S. 'Cloud' health-care workers. *Emerg Infect Dis* 2001; 7: 241–4.

HIV

Since the first description of the HIV immunodeficiency syndrome in 1981, the prognosis for individuals living with HIV infection in the Western world has transformed. In the early years of the epidemic, survival was <10yrs and the emphasis focused on palliative care. Now, however, most of the population living with HIV will survive for many years, providing they are able to access and adhere to highly active antiretroviral therapy (HAART). Previously, there had been a reticence to transfer individuals with HIV to more intensive/critical care settings due to the relatively poor clinical outcome. Admissions were often costly and unsuccessful. In the HAART era, with improvements in knowledge and management of HIV, this reticence has diminished.

The care of HIV patients

This should be provided by a multi-disciplinary team. Critical care provision should be no exception. Prescription of HAART may be complicated by factors including HIV resistance, drug administration and pharmacokinetics; thus, antiretroviral (ARV) regimens should not be altered without the advice of an HIV clinician and pharmacist. In areas where there is no direct access to a specialist HIV team, a network should exist to enable units to seek advice and support from a designated HIV centre.

As the prognosis for individuals living with HIV has improved, increasingly patients are affected by non-HIV co-morbidities including cardiovascular, hepatitis and chronic conditions, e.g. emphysema. The predominance of oncological diagnoses especially non-Hodgkins lymphoma in this population, and the subsequent chemotherapeutic regimens (which may be difficult to construct in the presence of HAART) may predispose to neutropenic sepsis, often requiring critical care support. The management of these conditions should not differ from that of the HIV-negative population. Within this chapter, we discuss the general management of HIV-infected individuals in the critical care setting, focusing upon opportunistic infections.

HIV testing in the critical care setting

A significant proportion of individuals admitted to the CCU/ICU are unaware of their HIV status. Obtaining informed consent is often impossible. HIV tests are often performed in 'the patients' best interests'. In practice, there are few situations where an HIV test result will alter a patient's immediate management but, where it may, testing should be performed. Low CD4 counts are often seen in the critically ill, irrespective of HIV status.

Antiretroviral therapy in the critically ill patient

There is limited information about the introduction of HAART in the ITU setting. There is concern regarding the immune reconstitution inflammatory syndrome (IRIS), a paradoxical worsening of an individual's clinical state as the immune system is restored. HAART administration is difficult as Zidovudine (AZT) is the only ARV available in IV form, and NG administration of ARVs may lead to inadequate plasma levels, fuelling the accumulation of HIV resistance. Drug interactions are common, e.g., co-administration of the protease inhibitor, atazanavir with antacids significantly reduces its plasma level. Renal or hepatic insufficiency may also contraindicate the use of ARVs.

In general, in individuals with non-HIV-related conditions and a CD4 count >200 cells/mm^3, ARV therapy can be deferred, as outcome will be related to the resolution of the non-HIV-related condition. In those admitted with an AIDS-defining illness or with a CD4 count <200 cells/mm^3, prophylaxis against opportunistic infections and, where appropriate, ARVs should be considered. If the individual develops IRIS, ARVs are usually continued. Corticosteroid therapy may be required.

Pneumocystis jirovecci pneumonia (PCP)

Historically, the most common reason for HIV-related critical care has been respiratory failure. Whilst bacterial pneumonia and TB are important causes of compromise in this population, PCP remains a major cause of morbidity, often requiring assisted ventilation. These patients are prone to pneumothorax, especially if pneumatocoeles are present, and ventilatory measures should be considered with care.

Presentation

Typically, dry cough, increasing dyspnoea and pyrexia. There may be few or no chest signs despite significant disease.

Investigation

CXR may be normal in up to 50% of individuals, or show perihilar shadowing with diffuse interstitial infiltration—'ground glass' shadowing. Pneumothoraces may be present. ABG indicates the disease severity and guides management. In the less sick, exercise oximetry is useful, and a drop in oxygen saturation to <90% after 10min on an exercise bicycle is suggestive of PCP. Induced sputum should be sent. If negative, consider bronchoscopy.

Treatment

If PaO_2 <8kPa, commence IV methyl prednisolone 40mg qds. First-line therapy is IV co-trimoxazole 3840mg bd (unless <60kg when dose should be adjusted to 60mg/kg bd) for 14–21 days. Side effects of nausea are commonm and pre-emptive antiemetics should be prescribed. Rash, bone marrow suppression (BMS), hepatotoxicty and nephrotoxocity may be observed. Monitor FBC, U&E and LFTs closely. Second-line therapy, instigated due to side effects or failure, comprises IV/oral clindamycin 600mg qds and oral primaquine 300mg od. Clindamycin is linked to diarrhoeal episodes (exclude *Clostridium difficile*) and hepatotoxicity. Primaquine may cause nausea, methaemaglobinaemia, haemolytic anaemia and BMS. Again, monitor bloods. Alternative agents include dapsone and trimethiprim, pentamadine and atovaquone Secondary prophylaxis is required post-treatment.

Cryptococcal meningitis

Presentation

Classically, headache and pyrexia. Meningism is present in <30%.

Investigation

Negative serum cryptococcal antigen (CrAg) excludes the diagnosis. Following a CT head, urgent LP, including measurement of CSF opening pressure (OP), should be performed. If the OP is >20cm H_2O, CSF should be drained until the OP is below this level. Daily LPs may be required, and a ventriculoperitoneal shunt may be necessary. CSF CrAg is positive in cryptococcal meningitis. Negative CSF

CrAg, with positive serum CrAg, indicates cryptococcosis, and individuals should be treated with fluconazole to prevent meningitis. Indicators of a poor prognosis include raised ICP, decreased level of consciousness, CSF CrAg 1:1024, low CSF WCC and positive serum cryptococcal culture.

Treatment
First-line therapy is IV amphotericin B. Give a test dose of 1mg in 100ml of normal saline and monitor for adverse events. Systemic symptoms such as fever, chills, myalgia and headache may occur. Chlorpheniramine 10mg IV, paracetamol and hydrocortisone 25–50mg IV given pre-emptively may alleviate these symptoms. Initial treatment is amphotericin 250mcg/kg/day following the test dose. Further side effects include nephrotoxicity, hypokalaemia, hypomagnesaemia, hepatotoxicity and thrombophlebitis. Again, blood parameters, including calcium and magnesium, should be monitored closely. Amphocil may be required in cases of nephrotoxicity. The use of additional flucytosine is controversial. Although there is a faster rate of CSF sterilization, this does not translate into a survival advantage, and the additional toxicity of flucytosine may not be warranted. Second-line therapy is comprised of fluconazole with or wiithout flucytosine. Secondary prophylaxis will be required following treatment.

Toxoplasmosis encephalitis

Presentation
Commonly headache, pyrexia, confusion ± focal neurology. The main differential diagnosis is primary cerebral lymphoma. In practice, diagnosis is often retrospective, indicated by a radiological and clinical improvement following 2 weeks of specific antitoxoplasmosis therapy.

Investigation
Negative serology (titre <1:16) implies that toxoplasmosis is unlikely but not impossible. Raised titres or presence of IgM are not diagnostic of acute infection, but indicate reactivation potential. MRI brain scan should be performed, classically revealing characteristic multiple ring enhancing lesions. Space-occupying lesions may preclude LP. If performed, results are often normal, or a slight elevation of protein ± mononuclear pleocytosis may be seen.

Treatment
Oral/IV sulfadiazine 2g qds (if patient weighs >70kg) with oral pyrimethamine 75mg od and oral folinic acid 15mg od support. Side effects include nausea, vomiting, rash, crystalluria, hepatotoxicity and BMS. Monitor bloods closely. Second-line therapy is oral clindamycin 600mg qds, oral pyrimethamine 75mg od and oral folinic acid 75mg od. Adverse events include rash, hepatotoxicity and BMS.

Approximately 80% of patients should respond to anti-*Toxoplasma* treatment. The majority will experience a radiological and clinical improvement within 14 days.

Further reading

Gottlieb M, Schroff R, Schanker H, *et al.* Pneumocystis carinii pneumonia and mucosal candidiasis in previously healthy homosexual men: evidence of a new acquired cellular deficiency. *N Engl J Med* 1981; 305: 1425–31.

Keiser O, Taffe P, Zwahlen M, *et al.* All cause mortality in the Swiss HIV Cohort Study from 1990 to 2001 in comparison with the Swiss population. *AIDS* 2004; 18: 1835–43.

Severe falciparum malaria

An estimated 300–500 million people contract malaria annually and 1.5–2.7 million die. Global travel has contributed to the increased incidence of imported malaria in developed countries, and the impact is compounded by the increasing incidence of drug-resistant *Plasmodium falciparum* malaria. Malaria is caused by obligate intraerythrocytic protozoa that are primarily transmitted by the infected female *Anopheles* mosquito.

Diagnosis

Malaria must always be suspected in any patient with unexplained fever or clinical deterioration who has returned from an endemic area within the past few years. The risk of severe falciparum malaria developing is greatest among young children and visitors (of any age) from non-endemic areas. There are four types of malarial parasite affecting man; however, severe malaria is caused almost invariably by *P. falciparum* infection. Patients are considered to have severe malaria if they have one or more of the underlying features:

- A parasitemia of >5%
- Altered consciousness
- Oliguria
- Jaundice
- Severe normocytic anaemia
- Hypoglycaemia
- Organ failure

In addition to the features cited above, other complications of severe falciparum malaria in adults include: seizures, acute renal failure, metabolic acidosis, ARDS, haemoglobinuria and bleeding. In adults, jaundice, pulmonary oedema, acute renal failure, and bleeding or clotting abnormalities are more common. In children seizures, other neurological sequelae, hypoglycaemia, cough and acidosis with respiratory distress are more frequent. While a parasite density >5% and the presence of schizonts in a peripheral blood smear are associated with severe disease, semi-immune individuals in highly endemic areas may have parasite densities of 20–30% in the absence of clinical symptoms, so clear correlation between counts and outcome is difficult to make. At any level of parasitaemia, the prognosis is worse in those with higher proportions of mature parasites (mature trophozoites or schizonts containing pigment).

Treatment

The parasite (and schizont) count should be monitored at least twice a day initially. Patients with severe malaria as well as those unable to tolerate oral therapy should be given parenteral treatment with either a quinine-based or an artesiminin-based regimen. Quinine-based alternatives include: IV quinidine gluconate 10mg/kg loading dose (maximum 600mg) over 1–2h, then continuous infusion of 0.02mg/kg/min **or** IV quinine dihydrochloride 20mg salt/kg loading dose over 4h followed by 10mg/kg over 2–4h every 8h (max 1800mg/day). Patients who received mefloquine or other quinine derivatives within the previous 12h should not receive a loading dose. Changes in the volume of distribution mean doses need to be reduced by 33–50% after 2 days. Some centres monitor quininine levels daily. Cardiac monitoring is required during IV infusion, and hypoglycaemia is a significant risk especially as malaria is associated with hyperinsulinaemia.

Although quinine is the current gold standard, artemisinin-based regimens may be better. Studies in Asia suggest that artemisinin derivatives reduce the mortality (15 vs 22%) in adults with severe malaria compared with quinine. Artesunate is well tolerated. Equivalent studies with artesunate from Africa are currently lacking, and good quality IV artesunate is unavailable or in short supply in many Western countries (IV artesunate is unlicensed in the EU), so quinine is often still used. Certainly quinine-resistant *P. falciparum* requiring IV therapy should be treated with IV artemisinin combined with tetracycline or mefloquine. If artemisinin is not available, IV quinine or quinidine plus tetracycline or doxycycline should be given.

Supportive measures

Patients with severe falciparum malaria must be admitted to HDU/ICU for full monitoring, including heart and blood glucose. If hypotension and hypoxaemia develop,then, as with all septic patients, appropriate filling guided by monitoring the cardiovascular state, stroke volume and mixed venous saturations should be undertaken. After early resuscitation (first 48h), a positive fluid balance should be avoided for any patients with ALI/ARDS. Intubation and mechanical ventilation may be indicated not only in those with respiratory failure but also as part of airway protection for cerebral malaria to prevent hypercapnia and a subsequent rise in ICP.

An LP should be performed in comatose patients to exclude bacterial meningitis. The OP is usually normal in adults; CSF is clear, with <10 white cells/μl and the protein is often slightly raised. Malaria itself is only associated with mild neck stiffness; neck rigidity and photophobia are absent. Other associated or nosocomial infections should also be looked for and treated; these are not uncommon and can lead to a picture of sepsis; shock can occur in malaria but is more often due to secondary infection.

Cerebral malaria is particularly serious but can resolve with support and treatment, although recovery can be slow. Convulsions and retinal haemorrhages are common; papilloedema is rare. A variety of transient abnormalities of eye movement, especially disconjugate gaze, may occur. Convulsions should be treated with diazepam. An NG tube should be inserted and the stomach aspirated unless airway protection has been secured.

Renal failure (usually oliguric) is virtually confined to adults. The mechanisms underlying renal failure are not well understood, although it is usually reversible. The old fashioned 'blackwater fever' with severe haemolosysis is now very uncommon. Treatment is supportive, maintaining a good fluid balance, ensuring no evidence of obstruction and commencement of haemofiltration if required. Hypoglycaemia is common and should be treated with 50% dextrose followed by a continuous infusion of dextrose, if required. Most patients can be established on eneteral nutrition early, and should be maintained on a regimen of tight glycaemic control. A very common finding is a low platelet count, usually without any bleeding. This typically recovers as the parasite count falls. DIC is uncommon.

Other treatments

Exchange transfusion is considered in *P. falciparum* infection when parasitaemia is >10% and in patients with coma, renal failure or ARDS, regardless of the level of parasitaemia although without a strong evidence base.

Studies of antipyretics, anticonvulsants (phenobarbital), anticytokine/anti-inflammatory agents (e.g. anti-TNF antibodies, dexamethasone, pentoxifylline), iron chelators and hyperimmune sera have all been disappointing. Steroids have been used in cerebral malaria but have been associated with a worse outcome than quinine alone. Heparin increases bleeding complications and should not be given.

Prognosis

Age <3yrs, seizures, papilloedema, deep coma, decerebrate or decorticate posturing, organ dysfunction, acidosis, respiratory distress and circulatory collapse are all associated with a poor outcome. The mortality of untreated falciparum malaria is close to 100%. The fatality rate for treated severe malaria is 10–40%. A lower mortality rate has been reported for patients with severe malaria treated in European ICUs which may be attributed to early admission to HDU/ICU; it may also be that this patient group selects out those prone to early cerebral malaria.

Further reading

Bruneel F, Hocqueloux L, Alberti C, *et al.* The clinical spectrum of severe imported falciparum malaria in the intensive care unit: report of 188 cases in adults. *Am J Respir Crit Care Med* 2003; 167: 684–9.

Dondorp A, Nosten F, Stepniewska K *et al.* Artesunate versus quinine for treatment of severe falciparum malaria: a randomised trial. *Lancet* 2005; 366: 717–25.

Lalloo DG, Shingadia D, Pasvol G, *et al.* UK malaria treatment guidelines. HPA Advisory Committee on Malaria Prevention in UK Travellers. *J Infect* 2007; 54: 111–21.

Pasvol G. Management of severe malaria: interventions and controversies. *Infect Dis Clin North Am* 2005; 19: 211–40.

WHO. Severe falciparum malaria, a practical handbook, 2nd edn. 2000. http://www.who.int/malaria/docs/hbsm.pdf

Vasculitides in the ICU

Introduction

Vasculitides are a heterogeneous group of relatively uncommon diseases characterized by destruction of the blood vessel wall and cellular inflammation. Systemic necrotizing vasculitides are potentially life-threatening conditions involving multiple organ systems. Their ICU outcome is poor, with in-hospital mortality of >50%.

Classification

Depending on the size of the vessels involved, the following disease entities of primary idiopathic vasculitis are recognised:

1 Large vessel vasculitis, e.g. giant cell arteritis, Takayasu's arteritis
2 Medium vessel vasculitis, e.g. classical polyarteritis nodosa (PAN), Kawasaki's disease;
3 Small vessel vasculitis, e.g. Wagner's granulomatosis (WG), microscopic polyangitis (MPA), Churg–Strauss syndrome (CSS), pauci-immune rapidly progressive glomerulonephritis (RPGN), isolated pauci-immune pulmonary capillaritis, Henoch–Schönlein purpura, etc. Small vessel vasculitides sometimes have medium vessel involvement as well, are most commonly associated with antineutrophil cytoplasmic antibodies (ANCAs; see below), are associated with high risk of glomerulonephritis and respond best to immunosuppression with cyclophosphamide.

Goodpasture's syndrome (primary immune complex-mediated vasculitis) and secondary vasculitis due to SLE, rheumatoid arthritis, ploymyositis, scleroderma, etc. are other vasculitic conditions.

Incidence, outcome and aetiology

Annual incidence of primary systemic vasculitides (WG, MPA, CSS and polyarteritis) in the UK is ~20 cases per million. They usually occur in those aged in their 50s and 60s (peak incidence in ages 65–74) with male preponderance. The incidence in the UK ICUs is ~0.07%, with ICU mortality of ~35% and hospital mortality of 55.2%; the majority of these cases are transferred to specialist centres for management.

Primary vasculitides (WG, MPA, CSS, etc.) arise *de novo*, but secondary vasculitides arise in association with an established disease such as rheumatoid arthritis, infections (hepatitis, HIV, syphilis), drugs (sulfonamides, penicillins, thiazides) and malignancy.

Presentation and diagnosis in ICU patients

A patient with known vasculitis may be admitted to the ICU as a consequence of their disease, e.g. respiratory failure due to diffuse alveolar haemorrhage (DAH) or acute renal failure. However, initial diagnosis of vasculitis may be made for the first time after ICU admission. In the critically ill, diagnosis is challenging because of variable and multifaceted presentation, low incidence of vasculitis in the general and ICU population, and overlap of signs and symptoms with a variety of common illnesses such as sepsis.

Signs and symptoms

Patients may present to ICU with respiratory failure and non-specific CXR changes rather than classical renal failure. Most of the signs and symptoms are non-specific and overlap with those of infections, sepsis, connective tissue disorders and malignancies. In patients with known vasculitis and who deteriorate clinically, identifying the cause of deterioration can be equally difficult. A high index of suspicion and awareness, combined with a thorough review of history and detailed clinical examination are a key to early diagnosis. History may highlight conditions such as hepatitis (associated with PAN), non-specific illness often diagnosed as infection, low grade fever, cough, breathlessness, anaemia, headaches, a previous history of vasculitis, etc. Clinical examination may reveal evidence of the vasculitic process: nail-fold infarcts, splinter haemorrhages, retinal haemorrhages, Roth spots (also seen in endocarditis), scleritis, episcleritis, palpable purpura, ulcerative lesions of the nose causing bloody or purulent nasal discharge, chronic otitis media, deafness and mononeuritis multiplex (sudden wrist or foot drop, paraesthesia, numbness, etc. occurring in two or more peripheral nerve distributions). There may be an unusual constellation of signs and symptoms involving multiple organ systems, either simultaneously or over time. Detailed clinical findings in each condition are given elsewhere.

Laboratory investigations

Routine blood tests show non-specific changes such as a normocytic or microcytic anaemia, a neutrophil leucocytosis and occasionally eosinophilia (in CCS). ESR (rarely measured in ICU patients) and CRP levels are both raised. Low serum albumin and raised alkaline phosphatase, urea and creatinine are usual. Urine examination may show blood and protein on dipstick test.

Serological, histopathological and radiological tests

ANCAs are important adjuncts in diagnosis of ANCA-associated vasculitides (WG, CSS, MPA, etc.) where ANCA positivity is common but not universal. Two types of assays for ANCA are in common use (indirect immunofluorescence and ELISA). Cytoplasmic ANCAs (C-ANCAs) are primarily associated with antibodies directed against proteinase 3 (PR3) found in azurophilic granules of neutrophils and lysosomes of monocytes, whereas perinuclear ANCAs (P-ANCAs) are commonly associated with those directed against myeloperoxidase (MPO), also found in azurophilic granules. ANCA binding to these molecules on activated neutrophils is thought to be an important mechanism of injury in these conditions. If immunofluorescence alone is used, then C-ANCA is more specific of vasculitis than P-ANCA. All serum that is ANCA positive should be tested in PR3 and MPO ELISAs as this increases their specificity. A negative ANCA does not exclude the possibility of vasculitis, as there are some small vessel vasculitides that are ANCA negative. Principles in relation to clinical utility of ANCA testing are:

- positive ANCA serology is extremely useful in suggesting the diagnosis
- positive immunofluorescence assays without confirmatory ELISA for PR3 or MPO are of limited value
- histopathology is the gold standard for diagnosis in most patients
- negative assays do not exclude vasculitis
- persistent ANCAs in the absence of clinical features of active disease does not mean continued treatment
- in ANCA-positive patients, persistent ANCA negativity during remissions is reassuring but no guarantee that the disease is inactive

- ANCA positivity, following a clinical quiescence (and ANCA negativity) means a risk of flare-up.

A plain CXR may show non-specific changes, nodular or cavitating lesions. Diffuse ground glass opacification should raise suspicion of DAH and vasculitis. High resolution CT may help, but features remain non-specific.

Where possible, biopsy of the lesions in the affected organs is desirable. Biopsies may be obtained from skin, nasopharyngeal lesions (if present) in WG and MPA. If no easily accessible lesions are seen, then the clinical picture present decides the next most appropriate site for biopsy. In most cases in ICU, a renal or lung biopsy may be most appropriate. Although features specific for vasculitis are rarely seen, percutaneous renal biopsy may show focal, segmental necrotizing glomerulonephritis without immune deposits (pauci-immune) and this generally reflects a systemic vasculitis. When lungs are involved, open lung or thoracoscopic biopsy provides a higher diagnostic yield than transbronchial biopsy.

No single test is capable of distinguishing between or even diagnosing various forms of vasculitides; a combination of history and clinical examination as well as serological, histopathological and radiological tests are required to make a final diagnosis.

Management

The mainstay of management is early and rapid identification of the vasculitic process and early treatment. The severity of disease dictates the intensity of initial treatment, which in turn is often directly associated with risk of treatment-related complications such as sepsis.

A combination of high dose corticosteroids and cyclophosphamide is the most commonly used first-line treatment for active generalized disease. Remission in WG and MPA has been reported to be up to 90%; this may be less so in the critically ill . Trial of corticosteroids alone can be considered for CSS, PAN and conditions that are not immediately life threatening. Although both drugs are usually given orally, in the critically ill, the IV route is preferred as there may be uncertainty about gastric absorption. There is evidence that pulsed IV cyclophosphamide is as effective in obtaining remission as oral therapy and may be less toxic. For the patient in ICU with fulminant multisystem disease, methylprednisolone is given IV in three daily doses (total daily dose of 0.25–1.0g) for 3–5 days followed by 1mg/kg oral prednisolone or equivalent. Cyclophosphamide (0.5–1g/m^2 body surface area) IV is given at the same time and repeated at 1–4 weekly intervals. Alternatively, 2–4mg/kg of oral cyclophosphamide is used, if gastric absorption is assured. Azathioprin may be substituted for cyclophosphamide at 3 months to reduce complications of therapy.

In addition to these therapies, plasma exchange may be used, though its role is far from clear. Because of the complications and morbidity associated with steroids and cyclophosphamide, alternative therapies with mycofenylate mofetil, levamisol and TNF-α inhibitors have been used recently. Many newer therapies and immunosuppressants are being trialled. There are several case reports of benefit of activated human factor VII in cases of DAH.

Specific ICU management

The management of these patients in the ICU is supportive in addition to specific immunosuppressive therapy. A few points are worthy of mention:

- WG involves the upper respiratory tract and patients may have subglottic stenosis making intubation potentially difficult. An ETT of smaller diameter may be needed, and tracheostomy may be required in many.
- DAH and massive pulmonary haemorrhage increase early mortality. Lung protective ventilation may reduce injury to lungs and allow DAH to resolve. Permissive hypercapnoea may be beneficial.
- Cardiovascular management may require invasive monitoring to keep patients on the 'drier' side while avoiding complications. This will reduce pulmonary oedema and may help in reducing DAH.
- Many patients will develop acute renal failure and will thus require renal support. This may be temporary, but the majority of patients will require long-term RRT and will progress to end-stage renal disease.
- Sepsis must be aggressively treated, as one of the common complications of immunosuppressive therapy is infection.
- Adequate nutrition, tight control of blood sugar, DVT prophylaxis, etc. will be required in managing these patients.

Conclusions

Vasculitides are very rare in the ICU and have a high mortality. Delays in diagnosis of vasculitis in a previously undiagnosed patient are due to a number of factors, not the least because of the rarity of the condition in UK ICUs. Nevertheless, prompt diagnosis is important for effective and aggressive therapy to be started. Unusual presentation, a high index of suspicion, detailed history and clinical examination along with serology in ANCA-associated vasculitides will speed the diagnostic process and start of therapy.

Further reading

Frankel SK, Cosgrove GP, Fischer A, *et al.* Update in the diagnosis and management of pulmonary vasculitis. *Chest* 2006;129: 452–65.

ICNARC case-mix programme database. ICNARC, UK. 2007.

Semple D, Keogh J, Forni L, *et al.* Clinical review: vasculitis on the intensive care unit—part 1: diagnosis. *Crit Care* 2004; 9: 92–7.

Semple D, Keogh J, Forni L, *et al.* Clinical review: vasculitis on the intensive care unit—part 2: treatment and prognosis. *Crit Care* 2004; 9: 193–7.

Seo P, Stone J. The antineutrophil cytoplasmic antibody-associated vasculitides. *Am J Med* 2004; 117: 39–50.

Source control

The reported incidence of severe sepsis in critical care units varies between countries, e.g. 11.8 per 100 ICU admissions in New Zealand/Australia, 27.1 per 100 in the UK. Such patients have an increased LOS and a higher mortality. A significant proportion of patients will be admitted because of their infection, whilst others will acquire it during their stay. Respiratory and abdominal infections are the most common cause of severe sepsis.

Surgery is not the only option when considering source control; the benefit of any intervention must be balanced against the inherent risk of performing the procedure itself and any associated complications.

Prophylaxis

Prevention is better than cure— the following (not exhaustive) should always be considered:

- Hand washing
- Aseptic technique
- Eradication therapy
  - MRSA to prevent colonisation
  - Selective decontamination of the digestive tract (SDD) to reduce risk of VAP
- Isolation of infected patients
- Closed suction of the respiratory tract
- Environment
  - Wall washing
  - Damp dusting
- Microbiological surveillance

These are usually incorporated into local policy. Some are common sense, some have strong evidence and some do not.

Treatment options

Any infective process may fuel an inflammatory response and may result in severe sepsis and MOF. The source may be an abscess, necrotic tissue, contamination secondary to a perforated viscus or an infected foreign body, e.g. in-dwelling catheter. In broad terms, source management may involve:

- Antibiotics
- Surgical/percutaneous drainage
- Debridement
- Catheter removal

Recent advances in imaging and interventional techniques frequently make percutaneous management an option with a better risk–benefit profile.

Antibiotics

The early use of appropriate antibiotics, i.e. within 1h of recognizing severe sepsis, is advised. This approach is associated with improved survival irrespective of whether infection is suspected or confirmed (the Surviving Sepsis Campaign guidelines). It also helps with source control. A knowledge of the local ecology and resistance patterns is essential in antibiotic choice; a good working relationship with the microbiology department is vital. Protocols may be in place but these need to evolve to fit the local ecology. If non-stock antibiotics are needed, then mechanisms to allow them to be rapidly dispensed from the pharmacy will minimize delays in administration.

Abscess

An abscess is a liquid-filled collection containing a variety of cells walled off from surrounding healthy tissue. It may drain spontaneously, to form a sinus or fistula, or as a result of surgical or radiological intervention. Imaging by ultrasound and CT are now both accurate and easy in competent hands and can easily proceed immediately to percutaneous drainage if possible. This reduces the risk of contamination, avoids the need for an operation and hence the complications associated with a surgical wound, e.g. wound infection, dehiscence and pain control.

The site of the collection and severity of illness of the patient will have some bearing on the method of control, e.g. an empyema can be identified with portable ultrasound and drained via a thoracostomy tube in the ward/ICU environment. More invasive radiological or surgical intervention will require transfer of the patient to another department with the additional risks that this entails. It is important to consider unusual sources of infection including sinus and dental collections.

Source control is secondary to appropriate resuscitation measures, but may have to occur concurrently and indeed may on occasion assist resuscitation. In dire circumstances where surgical drainage is necessary, then use of a temporary percutaneous drain could allow time for adequate resuscitation prior to definitive surgery.

The source of infection may be from a perforated viscus. This is likely to be identified clinically but aided by imaging. Management will be influenced by the severity of illness of the patient, the available surgical expertise and the site of the perforation. Options include:

- Surgery; removal of the damaged viscus, e.g. appendicectomy
- Drain insertion
- A proximal, defunctioning ostomy can be created
- Damage limitation surgery, i.e. doing the minimum to eliminate the source and allow recovery before returning for definitive treatment

Necrotic tissue

Dead tissue is an ideal medium to support the growth of microorganisms. Debridement, if possible, is the optimal management, and timing is critical; however, there are also a variety of potential approaches in different circumstances:

- Surgery
- The use of special dressings
- Applying enzymatic or other biological agents

Often a combination of the above is used. Typical radiological signs of necrosis will not always be evident, and in these circumstances, particularly when the patient is critically ill, surgery is the only safe option.

In most circumstances, debridement is not required immediately and therefore there will be time to resuscitate and stabilize the patient prior to surgery, e.g. debridement for necrotizing fasciitis should be performed within 12h, although as a general principle, the earlier the better. There are some situations where delay is beneficial and associated with better outcome, e.g. allowing clear demarcation between healthy and necrotic tissue to develop, during which time hyperaemia in surrounding inflamed tissue will reduce so there is less bleeding during surgery. It is for this reason that delayed pancreatic necrosectomy is associated with a better outcome.

The use of continuous peritoneal lavage may remove contaminated tissue and and reduce the risk of recurrent infection. Planned re-laparotomy can be facilitated by adopting an 'open abdomen' technique where mesh or another material is used to cover the defect temporarily. This avoids the risks associated with raised intra-abdominal pressure but can expose the patient to further infection and is labour intensive to manage.

Infected foreign body

The most common infected foreign body in ICU is the in-dwelling CVC. It always makes sense to remove an infected object. Occasionally this is not possible, e.g. endocarditis in a prosthetic valve.

When an in-dwelling vascular catheter is suspected as a source of infection, blood cultures should be taken from the line and via a peripheral stab. A new site is best, but if this is problematic then an infected line can safely be changed over a guide wire unless there is infection or inflammation around the entry site. Local guidelines should be followed. Tunnelled lines are less likely to become infected, and soft tissue infection can be managed with appropriate antibiotics.

There is debate as to when lines should be changed. Venous catheters should only be changed when there is evidence of infection.

Summary

1 Surveillance/prophylaxis

2 Early antibiotics/resuscitation

3 Source identification

- Imaging will depend on suspected site and severity of illness of patient. Seek advice from radiologist
- If collection identified, need to identify underlying cause. May require contrast studies

3 Source control

- Collection should be drained (percutaneous or surgical)
- Perforated viscus could be removed or defunctioned
- Extensive debridement within 12h of diagnosing necrotizing fasciitis
- Conservative/supportive management and/or peritoneal lavage if pancreatic necrosis
- Consider surgery if negative imaging confirmed by senior radiologist, dead tissue suspected as underlying cause and patient critically ill
- Only change invasive lines when they are suspected as the underlying cause or there is evidence of infection, e.g. inflamed/purulent entry site

Further reading

Jimenez MF, Marshall JC. Source control in the managament of sepsis. *Intensive Care Med* 2001; 27: S49–62.

Kunar A, Roberts D, Wood KE, *et al.* Duration of hypotension before initiation of effective antimicrobial therapy is the critical determinant of survival in human septic shock. *Crit Care Med* 2006; 34: 1589–96.

Selective decontamination of the digestive tract (SDD)

Philosophy

The key to SDD for infection control in the ICU is to consider that there are three different types of infection due to a limited range, 15 PPM, of potentially pathogenic microorganisms (PPMs): 6 'normal' and 9 'abnormal' organisms. Each requires a different prophylactic manoeuvre.

- Exogenous infections are controlled by a high level of hygiene
- Primary endogenous infections are controlled by the immediate administration of parenteral antibiotics.
- Secondary endogenous infections are controlled by the application of enteral antimicrobials in the throat and gut (See Table 27.7.1).

The terminology

Primary endogenous: infections caused by pathogens present on admission

Secondary endogenous: infections caused by pathogens not present on admission, but developing after acquired colonization in ICU

Exogenous: infections caused by pathogens not present on admission and developing without preceding colonization

Definition

SDD is a prophylactic protocol using hygiene, parenteral and enteral antimicrobials which aims to control exogenous, and primary and secondary endogenous infections, due to the 15 PPMs and hence reduce mortality.

Efficacy

There are 56 RCTs and 13 meta-analyses assessing the efficacy of SDD.

SDD reduces the OR for lower airway and bloodstream infections to 0.35 (95% confidence interval 0.29–0.41) and to 0.63 (95% CI 0.46–0.87), respectively.

SDD has the following effects.

1. Significantly reduces carriage and infection due to aerobic Gram-negative bacilli and yeasts (See Table 27.7.2).
2. Reduces Gram-positive lower airway infections (OR 0.52; 95% CI 0.34–0.78).
3. Does not reduce carriage due to Gram-positive bacteria (i.e. not significant).
4. Does not increase gram-positive bloodstream infections (OR 1.03; 95% CI 0.75–1.41).
5. Does not significantly reduce fungaemia (OR 0.89, 95% CI 0.16–4.95), due to the low event rate.

The most recent mortality meta-analysis including 4755 patients from 22 RCTs demonstrates that SDD reduces the OR for mortality to 0.71 (0.62–0.82) (See Table 27.7.2).

Safety

SDD does not increase the problem of antimicrobial resistance but rather solves the antibiotic resistance problem. An RCT of 1000 patients reported that carriage of aerobic Gram-negative bacteria (AGNB) resistant to imipenem, ceftazidime, ciprofloxacin, tobramycin and polymyxins occurred in 16% of patients receiving parenteral and enteral antimicrobials, compared with 26% of control patients receiving only parenteral antibiotics with an RR of 0.6 (95% CI 0.5–0.8).

Antimicrobial resistance as a long-term issue in SDD has been investigated in 11 studies over periods varying between 2 and 9 years, and bacterial resistance associated with SDD has not been a clinical problem.

Practical guidelines: how to do SDD

All ICU patients requiring >2 days of mechanical ventilation are given, on admission, parenteral cefotaxime in high doses, for 4 days. This targets mortality due to 'early' primary endogenous infections—'normal' PPMs such as *S. pneumoniae* and *S. aureus* (See Table 27.7.3)

Enteral antimicrobials are given throughout the treatment on ICU to control mortality associated with 'late' secondary endogenous infections.

A paste or gel is applied into the oropharynx to prevent or eradicate oral carriage of 'abnormal' PPMs, in the oropharynx. A suspension is administered via the NG tube to decontaminate stomach and gut.

Polymyxin and tobramycin are used to control carriage of 'abnormal' Gram-negative bacteria, in particular *Pseudomonas aeruginosa*. Enteral vancomycin is added to polymyxin/tobramycin in the case of MRSA endemicity. Enteral amphotericin B or nystatin is used to control yeast overgrowth.

'Exogenous' infections should be prevented by hygiene measures.

Regular surveillance cultures of throat and rectum are obtained to monitor efficacy and safety of the enteral antimicrobials.

SDD and evidence-based medicine

Five ICU interventions have been shown convincingly to reduce mortality (RCTs).

SDD has grade A recommendation and can be applied in all patients requiring long-term intensive care. It addresses the ever-increasing resistance problem. The same cannot be said for low tidal volume, APC, intensive insulin and steroids which have only been evaluated in specific subsets of ICU patients.

Conclusion

SDD is an evidence-based medical manoeuvre using parenteral and enteral antimicrobials which reduces morbidity by 65% and mortality by 29%. It is not associated with antimicrobial resistance emerging in unselected critically ill patients. It is a prophylactic method that costs 6 Euros a day.

Further Reading

Brun-buisson C, Legrand P, Rauss A, *et al.* Intestinal decontamination for control of multi-resistant Gram-negative bacilli. *Ann Intern Med* 1989; 110: 873–81.

Liberati A, D'Amico R, Pifferi S, *et al.* Antibiotic prophylaxis to reduce respiratory tract infections and mortality in adults receiving intensive care. *Cochrane Database Syst Rev* 2004; (1): CD000022.

Silvestri L, van Saene HKF. Survival benefit of the full digestive decontamination regimen. Systematic review of randomised controlled trials. *J Crit Care* 2008, in press.

Silvestri L, van Saene HKF, Casarin A, *et al.* Impact of selective decontamination of the digestive tract on carriage and infection due to Gram-negative and Gram-positive bacteria: a systematic review of randomised controlled trials. *Anaesth Intensive Care*, 2008; 36, 324–38.

Silvestri L, van Saene HKF, Milanese M, *et al.* Impact of selective decontamination of the digestive tract on fungal carriage and infection: systematic review of randomized controlled trials. Intensive Care Med 2005; 31: 898–910.

Silvestri L, van Saene HKF, Milanese M, *et al.* Selective decontamination of the digestive tract reduces bacterial bloodstream infections and mortality in critically ill patients. Systematic review of randomized controlled trials. J Hosp Infect 2007; 65, 187–203.

van Saene HKF, Silvestri L, de la Cal MA, *et al.* Selective decontamination of the digestive tract reduces lower airway and blood stream infection and mortality and prevents emergence of antimicrobial resistance. Microbes Infect 2006; 8: 953–4.

Table 27.7.1 Control of nosocomial infection

Infection	PPM	Timing	Frequency	Manoeuvre
1. Prim endog	6 'normal' 9 'abnormal'	<1 week	55%	Parenteral antimicrobials
2. Sec endog	9 'abnormal'	>1 week	30%	Enteral antimicrobials
3. Exogenous	9 'abnormal'	Any time during ICU treatment	15%	Hygiene
4. Monitoring efficacy/safety prophylaxis				Surveillance cultures Throat/rectum

PPM = potentially pathogenic microorganisms; Prim endog = primary endogenous; Sec endog = secondary endogenous.

6 'normal' PPM are *Streptococcus pneumoniae*, *Haemophilus influenzae*, *Moraxella catarrhalis*, *Candida albicans*, *Staphylococcus aureus*, *Escherichia coli*

9 'abnormal' PPM are *Klebsiella*, *Proteus*, *Morganella*, *Enterobacter*, *Citrobacter*, *Serratia*, *Acinetobacter*, *Pseudomonas* species and MRSA.

Table 27.7.2 Impact of SDD on carriage/infection due to Gram –ve, Gram +ve bacteria and yeasts

PPM	Type of patient	Sample size	Carriage OR (95% CI)	Overall infection OR (95% CI)
Gram –ve	All	9473	O. 0.13 (0.07–0.23) R. 0.15 (0.07–0.31)	0.17 (0.10–0.28)
Gram +ve	All	9473	O. 0.55 (6.30–1.02) R. 0.53 (0.12–2.43)	0.76 (0.41–1.40)
Yeasts	All	6075	0.32 (0.19–0.53)	0.30 (0.17–0.53)

PPM = potentially pathogenic microorganisms; O. = oropharyngeal; R. = rectal.

Table 27.7.3 Full four-component protocol of SDD

Target PPM and antimicrobials	Total daily dose (4 × daily)		
	<5yrs	5–12yrs	>12yrs
1. Enteral antimicrobials: 'abnormal' PPM			
A. Ooropharynx			
AGNB: polymyxin E with tobramycin	2 g of 2% paste or gel	2 g of 2% paste or gel	2 g of 2% paste or gel
Yeasts: amphotericin B or nystatin	2 g of 2% paste or gel	2 g of 2% paste or gel	2 g of 2% paste or gel
MRSA: vancomycin	2 g of 4% paste or gel	2 g of 4% paste or gel	2 g of 4% paste or gel
B. Gut			
AGNB: polymyxin E (mg)	100	200	400
with tobramycin (mg)	80	160	320
Yeasts : amphotericin B (mg) or	500	1000	2000
nystatin (units)	2×10^6	4×10^6	8×10^6
MRSA: vancomycin (mg)	20–40/kg	20–40/kg	500–2000
2. Parenteral antimicrobials: 'normal' PPM			
cefotaxime (mg)	150/kg	200/kg	4000
3. Hygiene			
4. Surveillance cultures of throat and rectum on admission, Monday, Thursday			

Markers of infection

The diagnosis of infection in the ICU patient may be obvious or extremely difficult. Infection, and especially sepsis, is a leading cause of death and the main cost driver in ICUs. Epidemiologic data show that sepsis is the third most frequent cause of death after coronary heart disease and MI in Germany. The first clinical signs of infection or sepsis are usually non-specific (e.g. fever or leucocytosis). More specific symptoms, such as arterial hypotension or raised lactate, often indicate progression to organ dysfunction associated with an increased mortality rate of 35–70%.

The ideal infection/sepsis marker has high sensitivity and specificity, easy handling and low costs. The marker should be able to indicate the stages of the disease and the prognosis of the patient.

The inflammatory reaction consists of humoral, cellular and molecular pathways. Changes in body temperature, leucocyte count, heart rate, blood pressure and respiration rate are clinical signs of systemic inflammation. They are neither specific nor sensitive for sepsis and also occur in non-infectious states. Generalized inflammation with organ dysfunction (systemic inflammatory response syndrome) may also result from pancreatitis, major trauma and burns. The American College of Chest Physicians/Society of Critical Care Medicine consensus criteria are not helpful for clinical differentiation at the bedside. Ideally, an infection marker should meet the following demands:

1 Shorten the time to and accuracy of diagnosis
2 Facilitate the differentiation between infectious and non-infectious causes of inflammation and its sequelae—organ dysfunction or shock
3 Allow differentiation between underlying viral and bacterial infections
4 Reflect the effectiveness of antimicrobial treatment and other measures of source control more accurately than conventional clinical and laboratory signs.

Clinical approach

Once infection is suspected in the ICU patient, the goal is to identify the infecting pathogen.

History: key points

- Past medical history to identify previous infections and co-morbidities) recently used antimicrobial therapy, recent medical interventions or the risk for colonization/infection with resistant organisms.
- Mental state. Septic encephalopathy is one of the most commonly missed initial signs of an infection.

Examination and investigation: key points

- Clinical opinion to confirm diagnosis by measuring temperature, respiratory rate, heart rate and blood pressure, examination of CNS, thorax, heart, lung, abdomen, kidney or any other susceptible area.
- FBC to measure the WCC.
- Blood specimen (2–3 blood aerobic and anaerobic cultures).
- Urine specimen to exclude UTI.
- Bronchoalveolar lavage (BAL) or tracheal secretions and direct examination of BAL specimen using Gram staining for the diagnosis of pneumonia.
- Faeces in the presence of diarrhoea,
- Other specimen (CSF, exudates, swabs of mucous membranes).
- Tips of in-dwelling catheters.
- Microbiological investigation of any drainage fluid available.
- Radiological investigation (CXR or a CT scan) searching a focus.
- Echocardiogram to exclude endocarditis.
- Dental status excluding an odontogenous focus.

Special investigations

- Procalcitonin (PCT): bacterial endotoxins are a major stimulus for PCT induction, but Gram-positive infections may also induce a PCT release and may be detected within 2h of endotoxaemia or bacteraemia. During severe fungal infections, PCT induction has been described in some patients. However, major surgery, severe trauma or burns may also induce an increase of PCT plasma levels, although usually not as high as in patients with severe sepsis or septic shock. A number of studies confirm PCT as a marker of severe infections and sepsis. Those with PCT levels ≤0.5ng/ml are unlikely to have severe sepsis or septic shock, whereas levels >2ng/ml identify patients at high risk. PCT concentrations >10ng/ml usually occur in patients with organ failure remote from the site of infection. When PCT is released non-specifically because of major surgery or severe trauma, daily monitoring may be helpful to detect supervening septic complications early.
- CRP is an acute-phase protein that is released from hepatic cells after stimulation by inflammatory mediators such as IL-6 and IL-8. The value of high plasma levels of CRP in diagnosing patients with infection and sepsis or the assessment of sepsis severity is controversial. CRP may not peak not till 48h. Circulating CRP increases during minor infections, does not correlate with the severity of host response and does not differentiate between survivors and non-survivors of sepsis. CRP plasma levels may remain elevated up to several days, and it is found in many non-infectious conditions, such as autoimmune and rheumatic disorders, ACS and malignant tumours, and after surgery.
- Endotoxin (LPS) is an essential structure in the outer cell membrane of Gram-negative bacteria. The Limulus amoebocyte lysate assay was problematic, with wide variation in value, low specificity (due to differences in the endotoxin structure in different bacteria) and interactions with plasma proteins and antibiotics. A new highly sensitive ex vivo biological assay will soon be available. It measures the zymosan antibody- and antiendotoxin antibody-elicited respiratory burst in a kinetic luminometric assay. It has a high negative predictive value for the diagnosis of Gram-negative infection and sepsis, with a sensitivity of 85.3% and a specificity of 44%. The endotoxin activity essay has promise for Gram-negative infection.

Clinical diagnostic difficulties to consider

In sepsis, blood cultures are positive in ~30–40% of those with sepsis and with false positives. Positive results may indicate colonization or contamination without pathophysiological relevance. Microbiological diagnosis may be difficult in patients with prior antibiotic treatment. In 35%, sepsis cannot be proved microbiologically despite the presence of clinical signs and suspicion of a focus.

Diagnosis of special infections

Ventilator-associated pneumonia

The diagnosis of VAP is difficult since there is no accurate diagnostic criterion which reliably differentiates pneumonia from non-infectious causes of pulmonary infiltration. Interpretation of microbiological findings is hampered by the high rate of colonization in mechanically ventilated patients. The International Sepsis Forum recommends the use of the Clinical Pulmonary Infection Score (CPIS) for the diagnosis of VAP (CPIS >6). The score is based on body temperature, WCC, volume and appearance of tracheal secretions, oxygenation (PAO_2/FIO_2), CXR and tracheal aspirate cultures. The CPIS allows for a standardized diagnosis by using simple clinical end-points. In a clinical study, the CPIS was able to diagnose pneumonia with a sensitivity of 93% and a specificity of 100%.

Catheter-induced infection

Again difficult. A catheter-induced infection cannot be diagnosed without the removal of the catheter. If a CVC is a potential source of infection, it needs to be removed to be tested. Blood cultures should be taken from the CVC before removal, plus a peripheral blood culture. Swabs should be taken from the insertion site. If infection is suspected, change of the CVC via the guide wire is not recommended. As routine change of CVC does not reduce the risk of bacteraemia, CVC change should be performed in the presence of suspected infection, not routinely.

Wound infection

In the presence of a wound infection, blood cultures are recommended. Ultrasonography-guided diagnostic puncture for fluid under a closed wound, or taking swabs from the suspected area enables microbiological diagnosis. A Gram stain, and aerobic and anaerobic microbiological cultures are recommended.

Intra-abdominal sepsis

Classical clinical and laboratory findings of intra-abdominal pathologies include fever, leucocytosis, elevated PCT and localized abdominal tenderness. Post-operative abscesses are difficult to diagnose because these signs are often present after abdominal surgery in patients without abscesses. Abdominal CT scan using contrast is the ultimate diagnostic intervention for diagnosis. Reduced mortality from intra-abdominal sepsis is attributed to early diagnosis using CT scanning rather than any improvement in the therapy of MOF.

Acute acalculous cholecystitis

Acute acalculous cholecystitis is marked by a very high mortality rate, but its relative rarity makes its features obscure to many physicians. The clinical findings can be subtle and misleading, contributing to delayed diagnosis. It must be excluded in all septic patients with an unknown focus presenting with right upper quadrant tenderness and pain and pathological cholestatic parameters. For the diagnosis, laboratory investigations (PCT), blood cultures, abdominal ultrasonography and abdominal CT scan are required.

Invasive Candida infection

The incidence of invasive *Candida* infection is ~1–2% in ICU patients. The gold standard for diagnosis of an invasive *Candida* infection is the histopathological or cytopathological proof in the suspected tissue areas or in usual sterile body fluids, but not the urine. Routine screening to identify *Candida* colonization, which is present in ~16% of ICU patients, is not recommended. Neutropenic, immune-compromised or immune-suppressed patient as well as patients after major abdominal surgery are at higher risk of developing a *Candida* infection.

Support group

German Sepsis Society <www.dsg.de.>, Tel. +49-3641-9323101.

Expert adviser

Professor K. Reinhart, Head of Department, Clinic for Anesthesiology and Intensive Care, D-07747 Jena, Germany

Further reading

Abraham E, Matthay MA, Dinarello CA, *et al.* Consensus conference definitions for sepsis, septic shock, acute lung injury, and acute respiratory distress syndrome: time for a re-evaluation. *Crit Care Med* 2000; 28: 232–5.

Clinical Pulmonary Infection Score (CPIS): *Am. J. Respir. Crit. Care Med.*, Volume 168, Number 2, July 2003, 173–179.

Engel C, Brunkhorst FM, Bone HG, *et al.* Epidemiology of sepsis in Germany: results from a national prospective multicenter study. *Intensive Care Med* 2007; 33: 606–18.

Meisner M, ed. Procalcitonin (PCT): a new innovative infection parameter. Biochemical and clinical aspects, 3rd revised and extended edn. Stuttgart; Georg Thieme Verlag, 2000.

Pugin J, Auckenthaler R, Mili N, *et al.* Diagnosis of ventilator-associated pneumonia by bacteriologic analysis of bronchoscopic and nonbronchoscopic 'blind' bronchoalveolar lavage fluid. *Am Rev Respir Dis* 1991; 143: 1121–9.

Ugarte H, Silva E, Mercan D, *et al.* Procalcitonin used as a marker of infection in the intensive care unit. *Crit Care Med* 1999; 27: 498–504.

Adrenal insufficiency and sepsis

Adrenal insufficiency is a condition in which cortisol synthesis, delivery and/or uptake by tissues is compromised. It is classified into:

1. Primary adrenal insufficiency when the adrenocortical cells are damaged or cortisol metabolism is altered.
2. Secondary adrenal insufficiency when corticotrophin releasing hormone or adrenocorticotrophin hormones synthesizing hypothalamic or pituitary cells are damaged.

A recent study in severe sepsis/septic shock suggested that adrenal insufficiency may reach 60%.

Mechanisms of action of glucocorticoids

Glucocorticoids act through genomic and non-genomic effects.

- Genomic effects: glucocorticoid is involved in regulation of gene transcription by nuclear receptors including genes for chemokines, cytokines, complement family members and innate immune-related genes, including scavenger and TLRs.
- Non-specific non-genomic effects: membrane effects of glucocorticoids in the hypothalamic synaptosomes affect sympathetic modulation of cardiac and blood vessel activity, as well as the potentiation of exogenous catecholamines.
- Specific non-genomic effects: enhanced endothelial NOS activation.

Main effects of glucocorticoids

Metabolic effects

Increase blood glucose concentrations by inducing systemic insulin resistance, liver gluconeogenesis and glycogenolysis. Enhance lipolysis and proteolysis, providing amino acids for neoglucogenesis.

Immune effects

- Innate immunity: increase neutrophils, promote apoptosis of eosinophils and basophils, improve opsonization and the activity of the scavenger system. Suppress the synthesis of inflammatory mediators such as cytokines, prostaglandins and leukotrienes.
- Adaptative immunity: prevent differentiation of CD4+ T cells into T helper (Th)1 lymphocytes, promote Th2 recruitment by increasing IL-10 secretion acting in synergy with IL-4. Thus, glucocorticoids induce a shift from a cellular toward a humoral immune response.

Cardiovascular effects

Maintain vascular tone, endothelium integrity, capillary permeability and myocardial inotropic activity. Synergistic with norepinephrine and angiotensin II. In catecholamine-treated septic shock, glucocorticoids improve SVR and hasten shock reversal.

Clinical approach

Examination: non-specific signs

- Hypotension, shock (90%)
- Fever (60-70%)
- Abdominal pain, distension (80–90%)
- Vomiting (50%).
- Confusion to coma (40–60%)

Special investigations

Random cortisol

If the serum albumin <25g/l, total cortisol levels may be unreliable; calculate free cortisol.

Random cortisol	
<3mcg/dl	Definite
<10mcg/dl	Maybe.
>44mcg/dl	Not

If cortisol levels are low, ACTH levels can discriminate between primary (high ACTH levels) and secondary adrenal insufficiency (low ACTH levels).

ACTH test

250mcg of synthetic corticotrophin.

cortisol levels >44mcg/dl or cortisol increment >16.8mc/dl rules out adrenal insufficiency.

Clinical consequences

Initial course of critical illness.

- Fluid and vasopressor unresponsiveness with low vascular resistance and high cardiac index
- Systemic inflammatory response syndrome with fever, tachycardia, tachypnea
- Multiple organ failure
- Increased risk of death from refractory shock

Late course of critical illness,

- Vasopressor dependency
- Ventilator dependency
- Multiple organ failure
- Increased risk of death from multiple organ failure

Management

Fluid and sodium losses should be managed with fluid and vasopressors, which should be titrated to restore SBP and tissue perfusion.

Practical modalities of hormonal treatment in sepsis

Steroids are indicated in adult septic shock patients whose blood pressure is poorly responsive to fluid resuscitation and vasopressor therapy. Not in the rest.

Treatment

- Hydrocortisone at a daily dose of 200–300mg.
- Treatment should be continued as long as the clinical consequences have disappeared. Prolonged treatment requires advice from an endocrinologist.
- Administration of fludrocortisone is optional and requires advice from an endocrinologist.

Surveillance

It is paramount that surveillance includes:

- blood glucose <150mg/dl
- serum sodium
- screening for infection. (hydrocortisone blunts the febrile response and interferes with WCC and inflammatory parameters.)

Further reading

Annane D, Maxime V, Ibrahim F, *et al.* Diagnosis of adrenal insufficiency in severe sepsis and septic shock. *Am J Respir Crit Care Med* 2006; 174: 1319–26.

Hamrahian AH, Oseni TS, Arafah BM. Measurements of serum free cortisol in critically ill patients. *N Engl J Med 2004*; 350: 1629–38.

Lipiner-Friedman D, Sprung CL, Laterre PF, *et al.* for the Corticus Study Group. Adrenal function in sepsis: the Corticus Retrospective Cohort Study. *Crit Care Med* 2007; 35: 1012–8.

Chapter 28

Trauma and burns

Chapter Contents

Initial management of major trauma

Major trauma remains a leading cause of death in both the developed and developing worlds, and has a significant impact on the workload of most critical care units. More people are disabled than killed, which has a significant impact on the economic potential of both the victims and society.

The most common method of initial management follows the principles espoused by the Advanced Trauma Life Support® (ATLS®) course of the American College of Surgeons. This course was started following an airplane crash in 1977 in which the family of James Styner (an orthopaedic surgeon working in Lincoln, Nebraska) was seriously injured. The management was so disorganized that, with colleagues, a course initially was devised to improve trauma care. This course, the ATLS® course, spread across the USA and then internationally.

The underpinning principle was the presumed tri-modal death distribution for major trauma, although this has been questioned in the UK where most trauma is made up of road traffic accidents. This concept proposes that there are a number of deaths immediately after trauma which are not amenable to medical intervention, a second peak of potentially avoidable deaths (the golden hour) and then those deaths occurring later, often in a critical care setting.

Predictors of death during the early period of trauma care include age of the patient, presence of isolated neurological damage, base excess, haemoglobin level and the triage revised trauma score. Trauma scoring is used as a means of describing injury severity, predicting patient outcomes and evaluating aspects of care. The scoring systems vary, with some using physiological variables (GCS, Revised Trauma Score), and others anatomical injury (Abbreviated Injury Score, Injury Severity Score). In the UK, the Trauma Audit and Research Network coordinates the audit of patient outcomes in a similar way to that of ICNARC and publishes outcomes on its website (www.uktarn.ac.uk).

Priorities in the golden hour revolve around the ABCDE resuscitation principles common to many of the life support courses.

In this context, ABCDE translates into:

1 **A**irway maintenance with cervical spine protection
2 **B**reathing and ventilation
3 **C**irculation with haemorrhage control
4 **D**isability: neurological status
5 **E**xposure/environmental control

In addition, the concept of primary and secondary surveys was introduced.

In the primary survey, the immediately life-threatening interventions are identified and dealt with using mainly clinical skills, with the addition of adjuncts. The management of the patient in the primary survey focuses on symptom and sign detection and their treatment, with less focus on the detail of diagnosis.

A

The airway is secured in a standardized way regardless of the underlying cause of obstruction. If the airway requires intubation to be performed, then capnography should be available to confirm tube placement.

The cervical spine is assumed to be injured in all victims of blunt trauma, and either the 'holy trinity' of hard collar, head blocks and tape/straps, or manual in-line immobilization until injury is ruled out.

B

There have traditionally been six 'immediately life-threatening' injuries taught using the acronym ATOM FC.

- Airway obstruction
- Tension pneumothorax
- Open pneumothorax
- Massive haemothorax
- Flail chest
- Cardiac tamponade

Thoracic trauma comprises 10–15% of all trauma and is the cause of death in 25% of all fatalities due to trauma. The mortality increases if there are>6 broken ribs, but this effect is reduced by the use of epidural analgesia.

Pulmonary contusion underlying a flail chest or in isolation is the most common injury requiring ongoing ventilation in a critical care unit, and is treated as for any other lung injury with appropriate use of PEEP.

C

By far the most common cause of haemodynamic disturbance in the early phase of trauma management is haemorrhage. Volume of blood loss can be assessed using the acronym one on the floor and four more; pelvis, chest, abdomen and long bones. The degree of shock in the early phase is often assessed using a grading system such as the ATLS® system that is based on the physiological disturbance related to the volume of estimated blood loss. Using this system, easily remembered from tennis scores, shock is graded from grade 1 (0–15% blood loss), through grade 2 (15–30%), grade 3 (30–40%) to grade 4 (>40% blood loss). Of note, SBP does not fall until grade 3 although the pulse pressure narrows as vasoconstriction raises the diastolic pressure. Both base deficit and lactate have been suggested as a monitor of the extent of shock.

Minimizing the time from injury to operative intervention has been shown to reduce the mortality in shocked trauma patients.

Adjuncts such as radiology of chest and pelvis and abdominal ultrasound (Focused Abdominal Scan for Trauma, FAST) for haemorrhagic shock may add diagnostic information, which mandates the patient going to theatre during the C of the primary survey. Using modern 16-slice CT scanners, total whole-body scanning time is ~120s. 64-slice CT scanners may reduce scanning time to <30s, although time to interpret the scans remains the same. If the scanner is adjacent to the emergency department, then CT scans provide more accurate diagnostic information, but unstable patients should go straight for operative intervention.

Bleeding from pelvic injury is best controlled with a combination of pelvic closure, using external fixators or binders, and angiographic embolization, although pelvic packing may also have a place.

Damage control laparotomy is increasingly employed to avoid the cold, coagulopathic and acidotic patient resistant to resuscitation. Control of bleeding and contamination is achieved and then the patient is admitted to the critical care unit to be fluid resuscitated, warmed and optimized with temporary closure of the abdomen. The patient is then returned to theatre for definitive repair of injury once stable.

There is an increasing drive for 'permissive hypotension' in the shocked bleeding patient, with the aim in the short term of resuscitation to maintain life but avoid excessive volumes and the risk of clot disruption until control of haemorrhage has been achieved. The only good evidence relates to penetrating truncal trauma in an urban setting, but the tendency is to resuscitate to an end-point of a palpable radial pulse until control of bleeding has been gained. Additional therapies such as early administration of clotting factors and other agents such as antifibrinolytics and activated VIIa may also have a place in the treatment of major haemorrhage.

D

Head injury accounts for 25% of trauma deaths. Morbidity and mortality are substantially increased by hypoxia and hypotension. Signs of an intracerebral haematoma such as unilateral pupil dilatation or lateralizing signs may be an indication for a CT scan for brain injury in D of the primary survey. This should only be performed if life-threatening haemorrhage has been treated or ruled out.

E

The final stage of the primary survey is complete exposure of the patient with care taken to not render them hypothermic.

Once the primary survey has been completed and the patient is improving, then a secondary survey is initiated with the aim of detecting all potential threats to life and any other injuries that may threaten the patient's return to full activity. In the context of critical care where the patient is usually sedated, the major missed injuries include ligament injuries in the knee, compartment syndromes and fractures of the small bones in the foot or hand. Some have proposed a tertiary survey to minimize these. Missed injuries are more common in those patients with a prolonged critical care stay.

Further reading

Bickell WH, Wall MJ, Pepe PE, *et al.* Immediate versus delayed fluid resuscitation for hypotensive patients with penetrating torso injuries. *N Engl J Med* 199427; 331: 1105–9.

Cales RH, Trunkey DD. Preventable trauma deaths. A review of trauma care systems development. *JAMA* 1985; 254: 1059–63.

Flagel BT, Luchette FA, Reed RL, *et al.* Half-a-dozen ribs: the breakpoint for mortality. *Surgery* 2005; 138: 717–25.

Janjua KJ, Sugrue M, Deane SA. Prospective evaluation of missed injuries and the role of tertiary trauma survey. *J Trauma* 1998; 44: 1001–6.

Lichtveld RA, Panhuizen IF, Smit RBJ, *et al.* Predictors of death in trauma patients who are alive on arrival at hospital. *Eur J Trauma Emerg Surg* 2007; 1: 46–51.

Mackenzie R, Bevan D. Is the 'golden hour' a prehospital event? *Emerg Med J* 2005; 22: e1.

Martinowitz U, Kenet G, Segal E, *et al.* Recombinant activated factor VII for adjunctive haemorrhage control in trauma *J Trauma* 2001; 51: 431–9.

Spahn CR, Cerny V, Coats TJ, *et al.* Management of bleeding following major trauma: a European guideline. *Crit Care* 2007; 11: R17

Ziegler DW, Agarwal NN. The morbidity and mortality of rib fractures. *J Trauma* 1994; 37: 975–9.

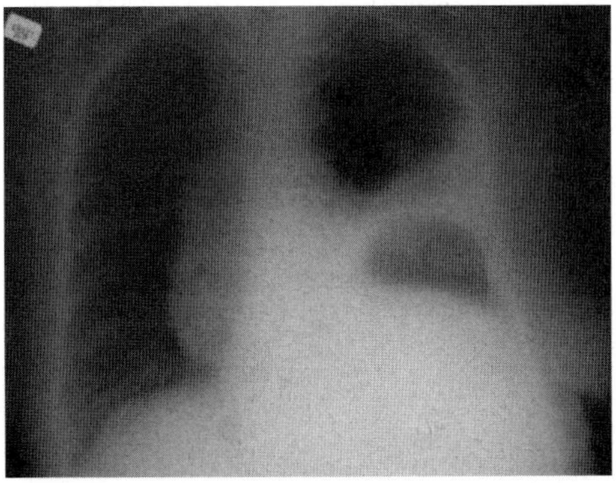

Fig. 28.1.1 Example of a ruptured diaphragm.

Head injury

Definition

Head injury is traditionally divided into mild, moderate and severe based upon the GCS (13–15, 8–13 and <8, respectively).

Incidence

The estimated incidence of major head injury, or traumatic brain injury (TBI) is between 100 and 400 per 100 000 capita. Worldwide that correlates with 1 in 8 deaths in men and 1 in 14 deaths in women.

Epidemiology

Head injury represents a major cause of death and long-term disability in young and old, with the subgroup of young men at a particularly high risk. The majority of severe head injuries in the UK are associated with road traffic accidents and commonly involve trauma to multiple organ systems.

Primary brain injury

The primary injury is caused by axial loading and shearing forces on the individual axons within the brain. This is referred to as diffuse axonal injury (DAI). Radiologically this appears as diffuse brain swelling and loss of grey–white differentiation on CT imaging. There may also be focal changes evident commonly in frontal, temporal and occipital regions, referred to as contusions.

Primary brain injuries may be associated with injury to the arterial, venous and capillary vasculature. This can cause extradural, subdural and intraparenchymal haematomas.

Secondary brain injury

There are several mechanisms by which the injured brain suffers a secondary injury. These can be divided into two categories.

The failure of adequate oxygen delivery

Brain oxygen delivery is governed by the following principles;

- Cerebral oxygen delivery = Blood oxygen content x Blood Flow ($\propto$PaCO2)
- Blood oxygen content = **haemoglobin level** x 1.32 x % **oxygen saturation**
- Cerebral perfusion pressure = **mean arterial pressure – intracranial pressure**

Manipulation of the parameters in bold will improve oxygen delivery to the cerebrum as a whole.

Cerebral blood flow *per se* will depend upon the resistance of the vessels in question and cardiac output, in addition to the CPP. It is the vessel resistance and capacitance that vary with fluctuations in $PaCO_2$.

Delivery must be equal to or in excess of oxygen consumption. The major determinant of consumption is the cerebral metabolic rate.

- **Cerebral metabolic rate**; increased with seizures and pyrexia, reduced with sedation.

At the cellular level, changes in oxygen uptake and utilization may be responsible for the ischaemic areas that are demonstrated despite optimization of global oxygen delivery.

Post-trauma, cell injury mechanisms

These include excitotoxicity, inflammation, pyrexia, hyperglycaemia, apoptosis and free radical damage.

Clinical management

Initial assessment and immediate management

This should be based upon ATLS principles. The assessment of disability should include the GCS, which provides a framework for assessment, and guides therapeutic management, further investigation and prognosis. Assessment of pupillary size and reactivity also gives valuable information on ICP and focal intracranial injuries.

The decision to intubate and ventilate will depend upon the GCS (including deterioration) and the need for airway protection, the extent of other injuries and the need for transfer for investigation/definitive management. As a general rule, failure to obey commands, to maintain good oxygenation and normocapnoea, or confused and combative behaviour should lead to a decision to intubate using a rapid sequence induction and manual in-line stabilization of the cervical spine.

Investigation, referral, transfer and surgical intervention

Early definitive imaging allows identification of acute traumatic intracranial injury and improves outcome. It also guides decisions about the intensity and length of observation in low risk cases. The decision to perform a CT scan in mild/minor head injury will depend upon local resources and protocols.

Transfer to a specialist neurological centre will provide access to the skills and facilities for intracranial surgery and the availability of advanced monitoring and guided medical management. Features mandating discussion with a neurosurgeon include:

- CT scan in a general hospital shows an acute intracranial lesion.
- When a patient fulfils criteria for a CT scan, but this cannot be performed urgently.
- When a patient has clinical features suggesting specialist care is appropriate (whatever the result of the CT scan). *These include;*
    - Persisting coma (GCS <9) and no eye opening after initial resuscitation
    - Confusion persisting >4h
    - Deterioration in conscious level
    - Persistent focal neurological signs
    - A seizure without full recovery
    - Compound depressed skull fracture
    - Definite or suspected penetrating brain injury
    - CSF leak or other sign of a skull fracture.

Intensive care

Neurological intensive care is based upon the optimization of physiological parameters. The goals are a CPP of >60mm Hg and an ICP of <20mm Hg.

Techniques for reducing ICP are considered double-edged swords, and pursuit of arbitrary levels has the potential to have a negative impact on brain recovery. It has been suggested that more advanced monitoring techniques could better guide therapeutic intervention and possibly reduce harm.

Monitoring

Intracranial pressure

A pressure transducer inserted into the non-dominant cerebral hemisphere (intraparenchymal) is the most commonly used site in the UK. This gives a continuous, reliable and rapidly responsive estimation of ICP. Intraventricular catheters are the gold standard and they allow sampling of CSF. However, they are associated with an increased risk of infection, particularly when used for periods >7 days.

Metabolic monitoring

Focal tissue oxygenation ($P_{BR}O_2$)

Continuous measurement of tissue oxygenation is available and in current use in some departments in the UK. $P_{Br}O_2$ gives an early warning of impending ischaemia and may allow for less vigorous treatment of ICP. It also can guide alternative therapies to improve oxygen delivery, such as red cell transfusion and inotropes. A limitation is that oxygenation in a single area of brain tissue may not reflect other areas of the brain, and that 'tissue ischaemia' may be due to mitochondrial failure. There is some evidence that directing treatment to $P_{Br}O_2$ improves outcome in comparison with ICP-directed treatment.

Jugular bulb oxygen saturation ($S_{jv}O2$)

$S_{jv}O_2$ is a global measure of brain oxygenation; however, it suffers from the same limitations as $P_{Br}O_2$ in that areas of the brain that are not extracting oxygen will falsely elevate readings.

Cerebral blood flow

PET scanning, perfusion CT scans and perfusion-weighted MRI techniques have all been used to estimate CBF. These techniques are not continuous, are technically difficult and are unable to predict what level of perfusion is required to match metabolic demands for individual areas of the brain. They are, however, useful as research tools.

Microdialysis

Future monitors may include microdialysis of glucose, pyruvate and lactate, indicating areas of brain with inadequate perfusion. Measurement of excitotoxic amines and inflammatory mediators may also be useful in the future; but this is still at the experimental stage.

General ICU care

The focus of care is the avoidance of medical complications and the provision of an environment optimal for brain recovery. The Brain Trauma Foundation (BTF) recommends;

- **Keep sodium >140mmol/l.** A decrease in serum sodium produces an osmotic gradient across the blood–brain barrier and aggravates cerebral oedema.
- **Avoid hyperglycaemia** (treat blood glucose >11mmol/l). Hyperglycaemia may aggravate ischaemic brain injury by increasing cerebral lactic acidosis.
- **Feed via orogastric tube and use motility agents as required**
- **Use TED stockings and avoid low dose heparin**
- **Apply 15–30° head-up tilt with head in neutral position**
- **No parenteral, non-ionic fluid to be given.**

Specific treatment of raised ICP

Hyperventilation

Prolonged hyperventilation is detrimental; however, there is controversy whether short-term hyperventilation in response to an acute rise in ICP is harmful. It is efficacious in reducing ICP; but there is doubt as to how quickly after hyperventilation CBF returns to normal, which may be up to 24h. The BTF guidelines recommend that hyperventilation is limited to short periods and only when response to other medical treatments for raised ICP have failed.

Recommended target $PaCO_2$ is between 4 and 4.5kPa.

Hypertonic solutions

Providing the patient is normocapnic and adequately sedated, hypertonic solutions are the first-line agents used to treat persistently elevated ICP. Promising level 3 evidence is emerging on the use of hypertonic saline, and this may provide a useful treatment in the future.

Boluses of 2ml/kg of a 20% mannitol solution provide rapid and effective reduction in ICP.

Metabolic suppression

Suppression of cerebral electrical activity produces significant reductions in ICP in patients who have intact coupling between cerebral metabolism and flow. This can be tested by $PaCO_2$ responsiveness or a test dose of hypnotic agent.

In resistant raised ICP, barbiturates are recommended. These are administered as boluses followed by an infusion, with continuous monitoring of brain electrical activity to achieve burst suppression.

Surgical intervention

Early surgical intervention saves lives after head injury. Indications include hydrocephalus, contusions, extradural and subdural haematomas.

In addition, the role of decompressive craniectomy is currently under investigation, with some promising pilot studies.

Cerebral protection

Hypothermia

Pyrexia is common in brain injury and is associated with a worsening of outcome. It may be centrally mediated and independent of an infective cause. Hypothermia has been shown to be effective in animal models; however, trials of therapeutic hypothermia have failed to show benefit.

Hypothermia is associated with an increase in need for support of the circulation, electrolyte abnormalities, a raised serum amylase, bleeding and arrhythmias.

Maintenance of normothermia is common practice either by active cooling or by pharmacological intervention.

The lack of evidence surrounding pharmacological neuroprotective intervention makes it unlikely that changes in care for patients with severe head injury in hospitals without neurological services would deliver outcome improvements of the magnitude that could follow significant expansion in neurological intensive care facilities.

Conclusion

It therefore remains the priority of neurointensive care to deliver the assured physiological parameters and prevent medical and surgical complications impairing the patient's recovery.

Further reading

`http://www2.braintrauma.org/site/Pageserver?pagename=guidelines`

Marshall LF. Epidemiology and cost of central nervous system injury. *Clin Neurosurg* 2000; 46: 105–12.

Ravussin P. Abou-Madi M, Archer D, *et al.* Changes in CSF pressure after mannitol in patients with and without elevated CSF pressure. *J Neurosurg* 1988; 69: 869–76.

Stieffel MF, Spiotta A, Gracias V, *et al.* Reduced mortality rate in patients with severe traumatic brain injury treated with brain tissue oxygen monitoring. *J Neurosurg* 2005; 103: 805–11.

Sahuquillo J, Arikan F. Decompressive craniectomy for the treatment of refractory high intracranial pressure in traumatic brain injury. *Cochrane Database Syst Rev* 2006; (4): CD003983.

Spinal trauma

Spinal injuries can lead to a poor quality of life, reduced functional independence and marked financial and social implications for ongoing care in survivors of major trauma. The severity of the sequelae of spinal cord injury has led to PHTLS® and ATLS® advocating the management of airway security with cervical spine control as a first priority. Cervical spine injury is associated with up to 10% of blunt polytrauma.

Annually, there are 1000 new cases of cervical cord injury in the UK.

The pattern of spinal injuries involves 55% in cervical, 15% thoracic, 15% at the thoracolumbar junction and 15% in the lumbosacral area.

With any injury involving the head, neck or upper torso, one should strongly suspect a cervical spinal injury. Pre-existing spinal disease (rheumatoid arthritis/osteoarthritis, ankylosing spondylitis, canal stenosis) increases the risk of potential spinal cord injury. Trauma patients are often obtunded and unable to give a complete history or be adequately examined neurologically in the resuscitation room.

C spine clearance

Initial management will involve the 'holy trinity' of semi-rigid collar, blocks (sandbags) and tape. If the spine is protected, then evaluation of the spine can be withheld, whilst resuscitation and primary survey concentrate on ABCDE. In the polytrauma patient, this is often deferred to the ICU. The ICS has produced guidance on spinal evaluation in unconscious victims of blunt polytrauma (Fig. 28.3.1).

The standard 3-view cervical (craniocervical to C7/T1) radiograph series in the emergency setting may miss 5–10% of cervical injuries in the unconscious patient, and additional helical CT scanning of this region is recommended. Plain radiographs have a higher rate of detecting ligamentous disruption and malalignment, but CT is better for detecting fractures.

Many trauma patients on the ICU will be sedated, ventilated and have a potentially unstable C spine. Prolonged immobilization is associated with significant morbidity, including airway and central venous access difficulties, pneumonia, skin ulceration and venous thromboembolism.

It is strongly recommended that the cervical thoracic and lumbar spine who remains unconscious be cleared within 48–72h.

The routine use of MRI is not recommended, but should be urgently considered for any patient with a neurological deficit which may be amenable to surgical intervention.

Victims of polytrauma, high velocity injury or fall from a height of >6ft, who are obtunded and cannot be assessed clinically must have their thoracolumbar spine imaged. If thoracic/abdominal helical CT scanning is performed as part of the assessment, then these can be reconstructed to assess the thoracolumbar spine. Ideally, scanning should be prior to admission to ICU to minimize the complications of transferring critically ill patients within the hospital.

After radiography, immobilization of potential C spine injuries should be undertaken with a semi-rigid collar (e.g. Philadelphia). Patients who are immobile (heavy sedation, paralysed) may have sandbags and tape to minimize movement.

Spinal cord injury (SCI)

The aim of immobilization is to prevent further SCI or any deterioration due to movement. SCI itself is associated with marked physiological sequelae, which are dependent on the level and extent of injury.

Acutely there is a flaccid paralysis below the spinal level, which after resolution of the spinal shock phase develops into spasticity.

Respiratory failure is more common in complete than incomplete SCI. Diaphragmatic supply is from C3–5, and injury above C3 results in apnoea. Injuries below C5 may have diaphragmatic function maintained. However, marked ventilatory dysfunction is apparent in the acute setting, with loss of intercostal muscle function; diaphragmatic contraction and descent occurs with chest wall indrawing rather than expansion. FVC and maximal inspiratory force are reduced by nearly 70%. Similarly, loss of abdominal wall contraction reduces expiratory effort. These result in atelectasis, hypoventilation and hypoxaemia.

Ventilator dependence correlates strongly with level of injury; C1–4: 65 days, C5–8: 22 days, thoracic: 12 days. One-third of patients with cervical injuries will require intubation within the first 24h of injury. Specific indications include:

- fatigue
- VC <1l
- rising PaCO2
- rising respiratory rate

It is better to be pre-emptive and undertake intubation in controlled circumstances, using manual in-line stabilization and a skilled anaesthetist. Suxamethonium can be used up to 4 days after injury, with risks of severe hyperkalaemia thereafter. VAP is a significant problem in this group of patients. In patients with injuries at C4 and below, the development of chest wall spasticity enables a significant number to be weaned from mechanical ventilation.

Quadriplegics display better respiratory function when supine. This enables abdominal contents to push the diaphragm into a more favourable position for contraction. Tracheostomy is often complicated by the site of cervical injury and potential surgical access for anterior approach stabilization. A delay of 2 weeks between surgery and tracheostomy has been suggested.

Patients with C1–3 SCI who cannot be weaned are ventilator dependent for life. These patients may be considered for home ventilation and/or phrenic nerve electrostimulation. This is a significant psychological and financial burden, and reiterates the need for careful spinal immobilization and handling during resuscitation and ongoing intensive care.

Disruption of sympathetic outflow and unopposed parasympathetic action due to cervical SCI invariably leads to cardiovascular instability. Bradycardias are common, though tachyarrhymias are also seen. These are most commonly seen in the first 2 weeks after injury. Tracheal suctioning can cause severe bradycardias or asystole, which may be preventable with atropine.

Adequate perfusion to the spinal cord must be ensured to prevent secondary SCI. The loss of arteriolar tone in the peripheries leads to pooling and hypotension. Initially IV fluid can restore BP. With the disruption of cardiac sympathetic accelerator outflow in lesions above T1, cardiac output cannot be augmented by heart rate and relies on stroke volume alone. Both vasopressors and chronotropes may be required to augment these respectively.

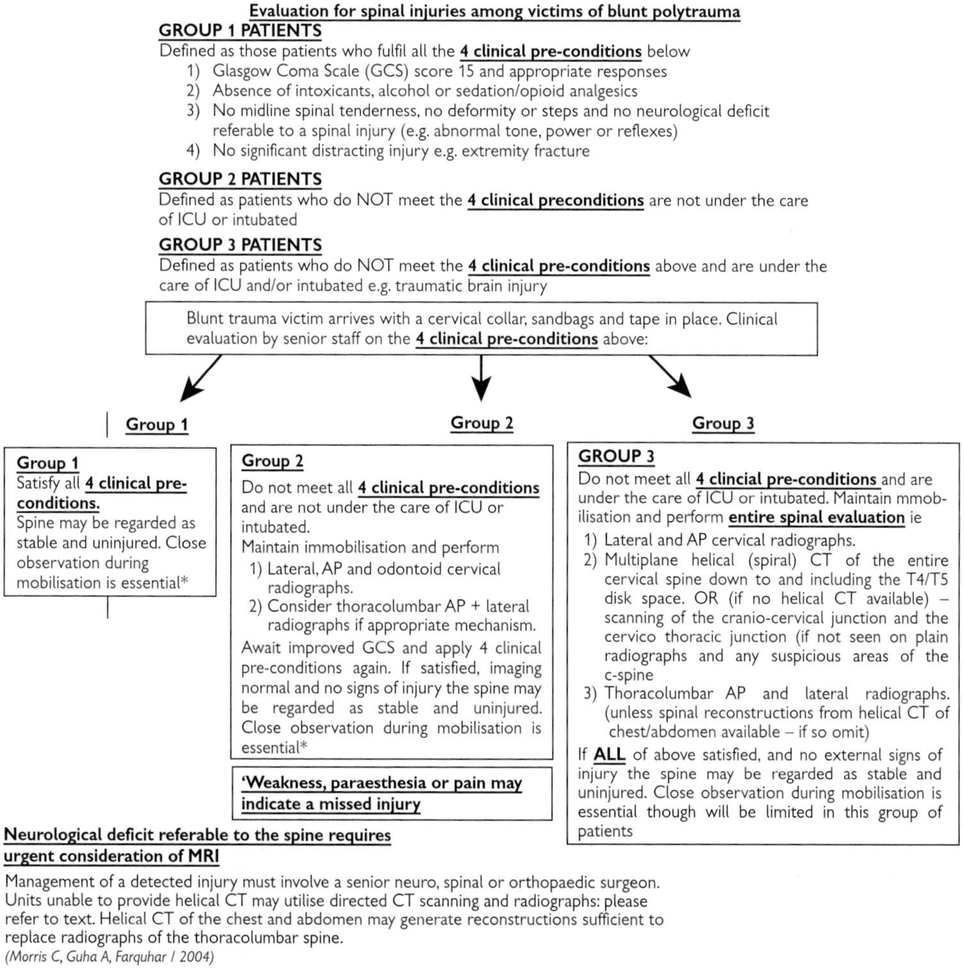
Evaluation for spinal injuries among victims of blunt polytrauma
GROUP 1 PATIENTS
Defined as those patients who fulfil all the 4 clinical pre-conditions below
1) Glasgow Coma Scale (GCS) score 15 and appropriate responses
2) Absence of intoxicants, alcohol or sedation/opioid analgesics
3) No midline spinal tenderness, no deformity or steps and no neurological deficit referable to a spinal injury (e.g. abnormal tone, power or reflexes)
4) No significant distracting injury e.g. extremity fracture
GROUP 2 PATIENTS
Defined as patients who do NOT meet the 4 clinical preconditions are not under the care of ICU or intubated
GROUP 3 PATIENTS
Defined as patients who do NOT meet the 4 clinical pre-conditions above and are under the care of ICU and/or intubated e.g. traumatic brain injury
Blunt trauma victim arrives with a cervical collar, sandbags and tape in place. Clinical evaluation by senior staff on the 4 clinical pre-conditions above:
Group 1
Group 2
Group 3
Group 1
Satisfy all 4 clinical pre-conditions.
Spine may be regarded as stable and uninjured. Close observation during mobilisation is essential*
Group 2
Do not meet all 4 clinical pre-conditions and are not under the care of ICU or intubated.
Maintain immobilisation and perform
1) Lateral, AP and odontoid cervical radiographs.
2) Consider thoracolumbar AP + lateral radiographs if appropriate mechanism.
Await improved GCS and apply 4 clinical pre-conditions again. If satisfied, imaging normal and no signs of injury the spine may be regarded as stable and uninjured. Close observation during mobilisation is essential*
'Weakness, paraesthesia or pain may indicate a missed injury
GROUP 3
Do not meet all 4 clincial pre-conditions and are under the care of ICU or intubated. Maintain mmobilisation and perform entire spinal evaluation ie
1) Lateral and AP cervical radiographs.
2) Multiplane helical (spiral) CT of the entire cervical spine down to and including the T4/T5 disk space. OR (if no helical CT available) – scanning of the cranio-cervical junction and the cervico thoracic junction (if not seen on plain radiographs and any suspicious areas of the c-spine
3) Thoracolumbar AP and lateral radiographs. (unless spinal reconstructions from helical CT of chest/abdomen available – if so omit)
If ALL of above satisfied, and no external signs of injury the spine may be regarded as stable and uninjured. Close observation during mobilisation is essential though will be limited in this group of patients
Neurological deficit referable to the spine requires urgent consideration of MRI
Management of a detected injury must involve a senior neuro, spinal or orthopaedic surgeon.
Units unable to provide helical CT may utilise directed CT scanning and radiographs: please refer to text. Helical CT of the chest and abdomen may generate reconstructions sufficient to replace radiographs of the thoracolumbar spine.
(Morris C, Guha A, Farquhar I 2004)

Fig. 28.3.1 ICS flowchart.

Autonomic hyper-reflexia

This starts within 6 months of SCI after the recovery from spinal shock. It is normally significant if the injury is above T6. Stimulation (e.g. bladder/bowel distension, cutaneous, surgery) below the level of injury leads to a supranormal autonomic response. Intense vasoconstriction causes severe hypertension as a result of an excessive sympathetic efferent response, increasing risks of cerebral events (stroke, seizures). Paraplegics may display reflex vasodilatation and bradycardia above the injury level.

Venous thromboembolism

There is a substantial risk of thromboembolic disease in SCI. Spinal fractures double the risk whilst SCI trebles it. The use of mechanical devices (TEDS, pneumatic compression systems) alone are insufficient to provide prophylaxis. In view of potential haemorrhage or urgency of surgery, there is often apprehension in starting anticoagulant therapy in patients with spinal fractures. The risk of developing DVT within the first 72h after injury has been shown to be low, and mechanical devices alone may suffice. Following this, anticoagulants, e.g. LMWH, should be considered for 8 weeks or until the patient is able to mobilize. If a PE is diagnosed with cardiovascular stability, anticoagulation should be commenced. Contraindications to anticoagulation may necessitate an IVC filter.

Drugs

The use of steroids in SCI has been studied. The series of NACSIS trials has shown some motor improvement with methylprednisolone started within 3–8h of injury.

Further reading

Ball PA. Critical care of spinal cord injury. *Spine* 2001; 26 (24 Suppl): 27–30.

Bracken MB, Shepard MJ, Holford TR, *et al.* Administration of methylprednisolone for 24 or 48 hours or tirilazad mesylate for 48 hours in the treatment of acute spinal injury. *JAMA* 1997; 277: 1597–604.

Jackson A, Groomes T. Incidence of respiratory complications following spinal cord injury. *Arch Phys Med Rehabil* 1994; 75: 270–5.

Morris C, Guha A, Farquhar I. Evaluation for spinal injuries among unconscious victims of blunt polytrauma: a management guideline for intensive care. *ICS*. 2005.

Chest trauma

Chest trauma can cause rapid deterioration and death from any part of ABC. 25% of all trauma deaths are caused by thoracic injury. 11% of pre-hospital mortality is due to penetrating chest trauma, often due to great vessel or heart injury, pneumothorax or airway obstruction. It is mandatory to be aware of the major life-threatening injuries and their subsequent management on the ICU.

The polytrauma patient is unlikely to have an isolated chest injury, so diagnosis and management of other injuries should be addressed.

The majority of chest injuries can be treated with simple interventions such as chest drainage. Only 15% of patients require surgical intervention (thoracotomy or sternotomy). Thoracotomy is still the preferred route for massive haemorrhage, but many procedures, particularly diagnostic, are now undertaken by video thoracoscopy.

Initial examination includes a CXR, but the nature of injuries often necessitates CT of the thorax. This accurately detects pulmonary contusions, pneumothorax, haemothorax, pneumomediastinum and great vessel injuries. There is increasing use of thoracic ultrasound in critical care, which may mean that pnemothoraces and other injuries may be detected more quickly.

Clinical approach

Tension pneumothorax

Life threatening—requires immediate treatment. An undiagnosed simple pneumothorax on admission may tension with IPPV on the ICU, with deteriorating hypoxia, tachycardia and high airway pressures. The presence of a chest tube does not guarantee protection against tensioning, as tubes may block or kink. The diagnosis is suggested by absence of ipsilateral breath sounds, hyper-resonant percussion note, trachea deviation (late) to the contralateral side and distended neck veins (which may not be present if the patient is hypovolaemic). Treatment is initially with a large bore, e.g. 14G, IV cannula inserted in the 2nd intercostal space mid-clavicular line (therefore converting to an open pneumothorax), followed by a chest drain.

Haemothorax

Blood collecting in the pleural space can result from both blunt and penetrating trauma. Initial treatment is with chest drainage. If the initial loss is ≥1500ml or ongoing haemorrhage of >200ml/h for 4h, surgical intervention is indicated. Prompt evacuation of haemothorax decreases later complications including empyema and entrapped lung. Beware intercostal tubes blocked by blood clot which may mislead as to bleeding rate.

Aortic injury

The thoracic aorta is fixed at 3 distinct points: aortic valve, ligamentum arteriosum and diaphragmatic hiatus. Sudden deceleration causes mobile parts of the aorta to move relative to fixed parts, leading to shear forces and tearing. The majority of traumatic ruptures occur at the isthmus. This is situated immediately distal to the origin of the left subclavian artery, at the junction of the fixed descending aorta and mobile aortic arch.

Widened mediastinum on CXR should raise suspicion of aortic rupture. Other radiographic features include:

- Left haemothorax
- Depressed left main bronchus
- Blurred outline of arch or descending aorta
- First rib fracture
- Left apical haematoma
- Right displacement of mid-oesophagus (detected by NG tube)

Either helical CT with contrast or aortography can be used to confirm aortic injury. TOE is useful in cardiovascularly unstable patients, and is more sensitive than CT in diagnosing intimal/medial layer injuries.

Treatment has recently moved away from timely surgery to non-surgical and delayed management. Major trauma patients have been seen to benefit from deferred repair. In injuries to the intima or media, medical management similar to descending thoracic aortic aneurysm may be employed: avoiding hypertension by maintaining MAP 60–70mm Hg with β-blockers and vasodilators. A thoracic surgical opinion is required to decide treatment options.

Flail segment

This is due to a considerable force applied to the torso causing ≥2 ribs to fracture in ≥2 places. Fracture of >6 ribs is associated with a steep increase in mortality, which may be reduced with epidural analgesia. The main problem caused by such a direct force is parenchymal lung injury beneath the flail segment, leading to pulmonary contusion.

Pulmonary contusion

Injury to the lung tissue increases pulmonary vascular permeability and protein-fluid leak into the alveolus, affecting the quality of surfactant. Reduced lung compliance and shunt lead to hypoxaemia. Contusions associated with major chest injury (multiple rib fractures, haemothorax, pneumothorax) are associated with increased mortality and are often underestimated on CXR.

Achieving adequate ventilation in these patients is often difficult. Alongside other injuries such as brain or spinal, a compromise has to be reached for instituting lung-protective strategies. Modes of ventilation may begin with NIV/CPAP and escalating through IPPV, individual lung ventilation, HFOV and ECMO. Additional therapies include proning (which may be impossible in this patient group). The treatment does not differ substantially from that of other form of restrictive lung injury such as ARDS.

Diaphragmatic rupture

This is uncommon and tends to occur alongside other thoracoabdominal injuries. The nature of the injury leads to a high morbidity and mortality. Diagnosis is usually through CT or ultrasound. Repair is surgical.

Air embolism

Air entering the vascular compartment is potentially fatal. It may present with sudden cardiovascular or neurological collapse. Clinical features also include retinal vessel air and haemoptysis. Positive pressure ventilation is detrimental and may worsen symptoms. One-lung ventilation may be utilized in unilateral injury. If both lungs are affected, low ventilation pressures should be instituted to reduce the possibility of further air entering the circulation. Negative pressure spontaneous breathing is ideal. HBO should be considered in cerebral air embolism or significant pulmonary air embolism, to reduce the size.

Cardiac tamponade

This should be suspected in any hypotensive patient with raised venous pressure following thoracic trauma, with pneumothorax ruled out. TTE or TOE is used for diagnosis. In the presence of a suitably qualified thoracic surgeon, limited left thoracotomy is the treatment of choice, but needle pericardiocentesis may buy time in other hands.

Myocardial contusion

Following chest trauma, myocardial contusions are relatively common. Clinical features include arrhythmias and cardiac failure. Following direct sternal force, the right ventricle is most commonly injured. Cardiac troponin assays (as opposed to CK-MB) are highly specific and sensitive for myocardial injury. However, non-cardiac injuries and severe shock may lead to increased levels. Whilst TOE is sensitive to identify areas of wall motion abnormality, it is not specific for myocardial injury. TTE is relatively insensitive. Patients who display ECG abnormalities should be observed and ECG monitored for at least 24h. Differentiating between contusion and MI can be difficult. It can be achieved by MRI angiography.

Oesophageal injuries

These tend to occur secondary to penetrating, rarely blunt, injury. The morbidity and mortality is due to the systemic response to GI contents in the mediastinum. Clinical features include retrosternal pain, dysphagia and subcutaneous emphysema. CXR features include pneumomediastinum, subcutaneous emphysema, mediastinal fluid levels, pleural effusions (more left sided) and pneumo/hydrothorax. Diagnosis is by contrast swallow or careful endoscopy, followed by surgical repair.

Further reading

Cain JG, Tesfaye Y. Pulmonary trauma. *Curr Opin Anaesthesiol* 2001; 14: 245–9.

Goettler CE, Fallon WF. Blunt thoraco-abdominal injury. *Curr Opin Anaesthesiol* 2001; 14: 237–43.

Kaye P, O'Sullivan I. Myocardial contusion: emergency investigation and diagnosis. *Emerg Med J* 2002; 19: 8-10.

Flagel BT, Luchette FA, Reed RL, *et al*. Half-a-dozen ribs: breakpoint for mortality. *Surgery* 2005; 138: 717–25.

Pelvic trauma

Pelvic fractures account for 3% of skeletal injuries. Stable fractures are low energy injuries which are not life-threatening, and will not be discussed. Unstable fractures are high energy injuries associated with major soft tissue damage, and frequently other injuries (abdominal, long-bone, spinal, thoracic and cranial). Pelvic trauma may also damage the urethra and genitalia, rectum, bladder, peripheral nerves and blood vessels Patients presenting with unstable pelvic fractures and shock (1–2% of all pelvic injuries) have a mortality of 50%, and require aggressive management. Open pelvic fractures are rare (2% of cases) but carry a high mortality.

Mechanisms

Unstable pelvic injuries may be suspected in the following: crush injuries, falls, pedestrians hit by a vehicle, motorcycle accidents and ejection from a vehicle. Since the pelvis is a ring, displacement requires 2 separate fractures. The Young–Burgess classification defines the following fractures as unstable:

- Lateral compression fractures (types II and III) break the ring at the weakest point, the pubic rami, in combination with iliac wing fractures and sacroiliac joint disruption (windswept pelvis).
- Anterior–posterior compression fractures (types II and III) separate the symphysis pubis and disrupt the sacroiliac joints (open book).
- Vertical shear forces fracture the pubic rami vertically, and separate the symphysis, and sacroiliac joints. Vertical fractures of the ilium and sacrum are rare,

Fractures which increase pelvic volume (vertical shear, open book) result in larger transfusion requirements. However, there is a poor correlation between the type of fracture and the need for emergency haemostasis.

Initial management

Initial management should follow ATLS principles.

Primary survey

Patients in shock require simultaneous fluid resuscitation and rapid identification of possible causes. Clinical signs of a pelvic fracture include obvious deformity, and shortening or rotation of the leg. Bruising of the external genitalia and loins, although specific, can be delayed.

In the absence of obvious signs of fracture, pelvic instability may be detected by applying anterior–posterior pressure, springing the iliac crests and pulling on the leg to detect axial instability. These manoeuvres risk exacerbating the bleeding, and should be performed only once, if at all.

An AP X-ray of the pelvis (and chest) is an essential adjunct to the primary survey. Separation of the symphysis pubis by >1cm implies serious disruption.

A rectal examination is essential to assess bleeding, perforation by bony fragments, a palpable pelvic haematoma or fracture, and anal tone.

Urethral injury is much nore common in men, but may occur in women. Signs include:

- Perineal bruising and scrotal haematoma
- Blood at the external urethral meatus
- High riding prostate

If urethral injury is suspected, urinary catheterization is contraindicated until a retrograde urethrogram has been performed.

Resuscitation

Fluid loading via two large bore IV cannulae should follow ATLS guidelines. Bleeding is venous in 80–90% of cases, from the fracture sites and damaged venous plexi. Such patients respond transiently to fluids. However, pressure-induced tamponade will not occur in the retroperitoneum, as the blood tracks cranially (chimney effect). Ongoing bleeding can result in progressive acidosis, coagulopathy, hypothermia and abdominal compartment syndrome.

In the emergency room, a folded sheet wrapped around the pelvis, and secured with a clamp, acts as an effective pelvic sling. By reducing of the fracture, and possibly by reducing pelvic volume, blood loss is reduced. Military antishock trousers are associated with significant complications, and are no longer recommended.

Stopping the bleeding

Once emergency measures have been instituted, the priority is to stop the bleeding. It should be remembered that massive bleeding from pelvic fractures is unusual compared with other sites, particularly the abdomen. Bleeding often occurs from more than one site.

External fixation

An external fixation device should be applied as soon as possible in patients with hypotension and unstable pelvic fractures. Blood loss is reduced by re-apposing the bony surfaces and controlling venous bleeding. Such a device should also be applied in patients with unstable pelvic fractures who require a laparotomy, prior to skin incision. A pelvic C-clamp gives improved stabilization of the posterior pelvis, but is not applicable to all fractures.

Laparotomy

Following external fixation, the next decision is whether a laparotomy is required. A laparotomy is indicated for intra-abdominal bleeding, perforated bowel and a ruptured intra-abdominal bladder. However, the diagnosis of abdominal bleeding is not easy in the presence of a fractured pelvis. The investigation of choice is a contrast CT scan, but many patients are too unstable for this to be performed safely. Ultrasound (FAST) scanning can exclude haemothorax and intraperitoneal fluid, but lacks sensitivity in this situation. The most reliable test is a supraumbilical peritoneal tap, which is positive if 5–10ml of frank blood or GI contents is aspirated. Microscopy of lavage fluid is often positive for red cells in the absence of intra-abdominal bleeding, and does not mandate a laparotomy. If a laparotomy is performed, pelvic packing (see below) can be undertaken at the same time.

Angiographic embolization

If a laparotomy is not indicated, but evidence of bleeding continues, pelvic angiography with a view to embolization can be considered. However, shock due to arterial bleeding accounts for only 10–20% of cases, and the type of fracture does not help predict the presence of arterial injury. One approach is to perform angiography in patients after external fixation, who can be stabilized, but continue to require blood transfusion at a rate of 1–2 units/h.

These patients can be safely transported to the angiography suite. The arteries most commonly damaged are branches of the internal iliac, the pudendal (anterior injuries) and the superior gluteal (damage to the sciatic notch). Angiographic embolization is unlikely to be practical in patients who are *in extremis,* losing up to 8 units/h. In these patients, pelvic packing at laparotomy can be considered.

Pelvic packing

Laparotomy has traditionally not been indicated for a fractured pelvis alone, and hypogastric artery ligation is known to be ineffective. More recently a combination of external fixation, or C-clamps, with presacral and paravesical packing has been employed in patients in severe shock, in whom the mortality is very high. Temporary aortic clamping can allow visualization and access. The rationale is that of 'damage control surgery'; performing rapid life-saving interventions without attempting definitive treatment.

Secondary survey

The secondary survey is undertaken once life-threatening injuries have been stabilized. The purpose is to identify all other injuries. The urethra, bladder, rectum and neurovascular structures may all be damaged by pelvic fractures due to deformity, tearing or penetration by bony fragments. In stable patients, a CT scan is the investigation of choice for defining the extent of these injuries.

Bladder, urethral and rectal injuries

Extraperitoneal bladder rupture (80%) is more common than intraperitoneal rupture (20%), and in the majority of cases resolves with drainage and irrigation. Intraperitoneal bladder rupture requires emergency laparotomy. One-fifth of patients with bladder lesions have urethral injuries. These are managed initially by suprapubic drainage, but complete tears will require subsequent urethroplasty. Impotence is associated with urethral injuries. Rectal perforation is associated with bladder and urethral injuries, and is most commonly extraperitoneal. A defunctioning colostomy may be required.

Nerve injuries

The sacral plexus or sacral nerve roots can be damaged by fractures of the sacrum or sacroiliac joints. This results in loss of anal tone and perineal anaesthesia. The sciatic nerve can be injured by fractures of the posterior acetabulum or greater sciatic notch. The L5 root may also be damaged with sacral fractures. Injuries to the obdurator nerve are easily overlooked.

Definitive care

Early internal fixation of unstable pelvic ring fractures with plates and screws allows more rapid mobilization, and reduces hospital stay and long-term disability. However, the surgery can be challenging and lengthy, and should only be undertaken in stable patients.

Complications

Sepsis

Haematoma resulting from pelvic fractures may become infected and form abscesses. Other local sources of infection include fixation devices and wounds. If undiagnosed, extraperitoneal rupture of the rectum may form a pelvic abscess and systemic sepsis.

Thromboembolism

Thromboembolism is a major risk following trauma, and particularly following pelvic fractures, due to immobility, and damage to blood vessels. Prophylaxis should be given depending on other injuries, according to local protocols. Doppler ultrasound will detect thrombi in the leg, but will not detect pelvic thrombi, which are more clinically significant.

Pain

Chronic pain syndromes may follow pelvic fractures, often due to damage to the sacroiliac joint, or leg-length discrepancies.

Prognosis

Mortality is primarily determined by the severity of the associated injuries, rather than the pelvic fracture *per se.* Mortality is low (3–4%) in the absence of shock. Mortality is increased in the presence of a head injury, shock on presentation and increasing transfusion requirements. Those presenting in shock have a mortality of 50%. Posterior pelvic fractures have higher transfusion requirements and a higher mortality.

Further reading

Advanced Trauma Life Support for Doctors, ATLS, faculty course manual. Chicago: American College of Surgeons, 2004.

Gansslen A, Giannoudis P, Pape H-C. Haemorrhage in pelvic fracture; who needs angiography? *Curr Opin Crit Care* 2003; 9: 515-23.

Incaglioni P, Viggiano M, Carli P. Priorities in th management of severe pelvic trauma. *Curr Opin Crit Care* 2000; 6: 401–7.

Shepherd C. eMedicine. Pelvic fractures. http://www.emedicine.com/emerg/topic203.htm.

Thornton DD. eMedicine. Pelvic ring fractures. http://www.emedicine.com/radio/topic546.htm.

Wheeles's textbook of orthopaedics.; pelvic fractures menu. http://www.wheelessonline.com/ortho/pelvic_fractures.

Burns—fluid management

Introduction

In the decades from 1930 to 1950 hypovolaemic shock and shock-induced renal failure were the leading causes of death following significant burn injury. It was then discovered that mortality could be improved by fluid resuscitation to replace the considerable post-burn intravascular fluid deficits. Since then, numerous fluid resuscitation strategies have been developed.

Pathophysiology

A burn injury results in an intense inflammatory reaction involving numerous inflammatory mediators including histamine and bradykinin. This is exacerbated by considerable endothelial oxidant damage (mainly of neutrophil origin), leading to increased capillary permeability that is exacerbated by localized (or systemic) hypoxia. Interstitial oncotic pressure is increased by macromolecular fragmentation (caused by direct thermal injury), and interstitial hydrostatic pressure plummets to negative values due to the sudden increase in osmotically active particles. These factors promote the rapid shift of fluid into the interstitial space. Oedema formation is most rapid in partial thickness burns, whereas in deeper injuries the oedema formation is slower, but of a greater magnitude. In burns >25–30% of total body surface area (TBSA), these effects cease to be confined solely to burned tissues, and oedema formation becomes systemic.

Leaking capillaries can allow molecules of up to 300kDa (cf. red blood cells which are 350kDa. Albumin (69kDa) escapes from the intravascular compartment, and experiments have shown that the entirety of the body's serum proteins can be lost from the circulation within 24h of a 20% TBSA burn. The increased systemic capillary permeability usually resolves between 8 and 24h post-burn, and is reflected by a reduction in fluid requirements.

Jackson classically, conceptualized three zones within a burn wound.

- Zone of coagulation (innermost)—comprising irreversible tissue loss
- Zone of ischaemia/stasis—an area of damaged but potentially salvageable tissue which may progress to necrosis if resuscitation is inadequate
- Zone of hyperaemia (outermost)—tissues on the periphery of the burn that are minimally damaged, and will survive, but are hyperaemic in response to inflammatory mediators

As well as preventing circulatory collapse, proper fluid resuscitation can help salvage potentially ischaemic tissues.

Intravenous access

Effective fluid resuscitation requires reliable IV access. In the first instance, two large bore cannulae will suffice, but major burns will often require central venous catheterization. Placing cannulae through burned skin is best avoided if possible, due to the heightened risk of infection and difficulty in siting and securing cannulae, but acceptable if there is no choice. Extensive burns may require a surgical cut-down. If a central line is deemed necessary, it should be inserted early, as the inevitable oedema formation will make insertion much more difficult later. The internal jugular and subclavian veins are the preferred routes for central venous access, as they give a more reliable CVP and carry a lower risk of infection than the femoral veins, but choice is generally dictated by the distribution of the burn. Full aseptic precautions are essential, and meticulous care of any central venous cannula is necessary to prevent infection. Ultrasound guidance is recommended because even at an early stage, constricting burns and oedema can distort the anatomy.

Urine output is an important indicator of adequate resuscitation, so all patients with burns of >20% or so TBSA should have a urinary catheter inserted early, as oedema formation can make insertion difficult later on.

Oedema formation can be extensive and progressive, so care must be taken when using any circumferential dressings (e.g. to secure IV access) to avoid any tourniquet effect. Progressive oedema formation can also kink or dislodge peripheral and central cannulae from the vein, so a high index of suspicion and regular assessments are necessary.

Fluid nanagement

Post-burn fluid requirements are highly variable because of factors relating to the patient, the presence of other injuries and those related to treatment, e.g. fluid requirements are increased by delayed resuscitation, inhalational injury and deeper burns. Predicting fluid requirements is not an exact science as in the last 60yrs or so numerous formulae have been derived to help in the estimation process. The main variables dictating volume requirements are TBSA burnt, patient age and weight, and their intubation status. None of the available formulae has been shown to be unquestionably superior, but the Parkland formula has been most commonly adopted worldwide.

The Parkland formula advocates a total of 4ml/kg/% TBSA burn of lactated Ringer's solution (similar in composition to Hartmann's solution) in the first 24h post-burn (half to be given in the first 8h post-burn, and half in the next 16h). It must be emphasized that all formulae only act as a rough guide. A patient's requirements will not always be accurately reflected by such formulae, and they present at various time points following burn injury and in various states of hypovolaemia. It is therefore essential to be guided by the clinical picture, as there are serious consequences to either over- or under-resuscitation, and since widespread adoption of crystalloid burns resuscitation, the global trend has been to over-resuscitation. This iatrogenic injury is as damaging to morbidity and mortality as under-resuscitation.

By convention, IV fluid resuscitation is given to all adults with burns >15% TBSA, and all children (≤6 years) with burns >10% TBSA. However, due to poorer compensatory mechanisms (primarily within the renal and cardiovascular systems), elderly patients with burns <15% TBSA may also benefit from parenteral resuscitation.

Recommendations regarding the fluid types to use have varied, but internationally, the most widely adopted stance is for crystalloids, at least initially, rather than colloid, for the following reasons:

- Macromolecules up to ~300kDa can leak from the circulation, negating the volume expansion benefit of colloids
- Colloids can accumulate in the interstitium, thus increasing local oncotic pressure and prolonging oedema
- Some colloids have been associated with significant pruritis

- Many colloids have additional adverse effects, e.g. with starches, the larger the molecular size, the greater the coagulopathy.

For these reasons, colloids are generally avoided for the first 12–24h post-burn. However, crystalloids have their own disadvantages, primarily the considerably heightened volumes required, whose corollary is increased oedema formation and its consequences, e.g. higher incidence of compartment syndromes, including in unburned limbs.

In the choice of crystalloid solution, iso- or hypertonic fluids are used, as they benefit from the greatest volume expansion properties. Solutions mimicking plasma electrolyte composition are favoured, e.g. Hartmann's solution, as they more closely reflect the composition of the lost fluid and, with their lower chloride concentration, present a lesser acid load compared with 0.9% sodium chloride.

Monitoring

Patients with major burns must be monitored closely and the fluid resuscitation altered according to individual patient response. It is essential to use a variety of monitoring methods to gauge overall response to fluid resuscitation, because numerous factors complicate their interpretation.

Urine output is probably the most useful parameter to guide resuscitation, and should be maintained between 0.5 and 1.0ml/kg/h (1–1.5 ml/kg/h in children <20kg). Note the recommendation of a target range, not merely a minimum target output. However, a physiological oliguria is to be expected after trauma and, also, haemochromogenuria and rhabdomyolysis are common in this patient population, which may compromise the utility of urine output as a monitoring tool. Treatment of the latter conditions normally involves maintaining a high urine output, but this necessitates over-resuscitation which may increase morbidity. We would, therefore, advise a low threshold for instituting haemofiltration rather than excessive crystalloid administration.

The pain and anxiety associated with burn injuries can cause heart rate and blood pressure to be misleading consequent to high levels of endogenous catecholamines. Trying to correct fully any 'swing' in the arterial waveform by augmenting preload can also lead to overadministration of fluids.

CVP may be misleading because of excessive catecholamines, pulmonary vasoconstriction and elevated abdominal compartment pressures. In major burns, the CVP has been found to correlate more closely with the latter than with intravascular filling, so a high CVP is of little value, but a low value remains likely to indicate hypovolaemia; trends rather than isolated absolute values should guide therapy.

Monitoring acid–base balance can be useful to reveal hypoperfusion-related acidosis, but interpretation may be compromised by exogenous organic or inorganic acids, poisoning by carbon monoxide and/or cyanide, ketoacidosis, poor renal function compromising clearance of acids, or even an occult compartment syndrome.

The haematocrit (and other indicators of haemoconcentration) also contribute a minor role in monitoring, but interpretation is compromised by haemolysis, haemorrhage, sequestration within burned tissues and rouleaux formation.

Cardiac output monitoring is not necessary for all patients, but is a useful adjunct if there is reason to suspect many of the above conventional methods of monitoring are unreliable or if the patient has either a huge burn injury or poor compensatory mechanisms, e.g. the elderly or those with heart disease. Monitoring trends is more useful than absolute numbers as cardiovascular haemodynamics can be grossly deranged, and achieving 'normal' physiological values may be either impossible or undesirable.

When it is thought that the patient requires more fluid, it is recommended to increase the rate of infusion rather than giving boluses (except in severe hypotensive episodes) because boluses transiently cause high venous pressures which increase capillary leakage and hence oedema formation.

When using crystalloid fluid resuscitation in major burns, abdominal compartment syndrome is a potential complication. In large injuries, it is therefore advisable to monitor intra-abdominal pressure (e.g. by transducing the urinary catheter).

After the first 24h, fluid requirements reduce, but remain elevated above usual maintenance volumes, and they are crudely predicted as 1ml/kg/% TBSA burn in 24h.

By this stage, colloids are usually better retained within the circulation and can now be added if required to enhance the intravascular colloid osmotic pressure and reduce the overall fluid volume.

Further reading

Arturson G. Microvascular permeability to macromolecules in thermal injury. *Acta Physiol Scand Suppl* 1979; 463: 111–2.

Baxter CR, Shires T. Physiological response to crystalloid resuscitation of severe burns. *Ann NY Acad Sci* 1968; 150: 874–94.

Jackson D. The diagnosis of the depth of burning. *Br J Plastic Surg* 1953; 40: 588–96.

Yowler CJ, Fratianne RB. Current status of burn resuscitation. *Clin Plast Surg* 2000; 27: 1–10.

Burns—general management

Epidemiology

Burns are injuries caused by exposure to heat (moat common) and electrical, chemical or radioactive agents. In the UK, ~16 000 burns per year require hospitalization, of which 1000 are major burns requiring fluid resuscitation (half are children).

National guidelines

All patients should be referred to the local Burns and Plastic Surgery Department (and, if being transferred, should arrive within 6h of injury). The regional Burns Centre will either take over care or assess and advise regarding ongoing management. Some offer a Burns Outreach Service to provide continuing support. If no specialist burns bed is available locally, the National Burn Bed Bureau can locate the nearest suitable bed nationally (Tel. 01384 215 576).

History

It is important to elicit an accurate history of events surrounding the injury: what happened, when and where?

- Did the injury occur indoors or outdoors? (*inhalation injury*)
- What was burning? (*toxic fumes*)
- Were they rescued or escaped independently? (*implications for duration of exposure*)
- Was there an explosion? (*blast injuries affecting lung, bowel, ears*)
- Where were they found? (*consider occult injuries, e.g. if found in front of house, did they jump out an upper floor window?*)
- Condition at scene? (*unconscious or CPR at scene explains failure to regain consciousness after several days treatment due to hypoxic brain injury*)

Assessment

As for any major trauma, an ATLS-style assessment is indicated in the initial evaluation of patients with burns. Severity of injury is mainly dependent on: anatomical site(s), burn size, burn depth, patient age and the presence of an inhalational injury.

Respiratory management

Burns to the head, neck or upper airways can cause considerable oedema, leading to airway compromise and a difficult (or impossible) intubation. Any patient with burns to such areas should be seen by a senior anaesthetist or intensivist to assess requirement for pre-emptive intubation. Significant upper airway burns swell rapidly and require prompt intubation. Delaying intubation may make it technically difficult, so a watch and wait strategy should be avoided. One of the most sensitive symptoms is development of a hoarse voice.

Intubation: if possible, in adults an ETT ≥8.0mm should be used to allow diagnostic and therapeutic bronchoscopy without significant ventilatory compromise. The tube should not be cut to less that 28cm (still allows use of a gum elastic bougie) since major swelling causes it to retract intraorally. If marked swelling is anticipated consider an armoured tube or bite block (jaws may otherwise progressively clamp the tube and occlude ventilation.

The lower airways rarely sustain thermal injury due to the effective heat exchange system in the upper airways. The lower airways are instead more commonly injured by contamination with particulate matter and chemical products of combustion (usually acidic in nature). Early bronchoscopy should be performed for diagnosis (document involved bronchi, mucosal injury (erythematous, pale, dry or ulcerated) and particulate contamination (percentage of mucosal surface coated). Endoscopic bronchial lavage (using 1.4% sodium bicarbonate solution) may help clear particulate matter and neutralize acidic particles. This may need to be repeated and should be supplemented with chest physiotherapy and 4 hourly nebulizers of 1.4% $NaHCO_3$ until soot has cleared from sputum.

Exclude carbon monoxide poisoning in all smoke inhalation injuries by measurement of carboxy-Hb levels. Normally this is <1.0%, though those living in urban areas or who smoke may have levels >5%. Treatment is with 100% oxygen until the carboxy-Hb level is <2%.

Cardiovascular management

Fluid requirements are highly variable as they depend upon many factors, including patient weight, injury size and depth, inhalational injury and type of fluid administered. Recent trends have been to use the Parkland formula to guide likely crystalloid requirements, but such formulae are a guide only. Over-resuscitation is as harmful as under-resuscitation, so consider defining upper as well as lower limits for urine output. Reliable IV access is essential, and can be placed through burns if options are limited.

Burn size

Burn size is quoted as a percentage of the TBSA, and should be assessed in hospital using a Lund and Browder Chart (Appendix 2). Areas of epidermal depth burn (erythema only, no blistering) are excluded from the size estimation. With early assessments, burns may not yet have developed blisters, so such areas should be rubbed with gauze to see if this causes epidermolysis. In burns are >25% TBSA, generalized oedema occurs.

Burn depth

Burn depth is defined anatomically (from superficial to deep): epidermal, superficial dermal (SD), deep dermal (DD) and full thickness (FT). Burn depth can be assessed by the appearance and texture of the wound plus its vascularity and sensation. Deeper burns exhibit more pallor, fixed dermal staining, decreased vascularity (blanching) and sensation. FT burns have a leathery texture from coagulated and contracted dermal macromolecules.

The burn depth has implications for healing times, scar formation and requirement for surgery—significant DD and FT burns require skin grafting. Burns extending into the dermis have some non-viable tissue, which must be removed before re-epithelialization can occur (either naturally by autolytic enzymatic debridement, or surgically). Its persistence on the body exacerbates the inflammatory response, releases toxins and is an infection risk. Early surgery is therefore generally advocated.

Escharotomies, fasciotomies and compartment syndromes

Dermal contraction in greater than hemi-circumferential DD and FT burns can cause vascular (or respiratory) compromise by a tourniquet effect upon limbs, neck or chest.

Treatment is by escharotomy (incisions through burned skin to release constrictions).

Swelling limbs (even if unburned) can develop compartment syndromes, requiring fasciotomy (incisions through deep fascia to release tight muscle compartments). Intra-abdominal hypertension (>12mm Hg) is common, and can progress to abdominal compartment syndrome requiring paracentesis, peritoneal drain or decompressive laparotomy. Maintain a high index of suspicion; consider monitoring compartment pressures and the intravesical pressure.

Dressings

Patients being transferred to a local burns service usually have only cling-film applied to all non-facial burns (acts as a barrier to environmental contamination, reduces pain and evaporation and allows the burns team to visualize wounds). Beware of cling-film rolling up and forming a tourniquet around the neck and limbs.

The main cause of mortality in burn injuries is infection, so treatment is focused upon maintenance of wound cleanliness and regular microbiological surveillance; prophylactic antibiotics are not recommended. Dressings are used to allow the moist environment required for optimum wound healing whilst absorbing wound exudates, delivering antimicrobials to the wound surface, avoiding wound contamination and maintaining comfort. Burns should not generally be left exposed.

Prior to the first formal application of dressings, wounds should be cleaned (soap and water will suffice), swabbed for organisms and blisters removed (not drained) to facilitate burn assessment, remove necrotic tissue and allow contact of topical antimicrobials directly with wounds. Burn wounds should be photographed on admission for medicolegal documentation and to avoid repeated dressing removal for different clinicians to visualize the extent of the burn, thus reducing pain, contamination and heat loss.

Many options exist for dressings, but traditionally they comprise: a non-adherent layer (e.g. paraffin tulle) with a topical antimicrobial applied (e.g. silver sulfadiazine or povidone-iodine), layers of absorbent woven gauze, then bandages. Dressings are changed daily or on alternate days, or if exudates penetrate through outer bandages since their absorbency has been lost and there is then an infection risk. Grossly swollen hands and feet may be placed in a polythene bag containing antimicrobials to avoid restrictive and constricting dressings and permit easy visualization.

Positioning

Head-up positioning can be used to reduce head and neck swelling, but a bed tilt may be required rather than breaking the bed, to minimize diaphragmatic splinting from intra-abdominal swelling. Long-term hand function can be improved using Bradford sling elevation, regular physiotherapy and often splinting.

Myoglobinuria

Extensive burns can result in haemoglobinuria from red cell destruction and, in deep burns involving muscle, rhabdomyolysis with myoglobinuria with the risk of acute renal failure. Measure serum creatine kinase and serum or urinary myoglobin soon after admission and, if elevated, maintain a good urine output ± urinary alkalinization; haemofiltration may be required.

Early management—don't forget

- Make an early accurate measurement of the patient's weight to guide fluid and nutritional requirements
- Consider potential self-harm, e.g. an overdose
- Insert an NG tube and start feeding within 6h of injury after adequate resuscitation
- Examine potentially injured eyes early, using fluorescein stain, before swelling prevents it
- Give tetanus toxoid booster if required
- Ensure good analgesia
- Monitor core temperature and prevent or correct hypothermia: nurse in a cubicle at ~30°C, warm all IV fluids, keep burns covered except whilst assessing to reduce latent heat of evaporation (eventually a physiological pyrexia will develop)
- Beware coagulopathies from consumption of platelets and clotting factors, and from hypothermia
- Involve the whole multi-disciplinary team early including Physiotherapist, Occupational Therapist, Dietician and Psychologist

Further information

The one day internationally recognized Emergency Management of Severe Burns Course (EMSB) is held at various UK centres (see `www.britishburnassociation.co.uk` for details).

Further reading

National Burn Care Review Committee. Standards and Strategy for Burn Care, A review of burn care in the British Isles. 2001.

Chapter 29

Physical disorders

Chapter contents

Hypothermia

Defined as core temperature <35°C

Mild 32–35°C; moderate 26–32°C; severe <26°C

Risk factors

Increasing age, abnormal mental state, immobility (orthopaedic, Parkinsonism), drugs (alcohol, barbiturate, major tranquillizers, antidepressants), endocrine (hypothyroidism, hyperglycaemia, adrenal insufficiency, hypopituitarism), autonomic neuropathy (diabetes mellitus, Parkinsonism), malnutrition, renal failure, sepsis (excessive heat loss from vasodilatation), exposure (inadequate clothing/eating, near drowning).

Presentation

Mild hypothermia

- Shivering—maximal at 35°C and decreases thereafter. Absent at <32°C.
- Mild confusion, weakness, fatiguebility, lethargy, ataxia, dysarthia

Progressive hypothermia

- Delirium, coma, bradycardia and low respiratory rate, cardiac arrhythmias, dilated unresponsive pupils and loss of reflexes
- EEG is flat at <20°C; asystole at <15°C

Immediate hypothermia

It has been suggested that very rapid hypothermia may occur in some cases of drowning where large volumes of cold fluid are aspirated into the lungs without immediate cardiac standstill. The ongoing circulation results in rapid central cooling and potentially protection. More often, glottic spasm or onset of VF preclude this speed of cooling in nature, although it can be done with an extracorporeal circulation.

Complications

VF, atrial tachy and bradyarrythmias, aspiration pneumonia, pancreatitis, bowel ischaemia, acute renal failure, rhabdomyolysis, DIC.

Investigations

- Check core temperature using a low reading rectal thermometer
- Urgent bloods: U&Es, CK (dehydration, rhabdomyolysis), glucose (usually high), amylase (pancreatitis)
- Routine bloods: FBC, phosphate (↓), magnesium (↑), blood cultures, thyroid function test, toxic screen, serum cortisol
- ABG: expect artefactual lower pH and higher PaO2 and PaCO2. Hence, to be corrected to 37°C
- ECG: prolonged PR and QT intervals, J-waves <30°C (see Fig. 29.1.1)
- Urine: microscopy, culture and sensitivity (MCS), dipstick (blood and protein), myoglobinuria

Treatment of severely hypothermic victims in cardiac arrest in the hospital setting should be directed at rapid

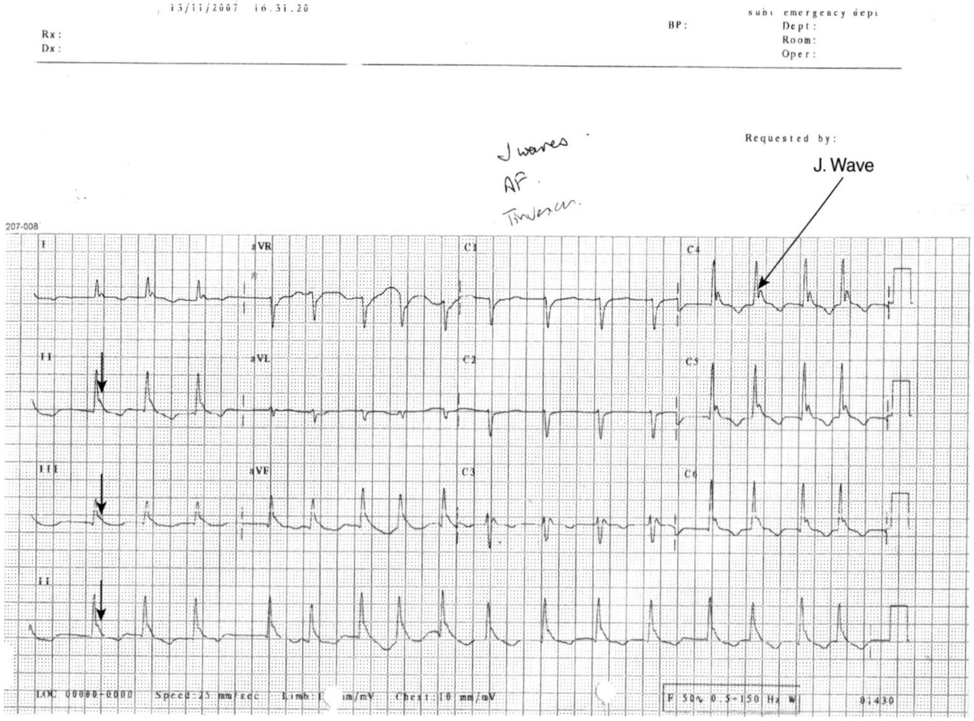

Fig. 29.1.1 In hypothermia, note the extensive J-waves; the patient is also in AF and has significant widespread T inversion.

core rewarming. Techniques that can be used include the administration of heated, humidified oxygen (42–46°C (108.7–115°F), warmed IV fluids (normal saline) at 43°C (109°F) infused centrally at rates of ~150–200ml/h (to avoid overhydration), peritoneal lavage with warmed (43°C (109°F)) potassium-free fluid administered 2l at a time, or extracorporeal blood warming with partial bypass. Pleural lavage with warm saline instilled through a chest tube has also been used successfully. The routine administration of steroids, barbiturates or antibiotics has not been documented to help increase survival or decrease post-resuscitative damage.

Prevention of hypothermia

Heat loss occurs by radiation (60%), convection (25%), and evaporation of body fluids (10%).

General anaesthesia typically results in mild core hypothermia (1–3°C). As with general anaesthesia, redistribution of body heat during spinal or epidural anaesthesia is the main cause of hypothermia.

There are three basic strategies for the prevention and treatment of mild hypothermia:

1. Minimizing redistribution of heat
2. Cutaneous warming during anaesthesia
3. Internal warming.

Cutaneous warming

- Passive insulation—a single layer of any insulator (e.g. space blanket) reduces cutaneous heat loss by ~30%.
- Active warming—warm air via a air mattress/blanket. Active warming by resistive heating (electric) blankets is a recent development
- Internal warming—fluid warming to body temperature prior to infusion. The administration of 1l of fluid at room temperature decreases core temperature by 0.25°C.
- Airway humidification—this contributes little to preservation of core temperature because <10% of metabolic heat loss occurs via the respiratory tract.

Invasive internal warming techniques

- Cardiopulmonary bypass
- Peritoneal dialysis

Very effective but neither technique is relevant to mild hypothermia.

Further reading

Hayward JS, Eckerson JD, Kemna D. Thermal and cardiovascular changes during three methods of resuscitation from mild hypothermia. *Resuscitation* 1984; 11: 21–33.

Kirkbride DA, Buggy DJ. Thermoregulation and mild peri-operative hypothermia. *Br J Anaesth CEPD Rev* 2003; 3: 24–8.

Drowning and near-drowning

Drowning is death from asphyxiation following submersion, usually in water. Incidents involving immersion or submersion may be referred to as 'near-drowning', a term which implies survival. Near-drowning is more common and many incidents are unreported. They tend to occur in childhood, early adulthood and in males, and are associated with the use of recreational drugs, especially alcohol. Epilepsy, heart disease, CVA and deliberate self-harm are less common associations. (The practical distinction between immersion and submersion may be unclear.)

Pathophysiological factors

Aspiration of water into the lungs

Aspiration of relatively small quantities of water alters surfactant activity, causes atelectasis and produces hypoxia within a few minutes. People rescued conscious and alert may become hypoxic soon afterwards and take several days to recover normal levels of oxygenation.

The effects of immersion in thermoneutral water

With the head above water, hydrostatic pressure to the chest and abdomen increases venous return and cardiac output by between 32 and 67%. Increased pulmonary blood volume, upward displacement of the diaphragm and compression of the chest wall combine to increase work of breathing by >60%.

The effects of immersion in cold water (<25°C): cold shock and the diving reflex

With the head above water, the cold shock reflexes are triggered by a sudden fall in skin temperature. Increasing respiratory drive can generate a 10-fold increase in minute ventilation in water at 10°C. Breath holding time is reduced to <10s. Peripheral vasoconstriction increases right atrial pressure and is accompanied by a tachycardia and an increase in cardiac output of between 60 and 100%, which significantly increases myocardial work. These effects prevent effective breathing and swimming even in the young and fit, and are sufficient to cause MI or dysrrhythmia.

The diving response, the purpose of which is to conserve oxygen, is activated by immersion of the face in cold water. It is well developed in diving animals but is less predictable in humans, although more marked in infants. It is characterized by apnoea, peripheral vasoconstriction and bradycardia, and is mediated via the ophthalmic division of the trigeminal nerve. In humans, the cold shock response is more marked than the diving reflex. About 15% of humans have a marked diving reflex which is accentuated in those wearing wet-suits or 'dry' immersion suits which leave only their face uninsulated against the cold environment.

Hypothermia and the value of a life jacket

Hypothermia is a core body temperature of <35°C. The rate at which an immersed body cools depends on water temperature, movement of water over the skin, body surface area:mass ratio, insulation, peripheral circulation, metabolic rate and injuries or illness which may affect these. The summer time seawater temperature in the UK is between 15 and 18°C.

Neuromuscular function

Peripheral cooling over ~30min affects neuromuscular activity leading to finger stiffness, poor coordination and loss of power, making it difficult to initiate or maintain activities to assist survival, such as catching a rope or clinging to a floating object. At core temperatures of 33–35°C, muscle temperature may be as low as 28°C, precluding any purposeful movement.

Consciousness

Consciousness is impaired as temperature falls, until coma supervenes at ~30°C. CBF is reduced and cerebral activity ceases at brain temperatures <22°C. In victims whose airway is protected from aspiration of water by a life jacket or suspension in debris, cooling to temperatures <28°C may result in VF or a profound bradycardia and, at 24–26°C, asystole. Children have a higher ratio of body surface area to mass, and cool faster than adults. It is likely that victims become hypothermic, lose consciousness and aspirate water before cooling to a temperature sufficiently low to provide cerebral protection.

Under favourable circumstances, hypothermia may exert a positive influence on survival through a cerebral protective effect. However, this depends largely on the preservation of cardiac output.

In practical terms, when submersion in water occurs, initial voluntary breath holding may be followed by components of the cold shock and diving responses. When breath holding is overcome, involuntary gasping occurs and aspiration of water leads to laryngeal spasm. Vomiting may occur. Unconsciousness and death are inevitable without rescue.

Rescue and subsequent management

It is important to ensure the safety of personnel involved in rescue. Surface tension and G-force are sufficient to cause circulatory collapse in conscious victims lifted vertically, especially by helicopter. Rescuers should anticipate other illnesses and injuries, especially of the cervical spine. Management should proceed along standard ABC guidelines with a view to transfer to an emergency department with access to an intensive care facility.

Categories of patient

1. Patients with no evidence of aspiration

This group may have recovered substantially by the time they arrive at hospital, make light of the event and ask to be discharged. They should be admitted and observed for 24h because of the risk of ALI and cerebral oedema. If they insist on leaving, they should receive instructions to return if they become unwell.

2. Patients with evidence of aspiration but without ventilatory compromise

Pulmonary oedema may develop several hours after aspiration with rapid deterioration of ventilatory function. Non-invasive or invasive ventilation may be required.

3. Patients with ventilatory compromise or hypothermia or both, but with a functional circulation

Hypothermic patients should be monitored in an ICU and actively warmed at ~1°C/h. NIV may not be practical because of reduced level of consciousness, shivering or cardiovascular instability, in which case tracheal intubation and ventilation using a protective lung ventilation strategy should be started without delay. At ~28°C there is a risk of ventricular arrhythmias.

4. Patients in cardiac arrest—the apparently dead

CPR may be required for several hours while the patient is warmed to 33°C by whatever means are available.

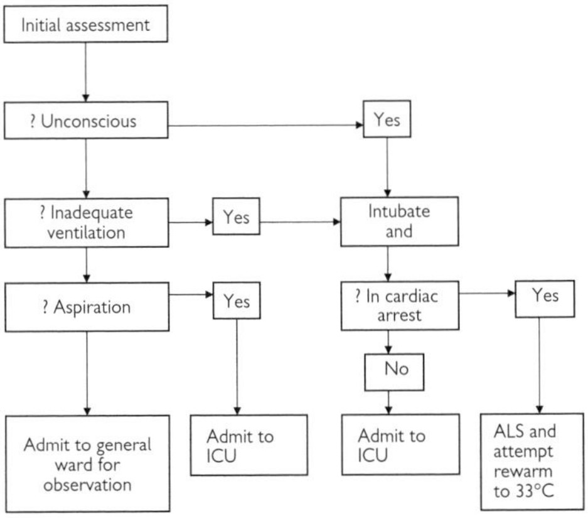

Fig. 29.2.1 Algorithm for the management of near-drowning.

The diagnosis of death may present a problem while the patient remains hypothermic.

General management

Respiratory

Hypothermia may cause rigidity unresponsive to neuromuscular blocking agents. Circulatory compromise may render these drugs ineffective. Mouth opening and tracheal intubation may be difficult. There is little practical difference between inhalation of fresh and salt water, but bacterial contamination may lead to unusual infections. Aspiration of gastric contents may occur at any time. Prophylactic antibiotics are usually omitted in favour of culture and active treatment of infection as it arises. ALI or ARDS may supervene. Radiographic abnormalities are common in patients without clinical evidence of aspiration.

Acid–base balance, blood gas analysis and metabolism

Metabolic acidosis is common. Persistent lactic acidosis raises the possibility of hypoxic liver or bowel injury. Hyperkalaemia is common during re-warming, re-perfusion and renal dysfunction. A potassium >10mmol/l with profound hypothermia is associated with asphyxial cardiac arrest and is not compatible with successful resuscitation. Hyponatraemia may occur as a result of fresh water absorption. Hyperglycaemia is common during initial resuscitation.

Cardiovascular

Hypothermia causes bradycardia with prolongation of the PR and QT interval, but a variety of supraventricular dysrhythmias may occur. J-waves appear below 33°C. Below 28°C the victim is likely to be in VF and requires re-warming to >30°C so that defibrillation has a reasonable chance of success. Defibrillation is hazardous to personnel in a wet environment. Troponin elevation may reflect global myocardial hypoxaemia and resuscitation rather than conventional MI. Pulse oximetry may be unreliable. It may be difficult to establish vascular access and the intraosseous route should be considered early, even in adults. When spontaneous output has been established, invasive monitoring is a priority for managing cardiac and circulatory function.

Renal

Renal failure is common. Rhabdomyolysis may occur.

Central nervous system

Hyoxic brain injury may develop over 24–72h and may not be immediately evident on CT scan. ICP is a better guide to its development.

Haematological

Aspiration of large quantities of fresh water into the circulation may cause haemolysis.

Re-warming

- Victims who are conscious and not in ventilatory distress may be warmed in a bath at 40°C. Surface warming devices are also useful.
- In patients with no cardiac output, warming is most effectively achieved using cardiopulmonary bypass, from which there are encouraging results. If this is not accessible, external cardiac massage must be continued while a variety of techniques are employed to elevate the victim's temperature to a level where spontaneous cardiac output returns or defibrillation is possible. None of these is efficient.
- Wet clothing should be removed, the skin dried, the victim covered with warm blankets and kept out of drafts. A number of devices are available for application to a patient's skin surface to control body temperature.
- Inspired ventilatory gases should be warmed to 45°C and humidified.
- IV fluids should be warmed to 40°C and administered through a warming device.
- Warmed water at 40°C may be instilled into the stomach and bladder.
- Potassium-free peritoneal dialysis fluid at 40°C may be instilled intraperitoneally with a short dwell time.
- Once cardiac output has been restored, an intravascular warming circuit may be installed. Devices for regulating body temperature following out-of-hospital cardiac arrest and in the management of traumatic brain injury can be used to elevate a patient's temperature and may have a role in the subsequent control of body temperature in this group of patients.
- A haemofiltration circuit at a pump speed of 200ml/min can deliver ~120kcal/h and also allows correction of acid–base and other metabolic abnormalities.

Prognostic indicators

Survival

Patients in categories 1 and 2 usually make good spontaneous recovery, but serious organ system dysfunction may follow in patients in category 3. Patients in category 4 rarely survive. Outlook worsens in patients whose GCS is <9 or who have sustained a cardiac arrest which has not been rapidly rectified.

Further reading

Golden F StC, Tipton MJ, Scott RC, Immersion, near-drowning and drowning. *Br J Anaesth* 1997; 79: 214–25.

Rhabdomyolysis

Rhabdomyolysis is disintegration of striated muscle. It is characterized by muscle necrosis leading to release of intracellular constituents into extracellular fluid and the circulation. Causes include trauma, overexertion, substance abuse, muscle enzyme deficiencies, electrolyte abnormalities, infections, drugs, toxins and endocrinopathies (Table 29.3.1). Mechanisms of injury include direct injury to the cell membrane, muscle cell or hypoxia, leading to ATP depletion and sodium–potassium pump failure. Extracellular calcium ions leak into the cell and increase free cytosolic ionized calcium with activation of calcium-dependent proteases and phospholipases, resulting in muscle destruction. Following muscle injury potassium, phosphate, myoglobin, creatine kinase (CK), creatinine and nucleosides (metabolized to urate) leak into the circulation. The muscle necrosis, inflammation and oedema lead to fluid accumulation in affected muscles and intravascular volume depletion.

Early complications (within 12–24h) include hyperkalaemia, hypocalcaemia and cardiac dysrhythmias, hepatic dysfunction and early compartment syndrome. Late complications (≥24h) include acute renal failure, DIC, late compartment syndrome and (following recovery) hypercalcaemia. Prompt recognition and early intervention are therefore vital.

Clinical manifestations

Clinical manifestations are varied, dictated by the underlying cause and by the ensuing complications. Classic triad—muscle pain, weakness and passage of dark urine. Muscles may be tender and swollen. The most frequently involved muscles are in the calves and lower back. Where pressure necrosis is part of the pathogenesis, there may be overlying skin changes. In >50% of cases these 'local' manifestations may be absent. Urinary myoglobin concentration provides coloration ranging from pink-tinged through to muddy-brown/black.

Systemic features include fever, malaise, nausea, vomiting, tachycardia, confusion and agitation. Oliguria/anuria may be apparent, and severe hyperkalaemia may lead to cardiac dysrhythmia and arrest.

Laboratory features

Laboratory findings confirm the diagnosis and to an extent predict the prognosis in terms of complications. CK levels are the most sensitive indicator of muscle damage and begin to rise within 12h of injury, peaking at 1–3 days and declining 3–5 days after injury. Supervention of compartment syndrome may lead to a secondary rise. The peak CK level is said to be predictive of acute renal failure, levels of >16 000U/l being more likely to be associated with acute renal failure.

Myoglobin has a molecular weight of 18 800Da and in serum is bound to haptoglobin. Normal plasma levels of myoglobin are very low (<30mcg/l). When >100g of skeletal muscle are damaged, haptoglobin-binding sites are saturated and myoglobin is filtered and appears in the urine. Normal urinary levels of myoglobin are <5ng/ml, visible myoglobinuria (tea- or coca-cola-coloured urine) occurs when levels exceed 250mcg/ml. Myoglobin has a very short half-life (2–3h) and serum levels return to normal within 6–8h. Therefore, although myoglobin may be measured in both blood and urine, the clinical utility of such measurements is questionable.

Electrolyte disturbance: hyperkalaemia, hypocalcaemia, hyerphosphataemia and hyperuricaemia. Creatinine levels are elevated out of proportion to urea levels and acidosis, and deranged liver function may also be apparent in 25% of patients.

Essential laboratory investigations

- CK
- Urea, electrolytes and creatinine
- Calcium, phosphate and urate
- Blood gases and urinary pH
- Clotting studies

Table 29.3.1 Causes of rhabdomyolysis

Trauma and compression	*Crush injury, road traffic accident prolonged immobilization, electrical injury*
Ischaemic limb injury	
Exertional causes	*Marathon running, status epilepticus*
Heat-related causes	*Heat stroke, malignant hyperthermia and neuroleptic malignant syndrome*
Substance abuse	*Alcohol, cocaine, amphetamine, lysergic acid, Ecstasy*
Toxins	*Carbon monoxide, heavy metals, snake & insect venom*
Drugs	*Antipsychotics and antidepressants, sedative hypnotics, statins and fibrates, theophyllines*
Metabolic and endocrine causes	*Hypo- and hypernatraemia, hypocalcaemia, hypophosphataemia, hypocalcaemia, hypo- and hyperthyroidism, hyperosmolar conditions (HONK)*
Infectious causes	*Viruses: influenza and parainfluenza, coxsackie virus, adenovirus, echovirus, herpes viruses, CMV, HIV, EBV* *Bacteria: Streptococcus, Legionella, Salmonella, Staphylococcus, Listeria, Tularaemia* *Other: Falciparum malaria, sepsis syndrome*
Genetic enzyme deficiencies	*Myophosphorylase, phosphorylase kinase, phosphofructokinase, phosphoglycerate mutase, lactate dehydrogenase, carnitine palmityl transferase, acyl-coenzyme A dehydrogenase, mycoadenylate deaminase*
Autoimmune causes	*Polymyositis, dermatomyositis*

Complications of rhabdomyolysis

Early complications

Potassium, phosphate, creatinine, organic acids, myoglobin and nucleosides are all released into the circulation. Severe hyperkalaemia may lead to cardiac dysrhythmias and even cardiac arrest, particularly in association with severe hypocalcaemia and acidosis.

Early or late complications
Compartment syndrome may occur either early or later in the course of rhabdomyolysis and may be exacerbated by hypotension. Fluid sequestration occurs and, as most muscles are within rigid compartments, this oedema leads to a rise in compartment pressure and impaired perfusion (compartment syndrome). Compartment pressures >30mm Hg produce clinically significant muscle ischaemia and secondary rhabdomyolysis. Prolonged pressure may also lead to nerve damage.

Late complications
DIC may develop following rhabdomyolysis, usually >72h following injury. Acute renal failure is the most serious complication, developing in 16.5% of patients. It results from a combination of renal vasoconstriction, hypovolaemia, mechanical obstruction by intraluminal cast formation and direct cytotoxicity from the haem moiety of myoglobin. In the presence of low urine flow rates and low urinary pH, myoglobin interacts with Tamm–Horsfall protein and precipitates, causing obstructive cast formation. Hyperuricaemia and urinary excretion of uric acid exacerbate tubular obstruction through formation of uric acid casts. Degradation of precipitated myoglobin initiates lipid peroxidation and renal injury, and release of free iron catalyses free radical production and further enhances ischaemic damage.

During recovery, hypercalcaemia may occur. Calcium that has accumulated in muscles at the time of initial muscle necrosis is released from storage sites during recovery, and this is enhanced if calcium supplementation has been administered during the hypocalcaemic stage This can be associated with hyperparathyroidism and hypervitaminosis D in some cases, leading to overt hypercalcaemia.

Management of rhabdomyolysis

Initial stabilization and resuscitation, and prevention of acute renal failure
As much as 10–12l of fluid may be sequestrated in damaged muscle, and IV hydration should be started as early as possible (Table 29.3.2). In patients with crush injury, this means implementation of IV therapy even whilst the patient is still trapped. The longer it takes for rehydration to be initiated, the more likely it is that acute rebal failure will supervene.

Rationale for mannitol and bicarbonate therapy
Mannitol is said to increase renal blood flow and the GFR, potentially suck fluid out of the interstitial compartment reducing muscle swelling and thus risk of compartment syndrome, promote a diuresis and prevent precipitation of obstructive tubular casts, and serve as a free radical scavenger.

Bicarbonate therapy is said to correct acidosis, reduces risk of hyperkalaemia and increases urinary pH, preventing precipitation and degradation of myoglobin in the urinary tubules.

Both mannitol and bicarbonate therapy are standard therapy, but neither has been subject to clinical trials. Observational data suggest that they provide no additional benefit over and above volume expansion with saline. Addition of mannitol and bicarbonate had no impact on development of acute renal failure, need for dialysis or mortality.

Table 29.3.2. Management of rhabdomyolysis

1. Obtain immediate IV access and start isotonic saline 500ml/h then titrate to maintain a urine output of 200–300ml/h
2. Consider CVP monitoring (elderly, presence of cardiac failure, renal failure)
3. Treat any underlying conditions where indicated
4. Add IV sodium bicarbonate and titrate to urinary pH >6.5 where metabolic acidosis and/or hyperkalaemia are present
5. Consider IV mannitol (test dose of 200mg/kg IV over 3–5min to ensure adequate renal function, then 10ml/h)
6. Monitor for, and treat, complications
7. Repeat CK assay to determine peak CK level
8. Consider fasciotomy in compartment syndrome

Compartment syndrome
Delay in management of compartment syndrome can lead to irreversible muscle and nerve damage. Neurological symptoms and signs may indicate the need for fasciotomy, but measurement of intramuscular pressure provides an objective guide. Pressures consistently exceeding 30mm Hg with no tendency to reduce are a clear indication.

Renal replacement therapy
Where acute renal failure is established, or in the presence of severe hyperkalaemia and acidosis, RRT may be required. Fluid overload is rarely an indication for RRT in rhabdomyolysis. Haemodialysis offers distinct advantages through its greater efficiency and lack of need for continuous anticoagulation. Peritoneal dialysis is the least desirable mode of RRT in patients with rhabdomyolysis due to inefficiency and difficulties with administration.

Adjuvants
Free radical scavengers and antioxidants and dantrolene sodium have all been used experimentally, but do not yet have a proven clinical role.

Further reading

Akmal M, Massry S. Reversible hepatic dysfunction associated with rhabdomyolysis. *Am J Nephrol* 1990; 10: 49–52.

Better OS, Stein JH. Early management of shock and prophylaxis of acute renal failure in traumatic rhabdomyolysis. *N Engl J Med* 1990; 322: 825–9.

Brown C, Rhee P, Chan L, *et al.* Preventing renal failure in patients with rhabdomyolysis: do bicarbonate and mannitol make a difference? *J Trauma* 2004; 56: 1191–6.

Gabow PA, Kaehny WD, Kelleher SP. The spectrum of rhabdomyolysis. Medicine (Baltimore) 1982; 61: 141–52.

Knochel JP. Mechanisms of rhabdomyolysis. *Curr Opin Rheumatol* 1993; 5: 725–31.

Lane JT, Boudreau RJ, Kinlaw WB. Disappearance of muscular calcium deposits during resolution of prolonged rhabdomyolysisinduced hypercalcemia. *Am J Med* 1990; 89: 523–25.

Orrell RW, Lane RJM. Myoglobinuria. In: Lane RJM, ed. Handbook of muscle disease. New York: Marcel Dekker, 1996: 607–11.

Ward MM. Factors predictive of acute renal failure in rhabdomyolysis. *Arch Intern Med* 1988; 148: 1553–7.

Zager RA. Rhabdomyolysis and myohemoglobinuric acute renal failure. *Kidney Int* 1996; 49: 314–2.

Pressure sores

Introduction

Pressure sores are a hazardous complication of ICU. They are defined as an area(s) of local tissue damage caused by pressure, shear, moisture and friction or a combination thereof. The incidence of pressure sores within the intensive care population has been reported to be between 3 and 29%. They are also expensive and can cost up to £40 000 to treat. They can appear anywhere on the body. They act as a reservoir for microorganisms and are often extremely painful. For reasons not yet clear, medical staff often leave the entire problem to nursing staff; a team approach must be adopted.

Identification

Identification of those at risk is problematic. Current scoring systems that attempt to identify patients at risk on ICU are often derivatives of those developed for ward patients. Their effectiveness is unclear. All have the ability to over- or underestimate the risk of pressure sore development. They must be used in conjunction with clinical judgement. Common scoring systems include:

- Waterlow
- Norton
- Braden

Risk factors

General

Exposure either on one or more occasion to the forces of friction, shear and pressure in the following context:

- Pressure occurs when the patient's weight on a support surface causes body tissue to become compressed against a bony prominence, resulting in poor capillary perfusion.
- Shear is the result of horizontal forces perpendicular to pressure, and is usually the end result of a combination of friction and movement. A common example of this occurs when a patient is sitting upright in bed but slides down, causing the sacral area to 'shear'.
- Friction occurs when two surfaces (usually the patient's skin and bed surface) move against each other in opposition.

ICU patients are generally at greater risk of pressure sore development due to prolonged periods of inactivity.

Specific

In one study of 283 ICU patients, the following risk factors were found to be significant in the development of pressure sores on ICU:

- Anaemia
- Noradrenaline infusion
- APACHE II score >13 upon admission
- Faecal incontinence
- Length of stay >3 days

Other

A plethora of intrinsic factors exist that usually exacerbate the condition. They include:

- Poor dietary intake
- Steroids
- General health
- Weight
- Continence
- Medications
- Age
- Diabetes

Achieving correct protein and calorific intake of ICU patients is particularly problematic. Tube feeding or TPN is often instigated despite their inherent risks. Knowing the patients weight is important as it allow the calculation of calorific input. The European Pressure Ulcer Advisory Panel (EPUAP) recommends that 30–35kcal/kg body weight per day, with 1–1.5g/kg/day protein required and 1ml/kcal/day of fluid intake serve as a minimum requirement.

A common mistake is to overlook the patient's bowel status. If the patient is suffering from perfuse diarrhoea, then it is unlikely that they will be absorbing their nutritional needs despite the calculation being correct.

Low serum albumin levels (<3.5g/dl) has been associated with an increase risk in pressure sore development. The pitfall here is to give IV albumin, raise the level and then assume the patient is no longer at risk. The correct approach is to treat the cause of the low serum albumin.

Prevention

In the ICU the most frequent method of prevention is a specialist bed or mattress. These have cost implications. There are also many different types, but all aim to:

- Provide a comfortable surface
- Redistribute pressure

The redistribution of pressure is achieved by either one of two methods:

- Pressure-reducing
- Pressure-relieving

An example of a pressure-reducing mattress is the standard hospital mattress. It reduces peak interface pressures by maximizing skin contact. It is of little use in very heavy patients—a specialist mattress will be required. A pressure-relieving mattress has the aim of removing all pressure. This is done in either of two ways:

- By suspending or raising vulnerable areas of the body by deflating special cells built into the mattress.
- By timed inflation and deflation of air-filled cells.

The latter method uses 5–10min cycles provided by a pump that is often located at the end of a patient's bed. Time cycles are of extreme importance, but optimal time cycles are difficult to achieve as the patient's condition changes.

Other forms of prevention

Frequent turning and repositioning (condition allowing) of the patient must be implemented even if they are on a pressure0relieving/reducing mattress. An unscientific 2-hourly turning regime is often quoted, but in all probability the frequency is proportionate to patient risk.

Treating the patient's underlying condition, addressing dietary requirements (the involvement of a dietician is mandatory), correcting of anaemia and early mobilization also fall into this category of prevention.

Grading

Several grading systems attempt to classify the extent and nature of a pressure sore. One of the better ones is that recommended by EPUAP. Pressure sores are graded into 4 types:

- Grade 1—non-blanchable erythema of intact skin. Discoloration, warmth, induration or hardness of skin may also be used as indicators, particularly in people with darker skin.
- Grade 2—partial thickness skin loss, involving the epidermis, dermis or both. The ulcer is superficial and presents clinically as an abrasion or blister.
- Grade 3—full thickness skin loss involving damage to or necrosis of subcutaneous tissue that may extend down to, but not through, underlying fascia.
- Grade 4—extensive destruction, tissue necrosis or damage to muscle, bone or supporting structures, with or without full thickness skin loss.

Frequent assessment and documentation of the pressure sore using this scale is mandatory in order to track wound progress.

A pressure sore can be likened to an iceberg in that despite the appearance of slight skin damage on the skin surface, the dermis and epidermis may have considerable damage. Any area of redness is a cause for concern.

Pressure sores can develop as a result of the use of equipment. Pressure sores developing on the bridge of patient's noses from CPAP masks is not uncommon, and have been the subject of successful litigation. Ventilator tubing, abandoned venflon bungs, drip and drain tubing, ECG dots and monitor wiring serve as other examples.

Wound treatment

ICU patients seem particularly vulnerable to developing pressure sores on their heels. If a pressure sore develops it will require treatment. Wound treatments exist that range from wound cleaning to surgical debridement. Grade 1 pressure sores seldom require pharmaceutical or surgical treatment, but for the other grades an expanse of creams, gels, pads, dressings and devices exist. Treatment is largely governed by the nature, location and type of pressure sore. In general:

- Dressings should not 'dry' the wound but maintain a moist environment.
- Do not use systemic antibiotics in an attempt to eradicate bacteria within the wound.
- Frequent removal of dressings could disturb the wound-healing process
- 'Hard' dressings or pads should not be used as they can exacerbate pressure.
- Handwashing and other infection control measures must be adopted to prevent wound contamination or bacterial spread.
- Dressings should remain in place as in accordance with the manufacturer's recommendations.

A large 'custom and practice' culture exists around the treatment of pressure sores. Expert advice from a tissue viability or wound care expert is mandatory. A positive wound swab will need the involvement of the microbiology team. There will be a difference as to whether the identified organism(s) are either 'colonizing' or 'infecting' the wound. An unnecessarily aggressive attempt to remove the organism(s) may result in delayed wound healing.

Wound healing

There are 3 distinct stages of wound healing:

- Inflammatory
- Proliferation
- Maturation and remodelling

The initial inflammatory stage lasts usually only for a few days. Blood vessels are constricted to minimize loss of blood; platelets and thromboplastin attend the affected area in an effort to form a clot. White cells then enter the area to clear it of organisms and debris. This process generates heat and redness which can be seen and felt at the wound site. Depending on the severity of the pressure sore, the next stage of proliferation lasts for ~3 weeks. Fibroblasts attend the area to make collagen. Collagen 'fills' in the wound and is assisted significantly by the formation of new blood vessels. The final stage of maturation and remodelling is the most protracted. It can take up to 2yrs to complete. A new form of collagen arrives and attempts to re-mould and strengthen the wound site. Scar tissue develops which although visibly appears stronger is, in fact, only 75% as strong as normal tissue.

There is a particular problem associated with chronic wounds in that the scar tissue cells can become unresponsive to growth markers and cytokines, thereby prolonging the above stages and delaying healing considerably.

Conclusion

The following serve as an *aide memoir* to the successful management of pressure sores:

- Do not use sheep skins, they do not work
- Do not leave pressure sores to nursing staff; you have a part to play
- Inspect skin areas frequently, particularly the sacrum and the heels.
- Document, and if necessary photograph, any pressure sores
- Ensure regular reviews of the patient's risk factors are performed
- Regularly inspect any pressure sores that develop
- Treat pressure sores appropriately; quality advice can be obtained from your local Tissue Viability Nurse.

Further reading

Theaker C, Mannan M, Ives N, *et al.* Risk factors for pressure sores in the critically ill. *Anaesthesia* 2000; 55: 221–4.

Chapter 30

Pain and post-operative intensive care

Chapter contents

Pain management in ICU

Introduction

Relief from pain is not only indicated on humanitarian and ethical grounds alone, but has medical and possibly cost benefits.

Terminology

- *Oxford dictionary*—sensation of physical suffering or acute discomfort
- *The International Association for the Study of Pain 1986*—an unpleasant sensory and emotional experience associated with actual or potential tissue damage or described in terms of such damage
- *Neuropathic pain*—seen in patients in the ICU due to nerve damage, herpes zoster, GBS; does not respond to conventional analgesics but may require combinations of drugs such as amitryptylline, carbemazepine, sodium valproate, gabapentin and ketamine.

Causes of pain in ICU patients

- Post-surgery
- Trauma
- Organ dysfunction: gut ischaemia, DVT, cardiac
- Treatment: procedures on ICU, change of dressings
- Pre-existing pain: vascular, neuropathic, rheumatoid
- Pain of terminal disease.

Adverse effects of pain

- Respiratory: atelectasis
- Cardiovascular: stress, MI
- Gut: ileus, nausea, vomiting
- Genitourinary: retention, agitation
- Endocrine: increased ADH, water retention
- Haematological: venous stasis, DVT
- Musculoskeletal: immobility, critical illness polyneuropathy and myopathy, pulse oximeter probe
- Neuropsychological: decreased sleep, agitation, delirium, post-traumatic stress disorder.

Assessment of pain in ICU

- Difficult if patient cannot communicate
- If in doubt assume they are in pain
- Use surrogate markers such as stress response, but this will be affected by β-blockers and inotropes, and anticholinergics.

Balanced sedation in the ICU

Traditionally, sedation as practised in UK, European and US ICUs has been based on hypnotic regimes. However, as intubated patients on ICU are unable always to communicate, it may be that they would benefit from an analgesic-based regime if pain is a feature of their disease and management whilst in ICU. There is an assumption amongst doctors, nurses and relatives that it is probably best that patients remember relatively little of their ICU stay, hence the widespread use of hypnotic regimes. However, when patients are recovering from critical illness, the absence of memory of events in ICU may lead to lack of understanding of why they are exhausted and psychologically disturbed during their rehabilitation phase. The emphasis these days is on trying to ensure adequate analgesia in order to ensure comfort and reduce the need for hypnotic drugs which may prolong the patient's time spent ventilated and their stay on ICU. In order to minimize this time, daily sedation holding is now a feature of the 'ventilator' bundle of care. The use of early percutaneous tracheostomy may also be a means of reducing weaning times.

Before resorting to hypnotic-based regimes for sedation, it is important that the patient is assessed regularly for pain and adequately treated. Patients' requirements for strong analgesic drugs may be modified or reduced by attention to:

- Reduce noise levels
- Change pulse oximeter finger regularly
- Reduce flatulence, nausea
- Immobilize fractures
- Establish sleep pattern

Despite ICU staff believing that pain is adequately treated, many studies have shown that at least 50% of ICU patients experienced moderate or severe pain during their ICU stay, and the CoBATRICE patient and relatives survey demonstrated that 76% of responders expected intensive care staff to do everything to control pain.

The use of analgesia-based sedation was described by Lane *et al.* in 2002, and has been responsible for a trend in the reduction of hypnotic-based regimes. There are concerns with hypnotic-based regimes particularly since 1984 when it was discovered that etomidate was associated with adenal gland suppression and increased mortality in trauma patients. However, it is only recently in 2005 that the continued use of etomidate has been questioned.

There is literature to demonstrate that propofol in children and in adults with head injury can be associated with an excess mortality.

Guidelines

The Fundamentals of the Critical Care Support (FCCS) manual outlines the use of drugs such as lorazepam, morphine and fentanyl for analgesia and sedation, and emphasizes the importance of not using these drugs as a method of restraint by staff (Federal Regulation 42 CFR 482.13), but points out that where it is thought that pain is the cause of agitation, then analgesia would be the appropriate initial therapy.

The Intensive Care Society Guidelines state that:

- All patients must be comfortable and painfree
- Anxiety should be minimized
- Patients sould be calm, cooperative and able to sleep
- Patients should tolerate organ system support and be able to synchronize with ventilator
- Patients must not be paralysed and awake

Thus both US and UK societies say the same thing, i.e. that analgesia and comfort must be the first aim of sedating patients in intensive care.

Methods of pain relief in ICU

Non-steroidal anti-inflammatory drugs (NSAIDs)

In view of important and frequent side effects, it seems prudent to avoid this class in the critically ill in the absence of any definite gain to be had.

Paracetomol

Now that it is available as an IV infusion 10mg/ml, this is becoming a popular choice for analgesia in intensive care practice.

Epidural

Epidural pain relief is especially useful for post-operative surgical management and for 'flail' chest injuries, but ideally patients need to be cooperative as there is controversy about the safe placement of epidural catheters in sedated patients and there are concerns about catheter placement in the presence of coagulopathy and sepsis.

Acupuncture, aromatherapy

These and other alternative methods may have a role.

Opioid analgesic drugs

These remain the mainstay of analgesia in the ICU. The minimum effective analgesic concentration for each patient will vary widely. In the frequent presence of organ dysfunction, pharmacokinetic considerations play the most important role in the choice of agent.

The ideal agent

This has the following properties:

- rapid onset
- predictable
- no active metabolites
- wears off quickly
- no cardiorespiratory depression
- no nausea, vomiting
- not addictive, no tolerance
- not affected by renal or hepatic disease
- wide therapeutic index

Remifentanil

This opioid has the properties above of an ideal agent, and is increasingly finding a role for sedation in UK intensive care practice. Many intensivists feel that it allows patients to be comfortable and cooperative. It has a licence for use up to 72h so may not be ideal for long-stay patients. Its rapid breakdown to remifentanil acid (with only 1/1460 potency of remifentanil) by non-specific esterases means that it cannot accumulate in the bloodstream; this is not the case with morphine, fentanyl or alfentanil. Studies to date demonstrate that with a remifentanil-based sedative regime patients can be extubated more quickly and leave ICU when compared with conventional regimes. Cost-benefit analyses to date make analgosedation with a remifentanil regime an attractive proposition.

Summary

- Opioids the most common method for analgesia
- Hypnotics associated with many unwanted effects
- Remember neuropathic pain
- Involve pain team if complicated.
- Regional techniques can improve outcome in high risk surgical patients
- Avoid NSAIDs
- Remifentanil shows promise and widespread use already in Neuro and Cardiac ICU

Further reading

Annane D. ICU Physicians should abandon the use of etomidate! *Intensive Care Med* 2005: 31: 325–6.

Bakker J, Mulder P. Remifentanil shortens duration of mechanical ventilation and ICU stay. *Intensive Care Med* 2006; 32(Suppl 13): S86.

Cohen A. http://www.ics.ac.uk/downloads/Sedation.pdf 2001

Cremer O, Moons K, Bouman E, *et al.* Long-term propofol infusion and cardiac failure in adult head-injured patients. *Lancet* 2001; 357: 117–8.

Jacobi J, Fraser GL, Coursin DB, *et al*; Task Force of the American College of Critical Care Medicine (ACCM) of the Society of Critical Care Medicine (SCCM), American Society of Health-System Pharmacists (ASHP), American College of Chest Physicians. Clinical practice guidelines for the sustained use of sedatives and analgesics in the critically ill adult. *Crit Care Med* 2002; 30: 119–41.

Lane M, Cadman B and Park G. Sedation and analgesia in the critically ill patient using remifentanil—frequently asked questions and their answers. *Care Crit Ill* 2002; 18: 146–7.

Parke J, Stevens J, Rice A, Greenaway C, *et al.* Fatal myocardial failure, metabolic acidosis. *BMJ* 1992; 305: 613–6.

www.cobatrice.org

Intensive care for the high risk surgical patient

Introduction

The majority of in-patient surgical procedures culminate in a good outcome, but low overall surgical mortality rates (<2% in the UK) disguise the presence of an important subpopulation of patients at significantly greater risk of complications and death. Up to 15% of in-patient surgical procedures may be classified as high risk, accounting for >80% of post-operative deaths. Around 10–15% of high risk patients die following surgery, and as many as 70% develop complications. The key features of the typical high risk surgical patient are listed in Table 30.2.1. Early identification and optimal care of the high risk patient may result in a substantial reduction in risk. This chapter describes a basic approach to the care of such patients.

Pre-operative assessment and care

Although the characteristics of the high risk patient are well described, many do not receive an appropriate level of perioperative care. New approaches to risk assessment may help to stratify patients to an appropriate level of care. An important example is the increasing use of submaximal exercise testing to measure anaerobic threshold. Where this is not possible, subjective evaluation of exercise tolerance will still provide a useful indication of cardiorespiratory reserve.

Table 30.2.1 Factors associated with an increased risk of post-operative complications and death

Patient factors
Ischaemic heart disease
Chronic obstructive pulmonary disease
Diabetes
Advanced age
Poor exercise tolerance
Poor nutritional status
Surgical factors
Emergency surgery
Major or complex surgery
Body cavity surgery
Large blood or insensible fluid loss
Prolonged duration of surgery
Perioperative care factors
Inadequate critical care facilities
Insufficient patient monitoring
Inadequate analgesia
Lack of early intervention as complications develop

Many high risk patients present on an emergency basis, leaving little time to adjust basic medical treatments. However, wherever possible, medical therapies should be optimized prior to surgery, particularly in the case of COPD, asthma, hypertension, ischaemic heart disease and diabetes. For those patients considered to be at high risk of perioperative myocardial ischaemia, prophylactic β-blockade may also prove beneficial.

Management during surgery

Critical care of the high risk patient should commence in the operating theatre. Standard anaesthetic and surgical care should be complemented by treatment approaches which are now considered standard in the ICU. These include appropriate antibiotic therapy, low tidal volume ventilation, restrictive red blood cell transfusion (maintain haemoglobin ≥8g/dl), maintenance of normothermia and tight glycaemic control. Recent developments in intraoperative fluid therapy may also offer an opportunity to improve outcome. Most high risk patients will develop some degree of circulatory dysfunction during or after surgery. Reduced fluid intake, haemorrhage and insensible losses will result in a variable degree of hypovolaemia. The resulting circulatory dysfunction may be further exacerbated by cardiac failure and sepsis. Optimal fluid therapy will require careful consideration of the risks associated with both inadequate and excessive IV fluid administration. However, precise estimation of fluid deficit may be difficult, particularly with patients undergoing GI surgery. Fluid therapy may be more effective when measurements of cardiac output and stroke volume are used as end-points. In this respect, the use of oesophageal Doppler monitoring may improve outcomes following cardiac, orthopaedic and abdominal surgery.

Post-operative intensive care

Close liaison with critical care unit staff is required to ensure a seamless transition into post-operative care. In the first few hours after surgery, a strong emphasis should be placed on maintaining the balance between oxygen consumption and oxygen delivery. Even brief admission to a critical care unit will allow the optimization of analgesia, body temperature and a gradual decrease in sedation (oxygen consumption factors). as well as adequate fluid, inotrope and vasopressor therapy (oxygen delivery factors). This approach may substantially decrease the risk of cardiorespiratory failure following extubation. In some institutions, overnight intensive recovery units facilitate this approach without the expense and complexity of a full-scale ICU.

Post-operative ventilation

Major surgery under general anaesthesia will result in a significant degree of respiratory compromise as a result of reductions in functional residual capacity which cause atelectasis and a reduction in minute volume. Post-operative pain may prevent full inspiration, preventing any correction of this process. Along with increases in oxygen consump-

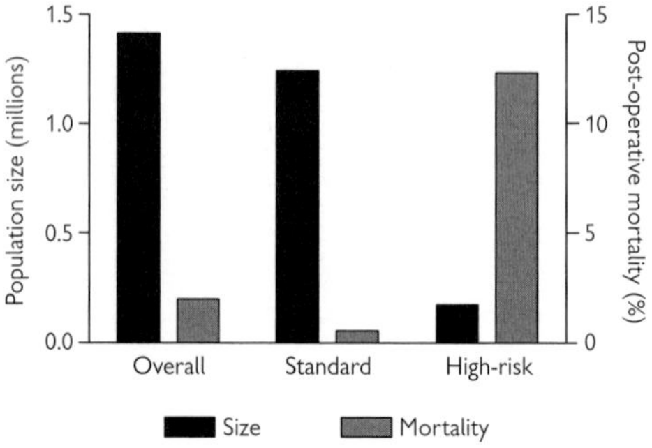

Fig. 30.2.1 Mortality rates for standard and high risk surgical procedures in the UK.

tion due to agitation, pain or shivering, these factors will predispose the high risk patient to respiratory failure and pneumonia. Early extubation after surgery may ease pressure on critical care resources, but for high risk patients it is preferable to wean sedation and invasive ventilation over a period of a few hours. This approach is an effective part of the routine care of cardiac surgical patients. CPAP or NIV may also be used to maintain and improve respiratory function in the hours after surgery. This approach can reduce the incidence of respiratory failure and subsequent re-intubation.

Post-operative haemodynamic therapy

Occult circulatory disturbances often persist after surgery. Minimally invasive cardiac output monitoring may also be used to guide haemodynamic therapy in the early post-operative period. This approach may be extended to include low dose inotropic agents in addition to fluid therapy. This technique, which is sometimes termed goal-directed haemodynamic therapy, improves tissue oxygen delivery, leading to a reduction in post-operative complications as well as duration of hospital stay.

Other important aspects of post-operative care

It is often preferable to commence enteral nutrition early (within 24h of surgery) via an NG tube, provided that any contraindications have been carefully excluded. Following surgery for bowel obstruction or perforation, for example, a more cautious approach may be preferable because of the risk of paralytic ileus. The typical high risk surgical patient will have a number of predisposing factors for venous thromboembolism. LMWH should usually be administered on a prophylactic basis. Other aspects of treatment which may potentially have an impact on outcome following high risk surgery include analgesia and early mobilization.

Summary

Post-operative complications and death are commonplace in the high risk surgical population. Perioperative critical care may substantially improve both short- and long-term outcomes for such patients. The most effective way of achieving this may be through the use of treatment protocols to standardize care during and immediately after surgery.

Further reading

Cullinane M, Gray AJ, Hargraves CM, *et al.* The 2003 Report of the National Confidential Enquiry into Peri-Operative Deaths. London: NCEPOD. 2003.

Pearse RM, Harrison DA, James P, *et al.* Identification and characterisation of the high-risk surgical population in the United Kingdom. *Crit Care* 2006; 10: R81.

Bersten A, Soni N, Oh T. Oh's intensive care manualn 5th edn. London: Butterworth-Heinemann. 2003.

The acute surgical abdomen in the ITU

Assessing the acute abdomen remains an art. The causes of the acute abdomen or intra-abdominal catastrophe are bleeds, infarctions, obstructions, leaks and inflammations. Clinical assessment is more difficult in ICU because of distractions such as sedation, ventilation or other organ support. There is heavy reliance on the history, imaging, measurable physiological parameters and, most importantly, changes thereof. An intra-abdominal problem increases the probability of mortality as predicted by the APACHE II score, in part because of delays in obtaining surgical assessment.

Early manifestations include pain and distension, and changes in measured inflammatory markers, acidosis, respiratory and renal function. A serially rising lactate in an apparently unremarkable abdomen, for example, is a seriously worrying feature of an impending problem. These signs and symptoms are non-specific and often occur without associated significant intra-abdominal pathology. Access to good quality imaging such as ultrasound is essential but, with the exception of biliary system pathology, CT scan is the imaging modality of choice.

Ideally the same surgical team should re-evaluate the patient.

Causation is often reflected in the recent history, such as recent abdominal surgery and the development of an intestinal leak or surgical bleed. The medical patient is also prone to secondary events giving rise to intra-abdominal problems, and the pattern of signs and symptoms is likely to be similar. Satisfactory outcome requires control of the initiating event, control of the intra-abdominal pathology and then management of the consequences of the systemic response to the intra-abdominal catastrophe.

Complications of abdominal surgery

Post-operative haemorrhage and intestinal leaks are the most common complications following abdominal surgery.

Haemorrhage

Distension and a precipitous fall in the haemoglobin and haematocrit. Fluid replacement, drugs and epidural analgesia may confuse the picture, and substantial blood loss can occur before being recognized. Drainage tubes should never be relied upon as a negative indicator for blood loss. Blood in the peritoneal space and especially in the retroperitoneum gives rise to pain and ileus. If bleeding is continuing, urgent surgical action to control the source or, if non-specific, such as following major retroperitoneal or pelvic resection, then packing of cavities and possibly the use of clotting factors locally and systemically might be required. Radiological embolization is rarely appropriate. For persistent or unusual bleeding response, a search should be made for inherited disorders of coagulation such as von Willebrand disease, and so on.

If bleeding stops spontanously

A small amount of intra-abdominal blood will cause a transient peritonitis and prolongation of the post-operative ileus. Intra-abdominal haematoma predisposes to infection, especially if there has been contamination with intestinal contents. If ultrasound or CT demonstrate substantial haematoma, early evacuation is preferable, but radiological drainage of haematoma is usually fruitless as the clot is too thick to pass through even the largest radiological drain. A smaller haematoma might be observed and followed for evidence of infection and abscess formation. Intervention at that time might be surgical or by radiological drainage if the collection appears to be predominantly liquefied.

Leaks

Peritonitis secondary to intestinal tends to present slowly and insidiously. The leak might not begin until a day or two after operation, with gradual onset of physiological disturbance. Drains may indicate bile or other fluids. Pancreatic effluent has a characteristic prune juice colour and can be confirmed by fluid amylase estimation, which in a leak is likely to be in the 10s of thousands but at least 5-fold greater than the serum amylase. A raised urea in the setting of normal cardiovascular and renal parameters should alert one to the possibility of a urinary leak if the surgical episode has involved bladder surgery. The negative predictive value of a drain is poor. Typical manifestations of secondary peritonitis are likely to be unaccountable elevation in inflammatory parameters such as CRP. Unexplained tachycardia and more diffuse features such as abdominal distension and ileus may be present. Whether a leak is dealt with by re-operation or not depends on many factors and requires early involvement of the surgical team and close serial assessment. As a general principle, if the leak is apparent early in the post-operative period and where it is safe to do so, re-operation is preferred to perform toilet and either repair the anastomosis or divert flow by defunctioning the stoma at or proximal to the anastomosis. However, when the leak manifests late or where repair or diversion are not feasible, e.g. in a leaking pancreatic or high bile duct anastomosis, then achieving a controlled fistula is more appropriate. This might still require operation to perform toilet and drainage, but radiological drainage should also be considered especially for very fluid leaks such as bile.

The natural history of fistulae is to close unless there is a distant obstruction, malignant or radiotherapy-treated tissues are involved or there is persistent local sepsis. There is some evidence that the use of octreotide to reduce secretions might reduce the time to closure of pancreatic, biliary and small bowel fistulae but not the rate of closure.

A substantial systemic inflammatory response is often exhibited. Unless and sometimes even despite early control of leakage, multi-system failure supervenes and systems support will be required. Attention should be paid to infection, including yeasts, BMS and nutrition. Enteral feeding is usually possible in most cases, even in upper GI tract problems. Care of the skin is essential in these patients as the fistula contents are corrosive.

Colorectal anastomoses represent an area of potential concern. Some surgeons prefer to 'defunction' their vulnerable anastomoses such as after low rectal surgery. Then, even if there is a leak, a clinically threatening situation should not ensue. Signs and symptoms of an intraperitoneal leak from a colorectal anastomosis are likely to be fever and rise in inflammatory markers. There may be urinary frequency and diarrhoea. Depending on the extent of contamination, there may be little in the way of abdominal signs until the collection is substantial. Suspicion and early evaluation are essential. CT scan will be required and, if the leak is detected early after operation, the surgeon might consider re-operation and lavage and drainage, or diversion by defunctioning the stoma or conversion to end stoma.

Leaks discovered later, after ~7 days, are more problematic as the hazards of re-operation are high, and in this setting drainage through the rectum or percutaneously might represent the best option.

Previously, secondary sepsis from intestinal perforation or anastomotic failure was often managed by serial re-laparotomy and surgical toilet every 2 or 3 days, but more recently the trend is for re-laparotomy on demand, only if there is evidence of surgically amenable collection or deterioration in general condition.

Summary

In summary, where a GI anastomosis has been carried out, and the patient appears not to be progressing as expected, has excessive fluid requirement, tachycardia or fever and unexplained or rising lactic acidosis, always suspect a leak until proven otherwise. Failure to show anastomotic contents leakage in the drains is not sufficient to rule out a leak. The patient should be considered for re-operation. Gaining control of the leak by exteriorization through drains or a diverting stoma is essential. Routine re-laparotomy is not advocated, but rather is a selective approach. Careful attention to all aspects and especially nutrition is key to the successful management of these patients.

Further reading

Crandall M, West MA. Evaluation of the abdomen in the critically ill patient: opening the black box. *Curr Opin Crit Care* 2006; 12: 333–9.

Evenson AR, Fischer JE. Evenson AR, *et al.* Current management of enterocutaneous fistula. *J Gastrointest Surg* 2006; 10: 455–64.

Frileux P, Attal E, Sarkis R, *et al.* Anastomic dehiscence and severe peritonitis. *Infection* 1999; 27: 67–70.

Fujii Y, Shimada H, Endo I, *et al.* Management of massive arterial hemorrhage after pancreatobiliary surgery: does embolotherapy contribute to successful outcome? *J Gastrointest Surg* 2007; 11: 432–8.

Hutchins RR, Gunning MP, Lucas DN, *et al.* Relaparotomy for suspected intraperitoneal sepsis after abdominal surgery. *World J Surg* 2004; 28: 137–41.

Lamme B, Boermeester MA, Belt EJ, *et al.* Mortality and morbidity of planned relaparotomy versus relaparotomy on demand for secondary peritonitis. *Br J Surg* 2004; 91: 1046–54.

van Ruler O, Lamme B, Gouma DJ, *et al.* Variables associated with positive findings at relaparotomy in patients with secondary peritonitis. *Crit Care Med* 2007; 35: 468–76.

The medical patient with surgical problems

In medical patients the incidence of a GI problem complicating an ITU admission is thought to be between 1 and 7%. This also applies to patients admitted following a non-abdominal major operation such as cardiac bypass or neurological surgery. The mortality hazard predicted by the admission severity risk scores is increased, and an abdominal complication is a substantial contributor to ITU mortality. Delays in diagnosis and surgical referral contribute to a deleterious outcome. High clinical suspicion and early reporting of abdominal signs or unaccountable deterioration in physiological parameters are fundamental to management of the critically ill patient in the ITU.

The background reason for admission, e.g. diabetic complication, respiratory failure, cardiovascular disease or treatment-related neutropenia, may determine the type of surgical problem that follows. Complications include GI bleed, perforation, cholecystitis, pancreatitis and intestinal ischaemia, the mortality for the latter being close to 100%.

Severe metabolic derangement such as uraemia and use of mechanical ventiliation and pressors quickly lead to erosive changes in the intestinal and gastric mucosa. Such patients are especially prone to GI haemorrhage and should have pharmacological prophylaxis. The bleeding is likely to be upper GI rather than lower GI, with a 2:1 ratio. Fresh red blood or blood clots passed rectally can be either a lower GI tract bleed or a brisk upper GI tract bleed. Melaena can only come from the upper GI tract (proximal to the ligament of Treitz) where the blood has been exposed to enzymic and acid action. The patient should be resuscitated, commenced on acid blockade and an upper GI endoscopy carried out. Bleeding from a gastric or duodenal ulcer may be seen and treated via the endoscope by injection. A more florid picture of a bleeding pan-gastritis is sometimes seen in the uraemic patient, and no local therapy is effective. For bleeding lesions not controlled by endoscopic means, the alternatives lie with surgery or with radiological embolization. The extensive blood supply of the stomach sometimes makes control of gastric bleeding by radiological embolization difficult. More difficult diagnoses such as gastro-oesophageal varices or a DieuLafoy abnormality obviously require the appropriate specialist input, as will unexpected findings such as a clinically occult cancer. Bleeding from the small intestine is very difficult to diagnose, and radiology by either CT or visceral angiography is often helpful here if it is active bleeding. Low volume bleeding might require deployment of wireless capsule endoscopy. Diverticular disease and the colitides cause bleeding from the colon, and the former usually presents with a substantial bleed of fresh blood that usually settles and does not re-bleed. Pancolitis tends to have a picture of small amounts of blood clot mixed with mucus, and is more difficult to settle. Colonoscopy should be considered and surgery for colectomy might be required.

Neutropenic colitis, a syndrome of non-specific nausea, abdominal swelling and pain, is seen ~7 days after administration of cytotoxic chemotherapy. Bleeding is not a feature. Fever may be absent and blood count shows leucopenia and a neutrophil count typically below 1.5×10^9/l. This problem is seen in patients having high dose chemotherapy such as for haematological malignancy, and is less common in chemotherapy for solid tumours. The chemistry shows a rising lactate and, in severe cases, liver and renal dysfunction. The colon is very soft, and instrumentation should be avoided as it may cause bacteraemia, haemorrhage or perforation. CT examination is most helpful in the diagnosis, and shows large bowel dilatation, bowel wall thickening and sometimes pneumotosis. Any part of the colon can be involved, but more typically the right colon and terminal ileum. Treatment is supportive with fluids and antibiosis, and surgery is rarely helpful. Early introduction of G-CSF to hasten haemopoietic cell recovery can be helpful. The patient may progress slowly to a palpable mass, but sometimes rapidly to a picture of sepsis and MOF. The differential diagnosis in these patients is usually between *Clostridium difficile* and CMV colitis.

Rare causes of abdominal pain such as porphyria cause great diagnostic difficulty, and the nature of the disease is such that occasionally these will surface on the ITU perhaps masquerading as an acute epileptic fit.

Spontaneous retroperitoneal haematoma in the anticoagulated patient is a rare but potentially life-threatening event for the patient in the ITU. The initial event is a fall in the haemoglobin, but compartment syndrome caused by the expansion of the haematoma and complications thereof require radiological evaluation and sometimes intervention. Radiological drainage is likely not to be effective, and open retroperitoneal drainage might be required. However, this tends to be a high morbidity procedure and potentially contaminates a sterile field, resulting in retroperitoneal abscess formation.

Obstructions

Acute colonic pseudo-obstruction (Ogilvie's syndrome) is seen in the chronically hospitalized or seriously ill patient. Spinal surgery and retroperitoneal bleeding or other space-occupying lesions are recognized causes. The syndrome consists of massive colonic dilatation in the absence of a mechanical obstruction, and is probably due to autonomic failure. The abdomen is distended and bowel sounds are tinkling. Imaging shows a massive dilatation of the colon with preservation of haustral markings and a thin wall, in contradistinction from dilatation of colitis. Unprepared enema with gastrograffin should be carried out to rule out a mechanical problem and is on its own sometimes therapeutic in relieving the problem. Ischaemia or spontaneous perforations occur in ~3% of cases, and in these the mortality is ~40%. Other causes of non-obstructed colonic dilatation such as *C. difficile* or CMV-related colitis should be excluded. Initial treatment consists of correction of electrolyte abnormalities, nasogastric aspiration and prokinetic therapy with erythromycin or sometimes neostigmine. Serial plain AXR is used to follow the patient, and a failure to settle on conservative therapies requires intervention; the patient should have decompression by colonoscopy. Repeat colonoscopy is required in some patients. Caecal dilatation of >10cm carries a risk of perforation, and surgery might be required if decompressive colonoscopy has failed.

True mechanical obstructions in the ITU patient are not common. Previously undetected pathology such as a bowel tumour or complications of existing disease such as diverticulitis or intestinal adhesions are the common causes. In the elderly patient, one should be aware of incarceration of hernia, and the groin and surgical wounds should be inspected carefully.

After initial conservative treatment, the solution usually lies with surgical intervention, the exact nature of which will depend on the site of obstruction. The more recent advent of colonic stents can avoid operation in some colon obstructions involving the left colon, but are more difficult to place in the more proximal colon. Definitive surgical solution is usually required at some time.

Ischaemia of the bowel

A secondary ischaemic event such as mesenteric infarction by occlusion of the visceral vessels as either a thrombotic or embolic event may occur. Cardiac, autoimmune and oncological diagnoses predispose to this complication. Conditions that cause splanchnic hypoperfusion such as mechanical ventilation or use of vasopressors may be complicated by non-occlusive ischaemia. Erosions can be detected in ITU patients 24h from admission, suggesting that stress-related mucosal ischaemia is an early event.

The mortality from ischaemic bowel complicating the ITU admission is high, ~60–70%. The patient usually presents with intense pain which appears to be out of proportion to the clinical signs in the abdomen. The abdomen is often diffusely distended with a doughy feel. The lactate is elevated and rises progressively, the abdominal signs of peritonitis become more obvious and extensive necrosis is present, and usually by this stage the patient is extremely ill and beyond the point of surgical salvage. Early diagnosis is difficult. CT may be helpful in showing wall thickening, lack of enhancement in the bowel wall, pneumotosis and possibly portal venous gas. Early surgical consultation should be sought. Failure to settle and a rising lactate should initiate further investigation by consideration of laparotomy or laparoscopy to examine the abdominal contents. In the past, we have favoured bedside laparoscopy, to avoid moving a potentially unstable patient, and transfer to theatre only for those few with ischaemic gut thought suitable for surgical salvage.

Acalculous cholecystitis (ACC)

ACC occurs with an incidence of 1% in the ITU patient. The aetiology may relate to end-organ perfusion. The clinical picture is of right upper quadrant pain and inflammation. The initial management is with antibiotics and then surgery if there is a failure of rapid resolution. In the unstable patient, percutaneous drainage should be carried out. While cholecystitis can be seen on CT scan, interrogation of the biliary system is often better with ultrasound and has the advantage of being available at the ITU bedside, obviating transfer to the radiology department of a sick patient.

Gall stone ileus

A rare cause of intestinal obstruction is a rare complication of a common enough condition. Gallstone ileus is occasionally seen in elderly patients. Following an attack of acute cholecystitis, a large (>2cm, <5cm) stone from within the gallbladder erodes through the gallbladder and into the adjacent gut (1% of cases of acute cholecystitis in the elderly), usually the duodenum, leaving a cholecystoduodenal fistula. Progess of the stone through the intestinal tract eventually leads to lodgement of the stone in the narrow terminal ileum, classically 60cm from the ileocaecal valve, and small bowel obstruction follows. Occasionally a very large stone may give rise to Bouvret's syndrome where the large stone lodges in the duodenum and causes a gastric outlet obstruction.

Classically imaging reveals Rigler's triad of intestinal obstruction, ectopic gallstone and pneumobilia; sometimes air can be seen in the gallbladder. Surgery is always required to salvage the situation.

Intra-abdominal hypertension

Primary raised IAP may occur because of an intra-abdominal pathology or be secondary to a non-abdominal event such as a major burn injury. Elevation of the IAP has adverse effects on pulmonary, cardiovascular, renal, splanchnic and neurological physiology.

The mortality varies from 10 to 60%. IAH can be said to exist when the normal IAP of ~7mm Hg is exceeded. A pressure >20mm Hg and with new organ failure is termed abdominal compartment syndrome.

An increase in abdominal pressure >15mm Hg reduces the pulmonary capacity, functional residual capacity and volume. Hypoventilation and increased PVR lead to hypoxia, hypercapnia and increased ventilatory pressue.

Similarly, reduction in venous return from compression of the IVC and portal vein results in a down and right shift of the Starling curve. Renal tamponade causes a reduction in renal blood flow at ~15mm Hg and results in anuria at an IAP >30mm Hg. Reductions in the splanchnic blood flow and reduction in liver and gut blood flow contribute to mucosal acidosis and breakdown of bacterial integrity. The increased intrathoracic and central venous pressure leads to rises in the ICP.

Intervention to relieve the pressure is required somewhere between an IAP of 20 and 25mm Hg. If intervention is early, the effects are reversible, but prolonged abdominal compartment syndrome leads to irreversible MOF regardless of decompression.

Decompression of the abdomen by laparostomy is carried out, and the open abdomen managed by covering with a clear non-adherent plastic sheet or by a vacuum dressing to aid collection of the exudates and promote tissue perfusion. Fluid losses after decompression to an open abdomen can be great, and require careful monitoring.

Soft tissue infections

Necrotizing fasciitis is a serious and potentially life-threatening infection more common in the severely ill patient. Predisposing factors include, peripheral vascular disease, liver disease, renal disease, malignancy, immunocompromise, diabetes, perianal sepsis, chronic skin disease and skin trauma, even of a minor nature. Classification is into three groups depending on the organisms involved. Type 1 results from a mixed aerobic and anaerobic flora found in sites of surgical trauma and in the perineum, typically group A β-haemolytic streptococci, *S. aureus*, *E. coli*, *Bacteroides* spp, *Pseudomonas* sp. and *Clostridia* spp. Type 2 is found typically in the extremities and ia infected with group A β-haemolytic streptococci and *S. aureus*. Type 3 is asscociated with *Vibrio vulnificus* and is caused by skin puncture from marine insects and fish.

Fournier's gangrene is a particular type 1 necrotizing fasciitis affecting the perineum and caused by perianal conditions or involving the genitourinary tract.

Mortality can be 20–50%, and is greatest in the elderly, obese, diabetic or immunocompromised patients.

The pathogenesis is by implantation of bacteria possibly from a remote site such as a Bartholin's cyst or an anocutaneous fistula into the subcutaneous tissue. Subsequent proliferation and release of bacterial toxins causes thrombosis of the microvasculature, lysis and necrosis of the subcutaneous tissues.

The clinical course is rapid and begins with painful oedema and erythema of the skin. There may be systemic disturbance ranging from flu-like illness to toxic shock syndrome in rapidly progressing patients. The local changes progress to bullae, and the skin colour changes from red to purple and then black. Crepitations might be felt if gas-forming organisms are present. A fulminant case may show spread of necrosis over a matter of hours, and so repeated clinical examination every few hours is essential.

Early recognition and initiation of treatment is essential. IV antibiotics should be commenced. If necrosis is evident then aggressive surgical debridement will be required, often serially.

If the patient survives, reconstruction by tissue flaps or skin graft might be required.

Further reading

Achyra PS, Lipson DA. Gastrointestinal complications of acute respiratory failure. *Clin PulmonMed* 2003; 10: 80–4.

Anaya DA, Dellinger EP. Necrotizing soft-tissue infection: diagnosis and management. *Clin Infect Dis* 2007; 44: 705–10.

Cheatham ML, Malbrain ML, Kirkpatrick A, *et al.* Results from the International Conference of Experts on Intra-abdominal Hypertension and Abdominal Compartment Syndrome. II. Recommendations. *Intensive Care Med* 2007; 33: 951–62.

Chou JW, Hsu CH, Liao KF, *et al.* Gallstone ileus: report of two cases and review of the literature. *World J Gastroenterol* 2007; 13: 1295–8.

De Waele JJ, Hoste EA, Malbrain ML. Decompressive laparotomy for abdominal compartment syndrome—a critical analysis. *Crit Care* 2006; 10: R51.

Edelman DA, Sugawa C. Lower gastrointestinal bleeding: a review. *Surg Endosc* 2007; 21: 514–20.

Fazel A, Verne GN. New solutions to an old problem: acute colonic pseudo-obstruction. *J Clin Gastroenterol* 2005; 39: 17–20.

Filsoufi F, Rahmanian PB, Castillo JG, *et al.* Predictors and outcome of gastrointestinal complications in patients undergoing cardiac surgery. *Ann Surg* 2007; 246: 323–9.

Masannat Y, Masannat Y, Shatnawei A. Gallstone ileus: a review. *Mt Sinai J Med* 2006; 73: 1132–4.

Salcido RS. Necrotizing fasciitis: reviewing the causes and treatment strategies. *Adv Skin Wound Care* 2007; 20: 288–93.

Saunders MD. Acute colonic pseudo-obstruction. *Gastrointest Endosc Clin N Am* 2007; 17: 341–60, vi–vii.

Williams N, Scott AD. Neutropenic colitis: a continuing surgical challenge. *Br J Surg* 1997; 84: 1200–5.

Chapter 31

Obstetric emergencies

Chapter contents

Pre-eclampsia

Pre-eclampsia is a common complication of pregnancy, UK incidence is 3–5%, with a complex hereditary, immunological and environmental aetiology.

Pathophysiology

Abnormal placentation is characterized by impaired myometrial spiral artery relaxation, failure of trophoblastic invasion of these arterial walls and blockage of some vessels with fibrin, platelets and lipid-laden macrophages. There is a 30–40%, reduction in placental perfusion by the uterine arcuate arteries as seen by Doppler studies at 18–24 weeks gestation. Ultimately the shrunken, calcified, and microembolized placenta typical of the disease is seen. The placental lesion is responsible for fetal growth retardation and increased risks of premature labour, abruption and fetal demise. Maternal systemic features of this condition are characterized by widespread endothelial damage, affecting the peripheral, renal, hepatic, cerebral, and pulmonary vasculatures. These manifest clinically as hypertension, proteinuria and peripheral oedema, and in severe cases as eclamptic convulsions, cerebral haemorrhage (the most common cause of death due to pre-eclampsia in the UK), pulmonary oedema, hepatic infarcts and haemorrhage, coagulopathy and renal dysfunction.

Risk factors include:

1 positive family history
2 pre-eclampsia in a previous pregnancy with the same partner
3 conditions associated with large placental mass, including obesity, diabetes, multiple pregnancy and hydatidiform mole.

Severe pre-eclampsia is defined by the degree of hypertension and proteinuria, and by the presence of epigastric pain, headache, visual disturbance, severe oliguria, convulsions, pulmonary oedema and HELLP syndrome. Precise criteria for severe pre-eclampsia vary between units, but most are based on the definitions of Davey and MacGillivray. Those shown below are used in the Yorkshire Pre-eclampsia protocol, and are widely accepted.

Clinical features

Rare before 20 weeks gestation, but early onset indicates poor prognosis. It is more common in young women, primiparas and women of poor socioeconomic background. It is vital to identify severe disease (mild disease does not indicate specific treatment), and failure to monitor adequately or to appreciate the significance of the symptoms of severe disease are consistent features of substandard care with its consequences.

History and examination: key points

Diagnostic criteria of severe preeclampsia are:

- Eclampsia
- Severe hypertension. SBP >170mm Hg or DBP >110mm Hg from 3 readings over 15min, with at least 1+ of proteinuria.
- Moderate hypertension. SBP >140mm Hg or DBP >90mm Hg from 3 readings over 45min, with at least 2+ of proteinuria.
- Plus any of the following: headache, epigastric pain, visual disturbance, clonus, papilloedema, liver tenderness, platelets <100 x 10^9/l, ALT >50IU/l.

Special investigations

- Haematology. Pre-eclampsia induces a hypercoagulable state, but can also cause thrombocytopaenia and coagulopathy. In mild disease, the FBC is normal. A platelet count <100 x 10^9/l is an indicator of severe disease, and should trigger full coagulation studies. The rate of decline of platelet count is more important than the absolute figure, with a rapid decline indicating aggressive disease. If anaemia is noted, tests for haemolysis should be performed and HELLP syndrome excluded.
- Biochemistry. GFR and renal perfusion both decline in pre-eclampsia, and mild elevations in urea and creatinine may be seen, but serious renal dysfunction is rare unless a second insult occurs, such as haemorrhage. If oliguric, it is important to monitor biochemistry, especially serum potassium. Obstetricians traditionally monitor serum urate levels as a marker of disease severity, but this is of no therapeutic relevance for anaesthetists. LFTs should be monitored for signs of HELLP syndrome.
- Radiology. Rarely indicated, but a CXR may be necessary if pulmonary oedema is suspected through hypoxia or crepitations. Neurological deficit after convulsions should raise the suspicion of cerebral haemorrhage. If a patient is intubated and ventilated after a convulsion, return of normal neurology cannot be clinically confirmed and CT scanning should be considered.
- Fetal studies. Cardiotocography, fetal growth, liquor volume and umbilical artery Doppler studies are all used to monitor fetal well-being. These will determine fetal indications for early delivery.

Management

Mild disease does not require specific treatment, but the mother and fetus should be regularly monitored for signs of severe disease. If there are signs of severe disease, the patient should be monitored in a high dependency setting with regular, 15min, blood pressure measurement till stabilized and then hourly. Fluid balance should be meticulously recorded, with urine output measured with an in-dwelling catheter. Proteinuria should be assessed hourly. Continuous oxygen saturation and hourly respiratory rate should be instituted to monitor for signs of pulmonary oedema. Central venous and pulmonary artery pressure monitoring are not required except possibly after significant haemorrhage, persistent pulmonary oedema or during ventilation on intensive care. Specific therapies include the following.

Antihypertensive therapy

The immediate goal is to treat extremes of systolic pressure, since it is most likely that shearing forces during systole are the precipitant for cerebral haemorrhage. There is no clear safe maximum pressure, but 160mm Hg has been suggested. There is also no clear evidence indicating the best antihypertensive regimen, and local familiarity and experience is probably more important than which drug is used. One example regimen is:

- Labetolol is a suitable first-line therapy, beginning with the oral route if tolerated. Initial administration of two doses of 200mg 1h apart is often effective. If not, or if the oral route cannot be tolerated, IV therapy should be instituted with a bolus of 50mg over 1min, repeated as necessary to a maximum of 200mg. This should be followed with a continuous infusion of 20–160mg/h as required.

- If labetolol cannot be tolerated because of asthma or bradycardia, or if labetolol has failed to control the hypertension, nifedipine 10mg 6 hourly is a suitable second-line agent.
- Ventilated patients will benefit from the hypotensive effects of sedative agents, sometimes obviating the need for specific hypotensive therapy. Rebound hypertension should be anticipated and prevented during weaning.

Fluid management

Here is the key: oliguria in pre-eclampsia can be due to volume depletion (pre-renal), glomerular capillary endotheliosis (renal) or a combination of the two. In the absence of a secondary pre-renal insult such as haemorrhage, the renal lesion is completely reversible and is not incipient acute tubular necrosis. In addition to this, severe pre-eclampsia damages the pulmonary capillary endothelium, lowering the pressure threshold for pulmonary oedema. These points mean that aggressive fluid therapy is both unnecessary and dangerous. Indeed, it is not long since pulmonary oedema (with a significant iatrogenic component) was the leading cause of death in pre-eclampsia in the UK

Women with severe pre-eclampsia in Yorkshire receive 80ml/h total fluids (plus replacement of extra losses through bleeding, vomiting, etc.) and a urine output of down to 80ml over 4h is tolerated. Cautious fluid challenges are used, and in some cases diuretics are used to restore urine output. This approach is contrary to the typical management of critical care patients with multi-system disease, but has reduced the incidence of pulmonary oedema and critical care admissions, without any concurrent rise in renal problems. However, few data or experience exist regarding fluid management in ventilated pre-eclamptic patients. If should be born in mind that if higher vascular filling pressures are used to improve renal perfusion during IPPV, pulmonary oedema can occur after extubation. In summary, the ventilated patient should have cautious fluid management, and typical critical care targets for CVP and urine output should be not be used.

Magnesium sulfate therapy

This should be considered for all women with severe pre-eclampsia as prophylaxis against eclampsia. It should be delivered as a loading dose, followed by an infusion for 24h, or until 24h after delivery, whichever comes first. The regimen consists of:

- Loading dose of 5g over 25min
- Continuous infusion of 1g/h

As deep tendon reflexes are abolished before magnesium levels reach cardiotoxic levels, blood level monitoring is not necessary with this regimen unless a patient is paralysed. If urine output falls below 100ml in 4h, levels can rise rapidly. In this situation, magnesium should be stopped until the urine output is restored. If signs of toxicity occur (loss of reflexes, respiratory weakness, dysrrhythmia), the antidote to magnesium is 10ml of calcium gluconate.

Thromboprophylaxis

Because of the hypercoaguable state induced by pre-eclampsia, LMWH, e.g. 40mg clexane, should be administered daily. Appropriate timing of regional anaesthesia and removal of epidural catheters must therefore be born in mind.

Timing and mode of delivery

The only indication for immediate delivery is severe fetal distress or abruption. In the presence of maternal indications for early delivery, such as severe hypertension or eclamptic convulsion, it is desirable to stabilize the woman's condition before delivery with antihypertensive therapy and magnesium. This may also allow enough time for steroids to be administered to assist fetal lung maturation. Before 32 weeks gestation, Caesarean delivery is indicated, but after 34 weeks vaginal delivery is considered. After delivery, uterotonic agents containing ergometrine should not be used, as these can exacerbate hypertension.

Anaesthetic care

Once coagulopathy has been excluded, regional analgesia and anaesthesia are appropriate techniques. Fluid preloading is inappropriate because of the risk of relative hypervolaemia and pulmonary oedema as regional blockade recedes. Pre-eclamptic women are resistant to the hypotensive effects of regional anaesthesia, so spinal anaesthesia is safe and vasoconstrictor requirements are usually reduced. If general anaesthesia or intubation are required, steps to prevent pressor responses should be employed. Bolus alfentanil of remifentanil infusion are suitable techniques. Post-operative recovery should take place in a high dependency setting.

Further reading

Clark VA, Sharwood-Smith GH, Stewart AVG. Ephedine requirements are reduced during spinal anaesthesia for caesarean section in preeclampsia. *Int J Obstet Anesth* 2005; 14: 9-13.

Davey DA, MacGillivray I. The classification and definition of hypertensive disorders of pregnancy. *Am J Obstet Gynecol* 1988; 158: 892–8.

Duley L, Hendrson-Smart DJ, Meher S. Drugs for treatment of very high blood pressure during pregnancy. *Cochrane Database Syst Rev* 2006; (3): CD001449.

Magpie Collaborative Group. Do women with pre-eclampsia and their babies benefit from magnesium sulphate? *Lancet* 2002; 359: 1877–90.

Why Mothers Die 2000–2002. Report on confidential enquiries into maternal deaths in the United Kingdom. www.cemach.org.uk

Why Mothers Die 1994–1996. Report on confidential enquiries into maternal deaths in the United Kingdom. www.cemach.org.uk

Eclampsia

Eclampsia is seizure activity in a pregnant or peripartum woman with pre-eclampsia, where no evidence of other cerebral conditions exists. It is more common in developing nations. UK incidence is 1 case per 2500 maternities, with a mortality of 1.8% (survey, performed by the British Eclampsia Survey Team), i.e. 1–2% of women with pre-eclampsia. Prophylactic magnesium sulfate therapy has become standard practice in severe pre-eclampsia, so the incidence of eclampsia may have fallen in the UK, but as 41% of cases of eclampsia in the survey presented before the diagnosis of pre-eclampsia had been made, magnesium prophylaxis will never abolish eclampsia completely.

The pathophysiology of eclamptic convulsions is unclear. Ischaemia, haemorrhage, infarct and oedema have all been identified by imaging and autopsy, and cerebrovascular endothelial damage is postulated to be the underlying pathology. The hydrostatic effects of hypertension may play a part, but many victims of eclampsia have only moderate hypertension before convulsing.

Teenage women are 3 times more likely to suffer eclampsia than their older counterparts, and multiple pregnancy increases the risk 6-fold.

Clinical features

Premonitory signs: headache, visual disturbance, followed by epigastric pain. Around 40% of cases will present without warning symptoms, and before hypertension and proteinuria are identified.

Presentation: Convulsions occur antenatally in 38%, intrapartum in 18% and postnatally in 44%. In 12% of postnatal cases, the convulsion occurred >48h after delivery. Convulsions usually last for 1–2min and are self-limiting, but a second convulsion can occur within minutes.

History and examination

Eclampsia can occur with no previous indicators of pre-eclampsia. After a convulsion, it is important to question relatives about any history of neurological disease and of the occurrence of symptoms of severe pre-eclampsia. Neurological examination should be performed at the earliest opportunity to exclude signs of cerebral haemorrhage, and regular monitoring for hypertension, proteinuria and pulmonary oedema should begin.

Special investigations

- The same haematological and biochemical tests used in severe pre-eclampsia should be performed.
- Radiology. A CT scan may be indicated to exclude cerebral haemorrhage. This should be suspected if focal neurological signs are found or if persistent unconsciousness follows a convulsion.
- Fetal studies. Continuous cardiotocography should be instituted in antenatal women.

Management of eclampsia

General

- maintenance of a clear airway
- ensuring adequate oxygenation
- protection against aspiration

Magnesium sufate; loading dose 4–6g over 20min amd infusion at 1–3g/h.

Terminating convulsions. Most eclamptic convulsions last <2min and are followed by a typical post-ictal phase, during which normal gross neurology can be confirmed, allaying fears of cerebral haemorrhage. Avoid general anaesthesia, where possible. Good conservative airway management in a lateral position and oxygen via face mask whilst awaiting rapid spontaneous resolution of the convulsion is ideal. Sedation and paralysis, which may be necessary, preclude this assessment, forcing clinicians to use imaging to exclude cerebral haemorrhage.

Anticonvulsant therapy

Magnesium sulfate is the most effective and safe therapy for eclampsia. Its role in reducing the incidence of re-convulsion is clear, but its value as an acute anticonvulsant is debatable. Most eclamptic convulsions have stopped spontaneously before the magnesium loading dose is given. In the presence of persistent or multiple convulsions, it is reasonable to add an easily titrated benzodiazepine such as midazolam. A second fit despite magnesium should prompt an increase of the infusion to 1.5g/h. If fits still persist or the airway and oxygenation cannot be adequately maintained, intubation and ventilation are justified.

Other therapies

Antihypertensive agents and fluid management should be instituted as for any woman with severe pre-eclampsia. Haematological and biochemical investigations should be performed to monitor for other features of severe pre-eclampsia and HELLP. Prior to delivery, fetal monitoring should be instituted immediately from the time of convulsion to monitor for signs of fetal distress.

Delivery

Fetal distress is common during a convulsion, and this may necessitate immediate operative delivery under general anaesthesia. However, if the fetal condition is acceptable, it may be possible to institute magnesium and antihypertensive therapy before delivery. Platelet and coagulation tests should be performed before regional anaesthesia is used.

Further reading

Douglas KA, Redman CWG. Eclampsia in the United Kingdom. *BMJ* 1994; 309: 1395–400.

Duly L. Which anticonvulsant for women with eclampsia? Evidence from the Collaborative eclampsia trial. *Lancet* 1995; 345: 1455–63.

HELLP syndrome

HELLP stands for **H**aemolysis, **E**levated **L**iver enzymes, and **L**ow **P**latelets, and is a severe variant of pre-eclampsia peculiar to humans. It occurs in ~20% of cases of severe pre-eclampsia, with a mortality of 1–3.5%. Its insidious presentation and potential for sudden exacerbation frequently catches clinicians unaware, and its management requires rapid, multidisciplinary input. 80% of cases present before term, but 1/3 of cases are identified after delivery. Premature delivery contributes to the very high perinatal mortality associated with HELLP syndrome.

Clinical features

While only 10% of cases present before 27 weeks, most do so before 36 weeks gestation. Symptoms and signs are common but non-specific, and do not fit the usual pattern of severe pre-eclampsia. In addition to this, hypertension and proteinuria are not necessarily severe. There is therefore great potential for diagnostic delay while simple malaise rapidly progresses to anaemia, coagulopathy and hepatorenal failure. There is also considerable risk of iatrogenic problems, largely through fluid overload during the treatment of haemolysis, thrombocytopaenia, coagulopathy and haemorrhage. As a final insult, recovery after delivery is much more protracted than simple pre-eclampsia, and indeed the condition may worsen for the first 48h. For example, women with a platelet count $<50 \times 10^9$/l may take 11 days to achieve a count $>100 \times 10^9$/l.

Of all pre-eclamptic patients, HELLP syndrome women are the most likely to require critical care, including renal support and possibly ventilation.

History and examination

- Symptoms: malaise (90%), epigastric pain (90%), nausea and vomiting (50%), and flu-like symptoms.
- Signs: right upper quadrant tenderness (80%), weight gain and peripheral oedema (60%). Hypertension and proteinuria may be mild or even absent.

Special investigations

There is disagreement over the specific haematological and biochemical criteria for the diagnosis of HELLP, but trends are more important than absolute figures.

- Haematology. Haemolysis can be identified with a blood smear, rising LDH and rising total bilirubin. A platelet count $<100 \times 10^9$/l is an agreed diagnostic criterion of HELLP. As liver function deteriorates, coagulation tests will also become abnormal. All haematological problems can be exacerbated by haemorrhage and dilution with IV fluids.
- Biochemistry. The levels of AST and ALT used to define raised liver enzymes vary widely between authors. Local laboratory normal values and trends should therefore be used. Serum albumin will also fall, especially in cases complicated by haemorrhage and multi-system failure.

Management

General

High dependency care and regular fetal monitoring are required once HELLP syndrome is diagnosed. Deterioration should be anticipated, and in advanced pregnancy it is advisable to proceed to early delivery before serious coagulopathy develops. In early pregnancy, risks to the neonate are obviously much increased by delivery, so sympathetic counselling is vital for both partners.

Glucocorticosteroids

Observations that glucocorticoids, given to stimulate maturation of the fetal lungs, were associated with improvement of some of the markers of HELLP syndrome, led to several clinical trials and a Cochrane Review. Whilst no clear improvements in maternal and perinatal mortality were found, higher platelet count, reduced hospital stay and higher birth weight followed steroid therapy. Prednisolone has limited placental transfer, so for benefits to mother and fetus, dexamethasone or betamethasone should be used.

Fluid management

Renal function is precarious, with the renal lesion of pre-eclampsia compounded by hepatic disease, third space losses and a high incidence of haemorrhage. However, pulmonary oedema is also commonly associated with HELLP. Careful fluid balance is therefore essential, but it can be easily derailed by the combination of haematological deficits and haemorrhage. Fluid overload may necessitate early dialysis if pulmonary oedema is to be averted, because the kidneys may not respond adequately to diuretics. In antenatal women, pulmonary oedema can precipitate the need for urgent Caesarean delivery in the face of coagulopathy, and a spiral of decline from massive haemorrhage to multi-system failure.

Key points

- Symptoms and signs are non-specific, so diagnosis depends on close attention and a low threshold for further investigation.
- Anticipate and plan for exacerbation to hepatorenal failure, haemorrhage and pulmonary oedema.
- The early input of senior haematology, critical care and renal support clinicians is vital.

Further reading

Martin JN Jr, Blake PE, Lowry SI, *et al.* Pregnancy complicated by preeclampsia–eclampsia with the syndrome of hemolysis, elevated liver enzymes, and low platelet count: How rapid is postpartum recovery? *Obstet Gynecol* 1990; 76: 737–41.

Matchaba P, Moodley J. Corticosteroids for HELLP syndrome in pregnancy. *Cochrane Database Syst Rev* 2004: (1): CD002076.

Sibai BM, Mabie BC, Harvey CJ, *et al.* Pulmonary edema in severe preeclampsia–eclampsia: analysis of thirty-seven consecutive cases. *Am J Obstet Gynecol* 1987; 156: 1174–9.

Sibai BM, Ramadan MK, Usta I, *et al.* Maternal morbidity and mortality in 442 pregnancies with haemolysis, elevated liver enzymes, and low platelets (HELLP syndrome). *Am J Obstet Gynecol* 1993; 169: 1000–6.

Postpartum haemorrhage

Major obstetric haemorrhage remains a leading cause of significant maternal morbidity and mortality. The latest Confidential Enquiry into Maternal and Child Health (CEMCH) revealed it to be the 2nd most common cause of direct maternal death, with a mortality rate of 8.5/1 000 000 maternities (17 deaths in total). This is a >2-fold increase from previous reports, the largest increase occurring in deaths from postpartum haemorrhage (PPH). PPH complicates 5% of deliveries.

Classification

1. Primary PPH. This is blood loss of >500ml from the genital tract within 24h of childbirth. Causes are discussed below.
2. Secondary PPH. This is abnormal bleeding between 24h and 6 weeks postpartum, usually due to retained products of conception and/or infection.

Causes

Uterine atony

- Most common cause of PPH.
- Risk factors include previous history of PPH, large placental site (e.g. multiple pregnancy), long or precipitous labour, prolonged oxytocin administration, grand multi-parity, macrosomia, polyhydramnios, retained products, inverted or ruptured uterus, drugs (volatile anaesthetics, tocolytics).
- Not excluded by absence of bleeding per vaginum as the atonic uterus may accommodate >1l of blood.
- Incidence reduced by prophylactic administration of oxytocic agents at delivery.

Retained tissue

- Retained products of conception, placental tissue or membranes.
- Cause bleeding themselves and uterine atony.

Trauma

- May arise anywhere in the genital tract.
- Includes lacerations in the perineum, vagina, cervix or uterus following vaginal or operative delivery.

Coagulopathy

- May be a cause or complication of PPH
- May be pre-existing or develop in pregnancy due to massive blood transfusion, HELLP, drugs or DIC (e.g. placental abruption, pre-eclampsia, amniotic fluid embolism (AFE), prolonged intrauterine death, massive transfusion).

Clinical approach

Blood loss is difficult to assess accurately and is commonly underestimated. It may be partially or completely concealed or a slow persistent trickle, which may go unnoticed for some time.

- Pregnant woman tolerate blood loss very well. They are usually young, fit and healthy, and the physiological changes of pregnancy mean that several litres of blood may be lost before the classical signs of hypovolaemia develop. Hypotension is a late and ominous sign.
- Uterine blood flow at term of 20% cardiac output gives rise to potential for massive blood loss. What appears to be initially inconsequential bleeding may progress rapidly to major life-threatening haemorrhage that proves difficult to correct.
- May follow antepartum haemorrhage (APH), especially placental abruption or praevia. In these circumstances, it is often poorly tolerated, especially if the degree of APH has been underestimated and the woman inadequately resuscitated.

Management

Early recognition of bleeding and mobilization of the team

Multi-disciplinary team working and communication are vital in the management of PPH.

- Call essential personnel once recognized: on-call and consultant anaesthetist and obstetrician, senior midwifery staff, labour ward operating department practitioner and theatre staff from outside of labour ward (for 'extra hands' and to bring equipment such as rapid infusers and cell savers), porters (for transport of blood samples, blood and blood products), haematology and blood transfusion staff (for analysis of blood samples and rapid provision of blood and blood products) and consultant haematologist (for advice regarding appropriate blood and product replacement).

Resuscitation and restoration of circulating blood volume

Rapid and effective resuscitation, following the standard ABC (airway, breathing, circulation) approach.

- High flow oxygen through face mask to a patent airway. Intubate and ventilate if reduced level of consciousness.
- Insert at least 2 large bore IV cannulae (14–16G) and take bloods for baseline U&E, FBC, coagulation screen, group and cross-match (>6 units). Head-down tilt to aid venous return.
- Restore circulating blood volume with warmed crystalloid and colloids, given rapidly via a pressure device until blood products are indicated or available. Vasoconstrictors may be necessary to maintain an adequate blood pressure.
- Red blood cell transfusion indicated if several litres of crystalloid or colloid given, estimated blood loss >1.5l, Hb <7g/dl or blood loss very rapid. Rapid provision of group-specific blood aided by antenatal screening of blood group and abnormal antibodies.
- Emergency group O Rhesus negative red cells from delivery suite blood fridge in life-threatening, dire emergency or if patient's blood group not known.
- Give blood products sooner rather than later. Be guided by clinical situation and blood results, but do not allow these to delay their administration. Give 2 adult therapeutic doses of platelets and 4 units (15ml/kg) of FFP for each 6-unit red cell transfusion or if indicated by abnormal blood results (platelets <75 x 10^9/l in acutely bleeding patient, higher if known abnormal platelet function, clotting deranged 1.5 × control). Cryoprecipitate if fibrinogen <1g/l.
- Avoid hypothermia (fluid warmer, forced warm air device, high ambient temperature).

Appropriate monitoring

- Standard monitoring including pulse, blood pressure, ECG, oxygen saturation, respiratory rate, urine output and temperature.

- Early invasive monitoring (arterial and CVP) if haemodynamically unstable, but without delaying resuscitation and definitive treatment.
- If coagulopathy, consider ultrasound guidance or antecubital site for CVP line.
- Delegate someone to document observations, along with timings and interventions, such as drugs and fluid input and output.
- Consider need for HDU/ICU.

Control of haemorrhage—treat cause and resultant complications

Exclude uterine atony. If the uterus fails to contract adequately and bleeding continues, massage the uterus to stimulate contraction and consider bimanual uterine compression.

Oxytocic agents

Consider if uterine massage fails, but remember will be of no benefit if the haemorrhage is not due to atony, and may be harmful, as all have potentially serious side effects.

- Oxytocin (Syntocinon®). Synthetic analogue of oxytocin. Short half-life of 10min. Given as slow IV bolus of 5IU and/or by infusion (40IU in 500ml of normal saline over 4h). It causes vasodilatation, which is compensated for by large increases in cardiac output by healthy women. In the presence of hypovolaemia, compensation is prevented and fatal cardiovascular collapse can ensue.
- Ergometrine. Ergot alkaloid given as IV or IM injections of 125mcg up to 500mcg. Smooth muscle constrictor causing increased uterine tone, peripheral and pulmonary vasoconstriction, bronchospasm. Also severe nausea and vomiting. Avoid in pre-eclampsia, asthma and some cardiac conditions.
- Carboprost (Haemobate®). Synthetic prostaglandin analogue given as a deep IM injection, or intramyometrially (but not licensed for this), at a dose of 250mcg every 15min, up to a maximum of 2mg. It has potentially serious side effects including bronchospasm, pulmonary oedema, hypertension and increased intrapulmonary shunting with hypoxia.

Surgical interventions 'examination under anaesthesia'

- Empty the uterus. Remove placenta or retained products of conception. Aids uterine contraction too.
- Repair of genital tract injury.
- Uterine tamponade. Intrauterine balloon catheter (e.g. Rusch balloon), uterine packing.
- Laparotomy. Compression of aorta to allow catch up for resuscitation, uterine haemostatic suture (e.g. B-Lynch suture), arterial ligation, repair of bleeding post-lower segment Caesarean section, hysterectomy.

Radiological interventions

- High success rates reported for uterine artery embolization.
- May avoid need for hysterectomy and preserve fertility.
- Practical difficulties include need for appropriately trained staff, equipment and facilities, and transfer of unstable patient to isolated radiology suite

Antifibrinolytic agents

- Tranexamic acid (cyklokapron®) up to 0.5–1g IV bolus up to 3 times a day, or aprotonin (Trasylol®) up to 2 000 000U bolus followed by infusion 50-100 000U/h. License suspended 2007. CEM/CMO/2007/23.
- Both inhibit fibrinolysis by enzyme inhibition
- Limited case reports of successful use in obstetric haemorrhage
- Possible thromboembolism risk

Cell salvage techniques

- Traditional concerns of iatrogenic AFE minimized by use of specific suction systems and leucocyte depletion filter.
- Avoids complications associated with blood transfusion.
- Consider in presence of life-threatening PPH when the rate of blood loss greatly exceeds that at which homologous blood can be supplied, and in the Jehovah's witness population.

Recombinant factor VIIa (Novoseven®)

- Prohaemostatic agent promoting local thrombin generation at bleeding sites.
- Several case reports of its successful use 'off licence' in obstetric haemorrhage.
- Should be used in combination with replacement of deficient red blood cells, clotting factors, fibrinogen and platelets, and attention to general measures such as surgical haemostasis, avoiding hypothermia and acidaemia. (Cannot work without fibrinogen.)
- Uncertainties remain about appropriate dosing regimens (possibly 90–100mcg/kg), how to monitor its effects and potential complications (DIC or thromboembolism, especially in the presence of sepsis).

General vs regional anaesthesia

- Regional anaesthesia is usually the technique of choice in obstetric patients because of the well documented risks associated with general anaesthesia.
- An epidural top-up or single shot spinal is usually a safe and acceptable technique where PPH is not life-threatening and the mother is not severely hypovolaemic and/or coagulopathic. It may unmask hypovolaemia, due to the loss of compensatory vasoconstriction with the onset of sympathetic blockade, especially when blood loss has been underestimated.
- General anaesthesia may be the technique of choice in the presence of severe, continuing blood loss, haemodynamic instability, life-threatening maternal compromise, coagulopathy or anticipated prolonged or difficult surgery. Caution with volatile anaesthetics reducing uterine tone.
- Be prepared for major blood loss whatever the mode of anaesthesia.

Further reading

Department of Health. Confidential Enquiry into Maternal and Child Health. Why mothers die 2000–2. The sixth report of the confidential enquiries into maternal deaths in the UK. London RCOG Press, 2004.

Grady K, Howell C, Cox C. Managing obstetric emergencies and trauma. The MOET course manual, 2nd edn. London: RCOG Press, 2007.

Amniotic fluid embolism

Amniotic fluid embolism (AFE) is a rare condition, with incidence varying between 1 in 8000 and 1 in 80 000 pregnancies. This wide range reflects the difficulty in confirming its accurate diagnosis. Despite its rarity, AFE remains a leading cause of maternal morbidity and mortality. The latest CEMCH report revealed it to be the 8th most common cause of direct maternal death in the UK, with a mortality rate of 2.5/1 000 000 maternities (5 deaths). The number of maternal deaths due to AFE has fallen significantly over the last 3 triennia, largely attributable to improved intensive care management and recognition of milder cases.

All cases of suspected or proven AFE, whether fatal or not, should be reported to the UK Obstetric Surveillance System (UKOSS). This national registry aims to study the incidence, risk factors, management and outcomes of AFE in the UK. Nineteen cases of AFE were reported to UKOSS during 2000–2002, giving a 25% mortality rate. Previous registries from the UK, the USA and Australasia, which have provided much of our current knowledge about AFE, reported much higher mortality rates of up to 80%, with only 15% of patients surviving neurologically intact .

Risk factors

- Increasing maternal age.
- Overactivity of the uterus/overuse of oxytocic drugs.
- Short and tumultuous labour.
- Multiparity.
- Large fetus.
- Increased gestational age.
- Placental abruption.
- Intrauterine death.
- Uterine rupture.
- Trauma.

Association of these risk factors with AFE has been inconsistent. Many patients who develop AFE have no risk factors. The classical 'hypertonic' uterus may be the result of, rather than the precipitant of, AFE.

Clinical features

Classical 'triad'—hypoxia cardiovascular collapse coagulopathy—presenting during labour, delivery or 30min postpartum, with no other clinical condition to explain signs and symptoms. It has also been reported to occur during or after Caesarean section, amniocentesis, first and second trimester abortions, abdominal trauma, artificial rupture of membranes and up to 48h postpartum.

- Acute hypoxia. Causes may be pulmonary vasospasm, ventilation–perfusion mismatch, bronchospasm or pulmonary oedema. This may present as cyanosis, dyspnoea, wheezing or respiratory arrest.
- Acute cardiovascular collapse. Hypotension, dysrhythmias or cardiac arrest.
- Coagulopathy. If rapid onset and deterioration, DIC or clinical haemorrhage may not have time to develop.

Less common presentations include chest pain, seizures, confusion and acute fetal distress.

The latest CEMACH report highlighted premonitory signs and symptoms such as restlessness, abnormal behaviour and respiratory distress occurring before collapse and haemorrhage. Earlier suspicion of AFE may then permit earlier involvement of intensive care and an improved prognosis. Despite this, the most severe, fulminant end of the disease spectrum may prove rapidly fatal despite optimal management, many deaths occurring within an hour of presentation.

Diagnosis

Clinical

AFE exists as a spectrum of disease, ranging from a subclinical entity to a severe and rapidly fatal event. The initial diagnosis is usually made on clinical grounds following the sudden onset of characteristic signs and symptoms as above.

Histological

Traditionally, AFE was a post-mortem diagnosis. Nowadays, the finding of amniotic fluid debris (fetal squames, epithelial cells, mucin, lanugo) in maternal lung tissue or pulmonary artery blood can be used to support the diagnosis of AFE, suspected on clinical grounds. These post-mortem findings alone, without a clinical suspicion of AFE, are no longer considered pathognomonic as small amounts of such elements can enter the maternal circulation without sequelae.

Investigations

No specific investigation can confirm the diagnosis of AFE, although some may be useful for diagnosis and management.

- *ABG.* Hypoxaemia and adequacy of ventilation.
- *FBC and clotting profile.* Diagnose DIC and manage haemorrhage and DIC.
- *Serum tryptase..*
- *CXR.* Pulmonary oedema.
- *ECG.* RV strain, arrhythmias.
- *TTE or TOE.* Assessment of ventricular function.
- CVP/pulmonary artery catheter blood sample. As with post-mortem, the presence of fetal squames and other debris supports a clinical diagnosis but is not pathognomonic.

Differential diagnosis

AFE is a diagnosis of exclusion from other causes of maternal collapse:

- Pre-eclampsia or eclampsia
- Pulmonary aspiration
- Pulmonary thromboembolism
- Placental abruption
- Air embolism
- Septic shock
- AMI
- Anaphylaxis
- Coagulopathy
- Uterine rupture
- Uterine atony and PPH
- CVA
- Anaesthetic toxicity

Pathophsiology

AFE was classically attributed to amniotic fluid and debris entering the maternal circulation. This needed a disruption of the normal barriers between amniotic fluid and the maternal venous circulation, and a pressure gradient allowing the entrance of amniotic fluid into the maternal circulation.

As fetal squames can be detected in the maternal circulation in normal labour, without AFE developing, their mere presence 'plugging' the pulmonary vasculature cannot account for the syndrome that develops in some women. It is still unclear whether abnormal factors in amniotic fluid, such as meconium, are responsible or whether the syndrome represents an anaphylactoid-type reaction to amniotic fluid in susceptible individuals. The latter is supported by the similar clinical, haematological and haemodynamic derangements found in both AFE and anaphylactoid reactions, suggesting common underlying pathophysiologic mechanisms, and a history of allergy and atopy in almost half of women who develop AFE. The variable clinical picture seen in response to fetal material in the maternal circulation would then be dependent on the nature and quantity of that material and the susceptibility of the mother.

A biphasic model has also been described. The initial phase develops following the entry of amniotic fluid into the maternal circulation. Pulmonary vasospasm with acute pulmonary hypertension and right heart failure follow, causing severe hypoxia and a fall in cardiac output. This initial phase is transient, lasting usually <30min, but the profound hypoxia that develops is responsible for most early AFE deaths and the permanent neurological impairment in survivors. During the secondary phase, RV function returns to normal but LV failure with pulmonary oedema and hypotension develop, secondary to hypoxia and direct depressant effects of amniotic fluid on the myocardium. Procoagulants in the amniotic fluid and widespread tissue hypoxia then trigger excessive coagulation in those women lucky enough to survive the initial insults.

Management

No specific pharmacological or other therapies prevent or treat AFE. Management is purely supportive to maintain oxygenation, restore normal blood pressure and cardiac output, and correct coagulopathy.

- Call for help, including senior anaesthetic, obstetric and midwifery colleagues. Inform ITU and haematologist.
- Rapid and effective resuscitation, following the standard ABC (airway, breathing, circulation) approach.
- Airway and breathing. High flow oxygen through face mask to a patent airway. Consider intubation and ventilation if reduced level of consciousness or severe hypoxaemia on ABG analysis. Oxygen is also an effective pulmonary vasodilator for the management of pulmonary vasospasm, although the latter is usually only a transient phenomenon. IV pulmonary vasodilators risk systemic vasodilatation and hypotension. NO or prostacyclin could be useful, but are unlikely to be available in the time they would potentially be beneficial.
- Circulation. Insert at least 2 large bore IV cannulae (14–16G) and take bloods for baseline U&E, FBC, coagulation screen (including fibrinogen and D-dimers), tryptase, group and cross-match (>6 units). Maintain cardiac output with IV fluids and inotropes as required. Caution with fluid loading in the presence of right, then left ventricular failure. *Remember uterine displacement if antepartum.*
- Standard monitoring including pulse, blood pressure, ECG, oxygen saturation, respiratory rate, urine output and temperature.
- Early invasive monitoring (arterial and CVP, under ultrasound guidance) if haemodynamically unstable, but without delaying resuscitation and definitive treatment. Consider pulmonary artery catheter or TOE to guide fluid resuscitation.
- If maternal cardiac arrest, follow standard ALS algorithms, including perimortem Caesarean section within 5min.
- Correct DIC with red blood cells, FFP, cryoprecipitate and platelets, under the guidance of a consultant haematologist.
- Manage the predictable massive obstetric haemorrhage resulting from DIC and uterine atony. Caution with oxytocic agents (see Chapter 32.4).
- Delegate someone to document observations, along with timings and interventions, such as drugs and fluid input and output.
- If survives, transfer to ICU.

Further reading

Burros A, Khoo S. The amniotic fluid embolism syndrome: 10 years experience at a major teaching hospital. *Aust N Z Obstet Gynaecol* 1995; 35: 245–50.

Clark SL, Hankins GDV, Dudley DA, *et al.* Amniotic fluid embolism: Analysis of the registry. *Am J Obstet Gynecol* 1995; 172: 1158–67.

Department of Health. Confidential Enquiry into Maternal and Child Health. Why mothers die 2000-2. The sixth report of the confidential enquiries into maternal deaths in the UK. London: RCOG Press, 2004.

Grady K, Howell C, Cox C. Managing obstetric emergencies and trauma. The MOET course manual, 2nd edn. London: RCOG Press, 2007.

Tuffnell DJ. UK amniotic fluid register. *Br J Obstet Gynaecol* 2005; 112: 1625–9.

UK Obstetric Surveillance System, National Perinatal Epidemiology Unit. Oxford.

Chapter 32

Death and dying

Chapter contents

Confirming death using neurological criteria (brainstem death)

The brainstem provides the anatomical link between the spinal cord and cerebral hemispheres relaying sensory and motor impulses between the periphery and higher cortical centres. It also contains cranial nerve nuclei, the reticular activating system and cardiorespiratory control centres, the destruction of which underlies the process of confirming death according to neurological criteria (brainstem death).

Background

Described in 1968 by the Harvard Medical Committee and adopted in the UK in 1976 following the Conference of the Royal Colleges and their Faculties, the permanent and irreversible loss of all brainstem reflexes equates to the death of an individual, with the permanent functional death of the brainstem constituting brain death; a position since adopted by the courts of England and Wales. The UK guidelines have been most recently published by the Department of Heath and Academy of Royal Medical Colleges in 2008.

Aetiology

Brainstem death may follow a severe global insult such as hypoxia or a direct insult such as trauma or focal ischaemia resulting from vertebral/basilar artery pathology. The most common causes of brainstem death are traumatic brain injury, CVAs (including SAH), cerebral tumours, meningitis and hypoxic brain injury.

The process of confirming death by neurological testing

Pre-conditions

Certain pre-conditions must be met before neurological testing can be undertaken:

- The cause of the coma must be established as an irreversible structural cause of brain injury.
- The patient must be deeply comatose, apnoeic and dependent on mechanical ventilation. The possibility of neuromuscular blockade should be excluded by means of a peripheral nerve stimulator or the eliciting of deep tendon reflexes. Ventilatory depression due to drugs or spinal cord injury must be excluded.
- The patient must be unresponsive with reversible causes of brainstem depression excluded: hypothermia (<34°C), sedative drugs, alcohol, circulatory, endocrine and metabolic disturbances. Deviations outside normal values that are clearly a consequence of brainstem death rather than its cause do not preclude the diagnosis.

Establishing the irreversible loss of brainstem reflexes

This may only take place in a setting where the above pre-conditions have been met

- The pupils are fixed with no direct or consensual response to light. The pupils need not be dilated or equal in size and shape for the diagnosis to be confirmed.
- The corneal reflex is absent.
- There is no motor response within the cranial nerve distribution to a painful stimulus applied centrally or peripherally. Spinal reflexes may persist in brainstem dead patients.
- The oculovestibular (caloric) reflex is absent. This is performed by injecting 50ml of ice-cold water over 1min into each external auditory meatus whilst the eyelids are held open. There should be no eye movement, principally nystagmus, during or after the injection, and the eyes should be observed for 1min after each injection. Direct access to the tympanic membrane must be confirmed on each side using an auriscope, and the head should be flexed at 30° to the horizontal plane. The diagnosis is not invalidated if it cannot be performed on one side due to localized trauma.
- There should be no gag reflex or cough reflex in response to a suction catheter being passed into the pharynx or down the ETT to stimulate the carina.

Apnoea testing

The responsiveness of the respiratory system to hypercarbia is the final test performed to confirm brainstem death, and should not be performed if any of the preceding tests confirm the presence of brainstem function. It is recommended that end-tidal carbon dioxide ($ETCO_2$) monitoring is utilized to minimize the risk of excessive hypercarbia and/or rapid changes in carbon dioxide tension, so limiting the risk of further injury to potentially recoverable brain tissue. The patient should be pre-oxygenated with 100% oxygen for 5min. With a SpO_2 >95%, minute volume ventilation is reduced and the $ETCO_2$ allowed to rise slowly. Once the $ETCO_2$ is >6.5kPa, a level high enough to exceed the normal threshold for stimulation of respiration, an ABG is taken to confirm that the $PaCO_2$ is >6.5kPa. If cardiovascular stability is maintained, the patient should then be disconnected from the ventilator for 5min. Hypoxia is prevented by insufflating oxygen at 10l/min via a suction catheter placed down the ETT with continual SpO_2 monitoring. Whilst disconnected, the patient should remain apnoeic and is continually observed for any respiratory effort (abdomen and chest exposed). If after the 5min there has been no spontaneous respiratory effort, a further confirmatory ABG is taken. The ventilator should then be reconnected and the minute volume returned to the setting that allows blood gases to return to the target value for the patient's further management. In patients with pre-existing chronic respiratory disease who rely on a hypoxic drive to respiration, a mild but significant acidosis should be achieved by allowing the $PaCO_2$ to rise to a point where the pH is <7.35.

Timing of testing

Testing should not be considered until at least 6h after the onset of apnoeic coma or, if the cause is presumed to be hypoxic injury following cardiac arrest, many would allow a minimum of 24h after the restoration of the circulation.

Conduct of testing

Neurological testing to confirm death should be performed by two medical practitioners both of whom should have held full registration with the General Medical Council for at least 5yrs. One should be an ICU consultant or the consultant in charge of the patient, and both should be competent in the procedure. Neither should have any connection to the transplant team. The doctors may perform the tests independently or together. There is no statutory time interval that must pass between the two sets of tests; it is a matter of clinical judgement to decide when sufficient time has elapsed between tests to satisfy all those involved. Two sets are undertaken to remove the risk of observer error and to reassure the family.

Other considerations

- Death may be confirmed after completion of the second set of tests.
- The time of death is then recorded as the time at which the **first** set of tests was completed.
- Documentation of the results should be on the appropriate form approved by the UK Department of Health.
- The coroner should be informed of most of these patients due to the underlying diagnosis, mechanism of injury or if organ donation is to take place.
- Effective communication with relatives enables understanding of the indications for and components of brainstem death testing and its implications, and may help to alleviate emotional distress.

Ancillary tests

No additional tests are required in the UK to confirm brainstem death, although ancillary tests such as four-vessel cerebral angiography, transcranial Doppler or radioisotope scanning may be used to establish the absence of CBF in cases of diagnostic uncertainties. EEG or brainstem evoked potential testing are not usually helpful in establishing the diagnosis.

Problems

- Depending on the underlying pathology, there may be uncertainty as to when the brain injury can be considered irreversible and brainstem testing can take place.
- With altered pharmacokinetics in critically ill patients, uncertainty may surround the length of time that has to elapse before the effects of sedative agents, e.g. thiopenton,e can be said to be negligible following prolonged administration.
- No specific ranges can be set within which biochemical variables must fall to be considered 'normal' and compatible with brainstem death testing, although recommendations as such have been made by the Academy of Royal Medical Colleges.

Subsequent actions

After the neurological confirmation of death, subsequent actions depend on whether the patient had expressed a wish to donate their organs after death. If so, the maintenance of normal physiological parameters is vital to ensure optimal organ viability. This includes correcting the physiological consequences of brainstem death including cardiovascular instability (hypotension and arrhythmias), hypothermia, diabetes insipidus, DIC, hyperglycaemia, acidosis and other metabolic and endocrine abnormalities. If donation is not an option, then following consultation with the relatives, withdrawal of respiratory support may take place at a time acceptable to all parties.

Further reading

Report of the Ad Hoc Committee of the Harvard Medical School to Examine the Definition of Brain Death. A definition of irreversible coma. *JAMA* 1968; 205: 337–40.

Conference of the Medical Royal Colleges and their Faculties in the United Kingdom. Diagnosis of brainstem death. *BMJ* 1976: 1187–8.

Department of Heath and Academy of Royal Medical Colleges. A code of practice for the diagnosis of death. 2008.

Withdrawing and withholding treatment

Across Europe, 13.5% of patients admitted to an ICU die. Of these patients who are going to die, 72.6% had limitations applied to their treatment. This equates to 10% of all ICU admissions in this study population. Therefore, decisions about withdrawing and withholding treatment are occurring constantly. In the European Society of Intensive Care Medicine (ESICM) 'Ethicus' paper, it was argued that there were 3 methods that could be adopted by intensivists, that could lead to a patient's death:

1. Withholding treatment was defined as a decision that was made not to start or increase a life-sustaining intervention.
2. Withdrawing treatment was defined as a decision that was made actively to stop a life-sustaining intervention presently being given.
3. Active shortening of the dying process was defined as a circumstance in which someone performed an act with the specific intent of shortening the dying process. This is unlawful in the UK, but not in certain jurisdictions in Europe and elsewhere in the world. Certain authors hold that the 'double effect' may fall into this category.

Generally (with some exceptions, e.g. the Jewish faith), it is argued that withdrawing and withholding treatment are morally and ethically the same.

In the USA, the President's Commission for the Study of Ethical problems in Medicine and Biomedical Research has said, '[The] healthcare professional has an obligation to allow a patient to choose from among the medically acceptable treatment options ... or to reject all options. No one, however, has an obligation to provide interventions that would, in his or her judgement, be countertherapeutic.' It is establishing whether treatment options are countertherapeutic, or futile, that is difficult.

Futility

One way of establishing whether a treatment is countertherapeutic is by using the concept of futility. Unfortunately, this is difficult to define, with the courts saying, 'Futility is a subjective and nebulous concept which, except in the strictest physiological sense, incorporates value judgements.' Futility can be defined in a number of ways, including (and modifying) Ardagh's definitions

- Physiological futility exists when a procedure cannot bring about its physiological objective. For example, it is physiologically futile if the administration of epinephrine to a hypotensive patient fails to result in an increase in blood pressure.
- Benefit-centred definition of futility has been defined as consisting of quantitative and qualitative considerations. First, the quantitative estimate of futility is one in which an intervention is considered futile if it has failed in the last defined number of times attempted. For example, should a condition produce a predicted mortality of 99.9%, then 1 patient in 1000 will live if treated. It is not possible to determine which patient will survive and which one will die in advance of treatment. In this example, treatment is futile for 999 patients, but not futile for one individual who could survive. The qualitative component is defined as occurring where the patient's resulting quality of life falls well below the threshold considered minimal by general professional judgement. Note that possible considerations of the patient may be ignored, which is precisely the situation that worried Mr Burke so that he brought a case against the GMC. Mr Burke requested a declaration that it would be unlawful to withdraw treatment (in the form of artificial nutrition and hydration) against his wishes. The Court of Appeal ruled against him saying, 'Ultimately, however, a patient cannot demand that a doctor administer a treatment which the doctor considers is adverse to the patient's clinical needs.'
- Operationalizing or cost-based futility. This definition of futility is when treatment is so unlikely to succeed that many people, both professional and lay persons, would consider it not worth the cost. Treatments which are now considered by many as mainstream can fall into this category, such as APC. Cost is relative and depends on society's needs and wishes, e.g. in the aftermath of the Ladbroke Grove rail crash, it has been estimated that the Train Passenger Warning System installed would save ~38 lives over 25yrs, at a cost of £15.4million per life saved. In the UK, case-law suggests that where a treatment is felt clinically appropriate, then it may not be withheld solely on the basis of that cost.

Doctors rarely use the physiological definition of futility in common practice. The latter two definitions of futility mentioned above follow utilitarian principles such as those espoused by Savulescu and Shaw and advocated by the US President's Commission (mentioned above), but incorporate value judgements. These value judgements may be subject to challenge by relatives, those with power of attorney and the courts. It has been argued that, 'The principle that each individual is entitled to an equal opportunity to benefit from any public health care system, and that this entitlement is proportionate neither to the size of their chance of benefiting, nor to the quality of the benefit, nor to the length of lifetime remaining in which that benefit may be enjoyed.'

Best interests

If futility is not as useful as it first appears, the best interests of the patient can be considered.

Competent patients

- A competent patient (see Chapter 33.1) should be involved with the decision and a discussion should be held with the patient. As Harris has said, 'Each person's desire to stay alive should be regarded as of the same importance and as deserving the same respect as that of anyone else, irrespective of the quality of their life or its expected duration.'
- There are some individuals who wish to die rather than continue treatment. Recent examples in medicine include the cases of Dianne Pretty and Ms B.
- In justification of this wish to die, consider Kuhse's thought experiment: 'A truck driver and his co-driver had an accident on a lonely stretch of road. The truck caught fire and the driver was trapped in the wreckage of the cabin. The co-driver struggled to free him, but could not do so. The driver, now burning, pleaded with his colleague—an experienced shooter—to take a rifle, which was stowed in a box on the back of the truck, and shoot him. The co-driver took the rifle and shot his colleague. Was what the co-driver did morally reprehensible? Did he act wrongly? Students who are presented with

this case will generally answer both questions in the negative. The reason for their intuitions are not hard to find. In this case, the agent was not motivated by personal gain, but by compassion.'

- If we accept this, then we can accept the underlying premise that it is sometimes in the best interests of the patient to die.

Patients who lack capacity

If the patient is not competent, then it is important to consult widely to discover the person's past and present wishes and feelings, the beliefs and values that would be likely to influence his decision, and any other factors that he would be likely to consider. Once this has been done, the doctor can then consider whether further treatment of this patient is justified, or whether it is in the patient's best interests to cease treatment and be permitted to die. The key is to consider the individual concerned, and not merely the pathology.

Process

Although every case of withholding or withdrawing treatment is different, it is sensible to have departmental guidelines drawn up to guide inexperienced practitioners. The emphasis of care changes from one of cure to one of symptom control. It is likely that analgesics and anxiolytics are continued. It is further likely that other agents such as antisialogogues are added. The precise treatment will vary according to the individual patient.

Penalties

If we get it wrong, then we risk the censure of the courts and the GMC.

- Dr Ann David withdrew ventilatory support from a patient and administered 20mg Diazemuls. The patient subsequently died. Consequently, on the 16th November 2005, Dr David was stuck off the medical register for gross professional misconduct. The Fitness to Practise Panel found proven that her actions were, 'clinically unjustified, inappropriate, premature and not in the patient's best interests'.
- Dr David came to the view that further treatment of the patient was futile because he was not responding to her treatment and his ventilatory requirements were increasing. Despite disagreement from the family, she withdrew treatment.
- Dr David discussed her opinion with the patient's family, but appears not to have discussed the matter with her patient. Yet, he 'was not in imminent danger of dying and was recorded as being conscious and orientated'. She knew, however, that the family did not wish treatment to be withdrawn. Family's requests are not binding on clinicians because doctors have to promote their patient's best interests. Nevertheless, the GMC specifically censured Dr David for her failure to treat the patient in his best interests.

Consider the busy hospital, with high pressure on beds; the consultant, unable to take time to establish a rapport with the family; working with limited access to an appropriate peer group. There are a number of factors that could help minimize the occurrence of unfortunate episodes.

- Doctors should establish local, regional and national networks of support to which to turn for advice.
- The counsel of a trusted colleague is invaluable in clinical practise.
- It has been suggested that the presence of a hospital-based clinical ethics committee would help clinicians and families in this terrible position. Such a forum would facilitate dialogue between the parties, but not provide a didactic answer.

Finally, there may be a way to resolve these conflicts through legislation. In the state of Texas, the Texas Advance Directives Act 1999 provides that there is a mandated period of 10 days in which care may not be withdrawn. During this time, doctors and relatives attempt to find an alternative hospital that would be prepared to continue treating the patient. Only if no medical facility is found can there be any consideration of withdrawal of medical care against the wishes of the family. The experience of this Act suggests that most disagreements between families and medical staff are resolved in the 10 day 'cooling off' period.

Conclusion

The pattern of death in modern society is changing from occurring at home to occurring in hospital. The general practitioner will refer the patient to hospital when the patient's condition is not able to be managed in a home environment. Once in hospital, should the patient's condition worsen, he or she becomes more likely to be referred to ICU. It is likely that more people will die on ICU as an ever-increasing number are referred. Death is traditionally perceived by the medical profession as a failure, as opposed to being seen as in the best interests of the patient. If death is accepted as a best interest, then the management of that death is paramount. Quality of death is as important as quality of life. Intensivists have been given a new goal: to provide excellence in end-of-life care. We must be ready to meet this challenge.

Further reading

Ardagh M. Futility has no utility in resuscitation medicine. *J Med Ethics* 2000; 26: 396.

Harris J. The value of life. London: Routledge, 1985.

Harris J. Justice and equal opportunities in health care. *Bioethics* 1999; 13: 392–404.

Kuhse H. Why killing is not always worse—and sometimes better—than letting die. Cambridge *Q Healthcare Ethics* 1998; 7: 371.

Savulescu J. Consequentialism, reasons, value and justice. *Bioethics* 1998; 12: 212.

Shaw AB. In defence of ageism. *J Med Ethics* 1994; 20: 188.

Sprung CL, Cohen SL, Sjokvist P, *et al.* End-of-life practices in European intensive care units: the Ethicus study. *JAMA* 2003; 290: 790.

R (on the application of Burke) v General Medical Council [2004] All ER (D) 588 (Jul) and [2005] EWCA 1003.

R v North Derbyshire HA, ex parte Fisher [1997] 8 Med LR 327

North West Lancashire HA v A,D and G [1999] Lloyd's Rep Med 399

Ms B v An NHS Hospital Trust. [2002] WL 347038

Case of Pretty v United Kingdom. (2002) 35 E.H.R.R. 1

The potential heart-beating organ donor

Organ transplantation is one of the most significant medical advances of recent times, with >90% of recipients surviving 1yr. This success has led to a situation worldwide whereby demand for organs outstrips supply. The transplantation of organs in suboptimal conditions is a significant cause of graft failure. It is therefore vital that comprehensive physiological support is given to a potential organ donor to ensure that donated organs reach the recipients in optimal condition. Clinicians caring for an organ donor have a duty of care and obligation to both the donor and the recipient to ensure that this is the case.

Identification of the potential organ donor

Organ donation is widely supported, with >14 million (23%) of the UK's population actively expressing a wish to donate their organs after death by registering on the UK Transplant's Organ Donor Register. Few of these people will die in an ICU and, of those who do, only 6% will have death confirmed using neurological criteria. To ensure that the wishes of dying patients are met, any patient under the age of 75 years who has been confirmed dead using neurological criteria should be considered as a potential heart-beating organ donor, and their relatives should be offered the option. There are very few absolute contraindications to organ donation:

- Presence of malignancy (except certain primary tumours of the CNS)
- Systemic sepsis
- Confirmed diagnosis of HIV
- Known or suspected classical or variant CJD

In order to avoid missing potential organ donors, all such patients should be discussed with the donor transplant coordinator regarding suitability, as 'marginal' organs may still be transplanted if the clinical situation of the recipient demands it. Until recently hepatitis B- or C-positive donors were not considered suitable for donation, but organs from these patients are now transplanted into hepatitis B- or C-positive recipients

Approaching a potential donor's family

Once a potential donor has been discussed with the donor transplant coordinator, the suitability of the patient can be determined, avoiding the situation whereby a patient's relatives are approached with a request for organ donation only to find subsequently that they are not suitable. They are also able to check with the organ donor register to see if the patient had registered their wish to donate their organs after death. An approach to the relatives requesting organ donation should be made by an experienced member of the ICU team with or without the transplant coordinator present. No member of the transplant team should be involved with the request for organ donation. There is some evidence to suggest that a collaborative approach to the family by the patient's clinician and the transplant coordinator achieves higher consent rates, although these findings need to be confirmed. Relatives should be fully informed of progress at every stage, and time taken to explain the need for ongoing therapeutic interventions aimed at optimizing the function of potentially transplantable organs after confirming death. Permission for donation may be required from the coroner or procurator's fiscal, depending on the circumstances of the death, and should be sought prior to approaching the donor's relatives.

Pathophysiological changes after death according to neurological criteria

Pathophysiological changes occur in all major organ systems after the irreversible loss of brainstem reflexes, all of which may jeopardize function in potentially transplantable organs (Table 32.3.1).

Table 32.3.1 Incidence of pathophysiological changes after death according to neurological criteria

Hypotension	80%
Diabetes insipidus	65%
Disseminated intravascular coagulation	30%
Cardiac arrhythmias	30%
Pulmonary oedema	20%
Metabolic acidosis	10%

Cardiovascular changes

Irreversible loss of brainstem reflexes is associated with intense autonomic activity and massive catecholamine release. The resulting increases in heart rate, blood pressure, cardiac output and PVR lead to widespread myocardial ischaemic damage. Impaired ATP production, increased free radical production and defective oxidative metabolism exacerbate the cellular damage and worsen myocardial function. ST segment and T wave changes are common, along with atrial or ventricular arrhythmias and conduction abnormalities. Multi-factorial in origin, these changes reflect loss of vagal tone, sympathetic overactivity, myocardial ischaemia, electrolyte abnormalities and/or the administration of exogenous catecholamines. As vasomotor control by the brainstem is lost, all sympathetic activity is lost, resulting in profound vasodilatation and myocardial depression with consequent hypotension. This hypotension may be potentiated by other factors (Table 32.3.2). Asystolic cardiac arrest is likely to occur within days if no other organ support except mechanical ventilation is provided.

Table 32.3.2 Causes of hypotension after death according to neurological criteria

Peripheral vasodilatation
Hypovolaemia
Diabetes insipidus
Osmotic diuresis (mannitol)
Hyperglycaemia
Therapeutic fluid restriction
Myocardial depression
Depletion of high energy phosphate
Mitochondrial inhibition
Possible reduction in T_3 production
Electrolyte disturbance

Pulmonary changes

Neurogenic pulmonary oedema resulting initially from elevated pulmonary capillary hydrostatic pressure caused by acute LV dysfunction followed by increased capillary permeability is common after a severe intracranial injury. Pulmonary dysfunction may also occur as a result of pneumonia, contusions, aspiration, atelectasis, fluid overload or as part of any other coincidental disease process.

Endocrine changes

Failure of the anterior and posterior pituitary leads to reduced circulating levels of ADH, cortisol, T_3 and T_4. Diabetes insipidus occurs in up to 65% of potential organ donors, and is characterized by diuresis, hypovolaemia and metabolic derangement (plasma hyperosmolality, hypernatraemia, hypomagnesaemia and hypocalcaemia). Lack of T_3 may compound cardiovascular collapse through depletion of high energy phosphates, whilst a reduced blood cortisol level impairs the donor stress response. Insulin secretion is reduced and contributes to the development of hyperglycaemia. This may be aggravated by the administration of glucose-containing fluids to manage hypernatraemia and of exogenous catecholamines to treat hypotension. Left untreated, hyperglycaemia leads to increased plasma osmolality, metabolic acidosis, osmotic diuresis and cardiovascular instability.

Temperature regulation

Hypothermia is a common feature and results from loss of hypothalamic temperature-regulating mechanisms, a reduction in heat production due to a decreased metabolic rate, and increased heat loss due to peripheral vasodilatation

Haematological changes

The release of tissue thromboplastin and other mediators from severely damaged brain tissue may cause a coagulopathy, DIC being present in 30% of organ donors.

Immunological changes

The process of brainstem death alters the immunogenecity of organs by a variety of poorly understood mechanisms. This may explain why acute rejection episodes are more frequent and more severe in recipients of organs from heart-beating donors compared with those receiving organs from living donors.

Clinical management of the potential heart-beating organ donor

Once death has been confirmed using neurological criteria, there is an alteration in the emphasis of patient care. Whereas therapies have previously been aimed at preserving brain function, they are now directed to optimize the function of transplantable organs. High quality routine general intensive care measures should continue, including strict asepsis, nutrition, regular tracheal suctioning, physiotherapy, turning and the active treatment of infection or arrhythmias. Additionally, specific therapies to control or reverse the pathophysiological abnormalities that may damage or impair the function of transplantable organs should be instigated. Invasive monitoring should be continued or commenced. If new lines are inserted, the arterial cannula should ideally be sited in the left radial or brachial artery and central venous or pulmonary arterial catheter in the right internal jugular vein as a result of the order in which the great vessels are ligated during organ retrieval.

Cardiovascular support

Early donor optimization increases the rate of successful organ retrieval. Suggested haemodynamic targets are:

- CVP 4–10mm Hg
- Cardiac index 2.2–2.5l/min/m^{-2}
- MAP 60–80mm Hg
- Pulse rate 60–100/m ideally sinus rhythm

Hypotension should initially be treated with fluids guided by CVP and/or cardiac output monitoring. Excessive fluid administration should, however, be avoided, particularly if the lungs are being considered for transplantation since they may have been damaged during the period of sympathetic hyperactivity and are susceptible to volume overload and capillary leakage. Measuring EVLW and maintaining it in the normal range may increase the rate of successful retrieval of the lungs for transplantation.

If hypotension persists despite adequate fluid resuscitation, then vasopressin is increasingly considered to be the vasoconstrictor of choice since, unlike other inotropes and vasoconstrictors, it does not deplete myocardial ATP levels whilst increasing blood pressure, maintaining cardiac output and reducing plasma hyperosmolality. Once a patient is considered suitable for organ donation, vasoconstrictors such as norepinephrine that had been used to maintain CPP should be stopped and vasopressin used instead. Dopamine or norepinephrine should be used when fluids and vasopressin fail to achieve the optimization targets. Prolonged administration of exogenous catecholamines should be avoided as rapid depletion of myocardial ATP stores and detrimental vasoconstriction in donor organs may result. If high doses of vasoactive drugs are required, 'hormone replacement' (see below) may be considered. Arrhythmias are common and should be aggressively treated along with any associated hypokalaemia or hypomagnesaemia.

Respiratory support

If the lungs are being considered for transplantation then, to minimize the risk of oxygen toxicity, the FiO_2 should be kept as low as possible to achieve a PaO_2 >10kPa. A ventilatory strategy aimed at protecting the lungs should be employed, with tidal volumes limited to 6–8ml/kg. A PEEP of 5–10cm H_2O will prevent alveolar collapse, whilst higher levels may induce hypotension in an inadequately fluid-resuscitated patient. Donor lungs are vulnerable to pulmonary oedema. and fluid loading to a CVP >6mm Hg (in the absence of PEEP) may worsen the arterial alveolar oxygen gradient.

Endocrine support

Diabetes insipidus: hypovolaemia and hypernatraemia should be corrected with appropriate IV fluid administration. Excessive polyuria should be managed with DDAVP which can be administered either as intermittent boluses or as an infusion. DDAVP is associated with a lower incidence of acute tubular necrosis and graft failure than vasopressin.

Hyperglycaemia should be treated with an insulin infusion according to usual intensive care protocols.

Other hormone replacement should be considered in organ donors with cardiovascular instability, escalating vasoactive drug requirements and a worsening acidosis.

- Some cardiothoracic transplant centres recommend using T_3 to reduce inotrope requirements and help restore cardiovascular stability, hoping that this will improving the function of the transplanted heart
- The administration of high dose methylprednisolone has been advocated to reduce vasoactive drug requirements, to attenuate the effects of proinflammatory cytokines, and to reduce the accumulation of lung water. It improves oxygenation in the donor and is associated with increasing likehood of successful retrieval and transplantation of the lungs.

On the basis of the failure of the hypothalamo-pituitary axis, others have suggested that 'hormonal resuscitation' with vasopressin, methylprednisolone and T_3 should be more routine since its administration has been associated with an increase in the possibility of the kidney, heart, liver, lung and pancreas being transplanted, along with an improvement in the short-term function of the donor heart. In practice whether it is used or not is determined by the preferences of the Transplant Centre involved.

Renal support

Renal perfusion pressure should be optimized by maintaining an adequate MAP with fluid resuscitation or vasoactive drugs as appropriate. Episodes of hypotension should be treated aggressively as they are associated with acute tubular necrosis and failure of the transplanted kidneys.

Haematological support

Any coagulopathy should be corrected with the administration of FFP and platelets. Four units of blood should be available prior to multi-organ procurement since the surgery may involve significant blood loss.

Temperature support

Normothermia should be restored and maintained using forced air warming blankets, IV fluid warmers, heated and humidified inspired gases and, if necessary, by increasing the ambient temperature

Other considerations

Documentation should be continued as for any critically ill patient. The time of death is recorded as the time that the first set of tests confirming death according to neurological criteria is completed. If a post-mortem is to be performed, local policy may dictate that intravascular cannulae, the ETT and urethral catheter are left in place, otherwise they may be removed. Last offices are performed by the nursing staff with help from the transplant coordinator, and the relatives should be given the opportunity to view the body after surgery if they wish to do so.

Meeting the wishes of individuals and their relatives to donate organs after death is an important aspect in bereavement care. The attitudes of medical staff in explaining the need for ongoing therapies despite the donor being declared dead will lead to greater understanding on the part of the relatives, many of whom gain comfort from following their relative's wishes after death and consolation in knowing that some good has come from their tragedy. Psychological and pastoral support offered to relatives by the ICU team and the transplant coordinator may help alleviate feelings of guilt, anger or remorse. They should be invited to return and discuss any issues with ICU staff or the coordinator in the future. It is common practic for relatives to be informed of the patients that benefited from the donation of their loved one's organs.

Further reading

Barber K, Falvey S, Hamilton C, *et al.* Potential for organ donation in the United Kingdom: audit of intensive care records. *BMJ* 2006; 352: 1124–6.

Pennefather SH, Bullock RE, Dark JH. Use of low dose arginine vasopressin to support brain dead organ donors. *Transplantation* 1995; 59: 58–62.

Pennefather SH, Bullock RE, Dark JH. The effect of fluid therapy on alveolar arterial oxygen gradient in brain dead organ donors. *Transplantation* 1993; 56: 1418–22.

Rosendale JD, Kauffman MH, McBride MA, *et al.* Aggressive pharmacologic donor management results in more transplanted organs. *Transplantation* 2003; 75: 482–7.

Shafer TJ, Ehrle RN, Davis KD, *et al.* Increasing organ recovery form level 1 trauma centres: the in-house coordinator intervention. *Prog Transplant* 2004; 14: 250–63.

Sque, M, Long, T. and Payne, S. Organ and tissue donation: exploring the needs of families. Final report of a three-year study commissioned by the British Organ Donor Society, funded by the National Lottery Community Fund. University of Southampton, 2003. http://eprints.soton.ac.uk/11140/

The Intensive Care Society's Working Group on Organ and Tissue Donation. Guidelines for adult organ and tissue donation, 2004. http://www.ics.ac.uk/icmprof/downloads/Organ%20&%20Tissue%20Donation.pdf

Non-heart-beating organ donation

Background

Organ transplantation offers patients with end-stage organ failure an improved quality of life and increased life expectancy. In non-heart-beating organ donation (NHBD), organs are retrieved form a donor following cardiorespiratory arrest rather than after the confirmation of death using neurological criteria. This is not a new concept. Prior to recognition in 1968 by the Harvard Medical Committee that death resulted from irreversible damage to the brainstem and the introduction in 1976 of clinical tests to confirm deaths using neurological criteria, organs for transplantation were routinely retrieved from NHBDs. After this declaration, transplant centres rapidly switched to transplanting organs from patients declared dead using neurological criteria, i.e. heart-beating donors, and the practice of NHBD declined rapidly. However, with the gap between organ supply and demand widening and the demonstration that kidneys retrieved from NHBDs have the same long-term outcome as those from brainstem dead donors, transplant centres are re-introducing NHBD schemes.

Rationale

In the UK, demand for organs continues to outstrip supply, with a record 7234 people listed as waiting for an organ transplant in March 2007. The disparity between the number of transplants performed and the number of patients on the waiting list continues to grow. Factors contributing to this disparity include:

- an ageing population
- an increase in the prevalence of renal failure
- advances in transplant technology

Whilst the demand for organs increases, the actual number of heart-beating donors is declining. This pattern is likely to continue for two reasons:

- Fewer young people are dying as a result of severe injury or catastrophic cerebrovascular events.
- Improvements in the ICU management and outcome of traumatic brain injuries means that fewer people fulfil neurological criteria for confirming death.

A 41% refusal rate amongst relatives approached with a request for organ donation, means that not all potential donors are converted into actual donors. One strategy to increase the number of organs available for transplantation is the introduction of NHBD schemes. Apart from the obvious benefit to transplant recipients, NHBDs also gives more families the opportunity to honour the wishes of a relative who had expressed a wish to donate their organs after death but who failed to fulfil the criteria for neurological death. NHBD meets the need of families to be with the deceased and to witness the observable ending of life as represented by the cessation of the heart beat.

Controlled non-heart beating organ donation

Classification

Potential NHBDs can be classified into 5 categories according to the modified Maastricht classification (Table 32.4.1). Categories I, II and V are described as 'uncontrolled' and categories III and IV as 'controlled', the main difference being that in controlled potential NHBD the patient's imminent death is expected and the donation process better planned. In the ICU setting NHBDs are usually controlled.

Table 32.4.1 The modified Maastricht classification of NHBDs

Category I	Dead on arrival
Category II	Unsuccessful resuscitation
Category III	Anticipated cardiac arrest
Category IV	Cardiac arrest in a brainstem dead donor
Category V	Unexpected cardiac arrest in an ICU patient

Potential NHBD

Patients suitable for NHBD are typically, but not exclusively, those who have experienced a catastrophic brain injury but who do not fulfil the neurological criteria for death. They are dependent on life-sustaining support, yet continued medical intervention is not considered to be in the patient's best interests. As a result, withdrawal of active treatment has been planned and it is anticipated that cardiorespiratory arrest will follow quickly and predictably. Patients with other diagnoses in whom treatment withdrawal is planned may also be suitable and should be discussed with the donor transplant coordinator to assess suitability. Absolute contraindications to NHBD are the same as those described for brainstem dead heart-beating donors.

Organs suitable for donation

The kidneys are relatively tolerant of warm ischaemia compared with other solid organs, and can achieve similar transplant outcomes to those retrieved from heart-beating donors. However, increasingly, other organs retrieved from NHBDs including the liver, pancreas and lungs are also being transplanted successfully with acceptable outcomes.

Withdrawal of active treatment

The decision to withdraw treatment should be made in consultation with the patient's relatives, the referring medical team and the critical care team in accordance with guidelines from the Intensive Care Society, British Medical Association and GMC, and must be made separate from any consideration of organ donation. To avoid a conflict of interest, no member of the transplant team should be involved in any aspect of the decision to withdraw treatment. Agreement on the exact timing of treatment withdrawal is then reached between the critical care team, patient's relatives and retrieval team. The dignity, well-being and comfort of the dying patient are paramount when withdrawing treatment, and the process itself should take place in line with local critical care unit policy; there should be no difference because organ donation is being considered. This may involve stopping mechanical ventilation, vasoactive drug support or supplementary oxygen and/or removing the ETT. The process should ideally take place within the ICU. In circumstances where the ICU is too distant from theatres for NHBD to be possible, treatment withdrawal may have to take place in the theatre complex if the wishes of the patient and relatives are to be met. This should not, however, be done routinely simply to reduce the warm ischaemic time. When treatment withdrawal does occur outside an ICU, the same degree of critical care nursing expertise in the management of the dying patient should be provided. Alongside treatment withdrawal, sedative or opioid infusions may be started as appropriate.

Once a decision to withdraw treatment has been made, the instigation of new therapies (e.g. the administration of heparin or vasoactive drugs) or the undertaking of invasive interventions (e.g. vascular cannulation to allow cold perfusion) that are of no benefit to the dying patient but are introduced specifically to improve organ viability are not recommended in the UK. With agreement from the relatives, blood samples may be taken from an in-dwelling intravascular catheter for tissue typing and serology purposes.

Once treatment is withdrawn, the transplant team need to be kept informed of any prolonged periods of hypotension (SBP <50mm Hg), hypoxia (SaO_2 <80%) or anuria, allowing them to decide whether organ donation remains a viable option. If cardiorespiratory arrest has not occurred within 2–3h following treatment withdrawal, organ donation is usually abandoned.

Communication

Discussion as to the suitability of the patient as a potential NHBD should take place with the transplant coordinator before approaching the relatives. This avoids the relatives agreeing to the patient becoming an organ donor only to then find that they are not suitable. Even if concerns exist about contraindications to the patient becoming an organ donor, all potential donors should be referred, leaving the decision about suitability to the transplant team. Agreement from the coroner/procurator's fiscal should also ideally be obtained where necessary before any approach to the family. The approach to the relatives offering NHBD should only be made once they have understood and accepted the futility of the clinical situation, the futility of continued treatment and the reasons for its withdrawal. The practicalities of NHBD should be explained, including, when appropriate, the requirement for post-mortem cannulation and perfusion to maintain organ viability. It is also important to explain that:

- Death may occur quickly after treatment withdrawal and that if organ donation is to be possible the time relatives can have with their loved one at this stage is limited.
- The dying process may be prolonged and therefore organ donation may not be possible due to an unacceptably long warm ischaemic time
- Retrieved organs may not always be suitable for transplantation if perfusion has failed or they are damaged during the retrieval process
- The relatives will have a further opportunity to spend time with their loved one after organ retrieval has taken place
- The relatives can stop the donation process at any stage.

The transplant coordinator has a central role in facilitating effective communication between the critical care team, retrieval team, operating theatre staff and the relatives. They are responsible for ensuring a smooth transition from withdrawal of active treatment to confirmation of death and organ retrieval.

Confirming death using cardiorespiratory criteria

Once cardiorespiratory arrest has occurred after the withdrawal of treatment, a member of the critical care team confirms death after observing a 5min period of continuous asystole, apnoea and unconsciousness as recommended by the ethics committee of the Society of Critical Care Medicine and adopted by the Intensive Care Society's Working Group on Organ and Tissue Donation. In the ICU setting these observations should be supported by the continued use of current monitoring including ECG and IAP monitoring. Any return of cardiac or respiratory activity during this period prompts a further 5min of observation from that point. After 5min, a lack of response to supraorbital pressure and the absence of papillary and corneal reflexes are confirmed.

Management of the NHBD after death

Once death has been confirmed, the opportunity to spend a further period of time with the patient should be available to the relatives. This period should necessarily be brief, usually ~5min, in order to minimize the warm ischaemic time of organs to be transplanted. Should relatives require a longer period of time with the patient then the donation process should be reviewed and, if necessary, abandoned. Procedures such as chest compressions and full cardiopulmonary bypass designed to reduce the warm ischaemic time, but that may inadvertently restore CBF should not be instituted post-mortem. Cannulation of the femoral vessels to allow cold perfusion of the intra-abdominal organs may take place in ICU whilst awaiting an operating theatre to become available. Alternatively the patient is transferred quickly to the operating theatre for organ retrieval to be undertaken. Once the retrieval process has been completed, relatives of the patient are given the opportunity to spend a further period of time with the deceased patient if required.

Care of relatives of the NHBD

It is central to the principles of organ donation that donation be carried out to meet the wishes of the deceased and also to bring comfort to the relatives. All medical staff have a role in offering support to the relatives of the donor before, during and after the process. Some relatives may wish to be present at the time of death following treatment withdrawal, and this option should be incorporated into NHBD protocols. Pastoral care and bereavement counselling should be made available to relatives if required.

Controversies

Despite the endorsement of the practice of NHBD by professional and regulatory bodies on both sides of the Atlantic, some intensive care practitioners remain concerned about the ethics and legality of NHBD. The areas of concern revolve around reaching a decision that continued treatment is futile, the associated potential for conflict of interest in the context of NHBD, uncertainties over the time at which death can be confirmed using cardiorespiratory criteria and the possibility of the spontaneous return of cardiac function after asystole (the Lazarus phenomenon).

Further reading

A definition of irreversible coma. Report of the Ad Hoc Committee of the Havard Medical School to Examine the Definition of Brain Stem Death. *JAMA* 1968; 205: 337–40.

American College of Critical Care Medicine. Position Paper by the Ethics Committee, Recommendations for non-heart beating organ donation. *Crit Care Med* 2001; 29: 1826.

Barber K, Falvey S, Hamilton C, *et al.* Potential for organ donation in the United Kingdom: audit of intensive care records. *BMJ* 2006; 352: 1124–6.

Clayton TJ, Nelson RJ, Manara AR. Reduction in mortality from severe heads injury following introduction of a protocol for intensive care management. *Br J Anaesth* 2004; 93: 761–7.

Conference of the Medical Royal Colleges and their Faculties in the United Kingdom. Diagnosis of Brainstem Death. *Lancet* 1976; ii: 1069–70.

Death rate trends for RTA's and CVA's, WHO European Health for All Database http://www.euro.who.int/hfadb

Dobson R. Number on UK transplant waiting list reaches new high. *BMJ* 2007, 334; 920–1.

Gardiner D, Riley B. Non-heart-beating organ donation—solution or a step too far. *Anaesthesia* 2007; 62: 431 1 –3.

Kootstra G, Daemen JH, Oomen AP. Categories of non-heart beating organ donors. *Transplant Proc* 1995; 27: 2893–4.

Patel HC, Menon DK, Tebbs S, *et al.* Specialist neurocritical care and outcome from head injury. *Intensive Care Med* 2002; 28: 547–53.

Ridley S, Bonner S, Bray K, *et al.* UK guidance for non-heart beating organ donation. *Br J Anaesth* 2005; 95: 592-5.

Sque M, Long T, Payne S. Organ donation: key factors influencing families' decision making. *Transplant Proc* 2005: 37: 543.

Weber M, Dindo D, Demartines N, *et al.* Kidney transplantation from donors without a heartbeat. *N Engl J Med* 2002; 347: 248–55.

Chapter 33

ICU organization and management

Chapter contents

Consent on the ICU

Definition

Consent is the giving of permission of a person for another individual, or group, to touch them. Although, the Law Commission has said that, 'if seriously disabling injury results, we will take the view that a person, who consents to it has made a mistake and that to be really disabled is against his or her interests'. Within the confines of a doctor/patient relationship, consent provides a 'Legal flak-jacket' protecting the doctor and the rest of the medical team from the charge of assault.

Consent for treatment can be withdrawn at any stage for any reason.

Consent does not have to be written. It can be verbal or implicit. The presence of a signed consent form indicates that the process of consent may have taken place, but does not imply that it has definitely taken place.

Who can consent on behalf of a patient?

Competent adults

All adults are presumed to be able to consent or refuse consent for themselves.

- No one else can consent or refuse consent on behalf of a competent adult. As Dame Butler-Sloss said, 'A competent woman who has the capacity to decide may, for religious reasons, other reasons, for rational or irrational reasons or for no reason at all, choose not to have medical intervention, even though the consequence may be her own death'. Further, if the woman is pregnant, then the unborn child has no rights in law until it is born.
- An example of what can happen occurred to Ms B whilst she was treated on an ICU for 10 months in 2001. Ms B repeatedly expressed a wish to be allowed to die, i.e. she refused continued treatment. The treating team did not respect her wishes and she brought a case against the hospital. The hospital was held to be treating her unlawfully. The trial judge said, 'The treating clinicians and the hospital should always have in mind that a seriously physically disabled patient who is mentally competent has the same right to personal autonomy and to make decisions as any other person with mental capacity.'
- Mental Health Legislation only applies to the treatment of mental health. Specifically, a person held under the terms of the Mental Health Act, may not be treated for a physical ailment without their consent

Incompetent adults

A person with a Lasting Power of Attorney (LPA), or Welfare Attorney (WA) in Scotland, may consent or refuse consent on behalf of the individual to whom the LPA/WA applies.

The Courts may grant or withhold consent

- The majority of patients presenting in an emergency to ICU fall into this group of temporary incompetence. Studies have shown that <5% of patients on ICU have the capacity to determine their own best interests. Unless an LPA or court deputy is available, no-one can grant or withhold consent on behalf of an incapacitated adult. Medical treatment can be undertaken in an emergency even if, through a lack of capacity, no consent had been competently given, provided the treatment was a necessity and did no more than was reasonably required in the best interests of the patient. This standard, of 'best interests', will be discussed later.
- The commonly held view that the next-of-kin has an intrinsic right to grant or withhold consent is wrong.
- If the incapacitated adult does not have any family or friends available to participate in discussions, NHS bodies are required to provide an Independent Mental Capacity Advocate. This person is mandated to participate in the decision-making process in such circumstances. In this situation, the doctor is not obliged to adhere to the opinions of the Advocate, although it would be wise to document the reasons for not doing so.
- When considering treating the incapacitated adult, it must be remembered that a major focus of that treatment must be to restore the capacity of the individual, so that they can make autonomous decisions. However, psychiatric pathologies may co-exist, or be precipitated by the physical illness. In the case of Ms B, mentioned above, it was successfully argued that she lacked capacity for some months, due to a depressive illness brought on by her physical illness. Therefore, if a patient on ICU who otherwise appears to have capacity expresses unexpected wishes, it is sensible to seek psychiatric review.

Children

- A 'Gillick' competent child
- A person or local authority with parental responsibility
- The Court of Protection
  - In treating children, consent from one valid source is all that is legally required to treat the child. A child's and/or parents' refusal can be over-ridden by another valid source. However, it is good practice to discuss the treatment decision with all concerned.
  - There have been cases where the Courts have insisted on the treatment of minors against their own and their parents wishes. These are few and far between, but the absence of a child's and parents' consent does not obviate a doctor against treating that child in what the doctor perceives to be their best interests. In these circumstances it is advisable to seek a second opinion and consult with the legal services department. This illustrates the point that 'Gillick' competent children have the right to consent, but not to refuse consent.

Capacity

A person must be assumed to have capacity unless it is established that he lacks capacity. She is not to be treated as unable to make a decision unless all practicable steps to help her to do so have been taken without success. She is not to be treated as unable to make a decision merely because she makes an unwise decision. To test to see if a patient has the capacity to consent, the following tests must be applied and should be documented in the medical notes. The patient should,

- Understand the information relevant to the decision. (The fact that a person is able to retain the information relevant to a decision for a short period only does not prevent him from being regarded as able to make the decision.)
- Retain that information.

- Use or weigh that information as part of the process of making the decision.
- Communicate his decision (whether by talking, using sign language or any other means).

What matters is that the doctors should consider, whether at the time of the decision, the patient had a capacity which was commensurate with the gravity of the decision which he purported to make. The more serious the decision, the greater the capacity required.

Best interests

With regards to the incompetent patient, who lacks the requisite surrogate, the principal that applies is that of 'best interests'. Best interests are not limited to best medical interests. The doctor must consider, so far as is reasonably ascertainable

- the person's past and present wishes and feelings (and, in particular, any relevant written statement made by him when he had capacity),
- the beliefs and values that would be likely to influence his decision if he had capacity and
- any other factors that he would be likely to consider if he were able to do so.

Further, in addition to the views of an LPA or the Court, the doctor must take into account, if it is practicable and appropriate to consult them, the views of

- anyone named by the person as someone to be consulted on the matter in question or on matters of that kind,
- anyone engaged in caring for the person or interested in his welfare.

Mental Capacity Act 2005

The Act creates a statutory framework in England and Wales based in large part on the common law that has developed over the last few years. Scotland passed the Adults with Incapacity Act (Sc) in 2001 which makes similar provisions. With respect to intensive care medicine, it has enabled

- Adults to appoint another individual as LPA. The LPA can make decisions on their behalf if they become incapacitated. The LPA document has to be signed in advance of the time the patient becomes incapacitated and has to state specifically that the LPA has powers to make healthcare decisions.
- The courts to appoint a deputy with similar powers to an LPA
- A requirement for NHS bodies to appoint an independent Mental Capacity Advocate to represent their interests, when there is no-one appropriate to represent their interests
- Statutory rules and safeguards on advance directives
- New criteria and safeguards for research involving incapacitated adults
- A new criminal offence of neglect
- The Court of Protection

Further reading

Mental Capacity Act 2005, http://www.opsi.gov.uk/acts/acts2005/20050009.htm

Mental Health Act 1983. Law Commission Consultation Paper No. 139

Re MB (Medical Treatment). [1997] 2 FLR 426

In re C (Adult: Refusal of Treatment). [1994] 1 WLR 290

In re T (Adult: Refusal of Treatment). [1993] Fam. 95

St George's Healthcare NHS Trust v S. [1998] 3 All ER 673

Ms B v An NHS Hospital Trust. [2002] WL 347038

Rationing in critical care

In the USA, 40% of health expenditure is spent in the last month of the patient's life, which amounts to ~1.5% of the GDP of the USA. At the pinnacle of high tech medicine is the critical care unit. It is hardly news that a limitation of healthcare expenditure coupled with temporary or permanent demand excess leads to an imbalance between available resources and expenditure. This imbalance has led to providers seeking to 'contain costs' in a wide variety of disciplines in medicine. In the UK, the use of the R word (Rationing) in conjunction with healthcare is politically and sociologically problematical, conjuring up images of the post-war period of austerity and conflicting with the concept of free access from cradle to the grave healthcare. It is, however, self-evident that those resources are not infinite. Coupling this fact with rising expectations amongst patients and increasing costs in critical care leads to a conflict between expressed needs and our ability to meet them. The ensuing balancing act may have untoward consequences; a systematic review of rationing of critical care beds in the UK has shown that people die that otherwise might have lived. For the most part, choosing between competing patients is often a matter of logistics as alternative arrangements can often be made. Notwithstanding that, at the bedrock of rationing and discussion thereof is the question that is health or life itself so special that we should improves its quality or longevity at any cost? This chapter examines the ethical and economic principles behind rationing in critical care.

Terminology—economics

In all but a perfect situation of unlimited supply of healthcare goods, every healthcare decision involves an economic trade-off. If supply of health goods is limited and demand (i.e. health needs) is not, then any decision of resource allocation is one of rationing. This maxim is true of any economic decision; an allocation of health dollars to one area inevitably involves a reduction in expenditure, current or future, in another area. As well as the cost of treating patient X, such allocation involves a cost of not treating patient Y or perhaps restricting the treatment of patient Y; this is the ***opportunity cost*** of treating patient X, or building hospital X. Decisions made about resource allocation may be related to hospitals or Primary Care Trusts, regionally or nationally; these may be considered as ***Macro*** economic decisions. Decisions may also be made about individual patients or patient groups when they can be described as **Micro** economic decisions. Rationing for a specific patient has also been described as ***bedside rationing***. It has been suggested that for bedside rationing to occur three conditions are met; doctors should have control over the use a beneficial service which they withdraw or withhold and that in so doing they act in the interests of someone other than the patient.

Decisions made about rationing healthcare often use ***cost-effective analysis*** (CEA). CEA is a methodology of maximizing health benefits within a given budget. At its simplest, it examines how a moderately expensive treatment bringing large benefits compares with a moderately expensive treatment bringing moderate benefits. Such analysis also uses concepts such as the ***quality-adjusted life year***, the QALY approach looks at cost-effectiveness aggregated over time to produce an integer—a quality-adjusted life year—with which to compare different healthcare interventions. In such an approach, the health needs of individuals do not determine benefit, merely the outcome of treatment. If we accept that expenditure is limited, CEA and QALY analysis may give us a means of deciding where to allocate resources and when it would be appropriate to stop. A much quoted example is the cost of increasing the number of faecal occult blood tests per patient in screening for colon cancer in the USA; extending the screening to six from five tests saves a year of life but at the cost of $26m, compared with $810 for mammography for women >50yrs.

Terminology—ethics

Any discussion of rationing must inevitably involve ethical principles. Deciding what ought to be done involves using principles of ethics or moral philosophy. Allocating resources may involve the use of ***utilitarian principles*** as mentioned in CEA analysis above, where resources are used to maximize the benefit for the greatest number of patients. Utilitarianism in this context articulates an important concept, that of **consequentialism**. That it is the consequences of actions that matter. When looking at rationing decisions using consequentialism, everybody counts equally. However, a pure utilitarian system may not necessarily produce a 'fair' result for an individual, indeed a rigid utilitarian might argue that it is right to harvest organs from one living person to save the lives of many others. This would clearly be unacceptable and to most people morally wrong.

Alternatively, resources may be allocated equally to all regardless of expressed need as in ***an egalitarian*** system, or the resources may be allocated in response to ***expressed health needs or capacity to benefit.*** Defining need, however, is complex; a critically sick patient with a very poor prognosis will still have healthcare needs. Using a concept of capacity to benefit raises the issue of unmeetable needs. If a healthcare need cannot be met,then it may be argued that there is no moral obligation to provide healthcare. This has particular resonance for critical care; using resources to attempt to meet an unmeetable need might be unethical.

Of particular recent popularity is the concept of the four principles of medical ethics:

- ***Autonomy*** (self-rule)—in the critical care setting most patients' autonomy is significantly impaired if not absent.
- ***Beneficence or doing good*** implies promoting what is best for the patient.
- ***Non-maleficence***—not doing harm, seems fairly straightforward as in the clinical setting most doctors strive to avoid harm. Avoiding harm at all costs, the old adage *primum non-nocere*, is impossible in practically all healthcare settings as all treatments have some associated risk. In the critical care setting, the concept of harm vs benefit may be more finely balanced.
- ***Justice*** or fairness forms the fourth principle. In critical care we are concerned both with fairness, which mandates that similar patients get equal access to healthcare, but also more with ***distributive justice***, i.e. fair allocation of resources. In the latter context, we are concerned with the effect of resource usage on other or future patients.

The American Thoracic Society has articulated this concept well, 'Marginally beneficial intensive care may be justifiably limited on the basis of societal consensus that its cost is too high in relation to the value of its outcome ... extraordinary expenditures of resources for marginal gains unfairly compromise the availability of a basic minimum level of health care services for all'.

Rationing decisions

Making difficult decisions that affect patients' lives is a day-to-day activity in critical care. Decisions as to triage, and withholding and withdrawing active treatment all involve some degree of resource allocation whether directly or indirectly. Interestingly critical care providers seem reticent to allocate resources purely on the basis of maximizing benefit. This may be in part due to the rule of rescue. Within Western societies there is a powerful sense of a 'rule of rescue', which obliges us to throw a rope to a drowning man for example. Rescuing a lone sailor from the Southern Ocean at immense expense would go against a utilitarian calculus but would certainly fit in with concepts of virtue, solidarity and duty. There is enormous symbolic and rhetorical force from rescuing identified persons or treating named patients in peril, but allocating resources to the sickest patient may not maximize outcomes. How can such decisions be made when none of the theories will give us an answer? Daniels has specified four conditions to implement what is described as ' accountability for reasonableness' in resource allocation;

- decisions should be publicly accessible
- the rationales should aim to provide a reasonable construal of how the organization should provide healthcare in terms of value for money
- there should be a mechanism for appeal
- there should be some enforcement procedure to ensure such conditions are met.

None of these conditions is easy to meet, not least in the charged atmosphere of a critical care unit. However, it seems reasonable to ask that clinicians consider rationing services that bring marginal benefit at great cost. CEA may guide us in concert with ethical theories to making good decisions, but there may be an innate tension between concepts of beneficence and cost-effectiveness values. Our shared normative values determine the sort of healthcare we provide and to whom we provide it. Doing well, albeit at times inefficiently in cost terms, may have a significant societal value.

Further reading

ATS Bioethics Task Force. Fair allocation of intensive care unit resources. *Am J Respir Crit Care Med* 1997; 156: 1282–301.

Daniels N. Accountability for reasonableness in private and public health insurance. In: Coulter A, Ham C, eds. The global challenge of health care rationing. Buckingham: Oxford University Press, 2000: 89–106.

Halpern NA, Pastores SM, Greenstein RJ. Critical care medicine in the United States 1985–2000: an analysis of bed numbers, use, and costs. *Crit Care Med* 2004; 32: 1254–9.

Sinuff T, Kahnamoui K, Cook DJ, *et al.* Rationing critical care beds: a systematic review. *Crit Care Med* 2004; 32: 1588–97.

Society of Critical Care Medicine. Attitudes of critical care medicine professionals concerning distribution of intensive care resources *Crit Care Med* 1994; 22: 358–62.

Tengs TO, Adams ME, Pliskin JS, *et al.* Five hundred life saving interventions and their cost effectiveness. *Risk Analysis* 1995; 15: 1-30

Ubel P. Pricing life. Cambridge, MA, MIT Press, 2001.

ICU layout

In the UK, critically ill patients are now regarded as Level 2 (HDU) or Level 3 (ICU) in the critical illness dependency spectrum. It is recognized that levels of dependency change rapidly, requiring facilities to be flexible and cope with changing demand. Most hospitals operate critical care facilities that admit both Level 2 and 3 patients, and the layout of the unit must reflect this. Design has become more patient focused, with attention to environmental aspects such as light, noise and space. The needs of relatives and families are incorporated to a greater extent.

General principles

Core requirements in the design of quality critical care facilities include:

- Fitness for purpose
- Preserving patient privacy and dignity
- Good infection control practices
- Security
- Health and safety requirements
- A quality patient environment
- A welcoming environment for visitors

ICU location

The location of the critical care unit in proximity to certain services is vital. Key adjacencies are the A&E department, operating theatres, diagnostic imaging (especially CT scanning) and acute wards. Patient 'journeys' from these locations should be as short as possible. Only some services can be co-located on the same floor, but other key adjacencies should be planned such that vertical transfers, via a lift, are as direct as possible. Routes between key areas should not involve more than one lift transfer. This may be avoided by detailed planning of patient journeys through the hospital, and location of services accordingly.

How many beds?

The UK critical care beds make up ~1–1.5% of the total bed numbers in most hospitals, or <1 bed/10 000 population. This proportion has increased in recent years and is likely to continue doing so with increased levels of acuity and demand. In the USA and many European countries, a far greater proportion of hospital beds are provided in critical care facilities (USA >4 beds/10 000 population).

Multi-bed areas or single rooms?

Ideally, every patient should be cared for in a single room to help maintain the patient's privacy and dignity and reduce risks of cross-infection. This is seldom a realistic option with the numbers of staff required to care safely for patients in such facilities. Most published guidance recommends increasing the proportion of single rooms, which are often in short supply. Current guidance in the UK recommends that 30–50% of bed space allocation in general critical care units should be single rooms, though many do not yet meet this standard. All single rooms should have a lobby, allowing them to function as isolation facilities. Paediatric patients admitted to adult ICU require single rooms.

Isolation facilities

All single rooms should be able to function as true isolation facilities, for either source or protective isolation. Single rooms should be provided with a lobby for hand washing, and gloving and gowning, which functions as an airlock. The ventilation system to allow isolation may be switchable positive or negative pressure ventilation, or a balanced supply and extract ventilation system that provides a 'constant' system of ventilation without the requirement to switch between pressure systems. Ventilation should be filtered by HEPA filters to prevent the spread of airborne pathogens

Bed space layout

Bed space layout, whether in multi-bed areas or single rooms, is designed to allow bed areas to 'flex' and accommodate any patient, from the lowest to the highest level of acuity. Patients may then be cared for in any bed space. With this in mind, most critical care bed space layouts now follow a generic template, replicated in each bed space

Bed space size

With increased acuity, bed spaces have increased in size. Current recommendations are that each bed space should have a floor area of at least $26m^2$ to allow sufficient space for equipment and clinical activity around the patient's bed and adequate space between each patient. In multi-bed areas, there should be a further unobstructed 2.5m of corridor space beyond the clinical area.

Bedside medical services

Traditionally, medical services such as piped gases, electricity, suction, etc. have been supplied at the patient's bed head via wall-mounted outlets. This restricts access to the patient's head, limits the flexibility to turn beds (e.g. to allow a conscious patient to face a window) and reduces available window area. Most ICUs are now adopting ceiling-mounted pendant service delivery. The most versatile solutions are double-articulated twin pendant systems that allow for separation of 'wet' and 'dry' services if required, and offer the flexibility to turn a patient's bed through 90–180° without compromising access or the delivery of care. While local requirements may differ, as a rule, each bed space will require the provision of at least:

- 28 power points, protected by a UPS (uninterruptable power system)
- Multi-parameter monitoring
- Infusion and syringe pumps
- At least two vacuum points
- At least two 4-bar oxygen outlets
- Two 4-bar air outlets
- Ventilation and humidification equipment
- Examination lamp

Additional services, such as a gas-scavenging system as well as sockets for television, telephone and nurse call, may be required at all bed spaces.

Bed areas should be rectangular in shape to maximize the utility of the clinical space provided. Each bed space must have a clinical hand wash basin sited at the foot of the bed and provision for the storage of drugs and supplies locally (see below). The layout of each bed area should follow a generic template that is designed to facilitate clinical care, patient comfort and good infection control practice. Published guidance has suggested generic layouts that are tried and tested.

At each bed space, there needs to be provision for charting and notes, which will be via a computer terminal accessing the electronic patient record.

Infection control

Good infection control practices are facilitated by good clinical design. Hospital infection control teams should be represented on project teams planning new facilities.

Adequate bed space separation (see above) is critical, as is the provision of clinical hand wash basins, gloves, aprons, etc. at the foot of the bed (on entry to the clinical area). Air conditioning should be zonal. Furnishings and fittings must be easy to clean. Horizontal surfaces in the bed area should be kept to a minimum as they harbour dust containing resistant organisms. While recognizing the need to keep equipment at the bedside, large quantities of disposables may hamper adequate cleaning. Small regularly re-stocked trolleys are a better solution than large quantities of bedside storage. Screening between beds may be better achieved by portable screens that can be wiped clean, rather than curtains and curtain rails which attract dust and are difficult to keep clean. Computer keyboards should be protected with plastic covers that are cleaned daily and disposed of when a patient is discharged.

Environmental conditions

It is accepted that a pleasant and appealing environment is of benefit to staff and patients alike. Critically ill patients benefit from the provision of natural light and the opportunities for views of nature. Full-length windows should be provided wherever possible, with due consideration given to the problems of glare and solar gain as well as privacy. Consideration must be given to noise reduction strategies.

Ventilation

All clinical areas should be fully air conditioned and provided with temperature and humidity control, the former being adjustable locally between the ranges of 16 and 27°C. Humidity should be controlled within the range 40–60% relative humidity. The frequency of air changes required to achieve environmental control will vary depending on unit design and size. Single rooms should comply with published standards for isolation facilities in this regard (usually a minimum of 12 air changes per hour).

Lighting

Bed spaces should be illuminated by luminaires above the bed. Luminaires should be individually controllable by dimmer switches to adjust illumination from low level night lighting to at least 400–600lux for clinical procedures. Additional lighting should be provided in the general circulation space and support accommodation, which should also be dimmable, such that safe low level lighting can be provided at night.

Clinical support accommodation

Staff base

A central staff communications base should have an unobstructed view of the clinical area. The base fulfils many functions and needs provision for computer terminals, radiology image viewing and telecommunications. It is busy and noisy, and consideration should be given to reducing noise transmission, e.g. by glazed screening.

Clean utility

Provides for preparation of trolleys for clinical procedures and for storage of sterile supplies. It should be readily accessible from all bed spaces and the central communications base. It may function as the drug storage and preparation area, or this may be provided separately. Clinical hand wash facilities are required.

Dirty utility

Provides for disposal of bedpans and other waste fluids and consumables. It should be sited near the clinical area. Clean disposables should not be stored here. Unit design and operational policy should ensure one-way flow from clean utility, to patient, to dirty utility. Contaminated equipment may also be held, pending cleaning.

Laboratory

Blood gas analysis and an increasing array of near-patient testing equipment is required and best sited in a dedicated area with a clinical hand wash basin and adequate storage space for reagents, specimens and gas cylinders. Space is required for use of computer equipment.

Other support areas required are equipment servicing/technicians room; clinical equipment store (haemodialysis, ventilators, monitoring, etc.); linen storage; disposal hold; and medical gas cylinder storage. The volume of consumables stored within a critical care area may be reduced by efficient 'just in time' material supply systems. There is rarely enough storage space for clinical equipment! Well planned support accommodation enhances the operational efficiency of the critical care unit and improves the working environment for staff.

Facilities for visitors

Sitting rooms should be comfortable and welcoming. They must be of sufficient size to accommodate groups of families who may spend many hours there. Security controls should prevent unauthorized access to any clinical area, but there should be means of communication with the clinical area. Separate interview rooms should be provided for breaking bad news and private discussions. In surveys, the poor quality of relatives' facilities is frequently noted and is unacceptable.

Facilities for staff

There should be provision of staff changing facilities, including showers. Staff rest rooms should allow space for staff to relax, prepare food and eat, and should receive natural daylight. On-call facilities may be required. Office accommodation and supporting interview space are best provided in an area adjacent to, but separate from, the clinical area. Some education and training facilities should be provided within the critical care complex, though larger groups may require the use of central facilities elsewhere within the hospital.

Further reading

HBN 57. Facilities for critical care. London: NHS Estates, The Stationary Office, 2003.

Medical staffing in critical care

Background

Over the last 3 decades, ICUs have worked through an evolutionary process that has transformed their role in hospital services. Once regarded as enigmatic, isolated, and intimidating 'end of corridor' areas into which many patients were perceived to be admitted on a 'one-way' journey, ICU services have become an established core of acute patient care infrastructures, with quality patient care now being increasingly dependent on critical care support. In many units that have driven this change in status, high levels of consultant presence and supervision have played a key role in developing cohesive working relationships with other specialities, as well as in improving patient outcomes. Strong commitments to education and training programmes, many of which have been developed locally to enhance trainee recruitment, have also been very significant.

Consultant input to patient care has evolved considerably. On-call rotas of 'one in two' or 'one in three' were accepted as an inevitable consequence of signing up to intensive care as a consultant specialist, often with insistence that they must be informed of all admissions irrespective of whether they were 'on-call' or not! With hindsight such dedicated attention to continuity may be viewed as bordering on the 'obsessive compulsive', but the reality is that the establishment of high standards in critical care was a crucial part of an essential development pathway; once these became accepted as the 'norm', even the most reluctant employers could not escape the fact that it was unreasonable to expect them to be maintained by a small number of consultants working excessively long hours. Consequently, consultant staffing has steadily increased to more acceptable levels in many units, with the European Working Time Directive and the New Consultant Contract having added strength to the case for this trend.

Despite this progress, there is undoubtedly still a wide range of variation in staffing structures and medical presence on ICUs. Anecdotal reports still suggest that in some units supervision of care of the critically ill patients is still shared with other responsibilities such as anaesthesia on-call, and that middle grade trainees may also be required to provide concurrent cover for both critical care and anaesthesia services. Such systems are likely to increase the risks to patients and also increase vulnerability of staff to professional criticism or even litigation if an adverse event occurs because of lack of immediate medical expertise when required. Although the NCEPOD report into emergency admissions to critical care led to an erroneous perception that delayed referrals tended to occur as a result of failures of intensive care systems, the time intervals to consultant review of patients admitted to ICUs also led to a number of relevant questions being raised about consultant staffing and availability. The developing new pathways for common stem training in acute care are also dependent on high levels of consultant input to critical care components. The inevitable conclusion therefore reached by many was that formalized standards for ICU medical staffing were overdue, leading to their joint production by the Intensive Care Society (ICS) and the Intercollegiate Board for Training in Intensive Care Medicine (IBTICM).

Setting the standards

Previous attempts have been made to develop standards for medical staffing in ICUs. In 1984, the ICS produced the first UK document, but its recommendations were necessarily limited by many organizational issues and the wide range of differing clinical practices throughout the country. The Faculty of Intensive Care of the Australasian and New Zealand College of Anaesthetists also produced standards for medical staffing, but these were limited to a degree by the need to incorporate both large centralized units (where full-time intensivists were an increasingly established normality) and small, rural-sited ones which were predominantly dependent on anaesthetic services.

The Medical Staffing Standards document is based upon the principle that critical care services should be delivered by appropriately and fully trained staff, but recognizes that deficiencies in consultant numbers will limit the time scale. It also recognizes that differing levels of consultant expertise and availability have to be supported depending on the size of the unit and the proportion of their clinical work that is committed to critical care, and defines training requirements on this basis.

Table 33.4.1 Summary of staffing standards

All newly appointed consultants with programmed activities (PAs) in intensive care medicine (ICM) should have acquired Step 1 competences, or an equivalent level of training.
All newly appointed consultants with >50% commitment to ICM should have acquired Step 2 competences, a CCT in ICM, or an equivalent.
All units must have a minimum of 15 PAs of consultant time committed to ICM each week per 8 Level 3 beds.
All consultants providing an 'on-call' service to the ICU must have PAs committed to ICM.
Consultants should not have any other clinical commitment when covering the ICU during daytime hours.
During working hours, the consultant in charge of the ICU should spend the majority of his or her time on the ICU and must always be immediately available on the ICU.
There must be 24h ICU cover by a named consultant with appropriate experience and competences.
A consultant in ICM must see all admissions to the ICU within 12h.

The document sets out standards for consultant staffing structure of critical care units, based on recommendations learned from the evolutionary process and from those who have worked through different methods of medical input. Although these may be viewed as challenging (or even unrealistic) by some units, it is recommended that for those that fall significantly short of achieving them they should be regarded as a lever that will assist in the process of increasing consultant staffing and improving quality of care. They will also help units to work towards supporting many of the other quality and patient safety initiatives currently being developed by organizations such as NICE, the National Patient Safety Agency, the ICS and the Paediatric Intensive Care Society.

Clinical management

Information from a number of sources, including the ICS, the Intensive Care National Audit and Research Centre (ICNARC), the Critical Care Patient Liaison Group (CritPal) and NCEPOD support anecdotal reports of wide variations in clinical practice and supervision of patient care throughout the UK. To improve consistency and upgrade quality of care where deficiencies exist, the Standards document logically outlines minimum recommendations for clinical management and care infrastructures that are based on existing best practice. These include requirements that:

- A medical practitioner of appropriate experience and training must normally be present on the unit at all times.
- There should be a minimum of two, and preferably three, ICU rounds every day at which a consultant is present (except if the round has been specifically delegated to a senior trainee for training purposes)
- There must be continuity of care in the consultant cover of the ICU, best achieved by a consultant managing the unit for a period of several days at a time.
- Sufficient time must be allowed in consultant job plans for effective handover of unit responsibilities.
- The number of beds managed by one consultant must be carefully considered and will depend on the number of other partly qualified staff available.
- All admissions/refused admissions must be discussed with the duty ICU consultant and management plans agreed.

Trainee staffing and training recommendations

Training in critical care medicine is undergoing a period of relatively rapid change as a result of the recommendations of the IBTICM, minimum critical care training requirements for anaesthesia and the recommendations for the Postgraduate Medical Education and Training Board (PMETB). Trainee staff numbers will vary according to the size of units, rotational arrangements, the availability of fixed-term specialist training attachments (FTSTAs) and the preservation (and longer term viability) of independent 'fellow' or 'middle grade' posts locally. However, there is increasing recognition that in addition to the competency-based assessments that are a key component of training requirements, there are other basic requirements for all staff working in critical care. These include;

- A documented induction programme for all new staff (medical, nursing and allied health professionals)
- Incremental training programmes for all staff
- Allocated time for training and assessments for speciality-specific and generic mandatory training programmes
- Access to online resources and appropriate e-learning packages

The evolution of the acute care common stem (ACCS) training programmes should lead to more consistent and better organized training for future trainees in critical care, and the associated rotational training programmes are likely to increase the numbers of trainees working in ICUs which have training approval. Trainee presence will also be dependent on the proportion of those wishing to undertake specialist training in critical care medicine to either Step 1 or Step 2 levels and the number of posts that can be supported by the unit levels of activity.

The role of trainees in critical care units is also evolving; historically, many ICUs were dependent on the presence of an anaesthetic middle grade trainee for 'round the clock' cover; such individuals often shared responsibility for intensive care patients with other commitments such as being 'second on-call' for anaesthesia or obstetric anaesthetics. In recent years many larger units have overcome the associated conflicts of such systems by creating dedicated critical care 'fellow' or 'middle grade' posts—often integrated with anaesthesia, Emergency Department or acute medicine training programmes—to ensure that there is 24h presence and support of individuals with appropriate skill levels. For such trainees, a careful balance between clinical responsibilities, training provision and consultant supervision/availability has been essential, and will become even more important as the skill mix of middle grade trainees from differing clinical backgrounds evolve.

Variations in local preferences may see a trend towards developing critical care practitioners or nurse-specialists who may undertake greater clinical responsibilities. There are also some who advocate that consultant staffing levels and rotas should be developed to provide 24h resident consultant cover. Although there may be theoretical benefits of such systems, the implications for the development of trainee independence and for future speciality recruitment also have to be taken into consideration, and there is no current consensus on the wider benefits of a resident consultant programme.

The role of clinical academics who specialize in critical care medicine is also changing, with refinements in job planning being required to ensure that valuable contributions made to both clinical and research activities are not eroded by speciality evolution. The importance of maintaining clinical academic posts within critical care units and training programmes is highlighted in the Medical Staffing Standards document. The document also recognizes that however sensible and desirable the recommended standards may be, in the continuously changing environment of the NHS it is unrealistic to expect these all to be achieved in the immediate future. Accordingly, a timetable for the implementation of these standards, which should be applicable to all units which provide care for Level 2 and Level 3 critical care patients, has been included.

The full version of the ICS/IBTICM Standards for Medical Staffing document is available on the Intensive Care Society website.

Further reading

FFANZCA. Minimum standards for intensive care units. `http://www.anzca.edu.au/jficm/resources/policy/icl_2003.pdf`

ICS. Standards for consultant staffing of intensive care units `http://www.ics.ac.uk/icmprof/`

Kmietowicz Z. Many trusts fail to monitor whether complaints have any effect, says watchdog. *BMJ* 2007; 335: 738–9.

National Confidential Enquiry into Patient Outcome and Death NCEPOD paper. http://www.ncepod.org.uk and `http://www.ncepod.org.uk/2005.htm` and `http://www.ncepod.org.uk/2007.htm`

ICU staffing: nursing

Volumes have been written about the provision of nursing care to the critically ill over the years. Nursing Managers have experienced financial glut, belt-tightening, the introduction of workload measurement systems, shortages of nurses, foreign recruitment and, most recently, Payment By Results. Hospital beds have decreased in numbers and patient LOS has shortened, compressing the acute/high intervention period of patients' hospitalization. Tensions have been created within critical care as the staffing expenditure comes under ever-increasing scrutiny.

Table 33.5.1 Competing factors affecting the provision and cost of critical care nursing staffing

Forces driving increased need for critical care beds and nursing	Forces opposing current staffing patterns
Technology	Payment by Results
Increased ageing population	Caps on spending/reduction of critical care budgets
Diagnostic-related groups and shortened LOS	Nursing shortage
Rapid interventions and improved pre-hospital care	Rising health care costs
Compressed acuity	Litigious society
Increased complexity of patient care	

Workload and acuity measurement systems

Current research

A large number of different systems have been set up to assess the amount and type of care required by the critically ill. Some quantify the amount of care required as a result of required medical interventions: APACHE II, TISS, SAPSII, GRASP, SOPRA and the recent AUKUH Adult Acuity and Dependency Measurement Tool. The patient classification systems ICU nurses are currently using lack precision and do not accurately quantify the amount and type of care required by patients. They fail to include indirect nursing activity, skill mix, the knowledge and skill required for competent and expert practice, and unit geography.

Nonetheless, some investigators are examining the relationships between nursing workload and clinical severity. Clinical severity as measured by APACHE II was found to explain 25.6% of the daily variability of nursing workload measured by PRN Rea. In a study of 99 ICUs in 15 countries, investigators were able to add 5 new items and 15 subitems describing nursing activities in the ICU. This new system is the Nursing Activity Score (NAS) and explains 81% of nursing time as compared with 43% with TISS-28. Another study attempted to validate a new Intensive Care Nursing Scoring System (ICNSS) by comparing it with TISS-28 as a predictor of mortality. The ICNSS demonstrated higher scores for patients undergoing emergency treatment than electively operated patients. Encouragingly, the ICNSS included care of relatives in the 16 variables. This single-centre study requires replication, paying particular attention to the growing number of ICUs where nurses work 12h shifts.

Comprehensive critical care suggests appropriate levels of care based on patient requirement for organ support. The report also recommends that critical care be considered a process rather than a place, and that care is provided as a continuum. Interpretation of this report has led to many organizations equating Level 3 care with intensive care, Level 2 care with high dependency care, and then a further assumption that Level 3 care should be based on 1:1 nursing ratios and Level 2 care based on 1:1.6 or 1:2 care. These assumptions become very problematic for clinical staff when patients require increased supervision when showing signs of agitation or delirium, or are recovering from acute head injury, and require high levels of expert nursing supervision.

It should be noted that there are variations in staffing skill mix when comparing urban and rural hospital/critical care settings. The nursing workforce tends to move to large cities early on in their clinical careers, for training and experience. Later there is a tendency to move away from large urban centres, and they often become more established in smaller centres as 'career staff nurses'. They comprise a stable workforce with differing impact on recruitment, retention and training needs. Nursing establishments may therefore be constructed to reflect this stable workforce.

International perspective

Critical care nursing varies from country to country, and this, too, must be taken into account when establishing nurse:patient ratios. In North America, skilled practitioners such as Respiratory Therapists add to the total complement of carers. In some European countries, nurse patient ratios of 1:2 exist, but the complement of medical practitioners is higher than in the UK. In the UK, nursing roles have expanded over time, taking on expert roles in communication, management and organization of patient care. Such national variations also mandate caution when comparing nursing establishments directly with other countries. There is also variation in the definition and staffing of ICUs. The UK had the smallest percentage of critical care beds (2.6%) per total hospital beds of any country in Europe, but also has the highest number of nurses per bed, the third highest use of mechanical ventilation (55%) during the first 24h, and a higher mean SAPS II score than other countries. Driving forces vary. In the state of California, public and nursing concern about safe care in acute hospitals resulted in the California Department of Health Services being directed to establish nurse-to-patient staffing ratios by January 2002.

Future directions for the establishment of appropriate nursing staffing levels

In a major departure from validation of nursing workload measure, Ball and McElligot conducted a study to make evident the complexity of issues associated with the delivery of care by nurses to the critically ill. Their analysis demonstrated that an effective nursing resource was dependent on knowledge, experience and exposure. The unit geography, case mix, activity level and skill mix also had a significant effect on the ability of the nurses to contribute to the recovery of critically ill patients. They devised a model which demonstrated the factors that optimized or compromised nursing care and its impact on patient progression and recovery, and concluded that

> 'the need to develop a valid and reliable tool which addresses patients' needs for nursing in terms of nurses' knowledge and experience, patient dependency and decreasing clinical risk across the continuum of care. Current nursing workload tools and patient:nurse ratios were seen to lack validity because they do not appraise the context in which the care is delivered, define all nurses as equal and concentrate on activity rather than the effect nurses can have on the outcomes of the critically ill. (Ball and McElligot, 2003, 226–7)

This has effectively moved the focus of nursing staffing levels from the activities "done" to patients to the outcomes of skilled nursing care. Further work must be undertaken to establish a patient dependency tool that addresses patients' need for nursing tools or formulae developed for ICUs, taking into account their specific patient types and geographical set ups. In addition, the prevention of risks to patients must be made explicit, when developing unit-specific staffing establishments. Clinical risks such as accidental extubation, nosocomial infection rates, complications, re-admission rates and medication errors have been associated with reduced nurse:patient ratios. The American Association of Critical Care Nurses' Synergy Model for Patient Care was developed to create a match between patients' need for care and nurses' competency to provide such care. Study of this model in the context of UK critical care may assist with the process of objective, measurable consumption of the nursing resource.

The role of non-qualified staff in intensive care units—healthcare asssitants (HCAs)

The British Association of Critical Care Nurses (BACCN) has developed key points for action reflecting the current evidence to support the use of non-qualified staff in ICUs. Significant issues identified are contained within Table 33.5.2.

Table 33.5.2 BACCN position statement on the role of HCAs.

Must benefit patient care
Need for a designated coordinator for training and role development
Registered Nurses assess, plan and evaluate direct patient care activities
Healthcare assistants (HCAs) must be trained and assessed by a qualified practitioner
HCAs must work under the supervision of a qualified practitioner
HCAs must work within a competency framework
Work should be undertaken to establish national competencies
A national database of education and training for HCAs should be developed.

Clearly there is much work to be done in order to prevent risks to patients, increased workload for individual Registered Nurses who are supervising HCAs, and job dissatisfaction for Registered Nurses who may believe that they are not providing quality care.

Making the best use of current establishments

ICUs vary greatly in size, complexity and case mix. It is logical, therefore, to expect that staff roles and work patterns will also vary. For example, a Cardiothoracic ICU in a Teaching Hospital with a predominance of elective cases and few emergency cases will have a much more predictable workload and therefore staffing pattern than will a general ICU in a large urban setting which deals with trauma, neurosciences and a busy Emergency Department. A general ICU in a District General Hospital will similarly have a different mix of elective and emergency patients. Recognizing these patterns is key to utilizing staff efficiently. The Intensive Care National Audit and Research Centre (ICNARC) provides data that can be invaluable in describing individual ICU work patterns. It is then possible to develop staff roles and work patterns/rosters that address the needs of patients in individual units (see Table 33.5.3)

In conclusion, nursing staffing has never been in a more dynamic situation. Health budgets are strenuously pushing for efficiencies, patients in acute hospitals have higher than ever acuity, and patients are demanding a better hospital experience. This is fertile ground for research which, by demonstrating the relationship of nursing to patient outcome, will help ensure nursing leaders are utilizing the nursing resource appropriately.

Further reading

Adomat R, Hewison A. Assessing patient category/dependence systems for determining the nurse/patient ratio in ICU and HDU: a review of approaches, *J Nurs Manag* 2004;12: 299–308.

Ball C, McElligot M. Realising the potential of critical care nurses: an exploratory study of the factors that affect and comprise the nursing contribution to the recovery of critically ill patients. *Intensive Crit Care Nurs* 2003; 19: 226–38.

British Association of Critical Care Nurses. Position Statement on nurse–patient ratios in critical care, BACCN Working Party, 2000.

British Association of Critical Care Nurses. Position Statement on the role of health care assistants who are involved in direct patient care activities within critical care areas, BACCN Working Party, 2002.

Kiekkas P, Brokalaki H, Manolis E, *et al.* Patient severity as an indicator of nursing workload in the intensive care unit. *Nurs Crit Care* 2007; 12: 34–41.

Tarnow-Mordi, WO, Hau C, Warden A, *et al.* Hospital mortality in relation to staff workload: a 4-year study in an adult intensive-care unit, *Lancet* 2000; 356: 185–9.

www.dh.gov.uk/en/Policyandguidance/Organisationpolicy/Financeandplanning/NHSFinancialReforms

Table 35.5.3 Factors to consider when constructing duty rosters

Rostering elements	Influencing factors
Establishment size	Is this reviewed yearly against patient care activity?
	Do nurses and finance managers review activity on a yearly basis?
Establishment skill mix	How stable is the staff group?
	What are their requirements for development?
	How much supervision of staff is required?
	Does patient acuity require senior staff on duty 24/7?
	Are senior nursing staff allocated management time? How much?
Day/night activities	High percentage of emergency patients and unpredictable workload will influence the need for equal numbers of staff on all shifts, all week
	Predictable workload may allow for fewer staff on nights and weekends
Annual leave	Agenda for Change allows for varying amounts of annual leave based on time worked in the NHS; have individual unit budgets been adjusted for this?
	Are staff asked to take annual leave in equal amounts across the entire year in order to avoid periods of short staffing?
Education and training	Do staffing budgets account for time spent in mandatory training? Is this time re-assessed each budget year?
	Are there new programmes (e.g. CRS) which require additional training?
	Has the Trust policy for study leave been accounted for in the allowance for study leave in individual unit budgets?
Staff input	Are staff involved in roster patterns such as fixed rosters, self-rostering, writing rosters?
	Do staff work flexibly?
	Does unit management work flexibly?
Part-time staff	Are family friendly policies in place?
	Balance between staff convenience and unit need
Absence management	Is there an absence management programme in place to improve attendance?
Managing staffing shortage during periods of high activity	Is there a system in place to obtain short-term help from unit staff, e.g. Cable/bank/on-call system?
	If temporary staff are required, are the agencies able to meet the need with appropriately trained/skilled staff?
Monitoring staff utilization	Are there systems in place (paper or electronic) to capture staff utilization, e.g. number of hours of 'bought' time, number of hours of all 'losses'

ICU staffing: supporting professions

Whilst the medical and nursing professions make up the bulk of the workforce, a variety of other professions are routinely integrated into critical care practice, bringing different sets of skills, perspectives and knowledge to the multi-disciplinary team for the benefit of patients. The following is a summary of roles and staffing levels.

Clinical pharmacist

Role

Clinical pharmacists optimize drug therapy, improve patient outcomes and reduce costs in critical care. This is achieved through a variety of activities, ranging from the drawing up of clinical guidelines, provision of general advice and teaching in drug utilization as well as through individualizing drug therapy to maximize benefits and reduce risks to patients. Pharmacists take into account side effects, interactions, pharmacokinetics (particularly with organ failures or artificial organ support), pharmacodynamics, available routes of administration, drug compatibilities, cost-effectiveness, allergies, drug history and a host of other factors on a policy or individual patient basis.

A career structure and comprehensive competency framework is available to inform critical care units about the level of service various grades of pharmacist can offer, from a minimal level service to that provided by a Consultant Pharmacist .

Staffing level

0.1 whole time equivalent for every Level 3 bed and 0.1 whole time equivalent for every two Level 2 beds. The grade of pharmacist is dependent on factors such as size of unit, required level of service and support available from more senior critical care pharmacists across institutes or networks.

Physiotherapists

Role

Physiotherapists working in critical care have become experts in managing the cardiorespiratory system, providing support and education to medical and nursing teams. Key aspects include the management of complications of ventilation, provision of weaning strategies, mobilization and facilitating the rehabilitation of patients throughout the critical care stay and beyond. Much of physiotherapy practice in the critically ill is based on common sense rather than a firm evidence base, but is nevertheless regarded as a core feature of the care of the critically ill .

Staffing level

0.2 whole time equivalents for every critical care bed. Consideration of skill mix and career progression should also be born in mind when formulating the structure of the service.

Dietitians

Role

Dietitians manage the nutritional needs of patients. They identify patients who are malnourished or are at risk of becoming malnourished, and ensure that strategies to optimize nutritional status are put in place. All aspects of nutrition composition are calculated, from major components (protein, energy, fibre, water) to micronutrients such as electrolytes, trace elements and vitamins. Delivery of expertise in other aspects such as choice of feeding route, types of enteral tube and impact of organ dysfunction on nutritional requirements allows the patient to receive optimal nutritional care.

Staffing level

0.1–0.05 whole-time equivalents for every critical care bed at a senior dietitians grade.

Speech and language therapists

Role

Speech and language therapists posses specialist knowledge and expertise about speech, language, communication and swallowing. They can assess and diagnose issues pertaining to swallowing and provide advice on the use of communication aids and speaking valves. Some also have experience of managing tracheostomies.

Staffing level

There are no recognized staffing levels for critical care, but ready access on an *ad hoc* basis to speech and language therapy services with formal referral is important.

Occupational therapists

Role

Occupational therapists facilitate the rehabilitation of critically ill patients after their acute illness. The groundwork for this activity can occur whilst the patient is still critically ill (e.g. through the use of splints to prevent contractures). Provision of advice and teaching to other critical care staff in these techniques may improve the patient's quality of life after critical illness.

Staffing level

There are no recognized staffing levels for critical care, but ready access on an *ad hoc* basis to occupational therapy services with formal referral is important.

Clinical psychologist

Role

Psychologists can identify patients with likely significant psychological morbity and put in place plans to manage the patient's (and relatives') psychological state through the critical illness itself as well as the rehabilitation phase. The psychological impact of critical illness is well described and can be long lasting. The involvement of clinical psychologists in follow-up clinics can be very useful.

Staffing level

There are no recognized staffing levels for critical care. 0.05 whole-time equivalent of a consultant grade has been suggested. Alternatively the use of a formal referral system may be deemed appropriate.

Podiatrists/chiropodists

Role

Prevention and management of lower limb wounds and pathologies. The podiatrist can assist in the rehabilitation of the critically ill patient to maximize their ability to fulfil every day activities.

Staffing level

There are no recognized staffing levels for critical care. The use of a formal referral system is appropriate.

Radiographer

Role

Radiographers use a variety of imaging techniques that may be performed in the imaging department, in theatre or at ward level. Increasingly the role is extending, and radiographers may provide interventional procedures. They can provide advice on the most appropriate imaging modality for a given clinical scenario and provide rapid reports on image appearance and evolution.

Staffing level

Dependent on case mix and type of critical care service; no specific recommendations are given. Clearly the service provided must be fit for purpose.

Critical care technologist

Role

Critical care technologists use, maintain, develop and teach other healthcare professionals how to use a variety of devices and technology utilized in the care of the critically ill patient (e.g. ventilators, haemofilters, blood gas analysers, IABPs, NO delivery devices and a range of other devices that monitor or alter patient parameters). The exact role varies from institute to institute.

Staffing level

There are no recognized staffing levels as the role is varied and still developing.

Healthcare scientists

Role

A huge variety of roles is included under this generic term. Broadly, they can fall into one of three areas, although there is considerable overlap:

1. Clinical scientists and biomedical scientists in pathology (Clinical Biochemistry, Microbiology, Blood Transfusion and Haematology), providing diagnostic and interpretive services
2. Clinical scientists and medical technical officers in medical physics and engineering departments
   Providing physiological investigation, monitoring and equipment management services.
3. Medical technical officers
   Providing clinical perfusion, respiratory physiology, neurophysiology, cardiology, vascular technology services as well as support to other services such as in pharmacy.

Staffing level

There are no recognized staffing levels for critical care. The service is largely determined outside of critical care, but must be influenced by the critical care team for efficient use of these resources.

Further reading

Department of Health. Making the change: a strategy for the professions in healthcare science. Lodon: DoH, 2001.

Department of Health. Adult critical care: specialist pharmacy practice. London: DoH,2005

Intensive Care Society/NHS Modernisation Agency. Allied Health Professionals (AHP) and Healthcare Scientists (HCS). *Critical Care Staffing Guidance.* 2003.

Intensive Care Society. Guidance on Comprehensive Critical Care for Adults in Independent Sector Acute Hospitals. London: ICS, 2002.

Jones C, Griffiths RD, Humphris G, *et al.* Memory, delusions and the development of acute post traumatic stress disorder-related symptoms after intensive care. *Crit Care Med* 2001; 29: 573–80.

Kane SL, Weber RJ, Dasta JF. The impact of critical care pharmacists on enhancing patient outcomes. *Intensive Care Med* 2003; 29: 691–8.

NHS Modernisation Agency. AHP and HCS Advisory Group. The Role of Healthcare Professionals within Critical Care Services. London: NHS, 2002

Stiller K. Physiotherapy in intensive care: towards an evidence-based practice. *Chest* 2000; 118:1801–13.

Fire safety

Fire in the critical care unit fortunately is rare. When it occurs, however, it can be both devastating and frightening. During the period 1994/5 and 2004/5, there were 10,662 fire incidents reported from within the NHS. The cost of these has amounted to £14.6 million, with 17 fatalities and 651 injuries. Fires involving critical care areas are particularly complicated by the high dependency nature of the patients, the open space nature of unit design and the equipment required for patient support. The infrequent nature of fires in critical care areas means that prevention and response relies heavily on structural design, operational policies and staff training, rather than real-life experience for most staff.

The principles of fire safety in an intensive care area are based on:

- prevention and early detection
- containment
- the fire service response
- evacuation and compartment isolation procedures.

Policies for critical care or high dependency areas form part of larger coordinated Trust-wide policies. Within the NHS, these are based on and conform to the Department of Health fire safety policy. This includes the Firecode suite of documents specifically covering fire safety in the NHS in England (see Further reading). It considers management, functional requirements and operational provisions, and should be viewed in conjunction with the HBN 57 document, the NHS estates Facilities for critical care for all design and building of critical care areas in England. Where an alternative solution to Firecode is proposed within the NHS, the designer must demonstrate that the approach does not result in a lower standard of fire safety than if Firecode had been applied.

The fire safety law regarding non-domestic premises in England and Wales changed in October 2006. The main effect of the change is:

- a greater emphasis on fire prevention and reducing risk and
- abolishing the need for fire certificates. Instead, each organization now must have a designated person responsible for fire risk assessment.

Fire safety in the critical care area is the responsibility of everyone; responsibility lies with government, Trust management, individual staff, general public visitors and patients alike.

Prevention and early detection

Central to reduced harm from fire is prevention and early detection. This requires

- building planning and design
- behavioural responsibilities, and
- the use of fire detection and alarm systems.

All NHS buildings are expected to conform to or exceed the building and design standards laid out in the Firecode suite of documents. These contain elements relating to building design and departmental physical relationships which minimize fire risk. All new electrical equipment introduced into service should conform to minimum electrical safety standards and also should be checked and approved by the relevant department in the Trust locally.

Staff should undergo regular fire safety training which should cover prevention strategies and early response procedures, as well as isolation and evacuation policies. There should also be appropriate rules for visitors as well as targeted notices clearly visible to assist visitors unfamiliar to the hospital. One example is smoking; smoking is now banned in most NHS buildings. Until recently, there were often designated smoking areas. More recently, many Trusts have moved to a total no smoking policy despite arguments surrounding individual human rights. Such a move has been for reasons of both health and fire safety.

Fire detection and alarm systems design and use is now covered by Firecode document HTM 05-03 (replacing HTM 82). This document describes differing alarm systems for areas containing dependent or highly dependent occupants, which applies to critical care areas, as compared with other areas which contain either ambulant independent patients or staff. The function of fire alarms in critical care areas is to give warning to staff in the event of a fire so that an early call to the fire and rescue service, first-aid fire-fighting and evacuation may be carried out. In contrast to most other areas, it may not be necessary, desirable or even possible to give warning to the patients themselves. Alarms for critical care areas should be two-stage alarms, i.e. a different indication for an evacuation requirement from an alert of a fire in a neighbouring compartment or subcompartment.

All fire detection systems used in NHS buildings housing a critical care area since the 1980s have used addressable rather than conventional systems. The central control panel of a conventional system could only identify the zone of activation. In the addressable system, the control panel can identify each and every detector. This aids in pinpointing the source, and better recognition of false alarms, leading to a more timely and targeted response. The detectors (or sensors) in addressable systems are usually analogue sensors rather than the older two-state devices; the sensors continuously transmit to the control equipment a signal level that represents the amount of heat, smoke or flame being sensed. The decision as to whether or not this constitutes a fire condition is taken at the control panel. A two-state device simply rests in the activated or inactivated state depending on a fixed threshold, which is less informative at the control panel.

Containment of fire by design

Building design for containment of fire in the NHS is described in Firecode document HTM 05-02. It is often neither possible nor desirable in critical care areas to undertake rapid and total evacuation. Restricted mobility and dependence on immobile support equipment prevents such a task. Location of critical care areas on the ground floor, although desirable, is not essential. If a ground floor location is not possible, it is recommended that such areas be no higher than 12m above ground floor (typically 3 floors). However, the preferred and initial basic strategy for fire evacuation for such areas should be to move them on their bed or in wheelchairs to a safer area on the same floor. Critical care areas should therefore be designed with such isolation and horizontal evacuation strategies in mind, rather than external evacuation in the first instance.

Critical care areas should be located away from high fire risk departments. These include flammable stores, kitchens, boilerhouses, the laundry and main electrical switchgear areas. The risk of fire in a compartment adjacent to the critical care area is thus reduced. Critical care fire compartments should also be more resistant to fire than other patient areas. This is achieved by enhanced fire-resistant separators, the use of protective lobbies, and specific air conditioning and heating requirements.

Critical care areas should be divided into at least two subcompartments; nursing or patient areas (such as bed areas and clean and dirty utility rooms) should be separated from utility areas (such as staff changing and rest areas, and equipment storage areas), and larger units should be divided into two patient areas to facilitate horizontal evacuation from one compartment to another while retaining full critical care facilities for patients not able to be safely evacuated to a non-critical care area. Enhanced fire-resistant separators demand the use of at least 60min fire-resistant imperforate construction, together with mechanical methods of fire suppression which are activated automatically in compartments adjacent to the critical care area. Such systems may include water sprinklers and CO_2 flooding systems.

Every door opening in the critical care compartment wall should be provided with a protected lobby. This comprises a double door system containing an area large enough to contain a bed and ancillary equipment and staff, with space for manoeuvring as necessary. The lobby doors should provide a minimum of 30min fire resistance each.

Heating, ventilation and air conditioning (HVAC) systems provided to critical care areas are designed so that the pressure within the department is maintained at a level slightly above that of the adjacent area. In a fire emergency, the continuing operation of these systems will assist in preventing smoke and other products of combustion from entering. Specifically, the HVAC systems should be designed so that they do continue to operate in a fire emergency.

Fire service response

The fire service takes time to arrive, and its purpose is to contain, limit or extinguish the fire for the purpose of primarily limiting personal injury and loss of life, and secondarily minimizing loss or damage to the building. The response time and the number of fire engines, or appliances, which are sent is pre-determined and pre-agreed, depending on the assessed risk and location of the building. This is the pre-determined attendance. In a city centre, the pre-determined attendance will usually require that three appliances attend, two within 5min, and a third within 8min. In a rural area, the response must be one appliance within 20min.

Evacuation and isolation procedures

All staff should receive mandatory training on local Trust fire policies and procedures. The response to a fire should be a coordinated one between hospital staff, the nominated local fire officer and the attending fire service. It is rare that any staff member has prior real experience of fire evacuation procedures; a smooth effective response is achieved by adequate training and a level-headed approach with clear leadership. The first step is alerting the local fire officers and activating the fire service. Most fires in healthcare settings are first detected by direct observation rather than mechanical devices. The intensive care staff should ensure that the hospital switchboard has raised the fire alarm. Once the fire service has been alerted, the principle for critical care areas is local containment with or without staged internal evacuation until the fire service has arrived and controlled the fire. There are three stages of evacuation described in the Firecode documents:

- Stage 1 is horizontal evacuation from a subcompartment where the fire originates to an adjoining subcompartment or compartment.
- Stage 2 is horizontal evacuation from the entire compartment to an adjoining compartment on the same floor, and
- Stage 3 is vertical evacuation to a lower floor substantially remote from the floor of origin of the fire (at least two floors below), or to the outside.

Critical care evacuations are almost always practically limited to stage 1 or 2. Stage 3 evacuations of the critically ill are particularly slow and difficult, and increase potential mortality of patient and staff. If the fire is small, staff should make attempts to control the fire with equipment available, provided they do not endanger themselves or others in the process.

There should be advance provision for horizontal evacuation procedures. These include availability of equipment stored within the critical care compartment, ideally within the patient subcompartment. Such equipment includes ready-packed transport equipment and drugs. Most critical care departments will already have this in the form of a transportable transfer bag or pack for intra-hospital movement of patients. Senior clinicians will have the job of leadership within the intensive care team and making triage decisions. If an alert is activated indicating a fire in a nearby compartment, but not in the direct vicinity of intensive care, patients should be prepared for evacuation but not actually moved. Staff should ensure that all fire resistance barriers are closed and that automatic closure devices have functioned correctly to seal off the critical care compartment. Aspects of patient management may have to be changed to render movement of the patient easier with least risk. This might include, for example, cessation of RRT or attempts at respiratory weaning. Transport equipment and drugs should be gathered, checked and distributed to the patient bedside. Senior clinical staff should establish a rank order for evacuation should this become necessary and make the coordinated plan clear to all staff. Of note, with the most common cause of death in a fire being inhalation of toxic gases or fumes, patients connected to a closed ventilator circuit may be better protected than a self-ventilating patient for longer, and this should be taken into account when planning evacuation. In general terms, patients closest to the source, those self-ventilating and those least dependent should be moved first. Those whose evacuation would be slow and where the patient's chance of survival may be significantly compromised by movement may be best left contained in the hope that the fire will be contained without the need for evacuation.

Further reading

NHS Estates. Firecode—fire safety in the NHS. Health Technical Memorandum 05-03: operational provisions Part L: NHS fire statistics 1994/5–2004/5. 2007.

NHS Estates. Firecode—fire safety in the NHS. Health Technical Memorandum 05-01: managing healthcare fire safety. 2006.

NHS Estates. Firecode—fire safety in the NHS. Health Technical Memorandum 05-02: guidance in support of functional provisions for healthcare premises. 2007.

NHS Estates. Firecode—fire safety in the NHS. Health Technical Memorandum 05-03: Operational provisions Part B: fire detection and alarm systems. 2006.

NHS Estates. Firecode—fire safety in the NHS. Health Technical Memorandum 05-03: operational provisions Part D: commercial enterprises on healthcare premises. 2006.

NHS Estates. Firecode—fire safety in the NHS, Health Technical Memorandum 05-03: operational provisions. Part E: escape lifts in healthcare premises. 2006.

NHS Estates. Firecode—fire safety in the NHS. Health Technical Memorandum 05-03: operational provisions Part F: arson prevention in NHS premises. 2006.

NHS Estates. Firecode—fire safety in the NHS. Health Technical Memorandum 05-03: operational provisions Part G: Laboratories on Healthcare premises. 2006.

NHS Estates. Firecode—fire safety in the NHS. Health Technical Memorandum 05-03: operational provisions Part H: reducing unwanted fire signals in healthcare premises. 2006.

Ridley SA, Parry G. Guidelines for fire safety in the intensive care unit. London: *Intensive Care Society*, 1998.

Legal issues and the Coroner

Doctors working in intensive care need a knowledge of the law in a number of circumstances such as:

- Working with HM Coroner
  - reporting a death
  - witness of fact
  - organ donation
- Contact with the police
- Civil action
  - as party to a civil action
  - as expert
- Consent
- End of life decision making
  - futility
  - autonomy
  - assisted suicide

A doctor has a duty to be aware of regulations relating to clinical practice such as the recording and use of controlled drugs. They may need legal advice when in court, appearing in front of the GMC and in dealing with ethical issues arising in clinical practice. The GMC document 'Fitness to Practice' lays down guidance for all doctors. Some of the guidance relates to legal and ethical issues. It is continually under review, and doctors should be familiar with it.

The Coroner

Reporting a death to the Coroner

A death certificate has to be issued prior to disposal of a body. When a doctor has been caring for a patient during a terminal illness, he is responsible for issuing a certificate. Under certain circumstances, it would be usual to discuss the case with the Coroner rather than issue a certificate. Sometimes the need to discuss the case is clear, such as violent deaths and deaths related to neglect, but other situations may be unclear. Local practice concerning the amount of time between admission or surgery and death can vary.

Coroner's officer

It is unusual to discuss a case with the Coroner personally; first contact is more likely to be with a Coroner's officer. This will be an experienced police officer who works closely with the Coroner. It is always safer to discuss a questionable case with the Coroner's officer, who can be relied upon to be a source of useful information, than to put the patient's family at the inconvenience of a certificate being rejected when presented to the registrar. It does not take long to become familiar with local practice following a few of these discussions.

Possible mishap resulting in death

When an intensivist suspects that an error in patient care may have resulted in admission and ultimately death, they must ensure correct procedures are followed by informing the Coroner as well as relevant personnel within their organization. They must also remember their responsibilities laid out in the GMC's Good Medical Practice. It is generally more useful for the Coroner to be contacted by the member of the clinical team most familiar with events of concern.

Coroner's witness statement

During the investigation of a death, the Coroner might become aware of your involvement in the case. This could be due to you having reported the case, being the responsible senior doctor, being mentioned in an entry in the record or as a result of a comment from relatives or other witnesses. The Coroner's officer might ask to speak to you to discuss the case, but more commonly you will be asked by letter to provide a statement. Often the only information you are given is the name of the patient whose death is being investigated; consequently you may not know why you were approached for a statement or the reason it is required.

The statement should be written in such a way that it tells of your involvement in the case. It is wise to avoid making comments that could be taken to be expert opinion except when needed to explain your management. An experienced secretary will help format the statement in an efficient way, making it easier for the court to use. It is helpful to use paragraph numbering. A doctor will often be asked to read their statement to the court providing additional detail where necessary, so arranging it in a chronological way is helpful. It is important to avoid the use of excessive jargon while not explaining every minor detail in a condescending way.

An intensivist may be asked for a statement when the event of concern occurred prior to the patient arriving in the ICU. This is to help the Coroner establish the sequence of events leading up to a death.

Senior intensivists who are familiar with the system can be helpful to the Coroner by explaining that the care on an ICU is team based and that although their personal involvement in a case was minimal, they have generated a report and present evidence using their own knowledge and information from the records. This pragmatic approach saves each team member having to provide a report and attend court.

It would be advisable for inexperienced doctors to obtain assistance with a Coroner's report. This can be obtained from senior colleagues, the Trust legal or risk management department or the doctor's defence organization. If there is any suggestion that the actions of an individual doctor are being called into question, then they should seek the advice of the body that represents their interests. This is their defence organization.

Coroner's post-mortem

Following a discussion with the Coroner's officer, a doctor may be asked to issue a death certificate. If the doctor does not feel able to issue a certificate or the Coroner is unhappy with the suggested entry, then the Coroner will take over the case.

When there is conflict between the hospital and bereaved relatives about any aspect of care, it is worthwhile discussing concerns with the Coroner, who may take over the case at this stage to avoid future problems.

Once the Coroner takes on the responsibility for a case, he may arrange a post-mortem. If relatives are unhappy to have a post-mortem, it remains for the Coroner to consider the issues and make whatever arrangements he feels necessary. The Coroner's pathologist is usually happy for clinical staff to attend a post-mortem as they can be a useful source of information about the circumstances preceding the death. If a clinician is not present during the examination, then the results of the post-mortem will be unavailable prior to an inquest.

Coroner's inquest

The Coroner often opens and adjourns a preliminary inquest to allow formalities relating to identification of the body to be considered, facilitating release of the body for disposal. The full inquest is then held some time later at the convenience of the Coroner.

Prior to the inquest there will be a request for details of the doctor's availability. The court is not interested in routine clinical appointments but will take notice of difficult to reschedule commitments such as foreign travel. If necessary, the Coroner can insist on attendance.

A Coroner's inquest is often the first time a doctor enters a court. There are significant differences between an inquest and a trial. An inquest is an enquiry into how the deceased died; there is no defendant and it is not about attributing blame.

There is often a single court reporter present but important cases will attract interest from larger numbers of the press. Due to the widely variable nature of Coroners' courts, doctors should be prepared to find themselves coming across relatives of the deceased around the court building prior to and after the case. When called to give evidence, the doctor will be questioned first by the Coroner and then by representatives of the relatives or other interested parties, which could include the doctor's own legal team. Any of the interested parties may have a solicitor or barrister in court. The Coroner should not permit inappropriate questioning, but it is vital to indicate clearly if you cannot answer because you are unaware of the facts or you are being asked for an opinion outside of your area of expertise. Following your evidence, you may be given permission to leave the court. Be warned—if you remain it is much easier to recall you.

There are a number of possible verdicts following an inquest, such as natural causes, unlawful killing, accident or misadventure (another way of saying accident). After delivering a verdict, the Coroner may take matters further by communicating concerns to a responsible body or referring a case for potential criminal proceedings.

Organ donation

The principle of brainstem death and testing is well recognized. Coroners need to be involved where a death is violent or other circumstance in which a death would be reported. The local transplant coordinator will be able to provide advice relating to organ donation and can facilitate contact with the Coroner if necessary. The human tissue Act 2004 made a number of changes that affect the process of organ donation, such as defining suitable qualifying relationships for those providing consent. Experience improves donation rates, and coordinators will make themselves available to help with the consenting process if required. They can also advise on practical problems relating to brainstem dead or NHBDs.

The doctor, patient and the police

At times the interests of patients, doctors and the police may clash. The GMC advises that doctors have a duty of care to their patient as a prime responsibility, but that they are also expected to act as responsible citizens.

When the police request access to patient information, it would be usual to seek patient consent. When patients are unable to give consent or refuse, then the doctor's responsibility to the patient may be over-ridden if *'there are grounds for believing that this is the public interest or disclosure is required by law'* (see Further reading)

Civil actions

Any doctor in clinical practice is at risk of becoming involved in a civil action. The complaint may or may not have originally been directed at the intensive care component of a hospital stay. The direction of a claim can change as the litigation progresses. Much has been done in recent years to speed up the process and reduce the confrontational nature of civil actions. Most doctors involved in these actions say how stressful the experience is. The best way to protect yourself is to become familiar with the system so you can more effectively influence proceedings.

Complaints

Often things start to go wrong when a complaint is received about patient care. The best way to deal with this is to talk to the complainant and be honest and open. In an attempt to make complaint handling appear important, most Trusts commit themselves to response letters being rapidly dispatched and signed by a senior officer. A final letter responding to a complex complaint is likely to be a montage of uncoordinated responses from clinicians. Relatives receiving such a letter not infrequently consider the response to be a deliberate process of deception and seek legal assistance to have questions answered.

Consultation with solicitor

Medical negligence cases can follow a number of different paths. Once a medical negligence solicitor considers there is a case to answer, he will request that the Trust release the records. He may also give the hospital the opportunity to provide additional detail about patient care.

Limitation

Generally a medical negligence claim will only be heard if the proceedings commence within 3yrs of the claimant becoming aware of a potential claim.

Expert advice

Prior to proceeding, the solicitor will seek expert advice. On the first attempt they may not instruct the correct expert, but eventually one will be found who can comment authoritatively on the merits of the case. Experts are usually instructed separately by claimant and defendant, but their reports should be non-partisan and directed to the court. The report must contain a declaration making this clear.

Following expert review, the action may be terminated because either the client accepts advice that the case is likely to fail or those funding the action withdraw support.

Letter of Claim

If the claim is to proceed a formal 'Letter of Claim' is constructed and sent to the Trust detailing aspects of care that are being questioned.

The Trust will then instruct its own legal team who will investigate the case and consult its own experts to determine how the allegations should be defended.

Conferences

A lot of decision making by both claimant and defence teams will be in conferences of solicitors, counsel, experts and involved parties. In this environment, barristers may explore the experts' opinions, help establish additional information that is required and ultimately form a view of the chances the case might succeed.

Defence

Eventually unless the case is to be settled, the Trust will produce a formal defence explaining events and admitting or denying allegations that have been made.

Timing

The conduct of the case such as the time allowed to pass between each of these processes is carefully controlled by the court.

Meetings of experts

Expert opinions often differ. When this is important to the case, the court will instruct that the experts meet for a discussion. Experts are asked to produce a joint report in response to an agenda agreed between instructing solicitors. It is frequently possible for cases to be settled following the meeting of experts.

Witness statement

Once a claim has been brought, it can be many years before it reaches court. If you feel there is a chance that you will be called upon to give evidence in a civil action, it is worthwhile making a record for future review. This may take the form of an entry in the patient record. Any such entry should be accurately dated and timed. Alternatively, it is reasonable to write an account for your own files. If you use a formal style, it may be accepted later by the court, if you wish.

Court

Many cases are settled between parties prior to appearing in court. If a settlement cannot be agreed, then a trial will be held. During the trial, a judge will be called upon to assess the merits of the case and to determine the amount of any damages.

Providing expert opinion

Intensivists are frequently asked for expert opinion. Any experienced clinician who has been instructed in the workings of the legal system can act as an expert. The responsibilities of an expert are onerous. Advice must be given within the expert's area of expertise. Opinions must be full and frank, and directed to the court irrespective of the side that is providing instructions. Experts must be reliable and make themselves available to support an ongoing case.

English law is influenced by precedent or previous court decisions. For example, a doctor is considered to have acted in a reasonable way if there is a body of opinion that would have acted in the same way. This is called the Bolam test after the trial where the precedent was set. Even though many precedents have been set, there is a need for lawyers to interpret them. For example, the Bolam principle will not apply if the judge considers that the actions of the body of opinion in question are not logical.

Consent

Generally it is not possible for an individual to give consent to treat an incompetent adult. Doctors are expected to consider the patient's best interests. It is good practice to keep close relatives informed of events and to encourage their support for the management plan. The next of kin may be able to contribute to patient care by informing the medical team of the patient's wishes. Doctors are bound to respect a patient's autonomy or right to self-determination. Assuming there is no reason to question information provided by relatives, this could help the clinical team devise a treatment plan that respects the patient's autonomy. In the case of young children, parents can give or withhold consent. If there is conflict between the clinical team and relatives, it is possible to ask the court for advice. If the issue relates to a child where consent is being withheld for a treatment considered in the best interests of the child, the clinical team has no choice but to apply to the court.

End of life decision making

Futility

If a treatment is not going to help a patient, then it is inappropriate to continue with it. There is no single critical care scoring system designed to predict outcome in an individual, so each decision must be taken by assessing the patient on their merits. It is good practice for decisions of this nature to be shared by another senior doctor and supported by the team and the patient's relatives. It may be necessary to allow time for the futility of the situation to be realized. Ideally relatives will be left with the feeling that they have been consulted and their views considered without considering that it was their decision to limit or withdraw therapy.

Patient autonomy

Patients have a right to accept or refuse treatment. It is important for the clinical team to be sure the patient is of sound mind and not undergoing any form of coercion. If this is the case, then a patient has the right to refuse treatment even though this may result in death. As in other cases involving end of life decisions, it is helpful for senior doctors to have support for their actions from colleagues or the courts if necessary. Failure to honour a patient's right to refuse treatment has resulted in a judge criticizing intensivists.

Assisted suicide

The law sees no resemblance between withdrawing life-saving treatment and agreeing to help a patient commit suicide, even if such a patient has a terminal condition. Assisted suicide is illegal.

It is increasingly important for doctors working in intensive care to have an understanding of the law relating to their practice. They should always be prepared to seek legal advice when issues are complex. There may be times when a doctor would be best advised by a lawyer instructed on their behalf. Generally this advice would be from their own defence organization.

Further reading

Braithwaite M. Law for doctors—principles and practicalities. *RSM* London: Press Ltd. 2000.

General Medical Council. Withholding and withdrawing life-prolonging treatments: good practice in decision-making. Appendix A: the legal background. London: GMC, 2002.

Singer P. Ms B and Diane Pretty: a commentary, *J Med Ethics*; 2002; 28: 234–5.

What happens if the patient refuses to talk to the police, or the patient is unconscious? http://www.gmc-uk.org/guidance/current/library/reporting_gunshot_wounds.asp#1

Patient safety

Introduction

Patient safety is now recognized as a major healthcare issue. The Institute of Medicine's report in 2000 estimated that between 44 000 and 98 000 patients in the USA might die each year from what was termed 'medical error'. Other countries report similar rates of error and avoidable harm, and many have established national agencies for patient safety coordinated by the World Health Organization's World Alliance for Patient Safety.

The narrow definition of safety as 'avoidance of harm' should be broadened to include reliability of care—the right actions at the right time to the right patients. Error is a problem for the entire healthcare system, not just for the terminal point in the chain of causation—the front-line doctors and nurses charged with the responsibility of making unsafe systems safer.

Reducing error and improving reliability require changes in behaviour and attitudes as well as resources; these changes must be focused on processes of care, teamworking, communication, partnership with patients, and life-long learning through competence assessment.

Taxonomy

Comparisons between publications are made more difficult by the variety of terms and methods used in safety research. A selection of definitions is offered in Table 33.9.1. More are available from: http://psnet.ahrq.gov/glossary.aspx

Epidemiology and impact

Reported rates of error and harm vary. Most errors do not cause harm, and most go unreported. Retrospective case note reviews are particularly susceptible to observer bias and interpretation; they rely on detecting adverse events, and then making a value judgement about avoidability. The classical Harvard and Australian studies reported adverse event rates of 3.7 and 16.6%, respectively, of which 69 and 51% were considered avoidable. Prospective observational studies suggest higher rates, with adverse drug events being the most common. Harmful consequences include emotional and physical suffering, and financial costs; hospital-acquired infections alone affect ~2 million patients and cause 90 000 deaths in the USA at an estimated additional cost of ~US$5 billion per year. Physicians, patients and the public want safer systems. Acutely and critically ill patients, the elderly and longer stay patients are most susceptible to error and its consequences. In the ICU, errors affect 20–30% of admissions, of which around half are avoidable; of these, a quarter cause significant harm to the patient. Reported daily error rates vary from 0.18 to 1.7 per patient, and adverse events from 13 to 40 per 1000 patient days.

Detection and monitoring

Effective detection, reporting, and taking action to learn from and prevent error requires a patient-focused culture throughout the organization. There are many methods but no single solution for detecting and reporting error, and the precise instrument used depends on the use to which the data will be put.

Patients' or relatives' complaints are important (the majority refer to suboptimal communication with staff), but imprecise and delayed. Adverse event reporting means that harm may already have occurred. Critical incident reporting suffers from selection bias. Retrospective case note review is laborious, subject to hindsight and interpretation bias, and relies on good note-keeping. Process measures rather than outcome are better for performance management, but require rapid feedback of data to the user. The fact that nurses and (to a lesser extent) junior doctors are the most likely to report error, and that nurses are major 'error interceptors' suggests the need for workplace-based data collection at the point of care, integrated

Table 33.9.1 Definitions of commonly used terms relating to patient safety.

Term	Definition
Accident	An event which damages a defined system and disrupts the continuing or future output of that system.
System	A set of interdependent elements, human or non-human, which interact to achieve a common aim.
Error	The failure of a planned action to be completed as intended (execution error), or the use of a wrong plan to achieve an aim (planning error). Errors of commission are faulty actions; of omission, faulty inactions.
Mistake	Wrong action plan properly conducted, resulting in an unintended outcome
Slip or lapse	Execution errors in which the action performed differs from that intended. Slips are observable, lapses are not.
Active error	A fault in performance at the level of the operator.
Latent error	A fault in design, installation, management or maintenance which may subsequently result in harm.
Critical incident	A pivotal event with the potential to cause an adverse event.
Adverse event	An injury caused by medical management that resulted in measurable disability.
Negligent adverse event	A preventable adverse event caused by medical management which did not meet the standard of care expected of that practitioner.
Failure modes effects analysis	Systematic risk analysis of how failures occur, and their consequences. Facilitates prioritization of risk, and methods of prevention.
Iatrogenic disease	Illness or injury caused by doctors. Often misused to mean 'healthcare-related'.
Patient safety	Freedom from accidental injury. The avoidance, prevention, and amelioration of adverse outcomes or injuries arising from the processes of health care.
Patient safety practice	A process or structure whose application reduces the probability of adverse events resulting from exposure to the healthcare system.
Root cause analysis	A process for identifying the most basic or causal factor or factors that underlie variation in performance.
Redundancy	Independent elements contributing to desired outcome.
Sentinel event	Any unanticipated event in a healthcare setting resulting in death or serious physical or psychological injury unrelated to the natural course of the patient's illness.

in routine activities and clinical decision support, and linked to professional development.

Causation

High reliability organizations recognize that systems must support individuals to prevent error (Fig. 33.9.1). Every individual in an organization must share the same goals. Two of the most reliable services, blood transfusion services and anaesthesia, have long-established systems of process control, safety checks and (in most countries) well structured systems of supervision, training and education, resulting in reliability levels approaching 4–5 sigma, but still well below perfection (6-sigma, 3.4 defects per million opportunities).

Common causes of error include active failures at the level of the individual (e.g. to apply knowledge, communication problems, technical incompetence) combined with latent conditions in the individual (fatigue, illness, attitudinal problems) or the system (working environment, poor organization). It is usually the combination of the two which results in patient harm. Errors of commission are generally easier to detect (IV administration of concentrated potassium solution causing cardiac arrest) than errors of omission (failure to correct hypokalaemia in a septic patient, contributing to AF, low cardiac output and MOD). Errors of omission may be more important, however, as they may also reflect a lack of care.

Management and prevention

When error results in harm, we have two professional responsibilities. One is to provide appropriate care for the victim(s)—the patient, the family and the staff involved. The second is to learn from the episode and to take steps to minimize the risk of repetition. This requires transparency, honesty and a supportive environment. Structured methods of investigation make it easier to learn from defects in healthcare and impose a necessary discipline on the less effective morbidity and mortality meeting.

Prevention is the essence of safety improvement efforts. However, too narrow focus on safety may have the unintended consequence of impeding efficacy of care, which is why safety is better subsumed under reliability. There are six elements for improving reliability:

- Standardization
- Simplification
- Redundancy
- Teamworking and communication
- Partnership
- Education

Application of these principles has been shown to reduce bacteraemias associated with central venous catheters effectively to zero.

Standardization: medical staff are better at creating guidelines and protocols than implementing them in their own practice. Individual variations in clinical practice increase the opportunity for error. The Surviving Sepsis Campaign provides an example of evaluating evidence and formulating clinical guidance.

Simplification: reducing complexity minimizes opportunity for error by removing additional or unfamiliar steps in the processes of care, e.g. by reducing the number of handovers ('hand-offs') and using common forms of information transfer. Sepsis Care Bundles simplify by aggregation. Electronic prescribing systems with forcing functions limit choices to correct actions.

Redundancy: means more than one way of achieving the correct goal. This includes reminders, prompts, multiple communication channels and empowering team members to draw attention to errors, and adequate staffing to reduce fatigue. One approach is to ask the question 'what are the main safety risks for this patient today?'

Effective teamworking and communication: encourages group participation, mutual performance monitoring,and explicit daily goals (e.g. on the ICU chart), as well as making time for listening to others.

Partnership: means shared goals. For example, involving close relatives in the bedside ward rounds can enhance shared purpose, enable families to feel that they are

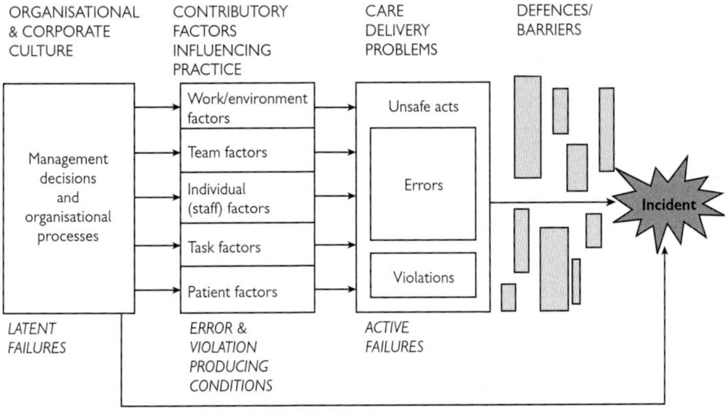

Fig. 33.9.1 A systems approach to analysing accidents (from Woloshynowych *et al.*, 2005).

contributing to care and improve the accuracy of information flows.

Education: in the clinical environment, safety, reliability and teamworking can be included in simulation-based learning. Learning from error must be embedded in undergraduate and postgraduate national training programmes (see www.cobatrice.org) and integrated across disciplines and over professional lifetimes.

Further reading

Bion JF, Heffner J. Improving hospital safety for acutely ill patients. A Lancet quintet. I: Current challenges in the care of the acutely ill patient. *Lancet* 2004; 363: 970–7. See also the subsequent four articles in this five-part series.

Blendon RJ, DesRoches CM, Brodie M, *et al.* Views of practicing physicians and the public on medical errors. *N Engl J Med* 2002; 347: 1933–40.

Brennan TA, Leape LL, Laird NM, *et al.* Incidence of adverse events and negligence in hospitalized patients. *N Engl J Med* 1991; 324: 370–6.

http://www.who.int/patientsafety/en/

Kohn LT, Corrigan JM, Donaldson MS, eds. To err is human: building a safer health system. Washington, DC: National Academic Press, 2000.

NICE guideline. Acutely ill patients in hospital: recognition of, and response to, acute illness in hospitalised adults. National Institute for Clinical Excellence 2007. http://www.nice.org.uk/CG50

Patient Safety Observatory. Safer care for the acutely ill patient: learning from serious incidents. National Patient Safety Agency 2007. http://www.npsa.nhs.uk/health/resources/pso

Reason J. Latent errors and system disasters human error. Cambridge: Cambridge University Press, 1990.

Rothschild JM, Landrigan CP, Cronin JW, *et al.* The Critical Care Safety Study: the incidence and nature of adverse events and serious medical errors in intensive care. *Crit Care Med* 2005; 33: 1694–700.

Weingart SN, Wilson RMcL, Gibberd RW, *et al.* Epidemiology of medical error. *BMJ* 2000; 320: 774–7.

Woloshynowych M, Rogers S, Taylor-Adams S, *et al.* The Investigation and analysis of critical incidents and adverse events in healthcare: a review of the literature. *Health Technol Assess* 2005; 9: 1–143.

Severity of illness scoring systems

The evaluation of severity of illness in the critically ill patient is made through the use of general severity scores and general outcome prognostic models.

1 Severity scores are instruments that aim at stratifying patients based on their severity, assigning to each patient an increasing number of points (or score) as their severity of illness increases.
2 Prognostic models usually use a given set of prognostic variables and a certain modelling equation.

- aim to stratify patients according to their severity of illness based in their respective risk
- aim at predicting a certain outcome—usually the vital status at hospital discharge.

Other outcomes, in both the short- and the long-term, can eventually be considered, but most of them are more prone to bias and manipulation or are of little interest for the patients, their families and the healthcare providers.

Available instruments

Several hundred severity scores have been proposed thus far. Most of them have been developed to be used in specific populations, such as children or infants, or patients with certain diseases (peritonitis, AMI). They can be divided in two broad categories:

Multiple organ dysfunction/failure scores

MOD scores have been designed to quantify organ dysfunction and organ failure in adult patients in ICUs. All these instruments have been developed with some similar principles in mind:

- Organ failure is not a simple all-or-nothing phenomenon, it is a spectrum or continuum of organ dysfunction from very mild altered function to total organ failure.
- Organ failure is not a static process and the degree of dysfunction varies with time during the course of disease.
- The variables chosen to evaluate each organ need to be objective, simple and available but reliable, routinely measured in every institution, specific to the organ in question, and independent of patient variables, so that the score can be easily calculated on any patient in any ICU.

There is no general agreement about how to assess organ dysfunction effectively, but all the widely used systems include six key organ systems (cardiovascular, respiratory, haematological, central nervous, renal and hepatic), evaluated through a combination of physiological (e.g. PaO_2) and therapeutic (e.g. use of vasopressor agents) variables.

Commonly used organ dysfunction/failure scores are the Multiple Organ Dysfunction Score (MODS). the Sequential Organ Failure Assessment (SOFA) score and The Logistic Organ Dysfunction System (LOD) score.

Usually these scores, describing a patient's progress, are registered at admission and then once a day until ICU discharge. Several derived measures are often computed such as the maximum score or the delta (maximum minus admission) score.

In Europe, the SOFA score is popular. It evaluates 6 organs/systems, with each scoring between 0 and 4. Zero is normal, 1–2 dysfunction and 3–4 failure. Individual organ function can thus be assessed and monitored over time, and an overall global score can also be calculated (see Table 33.10.1.

Table 33.10.1 Sepsis-related Organ Failure Assessment (SOFA) score

	0	1	2	3	4
Respiratory					
PaO2/FiO2, mm3	>400	≤400	≤300*	≤200*	≤100*
Hamatological					
Platelets (× 1000/mm3)	>150	≤150	≤100	≤50	≤20
Liver					
Serum bilirubin, mg/dl (μmol/l)	<1.2 (<20)	1.2–1.9 (20–32)	2.0–5.9 (33–101)	6.0–11.9 (102–204)	>12.0 (>204)
Cardiovascular					
Blood pressure	MAP ≥70	MAP <70	Dopamine ≤5 or dobutamine (any doses)	Dopamine >5 or epinephrine ≤0.1 or norepinephrine ≤0.1	Dopamine > 15 or epinephrine > 0.1 or norepinephrine >0.1
Neurological					
Glasgow Coma Scale	15	13–14	10–12	6–9	<6
Renal	0				
Serum creatinine, mg/dl (μmol/l)	<1.2 (<110)	1.2–1.9 (110–170)	2.0–3.4 171–299)	3.5–4.9 (300–440)	>5.0 (>440)
Urinary output (l/day)				<0.5	<0.2

Adrenergic agents should have been administered for at least 1h in continuous IV infusion. Doses are in mcg/kg/min.

*With ventilatory support

MAP = mean arterial pressure, mm Hg.

Severity of illness scoring systems

The most popular are described below.

Acute Physiology and Chronic Health Evaluation (APACHE)

The APACHE systems (versions I–III) have been described by Knaus in 1981 and there is now version IV. Designed and validated for use on, or within the first 24h of, admission and relating the calculated score during the first 24h of admission to the vital status at discharge from the hospital. They are not developed for repeated use at other time points during the patient's ICU stay (note: these scores are at entry to a clinical trial even if this is not at the time of ICU admission).

Developed and validated in the USA, the vaildity in other populations is questionable. A predictive model for risk-adjusted ICU length of stay is also available (`www.criticaloutcomes.cerner.com`).

A UK customization is available and was used as a first step in the development of the UK Intensive Care National Audit and Research Centre (ICNARC) score.

Simplified Acute Physiology Score (SAPS)

The SAPS system, originally from a simplification of the APACHE II model, is now a system based on a large multinational database intended to reflect the heterogeneity of current ICU case mix and typology all over the world, with customized equations described for major regions of the world. The original SAPS used data from the first 24h after ICU admission; the last version uses just data from the ICU admission (±1h).

For information and free software (allowing the calculation, storage and export of SAPS 3-related data), see `www.saps3.org`.

Mortality Probability Models (MPMs)

The MPM II used logistic regression techniques on a large international database of ICU patients There are two scores: the MPM_0 or admission model and the MPM_{24} or 24h model, There are equations to estimate the hospital mortality based on data from the 48h and the 72h after ICU admission. They are quick and easy to score.

MPM II models are no better than SAPS II and their use was always quite restricted. (MPM III has been described.)

Using a severity of illness scoring system

The ideal model must have been developed in a similar population, unless well done validation studies are available. Data collection should be as similar to the original model as possible. (This is specifically important when choosing the sampling rate for data collection and registry in patient data management systems. This problem compromises most severity of illness scoring systems based on data from the first 24h after ICU admission when using a patient data management system.)

Few studies have been published directly comparing the effectiveness of these scores at predicting mortality. More recent models have been shown to be better than their older counterparts.

These statistical models are of probabilistic nature. A well calibrated model, applied to an individual patient, may, for example, predict a hospital mortality of 48% for this individual; this, however, just means that for a group of 100 patients with a similar severity of illness, 48 patients are predicted to die; it makes no statement of whether the individual patient is included in the 48% who will eventually die or in the 52% who will eventually survive. Thus, application of these models to individual patients for decision making is not recommended.

Further reading

Harrison D, Parry G, Carpenter J, *et al.* A new risk prediction model: the Intensive Care National Audit & Research Centre (ICNARC) model. *Intensive Care Med* 2006; 32: S204.

Knaus WA, Draper EA, Wagner DP, *et al.* APACHE II: a severity of disease classification system. *Crit Care Med* 1985; 13: 818–29.

Le Gall JR, Lemeshow S, Saulnier F. A new simplified acute physiology score (SAPS II) based on a European/North American multicenter study. *JAMA* 1993; 270: 2957–63.

Lemeshow S, Teres D, Klar J, *et al.* Mortality Probability Models (MPM II) based on an international cohort of intensive care unit patients. *JAMA* 1993; 270: 2478–86.

Marshall JC, Cook DA, Christou NV, *et al.* Multiple organ dysfunction score: a reliable descriptor of a complex clinical outcome. *Crit Care Med* 1995; 23: 1638–52.

Vincent J-L, Moreno R, Takala J, *et al.* The SOFA (sepsis-related organ failure assessment) score to describe organ dysfunction/failure. *Intensive Care Med* 1996; 22: 707–10.

Zimmerman JE, Kramer AA, McNair DS, *et al.* Intensive care unit length of stay: benchmarking based on Acute Physiology and Chronic Health Evaluation (APACHE) IV. *Crit Care Med* 2006; 34: 2517–29.

Comparison of ICUs

Intensive care medicine is the science and art of preventing, detecting and managing patients at risk or with already established critical illness in order to achieve the best possible outcomes of care. It is a complex process, carried out on a heterogeneous patient population and influenced by several variables that include, but are not limited, to religious and cultural background, different structures and organizations of the healthcare systems. Major differences in the baseline characteristics of the populations, determined either by different genetic characteristics or by different lifestyles, are also important in the final result of the interaction of the patient with the healthcare system in general and with the ICU in particular.

This heterogeneity in patient characteristics depends on several factors, related to both the chronic health status and the degree of physiological reserve of the patient, but also on the acute insult or disease responsible for the acute situation and on the timing and characteristics of medical care applied until admission to the ICU. Consequently, any evaluation of the effects of any clinical or non-clinical practices in the critically ill patient must take into account the variability in the patient population characteristics. In other words, when we want to standardize different groups of patients, risk adjustment methods allow us to take into account all of the characteristics of patients known to affect their outcome, irrespective of the treatment received. This process is called risk adjustment.

Risk adjustment in the patient with critical illness

The risk of death in the patient is calculated using general severity scores and general outcome prognostic models (see Chapter 33.10). It is important to choose a model that can evaluate the risk of death in all the patients under analysis. In this process, several characteristics of the available models should be taken into account:

1 Can all the data needed for computation of the models be collected in a standard and reliable way?
2 Was the handling of data before analysis done according to the original description of the model?
3 Can the model be used in the large majority of the patients admitted to the ICU under analysis?
4 Does the model takes into account the differences in baseline patient characteristics known to influence mortality?
5 Was the reference population used to develop the model adequately chosen and is the model well calibrated on that population?
6 Is the dimension of the sample under analysis large enough to yield the power for detecting significant differences?

In this process, the evaluation of the applicability of the general outcome prediction model to the population under analysis is possibly the most crucial step. As stated by a recent Consensus Conference 'Mortality prediction models are almost always overspecific for the patient samples upon which they were developed, and thus performance usually deteriorates when models are applied to different population samples.... For this reason, we recommend that mortality prediction models always be tested in patient samples distinct from those in which the models were developed'.

Usually, three methods are used to test the adequacy of the model:

1 Calibration: evaluates the degree of correspondence between the estimated probabilities of mortality and the observed mortality in the sample under analysis. Four methods have been employed: overall observed/expected mortality ratios, Flora's Z score, Hosmer–Lemeshow goodness-of-fit tests and calibration curves.
2 Discrimination: how well the model can distinguish between observations with a positive or a negative outcome. This assessment can be done by a non-parametric test such as Harrell's c-index, using the rank of the magnitude of the assessment error. This index measures the probability that for two randomly chosen patients, the one with the higher probabilistic prediction has the outcome of interest. It has been shown that this index relates directly to the area under a receiver operating characteristic (ROC) curve and can be obtained as the parameter from the Mann–Whitney–Wilcoxon rank sum test statistic;
3 Uniformity of fit: or the performance of the model across major subgroups of patients.

The relative importance of calibration and discrimination varies with the utilization that will be given to the model. For research or quality assurance purposes (group comparisons), calibration is especially important; for decisions about individual patients both descriptors are very relevant. From a methodological point of view, the poor calibration of a model can be corrected. However, there is almost nothing that can adjust a model when it produces poor discrimination.

Computing and interpreting the standardized mortality ratio

If the answer to all these points is yes and an appropriate model identified, them we can proceed to the next steps of evaluating the risk-adjusted mortality of the ICU.

To achieve that aim, we must then:

- compute the predicted mortality for all patients admitted to the ICU during the period under analysis;
- count all non-survivals at hospital discharge
- compute the standardized mortality ratio or the ratio of the actual ICU mortality vs the predicted ICU mortality (additional computations can be done to compute the confidence intervals for this ratio.

As can be seen in Fig. 33.9.1, ICU A presents a standardized mortality ratio significantly lower than 1. This means that the number of observed deaths was significantly lower that the number predicted by the model. In other words, observed mortality, adjusted for the patient characteristics included in the model utilized for risk adjustment, was significantly lower than the mortality in the reference database utilized to calibrate the model. The reverse is true for ICU F.

Other methods have been proposed to compare the ICUs, with several advantages in terms of availability of the information, but more complex and difficult to use.

A word of caution

It is quite disputable that ICU performance can be evaluated exclusively by risk-adjusted hospital mortality.

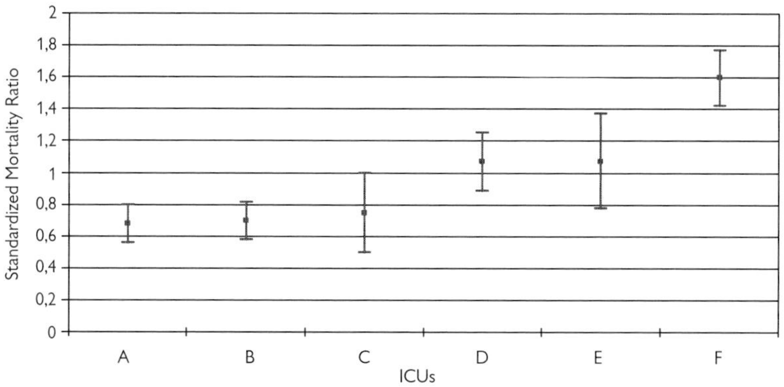

Fig. 33.11.1 Comparison of ICUs using a standardized mortality ratio. A–E represent ICUs. Unit A is well below 1, suggesting the mortality in that unit is less than predicted. Conversely, Unit F is well above 1, suggesting a greater mortality than would be predicted.

Other outcomes are certainly important to the patient and to the family (e.g. quality of life, long-term outcome) and also for the hospital manager (e.g. costs, effectiveness in the use of resources). Moreover, for quality improvement, process indicators are potentially more useful than outcome indicators.

Further reading

Hadorn DC, Keeler EB, Rogers WH, *et al.* Assessing the performance of mortality prediction models. Santa Monica, CA: RAND/UCLA/Harvard Center for Health Care Financing Policy Research, 1993.

Hanley J, McNeil B. The meaning and use of the area under a receiver operating characteristic (ROC) curve. *Radiology* 1982; 143: 29–36.

Moreno R, Apolone G, Reis Miranda D. Evaluation of the uniformity of fit of general outcome prediction models. *Intensive Care Med* 1998; 24: 40–7.

Randall Curtis J, Cook DJ, Wall RJ, *et al.* Intensive care unit quality improvement: a 'how-to' guide for the interdisciplinary team. *Crit Care Med* 2006; 34: 211–8.

Rapoport J, Teres D, Lemeshow S, *et al.* A method for assessing the clinical performance and cost-effectiveness of intensive care units: a multicenter inception cohort study. *Crit Care Med* 1994; 22: 1385–91.

Schuster DP. Predicting outcome after ICU admission. The art and science of assessing risk. *Chest* 1992; 102: 1861–70.

Critical care disaster planning

Introduction

A number of recent events have raised awareness of how the demand for critical care beds may rapidly exceed existing capacity. The first of these was the initial Department of Health publication on pandemic influenza which predicted >50 000 deaths in the UK. As a result of concerns raised by this estimate, and the prediction that significant numbers of affected patients may require respiratory support, the ICS accessed the Center for Disease Control Flusurge modelling program to predict the likely effect on UK intensive care bed requirements, and confirmed that existing capacity was likely to be rapidly overwhelmed during the peak of a pandemic. More detailed analysis by the Pandemic Influenza Scientific Modelling Committee confirmed this prediction, and helped to drive the multi-professional Critical Care Contingency Planning (CCCP) group that was established by the ICS and the Division of Emergency Preparedness, which has worked in conjunction with the Pandemic Influenza Group to coordinate contingency plans for expanding critical care capacity.

Shortly after the CCCP group was inaugurated, the July bombings occurred in London. Although the number of severely injured survivors who required critical care support was lower than might have been anticipated, the impact on several ICUs was dramatic, and many challenging problems had to be overcome, including cancellation of elective surgery and the transfer of existing patients. Many of the recommendations that had been included in the draft work undertaken by the CCCP group were enacted spontaneously by the clinicians faced with these problems, even though there had been no prior discussion, suggesting that the concepts being considered were logical. Later in 2006 the adverse drug trials reactions which led to the simultaneous requirement for ICU admission of 6 patients produced such pressure for beds that a major incident response had to be initiated.

Important points and lessons learned

- If/when a disaster event occurs, it is likely that existing critical care beds will already be occupied
- Professional responses of critical care staff are likely to result in extraordinary measures to try to ensure that patients receive prompt and appropriate treatment
- Sustaining such responses puts staff under considerable pressure, and team-supporting strategies are essential
- Equipment availability and supplies may be a problem
- The nature of the event may lead to previously unfamiliar and unpredictable injury patterns that can pose signficant challenges to critical clinicians and nursing staff
- Identifying patients and next of kin may be difficult
- Support of neighbouring units/specialist units is crucial
- The impact on elective surgery, waiting times and other patient services is likely to be significant

As a result of these lessons, and other work undertaken to plan for future eventualities, recommendations for critical care services have been made. Some of these may be more aspirational than achievable, and variations in infrastructures may mean that local solutions may result in a better likelihood of services coping. It is nevertheless important that all units should give consideration to expanding capacity, as even a relatively minor local event (e.g. train crash) could result in sudden excessive demand for critical care admissions. National requirements for NHS organizations to establish contingency plans for an influenza pandemic provides additional impetus for contingency planning.

Expanding critical care capacity

An information-gathering survey obtained responses from ~60% of UK units, and indicated that Level 2 and Level 3 ICU bed capacity could be escalated by 115 and 83%, respectively, of corresponding baseline totals. These estimates were based on the concepts of expanding critical care facilities into other clinical areas with appropriate resources (e.g. HDUs, theatre recovery areas, coronary care units, etc.), recruiting the use of all available ventilators, monitors and infusion devices, and the cancellation of elective surgical procedures to create additional resources and staff availability.

Recommendations to expand Level 3 ICU bed capacity

- Stocktaking should be undertaken to identify all available mechanical ventilators, monitoring equipment and infusion devices, recorded and updated annually.
- Clinical areas that can be upgraded to provide Level 3 care should be identified, and bed numbers calculated.
- Where new building (or upgrading of existing facilities) is being undertaken, consideration should be given to planning for the inclusion of piped air, oxygen and appropriate power supplies to allow capacity expansion
- If specialist units (e.g. cardiothoracic or neurosurgical ICUs) are available locally the planning process should include these resources whilst preserving sufficient capacity for urgent surgical procedures
- Planning strategies should also involve any independent sector facilities that might be able to provide 'step down' Level 2 care or provide support in other ways.
- Plans for transferring patients to other critical care units (or ward areas where appropriate) should be made, even though they are only likely to be of benefit if the increased demand is limited to a local geographical area.
- The CCCP guidance has suggested that a target level of 100% escalation of existing Level 3 capacity should be set. Although this figure exceeds the national survey estimates, a number of NHS units which have carried out their own planning exercises have indicated that expansion to this level (and in some instances considerably greater) is feasible.

Staffing

Critical care capacity expansion is more likely to be limited by staff availability than by equipment. One study suggests that, depending on the cause of the incident, up to 40% of healthcare staff may not be available to provide patient care. Infection/toxic events are more likely to produce staff absence; events that cause high levels of injury or trauma are more likely to be well attended. Staff availability may be compromised because of:

- Staff being affected/infected/injured by the event
- Need to provide care for children or relatives
- Transport availability
- Fear of disease transmission (to staff or their family)
- Communications failure

Principles to consider

- Operating theatre staff and those who work in areas such as HDUs or coronary care units are likely to be the most able to assist as reserve critical care staff.
- Trained critical care nurses (CCNs) should be able to oversee the care of several patients supported by reserve staff; the ratio of trained CCN to reserve staff/patients will depend on the severity of the event.
- Training programmes need to be developed to update reserve staff on the principles of critical care support; these should be maintained on a rolling basis.
- Teaching programmes should also be established to train staff in the use of personal protection equipment, infection control procedures, and other issues that relate to staff and patient safety.
- Robust mechanisms for support of staff morale should be developed; reassuring confidence and promoting teamworking will help to maintain staffing levels.
- Reductions/cancellation of elective surgery will mean that anaesthesia consultants and trainees may be able to assist in critical care expansion.
- The recruitment of senior staff/trainees from other clinical specialties may be feasible in the future as more trainees complete training modules in critical care. Basic critical care training programmes are also available online.

Standards of care

Although the aim should always be to maintain high standards of care, the need for pragmatism must be recognized. As the number of patients requiring mechanical ventilatory support rises and staffing ratios become more difficult, it is inevitable that the risks of adverse events will increase. When resources are significantly overstretched, interventions normally considered appropriate may not be achievable because of availability of staff, equipment or consumables. Staff who undertake responsibility for care of patients or procedures that are outside of their normal working practice need to have strong reassurance that they will not be vulnerable to professional criticism or litigation for doing the best that they can under difficult circumstances. Until this concept is formally supported nationally, the responsibility for providing adequate reassurance and support for staff must lie with local trust management and SHAs.

Supplies and disposables

Pandemic influenza planning has led to recognition that most NHS institutions depend on a 'just in time' supply system, and that mechanisms have to be refined to ensure that supply chains can be maintained during a major incident. Although a considerable amount of work has been put into this, it remains far from certain that supply systems will be sufficiently robust to maintain essential services, particularly as demand for some items may significantly exceed normal requirements. Cooperative networking arrangements will help units to cope with a local or even a regional major incident, but an event which results in simultaneous increased demand for supplies will pose a major challenge.

Triaging and ethics

These are the most complex problems that critical care staff may face, and many issues remain unresolved. In smaller incidents where local/regional expansion and networking will help to manage a surge of demand, it is less likely that treatment limitation decisions may have to be made. In a national crisis, however, where all critical care facilities may become rapidly overwhelmed, staff will be faced with very difficult decisions on which patients should receive mechanical ventilation and on escalation of treatment levels. Although recommended ethical principles have been made for pandemic influenza, concerns remain that these may not help clinicians faced with the reality of too many patients and not enough beds. Decisions to withhold or withdraw treatment that would not be considered in normal circumstances because of lack of resources may also have significant implications for intensivists. To address these concerns an extensive consultation process has been followed to produce guidance which emphasizes the importance of consistency of healthcare restrictions from primary to advanced secondary care, and includes triaging criteria based on the SOFA scoring system initially published by Canadian intensivists. Although the final Surge Capacity & Prioritisation document version is likely to help with many of the concerns raised, it also remains probable that in severe circumstances even more stringent triaging may be necessary because of the lower numbers of critical care beds per head of population in the UK. Accordingly local decisions on treatment restrictions—including the possibility of temporary ICU closure to new admissions—may have to be agreed with trust senior management and SHAs, the reasons being carefully documented and reviewed on a daily basis.

Paediatrics

Dealing with a significant number of infants and children who require critical care support will pose a major challenge. Paediatric ICUs already run at high levels of capacity and, even if escalation plans are enacted, will have limited ability to cope with increased demand. A local major incident could also produce the requirement for a number of children to receive critical care stabilization procedures prior to transfer to other centres. This reinforces the importance of preserving paediatric stabilization expertise in all hospitals where children may be admitted.

Further reading

Christian MD, Hawryluck, L, Wax RS, *et al.* Development of a triage protocol for critical care during an influenza pandemic. *CMAJ* 2006; 175: 1377–81.

http://www.aic.cuhk.edu.hk/web8/BASIC.htm

http://www.dh.gov.uk/en/Publicationsandstatistics/Publications/PublicationsPolicyAndGuidance/DH_073179

Menon DK, Taylor BL, Ridley SA. The Intensive Care Society, UK. Modelling the impact of an influenza pandemic on critical care services in England. *Anaesthesia* 2005; 60: 952–4.

Qureshi K, Gershon RRM, Sherman MF *et al.* Health care workers' ability and willingness to report to duty during catastrophic d isasters. *Bull NY Acad Med* 2005; 82: 378–88.

Suntharalingam G, Perry MR, Ward S, *et al.* Cytokine storm in a Phase 1 trial of the anti-CD28 monoclonal antibody TGN1412. *N Engl J Med* 2006; 355: 1018–28.

UK Department of Health. UK Health Department's influenza pandemic contingency plan. London: DoH, 2005.

www.dh.gov.uk/prod_consum_dh/groups/dh_digitalasets/@dh/@en/documents/digitalasset/dh_4137619.pdf (2006) Critical Care Contingency Planning.

Health technology assessment

Definition

'Health technologies' are broadly defined to include all interventions used to promote health, prevent and treat disease, and improve rehabilitation and long-term care. This may include drugs, devices, procedures (surgical techniques, screening and counselling) and even the settings of care, such as general practice, hospitals and care homes.

Background

The NHS Technology Assessment Programme was set up in 1993, and the findings and output from this Programme directly influence key decision-making bodies such as the NICE. Although the definition of health technology assessment (HTA) presents a wide spectrum of interventions, with the exception of drug based technologies, most of the principles involved can be considered with reference to medical devices.

The drug-based technologies and pharmaceutical industry are tightly legislated and require assessments ranging from animal studies to large interventional clinical trials. In contrast, medical devices have relatively little legislature surrounding clinical introduction, and there frequently may not be a consensus as to what constitutes adequate assessment. There is as a result a need for further developments of the science relating to HTA. This is especially pertinent when consideration of the escalating numbers of devices for which manufacturers make claims relating to patient care. The ensuing HTA exercises stipulate study design and assessment of these new technologies in an attempt to judge and evaluate short- and long-term benefits.

In effect, there are two questions to answer: does the device have a positive clinical impact and are the resultant economics affordable in the context of local/national healthcare funding? The requirement for a balanced approach of science vs economics ensures that the assessment design will draw on expertise from clinicians, engineers, statisticians, economists, ethicists and of course lawyers.

The assessment process

The HTA process has three core areas:

- device safety,
- device performance
- device cost.

Device safety

This is a complex area where there may be safety aspects related to using a device as well as the clinical process and context in which the device is used. Safety also encompasses accuracy of the device, as inappropriate clinical decisions can result from inaccurate measurements. Frequently overlooked is the obverse component of the assessment process which should scrutinize the impact of not using the device.

Assessing the safety of the device or box itself is a statutory requirement and includes elements of electrical safety, detailed multi-lingual instructions, packaging, conformation to environmental specifications and disposal instructions. All of these issues are dealt with using a European Standard, referred to as the CE mark (La Conformitee Europeenne), which certifies that technical manufacturing standards have been met. It is not a functional guarantee that the device or process will be of benefit or be safe in clinical use. In the USA, the FDA fulfils a similar role but, in addition, before granting approval for sale in the USA, has a remit beyond the technical qualifications of the CE mark and mandates some assessment of clinical operation. The FDA uses clinical experts to review investigational studies relating to the device to ascertain whether the product does what is claimed by the manufacturer and/or presents unreasonable risks to the patient. The FDA classify devices into three classes according to the risk of potential harm to the user, ranging from Class 1 devices that present minimal risk to the user, e.g. home blood pressure kits, to Class 3, e.g. dialysis machines or ICU ventilators

Device performance

Efficacy and effectiveness are used to assess device performance. The efficacy relates to the device performance under ideal conditions, and the effectiveness is the performance under normal clinical working conditions. This is an important distinction as efficacy ratings may indicate the necessity for 'experts' to operate the device, whereas effectiveness relates to the performance limitations under average clinical conditions. Overall, when reviewing technology, the new approach should offer improvement over current technologies. This may be because the device can obtain measurements with less risk to the patient, i.e. is less invasive, or has some other aspect which is advantageous.

Efficacy

Assessing efficacy usually means comparison of the device against a known 'gold' standard. When the measurement is well defined, e.g. cardiac output, the efficacy becomes the mathematical correlate of accuracy.

Accuracy is the closeness of the device measurement to the actual value and can be described by:

- Correlation (degree of association between readings)
- Precision (the closeness of repeated measurements)
- Bias (the difference between the means of the measurements)

The repeatability and inaccuracy of the gold standard is important as if it has a varying accuracy then the limits of agreement between it and the technology under scrutiny become wider and less meaningful, and this makes definitive comparisons difficult, e.g. thermodilution cardiac output vs other technologies

Where a gold standard reference does not exist, then it is necessary to show that the technology has a clinical utility, usually in relation to patient outcomes. This suggests that the monitor has to be able to detect a variable which when targeted will affect outcome. The efficacy assessment here, where there is not a gold standard, is the determination of the sensitivity, specificity and predictive values:

	Outcome improved	Outcome not improved
Positive	A	B
Negative	C	D

Sensitivity = A/A+C

Positive predictive value = A/A + B

Specificity = D/B + D

Negative predictive value = D/C + D

Effectiveness

Assessment of effectiveness requires clinical trials in which the technology is used as it would be under average conditions. Standard rules of engagement for conduct of comparative studies are important to produce valid results, and it must be appreciated that there may be issues related to study design.

The two obvious trials are a technology vs a control, or the technology with its measurement guiding subsequent therapeutic management. For the former type of trial, the data are usually comparative, whereas for the latter the results tend to be clinical outcome based. For outcome data, the ideal measurement is considered to be mortality but, because of the resource implications of numbers needed to power studies for mortality, the use of surrogates such as length of hospital stay or number of complications is common. If using a device to guide therapy, it is important to consider the relative contributions of the device being assessed as opposed to the therapeutic interventions of the protocol which may be the important determinant of the results.

Device cost

The economics related to health technologies is a key driver for HTA. These principles provide a safeguard for a finite and shrinking health budget and represent an attempt to ensure that resources and benefits are spread and do not favour one particular group. The area of cost containment is complex, as in many situations the only costs considered are 'direct' costs relating to the technology and disposables. Frequently the indirect costs such as training and storage are ignored, and these may represent a considerable financial load, e.g. a Clinical Information System may have a monetary cost per bed, but staff training, education and maintenance personnel may generate considerable additional add-on costs.

Practical use of HTA principles

In the hospital arena, the principles of HTA are used to enable decisions for device procurement. When purchasing a device, the functionality, i.e. safety and performance, has to be considered in relation to the cost. The selection criteria for the purchase and replacement of medical devices depends on cost and numbers being purchased. The selection process should also include an evaluation of the manufacturer/supplier in terms of track record, profile in the local and national healthcare market, company financial stability/survival, and service capability and response times.

The eventual procurement of technologies usually follows a defined process dependent on the size and cost of the intended purchase. High value public sector tenders are covered by special European Competition rules (OJEU). These rules are designed to guarantee open and fair competition across all EU states.

The tender process—the OJEU limits

The OJEU notice reflects business needs and priorities, and should achieve a realistic balance between a scope that is wide enough to encourage innovation and a statement of business need to which the market can make a meaningful response; it must also specify achievable timeframes within the EU Procurement rules. The rules prescribe how the tenders are advertised and awarded. Currently contracts over the following values are subject to these rules:

Type of contract	OJEU threshold
Supplies Contracts	£93 738
Service Contracts—Part A	£93 738
Service Contracts—Part B	£144 371
Works Contracts	£3 611 319

The tender is advertised in the Supplement to the *Official Journal of the European Union* (OJEU) and under the EU regulations there are three types of tender procedure available to buyers:

The open procedure

This is available in all circumstances and involves a single-stage approach, where all candidates may respond to the OJEU advertisement and all offers received must be considered.

The restricted procedure

This is available in all circumstances and involves a two-stage approach where candidates who respond to the OJEU advertisement will be considered to have expressed an interest. The buyer will shortlist a number of these, who will then be invited to submit offers.

Where the restricted procedure is used, the buyer must allow a minimum of 37 days from the date the OJEU notice was despatched to the closing date for receipt of expressions of interest. Once shortlisting has taken place, a minimum of 40 days must be allowed for offers to be returned

The negotiated procedure

This is only available in a very limited number of circumstances and is subject to strict conditions.

The most common tender used is the restricted procedure, as the open procedure is expensive and time consuming, and there is limited applicability surrounding the negotiated procedure.

Further reading

Critchley LAH, Critchley JAJH A meta-analysis of studies using bias and precision statistics to compare cardiac output measurement technologies *J Clin Monit* 1999; 15: 85–91.

Guyatt GH, Tugwell PX, Feeny DH, *et al.* A framework for clinical evaluation of diagnostic technologies *CMAJ* 1986;134: 587–94.

OJEU `www.ted.europa.eu`

Procurement Policies and standards `http://www.ogc.gov.uk/procurement`

Sibbald WJ,Inman KJ. Problems in assessing the technology of critical care medicine. *Int J Technol Assess Health Care* 1992; 8: 419–43.

Transfer of the critically ill patient

Primary transfer is from the scene of an incident.

Secondary transfer is between medical facilities or within the same facility for surgery or investigation. This chapter deals only with secondary transfer. Transfer either intra- or interhospital requires the same preparations. Patient transfers can and should be safe.

Components of a transfer

Patient

Reason to move

There must be a good reason to move, e.g. upgrade care, surgery, investigation, repatriation or because of lack of ICU beds. The reason should be documented. Moving one patient to make way for another when that move is not in the patient's best interests requires careful consideration at consultant level and consent from both patient and family.

Physiology of transportation

Acceleration and deceleration in an ambulance can cause profound shifts of fluid in the circulation, particularly in patients who are vasodilated, hypovolaemic or dysautonomic, with adverse effect on cardiac output and blood pressure. This affects both systemic and pulmonary circulations, worsening ventilation–perfusion matching and necessitating increased minute ventilation and inspired oxygen to maintain the same ABGs. Ideally patients would be placed across the direction of travel; however, this is rarely possible as the position of the trolley is determined by the ambulance layout.

Pre-transfer stabilization

The patient must be stable and well resuscitated.

- Endotracheal intubation is indicated if blood gases are poor, GCS <9, or a higher but declining score, or if there is airway compromise, e.g. burns or facial trauma. Intubation in a moving vehicle or in a lay-by at the side of the road may not be easy and should be avoided. The tube should be well secured.
- The patient should be attached and stabilized on the transport ventilator for a period prior to departure to allow blood gases to be checked and adequacy of ventilation established. Consider paralysis to facilitate ventilation and prevent unplanned self-extubation. Hand ventilation is unacceptable.
- Volume: full patients travel better than empty ones. Resuscitate using sequential fluid challenges accompanied by appropriate use of vasoconstrictors. Insert at least two large bore peripheral lines; central venous access may also be required for infusions. All lines should be well secured.
- Identify and drain pneumothoraces prior to transfer
- If patient has received thrombolysis for MI, remember reperfusion arrhythmias and consider delaying transfer.
- Electrolytes, if potassium <3 or >6.5mmol/l correct before transfer. Correct magnesium if low in the presence of rhythm disturbance.
- Fractures: splint to avoid pain and further injury. Pelvic fractures have significant blood loss—consider external fixation if possible.
- Urinary catheter and NG tube on free drainage.
- Ensure normothermia prior to transportl it's very easy to get cold in an ambulance.

Some patients should be transported without stabilization, e.g. those requiring urgent definitive surgical treatment for whom attempts at stabilization will compromise survival, such as leaking abdominal aortic aneurysm.

Surgical including burns

Leaking oesophageal varices—take appropriate advice on placement of a Sengstaken–Blackmore tube if patient must be transferred to another site for haemorrhage control.

Burns—if in doubt protect the airway; swelling can be severe and delayed intubation may be difficult. Use a high concentration of oxygen if carbon monoxide or inhalation injury is suspected until levels are established. For respiratory or limb circulatory problems, perform escharotomies prior to transfer; diagrams can be faxed from a burn centre to guide these. Fluid requirements can be large, and formulae especially in the presence of inhalation injury are only a guide; aim for urine output >0.5ml/kg/h. Maintain body temperature or re-warm; cold water immersion/irrigation and exposure can result in hypothermia. Cover burn with clean dry dressings or cling film.

Neurosurgical

Avoid secondary injury; maintain oxygenation and blood pressure. Treat other causes of haemorrhage, e.g. splenic rupture, prior to transfer to avoid hypotension. If patient is otherwise stable, aim for a prompt departure; early evacuation of blood clots leads to optimal outcome.

Equipment

Ensure competence with all devices before transfer.

All equipment used in an ambulance must be securely attached to the transport trolley and able to withstand a 10g force. The patient should be secured to the trolley with a 5-point restraint.

Monitoring

It is important to know your equipment and how and where it is stored. Monitors should be robust, intuitive and have an easily viewed screen, battery powered and kept charged. Need to know type of battery and whether it is susceptible to memory problems and poor charging. Batteries must be interchangeable in use without loss of monitoring.

- 5-lead ECG
- Preferably invasive blood pressure; non-invasive is more susceptible to movement interference and is expensive on battery power.
- Pulse oximetry
- Exhaled carbon dioxide
- If a pulmonary artery cather is used, the pressure must be continually monitored to avoid spontaneous wedging or it must be withdrawn into the SVC for transfer.
- Core temperature
- Airway pressure

Ventilator

Ventilators must be robust, have a wide range of settings for tidal volume, I:E ratio, rate and PEEP to accommodate most patients. Preferably battery powered and economical with oxygen—any gas used for the ventilator must be known and taken into account along with respiratory gas. It should have a disconnect alarm.

Oxygen

Calculate the amount of oxygen required for the projected transfer duration and include any driving gas for the ventilator. Take double this amount and at least an hour's supply in case of unexpected delays. If using the ambulance supply, check these cylinders contain enough for your projected journey time. Check connections are compatible. Take an ambu bag with reservoir and face mask in case of ventilator failure or unplanned extubation.

Volume of oxygen in standard UK cylinders in litres.

D size	340
E size	680
F size	1360

Infusion

All fluids must be administered via electronically controlled devices, avoid hanging bags of fluid; movement and transfer may result in air in the infusion tubing.

Drugs

Stop all unnecessary infusions before transport. Essential infusions should be made in a concentration such that syringe changes will not be required en route. If infusion concentrations are changed, allow a period of stabilization on the new concentrations prior to departure. Take spare pre-prepared syringes in case of problems. All syringes should be clearly labelled. Emergency drugs should preferably be in pre-loaded syringes.

Transfer team

Ideally all patients would be transferred by a specialized transfer team; in most cases this is not feasible for many reasons including cost, availability and the requirement for rapid treatment in, for example, head injury. All anaesthesia and critical care staff should undergo transfer training in the necessary skills and be competent in the use of all the equipment. It is not essential that all transfers are undertaken by doctors, but it is essential that the accompanying personnel are competent and have indemnity.

Whilst it is not acceptable to send the most junior inexperienced member of the hospital team on a transfer because they will be least missed, it is important to consider both the patient being transferred and those left behind, and distribute skills accordingly.

The team members have the ultimate veto on the transfer if they are unhappy that the patient, the equipment or they are not fit for the transfer.

The transfer team members should be involved in patient stabilization and the decision about fitness for and timing of transfer. It is inappropriate for someone who does not know the patient and their problems to be involved in a transfer.

Team members must be adequately insured and have suitable protective kit; they must have prior arranged transport back to base.

Communication

The referring hospital must ensure the recipient hospital is able to provide the care and treatment the patient requires before agreeing to transfer the patient. The recipient hospital must have spare capacity before accepting the patient. Whilst negotiating the transfer, the most senior clinician involved should provide a full and detailed verbal case summary including MRSA and *C. difficile* status. The clinician caring for the patient must give a detailed handover to the transferring team including all investigations and results. The transfer team should then give a full handover to the recipient team.

The team must have a means of communicating with their base whilst en route; mobile phones may be used.

The receiving hospital should be given an estimated time of arrival and informed when the patient is en route.

It is not appropriate for relatives to travel in an ambulance with the patient unless the patient is a child.

Documentation

The reason for transfer along with conversations with other teams, patient and family should all be documented.

Physiological observations should be charted during transfer. Many networks have multicopy transfer forms so that copies can be kept by the referring team and the network for audit, as well as a copy placed in the patient notes. Take all notes and X-rays on CD. Any critical incidents should be fully documented

Mode of transport

Aeromedical transport is covered in Chapter 33.15. Ambulances are not standard and vary considerably, so check you are happy with all the equipment before loading the patient. Many ambulances only have room for 2 rear passengers, in addition to the patient; negotiate in advance who will travel with the patient.

Patient and team safety

It is important to consider the safety not only of the patient but also that of the team. All members should wear seat belts. Protective reflective clothing should be available.

Each team member should be aware of his insurance status. Hospital Trusts may not arrange appropriate cover, and professional bodies may take out cover for their members.

Ethics of transfer

Transfer a patient because they will benefit from it, e.g. transfer to burns centre.

Protect and stabilize the patient so they do not come to harm.

If possible, discuss move with patient and seek their view.

In exceptional circumstances, a patient may be moved to free up resources for another patient, i.e. for the benefit of another.

Medicolegal aspects

Prior to transport it may be appropriate to take advice from the receiving centre on patient treatment; however, it remains the responsibility of the referring clinicians to decide if it is the correct advice.

Handover of responsibility follows formal handover; the transfer team accepts responsibility from the referring unit and then hands over to the receiving unit. Hospitals should agree lines of legal responsibility if a transfer team is used and they wish to stabilize a patient at the referring hospital where they are not employed.

Checklist system

Each unit or preferably network should establish a checklist which includes all of the above points; this should be with the patient documentation and should be formally worked through prior to every transfer and signed by the team members.

Further reading

Guidelines for the transport of the critically ill adult. Intensive Care Society 2002 http://www.ics.ac.uk/icmprof/standards.asp?menuid=7

Recommendations for the safe transfer of patients with brain injury. Association of Anaesthetists 2006

http://www.aagbi.org/publications/guidelines.htm#t

Aeromedical evacuation

Aeromedical evacuation is used to transfer critically ill patients over large distances or where road transfer would be impractical due to terrain, road condition, traffic etc. It comprises fixed wing aircraft or rotary wing (helicopters). Aeromedical transfer may be required to upgrade the level of critical care facility or to repatriate a patient from overseas.

The principles of patient transfer by air are identical to those for road inter-hospital transfer with the same level of monitoring and treatment and attention to patient and medical team safety. The peculiarities of the aeromedical environment need additional consideration.

Choice of aircraft

Speed and distance

Helicopters typically cruise at 120–150 knots (220–280km/h) with a useful radius of 50–300km. Time taken to prepare and launch the helicopter and also fuel endurance limit their advantages for very short or long distances, but the advantage over fixed wing aircraft is the ability to operate from a range of surfaces, e.g. dedicated helipads, parking areas, recreational parks and fields. Fixed wing aircraft benefit from increased cruise speed (from 300km/h for piston engine aircraft to 850km/h for jet aircraft) and are best suited for ranges of 200–2000km. They require prepared runways necessitating road or helicopter ambulance transfer between hospital and airport at each end.

Environmental factors

Helicopter

The internal noise levels are frequently >95dB(A) such that normal conversation is impossible. Auscultation is redundant, as is reliance on audible monitor alarms. Intercom headsets are required for crew communication. Earplugs are used for all patients regardless of conscious state to reduce hearing damage. Cabin lighting may be poor due to the dangers of distracting the aircrew and adversely affecting pilot night vision. Blue or red lighting may be used instead of white light, which may make monitors, cyanosis, veins and patient movement difficult to see.

Vibration is greatest at take-off and landing and may induce pain in unstable fractures, and makes accurate adjustment of fluid infusion rates difficult.

Fixed wing flights

Continuous noise, vibration, changes in temperature, cramped space, ultraviolet radiation and time zone changes contribute to high levels of fatigue. Limited chance for rotation of medical personnel en route may mean extended working hours; therefore, appropriate rest periods prior to and after flights should be scheduled in staff rosters. Staff should ensure they are physically fit to fly, not suffering from the effects of respiratory infections and be under the residual effects of neither medication nor alcohol. Neither helicopters nor small fixed wing aircraft have toilet facilities.

Axial tilt, acceleration and deceleration forces may be significant during take-off, landing and extreme turbulence in fixed wing aircraft. Adverse effects on haemodynamics and ICP may result. Altering patient orientation within the cabin during the flight to attenuate these forces is impractical.

Cabin heating may be poorly controlled or slow to respond to changes in temperature. Staff must be vigilant in monitoring the patient's temperature and avoiding hypothermia, and ensure they also wear suitable flight clothing.

Atmospheric pressure

Oxygen

Dalton's Law dictates that the partial pressure of oxygen decreases with altitude. Except for operations in high mountainous regions, this is not usually a problem for helicopters (typical cruise altitude 2000ft). Fixed wing jet aircraft fly at greater altitudes for reasons of aerodynamic efficiency and thus require cabin pressurization. According to the age and efficiency of the airframe and pressurization system, a set 'cabin altitude' can be achieved. Commercial aircraft fly at altitudes up to 40 000ft and typically achieve cabin altitudes of 7000ft. Atmospheric pressure at this altitude is 586mm Hg compared with 760 mm Hg at sea level. Corresponding PaO_2s are 73 and 103 mm Hg. Critically ill patients with high alveolar arterial gradients may become hypoxic at such cabin altitudes despite FiO_2 of 1.0. Prior consideration must be given to anticipated increased oxygen requirements at altitude. If necessary, the aircrew can be requested to provide sea level cabin pressurization. Typically this necessitates flying at altitudes of 20 000ft, which increases fuel consumption. Aside from cost implications, this may necessitate more frequent refuelling stops, which will significantly increase journey time with roll-on implications for patient safety, battery requirements, total oxygen requirements, fatigue, etc. Adverse meteorological conditions may on occasion prevent flying at lower altitude.

Pressure

According to Boyle's Law, as the atmospheric pressure falls, gas volume increases. At a cabin altitude of 7000ft this represents an increase of 27% as opposed to 8% at a typical helicopter altitude of 2000ft. Travellers will be familiar with expansion of air in nasal sinuses, the middle ear and the GI tract, but careful consideration must be given in disease states. Pneumothoraces, pneumocephalus, bubble emboli and trapped air in the abdominal cavity post-laparotomy will all expand proportional to the drop in cabin pressure. Consideration should also be given to splitting orthopaedic casts. Chest drains should be inserted where necessary prior to departure and left *in situ* for the duration of the flight. All surgical drains should be unclamped and patent.

ETT cuffs should either be filled with saline or have their pressure rigorously checked and adjusted in-flight. Ensure pulmonary artery catheter balloons are fully deflated.

Equipment: key points

Whilst the standard of monitoring needs to be equivalent to that in an ICU, aeromedical equipment needs to fulfil additional criteria:

- Portability and size. Each aircraft has a maximum permitted payload, and smaller helicopters are particularly limited in this regard. Trade-offs may have to be made with total fuel carried to allow additional weight, but this adversely affects flight endurance. Aircraft performance is significantly affected by ambient temperature and airfield altitude. Less payload can be carried when taking off from hot, high airfields.

- Sufficiently rugged to withstand knocks and falls.
- Reliable and extended battery life, with lightweight batteries preferably changeable without interrupting monitoring. Do not rely on being able to connect equipment to aircraft electrical supply.
- Clear backlit displays that can be easily read even in direct sunlight and with vibration.
- Ability to withstand acceleration/deceleration forces, vibration, extreme temperature changes, and not interfere with aircraft avionics or electrical systems (e.g. defibrillators).
- Ventilators should be oxygen efficient and deliver consistent tidal volumes irrespective of ambient pressure.
- Any integral on-board oxygen systems must be rigorously checked and maintained. Portable cylinders should be available in the event of systems failure, and for patient transfer at each end of the flight. Dedicated oxygen cylinders need to be carried on commercial aircraft as the integral passenger supply is for use in emergency decompression only. Oxygen is dangerous air cargo and needs official clearance for its carriage. Always plan sufficient oxygen in case of patient respiratory deterioration, aircraft delay or diversion. It is imperative that medical staff familiarize themselves with whichever oxygen system is used, and rigorously monitor consumption rate and contents. In-line oxygen analysers are recommended.
- Ideally the equipment can be neatly stacked to maximize access and minimize space occupied. Several organizations use specially designed equipment bridges to facilitate this.
- Drugs and consumable equipment need to be easily visualized and rapidly accessible. Thomas packs are popular as they are easily carried with rucksack straps, and have compartmentalized sections with clear pockets. Equipment should be arranged according to indication for use, e.g. airway equipment. There must be a system for regular checks to ensure all equipment is present and serviceable, and a system to restock equipment rapidly after use. Drugs must be within expiry dates and kept at the required temperature. Controlled drugs need written authority for carriage across borders.
- Transformers and adaptors will be required to ensure charging capability overseas.

Preparing the patient for transport

As far as possible the patient must be stabilized prior to transfer. Any necessary interventions and treatments need to be done prior to leaving the referring hospital e.g. chest drains, -rays, invasive pressure monitoring.

A formal handover of the patient by medical and nursing staff is essential, as are written notes, results of investigations and copies of imaging procedures. The referring medical staff should communicate directly with the receiving institution medical staff. The transfer team should speak directly with the receiving staff if further advice is required, and confirm an approximate arrival time. Recent blood results including biochemistry, glucose and haemoglobin are essential. ABGs must be examined after the patient has been stabilized on the transport ventilator. For anything other than short transfers, monitoring ABGs en route is recommended. The importance of rigorously securing the airway cannot be overemphasized. All IV access, infusion lines, monitoring equipment, drains, etc. must be checked, rechecked and secured. Spare IV access is essential. Arrange infusion lines and monitoring equipment such that they are free from tangling and lie in such a fashion that they will be accessible according to the particular aircraft used. Access to the patient's limbs, chest and abdomen may be restricted in flight, depending on the layout of the aircraft. Always plan for the worst case scenario, and consider how emergency re-intubation or CPR would be performed in the cabin.

Prior to moving the patient, all loose equipment around the patient should be safely secured to guard against downdraft from helicopter blades or wind when moving the patient around exposed airport areas. The patient must be secured onto the stretcher with a harness approved for aviation use.

Before leaving the referring hospital, a final check of the patient, equipment and team is performed and contact made with the aircrew to ensure the aircraft is fully fuelled, ready to receive the patient and there are no problems with the planned routing.

Safety

The aircraft is an unfamiliar environment for most medical staff. Safety of the patient and aeromedical team is paramount. Staff must undergo training in aeromedical evacuation and an orientation to the equipment and aircraft, with emphasis placed on common aircraft emergencies, emergency evacuation procedures, emergency depressurization, communication procedures and survival equipment. The tail rotor and main rotors of helicopters can be lethal, and even provide hazardous obstacles when motionless. Underwater escape training from a helicopter simulator is recommended where flights may take place over water.

Without proper training, disorientation and confusion are likely, and the ability for staff to provide the best patient care will be adversely affected. A study examining the ability of medical staff to provide CPR to mannequins during helicopter flight showed significant differences between those who had undergone training in aeromedical evacuation and those who had not.

No pressure must be put on the aircrew to alter their normal safety procedures. The captain has the final say on whether the conditions are suitable for flight, no matter what the condition of the patient.

Clinical governance mechanisms should be in place for reporting and investigation of critical incidents.

Further reading

Everest E, Munford B. Transport of the critically ill. In: Bersten AD, Soni N, eds. Oh's intensive care manual, Philadelphia, PA: Butterworth-Heinemann, 2003: 21–32.

Martin T. Aeromedical transportation. Aldershot, UK: Ashgate, 2006.

Outreach

The term outreach was first used in the 1999 Audit Commission report 'Critical to Success'. The UK Department of Health report 'Comprehensive Critical Care' (CCC) was published in 2000, and for the first time gave intensivists responsibility for critically ill patients wherever they were in the hospital. Patients' critical care needs were defined by levels from 0 to 3, and critical care outreach services were recommended as an integral part of each hospital's critical care services. CCC suggested that there were three main aims for outreach: to identify patients who are deteriorating to prevent admissions or ensure that the admission is timely; to enable discharges; and to share critical care skills with ward staff and the community. Outreach is therefore involved in identifying Level 2 and 3 patients who are on wards and should be in a critical care area, and in supporting Level 1 patients on the wards

Levels of care

Level 0: patients whose needs can be met through normal ward care in an acute hospital.

Level 1: at risk of their condition deteriorating, or those recently relocated from higher levels of care and whose needs can be met on an acute ward with additional advice and support from the critical care team.

Level 2: requiring more detailed observation or intervention including support for a single failing organ system or post-operative, care and those stepping down from higher levels of care.

Level 3: requiring advanced respiratory support alone or basic respiratory support together with support of at least two organ systems. This level includes all complex patients requiring support for MOF.

Background

Outreach came about as a response to a realization that there are many patients on hospital wards who are critically ill or at risk of becoming so. Care for these patients is often suboptimal and is associated with increased mortality. Critical care beds are a small proportion of acute hospital beds and have high rates of occupancy. With the move towards fewer hospital beds and shorter stays, ward patients tend to be sicker, and care has to be responsive to deteriorations that may occur over a short period of time. Changes in medical and nurse education have reduced training time in acute care, while key tasks such as measuring vital physiological signs are commonly delegated to untrained staff who may not understand the significance of abnormal values.

Previously, up to 30% of patients admitted from the wards to the ICU required CPR before ICU admission, and the longer they were on the wards before ICU the higher their mortality. In addition, ~25% of patients admitted to an ICU who die do so after they are discharged back to the wards following their first ICU admission. There is also evidence that premature discharges to the ward from ICU are associated with an increased mortality. It is therefore clear that the care patients receive on the wards, both before and after their ICU admission, can be an important determinant of outcome. These patients are already in hospital and are therefore easily accessible. Outreach is one attempt to address this problem.

In 1990 the concept of the medical emergency team (MET) was introduced in Australia (see Chapter 33.17). This began as an extension of the cardiac arrest team so that the MET responded not only to the need for CPR but to patients with gross physiological abnormality or other triggers including 'concern' on the part of the ward staff. In contrast, the initial philosophy behind the outreach concept was early recognition and intervention with the aim of preventing problems. Over time, the differences between the systems have somewhat blurred as METs have also focused on education, early recognition and prevention. There are now many models and a variety of terms for outreach services. Some organizations have enthusiastically embraced the concept while others have reservations. METs are usually physician led, while critical care outreach services are typically nurse led but may include other healthcare professionals, such as physiotherapists, as well as doctors.

All the systems share the following features

1 A mechanism for identifying ward patients who are acutely ill, or have the potential to become so
2 A trigger system to initiate a response
3 A prompt response from personnel with the required competencies, experience and resources

Recognizing critically ill patients

Critically ill patients are identified from their history, examination and investigations. Morbidity and mortality are associated with increasing age, co-morbidity and underlying pathology. However, physiological abnormality is central to any system for recognizing critically ill patients. A high percentage of hospital inpatients who arrest have abnormal physiological values in the hours preceding the arrest. The same has also been found in the hours before death on the hospital wards and also in patients admitted to ICU.

In all systems abnormal physiological values are used to trigger a response. These are incorporated into a variety of physiologically based early warning systems. The physiological variables are commonly blood pressure, heart rate, level of consciousness, respiratory rate, oxygen saturation and temperature. Other variables may be used, including urine output and biochemical or other investigations, events such as new seizures, or concern by the staff caring for the patient.

Scoring systems are based upon combinations of physiological variables and various trigger thresholds. These may use gross abnormality in a single variable, aggregated weighted scoring with points awarded to increasing degrees of abnormality, or combinations. METs tend to be based upon single parameter systems, whereas the aggregate scoring systems are much more common in the UK. One advantage of an aggregate multiple parameter system is that it aids tracking critically ill patients by changes in score as well as the ability to trigger a graded response depending on the score. For this reason, these scores may be called 'track and trigger' systems. However, aggregate scoring systems are more complex, and errors in data collection and calculating the score are more likely than with simpler scores. Another advantage of scoring systems in general is that they mandate a response where otherwise this might be dependent upon an individual's decision. In addition, they have been shown to increase the frequency of recording of physiological parameters on general wards. There is no evidence to support one score over another, and the sensitivity and specificity of the score depend crucially upon the trigger threshold.

The response

Nearly three-quarters of acute hospitals in England have a formal outreach service. There is a wide variation in the proportion of hospital wards covered, the size and composition of the team, and the balance between the provision of direct care and advice. Common interventions include changes in oxygen therapy, initiation of treatment limitation, adjustment to pain management, nutrition, medication or vasoactive drugs, changes in patient position and the use of NIV. Most of the evidence for the benefit of outreach systems and METs has come from papers looking at outcomes before and after the introduction of these systems. This evidence suggests that outreach may decrease cardiac arrests, ICU readmission rates and hospital mortality. To date there have only been two good quality prospective studies of outreach and METs. In both of these studies education was an important ingredient in delivering the change in service. It is possible that this may be the most important element of any outreach service. The UK study performed in a single hospital found that the outreach service reduced hospital mortality. The multi-centre randomized MERIT study in Australia found no difference in unexpected deaths, cardiac arrest rates or unplanned ICU admission between control and intervention groups.

A whole systems approach

Evidence suggests that physiological measurements may be taken infrequently, even in patients who are critically ill. When values are abnormal and fulfil the requirements to trigger a response, the appropriate teams is not always called. When teams are called, if they are to make a difference they must have the necessary competencies, experience and resources. Finally all outreach systems are based upon the presumption that early recognition and intervention will improve outcome for some patients. It should be recognized that death may be inevitable, but it should also be acknowledged that agreeing the limits to intervention or resuscitation is a legitimate and beneficial outcome that may involve the outreach service. There are, therefore, many elements which need to come together if outreach is to make a difference, and its effect depends crucially upon how well routine hospital care addresses the problems of critically ill ward patients.

The future

Outreach is one response to the perceived problem of critically ill patients on hospital wards. There may be other ways of addressing this problem including supporting the education and training of the primary team responsible, the intervention of acute physicians or expanding critical care beds to ensure that all who may benefit are admitted at the earliest opportunity. In the UK, the funding for outreach is uncertain, and is often taken from a stretched intensive care budget. NICE has published guidelines for the management of acutely ill adults in hospital. These recommend many of the elements of the outreach system including the use of a physiologically based track and trigger system, trained staff with competencies in monitoring, measurement and interpretation, and a graded response strategy which is to be agreed and delivered locally.

Further reading

Department of Health. Comprehensive Critical Care. A review of adult critical care services. London: DoH, 2000.

Gao H, McDonnell A, Harrison DA, *et al.* Systematic review and evaluation of physiological track and trigger warning systems for identifying at-risk patients on the ward. *Intensive Care Medicine* 2007; 33: 667–79.

Goldfrad C, Rowan K. Consequences of discharges from intensive care at night. *Lancet* 2000; 355: 1138–42.

Goldhill DR, McNarry AF, Hadjianastassiou VG, *et al.* The longer patients are in hospital before Intensive Care admission the higher their mortality. *Intensive Care Med* 2004; 30: 1908–13.

Goldhill DR, Sumner A. Outcome of intensive care patients in a group of British intensive care units. *Crit Care Med* 1998; 26: 1337–45.

Hillman K, Chen J, Cretikos M, *et al.* Introduction of the medical emergency team (MET) system: a cluster-randomised controlled trial. *Lancet* 2005; 365: 2091–7.

Intensive Care Society. Levels of critical care for adult patients. London: Intensive Care Society, 2002.

Lee A, Bishop G, Hillman KM, *et al.* The Medical Emergency Team. *Anaesthes Intensive Care* 1995; 23: 183–6.

McQuillan P, Pilkington S, Allan A, *et al.* Confidential inquiry into quality of care before admission to intensive care. *BMJ* 1998; 316: 1853–8.

Priestley G, Watson W, Rashidian A, *et al.* Introducing Critical Care Outreach: a ward-randomised trail of phased introduction in a general hospital. *Intensive Care Med* 2004; 30: 1398–404.

Medical emergency teams

A medical emergency team (MET) is a concept designed to identify and treat serious illness as early as possible. Sometimes called a rapid response team or, if the response is determined by different criteria, then the patient at-risk team (PART), or modified early warning score (MEWS) team. These teams can also be part of outreach initiatives which manage seriously ill and at-risk patients outside the ICU.

The seriously ill at-risk syndrome

It helps to consider the seriously ill at-risk patient in the same way as a patient with coronary artery syndrome. Irrespective of the cause of the illness, patients who have even minor degrees of hypoxia and/or ischaemia are at risk of potentially serious complications. Hypoxia and ischaemia can result in cytokine cascades and organ dysfunction, leading to MOF often requiring admission to the ICU.

More than half of all hospitalized patients who have serious adverse events such as cardiac arrests, unexpected deaths or unanticipated admissions to the ICU have marked abnormalities in vital signs or other observations such as coma or seizures for many hours preceding the event. Rather than wait until the patient develops MOD and requires admission to the ICU, even minor degrees of hypoxia and ischaemia should be detected and corrected as early as possible.

Reasons for the high incidence of serious and untreated events in hospitals world-wide include lack of knowledge and experience in the doctors first called to see the patient, often due to the failure to recognize a seriously ill patient until they are at the point of a cardiac arrest, a reluctance to call for help when advice is needed and a tendency for intensive care specialists to wait until the patient becomes ill enough to require multi-organ support or perhaps until their heart stops and they require CPR before seeing them.

Acute hospitals are generally focused around a medical team or a geographical site, and so the seriously ill at-risk patient can easily fall through the usual safety nets within these vertical constraints. This situation is compounded by the changing nature of patients now admitted to acute hospitals. They are generally older with multiple co-morbidities, having more invasive and complex procedures and therapies. They are more vulnerable to even minor degrees of acute deterioration and require earlier and more aggressive intervention in order to prevent serious organ dysfunction.

Defining the seriousy ill criteria

The MET criteria (Table 33.17.1) define the sort of patient who requires urgent attention. Most calling criteria rely on serious abnormalities in simple vital signs such as pulse rate, respiratory rate and blood pressure, as well as observational abnormalities such as seizures, obstructed airway and a decrease in the level of consciousness. Staff concern is usually added to the criteria as it empowers, especially nursing staff to seek immediate assistance from trained and experienced doctors when needed. Some criteria use a tiered response, using the home team or specially trained nursing staff to assess the at-risk patient initially. Some also use other criteria such as urine output levels, temperature and SpO_2. The exact levels of abnormalities are less important than providing all hospital staff with the general awareness of an at-risk patient who requires urgent attention.

Table 33.17.1 MET criteria.

Obstructed airway
Respiratory rate:
<4/min
>26/min
Heart rate
<40/min
>130/min
SBP <90mm Hg
Seizures
A sudden decrease in the GCS of >2
Staff concern

Defining the seriously ill patient is the first step in a system designed to minimize complications and adverse outcomes. It is sometimes called the afferent arm.

A major weakness in defining the seriously ill at-risk patient is the frequency with which we measure vital signs or observe patients in hospital general wards. Measuring the vital signs every 4h may be inadequate to detect acute and potentially dangerous early signs of deterioration. Respiratory rate, one of the most important early detectors of serious illness, is often not measured at all or is estimated inaccurately. More continuous, non-invasive measurement of vital signs in hospitalized patients on general wards should provide a safer environment.

The team

It has been clearly demonstrated that the existing system of home teams caring for patients does not provide adequate care for seriously ill at-risk patients. It is tempting to suggest that training every doctor working in acute hospitals in aspects of acute resuscitation would provide better care. There is no evidence, as yet, to support this and, even if there was, it would require significant resources and expense in order to achieve an adequate response to the seriously ill at all times in an acute hospital.

Rapid response teams and outreach programmes are constituted in many different ways. Some use nursing staff to assess patients initially and call on doctors if appropriate. Many teams are simply hospital cardiac arrest teams rebadged as a MET or MET-like team. It is important that each team has at least one person who is trained in all aspects of resuscitation and available at all times. Members of the team should be formally trained in advanced resuscitation and how to work effectively in teams. Simulators are useful for this purpose. The response to the seriously ill patient is often referred to as the afferent arm.

Implementation

The implementation of a new system such as the MET involves different and difficult challenges. Staff across the whole hospital need to be aware of the criteria for calling the team, and they must be and feel empowered to call the team at any time. Implementation is facilitated by auditing the effectiveness of the system by data collection. For example, information could be collected on all patients who die, have a cardiac arrest or are admitted unexpectedly to the ICU. Patients who have a 'do-not-resuscitate' order need to be excluded. Those who had MET criteria in the 24h before the event and where a call had not been made then need to be highlighted as 'potentially preventable'. These types of data are essential when implementing a MET system as they define whether the hospital has a problem and the extent of the problem. The data should be packaged in a simple and attractive way and distributed widely throughout the hospital, e.g. to all senior clinicians, all departments and patient areas, to the administration, as well as to hospital bodies and committees responsible for quality assurance.

Weekly hospital-wide meetings presenting the number of calls, reasons for calling, and outcomes also help in the effective implementation of a hospital-wide system. Possible barriers to implementation need to be identified before implementation. These may include the cost of initially establishing the system, such as data analysers and collators, staff to organize the meetings, and staff to follow-up implementation issues across the hospital.

Other factors which may assist in the implementation of a MET system include gaining leadership support from within the hospital, with administrative and clinical leadership concentrating on the benefits of early intervention. Establish a taskforce or committee to set up the system, develop written policies and procedures, promote education programmes and coordinate a pilot system. In any organization, there will always be individuals who will be threatened by change. The availability of data is the most powerful way around these problems. It is very difficult to argue against treating patients as early as possible rather than waiting until they die or have a cardiac arrest.

Evidence

There is evidence in before and after and case-controlled studies that the MET system reduces serious adverse events such as cardiac arrests, deaths and unexpected admissions to the ICU. Despite the fact that a larger cluster RCT was inconclusive and underpowered, many countries around the world now have a MET-type system in their hospital. It makes sense, and there are many other activities in healthcare which have no level 1 evidence but would be impossible to abandon, e.g. such as ICU or even hospital admission. Common sense dictates that in a patient with serious ischaemia or hypoxia, treatment should not be delayed until they became ill enough to require ventilation and dialysis or have a cardiac arrest, and no intensive care physicians would say otherwise. It is doubtful that the ethics committees would ever allow us to conduct the definitive trial by randomizing patients into early or late treatment of the seriously ill.

ICU without walls

As the specialty of intensive care has matured, the expertise of physicians working with the seriously ill within the four walls of the ICU is increasingly being utilized to advise on the care of at-risk patients in other parts of the hospital both before and after admission to the ICU. Many intensive care staff are now electively consulted on seriously ill patients long before they would require being admitted to the ICU. Intensive care nursing staff are often involved in outreach services, where they see at-risk patients, advise nursing colleagues on general wards and conduct educational programmes. Within this system, certain at-risk patients such as those recently discharged from ICUs are all electively seen.

Intensive care staff are also being increasingly involved in activities such as acute trauma management and early management of sepsis, both in the emergency department and in general wards. This is in response to increasing evidence that early management of critical illness results in improved outcomes.

Further reading

Bright D, Walker W, Bion J. Clinical review: outreach—a strategy for improving the care of the acutely ill hospitalised patient. *Crit Care* 2004; 8: 33–40.

Hillman K, Alexandrou E, Flabouris M, *et al.* Clinical outcome indicators in acute hospital medicine. *Clin Intensive Care* 2000; 11: 89–94.

Hillman K, Parr M, Flabouris A, *et al.* Redefining in-hospital resuscitation: the concept of the medical emergency team. *Resuscitation* 2001; 48: 105-10.

Lee A, Bishop G, Hillman KM, *et al.* The medical emergency team. *Anaesth Intensive Care* 1995; 23: 183–6.

MERIT Study Investigators. Introduction of the medical emergency team (MET) system: a cluster-randomised controlled trial. *Lancet* 2005; 365: 2091–7.

Critical care follow-up

Introduction

Research into outcome following critical illness has focused mainly on mortality after discharge from the ICU, but the focus is shifting to morbidity, rehabilitation and aiding patients to rebuild their health. Many ICU patients report physical, psychological and cognitive problems, which may require assessment and appropriate care planning. Early recognition of problems through formal follow-up, both ward and out-patient clinic based, allows the prompt referral of these patients for appropriate, timely help before the condition becomes chronic.

Long-term follow-up

There would seem to be little point undertaking longer term follow-up of ICU patients unless appropriate help can be offered where needed. For many patients, the simple provision of advice about the speed of recovery combined with a stepped care approach to assessment and care planning is sufficient to meet their needs. Physical recovery after discharge from the ICU is, on the whole, excellent. However, for some patients, particularly those aged >50yrs and those staying longer in ICU, physical recovery from critical illness is prolonged, in some cases taking >1yr. Loss of lean body mass, mainly skeletal muscle, occurs in the catabolic phase of illness, leading to profound muscle weakness; the diaphragm and other skeletal muscle of the respiratory system are not protected from this. Rebuilding of lost muscle occurs slowly and requires both physical activity and good nutrition. In addition, some patients may develop critical illness polyneuropathy (CIP), which is characterized by axonal degeneration of motor nerves.

Longer stay patients often report difficulty climbing the stairs even 2 months after ICU discharge. They may have difficulty walking outdoors and often tend to continue using a wheelchair. Poor muscle strength and easy fatigability account for some of the difficulty in getting up if they fall. This can lead to a feeling of vulnerability and fear of falling.

Psychological issues during recovery

The psychological sequelae of critical illness have only just begun to be recognized. There may be profound long-term psychological and psychosocial effects. An early questionnaire study of 3655 patients found a high incidence of psychosocial dysfunction, particularly in younger individuals. High levels of anxiety, depression, and post-traumatic stress disorder (PTSD) have also been reported. Such problems can have a significant long-term detrimental impact on both the patients' and their family's quality of life.

Many patients are amnesic for parts of their time in ICU, as well as regarding events prior to admission. A delusional memory of hallucinations, nightmares or paranoid delusions recalled from the time in ICU may be the traumatic event that precipitates the development of PTSD. Recall of delusional memories may be increased in patients who have a previous history of psychological problems before admission to ICU.

Cognitive deficits following critical illness

It has been shown that significant cognitive deficits may remain after critical illness. At present, it is unclear whether these cognitive deficits are permanent, due to neurological damage, or temporary due to sedative drugs, which may recover with time. One recent study suggests that although some patients improve with time, a significant number remain impaired and may have problems with tasks such as financial management and driving.

Interventions to aid physical and psychological recovery

Rehabilitation programmes

While there is increasing evidence of physical and psychological problems during recovery from critical illness, little work has been carried out on rehabilitation in this population, whilst rehabilitation programmes in other patient groups, with both acute and chronic illness, have shown improvements in physical functioning and reduced psychological distress.

To achieve successful rehabilitation of ICU patients, a multi-modal programme containing physical, psychological and cognitive elements would be needed. Patients do not necessarily follow a set chronological pathway, so any programme has to be individual with regular assessment of physical, psychological or cognitive problems.

The provision of a multi-modal self-help recovery package has been shown to accelerate the physical recovery of general ICU patients in an RCT, blinded at follow-up. The programme consisted of a 6-week rehabilitation manual that provided information on a wide range of topics, such as the possible physical, psychosocial and psychological problems after critical illness, and a comprehensive exercise programme. A total of 126 patients were randomized to receive either the ICU recovery manual programme or standard follow-up. At both the 2 and 6 month follow-up physical recovery was faster in the recovery manual patients than in the controls ($P = 0.006$). It also had an impact on smoking cessation, with significantly more intervention patients not smoking in the 6 months post-ICU compared with the control group (relative risk reduction 89%, 95% CI 98–36%). This has considerable importance as it improves the chance of lung recovery.

Psychological recovery was more complex, with a non-significant ($P = 0.06$) trend to a lower rate of depression at 2 months after ICU discharge (12 vs 25%). More importantly, there were no differences in levels of anxiety and PTSD-related symptoms between the groups at 6 months. Further analysis showed that those patients recalling delusional memories from their time on ICU were significantly more anxious and had higher levels of PTSD-related symptoms than those who did not have these memories, regardless of whether or not they had received the rehabilitation programme. Clearly, such patients need to be identified and referred for appropriate help.

At present, in the UK, the provision of specialist ICU rehabilitation after hospital discharge is almost non-existent. A recent survey of physiotherapists at 36 large UK hospitals showed that there was some ward rehabilitation, but that 93% of respondents felt there was a need for follow-up services to identify problems and to ensure that patients achieved their full recovery. Only a few hospitals were found to have a specific rehabilitation team for ICU patients.

ICU diaries

The patients' amnesia for the time in the ICU can hinder their recovery, as many patients do not understand how ill they have been and consequently the length of time it will take them to get back to normal. ICU diaries have become increasingly popular. These diaries are a day by day record of the patient's stay in ICU, written in everyday language by the ICU staff and the patient's family. It also includes photographs taken at points of change in the patient's illness. These diaries are popular with patients and seem to help them rebuild a memory of their illness. Where the patient has periods of agitation, confusion or seemed to be hallucinating, this is recorded in the diary and seems to help the patient to identify the point at which delusional memories may have occurred. An example of this is a patient whose memory for ICU was being in a fire and having to be rescued by firemen. This memory kept replaying as a flashback and hindering her recovery. When she read her diary she discovered she had gone to theatre urgently and she decided that this was where her delusional memory had come from. Each time she had a flashback of this memory she read her diary to put it in context. An ICU diary is a simple therapy that has the potential to reduce the psychological impact of such memories, and is undergoing further research to examine its impact on PTSD symptoms.

Treating PTSD

Patients can be overwhelmed by their PTSD symptoms and unable to engage with further medical care or return to their normal life. They usually do not seek help because of the overwhelming nature of their symptoms, and there is an onus on staff following-up these patients to recognize and refer patients for treatment. Although the incidence of PTSD amongst ICU patients varies considerably in different studies, possibly due to differences in case mix, and may have been exaggerated in some studies due to the tools used, it has a major impact on quality of life after critical illness. Two recent sets of treatment guidelines emphasize the need to screen individuals after a traumatic event and refer those with high levels of symptoms for further professional help. Where patients have moderate symptoms which they are coping with, 'watchful waiting' is recommended, as many patients will find their own way of working through their traumatic memories. Where PTSD symptom levels are very high or the patient is not coping, then they should be referred for professional help. Treatment guidelines published by the UK NICE make clear that individuals suffering from PTSD should be given information on common reactions to traumatic events, including the symptoms of PTSD, its course and treatment.

ICU patients should be screened for PTSD, and to facilitate this there may be a role for the use of PTSD screening tools, such as the Impact of Event Scale, the PTSS-10 or PTSS-14 (see www.i-canuk.org.uk for copies of questionnaires). However, it is important that staff have some training in PTSD assessment and can recognize how the patient is coping. Some individuals will be able to cope with quite high levels of symptoms, and feel that they can manage on their own. These individuals can be reassessed after ~1 month.

The provision of counselling, psychotherapy or psychology services targeted at post-ICU patients is almost non-existent in the UK. The growth of counselling services for patients diagnosed with cancer has arisen from the recognition of the psychological impact of such a severe illness. Perhaps critical care providers need to think along similar lines because of the high risk of psychological effects for both patients and families following an illness in ICU. The correlation between high levels of PTSD-related symptoms in patients and their families points to the need for family therapy.

Conclusion

The physical, psychological and cognitive sequelae of critical illness can be an enormous burden on both patients and their families. Care must continue long after discharge from the ICU, and a prolonged recovery time can be expected. The pathway of care offered to patients after such a severe illness needs to be improved to ensure that patients reach their full recovery potential. ICU physicians, nurses, physiotherapists and other professionals have important roles to play in the management of patients after discharge.

Further reading

Bäckman CG, Walther SM. Use of a personal diary written on the ICU during critical illness. *Intensive Care Med* 2001; 27: 426–9.

Hopkins RO, Weaver LK, Collingridge D, *et al.* Two-year cognitive, emotional, and quality-of-life outcomes in acute respiratory distress syndrome. *Am J Respir Crit Care Med* 2005; 171: 340–7.

Jones C, Backman C, Capuzzo M, *et al.* Precipitants of post-traumatic stress disorder following intensive care: a hypothesis generating study of diversity in care. *Intensive Care Med* 2007; 33: 978–85.

Jones C, Griffiths RD. Identifying post intensive care patients who may need physical rehabilitation. *Clin Intensive Care* 2000; 11: 35–8.

Jones C, Skirrow P, Griffiths RD, *et al.* Rehabilitation after critical illness: a randomized, controlled trial. *Crit Care Med* 2003; 31: 2456–61.

National Institute for Health and Clinical Excellence (NICE). Post-Traumatic stress disorder (PTSD): the management of PTSD in adults and children in primary and secondary care. Clinical Guideline 26. London: NICE, 2005. Available at: www.nice.org.uk/CG026NICEguideline

Managing antibiotic resistance

Resistance to antibiotics is an international concern and has been an increasing problem over years. Nowadays reistance is so high in several countries that some infections are becoming almost impossible to treat. The threat of returning to the pre-antibiotic area is greater than ever. The issue is even more critical in the intensive care setting. More than 60% of ICU patients receive antibiotics at some time during their stay, and cross-transmission of resistant microorganisms is difficult to prevent when patients are extremely sick and stay for long periods of time. When quality of care becomes suboptimal, in particular when ICU worker ratios are too low, the risk is considerably higher. Septic shock may be due to resistant strains, and mortality is heavily influenced by the delay in providing appropriate antibiotic therapy.

Multi-resistance to antibiotics in the ICU setting: epidemiology

Resistance to antibiotics is extremely high in the ICUs of many countries. This is the case for both Gram-positive cocci such as MRSA and Gram-negative bacteria. A serious concern is represented by community-acquired MRSA, highly prevalent in many countries, including the USA, as well as glycopeptide-intermediate *Staphylococcus aureus* (GISA) and VRE. This is also true for Gram-negative bacteria such as *E. coli* and other enterobacteriacae harbouring extended spectrum lactamases, or *Acinetobacter* or *Pseudomonas* spp. sometimes resistant to almost every antibiotic except colimycin. However, it is it of great interest, although imperfectly understood, that several countries, such as The Netherlands or the Scandinavian countries and to a lesser extent Switzerland and Canada, have been successful to date in maintaining very low levels of resistance, even in the ICU. MRSA remains very rare in those countries. It seems, however, that even in those few and 'happy' or clever countries some resistant strains, coming from outside, have been able to induce epidemic outbreaks and that the global level of resistance is increasing slowly.

The attributable mortality of resistance to antibiotics in the ICU remains a very controversial issue. It is, however, widely accepted that inappropriate initial antibiotic therapy is responsible for a dramatic overmortality. This supports the concept discussed further here that both optimizing the empiric antibiotic therapy and reassessing this therapy at day 2 or 3, when bacteriological data are back (sometimes called 'de-escalation' or 'streamlining'), is of paramount importance .

Surveillance of resistance in the ICU is more than ever a public health priority, and indicators should be decided in each hospital according to local epidemiology. MRSA is considered as the main public enemy in many countries.

The increasing description of virulent MRSA strains in the community, carrying the Panton–Valentine leucocidin toxin, and the presence of five strains of *S. aureus* fully resistant to glycopeptides are strong arguments for screening for MRSA at ICU admission and for implementing isolation procedures in a systematic way. The topic remains highly controversial, however, and European projects such as MOSAR are underway.

Acquisition of resistant strains in the ICU: mechanisms

Many factors explain that hospitals, in particular ICUs, are experimental factories for creating and amplifying resistance: widespread usage of broad-spectrum antibiotics, often in combination, in the presence of extremely sick patients who would have died 10 or 20yrs ago, with very severe underlying diseases or prolonged ICU stay, and/or very high and permanent risk for cross-transmission of the microorganisms via either the hands of the healthcare providers, frequent transportation to the X-ray department or the operating rooms, and the environment. The shorter the length of stay, the lower the incidence of nosocomial infections and antibiotic resistance.

It has been demonstrated that there is an 'inoculum' effect in ICUs regarding antibiotic-resistant microorganisms. When colonization pressure with resistant strains is above a certain level, then the risk of cross-transmission becomes extremely high and very difficult to overcome. Thus, in countries with a high endemic level of resistance, in particular for MRSA, *Acinetobacter* or *Pseudomonas* spp., there is a real risk of antibiotic 'spiral'. A very strong and sustained programme is mandatory to overcome this problem. Several countries, such as Denmark have been successful in slowly decreasing resistance levels.

Therapy for multi-resistant bacteria infections in the ICU

Treating infections due to multi-resistant bacteria is very difficult, and a strong cooperation with microbiologists or infectious disease specialists is key. A combination therapy is often helpful to widen the target of the chosen antibiotics. It is important to be active against both resistant microorganisms and sensitive ones. For example, it has been shown that vancomycin therapy was suboptimal to treat susceptible *S. aureus* infections. A combination of vancomycin and nafcillin could be necessary in those settings. The dosage of antibiotics must be carefully chosen. In general, initial doses must be high enough to provide appropriate serum and tissue levels. Regular assessments of plasma levels are often mandatory, for glycopeptides or aminoglycosides, but also for cephalosporins, quinolones, penicillins or penems in the most severe cases.

In some infections due to pan-resistant Gram-negative microorganisms responsible for recent epidemics in several countries, we have often come back to 'old' antibiotics such as colistin. This drug, as well as aminoglycosides, has been used in aerosols with promising results. There are very few new compounds active against very resistant Gram-negative bacteria, and this is very worrying. However, the real drama is that we have very few antibiotics in the 'pipeline' active against resistant Gram-negative organisms. If clinicians decide to use carbapenems to treat community-acquired infections due to *E. coli* because of the threat of ESBL strains, we will be left with nothing to treat nosocomial and resistant infections. Auditing the antibiotic usage in the ICU must be performed on a routine basis and should be used as a quality indicator.

Can we prevent resistance to antibiotics?

Two complementary programmes have to be conducted simultaneously: prudent and rational use of antibiotics and prevention of cross-transmission of resistant strains. This will be a real challenge for the next decades.

The programme should be hospital wide and not only localized in the ICU, because microorganisms have no boundaries. Guidelines are important but, even if international ones are sometimes useful, most of the time they should be tailored according to local epidemiology. It is a key element not only to optimize therapy but also to minimize useless antibiotic therapies and help people in reassessing and stopping therapy. Educational programmes and audit are important .

The way people that diagnose infections in critically ill patients can probably have a profound impact upon antibiotic usage and pressure. Any usage of useless antibiotics in the ICU setting can be considered as a non-quality indicator, as emphazised in the recent Surviving Sepsis Campaign Guidelines.

In the same way, duration of antibiotic therapy is very porbably a key component of resistance pressure, and everything must be done to keep therapy as short as clinically and scientifically possible. Data are still scarce in this respect, and new studies should be encouraged.

New diagnostic techniques, such as real-time PCR (or microarrays) might dramatically improve the time needed for diagnosis and thus the appropriateness of initial therapies, and might positively influence antibiotic usage in the very near future.

Cycling or rotation of antibiotics has been the subject of an extensive and controversial literature in the past few years. Recent papers indicate the efficacy of this strategy on the incidence of nosocomial infections and resistance to antibiotics in the short term, either in the ICU or even in non-ICU wards. Most people, at least in Europe, prefer treating patients 'à la carte', according to many factors such as pre-existing diseases (COPD), severity of illness, use of antibiotics in the past few days or weeks, length of stay in the hospital, long-term care facilities or the ICU, before the occurrence of infection.

We must both provide the best antibiotic up-front, in particular to the most severe cases, and minimize antibiotic resistance. The two objectives are not mutually exclusive and we can consider that quality of antibiotic therapy is a 'two-step contract'. The first contract is with the patient, the second with the ecology and with society. It is extremely urgent to implement the de-escalation strategy worldwide, and European or international professional societies have a special responsability to help in this respect.

Could the use of new antibiotics reduce antibiotic resistance in the hospitals?

Antibiotic 'monotony' has probably been an important factor in the increase in resistance, in particular regarding the extensive international usage of glycopeptides, both systemically and locally, and of quinolones. The widespread usage of third-generation cephalosporins has been accused of promoting VRE as well as MRSA, or resistant enterobacteriaecae. Hopefully, we have now a few new antibiotics to treat Gram-positive infections such as linezolid, synercid, ketolides, new penems and tigecycline. and several others will be introduced.

Thus, the armamentarium of effective drugs will be somewhat broader for therapy of resistant Gram-positive infections , and this, in principle, could decrease antibiotic monotony and pressure. We do not know for now if those antibiotics, in particular those which belong to the new classes, will exert less resistance than 'old 'compounds, over the short and long term. Unfortunately as mentioned above, we have very few new compounds to treat infections due to multi-resistant Gram-negative microorganisms, and it is more than likely that resistance to carbapenems, or even colistin will increase in the next few years. Antimicrobials involved with innate immunity, such as defensins, either systemically or locally, need to be tested, as well as vegetable compounds such as components of green tea which exert a marked antimicrobial effect.

Conclusion

Therapy of severe infections due to multi-resistant infections remain a real challenge.

Resistance to antibiotics in the hospital, particularly in the ICU, is a growing concern everywhere. Some countries have been able to maintain a very low level both in the community and in hospitals. In order to be successful, a strong and patient programme combining a prudent and intelligent usage of antibiotics and an 'obsessional' prevention of cross-transmission, in particular using hand decontamination with hand rub alcoholic solutions, is needed. Some controversies persist regarding MRSA screening. Regular symposia should be organized, and knowledge should be disseminated. Since resistance is now an international concern, a strong cooperation between countries is needed. We do not know if the availability of new compounds will help in overcoming this important public health problem. Initial empiric antibiotic therapy must be efficient. Combination therapy remains controversial. A systematic de-escalation strategy must be implemented in every hospital, and national or European professional societies have a special responsibility in promoting those programmes.

Further reading

Borg MA. Bed occupancy and overcrowding as determinant factors in the incidence of MRSA infections within general ward settings. *J Hosp Infect* 2003; 54: 316–8.

Chambers HF. Community-associated MRSA—resistance and virulence converge. *N Engl J Med* 2005; 352: 1485–7.

Cunningham R, Jenks P, Northwood J, *et al.* Effect of MRSA transmission of rapid PCR testing of patients to critical care. *J Hosp Infect* 2007; 65: 24–8.

Gillet Y, Issartel B, Vanhems P, *et al.* Association between Staphylococcus aureus strains carrying gene for Panton–Valentine leukocidin and highly lethal necrotising pneumonia in young immunocompetent patients. *Lancet* 2002; 359: 753–59.

Huskins WC, O'Grady NP, Samore M. Design and methodology of the Strategies to Reduce Trasmission Antimicrobial Resistant Bacteria in Intensive Care care Units (STAR-ICU) trial. *Infect Control Hosp Epidemiol* 2007; 28: 245–6.

Meyer E, Schwab F, Gastmeier P, *et al. Stenotrophomonas maltophilia* and antibiotic use in German intensive care units: data from Project SARI (Surveillance of Antimicrobial Use and Antimiocrobial Resistance in German Intensive Care Units). *J Hosp Infect* 2006; 64: 238–43.

Peres-Bota D, Rodriguez H, Dimopoulos G. Are infections due to resistant pathogens associated with a worse outcome in critically ill patients? *J Infect* 2003; 47: 307–1.

Vincent JL, Bihari DJ, Suter PM, *et al.* The prevalence of nosocomial infection in intensive care units in Europe. Results of the European Prevalence of Infection in Intensive Care (EPIC) Study. EPIC International Advisory Committee. *JAMA* 1995; 274: 639–44.

Appendix

Respiratory physiology

The symbols used in respiratory physiology are important in defining what they are describing. Please be aware that the literature is not as consistent as it might be in using these symbols.

1. Symbols.

Primary/large capitals for physical amounts/quantities

C Content of gas in blood
D Diffusing capacity
F Fractional concentration in dry gas
F Frequency of respiration (breaths/min)
P Pressure or partial pressure
$\dot{Q}$ Volume of blood
$\dot{V}$ Volume of blood per unit time
R Respiratory exchange ratio
S Saturation of haemoglobin with O_2

Secondary/ smaller capital (gas phase) is usually location and quantity

A Alveolar
B Barometric
D Dead space
I Inspired
E Expired
T Tidal

Examples. Arterial oxygen saturation SaO_2 . Alveolar partial pressure of oxygen PAO_2. Fractional inspired oxygen FIO_2

Secondary symbols for blood phase

a arterial
c capillary
c′ end-capillary
i ideal
$\bar{v}$ venous mixed venous
– above any symbol denotes a mean value
. above any symbol denotes a value per unit time
f frequency

Examples. Arterial oxygen saturation SaO_2. Alveolar partial pressure of oxygen PAO_2. Fractional inspired oxygen FIO_2

2. Lung volumes
   Adult values
   - Tidal volume 6 ml/kg (420 ml)
   - Functional residual capacity 2.4 litres
   - Residual volume 1.2 litres
   - Total lung capacity 6.0 litres
   - Vital capacity 4.8 litres
   - Peak expiratory flow rate : 450–700 l/min (males)
   - Or 300–500 l/min (females)
   - Forced expiratory volume in 1 sec (FEV1) 70–83% of vital capacity 3.5 litres

3. Criteria for acute lung injury;
   1. Acute onset of impaired oxygenation
   2. Severe hypoxaemia defined;
      PaO_2 to FIO_2 ratio of ≤ 40 (using kPa) or ≤ 300 (in mmHg)
   3. Bilateral diffuse infiltrates on chest Xray
   4. Pulmonary wedge pressure ≤ 18 mmHg to exclude a cardiogenic cause.

4. Bohr's equation defines physiological dead space.

$$\frac{VD}{VT} = \frac{PaCo_2 - P\bar{E}CO_2}{PaCO_2}$$

5. Alveolar PO_2 in its simplest form is

$$PAO_2 = PIO_2 - \frac{PaCo_2}{R}$$

where R is the respiratory quotient usually around 0.8.

From this the alveolar arterial gradient (A-a gradient) can be derived if te arterial oxygen is known.

6. Poiseuille equation; laminar flow through a tube.

$$P = \frac{\dot{V} \times 8l \times \mu}{\pi r^4 \times 980}$$

Where P = pressure drop, $\dot{V}$ = volume per unit time, l is length, r radius, μ viscosity

7. Minute ventilation

This comprises alveolar and dead space ventilation.

$$\dot{V}E = \dot{V}A + \dot{V}D$$

Index

N.B. 'f' following a locator indicates a figure and 't' indicates a table.

A

D

Q

R

S

W

X